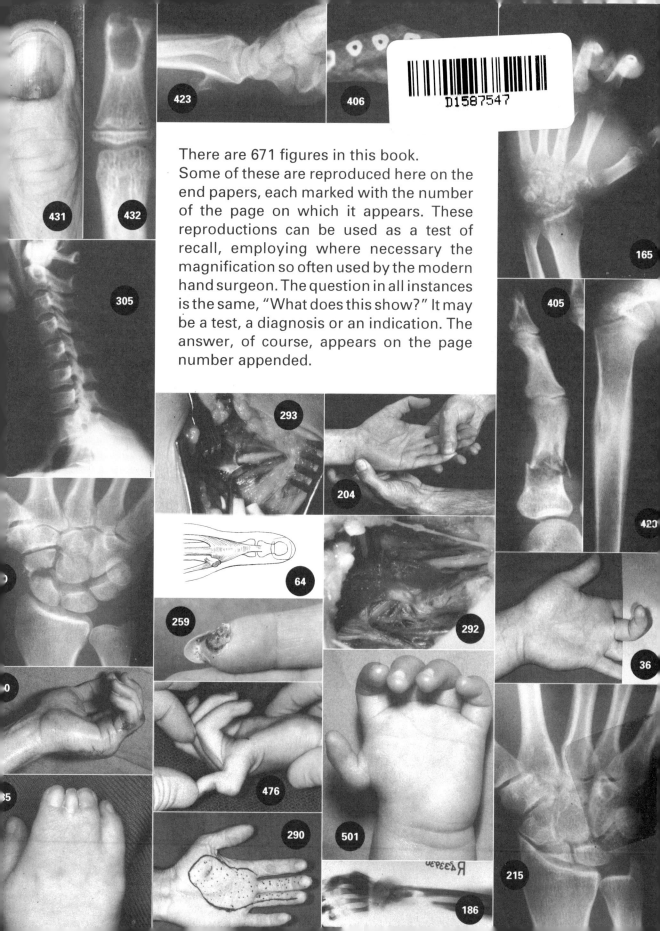

There are 671 figures in this book. Some of these are reproduced here on the end papers, each marked with the number of the page on which it appears. These reproductions can be used as a test of recall, employing where necessary the magnification so often used by the modern hand surgeon. The question in all instances is the same, "What does this show?" It may be a test, a diagnosis or an indication. The answer, of course, appears on the page number appended.

The Hand: Diagnosis and Indications

For Churchill Livingstone

Publisher: Mike Parkinson
Copy Editor: Paul Singleton
Indexer: Laurence Errington
Production Controllers: Neil Dickson, Mark Sanderson
Sales Promotion Executive: Kathy Crawford

The Hand:
Diagnosis and Indications

Graham Lister

THIRD EDITION

CHURCHILL LIVINGSTONE
EDINBURGH LONDON MADRID MELBOURNE NEW YORK AND TOKYO 1993

CHURCHILL LIVINGSTONE
Medical Division of Longman Group UK Limited

Distributed in the United States of America by Churchill
Livingstone Inc., 650 Avenue of the Americas, New York,
N.Y. 10011, and by associated companies, branches and
representatives throughout the world.

First edition 1977
Second edition 1984
Third edition 1993

ISBN 0-443-04545-3

British Library Cataloguing in Publication Data
A catalogue record for this book is available from the British
Library.

Library of Congress Cataloging in Publication Data
Lister, Graham.
    The hand, diagnosis and indications/Graham Lister. — 3rd ed.
        p.   cm.
    Includes bibliographical references and index.
    ISBN 0-443-04545-3
    1. Hand—Wounds and injuries—Diagnosis.   2. Hand—Diseases—
Diagnosis.   3. Hand—Surgery.   4. Surgical indications.   I. Title.
    [DNLM: 1. Hand—Surgery.   WE 830 L773h]
RD559.L57   1993
617.5'75—dc20
DNLM/DLC
for Library of Congress   92-49326
                                                                    CIP

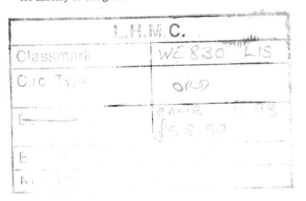
Produced by Longman Singapore Publishers (Pte.) Ltd.
Printed in Singapore

The
publisher's
policy is to use
**paper manufactured
from sustainable forests**

Contents

Preface to the Third Edition

A third edition? Worth buying?? A combination of simple arithmetic and a hidden talent of my word processor, which records the time spent and the keystrokes made on each document, allows me to offer the following statistics to the reader, understandably cautious in these stringent economic times.

Chapter	Figures 2nd Ed	Figures 3rd Ed	References 2nd Ed	References 3rd Ed	Time spent on 3rd Ed in hours	Keystrokes in thousands
1	176	203	271	696	100	337
2	137	151	205	654	65	156
3	57	58	165	271	8	38
4	37	37	131	256	19	101
5	75	82	95	161	21	57
6	38	77	226	380	54	248
7	48	63	87	200	27	94
Total	607	671	1180	2618	294	1031

At the least these numbers record that, in preparing this revision, and disregarding the time expended on research, I put considerable effort into trying to clarify the obscure and update the obsolescent. But actually they reveal more. For example, someone who has read the second edition can determine by looking at the right hand column that the amount of work devoted to each chapter rose from Compression (38K) to Injury (337K) and thereby decide how his time might be most profitably spent.

Where are the major revisions? While making significant changes elsewhere, I have added major sections on the wrist, on surgical indications in fractures and dislocations and on bone tumours. The 122% increase in the number of references only hints at the volume of publication on hand surgery during the past eight years. When the first edition was written sixteen years ago, I had to hunt out references to support my text. Now, in order to limit the bulk of this book, it has been necessary to review with a critical eye the available volume of written material. By and large, all references come from the ten journals most concerned with surgery of the hand. Readers are encouraged to consult the articles quoted, for the bibliography they will find there offers a portal to a much wider field of reading. But why do I even include all these when, as my friends tell me, literature reviews are readily available by electronic means? Why do I not keep this volume manageable as it used to be?

The book, as stated in the first edition, is intended to '... detail the techniques of diagnosis ...' and to help those who search for answers in that field (hence the 2618 references). Our diagnostic knowledge and the ancillary services available to help us have grown dramatically in the past decade and this volume must grow also if it is to serve its declared purpose. Those who seek a pocket book are recommended to the excellent paperback of similar name published by the American Society for Surgery of the Hand.

This is *not* a treatise on surgical technique. It *is* intended to take you to the point at which I pick up the knife knowing exactly *what* I am going to do, but I do not tell you *how* I do it. I do show photographs taken during surgery to illustrate anatomy or demonstrate findings. I do show selected results, for the reader should know something of the outcome of recommended procedures. By arrangement with David Green, the reader is referred to specific pages on technique in the third edition of *Operative Hand Surgery* from the same publisher.

As I said in the Preface to the second edition, I hesitate to offer acknowledgements, not because they are not richly deserved, but because I fear to offend those unintentionally omitted. Some, however, are mandatory. Bud Wheeler, whose angiograms I continue to use, is deceased. His friends, amongst whom I count myself, mourn the passing of a sensitive and intelligent colleague. The drawings of Grace von Drasek Ascher remain, for they cannot be improved. I would not have presumed to insert even the cryptic comments on bone tumours contained here-in without the guidance provided by Dr Sherman Coleman, who has a reputation richly deserved as a teacher of bone oncology. Any wisdom displayed in that part of Chapter 6 is his, any errors mine. Derek Priest read the section on non-invasive vascular studies and offered valuable advice and reassurance. Danny Smith, once again, has demonstrated his talents not only in taking the original color slides (of which more below) but also in converting them to the prints which so handsomely illustrate this work. Bruce Johnstone and Bruce Peat, my first two overseas hand fellows in Salt Lake City, both from Australasia, scrutinized the first two chapters and politely pointed out flaws I had sworn they would not find. Lois Thompson, who rode the wagon West with me, prepared and annotated all the references, both those included and those set aside, and retyped major portions of the text. To all of these and many others I am grateful.

I have enjoyed preparing this third edition, not least because it has made me run harder in the race to keep up with our expanding specialty. I hope that you gain equal pleasure and education.

Salt Lake City, 1993   G.L.

Note: *Most of the illustrations in this book are available as colour slides. Details can be obtained by writing to the author at the Division of Plastic and Reconstructive Surgery, University of Utah Medical Center 3C127, Salt Lake City, Utah 84132*

Preface to the Second Edition

Being a confessed cynic, I have always believed that second editions are inspired more by the publisher's avarice than by the author's greater enlightenment. It was therefore with the bitter satisfaction which comes with confirmation of a suspected fault in an otherwise perfect acquaintance that I received the request for this volume from Churchill Livingstone. I did not go beating on *their* door with inkstained hands.

But I should have done. As I reluctantly reviewed the first edition, which with groundless conceit I had believed to be carved in stone, I found more than sufficient cause to kindle embarrassment—and enthusiasm. Certain omissions had been detected by reviewers, notably Barton[1]. Some were intentional, glibly rationalized at the time, but in retrospect clearly due to ignorance. Thus the second edition contains a chapter on congenital anomalies, that most complex of therapeutic decisions, and new or expanded sections on quadriplegia, cerebral palsy, compartment syndromes, fractures new and old, frostbite and other topics previously sidestepped or only lightly brushed. Other portions of the first edition were sufficiently unclear that even I found myself confused! These have been reorganized and include amongst others the texts on sensory examination and the selection of skin cover. Advances in knowledge have occurred in hand surgery during the past six years, both general and personal, and these have been incorporated throughout, but most notably in carpal injuries, in the detection of the malingerer and in those problems which cause almost daily encounters between the surgeon and the microscope. The courteous criticisms of Linscheid[2] and Albright[3] have been heeded, most obviously in the section on muscle testing, which has been clarified and enhanced, as has the entire volume, by the drawings of Grace von Drasek Ascher, drawings which carry a unique blend of art and information. Furlow[4] politely hinted at a significant weakness of the first edition: references which are not annotated in the text are of much less value than those which are. This mistake has been corrected. In addition, classified references to the more esoteric infections, swellings and causes of nerve compression have been added to each chapter.

Giving thanks has similarities to throwing a party, one probably generates more resentment from those unintentionally omitted than appreciation from those justly included. Therefore, while recognizing and being grateful for all the help given by the office staff of Hand Surgery Associates of Louisville, I will confine my acknowledgements to the following: Dr C. S. Wheeler who provided the arteriograms together with clear and often justifiably caustic elucidation; Drs Alain Carlier and John Stilwell and Ms Irene Ward who read and kindly criticized the text; Gloria Troutman and Cara Heybach who helped to type it. Most of all, my thanks are extended to Danny Smith and his Photographic Department, to the quality of whose work the following pages testify, and to my secretary Carol Smith, who under another name also converted the first edition from illegible manuscript to impeccable type.

Louisville, Kentucky, 1984   G.L.

REFERENCES

1. Barton N 1978 The Hand 10: 110–111
2. Linscheid R L 1977 Mayo Clinic Proceedings 52: 671–672
3. Albright J A 1977 Archives of Surgery 112: 1506–1507
4. Furlow L T 1978 Plastic and Reconstructive Surgery 62: 443

Preface to the First Edition

Most texts on hand surgery, while not ignoring diagnosis, concern themselves more with the technicalities of a surgical skill only now achieving recognition as a specialty in its own right.

By contrast, the purpose of this book is to describe in detail the techniques of diagnosis applicable in the various disorders of the hand and to indicate how different findings influence the choice of treatment.

Standard nomenclature has been adopted in the main. 'Medial' and 'lateral' lie uneasily on the hand, which is probably less used in the anatomical position than in any other. They have therefore been discarded in favour of 'ulnar' and 'radial'. 'Lateral', freed from the possibility of ambiguity, has been retained to refer to the side of the digit where *which* side is immaterial to the point under discussion. 'Middle' and 'small' have been used to refer to the third and fifth digits rather than 'long' or 'little', allowing initial letters to be used in clinical records as clearly understandable abbreviations for the fingers.

Fractures of the forearm and wrist are omitted for they clearly lie in the province of the orthopaedic surgeon and present no diagnostic problems to be considered in this text. By contrast, the chapter on compression wanders far from the hand for symptoms therein may have their origins as far proximal as the cervical spine and even beyond. Repetition is used throughout, I hope judiciously, and I make no apologies for its presence. It is valuable to the writer to aid in clarity and convenient to the reader as it eliminates irritating references to other parts of the book.

When first I heard of them, I searched unduly long for a description of the Allen or the Adson test, the Phalen or the Spurling. How to test for the superficialis of the index finger or the independent action of pronator quadratus; how did one reveal intrinsic tightness or distinguish a tendon adhesion from a joint contracture? These and many other questions fascinated and frustrated my study of the hand. If this book helps those like me, then it serves its purpose. If in the process it conveys my enthusiasm for the study then that would give me great personal satisfaction, for, as Ian Donald declared in the first sentence of his text on obstetrics: 'The art of teaching is the art of sharing enthusiasm'.

Louisville, Kentucky, 1976   G.L.

1. Injury

One-third of all injuries involve the upper extremity. Each year in the United States of America there are 16 million upper extremity injuries sufficiently severe as to restrict activity[1]. Hand injuries result in more days lost from work annually—again, some 16 million—than any other form of occupational accident.

In 1987 in the United States the total cost of upper extremity trauma was $42.4 billion[2]. This represents 20% of all compensation payments. Using the Abbreviated Injury Scale severity score[3], in which 5 represents the most severe, in one series[4] the average charge for extremity injuries with a score of 1 or 2 was $7332, and $26 686 where the score was 3.

The injury with which patients present may be deemed *major* or *minor*. A common criterion for separating the two is whether or not they require to be taken to the operating room.

The injury may be *open* or *closed*. That is to say, there may or may not be a wound. This is a significant distinction for several reasons. The former is more apparent and more likely to be contaminated, and to become infected. It will require anaesthesia and sterile technique. This permits exploration — the second examination detailed below — and therefore, to a varying degree, postpones the final decision regarding the indications for management. By contrast, the closed injury is more subtle, and hence more prone to be missed. To open the hand increases the chance of infection, removes to a great degree the soft tissue splint, and in itself constitutes a decision of such magnitude that it should be undertaken only after the indications are clear in the surgeon's mind. While added decisions may be made on the basis of what is found at exploration, conclusions regarding the indications in closed injuries should for this reason be made during the initial examination. This is given further emphasis by the fact that, in many closed injuries, there may be no urgent need to operate. While early surgery is, in general, always desirable, the demands placed upon the operating room and the surgeon may be such that it is not practi-

cable. Triage dictates delay. The following text is organized with this in mind. Indications in closed injuries are decided after the initial examination, those in open wounds after exploration. In more extensive injuries, compassion may dictate that most of the inspection be moved to that second examination.

Like facial wounds, those of the hand are gory and obvious. This may mislead the harassed casualty officer into passing the patient on to a specialist surgeon without first excluding other hidden, more critical, damage. In turn, the specialist may assume that other injury has already been excluded and proceed with treatment, at worst under general anaesthesia where visceral or cranial complications may develop unheralded by symptoms. The first responsibility of any physician is that the patient should suffer no added harm through either his attention or neglect. It is therefore essential that every doctor who sees the patient should ensure that no other more urgent injury has been sustained than that to the hand. The patient with a hand injured beneath a car or through a windscreen may have sustained steering wheel injuries to thoracic and abdominal viscera. The patient with a gunshot wound of the hand may have sustained penetrating injuries to major vessels. The patient with a traction injury to the brachial plexus may have a middle meningeal haemorrhage. With one exception, hand injuries are never fatal and that fact should dictate their priority in management.

In all that follows, it will be assumed that other injuries have been excluded, or their care planned.

HISTORY

In assessing the injured hand, two matters concern the examiner. In being assessed, two matters concern the patient.

The examiner must establish, comprehensively and precisely, what structures have been injured. Secondly, he must decide what immediate steps he should take towards restoration of full function. Several factors play a part in making this latter decision. These are:

the number and nature of structures damaged
the irreversible loss of viability of any tissues
the precision with which the extent of this loss
   of viability can be determined
the time between injury and repair
the surgeon's expertise.

By contrast, the patient has two different preoccupations. Firstly, what effect will his injury have on his everyday life, both immediately and in the long term? Secondly, what is to be done to his hand and will it be done competently? In short, he requires information and assurance.

At this initial contact between surgeon and patient there are only a few highly significant facts which the examiner needs to know from the patient. A long and formal history is not required, for this makes only a minor contribution to resolving the prime concerns both of the examiner and of the patient. After preliminary introductions, the history, still systematic and exhaustive on significant points, should be taken while examining the injured hand.

Later, once preliminary decisions have been made with respect to the injury, a detailed history and examination of other systems should be undertaken by the hand surgeon or by a member of his team. In major open injuries to the extremity, particular attention should be paid to ensure that no more proximal closed injury is overlooked. Shoulder dislocation, brachial plexus avulsion and cervical spine injuries may all be present yet asymptomatic. The decision to undertake major distal reconstruction must be taken with the knowledge that a proximal injury exists, not in ignorance of it.

Nature of injury

Assuming that the surgical care offered is of good quality, during both operation and rehabilitation, nothing influences the eventual recovery of hand function more than the mechanism and the force of the injury.

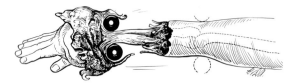

Fig. 1.1   Roller avulsion injury. The arm is drawn in by the rollers which, as the victim attempts to withdraw the limb, tear off distally based avulsion flaps.

What happened to your hand?
This first question is likely to elicit a general statement of the incident and will usually indicate the region of the hand injured and the nature of the injuring force. This may well require to be clarified by supplementary questions before the mechanism of injury is fully understood. For example, workers will tend to use technical jargon in referring to machinery, and the examiner must not let this pass if he is uncertain of the implications. As the answers are received, the surgeon mentally catalogues the probable damage he will encounter.

Does it have rollers?
What are they surfaced with?
What normally passes through them?
Do they have an automatic release mechanism?
How quickly were they stopped once your hand was caught?
Are they hot?

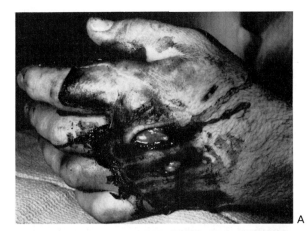

A

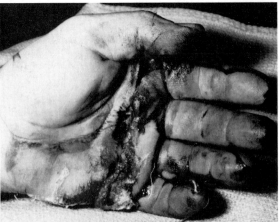

B

Fig. 1.2   A, B. Where the rollers come to rest and continue to rotate a full thickness burn is produced, the margins of which are undermined to a varying degree.

Roller injuries[5,6] (Fig. 1.1) commonly produce avulsion flaps, usually distally based, and of questionable viability. The viability will be further compromised by burns, either from heat or from the friction of rollers with no automatic release or arrest (Fig. 1.2). Depending on the hardness of the rollers and on the size of the gap between them, transverse or comminuted fractures of the phalanges, usually proximal, or metacarpals may or may not be present. Tendons and nerves may be intact and contused, although either may be avulsed from proximal or distal. Vessels are likely to be disrupted or thrombosed, requiring interpositional grafts to restore flow. If the gap between the rollers is small, distal crush may be so severe that it precludes successful revascularization (Fig. 1.3).

What roughly is the area and shape of the punch press? What does it make?

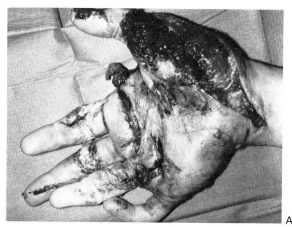

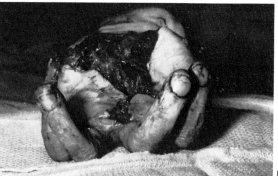

Fig. 1.4 A, B. Large area punch presses generate such great force that they totally disrupt the skeleton and all soft tissues.

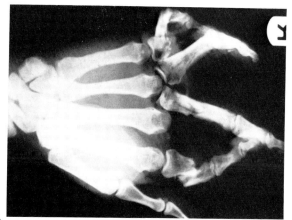

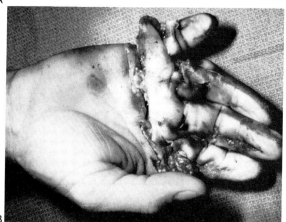

Fig. 1.3 A, B. The damage to the fingers distally may be so severe as to preclude revascularization.

How thick is that when it is complete? (i.e. What is the narrowest space in which your hand was compressed?)

Punch presses, depending on what they produce, can inflict moderate to very severe injuries, more commonly the latter. Comminuted fractures, carpal disruption and soft tissue crush are the rule in the large area injuries (Fig. 1.4). In the smaller, more defined injuries there is a greater likelihood of division of tendons and nerves than in roller injuries, and this often at two levels, corresponding with either side of the recess in the punch.

What kind of saw?

What's the set on that blade? (Set = amount of deflection in the saw's teeth from a straight line)

What were you cutting?

Saw injuries resulting from a high-speed metal saw with a narrow set will approximate to a knife cut. By contrast, table rip saws and chain saws used for heavy timber remove a 'kerf' from the wood which is wider than the blade itself and therefore destroys a swathe of

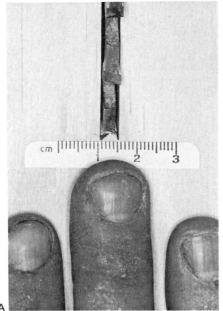

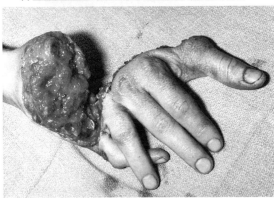

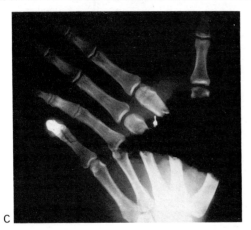

Fig. 1.5 A. Large table ripsaws have a wide set which removes a swathe of tissue and precludes exact matching of structures in repairing incomplete amputations (B, C).

all structures (Fig. 1.5), which precludes anatomical reduction of fractures and may dictate the use of grafts for all injured tissues. In addition, wide-set saws avulse as well as cut, producing damage distant from the skin wound which, in particular, makes revascularization and replantation difficult.

Woodworking accidents cause 720 000 hand injuries per annum in the United States. In one survey[7], 60.5% were incurred by amateur craftsmen; 42% involved the table saw.

Does that have a sharp or a dull blade?
Did it come down squarely on your wrist or did it slice across it?
Show me the position of your hand when it slipped on the knife.

Lacerations of the hand may be produced by slicing with sharp instruments, little force being generated, or by the guillotine effect of heavy objects with a narrow edge. Lacerations both of the slicing and of the guillotine variety commonly divide tendons, which are usually under tension at the time of injury. Major nerves will be divided by a slicing wound, but as they are not taut they may sustain no injury or only injury in continuity in guillotine lacerations, being pushed but not divided by the leading edge of the injuring agent.

The relationship of the distal cut end of the long flexor tendons of the fingers to the skin wound varies according to the posture of the hand at the time of injury (Fig. 1.6). Where wrist and fingers were fully

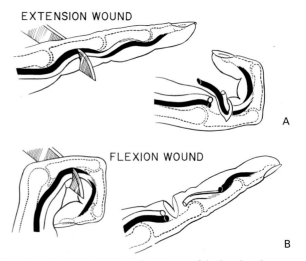

Fig. 1.6 Depending upon the posture of the hand at the time of the injury, the distal tendon ends may be at the wound itself when the finger is extended on the operating table. Alternatively, if the finger was fully flexed, then the distal tendon ends will be far removed from the skin laceration.

extended, as in falling to the ground or warding off a stabbing attack, the free distal end will be level with the skin wound, even a little proximal to it. Where the fingers were firmly flexed, as in holding a narrow-bladed knife which subsequently slipped, the cut distal end will lie *distal* to the skin wound by a distance which may be as great as the maximum excursion of the tendon. Depending on age, sex, level of the wound and the finger involved, this excursion may be as much as 4 cm.

In carrying out primary tendon repair, the cut distal end should be exposed and the proximal end retrieved to approximate to the distal end. The posture of the hand at the time of injury is therefore important in planning any incision to extend the skin wound.

What stuck into your hand?
What sort of an end does that have?
In what direction was it pointing?
Show me how it happened?

Penetrating injuries of the hand carry the same sinister implications of deep damage as do similar injuries to the abdomen or neck. An unimpressive skin wound may hide a remarkable amount of damage to deep structures[8]. Exploration in such situations is the absolute rule. What is to be found can often be predicted by knowing the site and direction of the injury and the nature of the wounding agent (Fig. 1.7). Tapered, blunt-pointed objects may cause little damage to structures deep to the skin, whereas the thin slivers of glass[9] which produce an unimpressive wound on the skin of

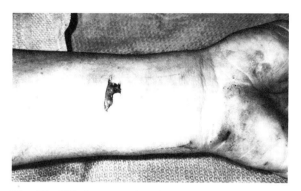

Fig. 1.8 This 2 cm wound on the anterior aspect of the forearm concealed a laceration of all eight flexor tendons of the fingers, of flexor carpi radialis and of the median nerve.

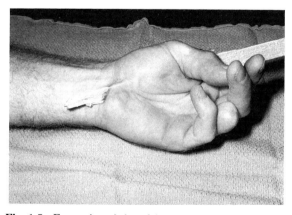

Fig. 1.7 From a knowledge of the anatomy, it is evident that this penetrating wound may well have damaged the structures in the first web space and the carpal tunnel. As in other circumstances in which a penetrating foreign object threatens vital structures, blind withdrawal of the penetrating instrument may inflict additional damage. Rather, it should be removed by careful incision and dissection away from vital structures.

the forearm commonly divide all flexor tendons and both major nerves (Fig. 1.8). Where the stab wound is inflicted by a sharp, narrow blade held in the dominant hand while working on an object held strongly in the injured, non-dominant hand, tendons are at much greater risk than are nerves (Fig. 1.9). This is better understood if one recalls the ease with which a sharp blade will cut a cord under tension as opposed to one which is slack. The damage to deep structures in stab wounds may be remote from the skin wound. Short, punctured lacerations over the knuckles should be the subject of deep suspicion. They are most likely to have been inflicted by a human tooth, but the victim may be unwilling to admit the fact. Such injuries are often the precursor of infection resistant to treatment (p. 331).

Pressure gun injuries (p. 107) should receive great respect. Depending upon the agent injected, they may or may not be painful immediately[10]. Whatever the patient's complaints, exploration should be undertaken and will often reveal a startlingly wide distribution of material (Fig. 1.10).

Shotgun, revolver or rifle?
Range and calibre?

Gunshot wounds. The damage caused by a *missile*[11-15] is related to the kinetic energy at the time of impact, which is equivalent to $MV^2/2$, where M = mass and V = velocity. Thus, a high-velocity weapon will cause more damage than a low-velocity one (a muzzle velocity of 2000 ft/sec being the dividing line), if range and calibre are equal (Fig. 1.11). Similarly, a large mass at a short range will cause a devastating injury even from a low-velocity weapon — the shotgun is the prime example (Fig. 1.12). With a high-energy injury one should expect comminution and loss of bone, significant skin defects and a high incidence of vascular and nerve

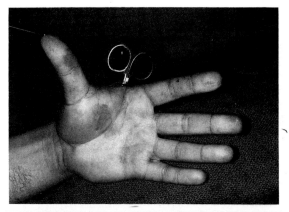

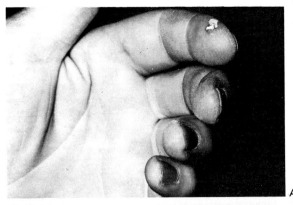

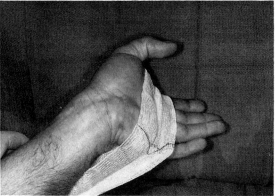

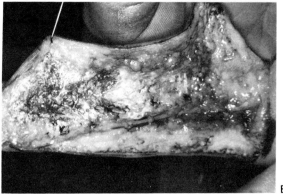

Fig. 1.9 A. Through an entry wound in the first web space, a sharp blade came to rest with its tip in Guyon's canal. B. With full wrist extension, the posture of the fingers reveals that all eight finger flexor tendons were divided. By contrast, all nerves and vessels were spared. Note the flexion of the interphalangeal joint of the thumb, indicating an intact flexor pollicis longus.

Fig. 1.10 A. This characteristically inconspicuous wound on the pulp of the left index finger was inflicted by a high pressure paint gun. B. Immediate exploration revealed that the paint had dissected along both neurovascular bundles of the index finger down as far as the distal palmar crease. Early debridement resulted in a vital digit with moderately good function.

injury often in continuity. Low-energy wounds, in contrast, often present as little more than a foreign body in the tissues (Fig. 1.13).

What height did you fall from?
Was there a lot of force behind it?
Did you realise you had broken something?
Did you have to stop what you were doing?

Blunt injury, including falls. Very heavy falls on an outstretched hand are commonly associated with supracondylar fractures in children, carpal injuries in young and middle-aged adults (see p. 75) and Colles fractures in older persons. Considerable direct force from a blunt object will produce a comminuted fracture, whereas mallet finger fractures and pathological fractures — most commonly through enchondromas in the hand — require very little force. The patient is often unaware in such circumstances that he has sustained

an injury. Even when the patient has enough pain to make him aware, he may elect to wait, because the injury is often closed. In these circumstances, both the unrecognized and the neglected, the patient may never be seen in an emergency room, presenting rather at a later juncture in the office.

These and other mechanisms of injury have received individual study. A representative, but not exhaustive, list is shown below, and the interested reader is referred to the appropriate paper.

Corn-picker[16-18]
Auger[19, 20] (Fig. 1.14)
Wood-splitter[21, 22]
Wool-carder[23]
Snow-blower[24-26] (Fig. 1.15)
Lawn-mower[27, 28]
Sodium chlorate bomb[29] (Fig. 1.16)
Escalator[30]
Automobile roll-over[31-33] (Fig. 1.17)

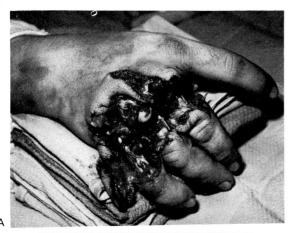

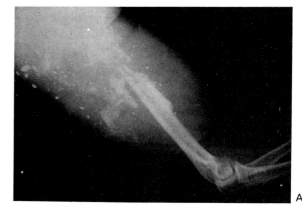

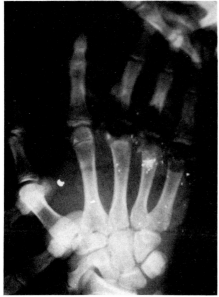

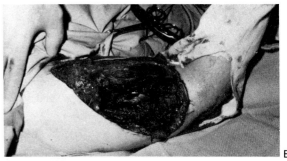

Fig. 1.11 A, B. This wound was inflicted by a large calibre revolver. It has removed a block of tissue from the region of the metacarpophalangeal joints.

Fig. 1.12 A. This exploded, comminuted fracture of the humerus was inflicted with a shotgun. B. After debridement, the resultant soft-tissue defect extended from the shoulder nearly to the elbow.

Woodworking tools[34]
X-radiation[35]
Electromagnetic radiation[36]
Drug addiction[37-40]
Snakebite[41-44]
Spider bite[45]
Karate[46-48]
Soccer[49]
Meat mincer[50]
Winches[51]
Roping[52, 53]
Pay-phone receiver cords[54]
Microwave[55-57] (see thermal injuries, p. 126)

With experience, the surgeon learns to expect more lawn-mower injuries on the first fine day after a period of spring rain, and more snow blower accidents when a heavy fall occurs while temperatures are relatively warm — both circumstances repeatedly clog the machines. He or she appreciates the great importance of clothing in corn-picker and wood-splitter accidents, where the severity of the injury is multiplied geometrically if gloves are worn — the surgeon only has to recall a gauze sponge caught in a drill bit to understand this fact. With experience, the surgeon understandably asks fewer questions of the kind detailed above. He or she knows the distance between the multi-level mutilations of the grain auger, and that the apparently 'clean' amputations inflicted by heavy wood-saws and mowers have zones of microvascular injury which extend at least 2 centimetres[58] on either side of the injury. This information, be it gleaned from questions or experience, is vital for the uncomplicated management of the case: vital in the true sense, for the knowledge sought is to a large degree intended to reveal implications of hidden injury not evident on wound inspection or radiological examination. Such injury may well impair the vitality, or viability, of the tissues. If not recognized, and in most

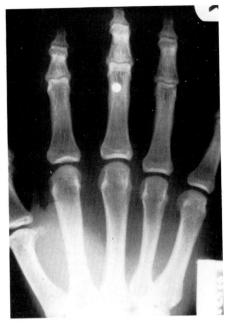

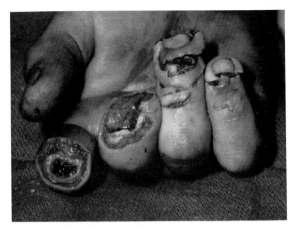

Fig. 1.15   Snow-blowers and lawn-mowers being of similar mechanism, produce similar injuries. The wounds are multiple, parallel, and separated by a distance which depends upon the speed both of the blade and with which the fingers were inadvertently put into the machine. Although they appear to be clean cut, there is an area of high pressure on either side of the blade which produces adjacent soft-tissue damage.

Fig. 1.13   By contrast with the high-kinetic-energy wounds of Figures 1.10 and 1.11, this patient, who had sustained a gunshot injury, presented with a small puncture wound, no loss of function and a pellet seen on the radiograph.

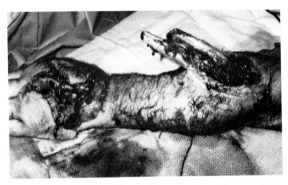

Fig. 1.14   Augers used for raising grain cause characteristic injuries which typically are multiple and separated by a distance which equals that between the spiral turns of the auger blade.

instances removed, such relatively avascular tissue will lead to infection, scar, and failure to attain the functional objectives of primary repair.

Time and injury

The time at which the patient was injured and at which the patient presented should be noted. Certain injuries

require unusual expedition and should be treated as soon as they are recognized — *in order of urgency*:

1. vascular injuries producing significant haemorrhage
2. major vascular injury or compromise (due to fracture or dislocation) producing doubtful viability
3. compartment syndrome (p. 40)
4. macro-replantation, that is, where the amputated part contains significant muscle bulk
5. hydrofluoric acid burns (p. 128)[59]
6. pressure gun injuries (p. 107)

   It is now recognized that there is no extreme urgency to replant parts containing little or no muscle. These have been designated *micro-replantations* and have been successfully performed in several replantation centres after more than 24 hours certainly of *cold* and even of warm ischaemia[60].

   As emphasized earlier, hand injuries should take the place in operating room priority appropriate to their urgency. However, since 30% of the injuries seen in the emergency room are to the upper extremity[1], it makes good sense for management to keep at least one room staffed and free for hand surgery if the hospital has a significant emergency commitment.

   If left untreated, the hand will undergo certain changes which may influence its eventual recovery of function:

1. Vessels occluded as a result of unstable fractures sustain permanent intimal damage at the site of

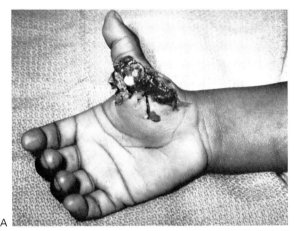

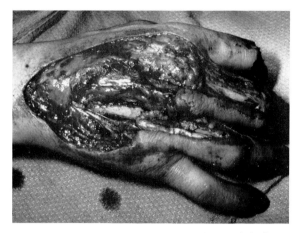

Fig. 1.17 Automobile roll-over injuries characteristically inflict deeply abrading wounds of the dorsum of the hand. The abrasion usually removes a large area of skin, underlying tendons, and the dorsal surface of the metacarpals and phalanges. This wound has been debrided, and repair of the extensor digitorum to the small finger already undertaken.

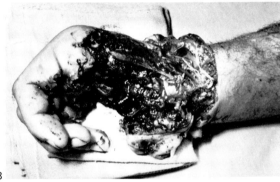

Fig. 1.16 Explosion of hand-held devices, be they fireworks or bombs, produces a characteristic injury which is located primarily on the radial side of the hand. With smaller force the thumb is dislocated dorsally (A), whereas with more powerful explosives (B) the thumb is completely removed, and the radial and palmar aspect of the hand is severely mutilated.

occlusion and may require replacement; the ischaemia in the area they serve may become irreversible; if this includes muscle compartments, necrosis and contracture may result.

2. Contaminants become incorporated in the tissues.
3. Infection may become established.
4. Oedema in the hand increases, leading to:
   (a) rise in intracompartmental pressures, with the consequences outlined in 1.
   (b) adoption of joint positions dictated by maximum laxity of the ligaments, namely wrist flexion, metacarpophalangeal joint extension, interphalangeal joint flexion and thumb adduction. If permitted to remain in this position, joint contractures will occur (p. 191) — an avoidable, and in truth iatrogenic, disaster.

(c) friability of tissues, which will particularly hinder tendon, nerve and vessel repairs.
(d) difficulty in skin closure, to the point of impairing skin circulation.

General health, current therapy, known allergies

Apart from scrupulously eliminating associated injuries, a brief general medical history should be obtained and examination performed, both aimed at discovering any cardiac or respiratory problems which may influence the choice of anaesthesia. Few, if any, medical conditions or drug therapies will interfere with adequate healing, but uncontrolled *diabetes*, certain *skin conditions*, and *steroid intake* are associated with an increased sepsis rate, while psychiatric disorders or mental defect may severely limit postoperative co-operation. Known allergies should be recorded.

Social history

Much emphasis has been laid by some on the importance of occupation in choosing the operative procedure. This is true in reconstructive surgery of the hand and will be discussed more fully there. In the acute situation it is of less significance, for the aim must always be to restore maximum function to the hand and to do that in the shortest time.

However, with the great increase in digital replantation and revascularization in the past ten years, the social history has assumed unaccustomed importance.

The functional, economic and cosmetic factors involved in replantation must be discussed with the patient and his relatives, and must be related to his or her individual situation. They must be told that:

1. The average time off work is 7 months.
2. They have a 36–77% chance of having only protective sensation and the mean speed of recovery of sensation is 1.4 cm per month.
3. Cold tolerance is directly related to recovery of nerve function.
4. Motion in the joints of the replanted part will average 50% of normal.
5. Some 60% of patients require an average of 2.5 further operations.
6. The total cost of replantation exceeds that of revision of the amputation by a factor of 5 to 10 for a wrist amputation, and 10 to 15 for a digital amputation.
   (These results are averaged from personal unpublished data and from reports available in January, 1991[61-68].)

Armed with the facts above, a self-employed person or one with a non-compensation injury (58% of amputations occur in the workplace[69]) may well elect not to undergo replantation, while a child or a young woman may choose to do so.

To replant all amputated parts without concern for factors other than survival is a mechanical exercise, the work of a technician. To inform and discuss with the patient, covering all implications, even to the point of making the always arbitrary decision *not* to attempt replantation requires knowledge, time and tact. It is rightly the work of a physician.

Replantation referral

An increasing number of patients are referred for replantation over long distances involving expensive private air transport. The contraindications to replantation[70] should be carefully sought *before transfer* to ensure that no patient, insurance carrier or Health Service incurs this expense in an ill-informed search for ill-advised treatment. The contraindications are detailed on page 24.

The statements made to, and the questions asked of, the caller wishing to refer a candidate for replantation are:

We will be pleased to take the patient, but would like to ask a few questions.
What is your name, that of your facility and the telephone number?

How did the amputation happen?
Are there other injuries elsewhere in the body?
How old is the patient and is he generally healthy?
Is that limb otherwise intact? How about the radiographs?
How will you prepare the limb for travel?

With respect to the amputated part:
Are there other injuries?
Is there bruising and where is it?
When you wash off the wound, are there structures dangling from the part?
Tell me about the radiograph of the part.
How will you transport it?

There is a good/fair/poor chance of replantation.
We will be glad to see the patient but please emphasize to him/her and the family that even the decision to try replantation can only be made here and, of course, success cannot be guaranteed. I can hold on, or you can call back, if you wish to discuss whether or not they wish to come.
How will the patient be transported?
Can you give me an estimated time of arrival?

As the process of taking the history has been accompanied by the initial examination of the hand, a diagnosis accurate in general terms will have been made on conclusion of the dialogue with the patient.

COUNSELLING

Information sufficient to address the four concerns detailed on commencement of the history-taking will have been gleaned. The surgeon will know what structures are injured and what needs to be done. Some estimate can be made of the impact on the patient's way of life. From the surgeon's demeanour, the manner in which the examination has been conducted, and the care displayed in the counselling which follows, the patient will be reassured that he is in competent hands. Contrary to widespread practice, it is at this juncture, even more perhaps than in the operating room, that the attending or consultant surgeon can help the patient. Especially in major injuries, and certainly in those where amputation may be necessary or where it has been deemed compassionate to await full examination until the patient is anaesthetized, the patient is reassured if there is present one whose thin and greying hair and facial wrinkles suggest experience and knowledge to a degree which cannot be conveyed by the best educated but fresh-faced resident or registrar. The nature of the injury should be explained in simple terms. By and large, patients understand the words 'skin' and 'bones', but not 'joints', 'tendons' or 'nerves'. They do, however, generally understand hinges, ropes, and electrical cables, and these can serve as useful analogies. Not only should the injury be described in outline but so also should the intended treatment, both immediate and secondary, and, where it is to be employed, the technique of regional block. While any proposed line of treatment should be made clear to the patient, particular care should be taken to ensure that he fully understands the need for amputation, free skin grafts or distant flaps. Whenever possible, decisions regarding amputation should be taken on the day of injury. Any temporizing by inadequate debridement, splintage and a proposed 'second look' only raises false hope in the patient and the family that the limb or part may be saved. It makes any later announcement that the limb must go that much more tragic, and one that is likely to raise doubts regarding the competence of care, with resultant loss of rapport. For these and other reasons, that later announcement is often never made, and the patient's hopes maintained without any reasonable chance of fulfillment. He is condemned to multiple surgeries over a prolonged period with little gain, by the completion of which he will have become dependent to an irreversible degree. By contrast, the patient confronted with an immediate and well-reasoned decision to ablate a worthless extremity will invariably accept it with courage and often with the comment that he had thought it hopeless when he first saw the injury. After an appropriate period of grieving, which can be shortened by vigorous rehabilitative efforts, he can resume a modified but useful place in the community at a much earlier stage than his less fortunate peer — who was ironically thought initially to be *more* fortunate — who encountered indecision at the outset. For the reasons stated previously, the decision is best made by, or in the presence of, a senior surgeon. The length of the patient's stay in hospital should be given, declared as an estimate assuming no complications. Possible complications and their management should be briefly touched upon, though not stressed unduly.

Where possible, the time before he is able to return to full employment and recreation should be given in very approximate terms. The major difficulty in making such an estimate is doubtful viability. This is most likely where crush, electrical burning or pressure gun injury exists.

Where the injury is so severe that the patient is unlikely to be able to resume his former employment or recreations, this news should probably be withheld until that outcome is virtually certain and until the patient has adjusted to some extent to the fact that he has been injured.

This whole dialogue, and the preliminary examination yet to be described, usually takes no more than ten minutes. At the end of that time the diagnosis has been made, appropriate treatment chosen, and in certain instances commenced, the patient has been informed and his anxieties allayed as far as possible. Where significant decisions are to be made with rational participation by the patient, the difficulties presented by excessive prior medication are evident. If it can be limited to that which will relieve without clouding the senses until after discussion, the patient will gain in the long term. In return for the added suffering, he should receive an explanation and prompt attention.

SURFACE ANATOMY

At this juncture, when the hand is to be inspected and palpated, it is appropriate to consider where certain structures lie in relationship to surface marking and bony points. When the position of the skin wound is then considered in conjunction with the nature of the injury, suspicions will be aroused that specific deep structures may have been damaged.

The flexor surface of the wrist

There are two skin creases at the wrist. The distal crease overlies the proximal margin of the flexor retinaculum and the proximal carpal row (Fig. 1.18). The flexor retinaculum is a strong fibrous band some 3 cm wide proximal to distal, which, by providing the roof of the canal formed by the carpal bones, completes the carpal tunnel. Into its superficial surface inserts the tendon of palmaris longus, and from its superficial surface arise, in part, the origins of the thenar and hypothenar muscles.

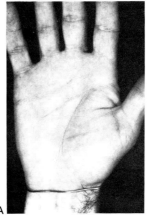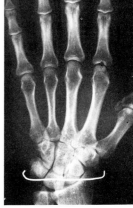

A B

Fig. 1.18 A wire had been laid on the distal wrist crease. Radiologic examination reveals the relationship of the crease to the carpus.

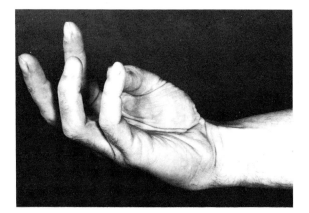

Fig. 1.19 If the wrist is gently flexed with the thumb in contact with the tip of the small finger, the tendon of palmaris longus, if present, will stand out clearly.

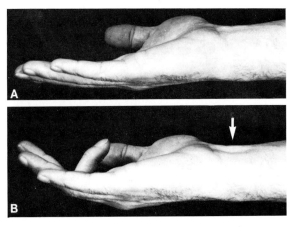

Fig. 1.20 A, B. When the proximal interphalangeal joint of each finger is flexed in turn, it will be seen that all movement occurs on the ulnar side of the palmaris longus tendon producing a depression in that situation.

The synovial sheath enveloping the flexors of the digits in the carpal tunnel extends to a point 2–3 cm proximal to the distal wrist crease.

If the thumb is brought to touch the tip of the small finger, and the wrist is then gently flexed, the tendon of palmaris longus stands out clearly (Fig. 1.19). This tendon lies superficial to the deep fascia of the forearm. It is absent in both hands in approximately 16% of subjects, and is present in only one or other hand in a further 14%. The median nerve lies beneath the fascia immediately deep to the tendon of palmaris longus, running parallel to it. The flexor carpi radialis lies deeply to the radial side of palmaris longus in its own tunnel of deep fascia.

With the hand open, the proximal interphalangeal joint of each finger should be flexed in turn while observing the wrist (Fig. 1.20). It will be seen that the movement of all tendons of flexor digitorum superficialis occurs on the *ulnar* side of the palmaris longus and therefore of the median nerve. The movement of flexor digitorum profundus tendons produced by flexing the distal interphalangeal joints is less easily observed but it can be palpated convincingly. Once again all movement is to the *ulnar* side of palmaris longus. Thus, *all flexor tendons to the fingers lie in the ulnar half of the wrist, together with the median and ulnar nerves and the ulnar artery.* Thus the majority of vital structures lie in the part of the wrist which is most vulnerable in falls on to sharp objects.

While attempting to flex the distal interphalangeal joints individually, a further fact will have been noted. It is not possible to flex the distal interphalangeal joints of the middle, ring and small fingers independently. This is because the flexor digitorum profundus tendons

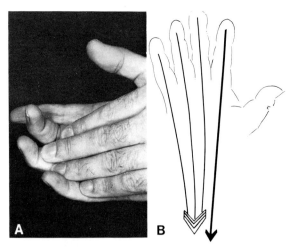

Fig. 1.21 A. With the motion of the proximal interphalangeal joint blocked, flexion of the distal interphalangeal joint is produced by flexor digitorum profundus. This motion is invariably accompanied by involuntary flexion of the distal interphalangeal joints of the adjacent fingers. B. This is due to the fact that the tendons of these three ulnar fingers all originate from a common muscle belly.

which produce this movement have a common muscle belly (Fig. 1.21). If the fingers are now strongly *extended* and the wrist *flexed* against resistance, flexor carpi radialis and flexor carpi ulnaris together with palmaris longus can sometimes be seen and always palpated (Fig. 1.22). Flexor carpi ulnaris lies to the ulnar side of the finger flexor tendons and on its deep, somewhat ra-

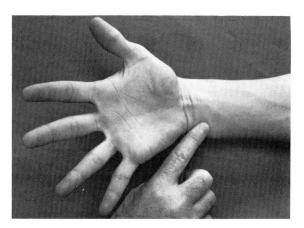

Fig. 1.22 Strong extension of the fingers produces powerful contraction of the flexor carpi ulnaris to stabilize the wrist. Since the long finger flexors are relaxed they do not obscure the wrist tendon.

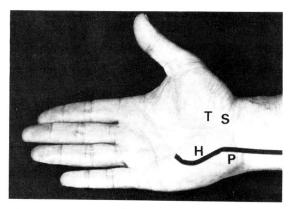

Fig. 1.23 The course of the ulnar artery and nerve can be deduced by palpating the pisiform P and the hook of the hamate H. The flexor retinaculum attaches at its ulnar end to these two bony prominences and at the radial margin to the tubercle of the scaphoid S and the ridge on the trapezium T.

dial, aspect lie the ulnar nerve and artery. The dorsal sensory branch of the ulnar nerve arises some 4–6 cm above the wrist and winding around the ulna deep to flexor carpi ulnaris it pierces the deep fascia to gain the subcutaneous tissue overlying the ulnar head against which it can often be rolled beneath the finger. It proceeds distally to serve the dorsum of the hand and of the proximal phalanges of the small and ring fingers. It is at risk during excision of the ulnar head.

The tendon of flexor carpi ulnaris can be traced distally to its insertion into the pisiform bone which can be palpated at the extreme ulnar end of the distal wrist crease. The pisiform in the relaxed hand can be moved in a radial direction by the examiner's thumb. This movement occurs in the piso-triquetral joint. Two centimetres distal to the pisiform, and somewhat radially, the hook of the hamate — also called the hamulus — can be felt as a well-padded ridge proximal to the soft hollow of the palm. It lies beneath the broken crease line which runs from the junction of the palmaris longus with the wrist crease towards the small finger and which demarcates the ulnar margin of the palmar fascia and the radial aspect of the hypothenar muscles. It lies at the bissection point of lines drawn along the ulnar side of the abducted ring finger and along the flexor surface of the radially abducted thumb — the cardinal line of Kaplan[71]. The ulnar attachment of the flexor retinaculum is to the pisiform and the hook of the hamate and therefore, all the flexor tendons lie on the radial side of these two landmarks. The ulnar nerve and artery in contrast, coming to lie on the radial side of the pisiform from their course beneath flexor carpi ulnaris, pass to the *ulnar* side of the hook of the hamate lying between

these bony prominences in a separate canal named after Guyon[72-75] (Fig. 1.23). The *floor* of the canal is formed by the flexor retinaculum (the roof of the carpal tunnel) and by the piso-hamate ligament. The *roof* consists of the superficial part of the flexor retinaculum, which is a localized thickening of the investing layer of the antebrachial fascia, and distally the aponeurotic origin of the hypothenar muscles, both covered by the palmaris brevis. Over this roof run the terminal branches of the palmar cutaneous branch of the ulnar nerve[76]. The ulnar nerve separates in the canal, and if palpation of the hook of the hamate is repeated using a firm rolling motion of the pulp of the examiner's thumb, the deep motor branch of the ulnar nerve can be felt moving from side to side over the hook. Accompanied by the deep branch of the ulnar artery which goes to complete the deep palmar arch deep to the flexor tendons, the deep motor branch of the ulnar nerve passes between the flexor and abductor digiti minimi and perforates the opponens digiti minimi, to follow the deep palmar arch to supply the muscles of the first web space, adductor pollicis and the first dorsal interosseous. The ulnar artery leaves the nerve just beyond the hook of the hamate, turning radially just distal to the flexor retinaculum and superficial to the flexor tendons to form the superficial palmar arch from which arise the common digital arteries of the second, third and fourth web spaces. The vascular anatomy of the hand is subject to considerable variation[77, 78].

The tendon of flexor carpi radialis can be seen to the radial side of palmaris longus and traced out to the most obvious bony landmark on the flexor aspect of the wrist and hand, the tubercle of the scaphoid which marks the

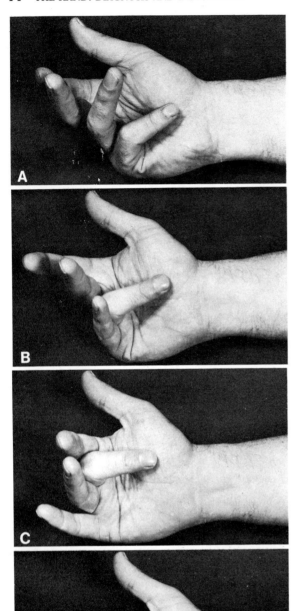

Fig. 1.24 A–D. All fingers on flexion at the metacarpophalangeal and proximal interphalangeal joints point to the tubercle of the scaphoid. This fact is of assistance in maintaining the correct rotation in fractures of the metacarpals and phalanges.

distal pole of that bone. The flexor carpi radialis tendon passes to the ulnar side of the tubercle, in its own compartment formed by two layers of the flexor retinaculum, then beneath the overhang of the ridge of the trapezium to insert into the bases of the second and third metacarpals. This last stretch of tendon distal to the scaphoid Verdan has been referred to as the 'forgotten tendon' and is the seat of inflammation in flexor carpi radialis tendinitis. It is to the scaphoid tubercle that all fingers point on flexion (Fig. 1.24). Immediately distal and somewhat radial to the tubercle lies the scapho-trapezial joint. The radial attachment of the flexor retinaculum is to the tubercle of the scaphoid and the ridge of the trapezium. The motor branch of the median nerve, which is subject to many variations[79,80], in most cases turns around the distal margin of the flexor retinaculum into the thenar muscle mass which overlies the scaphoid tubercle, trapezium, trapezoid, first metacarpal and the intervening joints. This it does at the point at which a line drawn distally from the scaphoid tubercle bisects Kaplan's cardinal line. The axis of the belly of the abductor pollicis brevis, the most important thenar muscle functionally and innervated solely by the median nerve in 95% of hands, runs from the tubercle on the scaphoid to the metacarpophalangeal joint of the thumb. Between the tendons of palmaris longus and flexor carpi radialis the palmar cutaneous branch of the median nerve[81] emerges through the deep fascia some 5–6 cm proximal to the distal wrist crease to pass down superficial to the radial margin of the flexor retinaculum to serve the skin of the palm (Fig. 1.25) often as far distally as the proximal phalanges. This nerve is commonly injured in release of the carpal tunnel, although it has been shown never to pass to the ulnar side of a line drawn through the midline of the ring finger[82]. Equally prone to injury, if present, is a communicating branch which runs from the (median) third common

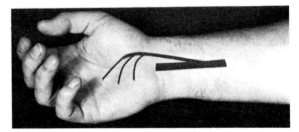

Fig. 1.25 The palmar cutaneous branch of the median nerve arises from its radial aspect some five to six centimetres proximal to the wrist, passes between the palmaris longus and flexor carpi radialis, crosses the base of the thenar eminence, and then gives numerous branches to serve the 'palmar triangle'.

digital nerve to the (ulnar) fourth at the level of the superficial palmar arch[83]. Beneath the flexor carpi radialis runs the tendon of flexor pollicis longus. It can be felt at this site if the wrist is relaxed in flexion and the thumb is actively flexed and extended. With this action, the muscle belly of flexor pollicis longus can be seen moving in the hollow to the radial side of flexor carpi radialis. On the belly the pulsations of the radial artery can be palpated. To the radial side of the artery the radius lies immediately beneath the skin. The insertion of brachioradialis can be felt to tighten along the border of the radius just proximal to the styloid if the elbow is flexed against resistance in the neutral position between pronation and supination.

The extensor surface of the wrist and hand

Distal to the insertion of the brachioradialis on the subcutaneous area of the radius a ridge can be palpated to which the extensor retinaculum attaches in part[84]. It passes around the dorsal aspect of the wrist to be attached on the ulnar border of the carpus to the triquetral and the pisiform, and distally to the abductor digiti minimi and the base of the fifth metacarpal, thus enclosing considerably more than half of the circumference of the wrist. The main bony landmark on the dorsum of the wrist is the ulnar head, while on the dorsum of the radius midway between the ulnar head and the ridge on the radial side of the wrist to which the extensor retinaculum gains attachment, a bony tubercle can be felt. Three centimetres distal to this radial tubercle in the adult hand a further bony prominence is evident. This is the base of the third metacarpal, and between it and the dorsal tubercle lies the carpus. When the wrist is in the neutral position with respect to ulnar and radial deviation, the radial tubercle aligns with the scapholunate joint lying just distally.

The scaphoid lies to the radial, the lunate to the ulnar side of this joint. Distal to lunate lies the capitate which articulates distally with the base of the third metacarpal. The trapezoid is found proximal to the base of the second metacarpal, articulating also with the capitate ulnarwards, the trapezium to its radial side and — together with the trapezium — the scaphoid proximally in what has become known as the 'triscaphe' joint. The third and fourth metacarpal bases both articulate with the hamate, which, in turn, articulates with the capitate on its radial aspect and the triquetrum proximally. Inspecting the wrist on both aspects during ulnar and radial deviation, it will be seen that one bone on each surface, the triquetrum dorsally and the tubercle of the scaphoid anteriorly, becomes more prominent in radial deviation, less so in ulnar. This can be explained in simplistic terms. In radial deviation, the base of the first metacarpal comes closer to the radial styloid. An intervening bone must therefore shorten. This the scaphoid does by flexing, reducing its vertical height by this polite gesture. Its 'bowing head', the tubercle, becomes more prominent anteriorly. In ulnar deviation, similarly, the fifth metacarpal base approximates to the ulnar styloid. Again, the intervening bones must somehow reduce in height. The hamate glides down the distal surface of the triquetrum, thereby exposing less of its ulnar vertical dimension. As this occurs, the triquetrum steps forward, eased there smoothly but firmly by its helicoid articulation with the hamate; hence the prominence of these two bones, the scaphoid and triquetrum, in radial deviation, their relative insignificance in ulnar deviation. These unfailingly fluid movements are achieved by the ligamentous attachments joining the carpal bones, for no tendons attach to the carpal bones, excepting the pisiform. Should the ligamentous attachments of the carpus be disrupted, instability results (pp 81 and 217).

Thirteen tendons — on average, for there may be less, or many more[85] — pass beneath the extensor retinaculum in six synovial compartments. Their compartments and positions are detailed in Table 1.1.

The position of all these tendons can be confirmed by palpation during movement. It is especially difficult to distinguish the extensor pollicis brevis from the abductor pollicis longus. The former is a much narrower tendon than the latter and can be palpated on the first metacarpal just beyond its base to which abductor pollicis longus is inserted. The abductor pollicis longus invariably has several tendons. One or more of these, or the tendon of extensor pollicis brevis, may lie in a separate unnamed compartment — 1A, perhaps? — which may be missed in releasing, and result in recurrence of, de Quervain's disease (p. 343). Such a septum creating an additional compartment was found in 34% of one cadaveric study[86]. An anomalous muscle has also been described in the first compartment[87], in association with similar tendinitis.

In the floor of the anatomical snuff box from proximal distally can be palpated the radial styloid, the scaphoid, the trapezium and the base of the first metacarpal. Palpation of the scaphoid should be practised by the examiner on himself, for the act is mildly painful in the uninjured. If this is not realized, an erroneous diagnosis of scaphoid fracture may be made on the evidence of normal tenderness. Across these structures the radial artery winds from the flexor aspect of the wrist beneath the tendons which define the snuff box to gain the space between first and second metacarpals. Overlying the artery lies the cephalic vein, and bleeding

Table 1.1

Synovial compartment	Tendons	Situation
1st compartment	(1)st two tendons of 'anatomical snuff box', *abductor pollicis longus* and *extensor pollicis brevis*	Palpable as the palmar boundary of the snuff box
2nd compartment*	(2)radial wrist extensors, *extensor carpi radialis longus* and *extensor carpi radialis brevis*	These pass beneath extensor pollicis longus just distal to radius and can be palpated there with the wrist in resisted dorsi-flexion with the thumb relaxed
3rd compartment	(3)rd tendon of 'anatomical snuff box' *extensor pollicis longus*	Palpable as the dorsal boundary of snuff box; passes to ulnar side of the radial tubercle
4th compartment	(4)finger extensors, i.e. *extensor indicis* and 3(±1) tendons of *extensor digitorum*[†]	On the dorsum of the radius, between the radial tubercle and ulnar head
5th compartment	(5)th finger extensor, *extensor digiti minimi*, which usually has two tendons	In the groove between ulnar head and radius
6th compartment	*Extensor carpi ulnaris*	On ulnar aspect of the ulna, can be palpated just distal to the ulnar head with the wrist in resisted ulnar deviation

* *Extensor carpi radialis intermedius* is present in 12% of hands in this compartment[91]; a valuable tendon in severe quadriplegia.
* The tendon of *extensor digitorum* to the small finger is absent more often than not, arising as an intertendinous connection from the ring finger tendon on the dorsum on the hand.

from a wound in this region may be from this substantial channel rather than from the radial artery.

Running in the subcutaneous tissue overlying the snuff box and its tendons are the terminal branches of the superficial radial nerve of which there may be several, serving the dorsal surface of the thumb and, to a varying degree, the dorsum of the hand and of the proximal phalanges of the index and middle finger. One or more can commonly be palpated by rolling the finger over the radius proximal to the styloid process (Fig. 1.26). The radial nerve here is especially prone to injury during release of the first compartment for de Quervain's disease.

The extensor pollicis longus is clearly seen when the thumb is raised with the palm of the hand on a table. It lies to the ulnar aspect of the adducted thumb, but over the first metacarpal when the thumb is abducted. Thus, in ulnar nerve palsy it can act as a weak but effective adductor of the adducted thumb, but not the abducted. No intertendinous connection (juncturae tendinum) exists between the extensor pollicis longus and the other extensors, except in one reported case[88], or between the

digital and other extensors, except in three[89]. Such connections do exist routinely between the tendons of extensor digitorum over the dorsum of the hand, accounting for the inability to extend the ring finger when the middle is flexed. One of the earliest hand operations, in harpsichord players, was to release this intertendinous connection. A similar operation on the connection between the index and middle fingers has recently been published[90]. When the fist is clenched, the 'knuckles' become prominent. These are, of course, the metacarpal heads, a fact to be remembered in understanding human bite injuries (p. 331). The heads are prominent also in the somewhat ineffectual extension attempted by rheumatoid patients whose joints have subluxed. The prominences should not be mistaken for synovial bulging. Over the knuckles in the clenched fist, the extensor tendons can be seen to ride in a slight, but definite, radial shift. An early sign of impending ulnar drift in rheumatoids is a change in this movement of the tendons to an ulnar direction. When the index finger is deviated radially against resistance, the first web space fills with the contracting muscle of the first dorsal inter-

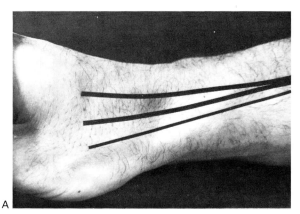

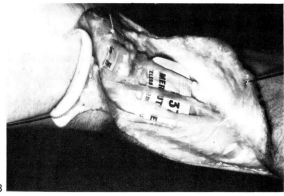

Fig. 1.26 A. The two or three branches of the superficial radial nerve can be rolled beneath the examiner's digit over the radial styloid beyond which the branches cross the snuff box to serve the skin of the dorsum of the first web space. B. These various branches of the radial nerve are seen together with the cephalic vein in the course of dissection of a neuroma resulting from their division during release of a de Quervain's tenovaginitis.

osseous, which arises by two heads from the first two metacarpal shafts. This is the last muscle supplied by the ulnar nerve and that which most rapidly shows wasting in injury or compression.

The palmar surface

SKIN CREASES AND JOINTS

Inspecting a finger from its lateral aspect, it will be appreciated that the flexor surface is relatively flat, with a slight protrusion of the fat over the phalanges between the creases. A lateral view of the skeleton has a quite different configuration, the prominent joints being separated by a relatively narrow waist or saddle at the diaphysis of the phalanges. Firm, subcutaneous fat fills the saddle and creates the final contour over the

phalanges. By contrast, there is no fat beneath the distal and middle digital creases which attach to the cruciate portion of the flexor tendon sheath, which is thin and diaphanous. This permits free flexion of the underlying joint, and also serves to create an even cushion of fat between the skeleton and objects grasped in flexion. Puncture wounds of the finger which introduce infection produce different pathology according to their location. If the wound is directly into one or other of the two creases mentioned, the resultant infection will be a flexor tenosynovitis, extending into the hand along the sheath. That into the pulp will remain localized to that compartment as a felon (Ch. 4).

A radiograph can be used to demonstrate that the distal and middle digital creases approximate closely to the underlying interphalangeal joints, the distal tending to be just proximal to the distal interphalangeal joint, the middle immediately overlying the proximal interphalangeal joint (Fig. 1.27A, B). By contrast, the proximal digital crease corresponds to no joint, overlying the A2 pulley on the proximal phalanx. Firm palpation, especially over the middle digital crease, detects a firm structure which can be rocked laterally. This is the flexor tendon, which can also be felt, less well, beneath the other digital creases. Its *absence* can also be palpated following laceration or rupture. Beneath it lies the glenoid, or fibrous, part of the palmar plate. To either side a smaller, more mobile, cord-like structure can be felt, the digital nerve, with the artery immediately posterior to it. Returning to the flexor tendon, and progressing just proximal to the prominence of the phalangeal head, one can feel a recess which corresponds to the neck of the phalanx. Here lies the membranous part of the palmar plate with, beneath it, the transverse palmar arterial arch[92], from which arise the vincula to the flexor tendons.

The flexor creases for the metacarpophalangeal joints are the proximal and distal palmar creases, and the surface marking is a line joining the ulnar end of the distal crease to the radial end of the proximal palmar crease. This can be easily confirmed by flexing the metacarpophalangeal joints with the interphalangeal joints straight (Fig. 1.27C).

The A1 pulleys which constitute the proximal ends of the fibrous flexor sheaths arise from the palmar plates of the MP joints[93]. The pulley and its contained tendons can be palpated here as at the middle digital crease. The palmar plates of the metacarpophalangeal joints are joined one to another across the hand by the deep transverse metacarpal ligament which separates the interossei dorsally from the lumbricals on its palmar aspect. Lying on the lumbrical muscle, which here is slender, approaching its musculotendinous junction, is

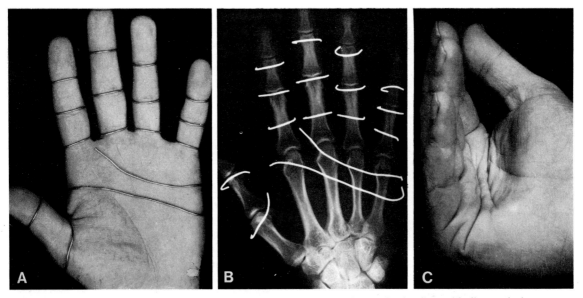

Fig. 1.27 A, B. Wires placed on the creases of a hand which was subsequently examined radiographically reveals the relationship of those creases to the various joints. It will be noted in particular that the proximal digital creases do not correspond to any joint, and that a line joining the ulnar end of the distal palmar crease to the radial end of the proximal palmar crease most closely approximates to the metacarpo-phalangeal joints. C. Flexion of the metacarpophalangeal joints illustrates that their corresponding 'skin joints' are the proximal and distal palmar creases.

the neurovascular bundle, nestled between the flexor tendons. At this level, beneath the palmar creases, the common digital nerve starts to divide into its two component proper digital nerves, having come to lie anterior to the common digital artery. Proximally, at the superficial palmar arch, which is located beneath the palmar triangle in the line of the palmar aspect of the fully abducted thumb, the arterial system lies superficial to the branches of the median and ulnar nerves. The common digital artery divides more distal than does the nerve, roughly midway between the distal palmar crease and the margin of the web. The flexor digitorum superficialis divides and starts to wind around the flexor digitorum profundus at the proximal end of the fibrous sheath, that is, deep to the palmar crease (Fig. 1.28). At the proximal digital crease, level with the free margin of the finger webs, the flexor digitorum profundus is already becoming the more superficial of the tendons. The palmar fascia, or aponeurosis, lies superficial to these structures, deep to the skin which is attached to it by multiple fibrous septa. The palmar fascia in turn is attached to the metacarpals by firm septa which pass between the tendons and neurovascular structures just proximal and distal to the transverse fibres of the fascia. These transverse fibres lie beneath the palmar creases. In the normal hand, the main substance of the palmar fascia is found beneath the palmar triangle, which is that

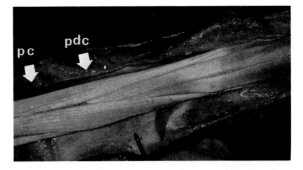

Fig. 1.28 The flexor digitorum superficialis divides beneath the distal palmar crease (pc) and the tendon of flexor digitorum profundus starts to become the more superficial of the two tendons at the level of the proximal digital crease (pdc). This relationship moves proximally when the fingers are strongly flexed. (Dissection by Dr. D. C. Riordan.)

area bounded by the distal palmar crease, the broken hypothenar crease referred to above and the thenar crease.

The long, curved thenar crease represents the skin joint which corresponds to the basal joint of the thumb, and, for that reason, should be seen along its full length clear of the margin of any splint in which full movement of the thumb is intended.

PALPABLE DIGITAL NERVES

With greater ease than those mentioned already, both digital nerves to the thumb can be palpated at the palmar surface of the metacarpophalangeal crease of the thumb — they lie close together over the sheath of flexor pollicis longus where they can be rolled beneath the examiner's thumb (Fig. 1.29) and may be damaged during release of a trigger thumb.

The radial digital nerve to the index finger can be palpated where it lies over the metacarpal head at least one centimetre ulnar to the radial end of the proximal palmar crease (Fig. 1.30).

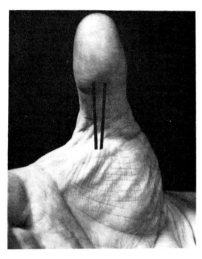

Fig. 1.29 The two digital nerves of the thumb can be palpated by the examiner in close proximity to one another on the palmar aspect of the metacarpophalangeal crease.

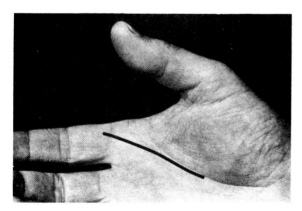

Fig. 1.30 The radial digital nerve to the index finger lies in a more ulnar position than might be supposed and can be palpated where it lies over the metacarpal head 1 cm from the radial end of the proximal palmar crease.

These three digital nerves are the most important in the hand. Ironically, they are also the most vulnerable, lying on unyielding structures and being devoid of the protection offered to the other digital nerves by the palmar aponeurosis. They are, in addition, those most at risk when sharp objects are grasped in the hand.

INITIAL EXAMINATION (Fig. 1.31)

(Note that this is the first stage of examination, as performed in the emergency room or casualty department; the second is exploration, done under aseptic conditions, (see p. 89). Final decisions regarding management — indications — will be made during this first stage only in closed injuries, being left in open wounds until exploration.)

As already suggested, examination should commence shortly after starting the dialogue with the patient detailed above. In children and in patients with more massive injuries, dressings may be left in place until after anaesthesia has been achieved, for in such cases the initial examination yields no subtle information. In such instances, a rough assessment of the magnitude of some injuries can be made by radiographs taken through splints and dressings. Again, definitive radiologic examination will be done under anaesthesia when positioning and distraction can clarify a confusing initial study. In these circumstances, where dressings are left in place, circulation and sensation should be assessed on the protruding fingertips. In other cases, where the patient, witnesses or the dressing testify to previous brisk haemorrhage which may recur, much information may be obtained by examination before

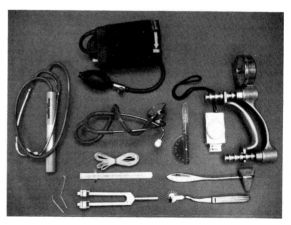

Fig. 1.31 The basic armamentarium for examination of the hand. All will be easily recognized with perhaps the exception of the instrument on the extreme left, which is a Doppler flow meter, and the instruments on the extreme right, which are the grip and pinch dynamometer, respectively.

removing that dressing. However, the bandages applied as a first aid measure should be gently removed in all except these special cases, for knowledge can be gained from the site, configuration and appearance of the wound.

Features of the wound

This has largely been determined during the history and this is confirmed and refined during examination. A classification is helpful in separating those wounds likely to show healing by primary intention from those likely to pursue a more complicated course:

Tidy wounds
   incised
   sliced
      (a) with tissue loss
      (b) with flaps

   puncture

Untidy wounds
   crush
   avulsion   } usually qualified by mechanism
   injection

Finger tip (see p. 117)
   nail bed
   pulp

Amputations
   complete
   incomplete — this implies an injury through bone and more than 50% of the skin circumference, viability doubtful or not

Tidy wounds are inflicted by sharp instruments and have well-defined edges. They are associated with little destruction of tissue, and primary healing with minimal scarring results. Tendons, arteries and nerves are commonly injured, but cleanly, so that primary repair is easily achieved. Fractures are uncommon in such injuries. If they *are* present they tend to be transverse and not comminuted.

Multiple, parallel, tidy lacerations, especially on the wrist suggest a self-inflicted injury[94]. A number of small cuts beside one deep laceration suggests the same mechanism; such cuts are called 'hesitation marks' (Fig. 1.32). Indeed, in any circumstance where the history does not fit the injury, the physician must pursue the truth. If he does not he may undertake inappropriate surgery and fail to offer appropriate ancillary treatment. Psychiatric consultation is required on all patients who injure themselves, for they need help. It

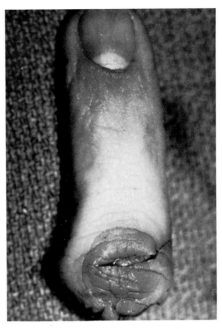

Fig. 1.32 This amputated digit arrived with a patient who, it was stated, had sustained an accidental amputation while alone chopping wood. Examination of the amputated part revealed a hesitation cut just distal to the point of amputation. Questioning revealed that this was a self-inflicted injury.

may also be true that the more they object and protest, the more they need that help.

The *site*, especially of tidy wounds, leads the examiner with a good knowledge of surface anatomy to suspect which structures may be involved.

The *configuration* of lacerations can also give information (Fig. 1.33A, B). Where a slicing injury has been inflicted by a flat blade with a straight cutting edge, the wound will be more curved the more acute the angle of incidence of the blade to the skin. Thus, a cut directly perpendicular to the skin will be straight, and one virtually parallel to the skin will be almost a full circle, to the point of actually removing a piece of skin. Further, by mentally drawing a straight line joining the ends of the wound, the surgeon can deduce which deep structures are likely to be involved. With a straight blade, it can be generalized that the more curved the cut the longer the wound and the less deep the damage. He can also draw conclusions regarding the location of these structures relative to the wound since deep injury will always lie to the concave side of a curved wound.

After stabbing or laceration with an irregular flat instrument, such as a piece of glass, *no* prediction can be made regarding depth or extent of injury, but the direction is still indicated by the shape of the wound. This

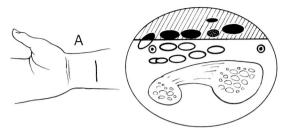

FDS to ring & middle
FCR, PL, partial FCU
Median n.

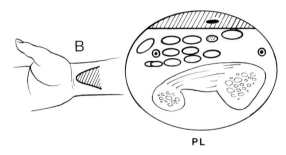

PL

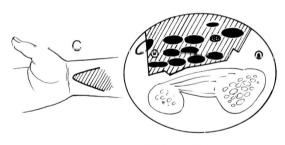

FDS to all
FDP to all
FCU, FCR, PL
Median n., Ulnar n.
Ulnar a.

Fig. 1.33 Depending upon the nature of the cutting agent, that is, whether it has a straight or a ragged edge, some conclusion can be drawn as to the nature of possible deep damage. A. If it has a straight edge and the laceration is transverse, by mentally joining the two ends of the wound the surgeon can deduce which structures will be lacerated. B. If the cutting edge was straight, but the wound V-shaped, then the laceration is likely to be fairly shallow. Once again, by joining the two ends some conclusion can be drawn as to the deep damage. C. If the weapon has been ragged, such as a piece of glass, or pointed, such as a knife blade, then no firm conclusion can be drawn since many structures can be damaged by the points of the instrument.

helps appreciably in planning extending incisions. The different potential of a slicing straight knife and a stabbing irregular piece of glass cannot be overemphasized and is shown in Figure 1.33C.

The *appearance* of the wound may reveal damage to deep structures either by their presentation in the wound or, much more commonly, by the presence of dark red, gelatinous blood clot, *always* an indicator of injury to tendons, nerves, or vessels.

A point of management during examination arises. While it is probable that free arterial bleeding will not be evident on removing the dressing, the skin wound being filled with clot, it will occasionally be present. When free bleeding does occur it is probably due to a *partial* laceration of a major vessel (p. 45) and, as such, constitutes the only potentially fatal injury of the upper extremity (Fig. 1.34). The choice of action to control such haemorrhage which has been recommended variously is fourfold:

1. carefully ligate the very end of the vessel
2. apply an upper-arm tourniquet
3. control the appropriate arterial pressure point
4. apply local pressure.

Careful ligation of the very end of the vessel is a solution made attractive by its implied precision, but only to those who have never dealt with such a situation in the hand. Exposure of a bleeding vessel in the examination room sufficient to ligate it precisely requires quite unjustified exploration of the wound in conditions far from ideal and will probably result in excessive blood loss. Were it exposed, ligation could then only be achieved by the destruction of the ends of the artery. That portion may be essential for a straightforward tension-free anastomosis.

The application of an upper-arm tourniquet in even the best ordered emergency room is fraught with the hazard of neglect and should for that reason be condemned. The tourniquet is acceptable only in that case where a collapsed patient is bleeding from a major vascular injury and is to be taken forthwith to the operating room. If a tourniquet is deemed essential, the person who applies it *must note the time and remain with the patient until it is removed.* This is not only to ensure that the cuff is deflated before ischaemia causes irreversible damage, that is, after at most two hours, but more frequently, to ensure that the pressure in the cuff remains above the patient's systolic pressure. That pressure may well be rising as resuscitative efforts succeed, while many cuffs and connections leak. If the pressure falls below systolic, the bleeding will be worse than that which would have occurred with no cuff at all, since it will be from both the arterial and the occluded venous systems.

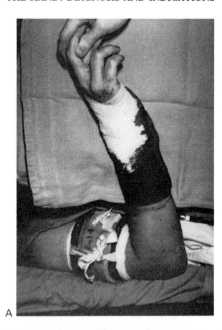

A

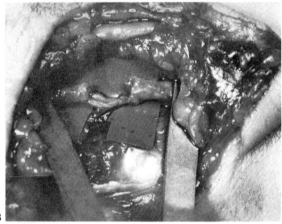

B

Fig. 1.34 A. Heavy bleeding through a compressive dressing suggests a partial laceration of a major vessel. Control of this wound required application of a tourniquet and immediate transportation to the operating room where, indeed, a partial injury of the ulnar artery (B) was found.

To control bleeding by *digital pressure* on the appropriate pressure point — the brachial artery at mid-humerus — is acceptable and permits adequate examination preoperatively. It is not practicable or reliable during the time between examination and surgery.

Once the examination has been completed using pressure point control, the bleeding should thereafter be controlled by a *local pressure dressing* supplemented by *elevation of the arm*. This should be maintained under frequent supervision until the hand is being prepared in

the operating room, when excessive blood loss can be prevented by the use of an upper-arm tourniquet. If pressure and elevation fail, as evidenced by bleeding through the dressing, a tourniquet *should* be applied and surgery expedited.

Untidy wounds result from tearing or bursting of the skin. They are caused by crush injuries, explosions, and by such as rollers, power-saws, industrial and farm machinery. The edges of the skin are irregular, with many flaps of doubtful viability. Primary healing is less likely than in tidy wounds, and extensive scarring tends to result. The full extent of injury to such patients is rarely clear until exploration, and indeed may not be evident until days or even weeks after the accident. The nature of damage in untidy injuries is:

Skin   indeterminable loss of viability

Skeleton   fractures common, usually multiple and
              comminuted, with joint disruption

Tendon   avulsion with or without loss of substance
              abrasion

Nerve   avulsion
              crush
              burn
              traction } often in continuity

Vessel   injury common, including
              avulsion
              partial tear in continuity
              thrombosis due to compression,
              torsion or traction.

Viability

In *tidy lacerations* this is less likely to be in doubt than in injuries resulting from crush or avulsion. Depending upon the quality and integrity of collateral circulation, division of the brachial artery or of *both* radial and ulnar arteries may or may not result in insufficient perfusion of the distal limb. Where *either* radial *or* ulnar arteries have been divided at the wrist, the viability of the hand is not compromised. Lack of frank vascular inadequacy should by no means imply that the vessels sho   t be repaired, for otherwise late problems with n... function may arise from ischaemia (p. 258).

In the finger, division of both digital arteries proximal to their dorsal branches will be evident from the greyish lividity of the pulp and even more of the nail bed. Vascular repair is necessary for survival of the digit. Since the digital artery lies dorsal to the nerve in the finger, division of the artery in palmar wounds is strong prima facie evidence that the nerve also has been divided.

The *non-viable digit* in incomplete amputation, where both arterial and venous flow is compromised, is characteristically very white in colour with areas of pale violet. The pulp is collapsed, and its temperature palpably lower than adjacent digits. With fingertip pressure it does not blanch and refill. Rotating the digit which is hanging loosely will not aid in determining whether or not vascular torsion or frank division is the cause of the pallor. Only exploration and fracture fixation can do so. In certain cases, however, flow *will* be improved by adjustment in the emergency room. This is especially true of the ring avulsion, and the degloved skin should be repositioned pending formal exploration.

In *untidy injuries* the paramount question, and often the one most difficult to answer is 'What tissues are viable?' No final decision regarding viability should be made until fractures are reduced and immobilized (Fig. 1.35). Torsion and compression of otherwise un-injured vessels may well arise through the instability of fractures, and apparently non-viable parts may be amputated needlessly if this is not appreciated.

Amputation and replantation

Replantation of totally severed parts and *revascularization* of incomplete amputations is becoming possible in an increasing number of centres.

There are two distinct groups of limb amputation requiring quite different care:

Macro-replantation, in which the amputated part contains muscle bulk; speed is important; a high level of microsurgical skill and unlimited surgical time are *not* necessary (Fig. 1.36). In these amputations, significant force has been involved, and other severe, but often obscure, injuries are likely[95]. Even in their absence, hypovolaemic shock is probable. These patients are at risk during long journeys.

Micro-replantation, in which the amputated parts are usually digits; speed is of secondary significance; a high level of microsurgical skill and unlimited surgical

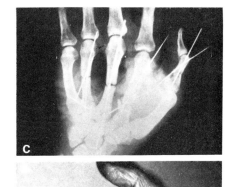

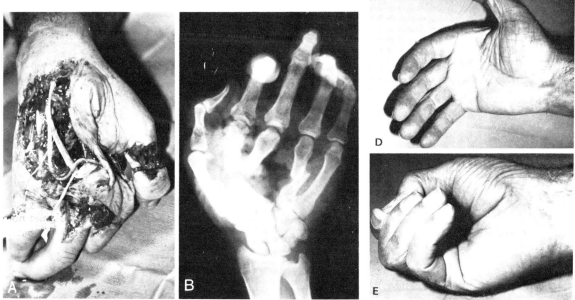

Fig. 1.35 A. This patient sustained a massive crush injury beneath the platform of a tip-up dumper truck which resulted in extensive metacarpal fractures and carpal–metacarpal dislocations. B. On initial examination, all of the digits appeared to be non-viable. C. After internal fixation of the fractures, however, flow returned to all digits without vascular repairs, and two years later it can be seen (D, E) that the four digits survived with a reasonable return of function.

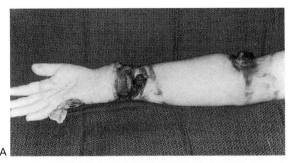

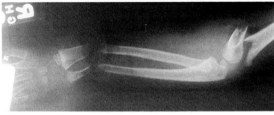

Fig. 1.36 A, B. This child, with a double-level incomplete amputation sustained in an auger, was transported for several hours before reaching the primary care facility. Further delay ensued before the child was transferred to a replantation centre where flow was re-established at the brachial artery level ten hours after injury. No muscle perfusion whatsoever was seen in the forearm, and above-elbow amputation was therefore obligatory. Macro-replantation at the brachial artery level requires haste, while replantation at the level of the wrist could wait, with cooling, without major loss of eventual function.

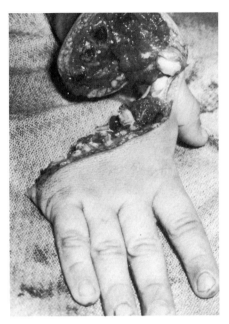

Fig. 1.37 The disc of a harrowing plow virtually amputated the right hand of this child. On arrival for replantation he was moribund, on account of an unsuspected fracture of the pelvis and retroperitoneal haematoma sustained when his body passed beneath the tractor wheel.

time are essential. In cases selected by the process detailed on p. 10, time-consuming travel to reach a microsurgical team is both acceptable and desirable, especially when multiple digital amputations have occurred[96].

Certain factors, given below, have come to be recognized as *contraindications* to replantation[70].

Strong contraindications
1. Significant associated injuries to torso and head; common in macro-replantation candidates (Fig. 1.37)
2. Extensive injury to the affected limb or to the amputated part — multiple level (Fig. 1.38); degloving; widespread crush
3. Severe chronic illness, such as to preclude transportation or prolonged surgery.

Relative contraindications
These are often present in combination and are then more discouraging.

1. Single digit amputation, especially proximal to the insertion of flexor digitorum superficialis (Fig. 1.39)

2. Avulsion injuries, as evidenced by:
   (a) mechanism
   (b) structures dangling from the part, usually nerves and tendons; this often indicates vessel avulsion *from* the part (Figs. 1.40, 1.41)
   (c) 'red-streak' — bruising over the neurovascular pedicle, indicating vessel disruption
3. Previous injury or surgery to the part
4. Extreme contamination
5. Lengthy warm ischaemia — in practice applicable only to macro-replantation[97]
6. Age — increased chance of vessel disease and systemic illness

Distal single digit replantation
Replantation of single digit amputations distal to the superficialis insertion is worthwhile. Two reports[98,99] involving 129 digits show over 80% survival with average two-point discrimination of 10 mm in one series. Such surgery is justified when common sense rules are applied:

1. The disadvantages, already detailed, are discussed with the patient.
2. Only one attempt is made with a time limit of 5 hours of surgery.

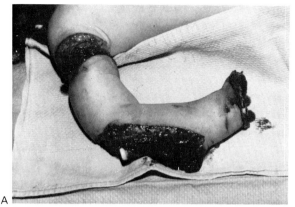

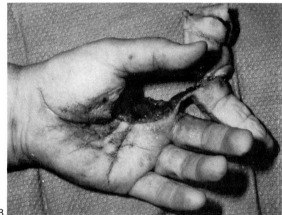

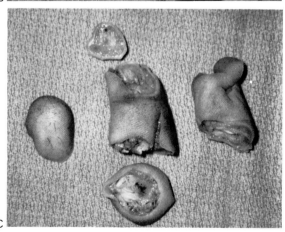

Fig. 1.38 A. This child sustained multiple-level amputations and partial amputations when she fell beneath a lawn mower. B. Double-level amputation of a single digit such as that shown here is a contraindication to replantation. C. A common sight after lawn mower injury. These multiple amputated parts are none of them fit for replantation. When multiple parts present they should all be inspected carefully, because transplantation from one digit to another may provide function which could not be gained by any other means.

3. No drugs, other than aspirin, are given.
4. The patient is not admitted postoperatively.

Rules 2 and 3 make admission unnecessary, and in the face of rising costs such management makes economic sense. In the admittedly small series with which the author has had experience, such outpatient replantations have all survived, provided they were viable at the end of surgery (Fig. 1.42).

Salvage replantation
Despite much of the above, replantation should be attempted in children, in whom 93% of normal growth can be expected in replanted digits[100], or following amputation of the thumb[101] or more than two fingers.

Ring avulsion injuries
Other classifications of ring injuries are available[102], but that of Urbaniak et al[103] is best related to current microsurgical capabilities:

Class I — circulation adequate (Fig. 1.43)
Class II — circulation inadequate: microvascular reconstruction will restore both circulation and function (Fig. 1.44)
  Subclassifications have been suggested: IIA, in which only digital arteries require repair; IIB in which arteries and bone, tendon and/or joint are involved[104], and IIC, in which only veins are involved[105]
Class III — complete degloving of skin or complete amputation of fingers (Fig. 1.45); microvascular reconstruction will restore circulation but only *poor* function; revision of the amputation is recommended, with or without a cross-finger flap to maintain competent length (Fig. 1.46).

(One group has reported acceptable results in Class III injuries and recommends replantation[106, 107].) In all cases, the final decision regarding replantation is made once the limb and the part have been explored under sterile conditions and with magnification (p. 106). The part(s) can be explored immediately while the patient is prepared for surgery, with resulting economy of time.

Systematic examination of each tissue will be discussed in turn. The order selected here, as in later exploration where it differs, is that employed in practice. The extent of assessment, and the decisions made, at first and second examination differ greatly from tissue to tissue, as previously emphasized.

Skin

Clean skin defects produced by tidy, slicing wounds can be evaluated in the emergency room.

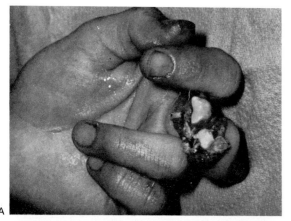

A

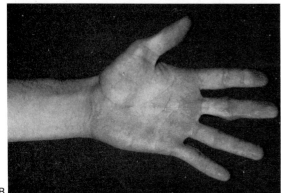

B

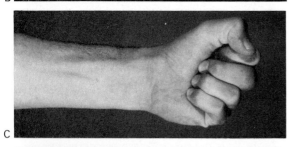

C

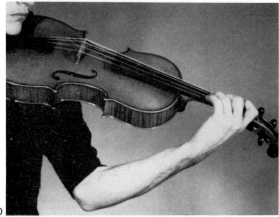

D

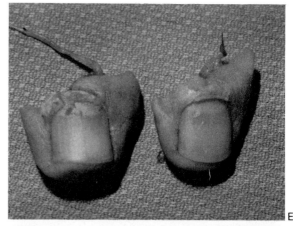

E

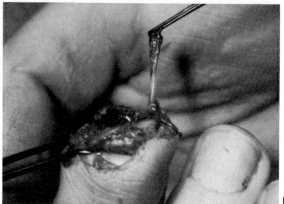

F

Fig. 1.40 A. The presence of dangling nerves from these amputated parts suggests avulsion. This not only means that the eventual recovery of sensation would be unsatisfactory, but that it is probable that the digital arteries were avulsed from distally. B. This was evident on exploration of the digit itself.

The choice of skin graft and flap are considered in more detail in the section on exploration (p. 111).

Untidy wounds are much more difficult to evaluate since undermining causes both retraction of skin edges and impairment of their blood supply. Thus, the skin loss resulting from the injury and the skin excision necessary for adequate debridement must be finally assessed in the operating room (p. 108). Where the

Fig. 1.39 A. Single digit amputation, both complete and incomplete, is usually a relative contraindication to replantation; however, this teenager was not only skilful with a saw — as can be seen by the fact that he went through the proximal interphalangeal joint without damaging either articular surface — but was also a very competent violinist. His determination to recover resulted in perfect function (B, C, D).

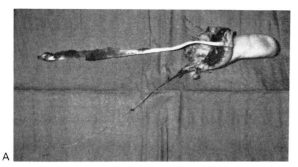

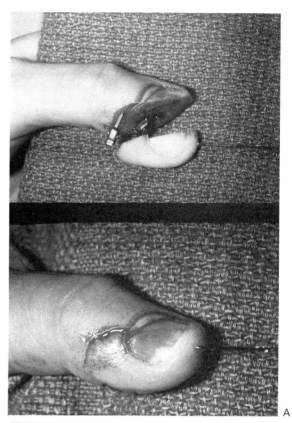

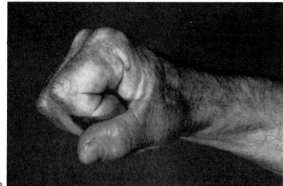

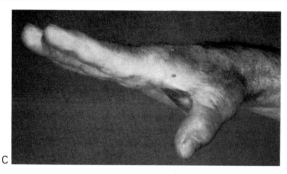

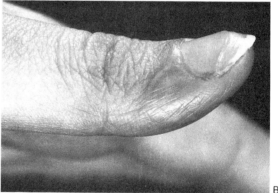

Fig. 1.41 A. This thumb was avulsed by a zoo animal, and the long strands of digital nerve can be seen in the upper and lower parts of the photograph. B, C. Because it was a thumb avulsion, it was nonetheless replanted employing long vein grafts. The patient at no time recovered normal sensation or motion; however, the thumb functioned adequately.

Fig. 1.42 A. Distal digital replantation. B. The result.

possibility exists, the patient and family must be prepared for distant flap procedures.

Those wound margins and skin flaps which are of doubtful viability can be distinguished by:

1. *Colour.* The flap may be white or may show purplish lividity if there is an element of venous congestion. (In the congested dorsal flap, formerly doomed, a significant increase in survival has been achieved by microvascular venous repair).

2. *Design.* If the flap clearly has only a narrow pedicle it is unlikely to survive. Experience has shown that random pattern flaps raised on the limbs *surgically* have a precarious blood supply, and certainly that proportions of length/breadth of 1/1 cannot be exceeded without risk of skin necrosis.
   Traumatically avulsed flaps have not been raised under such conditions, and, as a result, those which

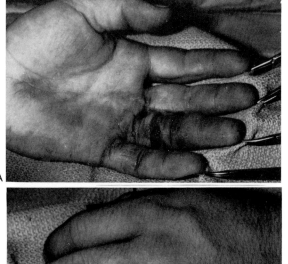

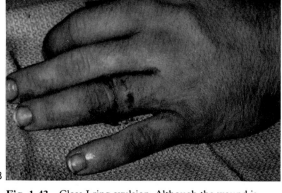

Fig. 1.43 Class I ring avulsion. Although the wound is circumferential, the circulation is identical to that in adjacent digits, and there was no damage to deep structures.

exceed or even equal those proportions rarely survive. It is very important that the extent to which a flap is undermined is accurately assessed. This is especially true in roller and run-over injuries where the flap may not be recognized as such, but where undermining may be very extensive, and, if left, much of the skin will die. The true state of affairs should be deduced from

history	run-over
examination	gaping wound, the edges of which do not bleed
	loss of skin sensation
exploration	widespread undermining of skin edges

3. *Return of flow after exsanguination.* This is the most common clinical test of blood flow which is applied; it involves observation of blood returning to the skin after its expression by the examiner's finger:

Slow return to an area of pallor suggests inadequate arterial supply

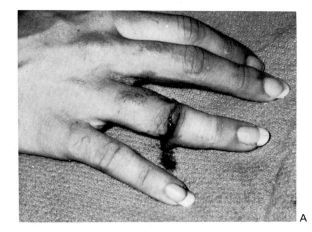

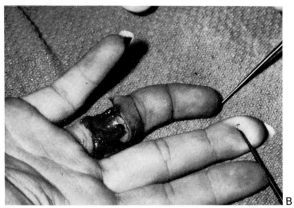

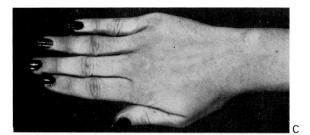

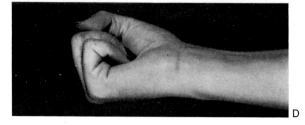

Fig. 1.44 A, B. Class II ring avulsion. Here there was dislocation of the distal interphalangeal joint, and, in addition, the vascularization of the digit was compromised. C, D. Very satisfactory function was achieved after revascularization.

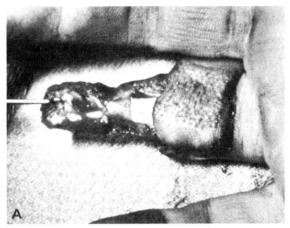

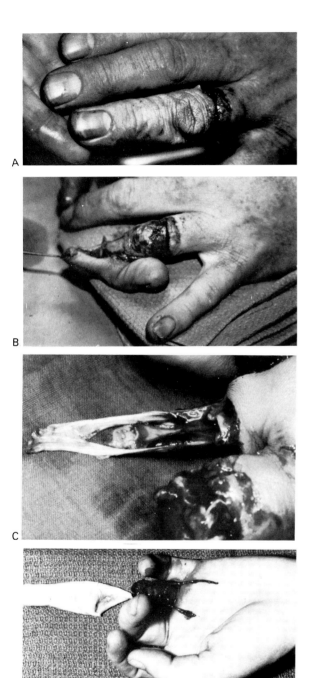

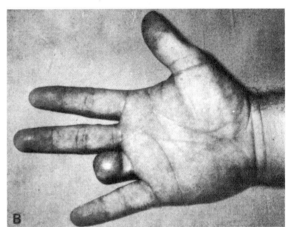

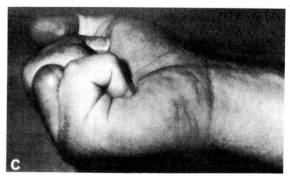

Fig. 1.45 Class III ring avulsions. A, B. Although not completely removed, all of the skin of this digit has been avulsed, and there is a complex injury to the underlying skeleton. Largely due to devascularization of the underlying skeleton, the eventual functional result would be poor. C. In this totally avulsed digit — one of two adjacent fingers damaged by rings — the entire extensor apparatus has been avulsed from the missing digit. D. Total avulsion — note long neurovascular structures.

Fig. 1.46 A. A ring avulsion resulted in total loss of the skin of this construction worker's ring finger, the palmar defect being larger than the dorsal, as is commonly the case. A cross finger flap was raised from the dorsum of the adjacent finger and is seen here covering the proximal part of the palmar defect. Partial amputation was performed. This gave a competent hand (B, C).

Swift return to a purple, swollen area suggests inadequate venous drainage

Swift return to a pink area indicates adequate blood flow.

This test in used even more effectively in the operating room (p. 109).

Untidy hand injuries are often grossly contaminated, and because of this it may not be possible to assess the skin viability with any accuracy. It may be necessary to wait until the limb has been anaesthetized and cleansed (Fig. 1.47). For skin exploration, see p. 107.

Tendon

HAND POSTURE

If the completely relaxed or anaesthetized normal hand is raised, with forearm supinated (Fig. 1.48), the weight of the hand causes the wrist to fall into some 30° of dorsiflexion. The metacarpophalangeal joints lie in increasing flexion from 40° in the index finger to 50° in the middle, 60° in the ring and 70° in the small, and the proximal and distal interphalangeal joints adopt a similar posture. Thus, the distance from the digital pulp to the palmar crease decreases in smooth progression from the index to the small finger — the so-called 'cascade'. The metacarpophalangeal and interphalangeal joints of the thumb both lie in 30° flexion, the thumb abducted to the extent that the pulp lies closely adjacent to the pulp of the index finger.

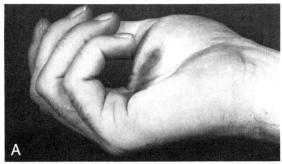

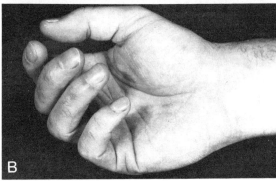

Fig. 1.48 A. A completely relaxed hand in the fully supinated position lies with the wrist in some 30° of dorsal flexion and with a 'cascade' of flexion in the fingers increasing from the index finger to a maximum at the joints of the small finger. B. The thumb lies gently flexed so that its pulp comes to lie in close approximation to that of the index finger.

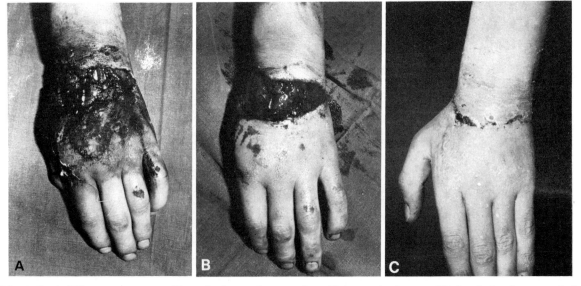

Fig. 1.47 A. This twenty-one-year-old sustained a grossly contaminated injury to the dorsum of his hand when it was caught in a coal conveyer belt. It was not possible to assess the viability of the skin margins until after cleansing (B), when it became evident that skin viability was good. Suture resulted in primary healing (C).

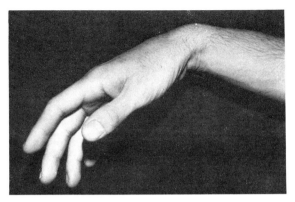

Fig. 1.49 With the arm in pronation, the wrist falls into palmar flexion and the fingers and thumb all extend.

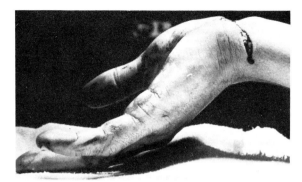

Fig. 1.50 Complete laceration of all flexor tendons at the wrist results in flaccid extension of all fingers in the supinated limb.

When the unsupported, relaxed arm is then turned into pronation, the wrist falls into 40–70° of palmar flexion, depending on whether the elbow is extended or flexed, and the fingers and thumb all extend, the thumb fully and the finger joints to within 20° of the neutral position (Fig. 1.49).

These postures in the relaxed hand are determined by the balance between the resting tone in the flexor and extensor tendons. The mechanism by which the posture of one joint is influenced by that of another via the passive tension in tendons which cross both joints is called the *tenodesis* effect. Any change in the condition of the tendons will therefore appreciably alter the resting posture of the hand, assuming the absence of pre-existing pathology.

Complete division of all flexor tendons at the wrist (Fig. 1.50) results in full extension of all fingers in the supinated limb.

Complete division of both flexor tendons to one finger results in that finger lying in full extension, in marked contrast with the normal posture of those adjacent (Fig. 1.51). Division of the flexor digitorum profundus alone will result in loss of flexion at the distal interphalangeal joint. This will cause the finger tip to fall out of alignment with the others if it is an isolated injury. Lacerations of profundus do not produce hyperextension because the presence of the intact short vinculum prevents it. Hyperextension of the distal interphalangeal joint suggests that the profundus tendon has been avulsed from its bony insertion.

Division of flexor pollicis longus results in full extension of the interphalangeal joint of the thumb which, depending upon the normal range of the joint, may appear hyperextended (Fig. 1.52).

It is important to appreciate, despite all that has been said about reaching a diagnosis on the basis of posture,

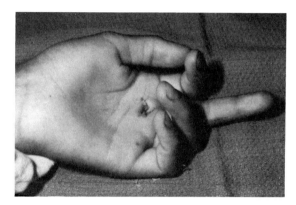

Fig. 1.51 The posture of the middle finger in this anaesthetized hand reveals division of both flexor tendons to that digit.

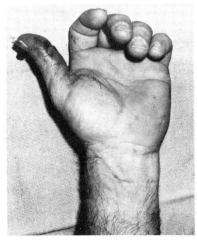

Fig. 1.52 Division of flexor pollicis longus, as has occurred in this patient, is shown by hyperextension of the interphalangeal joint.

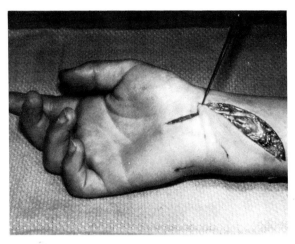

Fig. 1.53 No appreciable alteration in the posture of the fingers occurs when all the superficialis tendons are divided at the wrist but the profundus tendons remain intact, with the exception of that to the index.

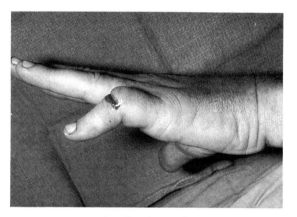

Fig. 1.54 A laceration directly over the proximal interphalangeal joint produces an immediate extensor lag.

that *partial division* of any tendon and *division of superficialis tendons without injury to profundus* will result in *no* detectable change in posture (Fig. 1.53).

The extensor tendon division is less distinct in its effect on posture because the intrinsic muscles are responsible for much of the extensor contribution to the normal balance at the interphalangeal joints, and because of the intertendinous connections of the long extensor tendons. However, in an isolated injury on the dorsum of the hand the metacarpophalangeal joint may fall into more flexion than its neighbours.

Division of the long extensor tendon over the proximal phalanx will produce no postural change and little if any functional loss, as the long extensor will continue to

extend the metacarpophalangeal joint, acting through the sagittal bands, while the lateral bands will extend the proximal interphalangeal joint.

Open injuries over the proximal interphalangeal joint will often result in an immediate boutonniere deformity (Fig. 1.54). A closed injury may not present until late (Fig. 1.55).

Likewise, where the extensor tendon has been divided or avulsed at its insertion into the terminal phalanx, the characteristic mallet finger deformity may not be obvious in the acute situation, developing some time later. (Fig. 1.56).

Postural changes in tendon injuries, though frequently diagnostic, are not always accurate for a variety of reasons:

1. Previous injury or disease
2. Partial tendon division
3. Tendon division proximal to a link with another intact tendon. This commonly occurs with:
   (a) divisions of the extensors of the middle, ring and small fingers proximal to their linking intertendinous connections
   (b) isolated division at the wrist of flexor digitorum profundus to any of the middle, ring or small fingers, as these tendons are only fully independent of one another distal to the carpal tunnel.

With any sharp injury over a joint with tendon involvement, one must *always* suspect and look for articular damage (Fig. 1.57).

TENDON TENSION

Gentle pressure exerted on each finger tip in turn is a surprisingly sensitive index of the integrity of tendons. Differences between the resistance encountered in adjacent fingers or between those in the injured and uninjured hands will certainly reveal complete division and may also indicate when incomplete division is present. In the latter case, there is inhibition of normal muscle tone and the movement caused commonly proves painful. The test differs only in degree from resisted active motion described below.

Nerve injuries are *not* associated at the time of injury with an appreciable change in muscle tone. The tension in a tendon is therefore not altered by division of its nerve supply.

PASSIVE MOTION

Where doubt still exists regarding tendon injury, and the patient cannot co-operate in active motion, it is

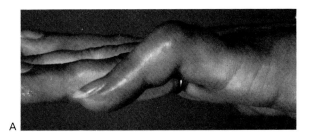

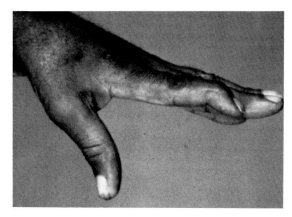

Fig. 1.56 A mallet finger deformity which developed gradually after a small laceration over the dorsum of the distal interphalangeal joint.

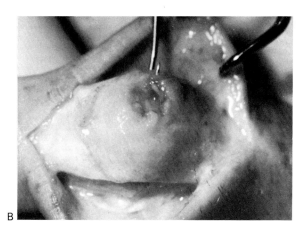

possible to produce passive tendon movement in the flexor tendons. Especially useful in children, this is done by pressing firmly on the junction of the middle and distal thirds of the ulnar half of the anterior aspect of the forearm. If the tendons are intact or partially so this results in flexion through 1 to 2 cm and is most marked in the ulnar three fingers (Fig. 1.58)[108]. If flexor pollicis longus is uninjured, when the pressure is exerted with one finger a little more distally over the anterior surface of the radius, the interphalangeal joint of the thumb will flex. In practice this is a test little used, and then only to supplement harder evidence.

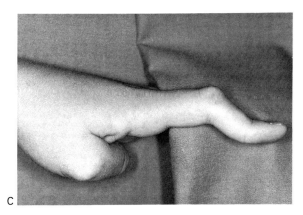

ACTIVE MOTION

Active motion can be assessed in any one of three ways: by asking the patient to perform the movement; by demonstrating what the examiner wishes him to do; by placing the appropriate joint in the position normally produced by the muscle being tested and asking the patient to maintain it.

'*Put your finger like that. Hold it there. Now, keep it there! Don't let me move it!*'

In all instances, resistance should then be offered to the motion since pain and even sudden release will clearly demonstrate the presence of a *partial tendon division*.

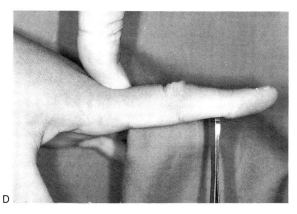

Fig. 1.55 This patient presented five weeks after a small laceration over the dorsum of the proximal interphalangeal joint. A. Maximum extension. Exploration of the finger (B) revealed an irregular injury to the central slip of the extensor apparatus. C, D. This patient had sustained a closed injury and presented six months later with a classical boutonniere deformity, which was passively correctable and therefore deemed appropriate for reconstruction.

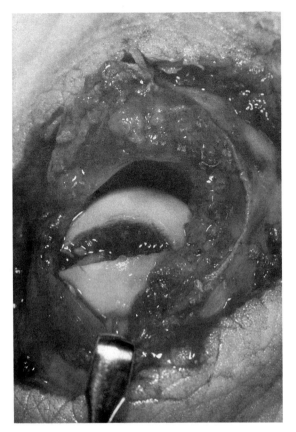

Fig. 1.57 A laceration over the metacarpophalangeal joint with loss of extension. The radiograph was deemed to be normal. Exploration of the joint revealed significant articular damage.

Flexor carpi radialis and flexor carpi ulnaris
With the fingers actively extended if possible, flexion of the wrist against gentle resistance will allow the examiner to palpate the tendons of the primary wrist flexors to ensure their integrity.

Fig. 1.58 A, B. In this child with intact tendons, it can be seen that firm pressure exerted over the anterior aspect of the forearm with the examiner's thumb results in flexion of all the digits leading to the conclusion that at least the profundus tendons are partially intact. C. The posture following this wrist laceration suggests that all flexor tendons are divided with the exception, perhaps, of the thumb. When the thumb is supported (D) and then pressure exerted over the anterior aspect of the wrist (E) it can be seen that flexion occurs in the thumb, suggesting that the flexor pollicis longus is intact, but that none of the fingers move, indicating that all digital flexor tendons have been divided.

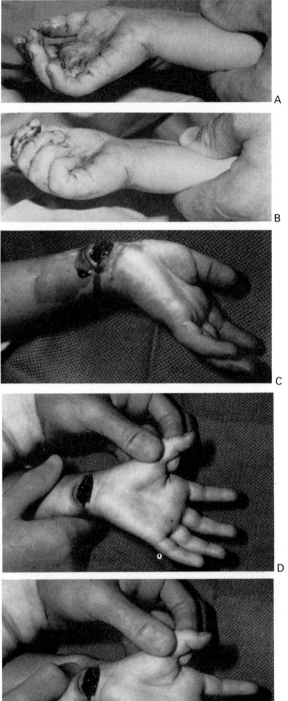

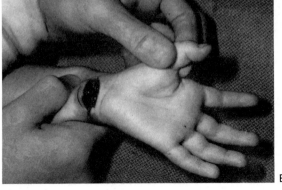

Flexor digitorum profundus and flexor pollicis longus

The examiner should immobilize in turn the middle phalanx of each finger and the proximal phalanx of the thumb and either ask the patient to flex the digit or passively place it in flexion and ask the patient to maintain that posture. Flexion at the distal interphalangeal joint will confirm the integrity of the flexor digitorum profundus and, at the interphalangeal joint in the thumb, of the flexor pollicis longus (Fig. 1.59).

If the patient is unable to flex with tendons which have been shown to be intact by the passive motion test described above, this is evidence of loss of innervation to the muscles in question. Such loss is probably due to nerve injury in the forearm or upper arm as follows:

Ulnar two fingers	Ulnar nerve *or* isolated injury to branch serving flexor digitorum profundus
Radial two fingers or the thumb	Median nerve above the antecubital fossa *or* anterior interosseous nerve in the forearm

Flexor digitorum superficialis[109]

As already discussed, it is not possible to flex the ulnar three distal interphalangeal joints independently of one

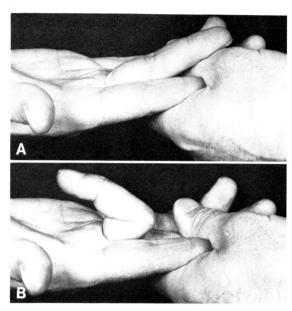

Fig. 1.60 A. If two of the three ulnar digits are held firmly in extension, flexion of the remaining digit (B) can be produced only by the action of the flexor digitorum superficialis. That this is the case can be confirmed by passive motion of the distal interphalangeal joint which will be found to be completely mobile.

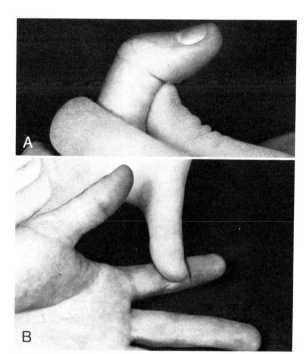

Fig. 1.59 Flexion of the distal joints of the thumb and finger respectively confirms the integrity of the flexor pollicis longus and flexor digitorum profundus.

another on account of the common origin of the profundus tendons (p. 12). It follows that if two of the three are fixed in extension by the examiner and the patient is asked to flex the third, this movement will be produced by the flexor digitorum superficialis and will occur at the proximal interphalangeal joint (Fig. 1.60). That flexor digitorum profundus is not responsible for any flexion during this test can be confirmed by passively moving the relaxed distal interphalangeal joint. The integrity or otherwise of flexor digitorum superficialis to the ulnar three fingers can thus be demonstrated. It should be noted that in one-third of normal patients the superficialis cannot achieve flexion of the small finger — in approximately half of those it will do so if the ring finger is permitted to flex simultaneously[110, 111]. In others, more rare, there is no profundus to the small finger, the superficialis inserting to both middle and distal phalanges[112, 113].

This test *cannot* be applied reliably to the index finger, the flexor digitorum profundus to it being independent (Fig. 1.61). To test the flexor digitorum superficialis to the index, the patient is asked to perform pulp-to-pulp pinch with the thumb and index finger as, for example, by gripping a piece of paper taken from the dressing pack. The more strongly this is performed by

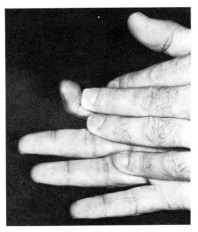

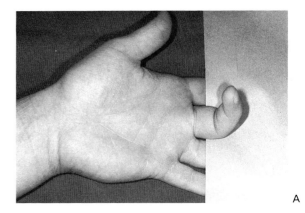

Fig. 1.61   The flexor digitorum profundus to the index finger, having a separate muscle belly, can act quite independently. The test previously described for superficialis of the ulnar three fingers cannot therefore be reliably applied to the index finger.

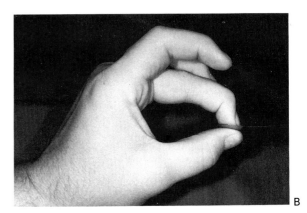

the uninjured hand the more it becomes an action of the flexor digitorum superficialis to the index finger with flexor digitorum profundus relaxed, as is shown by the hyperextension of the distal interphalangeal joint — a 'pseudo-boutonniere' posture (Fig. 1.62). In contrast, if this test is performed in the presence of flexor digitorum superficialis division, the distal interphalangeal joint becomes progressively more flexed as flexor digitorum profundus substitutes for flexor digitorum superficialis — a 'pseudo-mallet' (Fig. 1.63).

Closed flexor tendon injuries
In contrast to the extensor apparatus, the flexor tendons rarely rupture in the absence of disease (most commonly rheumatoid) or of a fracture of one of the bones over which they run, most commonly of the hamate, which may wear on profundus to the small finger. In those instances in which flexor tendons do rupture apparently spontaneously they do so in the palm of the hand[114-117].

Avulsion of the flexor digitorum profundus is a common injury sustained by players of rugby or American football, the ring finger being most often involved. This predilection has been shown to be due to a significantly weaker insertion of the profundus tendon there than in the middle finger[118] or to its greater length in flexion[119]. Rarely, it may be due to a pathological fracture of a distal phalanx which is the seat of a tumour, such as an enchondroma[120]. The tendon frequently takes a fragment of bone from the distal phalanx. The size of the fragment is inversely proportional to the distance by

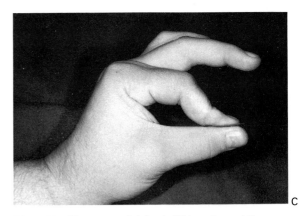

Fig. 1.62   Absent superficialis. A. This patient, while undertaking the test demonstrated in Fig. 1.60, has the capacity to flex independently the middle finger with the flexor digitorum profundus, as shown by the flexion of the distal joint. B. Asking the patient to pinch a thin object as it is withdrawn causes the middle finger to adopt a *pseudo-mallet posture* as opposed to the normal posture adopted by the index finger which has an intact superficialis (C) in which the profundus is relaxed and the superficialis contracted (pseudo-boutonniere).

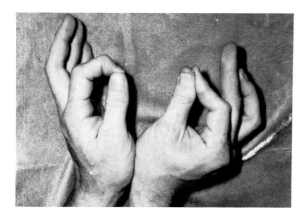

Fig. 1.63 The patient in this photograph is attempting to reproduce the posture achieved on his right hand with the one on the left. He fails to do this because of a previous division of his flexor digitorum superficialis, which was subsequently demonstrated at exploration.

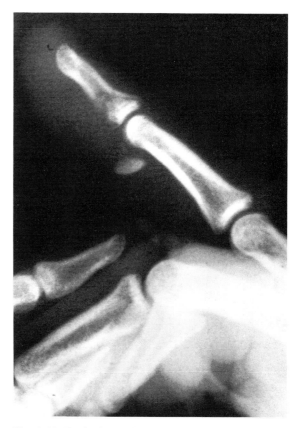

Fig. 1.64 Profundus avulsion. On lateral radiograph the fragment of distal phalanx avulsed by the flexor digitorum profundus can be seen.

which the tendon will retract, for, if large, it will hang up on the A4 pulley, if smaller, on the A3, the A2 distal margin or the division of the superficialis tendon. Lateral radiograph may reveal the location of the fragment (Fig. 1.64), and hence of the distal tendon end, although rare separation of tendon from fragment has been reported[121]. An unusually large fragment may cause vascular compromise of the digit which will be relieved by its reduction[122]. Avulsion of flexor digitorum superficialis is very rare[123], while avulsion of both may occur when hand-held devices explode.

INDICATIONS IN CLOSED AVULSION

Unfortunately, patients often present late with this injury, on average over 2 months after the event[124]. If the tendon has retracted into the palm, it should be repaired within the first week but if the end remains distal to the superficialis insertion, it can be repaired successfully even after several months[125]. Later cases should have the distal interphalangeal joint fused.

See Green D P 1993 Operative Hand Surgery, 3rd edn. Churchill Livingstone, New York, p. 1841.

Extensors
The long and short extensor and long abductor of the thumb can be tested by asking the patient to extend his thumb against gentle resistance applied to the nail (Fig. 1.65), while the tendons are palpated. Unresisted extension alone may provide false reassurance regarding the integrity of extensor pollicis longus since the adductor pollicis and abductor pollicis brevis each contribute through the dorsal expansion to extension of the interphalangeal joint.

Extensor pollicis longus rupture occurs as a result of:

1. An extreme hyperextension injury in which it is crushed between the radial tubercle, which may be fractured[126], and the base of the third metacarpal[127]
2. A direct blow, with delayed rupture[128]
3. Chronic attrition through excessive use, or more commonly, over an old Colles fracture, which need not be displaced[129] (a similar mechanism of rupture of the extensor digitorum[130, 131] and of the flexor tendons[132,133] has also been described)
4. Attrition and synovitis in rheumatoid disease (Ch. 5)
5. Secondary hyperparathyroidism, especially following chronic renal dialysis[134]
6. Surgery on the distal radius[135] or plate arthrodesis of the wrist joint.

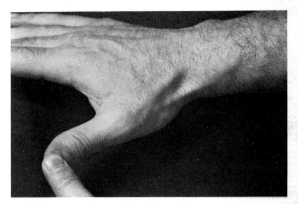

Fig. 1.65   The extensors of the thumb and the long abductor are tested by asking the patient to extend against resistance, when the tendons can be both seen and palpated.

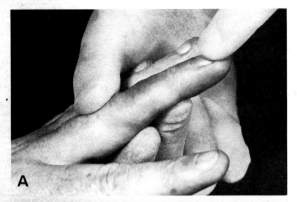

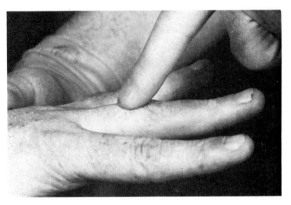

Fig. 1.66   The long extensor of the finger is tested by asking the patient to extend the metacarpophalangeal joint against resistance.

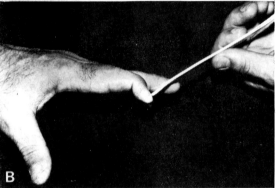

Fig. 1.67   A. Supporting the middle phalanx, the ability of the patient to extend the distal interphalangeal joint against resistance will eliminate the presence of a mallet finger (B).

The long extensors of the fingers are tested by asking the patient to extend against gentle resistance applied firstly to the dorsum of each proximal phalanx (Fig. 1.66) and secondly, with the middle phalanges supported on their palmar aspect, to the tips of the fingers (Fig. 1.67A). The second manoeuvre detects the presence of a *mallet finger* (Fig. 1.67B). With the use of gentle resistance to extension, division will be revealed by some lag in extension when compared with adjacent fingers and by pain over the site of division. This is particularly so in testing for both mallet finger and latent boutonniere deformity if the test is conducted with the wrist and metacarpophalangeal joints in full flexion[136]. If the patient with division of a long extensor is asked to extend fully the metacarpophalangeal joint with the interphalangeal joints flexed a quite

anomalous position will result in the affected finger, with the metacarpophalangeal joint flexed and the interphalangeal joints extended. When the extensor digitorum does not function but extensors indicis and digiti minimi are intact, the 'sign of the horns' will result[137] (Fig. 1.68). Other than direct laceration, this can also result from involvement in fractures of the radius[138], congenital absence of the muscle, selective injury or compression of the posterior interosseous nerve or its branches, or from chronic lead poisoning (see p. 311).

Traumatic dislocation of a digital extensor, usually the long[139], results from a tear of the radial transverse fibres of the extensor hood over the metacarpophalangeal joint, permitting ulnar dislocation of the long extensor tendon. The occurrence is acute, associated with pain and a snapping sensation. The result is chronic dislocation with pain but normal extension.

Active extension of the wrist against gentle resistance will allow the tendons of intact primary wrist extensors to be palpated. The radial wrist extensors are subject to common variations[140].

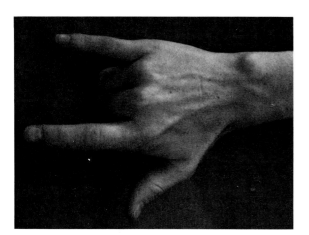

Fig. 1.68   The 'sign of the horns', evidence of intact extensor indicis and extensor digiti minimi.

Ancillary studies in closed extensor injuries
Lateral radiograph of the digit, readily and with advantage taken on dental films, may well show a fragment of bone avulsed from the dorsal base of the distal or middle phalanx in closed mallet and boutonniere injuries.
Arthrography of the interphalangeal joint has been reported to show leaks in the extensor apparatus in recent injuries[136].

INDICATIONS IN CLOSED EXTENSOR INJURIES

Mallet finger (and thumb). It is important to distinguish between pure rupture of the conjoined tendon and a mallet fracture, in which the tendon avulses a fragment of bone. It is important in the fracture to determine whether there is involvement of a significant portion of the articular surface and, if so, whether there is displacement between the fragment and the main portion of the distal phalanx, which may itself be subluxed. If the phalanx is subluxed, or if there is displacement of a significant avulsion fracture, *open reduction and fixation* of the phalanx and fragment are preferable[141]. If there is no fragment, or what fragment present is an insignificant sliver, or is undisplaced, then *closed splinting* in extension for six uninterrupted weeks will suffice[142-144]. Where doubt exists regarding the reliability of the patient, *closed pin fixation* of the distal interphalangeal joint, supplemented by splinting may be required. Treatment of mallet finger is not without complications, including skin necrosis consequent upon excessive hyperextension in a splint[145]. Skin problems occurred in 45% of one series following splintage, but most were transient and compared well with 53% complications following surgical treatment, three-fourths of which persisted for three years[146]. Clearly, management

should not be taken lightly, should not be left to the inexperienced, and the patient should be reviewed 48 hours after treatment.

Boutonniere injuries of the central slip are treated according to a similar protocol. However, it is much more difficult to maintain the splint on the proximal than on the distal interphalangeal joint, and it is much more difficult to treat the much more significant late deformity. For these reasons, the surgeon should be more ready to undertake *open repair* with pin fixation of the joint in pure tendon ruptures if he suspects poor patient compliance either immediately or at any of the initially frequent office visits.

Traumatic dislocation of the extensor at the metacarpophalangeal joint has been treated closed[147], but *open repair* is favoured by the majority[139,148,149], including the author.

Rupture of extensor pollicis longus can be treated with equal efficacy with an intercalated *tendon graft*[150] or *transfer* of extensor indicis.

See Green D P 1993 Operative Hand Surgery, 3rd edn. Churchill Livingstone, New York, pp. 1937 and 1943.

RESISTED ACTIVE MOTION

All of the active movements described above should be repeated. The examiner should then attempt to overcome the motion by applying gentle resistance. Where partial tendon lacerations are present, or where the division is complete and the active motion is spuriously produced by traction on an intact vinculum, the patient will experience pain and quickly release the digit. This test is important.
The conclusions to be drawn from movement or lack of it in the untidy injury, or that accompanied by a fracture, must be much more guarded than in the uncomplicated tidy injury. Active movement may be inhibited or absent in the presence of intact tendons because of pain, oedema, joint injury or fracture. Movement may, on the other hand, be produced by tendons which will not function in the long term for any of four reasons:

1. Partial division ⟶ late rupture
2. Loss of blood supply
   (a) avulsion ⎫
   (b) crush ⎬ ⟶ necrosis
   (c) burn ⎭
3. Abrasion ⟶ late rupture
   ⟶ late adhesions
4. Severe peritendinous
   damage ⟶ late adhesions

(For tendon exploration, see p. 99.)

Muscle

Lacerations of muscle are detected by the techniques described above for tendon injuries, especially resisted active motion.

COMPARTMENT SYNDROMES

'A compartment(al) syndrome is a condition in which increased pressure within a limited space compromises the circulation (by lowering the arteriovenous gradient) and function of the tissues within that space. Hypotension, haemorrhage, arterial occlusion, and limb elevation all appear to reduce the tolerance of limbs for increased tissue pressure' (Matsen, 1980[151]).

The investing fascia of the muscles of the extremities is firmly attached to bone by means of intermuscular septa. The fascia has very limited elasticity. It follows that any accumulation of additional fluid within the fascial compartment will soon result in a rise in pressure, increasing *tension in the compartment*. The critical closing pressure of the vessels serving the muscles is 40 mmHg. Should the pressure exceed that level, muscle ischaemia will result with the onset, initially, of *pain* followed within two hours by the spotty but spreading development of irreversible muscle necrosis — *Volkmann's ischaemia*[152,153]. Pain may well regress with this development. Nerves passing through the compartment are affected only a little later, with the onset of *paraesthesia and hypaesthesia*. By contrast, major vessels contain a pressure equal to the systolic pressure of the patient. Flow through these vessels will continue unimpaired, with palpable distal pulses, long after muscle necrosis has become irreversibly established. As the fascial compartment attempts to accommodate the increased fluid volume it approximates as far as it is able to the configuration which contains the largest volume in the smallest area — a sphere. This 'balling up' of the muscles adds to the initial pain and also pulls on the tendons which arise from them. Thus, in the most common anterior forearm compartment syndrome, the digits become flexed and resistant to any attempts to extend them — *the passive stretch test*, which will be positive whether or not the patient is conscious. The course of events described may arise with any injury likely to produce increased pressure, either by bleeding or by the accumulation of oedema fluid:

vascular injury	burns
fracture	prolonged ischaemia
crush injury	

The physician may unwittingly compound the problem by fracture manipulation, the application of external splints, or — worse — casts[154], by elevation of a limb at risk or by failing to correct hypovolaemia[155].

Less common causes have been described, including tourniquet malfunction[156], intravenous regional anaesthesia[157], leukaemic infiltrates[158], a traumatized vascular hamartoma[159], necrotizing fasciitis[160] and strenuous exercise[161].

Compartment syndrome in the upper extremity is most likely to afflict the flexor compartment of the forearm and the interosseous spaces, but can also occur in the dorsal compartment. The symptoms and signs as explained above are, in sequence:

1. *Pain* out of proportion to the injury
2. *Weakness* of the compartment muscles
3. *Increased tenseness* of the compartment envelope
4. *Hypaesthesia* in the sensory distribution of nerves which pass through the compartment.

Pain on passive stretch of the muscles of the compartment, with both voluntary and involuntary resistance to extension, will be present to an increasing degree from the onset.

Flexor compartment in the forearm
Increasing pain and progressive weakness should alert the surgeon to the possibility of a compartment syndrome. Palpation of the forearm will reveal increased tension and will probably be very uncomfortable to the patient. Hypaesthesia should be sought in all digits, although it will be most evident in the median nerve distribution.

Passive stretch test. With the fingers fully extended, if possible, the wrist should be gently and progressively extended also. Pain will result earlier in this sequence the more severe the condition. In fully established cases it is not possible to extend the fingers at all, let alone the wrist. (Fig. 1.69).

Interosseous compartment[162]
This is more difficult to detect than forearm compartment syndrome, for several of the criteria do not apply: inappropriate pain may pass unheeded in the injured hand; hypaesthesia does not occur; weakness of the muscles and raised compartment pressure are difficult to detect. Diagnosis therefore rests heavily on the passive stretch test.

Passive stretch test[163]. The metacarpophalangeal joint of each finger in turn is held in hyperextension, the interphalangeal joints are flexed, and the finger is then

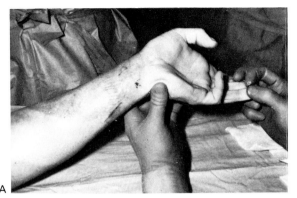

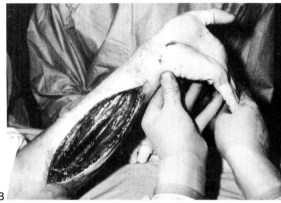

Fig. 1.69 A. Even under anaesthesia it is not possible to fully extend the wrist and fingers in this patient who sustained a closed roller injury to his forearm. B. After decompression of the forearm muscular compartment, full extension was achieved with relative ease.

deviated both radially and ulnarwards (Fig. 1.70). If pain is elicited, decompression is required. The interosseous compartments may be involved individually or, more often, in combination, thus:

2nd compartment — 1st palmar and 2nd dorsal interosseous
3rd compartment — 2nd palmar and 3rd dorsal interosseous
4th compartment — 3rd palmar and 4th dorsal interosseous

It should be reiterated that *the pulse is not lost* in either forearm or interosseous compartment syndrome since main arterial pressure is well above the critical closing pressure of vessels supplying the compartment tissues. If it is absent, that is probably evidence of major vascular impairment, which will coincidentally worsen the compartment syndrome by lowering the arterial pressure. Both require urgent attention.

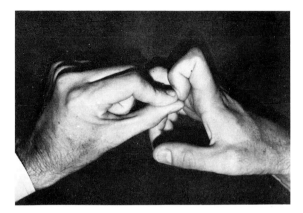

Fig. 1.70 Increase in the pressure within the intrinsic muscle compartments can be tested by placing each finger in turn in the intrinsic minus position as shown. If this manoeuvre cannot be undertaken without pain, it is an indication of a rise in intracompartmental pressure.

Angiography
In most circumstances where a probable compartment syndrome is accompanied by an absent pulse, exploration is urgently indicated and will reveal all pathology. Angiography is a waste of valuable time. Where, however, the patient's condition is critical for other reasons or there is significant doubt regarding the level of vascular injury, then angiography may be justified. The compartment syndrome which has advanced so far as to arrest flow will be revealed by a smooth tapering of the main vessels with absence of filling of small side branches as opposed to the sharp cut off in the main vessel which is evidence of arterial injury.

Electrical stimulation[164]
Occasionally no active function is detected in the muscles of a compartment; this may be due either to nerve injury more proximal or to raised compartment pressure. Electrical stimulation of the nerve close to the muscle will solve this dilemma:

Stimulation	contraction	proximal nerve injury
Stimulation	no contraction	compartment syndrome

Compartment pressure recording
When the signs are equivocal, the first requirement is for *frequent, regular, well-recorded reviews* of the patient. These will often reveal a deteriorating situation. When this is not so, or when examination is complicated by other injuries or by a combative patient, or when decompression is contraindicated unless absolutely necessary, then compartment pressure recording either with a

wick catheter[165] or by the continuous infusion technique becomes valuable. If the tissue pressure is above 40 mm Hg, then decompression is indicated. The technique of pressure recording must be impeccable and should be perfected on normal volunteers undergoing elective surgery. An erroneous reading is worse than no reading at all, since it will tend to supersede clinical signs.

Indications
Unequivocal cases, and those confusing ones with tissue pressure over 40 mm Hg, should be submitted to effective release of dressings[166] and then to wide release of the tissue envelope — fasciotomy — of the forearm compartments or the interosseous spaces[167] (Fig. 1.69). It must be remembered that significant post-ischaemic swelling may occur after release[168], and Matsen has drawn attention to the dangers of 'rebound' compartment syndrome. Vigilance must be maintained.

Three points concerning compartmental syndromes should be stressed:

1. The disappearance of pain after time may indicate necrosis, *not* recovery.
2. The syndrome may arise at any time during the first three days, and sometimes six, following an appropriate injury. The tests must therefore be repeated regularly until the surgeon is confident that danger has passed.
3. No surgeon or patient has ever regretted the performance of a fasciotomy, only the failure to do so. Therefore, if the surgeon feels that it *might* be necessary, it should be done. If decompression is not performed, muscle ischaemia will proceed to necrosis and, in time, to fibrosis — Volkmann's ischaemic contracture[152].

See Green D P 1993 Operative Hand Surgery, 3rd edn. Churchill Livingstone, New York, p. 670.

Nerve

Nerve injuries have been classified by both Sunderland[169] and Seddon[170] (p. 241) (Table 1.2).

SENSORY LOSS

Sweating is lost in the distribution of a divided peripheral nerve. An initial determination that a nerve injury is present or not can be made simply by stroking lightly with the examiner's own hand a digit on both the injured and the uninjured hand, each in the same dermatome. Frequently a distinct difference will be de-

Table 1.2

Sunderland[169]	Seddon[170]	Injury	Recovery potential
I	Neurapraxia	Ionic block; possible segmental demyelinization	Full
II	Axonotmesis	Axon severed; endoneurial tube intact	Full
III		Endoneurial tube torn	Slow, incomplete
IV		Only epineurium intact	Neuroma-in-continuity
V	Neurotmesis	Loss of continuity	None
VI		Combination of above	

tected, the digit in the denervated region being smooth and dry by comparison with the slightly adherent and moist finger in the uninjured. While doing this, the examiner can ask the alert patient whether the touch is perceived and whether or not it differs between the *two* sites. Where doubt still exists, a simple alternative remains.

The *tactile adherence test* will frequently reveal the pattern of nerve loss (p. 230). A plastic pen is held lightly by the examiner. Its smooth surface is passed gently but firmly back and forward repeatedly through an amplitude of 1 to 2 cm across the pulp on each side of each finger. This should be tried first on the uninjured hand to determine how much pressure is necessary to demonstrate adhesion between the pen and the finger. Adhesion is shown by slight but definite movement of the finger and is due to the presence of sweat. It will require somewhat firmer pressure in a cold hand than in a warm hand. An insensate pulp will have no sweating and will therefore show no 'tactile adherence' and therefore no motion.

The nerves divided can then be deduced, knowing the site of the wound, and that usually the ulnar nerve serves the small finger and the ulnar half of the ring, and the median nerve the remaining digits.

These simple tests have several advantages: they require no patient co-operation and can thus be used with equal benefit in the young, the inebriated and the unconscious; they require no special instruments; they inflict no pain and therefore do not disturb early rapport.

In the conscious and co-operative patient numbers should be recorded from the following test.

Two-point discrimination
Each side of each digital pulp and the dorsum of the metacarpal region of the thumb should be tested for *moving*[171] *or static two-point discrimination*[172] (12PD) using a paper clip twisted to appropriate shape[173] or a calibrated two-point discriminator[174] (p. 232). Both have been shown to be highly reproducible[175,176]. This should be done in a definite sequence.

1. The ends are shown to the patient to reassure him that they are *not* sharp.
2. The patient should be asked to observe the difference between one point and two points on the uninjured hand.
3. The ends should be set 5 to 8 mm apart for pulp testing and over 15 mm for dorsal testing.
4. The test should be performed holding the points in alignment along the axis of the digit and moving transversely across the axis. Pressure should be sufficiently light as to avoid blanching of a normal finger and thereby avoid overlap or recruitment. In heavily callused skin this is difficult, and the examiner should move away from the high contact area of the pulp.
5. Each side of each digit should be tested until any clear difference is shown between different areas on the same hand or between the two hands.

Certain sources of difficulty may arise:

1. *Patient error.* This may be due to the patient being too young, too old, too confused, too inebriated or too disturbed by his injury to co-operate. If completely relaxed, children can co-operate from the age of three. If the patient is frightened, shocked or overawed, this age of co-operation may rise into the early teens. In any event, concentration swiftly flags and examination should be abbreviated accordingly by testing only appropriate areas of absolute sensory loss, or by accepting the results of tactile adherence.
2. *Anomalous sensory loss*
   (a) Ulnar and median nerves.
      The number of fingers served by each nerve may vary. As an almost absolute rule, however, the palmar surface of the index and small fingers is served by the median and ulnar nerves respectively.

   (b) Radial nerve.
      Not infrequently the radial nerve distribution does not extend on to the thumb. On occasion, the lateral cutaneous nerve of the forearm entirely replaces the radial nerve in carrying sensation from the hand[177,178].
3. Congenital insensibility[179,180] very rare.

Many other methods of sensory evaluation have been described, and some are detailed in the next chapter (p. 227). All are either too painful, time-consuming or esoteric for routine use in the emergency room. The two described above are painless, swift, require no special equipment and give clear results in the great majority of patients. The remainder will be diagnosed by exploration.

POSTURE

The deformities associated with nerve injuries (p. 223), so characteristic particularly of ulnar nerve loss, are not seen in the acute situation.

PARALYSIS

The ulnar nerve in the hand usually serves the hypothenar muscles, all the interossei, the ulnar two lumbricals, the adductor pollicis and the deep head of flexor pollicis brevis. The median nerve in the hand serves the abductor pollicis brevis, the opponens pollicis, the radial two lumbricals and the superficial head of flexor pollicis brevis. This is a lengthy list for the trainee casualty surgeon to commit to memory and for the occasional examiner of the hand to recall. When this list is then qualified by the frequent variations which occur in the innervation of the lumbricals and of the thenar muscles, confusion arises or the attempt at recall is abandoned. For quick diagnosis of motor nerve injury at the wrist, *one muscle only* need be tested for each nerve:

Median — abductor pollicis brevis. With the hand flat and the palm up, the patient is asked to touch with his thumb the examiner's finger held directly over the thenar eminence and some 6 cm above it. If the patient is then asked to maintain this position against pressure from the examiner, the muscle belly can be seen and palpated between the scaphoid tubercle and the metacarpophalangeal joint of the thumb (Fig. 1.71).
Ulnar — flexor digiti minimi. In the same position, the patient is asked to raise the small finger vertically, that is, flex the metacarpophalangeal joint to 90° with the

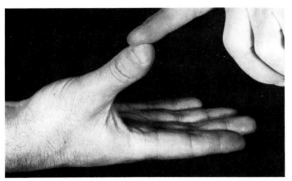

Fig. 1.71   The abductor pollicis brevis is innervated by the median nerve in the majority of cases. The integrity of the nerve therefore can be tested by asking the patient to reach up to meet the examiner's finger held over the hand in the line of the index finger.

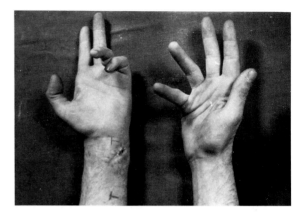

Fig. 1.73   This patient has sustained a division of the ulnar nerve at the left wrist. It can be seen that the action of his flexor digiti minimi in the normal hand produces the posture described in the previous figure, but that he cannot achieve this on the injured side.

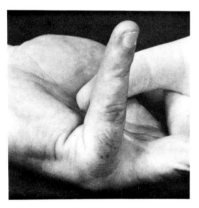

Fig. 1.72   The ulnar nerve invariably serves the flexor digiti minimi and this can be tested by asking the patient to flex the metacarpophalangeal joint of the small finger to 90° with the interphalangeal joints straight.

interphalangeal joints straight (Fig. 1.72). This posture cannot be achieved in ulnar nerve lesions (Fig. 1.73).

When a patient is unable to co-operate with even these simple motor tests, some indication may be given by asking him:

(i) to snap his fingers   — abductor pollicis brevis — median

(ii) to cross his fingers   — 1st palmar and 2nd dorsal (middle over index)   interosseous — ulnar[181]

This simplification of the examination of the hand for motor nerve loss does not release the surgeon from the responsibility of carrying out the full muscle test described in the Appendix (p. 513). This is especially necessary in multiple penetrating injuries, such as are sustained when the arm is put through a sheet of glass, since several injuries to both main nerve trunks and

their branches are not uncommon. It is also desirable as a routine in all hand examinations as the surgeon thereby becomes more familiar with the full test. With practice, all muscles in the upper extremity can be tested in little over one minute (see p. 234). The routine also eliminates the presence of pre-existing muscle loss which might be the subject of later dispute. In high or proximal injuries the most significant sensory loss is still in the hand itself. By contrast, proximal motor loss must be detected for all the reasons listed above and also to determine the precise level of the nerve injury and to distinguish between complete and partial nerve lesions. This is particularly important in patients with fractures and gunshot wounds where neurapraxia is common. The preliminary examination draws the baseline from which future recovery is measured. If open reduction and internal fixation are performed, a complete record eliminates any embarrassing doubt as to whether a palsy arose after injury or after surgery.

The inability to initiate movement is not absolute evidence that the muscle or its nerve supply is divided. Pain in the hand or nervousness may well inhibit motion. It is better therefore to test the patient's ability to resist movement as described previously. This requires the examiner to place the limb in the position which the muscle being tested normally produces and then to instruct the patient to *'Keep it there! Don't let me move it!'*

CLOSED NERVE INJURY

Peripheral nerve function may be impaired following closed injuries, most commonly fractures and dislocations, or penetrating injuries, most commonly gun shot wounds. Of such traumatic neuropathies, the most frequent is that of the radial nerve in association with fractures of the humerus.

Acute carpal tunnel syndrome (p. 285)
This may arise either as a result of oedema or because dislocation or fracture has directed a bone fragment into the tunnel. The features characteristic of chronic median nerve compression are present but may be obscured by the symptoms and signs of the injury. The diagnosis is made on the basis of:

an appropriate injury
a high level of suspicion
reduced sensation in median nerve distribution
a positive Tinel sign proximal to the wrist crease
weakness in abductor pollicis brevis.

Phalen's test usually cannot be applied because of discomfort. If the injury is complex and the diagnostic signs confusing, *nerve conduction studies* will help, an increased distal motor latency in excess of 4.0 ms being diagnostic. Like other compartment syndromes, if the potential is there but the findings equivocal, then the patient should be re-examined regularly for 3 to 6 days after the injury or until conditions have improved.

Indications in closed nerve injury
Where surgery is undertaken for other reasons, the nerve should be inspected to ensure its integrity. It should be palpated, and where a region of induration is encountered, epineurotomy performed. It may be found to be intact but lengthened, a sure sign of a Sunderland IV lesion (see above) which will require later excision or graft. Rarely the nerve will be disrupted[182] — later grafting will again be required.

Where surgery on a closed injury is not planned for repair of another structure, an expectant course is usually pursued, followed by repeated examination (p. 242). If no recovery is observed within six weeks employing electrical studies in addition to clinical examination, exploration should be performed. The exception to this policy of delay is in established acute carpal tunnel syndrome where release of the retinaculum is performed immediately.

Vessel

OPEN INJURIES

Arterial lacerations which are *complete* are distinguished by a history of dramatic blood loss at the time of injury, sometimes described as pulsatile, which has ceased by

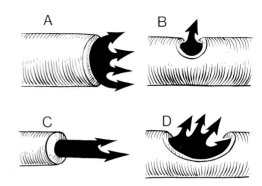

Fig. 1.74 A, B. In complete division of a major vessel, longitudinal and circumferential retraction results in dramatic reduction in blood loss. C, D. The same factors after partial injury tend to make the laceration in the wall of the artery wider, and therefore blood loss tends to be increased by the normally haemostatic mechanisms.

the time of examination due to longitudinal and circumferential retraction of the arterial wall. The wound is filled with thick, shiny, gelatinous, dark red clot which may be oozing somewhat. Examination of the peripheral *pulses* is worthless[183] since retrograde flow may fill the lacerated vessel from distally. If the suspected laceration is in the radial or ulnar artery, obliteration of the other may eliminate the pulse spuriously present. In theory, the Allen test (p. 259) could reveal an injury of either forearm vessel. In practice, this manoeuvre is often too painful and may also provoke renewed bleeding, and exploration of all likely wounds becomes the rule.

Partial lacerations of a major vessel may be associated with continued arterial haemorrhage since the normally haemostatic retraction serves to *increase* blood loss (Fig. 1.74). Such lacerations are the *only cause of death in the upper extremity* and should be treated as such an emergency. They *may* present with no active bleeding, a large wound clot, and distal pulses present due to occlusion of the defect in the wall by the clot, thereby re-establishing the vascular conduit. That is, flow continues past the expanding traumatic aneurysm.

Lacerations in the correct site, and of sufficient depth to have produced an arterial injury, require prompt exploration.

CLOSED INJURIES (including penetrating wounds)

In open injuries, the surgeon need only speculate on what the necessary exploration will reveal. By contrast, potential arterial injury in relatively closed spaces presents a much greater diagnostic challenge for h(must decide whether or not exploration is necess;

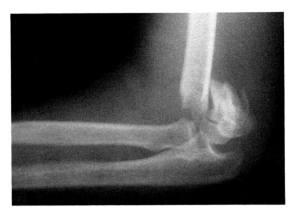

Fig. 1.75 Supracondylar fracture associated with vascular impairment and a forearm compartment syndrome.

Arterial compromise may result from several mechanisms:

1. Gunshot wounds[184,185]
2. Fractures: humerus[186,187] (Fig. 1.75); clavicle[188] and phalanges
3. Dislocations: elbow[189]; shoulder[190]

producing either:

(a) partial division ⟶ false aneurysm

or

(b) extensive intimal disruption ⟶ thrombosis[191]

The findings in the acute situation[192], in the upper extremity may be remarkably few. This is especially so and particularly hazardous in injuries to the subclavian and axillary arteries, where a neglected false aneurysm may result in later brachial palsy with less than a 50% chance of recovery[193]. In order of appearance, the signs of major arterial trauma in the arm are[194]:

1. Diminution or absence of distal *pulses* — in the swollen limb or in the ischaemic digit the use of the Doppler flowmeter to check pulses is valuable[195,196] (see below).
2. *Pallor*, especially evident in the nailbeds which show very poor refill after blanching.
3. *Pain*, most evident on handling the limb.
4. *Paraesthesia*, hypaesthesia and anaesthesia.
5. *Paralysis* – when this degree of muscle ischaemia is present, compartment syndromes are inevitable; correction of the vascular interruption may increase the problem by inducing post-ischaemic oedema (p. 40) — it should be accompanied by fasciotomy.
6. *Cold* — when the temperature of the involved limb or part is compared by simple touch with that of

other extremities, the contrast is often striking; as the examiner's hand progresses from distal to proximal a distinct change from cold to warm may be detected which gives evidence of the level of occlusion; the exact temperatures can be recorded with a thermocouple — any temperature below 30°C is suspect.

It should be re-emphasised that many of these peripheral signs may be absent. Delay may be disastrous, so, if suspicions remain, further steps must be taken, either by arteriography or exploration.

Arteriography is not indicated in open injuries since exploration can answer questions more directly with no loss of time. The value of arteriography in closed injuries has been questioned on similar grounds. However, exploration simply because major vessels may be injured is unnecessary surgery which may also be undesirable if other injuries or illnesses are present. Physical findings have been found to be unreliable, giving false-negative indications in 20% and false-positive in 42% of 86 patients subsequently evaluated by angiography[197].

Transfemoral subclavian arteriography is a swift, safe procedure. If it is undertaken to demonstrate the smaller, more distal vessels (p. 261) or prior to exploration to be done under axillary block, there is clear advantage and significant compassion in giving that block before the dye injection. The arteriogram may reveal:

1. False aneurysm (Fig. 1.76)
2. Thrombosis
3. Intimal flap formation — seen either as a dissection of dye beneath the intima (Fig. 1.77) or suggested by an abrupt, sharp occlusion without haemorrhage (Fig. 1.78)
4. Extrinsic compression
5. Acute arterio-venous fistula (Fig. 1.79)[198].

Spasm[199] in terms of angiography is now a largely discredited word. It was used to imply a transitory constriction of a vessel following trauma, which may produce clinical signs and angiographic changes, but which would resolve spontaneously. All such cases should be explored — all will reveal vessel pathology.

Arteriography is commonly employed in investigating all patients who *may* have sustained an arterial injury from blunt trauma or a proximate penetrating injury, even if they have no peripheral evidence of arterial occlusion. Such studies may reveal intimal fractures, pseudoaneurysms or mural stenoses which do not impede flow — a positive study in an asymptomatic patient.

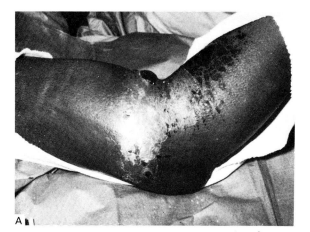

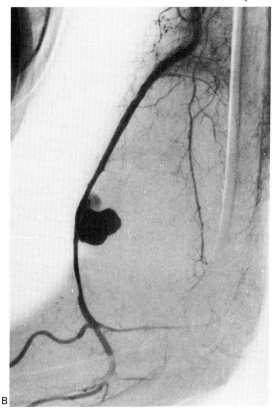

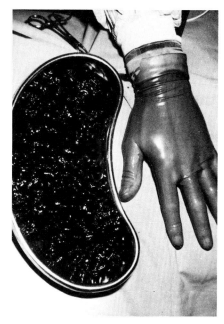

Fig. 1.76 A. This patient presented with a massive swelling in his upper arm, but with good circulation to the hand and normal pulses. B. Arteriography revealed a false aneurysm which (C) contained almost 3 units of blood.

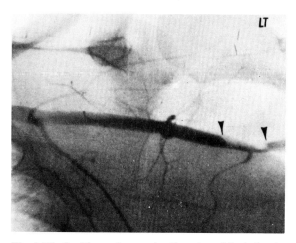

Fig. 1.77 In this arteriogram the dissection of the intima is revealed by a sudden narrowing of the vessel indicated by the arrow heads.

Colour duplex ultrasonography, in centres where it is available, challenges the need for arteriography. It can identify all forms of vascular trauma detailed above, including thrombus, aneurysm and stenosis. Its relatively low cost and portability, allied to the fact that it is non-invasive, makes ultrasonography an attractive alternative to angiography.

Doppler studies. The full range of non-invasive vascular studies (p. 261) are not customarily used in the emergency room. However, the simple Doppler pencil probe is valuable because it permits detection of flow in vessels which cannot be readily palpated because of pain, swelling or their relatively small calibre. Closed

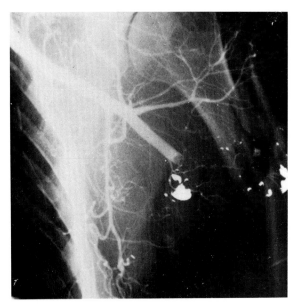

Fig. 1.78 An intimal flap is suggested by the sudden occlusion of the brachial artery following a gunshot wound without any evidence of haemorrhage.

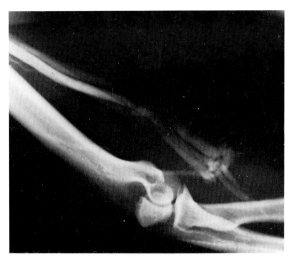

Fig. 1.79 An arteriovenous fistula is present here between the brachial artery and basilic vein.

injuries of digits may produce sufficient swelling to reduce arterial flow to the point where survival of the digit is in doubt. Such injuries may also have eliminated flow by damage to the vessel over such an extent as to render doubtful one's ability to restore flow. Both circumstances will have the same presentation. If the vessel can be followed into the digit with the Doppler, the problem

can be deemed to be one of compression. If there is clear loss of the signal proximally in both digital vessels, then occlusion or disruption exists. When available, colour duplex ultrasonography can give more detailed information regarding flow and vessel calibre in the emergency room or at the bedside.

Dynamic radionuclide imaging, especially in the first 'blood pool' stage, provides evidence of relative blood flow and preferential perfusion[200].

Iatrogenic

A small but worrisome group of patients arise as a result of arterial puncture, intentional or otherwise[201]. This may occur in the course of cardiac catheterization (Fig. 1.80), radial cannulation[202] for arterial blood gases — where the incidence of ischaemic complications in one series was 10%[203,204] — or misplaced intravenous lines[205]. The presentation may range from acute ischaemia, as detailed above, to compartment syndromes, to intermittent claudication. Prevention requires avoidance of these techniques in anticoagulated patients[206] and careful evaluation of the arterial tree by Allen's test and Doppler studies before inserting radial lines.

NON-TRAUMATIC VASCULAR EMERGENCIES

A relatively small group of patients will present as emergencies due to vascular compromise of an acute nature not related to injury. Severe upper limb ischaemia may arise from a number of causes[207] including embolization, thrombosis[208,209] arising from atherosclerosis and small vessel occlusion resulting from Raynaud's phenomenon or disease (p. 263)[210]. Regardless of the site, these patients present because of pain and changes in colour and temperature.

Examination reveals the classic features[211] detailed above:

pain
pulselessness
pallor and mottling of the skin
coolness of the part
paraesthesia, hypaesthesia and analgesia
paralysis, primarily in the intrinsic muscles and only if the occlusion is at or above the elbow.

If the patient presents later,

ulceration will appear in digital occlusion, *gangrene* in forearm occlusions, with the addition of *compartment syndromes* in more proximal blockage.

Emboli[212] usually arise from the heart, or more rarely from aneurysms, lodging either at the origin of the profunda brachii (Fig. 1.81) or at the bifurcation of the brachial artery into radial and ulnar.

Thrombosis occurs in previously diseased vessels and is diagnosed partly by exclusion of a source of embolus

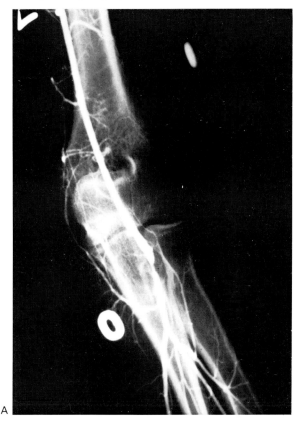

and partly by evidence of peripheral vessel disease on examination, arteriography and exploration.

Primary deep vein thrombosis (= effort thrombosis = Paget–Schroetter's syndrome)[213] arises as a result of a direct blow, prolonged pressure (as in sleep), adjacent major surgery or excessive stretch as in raking leaves, chopping wood or playing baseball, football or handball. It affects the subclavian or axillary veins and is characterized by swelling of the limb to a very variable degree, cyanotic discoloration, and a feeling of discomfort and heaviness. A prominent venous pattern develops over the shoulder due to distension of collateral venous circulation. The limb may be anaesthetic and cooler than the contralateral one, but *all pulses are present*. The thrombosed vein may or may not be palpable on the inner aspect of the arm or in the axilla. *Venography* or *colour duplex sonography* will reveal the venous thrombosis and the marked collateral flow (Fig. 1.82). More severe cases may progress to venous gangrene[214] or may be complicated by pulmonary embolism.

INDICATIONS IN CLOSED VASCULAR INJURIES

Closed injuries or occlusions of the vascular tree which are causing peripheral symptoms require *exploration*, as do asymptomatic extremities which, on angiography, show complete occlusion or a traumatic aneurysm. The management of non-occlusive angiographic findings in asymptomatic extremities is more controversial, for at least one series indicated the efficacy of observation

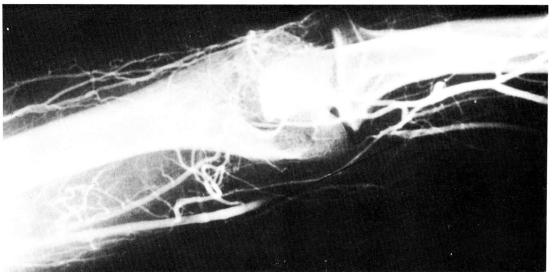

Fig. 1.80 A, B. These occlusions, complete and partial, both resulted from cardiac catheterization.

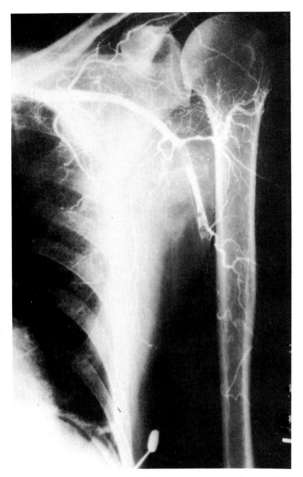

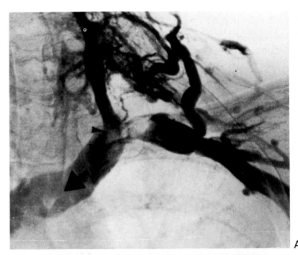

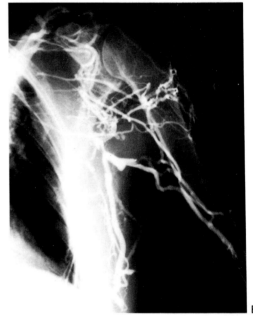

Fig. 1.81 This arteriogram shows the presence of emboli in the brachial artery just proximal to the origin of the profunda brachii artery, in the brachial artery just distal to the circumflex humeral artery and also small emboli in the circumflex humeral artery itself.

Fig. 1.82 A, B. Both of these venograms show evidence of thrombosis in the main venous stream. This has completely occluded the axillary vein in (B) and in both there is evidence of unusual filling of the collateral venous system.

and serial angiography[215]. At exploration, *embolectomy*[216] may suffice, but more commonly resection of the injured or occluded segment and interpositional *vein grafting* will be required. Such grafts may be taken as far as the superficial palmar arch[217] and beyond, with benefit. In those digits where the Doppler has indicated occlusion, mid-lateral *fasciotomy* is performed and peripheral flow re-examined. Where it has indicated occlusion or disruption, a *microsurgical vascular graft*, venous for short, arterial for long defects[218] (see Fig. 1.157) is required. The fear in all vessel explorations, proximal or distal, is that the damage inflicted by the injury extends further into the tree than can be determined or corrected, or that thrombus or additional emboli have propagated distally. If this has occurred,

the poor run-off will inevitably lead to thrombosis at the anastomoses already performed. *Microvascular exploration* further distally is then indicated[219]. An alternative, or adjunctive, technique is the use of *thrombolytic agents*[220]. These remain controversial, with some centres in favour[221], some sceptical[222]. Where surgery is unlikely to be of help because the occlusion is distal or the angiogram shows no distal refill of vessels to which the surgeon can hope to graft, or where surgery has failed, thrombolytic therapy should be attempted. It is by far best performed in the vascular radiology department, controlled by the haematologist and the vascular radiologist. It requires large volumes of thrombolytic agent — 100 000 units of streptokinase as a loading dose and 5000 units per hour — which is expensive. One study reported that complete success cost an average of $39 200[223] per case.

Major veins, be they occluded or disrupted, should also be reconstructed, for simple ligation has been shown to have significant consequent morbidity[224].

Routine intraoperative *angioscopy*[225] has been shown to aid significantly in decision making in the lower extremity. With the development of fibreoptic elements less than 1 mm in diameter, this tool will surely have a role in upper extremity surgery in the near future.

Vascular shunting is rarely indicated but should be employed where limb ischaemia has exceeded 6 hours, and significant surgery, such as complex fracture fixation, is to be performed before vascular reconstruction can be done.

Fasciotomy should be considered in *all* major closed vessel injuries and should certainly be done if the standard indications are present (p. 40) or if ischaemia has exceeded 6 hours — less if the patient has been hypotensive for much of that time. It should be done as a preliminary step if delay is anticipated[226].

See Green D P 1993 Operative Hand Surgery, 3rd edn. Churchill Livingstone, New York, pp. 2263 and 2274.

Bone and joint

Bone and joint are considered together here for two reasons: firstly, the injuring forces in the more common indirect injuries to skeleton and ligament are often identical; secondly, so many injuries in the hand involve both structures.

Open injuries play a minor role in this segment, for examination of fractures and dislocations which coexist with wounds, which require exploration in any event, consists largely of ordering and viewing all the appropriate radiological studies, which are the same as those employed in making decisions about closed injuries. A word of caution is appropriate, however. Major open injuries of the extremity have been inflicted only as a result of great force. Such force not uncommonly inflicts significant indirect, but closed, injuries more proximally in the limb. The patient, being in considerable pain from the obvious, will rarely have complaints related to the obscure. Radiologic assessment in such cases must include the humerus, the shoulder girdle and the cervical spine.

Fractures of the long bones can be classified according to their location and subclassified according to their configuration:

Head	— condylar – if both = 'T-condylar'
Diaphysis	— transverse
	— longitudinal
	— oblique
	— spiral
	— comminuted
Base	— palmar
	— dorsal
	— lateral

Physis (see p. 55)

The surgeon should be alert for the presence of underlying tumour or disease, leading to *pathological* fractures (Ch. 6).

The skeleton is injured by force, either direct or indirect. *Direct* blunt force to long bones, such as metacarpals and phalanges, produces transverse or comminuted fractures. The majority of the injuries sustained by the skeleton of the hand are, however, inflicted by *indirect* force, transmitted (i) *axially*, often causing articular fractures; (ii) by *leverage*, producing a ligament injury, a condylar fracture or an oblique diaphyseal fracture; or (iii) by *torsion*, which results in a ligament injury or a spiral diaphyseal fracture.

EXAMINATION — GENERAL COMMENTS

Certain symptoms and signs are common to all fractures and dislocations— *swelling, deformity, loss of motion,* the presence of *abnormal motion* and *tenderness*. Certain observations to be made on the standard radiographs are also universal. All these will be discussed initially, followed by considerations specific to the regions of the hand, progressing from distal to proximal. Diagnosis of the *complicated* fracture — one in which there is disturbance of *sensation, circulation* or *soft-tissue cover* — is highly significant in the eventual outcome, and is covered in the relevant sections (pp. 25, 42 and 45).

Describing fracture angulation in the antero-posterior plane is, by convention, done by referring to the direction in which the fracture itself moves. To avoid confusion, in this text the fracture will be termed the 'apex'; thus, an 'apex-palmar' angulation means that the angled fracture lies palmar to the line between the base and the head of the bone.

It is useful to remember, in considering fractures of the middle and proximal phalanges, and of all the metacarpals, that the dorsal surface is *flat*. The diaphyseal waist is created by significant curvature on the palmar aspect and gentler curves of the lateral cortices.

DEFORMITY

Significant swelling around a bone or joint is in itself sufficient to arouse suspicions of underlying skeletal injury. Any *bruising* beneath the skin, following an appropriate injury and in the absence of any other cause, is pathognomonic of fracture or ligament tear. Some general rules can be stated regarding angular deformity following fracture or dislocation in the hand:

1. Deformity is more evident in the phalanges than in the carpus. This is partly because soft-tissue coverage is thinner in more distal parts and partly because the force required to disrupt the skeleton is greater the more proximal the injury — there is therefore a greater accumulation of obscuring oedema.
2. *Fractures* angled in the line of digital motion, that is, antero-posterior, are less evident than those angled laterally or rotated.
3. *Joints* dislocated in the line of digital motion are more likely to remain so, and are therefore *more* evident than those dislocated laterally — which will often have reduced spontaneously.
4. A joint will remain in the dislocated position only if some element of the joint capsule either (i) remains intact and locks the bone ends in abnormal relationship, or (ii) tears, and becomes interposed between the bone ends[227-230]. Such locking is more likely to occur in antero-posterior dislocations, while tending to restore lateral dislocations to proper alignment.
5. However tempting, no deformity should be corrected before thorough clinical and radiological evaluation. Nerve dysfunction, circulatory embarrassment and fractures should all be documented *before* any treatment is offered.

LIMITATION OF NORMAL MOTION

Active. The probable absence of injury to skeletal structures is most speedily checked by asking the patient to put each joint through a normal range of motion. Apart from direct injury to the joint under examination, or to the bones which form the joint, limitation or lack of active motion may be due to:

tendon injury
paralysis
oedema
pain
significant injury proximally
lack of patient cooperation — age, anxiety, intoxication.

Where *pain* limits active motion note should be taken of its location and at what point in the joint range it occurs.

The *stability* of fractures already suspected or later revealed on radiographs will be shown by a relatively normal range of motion. Conversely, the more unstable the fracture — suggested by *severe initial deformity*, reported or observed — the more limited will be the motion.

Passive. Where active motion is absent or limited, the examiner should attempt gentle passive motion both to detect any injury sustained and also to place on record any limitation of normal range present *before* the injury in joints clearly not involved in the current accident. Such limitation may influence treatment and postoperative care. The record also refutes any subsequent charge that the limitation arose as a result of the injury or treatment. Injury will become evident during passive motion by the presence of painful limitation of range.

In recording joint range[231], the convention approved by all English-speaking Orthopaedic Associations, detailed later (p.190), should be employed. Basically, this dictates that all neutral joint positions — that is, when the two bones forming the joint are in line with one another — are recorded as 0°.

PRESENCE OF ABNORMAL MOTION

Stress is placed on periarticular structures which normally prevent abnormal motion, such as the palmar plate, the collateral ligament and the extrinsic carpal ligaments, all of which will be described in greater detail below. In the presence of injury this will elicit pain, and if the patient is stoical and the injury total, abnormal motion. If protective spasm or undue discomfort prevent a certain diagnosis, the test should be repeated under regional or local block, at which time stress radiographs should be obtained (Fig. 1.83).

The practice of moving broken bones to confirm the presence of a fracture is painful, unnecessary and not without risk, for, especially in the upper arm, major nerves and vessels lie close to the bones and may be damaged during such a manoeuvre.

TENDERNESS

Tenderness elicited by the palpating finger can be a guide to the site and extent of injury. All such tenderness should be compared to the opposite, uninjured hand to ensure that it is different and therefore significant.

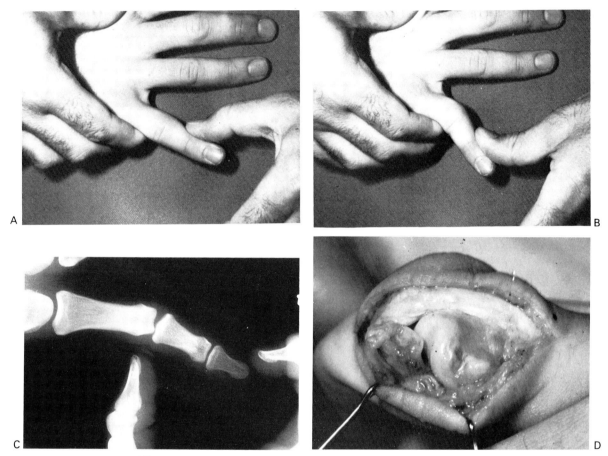

Fig. 1.83 A. The collateral ligament of the proximal interphalangeal joint is stressed, and in this case (B) reveals laxity to this true lateral stress which can only be due to a tear of the true collateral ligament. C. Radiograph. D. Exploration revealed this to be true, the collateral ligament being torn from its attachment to the proximal phalanx. (Note that the mechanism is different from that in gamekeeper's thumb, in which the ulnar collateral ligament is usually torn from its distal attachment.)

1. *Bone.* The fracture site will be tender, even on gentle pressure, and in some sites, e.g. the scaphoid, this is an important diagnostic test.
2. *Periarticular* structures. Where the joint range is limited by pain, rupture of the capsule, collateral ligament or palmar plate is one cause. The precise location of the tear can sometimes be determined by careful pressure around the joint applied by the examiner's finger nail.

RADIOLOGIC EXAMINATION — GENERAL COMMENTS

All injured hands should be radiographically examined, not only for reasons of litigation, but also because pre-vious injury should be recorded and because the most confident clinical exclusion of fractures can be wrong. More than one view is always necessary (Fig. 1.84) and the surgeon and radiographer should ideally study the films together to determine whether further views will aid in diagnosis.

While all bones should be scrutinized, particular attention should be paid to the following:
Points of insertion of ligaments and tendons (Fig. 1.85)
Even a small flake of bone at a point where it is known that a ligament or tendon is attached should command attention, otherwise an unstable joint or tendon imbal-ance may result. The mallet finger and post-traumatic boutonniere deformity (p. 38) may both result from such flake fragments.

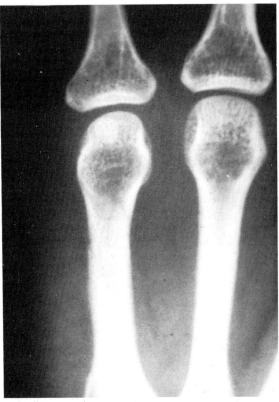 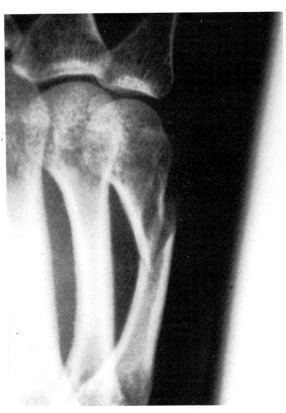

A   B

Fig. 1.84   A. An anteroposterior radiograph yielded no clear evidence of a fracture of the fifth metacarpal. B. In a lateral view supinated by 30° the fracture of the shaft was clearly evident.

Alignment of articular surfaces (Fig. 1.86)
If intra-articular fragments are displaced even minimally, accurate reduction is imperative otherwise early osteoarthritis will be likely. Such reduction commonly requires operative intervention in a closed fracture (Fig. 1.140). Many intra-articular fractures have ligaments or tendons attached to one or more of the fragments. This makes any reduction inherently unstable and internal fixation therefore necessary after reduction.

The alignment of articular surfaces in a different sense is important in avoiding minor degrees of lateral angulation in phalanges. On postero-anterior views of any phalanx the articular surfaces at either end should be parallel to one another. In the presence of swelling, some angulation may be obscured clinically but can be

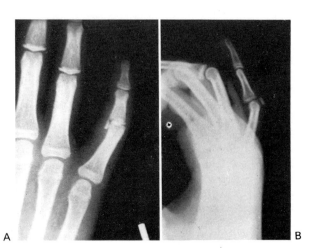

A   B

Fig. 1.85   This patient sustained an injury to his small finger while playing softball and presented with a swollen but clinically stable proximal interphalangeal joint. Radiographical examination revealed, however, that the central slip of the extensor tendon had avulsed a small fragment of bone from the middle phalanx and likewise the collateral ligament a small fragment on the radial aspect. Open reduction of these fragments ensured stability of the joint and prevented the development of a subsequent post-traumatic boutonniere deformity.

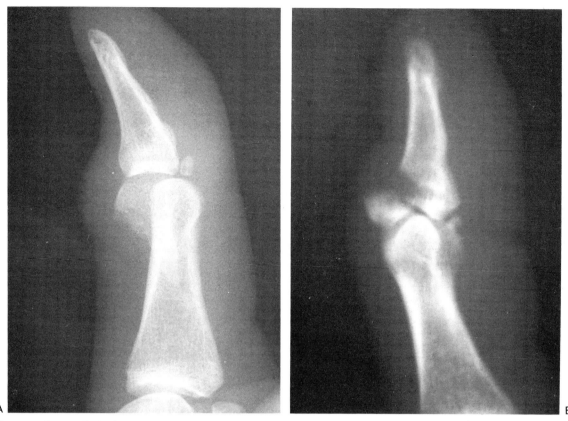

Fig. 1.86 Intra-articular fractures. The intra-articular fracture of (A), the head of the proximal phalanx, and (B), the base of the distal phalanx, were both poorly visualized on the postero-anterior view of the joint, but well seen on these true lateral views taken on dental films. Accurate reduction was necessary to preserve motion in the joint.

readily detected by drawing lines on the radiograph joining the condyles in each joint. (Figs 1.93 and 2.43, pp. 58 and 189).

Fractures confined entirely to the cartilage can occur and, of course, do not show on any radiograph. If the

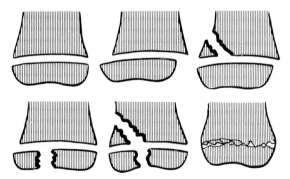

Fig. 1.87 The Salter classification of epiphyseal fractures (see text).

injury is closed, such patients usually present late with persistent swelling and pain (p. 196).

Epiphyseal fractures
Fractures which encroach on the epiphyseal plate have been classified by Salter and Harris[232] into five categories (Fig. 1.87), as follows.

Type I   Separation of the epiphysis from the metaphysis through the plate in a shearing manner (Fig. 1.88).

Type II   Separation of the epiphysis, a small angle of metaphysis being broken off with it (Fig. 1.89).

Type III   An intra-articular fracture of part of the epiphysis without interference with the epiphyseal plate (Fig. 1.90).

Type IV   A vertical, displaced fracture passing from the articular surface through epiphysis, plate and metaphysis.

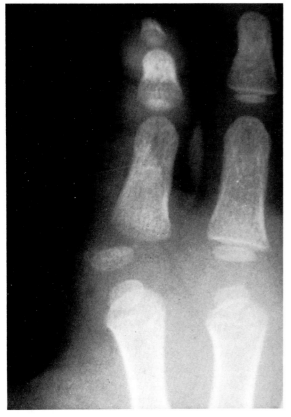

Fig. 1.88   Salter type I.

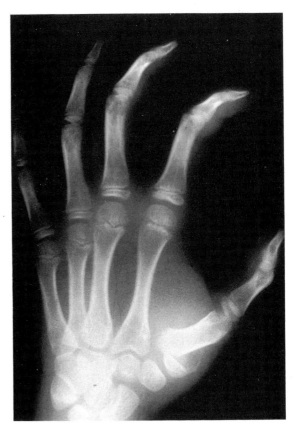

Fig. 1.89   Salter type II.

Type V   A compression fracture of the cartilaginous plate with no evident injury of epiphysis or metaphysis.

Type I injuries of the distal phalanx commonly produce a mallet finger appearance in the child, the extensor tendon being attached to the epiphysis, the flexor profundus to the metaphysis.

Types I and II remodel well but reduction should be attempted. Provided they are accurately reduced, type III fractures carry a good prognosis as they do not interfere directly with the epiphyseal plate. Types IV and V, which do, may arrest growth of all or part of the bone with consequent shortening or angulation (Fig. 1.91). The surgeon should recognize this and warn the parents of the possibility.

Fractures in children are often underestimated[233]. Remodelling can occur only in those fractures angulated in the line of pull of the tendons, that is, antero-posterior, and then best at the metaphysis. Lateral angulation and rotational malalignment will *never* remodel and require accurate reduction (Fig. 1.92).

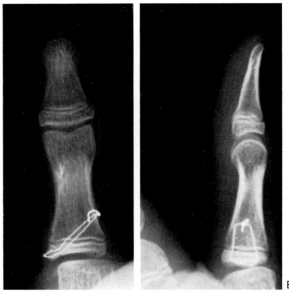

A   B

Fig. 1.90   Salter type III. Here the fragment is held in place with an interosseous wire.

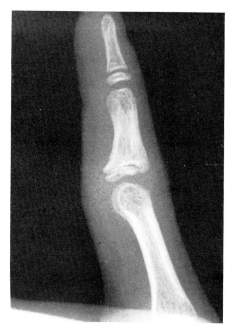

Fig. 1.91 Arrest of growth has occurred in the epiphysis of the middle phalanx consequent upon a type V Salter fracture.

INDICATIONS — GENERAL COMMENTS

In the ideal circumstance, if an unlimited range of fixation devices and sufficient technical skill to apply them were available, the aims should be those stated by the AO group:

1. Accurate anatomical reduction
2. Rigid internal fixation
3. Early, active motion of the adjacent joints.

In the fingers, the most significant of these aims is the early institution of motion in the joints. With this in mind, the fracture should be studied in a set sequence with the following questions in mind:

Is the fracture reduced?

If displaced, is the displacement acceptable? If not, can it be reduced closed?

If it is reduced, or can be, or is acceptable, is it then stable?

If it is not stable, can it be made so, closed?

If the fracture cannot be reduced or made stable without surgery, what procedure will be necessary to make it so? Is that surgery justifiable?

Is it possible with a high level of confidence?

The questions detailed above can be presented as an algorithm.

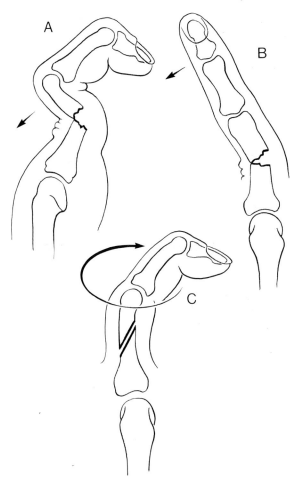

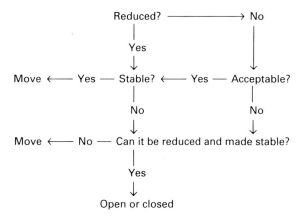

Fig. 1.92 Of the three malalignments of a fractured phalanx in a child only one will remodel, namely true palmar angulation (A). Lateral angulation (B) and rotatory malalignment (C) will not model with time and should therefore be corrected at the time of injury.

FRACTURE ANALYSIS

```
                    Reduced? ──────────→ No
                        |                 |
                       Yes                |
                        ↓                 ↓
Move ←── Yes ── Stable? ←── Yes ── Acceptable?
                        |                 |
                       No                No
                        ↓                 ↓
Move ←── No ── Can it be reduced and made stable?
                        |
                       Yes
                        ↓
                 Open or closed
```

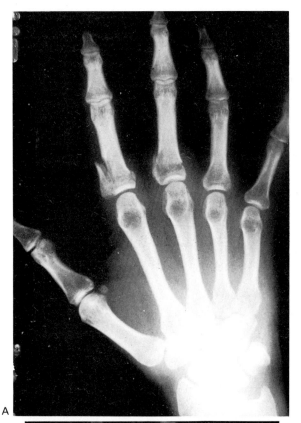

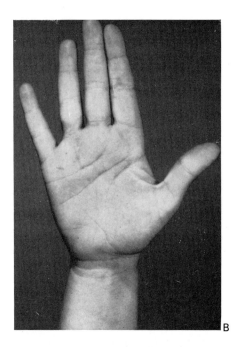

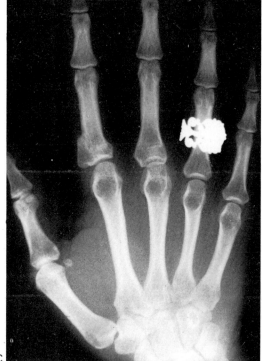

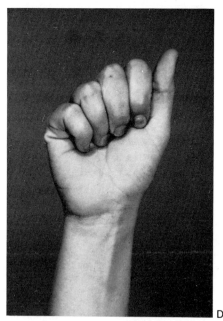

Fig. 1.93   A. This patient sustained closed comminuted fractures of the bases of the proximal phalanges of the index and middle fingers. Scrutiny of the radiographs suggested that it would not be possible to reduce and fix all of the fragments were surgery to be undertaken. For this reason, the patient was commenced on early, active, protected motion. B. This resulted in union of the phalangeal fractures with a full range of motion (C, D). (Note that the articular surfaces after healing at either end of each proximal phalanx are *not* parallel to each other in index and middle but are in ring and small.)

'*Acceptable*' fractures are important to recognize for they require no treatment. Acceptably displaced fractures, provided they are stable, include:

tuft of the distal phalanx

chips, if minimally displaced

antero-posterior angulation in metaphyseal fractures of children

non-articular comminution with minimal angulation (Fig. 1.93)

metacarpal neck — 15° angulation in index and middle
— 20–70° in ring and small (p. 74)

non-articular metacarpal base — 20° angulation in adults
— 40° in children

See Green D P 1993 Operative Hand Surgery, 3rd edn. Churchill Livingstone, New York, p. 695.

PHALANGEAL INJURIES

Distal phalanx

The most common fractures[234] of the distal phalanx[235] are:

(a) *Comminuted* — due to direct crushing force; these are almost invariably associated with injuries of the nailbed and are often confined to the '*tuft*', or distal margin of the phalanx.

(b) *Intra-articular*[236] — these are mainly avulsive injuries, including the mallet fracture due to traction by the extensor tendon (p. 38) (Fig. 1.94), the fracture of profundus avulsion (p. 36) and, less common here than in the proximal interphalangeal joint, a condylar fracture in which the fragment remains attached to the collateral ligament.

(c) *Transverse* — through the waist of the distal phalanx, this invariably adopts an apex-dorsal configuration; the key point is that the entire nailbed rides with the distal fragment, and the proximal edge of the germinal matrix often dislocates on to the superficial surface of the eponychial fold — it must be replaced to achieve, indeed to permit, fracture reduction.

Middle and proximal phalanges

Setting aside for the moment the *intra-articular* fractures which will be considered separately below with injuries of the proximal interphalangeal joint, fractures to the middle and proximal phalanges are either *spiral*, produced by torsion of the digit, or due to direct blows, which, depending on the force, and the quality of the bone, will result in either *transverse diaphyseal* or *comminuted* (Fig. 1.95A) fractures. While some may be

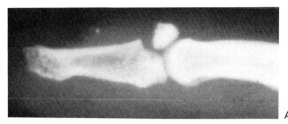

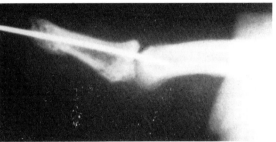

Fig. 1.94 A. Radiograph reveals a displaced mallet type fracture of the distal interphalangeal joint. B. Open reduction and transfixtion with a single Kirschner wire provide both reduction of the articular fragment and also the necessary splintage.

open fractures, the majority are closed. It is imperative to be aware that these are often *complicated* by soft-tissue injury, especially to the digital arteries which may be distorted, thrombosed or avulsed (Fig. 1.96). Failure to recognize and attend to the vascular element (p. 105) may result in loss of the finger.

Transverse fractures of the middle and proximal phalanges adopt an apex palmar angulation (Fig. 1.95B, C), due to the forces of the superficialis and interosseous insertions respectively. Failure to correct this angulation will not only threaten the flexor tendon, which may be impaled, but will result in a 'zig-zag' deformity whereby the change in pull on the long extrinsic tendons will produce a flexion deformity of the joints at either end of the broken bone. This deformity will at first be mobile but will later become a fixed contracture, often blamed unjustly on the innocent proximal interphalangeal joint (p. 192).

Interphalangeal joints (and the metacarpophalangeal joint of the thumb). The most commonly injured joints in the hand are the ginglymus, or hinge joints, probably because they are restricted to only one plane of movement. These ginglymus joints include all of the interphalangeal joints[237] and the metacarpophalangeal joint of the thumb. The latter is considered here rather than with the other metacarpophalangeal joints because it differs markedly in anatomy and mechanisms of injury. All have a similar structure[238]. The true and *accessory*

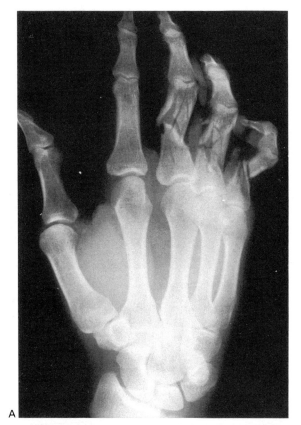

A

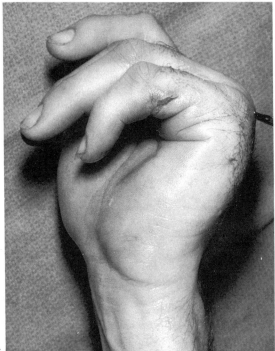

C

collateral ligaments together form a fan of fibres which radiate out from a recess on the lateral aspect of the head of the proximal bone. These fibres insert, the true collateral into the bone of the base of the distal bone, the accessory into the lateral aspect of the palmar plate. In children the ligament attaches to both epiphysis and metaphysis in the phalanges[239, 240]. The fibres are tight in all positions of the joint, which shows no freedom for lateral motion. The palmar plate has two distinct portions[241, 242]. The glenoid or fibrous part attaches to the palmar aspect of the base of the distal bone and by proximal lateral extensions to the margins of the anterior surface of the proximal bone. These extensions — following injury called check-rein ligaments — when viewed anteriorly give the appearance of a swallow-tail. The fibrous palmar plate serves both to restrict hyperex-

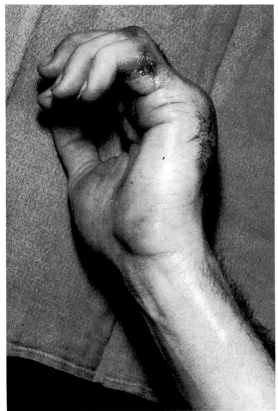

B

Fig. 1.95   A. Closed comminuted fractures of the proximal phalanges resulting from a crush between two heavy pipes show apex palmar angulation. B. The angulation is evident in the examination of the hand, the normally flat dorsal surface of the proximal phalanx having been compromised. C. This is restored by closed reduction and percutaneous fixation (p. 66).

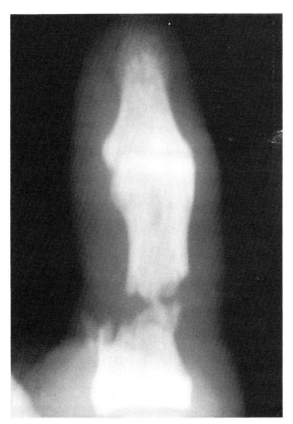

Fig. 1.96 A diaphyseal fracture of the proximal phalanx of the thumb caused by a circumferential rope injury. Such fractures are commonly complicated by disruptive injuries to both digital arteries as in this patient. If this is not recognized and corrected, distal necrosis can ensue.

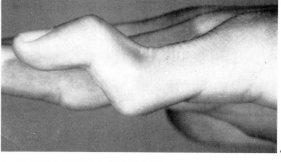

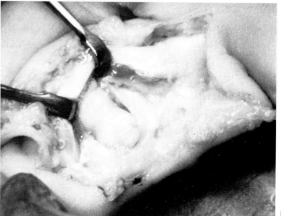

Fig. 1.97 A. A typical hyperextension deformity resulting from tear of the fibrous part of the palmar plate to the proximal interphalangeal joint. B. Exploration shows that the head of the proximal phalanx is protruding between the remnant of the fibrous portion distally and the major portion of the palmar plate proximally.

tension of the joint and as an extension of the articular surface of the base of the distal bone — hence glenoid. It is through the fibrous part that tears of the palmar plate occur (Fig. 1.97). Such tears extend to a varying degree into the collateral ligament, splitting between the fibres of the true and accessory elements (see Fig. 1.102). The membranous part of the palmar plate lies between the check-rein ligaments and serves to transmit blood vessels to the vincular system of the flexor tendons. The arterial arch on the neck of the proximal bone from which these arise is of particular importance at the metacarpal of the thumb as it may be the sole source of the radial digital artery in that digit. The extensor tendon closes the circle of attachments to the base of the distal bone, and in some joints is thickened to the extent that it has been referred to as a dorsal plate. If all the attachments are cut proximal, as in doing an arthrodesis, it can be seen that the base

of the distal bone is indeed encircled by the attached structures with no bare areas (Fig. 1.98). The head of the proximal bone is enveloped by these structures through which it tears in dislocation.

True lateral dislocations of the hinge joints of necessity tear the true collateral ligament. Hyperextension injuries and dorsal dislocations[243] tear the palmar plate but need not tear all of either collateral ligament, even when completely dislocated dorsally. Such hyperextension injuries commonly occur in sport when the tip of the finger is struck by the ball. The axial load tears the palmar plate or avulses its bony attachment, the palmar aspect of the base of the middle phalanx. If this injury is at the proximal interphalangeal joint, as is most frequent, the middle phalanx is often subluxed by the pull of the extensor. In the fracture illustrated in Figure 1.99 the central slip of the extensor tendon is attached to the larger portion of the middle phalanx and only wiring

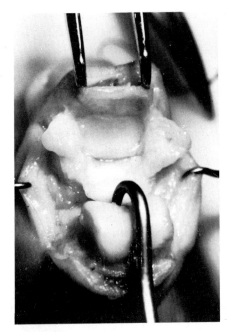

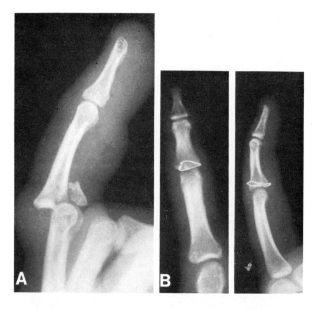

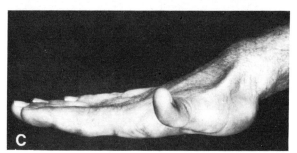

Fig. 1.98 Here, in a patient undergoing distal interphalangeal joint arthrodesis for an old avulsion injury of the flexor digitorum profundus, the structure of the ginglymus joint is demonstrated. All margins of the base of the distal phalanx have attachments, the palmar plate below, the extensor tendon above, and the collateral ligaments on either side. In addition, the accessory collateral ligament can be seen attaching to the palmar plate, the whole forming 'a chair in which the head of the proximal bone will sit' (J. W. Littler).

prevented recurrent dorsal subluxation of the middle phalanx. This injury is often disregarded, often with the urging of athletic staff, and is therefore referred to as a *'coach's finger'*. With use, the joint rapidly deteriorates (p. 200 and Fig. 2.63). The injury may also be open, with reportedly serious potential[244]. Oblique dislocations tear *between* the fibres of the collateral ligament and through the palmar plate, but often only partially. Anterior dislocations[245,246] tear the palmar *and* one or other or both collateral ligaments (Fig. 1.100). In all these ginglymus joints in the hand, the ligaments and tendons tear much more often from their distal attachment, frequently taking with them a fragment of bone of varying size[247,248]. The larger the bone fragment the more likely will it be that the phalanx from which it is torn will sublux from its proper articulation with the head of the proximal bone (Fig. 1.99).

The palmar plates are tested by hyperextension. All collateral ligaments should be stressed by lateral angulation of the joint (Fig. 1.101). Angulation of more than 20° indicates a complete tear[249]. Those especially prone

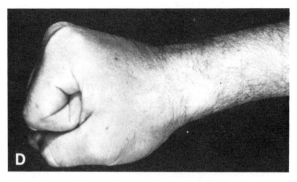

Fig. 1.99 A. This radiograph shows a relatively common intra-articular fracture of the proximal interphalangeal joint. The small palmar fragment is still attached to the palmar plate and its relationship to the proximal phalanx is not markedly changed. The remainder of the middle phalanx is, however, dorsally dislocated. If this fracture is not accurately reduced, subsequent function in the joint will be compromised and early osteoarthritis assured. B. Accurate reduction was obtained and maintained with intraosseous wiring through the triangular ligament region dorsally. This resulted in a full range of motion at eight weeks (C, D).

to injury are the collateral ligaments of the proximal interphalangeal joints and the ulnar collateral ligament of the metacarpophalangeal joint of the thumb, injured in forced abduction (gamekeeper's thumb, see below)[250] If a proximal interphalangeal joint cannot be fully extended, lateral stress may erroneously reveal apparent instability. This is due to the normal *rotation* of the proximal phalanx permitted by the normal laxity in extension of the collateral ligament of the metacarpophalangeal joint. This spurious motion can be eliminated by firmly *flexing* the metacarpophalangeal joint while testing interphalangeal joint stability.

In many instances true lateral and true antero-posterior stress will show *painful stability*. In such cases, the joint should be stressed obliquely, placing tension on the accessory collateral ligament. Tears between the accessory and true collateral ligaments extending partially into the palmar plate are not uncommon and will be revealed by *severe pain and potential instability* on such oblique stress (Fig. 1.102). All of these manoeuvres are painful in the presence of injury and should be done with this knowledge.

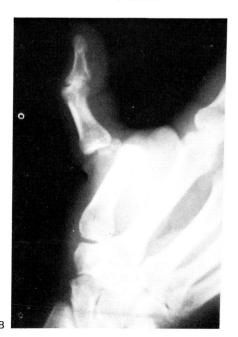

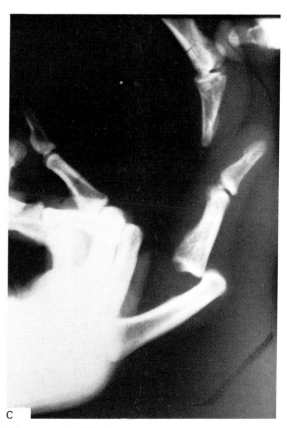

Fig. 1.100 A. This diagram illustrates the ligamentous damage which results from dislocation of a hinge joint. B. Although the bones in this dislocation appear to be widely separated, when the joint was explored it was found that both collateral ligaments were intact. C. Although the bones are apparently much closer together than in (B), exploration of this anterior dislocation revealed a complete tear of the palmar plate and of one collateral ligament.

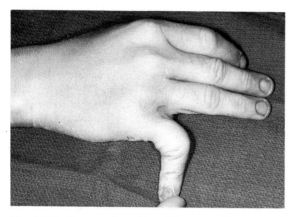

Fig. 1.101 A torn radial collateral ligament of the proximal phalangeal joint.

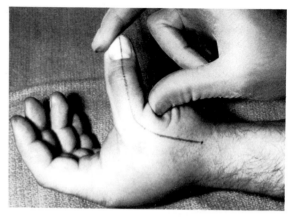

Fig. 1.103 By marking the mid-points of the adjacent joints, angulation on stress, even when it is of a much less significant degree than in this tear of the ulnar collateral ligament, is more readily appreciated.

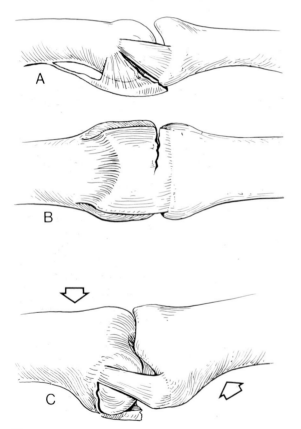

Fig. 1.102 Obliquely oriented injuries to a hinge joint tear between the fibres of the true and accessory collateral ligaments and part way across the palmar plate. Direct lateral and hyperextension stress fail to reveal instability. If, however, the stress is applied obliquely then the mechanism of injury is reproduced, and pain and instability are elicited.

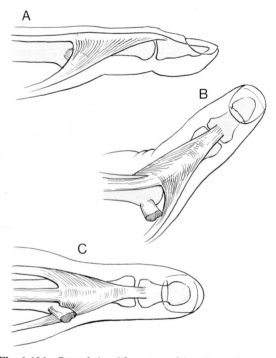

Fig. 1.104 *Stener lesion.* After a tear of the ulnar collateral ligament of the metacarpophalangeal joint of the thumb from its distal attachment, the ligament may come to lie outside the adductor contribution to the extensor expansion. Thus healing cannot occur.

Gamekeeper's thumb[251-255] (= ski-pole thumb). Tears of the ulnar collateral ligament of the metacarpophalangeal joint of the thumb are common and disabling. The injury was said to be sustained by keepers while breaking the necks of small game — hence the name. Now the injury most commonly results from falling on the outstretched hand — a combined extension and radially deviating stress — often with some additional force applied by something wrapped around the thumb itself. (Cut the straps from your ski poles[256] until you reach black diamond!) The injury involves avulsion of the collateral ligament from the base of the proximal phalanx with or without a fragment of bone[257] together with tearing of the palmar plate and accessory collateral ligament (Fig. 1.103). This differs from the proximal interphalangeal joint where collateral ligament rupture is more common proximally[258] (see Fig. 1.83). The torn ligament in the thumb may come to lie superficial to the adductor expansion, which normally overlies it, eliminating any chance of healing — the Stener lesion[259]

(Fig. 1.104) (described also in the proximal interphalangeal joint[260]).

Radiologic examination

True lateral, anteroposterior and oblique views. Standard radiographs of the hand will not give true views of any of the phalangeal bones or joints. These must be sought, and can often, with both economy and benefit, be obtained on *dental films.*

Simple fractures, that is, ones which are single and do not involve an articular surface, should first be examined closely to ensure that they are truly so. Quite commonly, after a direct injury, an apparently simple fracture will be seen to have undisplaced cracks running from it, often into the joint (Fig. 1.105). Such cracks will complicate fixation. *Displacement* should be categorized and a determination made whether or not it is *acceptable.* A wide gap between fragments should suggest the possibility of *interposed soft tissue.* The examiner should consider what structure it may be. The *stability*

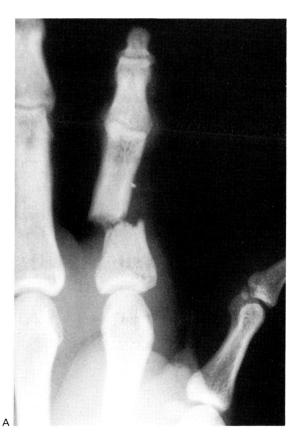

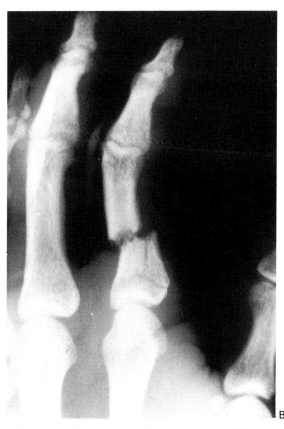

Fig. 1.105 A. This apparently simple displaced transverse diaphyseal fracture of the proximal phalanx was seen on a different view (B) to have a further fracture line which extended towards the metacarpophalangeal joint.

or otherwise of the fracture will have been determined in part by the limitation of active motion (above) but can be further estimated by the location of the fracture, the degree of displacement and by knowledge of the motors attached to each fragment. Angled fractures should be studied to determine whether they are *oblique* or *spiral*. The latter tend to be longer and they show apparent overlap of one fragment on the other, due to one cortex being fractured in a different line than the opposite cortex at the same level ('same' being in a proximo-distal sense).

Comminuted fractures require examination in several views, for there are invariably more fragments than one initially detects. Extension into joints should be suspected.

Articular views should be studied first to determine that they are indeed '*true*' — this is the case when the two condyles of the head are accurately superimposed one on the other yielding one crescentic image, not two (see Fig. 1.86).

Articular congruity should be ensured. There must be no '*open wedge*'[261] between the images of the two bones which would indicate subluxation.

Fragments of bone should be examined to determine their displacement and its degree. A conclusion should be drawn regarding the ligamentous or tendinous structure to which the fragment is most likely attached.

Stress views are of value in assessing dislocations and fracture–dislocations involving the collateral ligaments of the proximal interphalangeal joint and the metacarpophalangeal joint of the thumb (Fig. 1.106). While these can in some instances be taken without anaesthesia, infiltration or regional block is both kind and help-

ful, for full unresisted stress may reveal a greater degree of disruption than had been suspected.

In open injuries, many or all of the views outlined may be repeated under anaesthesia when distraction and positioning may provide superior radiographs. At that time it will be possible to assess whether or not bony fragments are missing, and to what extent.

Indications in closed phalangeal injuries

Certain closed fractures can only be reduced and made stable by complex surgery involving wide dissection, extensive use of fixation techniques and even requiring supplementary bone graft and transfixion of both adjacent joints. In some cases this may be justifiable. In others, however, non-operative management, consisting of initial *rest and elevation* for five days, followed by *early active motion* allied with the use of a *splint for rest and protection*, may effect an equally good result (see Fig. 1.93).

Angulated, rotated or shortened non-articular phalangeal fractures, be they spiral, oblique or transverse, should be reduced and fixed. This is necessary regardless of the direction and degree of the angulation, for the reasons previously stated. The single exception is modest antero-posterior angulation in the child — one in which the child can obtain full interphalangeal extension. This will remodel.

Closed reduction and percutaneous fixation[262] can be achieved in some — especially spiral — fractures and with the help of the image intensifier. This should be done under sterile conditions, preferably in the operating room, and the number of attempts should be strictly limited to three or unacceptable damage will be done to both soft tissues and bone. The transverse, sometimes comminuted, fracture of the diaphysis of the proximal phalanx which results from a direct and very heavy blow and which frequently breaks all four proximal phalanges is often closed, but is associated with severe soft-tissue trauma. If the circulation is intact there is merit in avoiding further injury to the soft tissue which would result from incision and dissection. Closed reduction can be obtained by firmly flexing the metacarpophalangeal joint by pressure on the head of the proximal phalanx. This pressure will also correct the apex-palmar deformity, but the extensor apparatus will prevent overcorrection. With the reduction so maintained, it can be fixed by driving a Kirschner wire through the dorsal aspect of the metacarpal head, across the metacarpophalangeal joint and along the medullary cavity of the phalanx to come to rest in the subchondral bone of the head[263]. If revascularization is required (Fig. 1.107), the pin(s) can be temporarily driven further distally until the metacarpophalangeal joint is free and can be

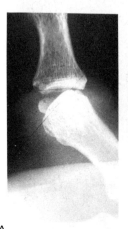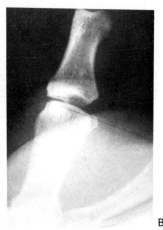

A   B

Fig. 1.106 Here the stress films of right and left thumb metacarpophalangeal joints are compared. That on the left opens to an angle of 45° compared with 10° on the right due to an ulnar collateral ligament tear — 'gamekeeper's thumb'.

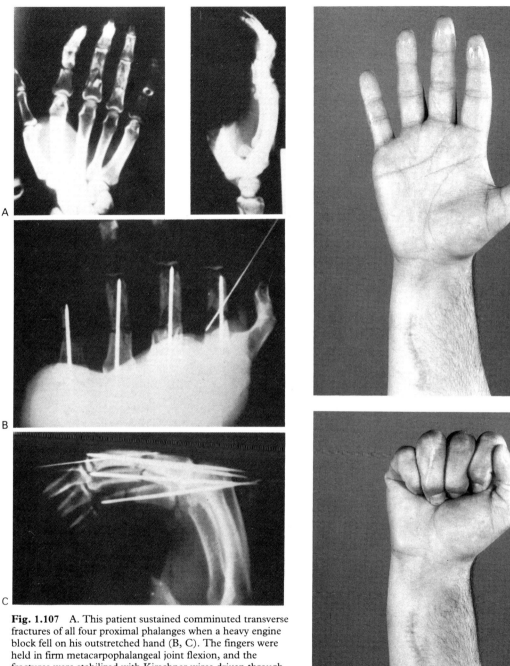

Fig. 1.107 A. This patient sustained comminuted transverse fractures of all four proximal phalanges when a heavy engine block fell on his outstretched hand (B, C). The fingers were held in firm metacarpophalangeal joint flexion, and the fractures were stabilized with Kirschner wires driven through the metacarpal head passing down along the shafts of the proximal phalanges. The comminution in the index finger was such that an additional oblique pericutaneous pin was added to control rotation. It can be seen that this maintains the hand in the 'safe' position. Revascularization of the middle finger required a vein graft. Probably because of the soft-tissue injury and the comminution, union of the fractures took fully eight weeks. Despite that, on removal of the pins, physical therapy very quickly restored full motion (D, E).

extended for microsurgical repair. Once that repair has been completed, the metacarpophalangeal joints are flexed while observing flow and the pins driven retrograde to immobilize them in the safe position.

Many non-articular fractures will require *open reduction and internal fixation*[264]. Various fixation techniques are meritorious[265,266], but the author has the following preferences: *screw fixation* of spiral fractures long enough to permit correct placement of two screws (Fig. 1.108B); *type A intraosseous wiring*[267] (Fig. 1.108C) and its variants[268] of other simple fractures; *intramedullary Steinmann pin fixation* of comminuted fractures, provided they have no intra-articular extensions (Fig. 1.109).

Despite isolated reports of their conservative treatment[269,270] *intra-articular fractures* must be reduced and fixed with absolute precision. While this *may* be achieved closed, the author always prefers direct visualization of the articular surface (see Fig. 1.140), fixation being achieved by a *screw*, two *Kirschner wires* or *type B*

intraosseous wiring[267] (Fig. 1.108B). Where the fragments in palmar plate avulsion fractures are too comminuted to fix, dynamic traction with early passive motion[271] is cumbersome and difficult to manage, and the author prefers excision of the fragments with *palmar plate advancement*[272] (Fig. 1.110).

Ligamentous tears following dislocation may be

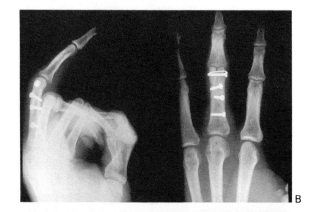

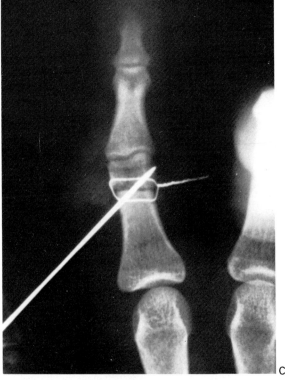

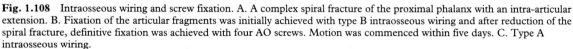

Fig. 1.108 Intraosseous wiring and screw fixation. A. A complex spiral fracture of the proximal phalanx with an intra-articular extension. B. Fixation of the articular fragments was initially achieved with type B intraosseous wiring and after reduction of the spiral fracture, definitive fixation was achieved with four AO screws. Motion was commenced within five days. C. Type A intraosseous wiring.

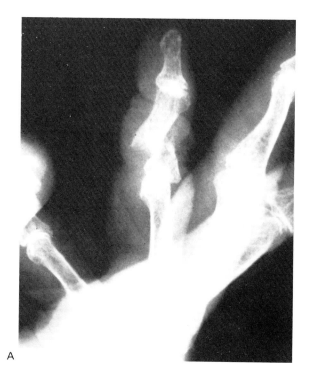

A

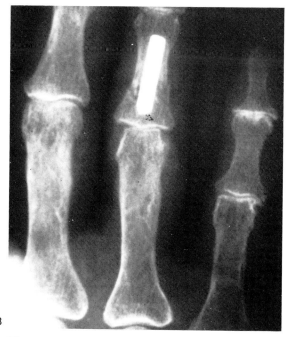

B

Fig. 1.109 A, B. A comminuted fracture in a 93-year-old lady with significant osteoporosis was effectively fixed using an intramedullary Steinmann pin. She proceeded to retrieve full motion in this digit.

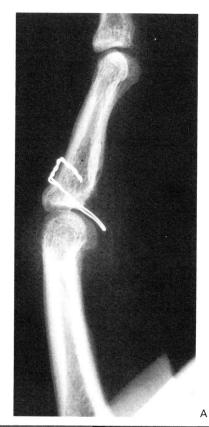

A

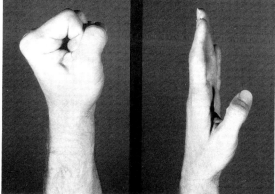

B

Fig. 1.110 A. Palmar plate advancement. B. Range of motion shows extensor lag of 15°.

managed by *protective splintage* or *open repair. Extension block* splinting[273] will protect the palmar plate, and *buddy* splinting the collateral ligament of the proximal interphalangeal joint, in the co-operative patient, but should not be applied until five days after injury to permit swelling to settle, during which time the hand and wrist should be supported in an anterior splint.

Open repair is indicated in both instances where patient compliance is in doubt.

Although methods have been reported by which to diagnose the presence of a Stener lesion in *ulnar collateral ligament* injuries of the metacarpophalangeal joint of the thumb by palpation[274] and by magnetic resonance imaging[275], they have not gained widespread acceptance. Functional bracing has been reported to yield acceptable results[276], but it also is not widely used. The author therefore opens all where the history is right and there is bruising over the appropriate region. The ligament is re-attached with *type B intraosseous wiring* and the metacarpophalangeal joint immobilized with a Kirschner wire. There are two important points:

1. The tension which tore the ligament on the ulnar aspect was accompanied by compression on the radial. The joint surfaces on the radial side of the joint should always be examined for articular fractures which will not be evident on radiographic examination. The patient should always have been warned of the possibility of *arthrodesis*, which is the correct treatment for such articular damage (see Fig. 1.144).
2. The thumb requires to be *stable* — it therefore should be immobilized for 6 weeks after ligament repair. The fingers require to be *mobile*; regardless of the injury and its management, all phalangeal skeletal injuries should be mobilized regularly, although still protected, by the fifth day following injury.

See Green D P 1993 Operative Hand Surgery, 3rd edn. Churchill Livingstone, New York, pp. 721, 735, 771 et seq., 783.

METACARPOPHALANGEAL JOINT INJURIES (OF THE FINGERS)

The metacarpophalangeal joint of the fingers is classified as ellipsoid. The head of the metacarpal is narrower on its dorsal surface than on its palmar surface. Viewed end on, the head therefore has the appearance of the letter 'A' with the apex removed — geometrically the shape of a trapezoid in America, a trapezium in Britain. The shoulders of the metacarpal lie closer to the dorsal portion of the articular surface than to the palmar. Since the *true collateral ligament* attaches to the recess created by the junction of shoulder and head — unlike the human body, the metacarpal has its neck below the shoulder — the distance from its attachment to the palmar surface of the head is greater than to the distal surface, with which the base of the proximal phalanx articulates in extension. As a result of these two facts — the wider palmar aspect of the head and the differing tension in the true collateral ligament — the ligament is tight and unyielding when the metacarpophalangeal joint is flexed. When the joint is extended, it is loose and the proximal phalanges have considerable lateral play into abduction and adduction. This movement is achieved by the action of the interosseous muscles, the dorsal abducting, the palmar adducting. This lateral movement in extension is used daily in actions such as typing and grasping large spherical objects. The fixation of the head in flexion serves to stabilize and strengthen the grip. In injury, oedema fluid in the joint and the periarticular soft tissues tends to force the metacarpophalangeal joint into extension. If left in that position, the collateral ligament shortens, producing an extension contracture (p. 195). The palmar plate is similar in construction to that of the proximal interphalangeal joint. It is connected to adjacent plates by the deep transverse metacarpal ligament (p. 17). Sesamoid bones are always present in the palmar plate of the thumb (their fracture may be an obscure source of pain[277]), often in the index and less commonly in the other fingers.

Because of the laxity of the collateral ligament compared with that of the proximal interphalangeal joint, it avoids frequent injury[278]. When torn it may be so in a variety of ways: totally or partially; in its substance or by avulsion of bone; the bone avulsed from either the shoulder of the metacarpal or the base of the proximal phalanx. The collateral ligaments of the metacarpophalangeal joints of the fingers can be tested for integrity or injury only by lateral stress on the proximal phalanx with the metacarpophalangeal joint in maximum *flexion*. A recognized *dislocation* of the metacarpophalangeal joint of the fingers is relatively uncommon[279], may rarely involve several joints[280-282], affects the index finger most frequently, and takes two distinct forms:

Simple. A posterior dislocation which can be readily and effectively reduced in closed fashion; indeed, the majority of patients present with a history of angulation reduced spontaneously, personally or by someone present at the accident.

Complex[283-285]. Posterior dislocation in which the metacarpal head becomes trapped between the palmar fascia on its palmar aspect and the displaced and ruptured palmar plate on its dorsal aspect, between the flexor tendons on its ulnar side and the lumbrical muscle on its radial side (Fig. 1.111).

The posture of the dislocated finger is distinct for each of these two types of dislocation. In the simple dislocation the proximal phalanx tends to lie in almost 90° of hyperextension while in the complex dislocation, the

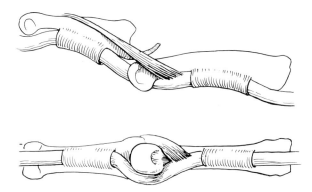

Fig. 1.111 This diagram illustrates the mechanism of a complex dislocation of the metacarpophalangeal joint. In the upper, lateral diagram it can be seen that the palmar plate is locked between the head of the metacarpal and the base of the proximal phalanx. In the lower diagram, an anterior view, the head of the metacarpal can be seen trapped between the flexor digitorum profundus on one aspect and the lumbrical on the other.

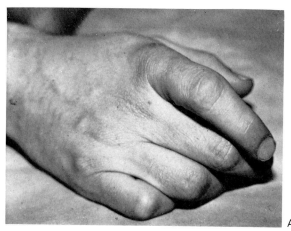
A

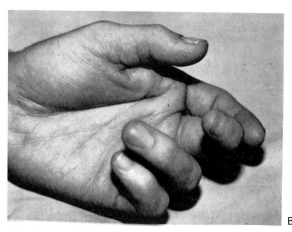
B

Fig. 1.112 A. The typical posture of the complex dislocation is seen, the index finger being locked in some 30° of hyperextension. B. The typical deep puckering at the palmar crease is evident, due to the traction on the palmar fascia and so, through its skin attachment, on the skin itself.

angle of hyperextension is appreciably less. In the complex dislocation, the displaced metacarpal head forms a marked prominence in the palm, which also shows deep puckering of the proximal palmar crease due to traction on the skin attachments of the palmar fascia (Fig. 1.112). In some cases of complex dislocation the circulation to the index finger may be embarrassed, as the neurovascular bundles are stretched and trapped by the displaced metacarpal head. Complex dislocation may, more rarely, occur in the thumb[286] and other fingers.

Human bite injuries are usually sustained by the metacarpophalangeal joint, usually of the middle finger (p. 331).[287] It is at this joint also that chondral fractures most commonly occur (p. 196). Capsular rupture and tears of the sagittal band of the extensor apparatus[288] may also result from direct blows to the metacarpal head.

Radiologic examination
Fractures of the head (see below) or base should be sought, recognizing that they may be avulsion fractures attached to the collateral ligament.

In *complex dislocation*, an increased joint space results from the presence of the entrapped palmar plate. If the plate contains a sesamoid bone, its appearance in the widened space is pathognomonic.

Brewerton view (see Fig. 5.79, p. 394) — taken with the fingers on the film and the metacarpophalangeal joints flexed to 65°, the tube at 15° ulnar to the vertical

— may reveal fractures of the metacarpal head[289] (Fig. 1.113).

Indications in the metacarpophalangeal joint of the fingers
Simple dislocations can be readily reduced, usually in the emergency room, often without anaesthesia. The hand should then be placed on an anterior *rest and protection* splint, with the commencement of early motion sessions protected by a *buddy* splint between the injured and an adjacent finger. By contrast, reduction of the complex dislocation requires anaesthesia. The finger may then be reduced closed by wrist flexion and traction on the digit, but often the joint must be opened, from a *dorsal* approach as opposed to the palmar previously recommended.

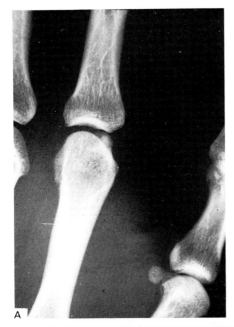

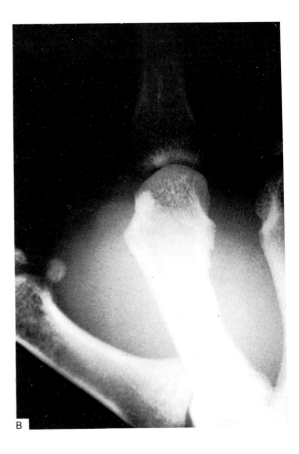

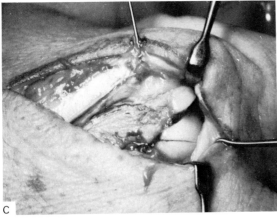

Fig. 1.113   A. An anteroposterior view of this metacarpal head failed to reveal a fracture. B. It was, however, evident on a Brewerton view. C. Exploration revealed the degree of displacement in this comminuted fracture of the metacarpal head.

Ligament tears are treated by protected mobilization after an initial brief period of rest. Chip fractures attached to the ligament can be ignored. Their reduction and internal fixation is a difficult — though interesting, but unnecessary — undertaking. If pain troubles the patient later, due to partial healing of a partial tear, it can be relieved by simply dividing the collateral ligament from its metacarpal attachment. Complete divisions are not troublesome and are performed routinely in releasing joint contractures (p. 200).

See Green D P 1993 Operative Hand Surgery, 3rd edn. Churchill Livingstone, New York, p. 778.

METACARPAL AND CARPOMETACARPAL INJURIES

Metacarpal head fractures are primarily intra-articular and include (i) the human bite injuries and chondral fractures mentioned above, (ii) ligament avulsions, (iii) epiphyseal injuries, which may go unrecognized and result in brachymetacarpia[290], (iv) single fractures in any plane, and, most frequently, (v) comminution[291].

Neck fractures are common, resulting from the fist striking a relatively immovable object — *boxer's fracture*. The anterior cortex proximal to the articular surface is comminuted, resulting in apex-dorsal angulation —

which is recognized clinically by loss of the prominence of the metacarpal head dorsally and its appearance in the palm of the hand.

Shaft fractures may be transverse, comminuted, or, frequently, spiral, for the diaphysis of the metacarpal is the frequent target of torsional forces on the finger. Deformities of *angulation, shortening* and *rotation* are common.

Fractures of the *base* are intra-articular and are an integral part of a complex which includes *dislocations* and *fracture–dislocations* of the carpometacarpal joints most frequently found in, but not limited to, the thumb[292,293]:

1. *Bennett's fracture*[294, 295] of the first metacarpal is the most common; due to traction of the abductor pollicis longus, which attaches to the base, the main portion of the metacarpal subluxes, leaving the anterior beak of the base, which is attached to the ulnar or palmar collateral ligament, in its correct anatomical position.
2. A similar fracture–dislocation of the *fifth metacarpal* is sometimes called a *reversed Bennett's*, for the displacement is similar and has a similar cause, the extensor carpi ulnaris subluxing the main portion of the fifth metacarpal as does the abductor pollicis

longus the first; damage to the deep motor branch of the ulnar nerve has been reported in this injury[296].

3. The *Rolando fracture*[297] resembles the Bennett's, differing from it only in the addition of a fracture of the dorsal portion of the base to which the abductor pollicis longus attaches, thus creating a so-called 'T-condylar fracture' (Fig. 1.114).
4. *Hamatometacarpal fracture dislocation* involves a fracture of the fourth metacarpal and dislocation of the fifth hamatometacarpal joint, with or without a coincident fracture of the hamate, a fracture which varies in pattern[298, 299].
5. *Carpometacarpal dislocations* (Fig. 1.115) have been reported of all the rays, in varying patterns[300-305], usually with the base dorsal, but occasionally palmar in location[306] and with the tendon of extensor carpi radialis brevis interposed in one dislocation of the second ray[307]; the diagnosis is

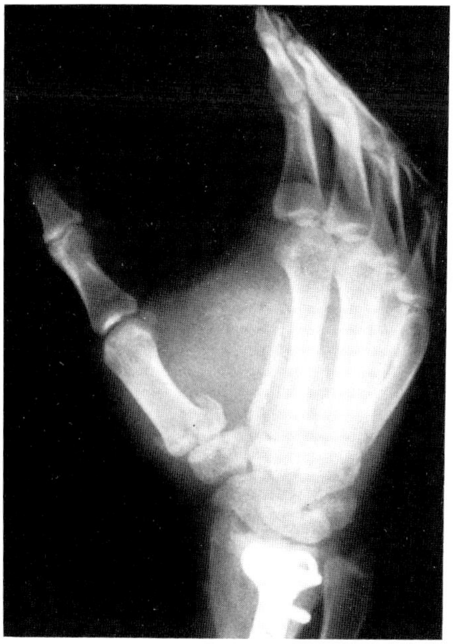

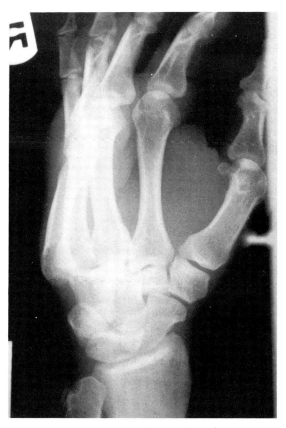

Fig. 1.114 This patient, who is clearly accident prone (evidence the plate on a Smith fracture of his radius), has sustained fractures of the metacarpal shafts and a Rolando fracture of the base of the thumb.

Fig. 1.115 A lateral pronated by 30° shows the carpometacarpal dislocation of the ring finger.

readily overlooked[308, 309], due largely to the significant swelling which accompanies the considerable force required to produce the injury. Pure dislocation of the first ray is uncommon, but is a variant of the Bennett's fracture differing only in that the ulnar (or palmar) collateral ligament has torn in its substance rather than avulsing the palmar beak of the metacarpal.

Radiologic examination
The standard postero-anterior and lateral view of the hand may show some injuries, especially dorsal carpo-metacarpal dislocations, but additional special views are required to reveal all lesions.

Modified lateral views of the metacarpals are necessary since little of the shaft or head can be seen on a true lateral of the hand. To study the index and middle the hand should be pronated 30° from lateral, for the ring and small supinated 30° (Fig. 1.115; see also Fig. 1.84).

Brewerton view (p. 394) to better visualize the meta-carpal head.

Robert view[310] — taken with the arm fully pronated, the shoulder internally rotated and the thumb abducted — shows all articulations of the trapezium and first metacarpal (Fig. 1.116).

Stress films[311] under anaesthesia. Where instability of the basal joint of the thumb is suggested, the stress is achieved by pushing the tip of one abducted thumb against the other, taking a simultaneous comparative view of both first carpometacarpal joints.

Indications in metacarpal and carpometacarpal injuries
Fractures of the *head*, being intra-articular, demand precise open reduction and internal fixation with insti-tution of an early motion programme[312] (see Fig. 1.113).

Fractures of the *metacarpal neck*. Since the second and third have virtually no motion at their carpo-meta-carpal joint, no angulation can be accepted, otherwise the anterior displacement of the metacarpal head may produce a painful grasp. By contrast, since there is mo-tion in the basal joint of the fourth and fifth metacarpals, some angulation can be accepted. In the common *boxer's fracture* of the fifth metacarpal neck, 40° of angulation is widely recommended as acceptable, and by some as much as 70°[313-314] (Fig. 1.117). Rather, hand function should dictate management. If the pa-tient can fully flex and fully extend his small finger, *without any tendency to claw*, then the angulation should be corrected closed as best as possible and immobilized in a splint[315, 316]. If motion is abnormal, reduction and fixation will be necessary. The technique of fixation where reduction of neck fractures is deemed desirable is another matter! Two *Kirschner wires* inserted through the shoulders of the metacarpal beneath the collateral ligament like Rush rods may work, as may an *intramed-ullary pin* supplemented by a *tension band wire*. *External fixation* has been shown to be effective[317].

Shaft fractures can be treated closed, simply with a protecting splint, provided that (i) there *is no rotation*, for as little as 5° rotation produces 1.5 cm overlap in the fingertips on flexion[318] (Fig. 1.118), and (ii) the shortening and angulation are deemed acceptable — what is acceptable varies widely between authors[315-320]. However, mobilization early enough to maintain full metacarpophalangeal joint function is likely to lead to

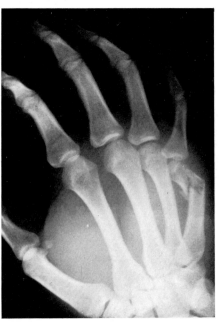

Fig. 1.117 Comminuted boxer's fracture of the head of the metacarpal.

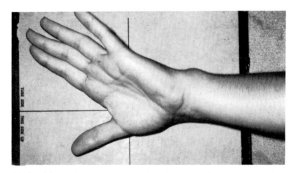

Fig. 1.116 The Robert view is taken with the forearm fully pronated, the shoulder internally rotated and the thumb abducted.

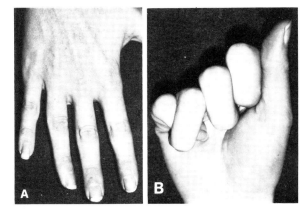

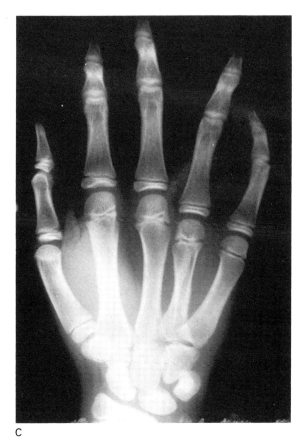

C

Fig. 1.118 A, B. This patient had sustained a fracture of the metacarpal of the right ring finger and insufficient attention was paid to obtaining the correct rotational alignment. This resulted in a deformity functionally and cosmetically unsatisfactory to the patient and embarrassing for the surgeon. C. Although the spiral fracture of the fourth metacarpal is not easily seen, the entirely unsatisfactory rotation in the finger can be readily appreciated. This must be corrected.

delayed union or non-union. The author's preference is for open reduction and internal fixation, followed by early protected motion. *Screw* fixation for spiral fractures (Fig. 1.119), and *plate and screw* for transverse fractures are preferred. If comminution exists, the fracture should be treated closed, but if open management is necessary, *external fixation* or an *intramedullary Steinmann pin* with a *tension band wire* are the main alternatives.

Carpometacarpal fractures and dislocations should be reduced, although different views have been expressed on both Bennett's[321–323] and Rolando fractures[323–325] In many instances reduction is done closed but often proves unstable, being overcome by percutaneous Kirschner wire fixation of the reduced metacarpal to the carpus. This is a method commonly used in the management of Bennett's fracture. However, a review of the literature[326] shows nineteen methods reported for management of this common fracture. *Open reduction and internal fixation* offers the attractive possibility of instituting early motion and, with the development of more sophisticated plates and screws, seems likely to become the method preferred by those skilled in their use[327,328].

See Green D P 1993 Operative Hand Surgery, 3rd edn. Churchill Livingstone, New York, pp. 696, 701, 708 and 713.

CARPAL INJURIES

Anatomy and biomechanics

The surface markings of the carpus have been reviewed (p. 15). There are eight carpal bones arranged in two rows of equal number, referred to as proximal and distal. The proximal row creates the distal surface of the radiocarpal joint, there being two shallow depressions on the distal radius, which are articular facets: the larger radial, lateral, facet is for the proximal pole of the scaphoid; the smaller surface which occupies the ulnar portion of the distal end of the radius articulates with the lunate. To the ulnar, medial, side of the lunate lies the triquetrum, or triquetral, which articulates proximally with the triangular fibrocartilaginous complex (TFCC). This ligamentous structure joins the fovea at the base of the ulnar styloid to the distal margin of the sigmoid notch of the radius. The head of the ulna articulates with the sigmoid notch as the inferior radioulnar joint. The TFCC separates this joint from the radiocarpal joint. Its distal surface creates a smooth glenoid extension of the distal end of the radius. In both coronal and sagittal planes, the radiocarpal joint creates a shallow 'U'. This 'U' is readily seen on both radial and carpal aspects of the joint in the lateral radiologic

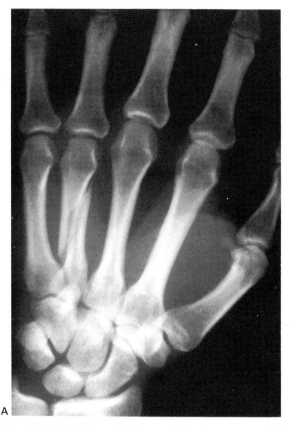
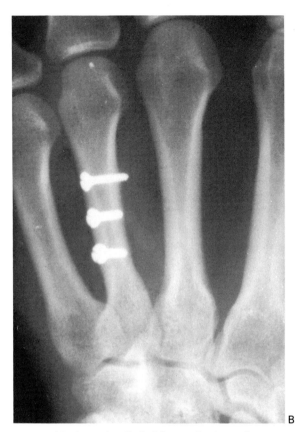

A

B

Fig. 1.119   A. A long spiral fracture of the ring metacarpal shows unacceptable shortening. B. Satisfactory fixation such as to permit immediate motion is achieved with three AO screws.

view, but in the postero-anterior view its full length is appreciated only on the carpal aspect, since the ulnar segment of the proximal surface in composed largely of the TFCC, which is radiolucent. The entire radiocarpal joint *is* outlined on a posteroanterior arthrogram (Fig. 1.120). The joint, thus curved in two planes, permits free extension and flexion, radial and ulnar deviation, and any combinations thereof. The last of the four bones of the proximal carpal row, the pisiform, plays no part in the radiocarpal joint, lying on, and articulating with, the anterior surface of the triquetrum. The contiguous surfaces of the scaphoid and the lunate, and of the lunate and the triquetrum are not only absolutely congruent, but, unlike many other joints, are of virtually equal area in each articulation and are bonded together by interosseous ligaments (S-L and L-T respectively) (see below). There are two consequences: (i) there is normally limited motion in the scapholunate and lunatotriquetral joints; (ii) the distal surfaces of the three bones together present a regular, unbroken articulation which forms the proximal facet of the mid-

carpal joint. This facet creates an additional 'U' or 'cup', again in both sagittal and coronal planes. The latter, that which is viewed on postero-anterior films, is deeper than that of the radiocarpal joint. Stated another way, it is a segment of a smaller circle. This cup articulates with the proximal surfaces of the capitate, which in the neutral position contacts the scaphoid and lunate, and the hamate. (Burgess[329] has described a 'type II' articulation in which a small hamato-lunate facet exists between the hamatotriquetral and capitolunate joints; he believes it to be significant in lunatotriquetral ligament tears (p. 220)). The hamatotriquetral joint has a spiral, or helicoid, configuration. As the hamate slides down the surface of the triquetrum with ulnar deviation, this helicoid orientation moves the triquetrum anteriorly, rotating its distal facet dorsally so that the entire proximal row points dorsally by virtue of the force transmitted through the strong L-T and S-L ligaments. That is, the proximal row is dorsiflexed. The proximal row is also called the intercalated segment, positioned as it is between the radius proximally and

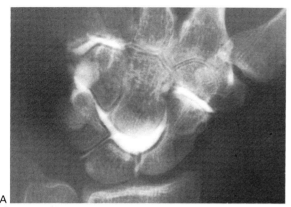

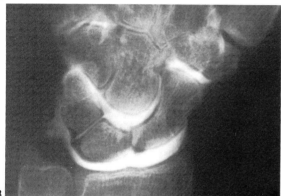

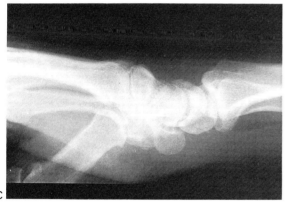

Fig. 1.120 A. Distraction midcarpal arthrogram. B. Distraction midcarpal and radiocarpal arthrogram (note the step-off in the scapholunate joint due to distraction). C. True lateral view of the wrist with mild DISI deformity (see text).

the carpometacarpal complex distally, both of which are relatively fixed when compared with the mobile proximal row[330]. The distance by which the hamate slides down the triquetrum as the wrist passes from extreme radial to extreme ulnar deviation is in no way equalled at the radial end of the midcarpal joint. This

apparent paradox is explained by the fact that the scaphoid rotates at its articulation with the capitate around an axis which runs approximately from the radial styloid to the centre of the capitate, the scaphoid becoming oriented longitudinally — or extended — in ulnar deviation, shortened or more horizontal — flexed — in radial. As the scaphoid flexes and extends it carries the proximal row with it through the interosseous ligamentous link[331]. Thus the whole row adopts a dorsiflexed posture in ulnar deviation, palmar flexed in radial. The two remaining bones of the distal carpal row, the trapezium and the trapezoid, articulate proximally with the distal pole of the scaphoid. Although this articulation can be considered as an extension of the midcarpal joint — and indeed communicates with it — it moves much less than does the midcarpal articulation. The reason in ulnar and radial deviation has been explained above — scaphoid extension and flexion, which the trapezium and trapezoid largely follow, due to the scaphotrapezial ligament complex[332], which is most strong on its palmar aspect, stabilizing the scaphoid link between the carpal rows. In wrist palmar and dorsiflexion, due to this relatively rigid ligament complex and scaphoid link, the ulnar side of the hand moves through a greater arc than does the radial. Thus the palm of the hand is supinated somewhat in wrist extension relative to the forearm, pronated in wrist flexion. The effect also contributes to bring the thumb passively into greater opposition in dorsiflexion, into more palmar adduction in palmar flexion. This facilitates grasp and release.

Carpal bones may be absent or fused from birth. The former occurs most often in conjunction with longitudinal absence (p. 465), but may occur in isolation[333]. Carpal fusion, synostosis or coalition, as it is variously called, occurs in 0.1% of the white population, but in 9% of the population in some West African tribes. Lunatotriquetral coalition is most common, followed by capitate-hamate. Coalition between the two rows is extremely rare. Coalitions are invariably asymptomatic, but if incomplete, have been reported to be symptomatic[334].

When rotation of the forearm is included, the wrist has three degrees of freedom with a significant range in each (p. 205), although in performing 52 standard tasks, the functional range was 5° of flexion, 30° of extension, 10° of radial and 15° of ulnar deviation[335]. The ability strongly to stabilize the hand in any of the positions this freedom permits exists despite the fact that no muscles or tendons insert into any of the seven carpal bones engaged in wrist motion. All of the wrist motors, with the exception of flexor carpi ulnaris, insert beyond the carpus. It follows that the ligaments which connect the metacarpus to the carpus and the carpal bones to one another are indispensable to wrist stability.

Several detailed descriptions of these ligaments exist, but in their admirable and successful attempts to be exhaustive, they can also be exhausting. Stated as simply as is necessary to comprehend the more common wrist instabilities, there are interosseous and 'transosseous' or extrinsic ligaments.

1. The *interosseous* ligaments joint adjacent bones, and there are three significant groups:
   (a) Those which join the lunate to the adjacent triquetrum and scaphoid; they are U-shaped, continuous from dorsal to proximal to palmar, thus permitting fluid to enter only from the midcarpal joint (see Fig. 1.120); they are very short as befits ligaments connecting bones

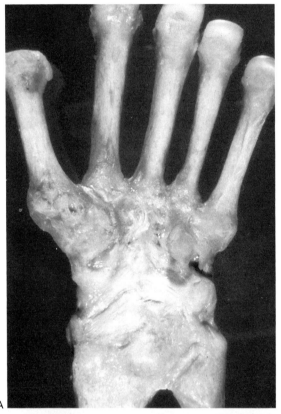

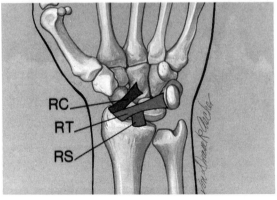

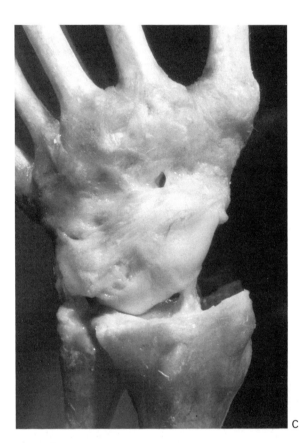

Fig. 1.121 A. Dissection of the extrinsic transosseous ligaments of the anterior surface of the wrist. B. Diagrammatic representation of the major ligaments. RC = radioscaphocapitate ligament; RT = radiolunatotriquetral ligament; RS = radioscapholunate ligament of Testut. C. Viewed from dorsally with distraction of the radiocarpal joint after removal of the dorsal capsule, the radioscapholunate ligament of Testut can be seen. In addition, the virtually uninterrupted surface created by the scaphoid, the lunate and the intervening interosseous scapholunate ligament is shown. (Dissections by Dr Douglas Hanel; artwork by Grace von Drasek Ascher.)

which move largely in unison; their surface, which forms part of the radiocarpal articulation, is covered with hyaline cartilage such that it is difficult to detect the line of the joints they connect (Fig. 1.121C).

(b) Those which join the four bones of the distal row; by contrast with the first group, dorsal and palmar are distinct, so that again fluid from the midcarpal joint can enter the intervening joints (see Fig. 1.120).

(c) Those joining the forearm bones to the proximal carpal row; of these the most significant are the *radioscapholunate* (RSL) — the ligament of Testut — and the *ulnolunate* (UL) on the palmar aspect (Fig. 1.121) and the various components of the dorsal *radiocarpal* (DRC) ligament (Fig. 1.122).

2. The *transosseous* ligaments, as the name (which is unique to this text!) implies, cross bones and attach to them. Some are especially important but simple to remember using the following personal logic:

(a) The radius and the carpus rotate around the ulna, therefore the main transosseous ligaments must tie *radius to carpus*, leaving the ulna as a free axis.

(b) Most loads are applied in dorsiflexion, therefore the main ligaments must be on the *palmar* aspect.

(c) Those loads, for reasons partly explained above, drive the carpus into ulnar deviation and supination relative to the forearm, therefore — to resist excesses in those movements — the ligaments must run from the *radial side of the radius* to the *ulnar side of the carpus*.

Two ligaments meet these criteria:

(i) The *radioscaphocapitate* (RSC); this passes from its attachment to the palmar aspect of the radial styloid, across the waist of the scaphoid to which it has a loose attachment, to the centre of the palmar aspect of the capitate. It is the 'sling' ligament over which the scaphoid bows in flexing during radial deviation.

(ii) The *radiolunato* (*triquetral*) (RL[T]); arising from the radial styloid just medial to the previous ligament, this pursues a more transverse course and has strong attachments to the lunate and, it was formerly believed and still widely taught, to the triquetrum. The reason for the brackets around triquetral is that it is probable (and the dissection in Fig. 1.121 supports that probability) that this will become the long radiolunate ligament (as opposed to the short radio(scapho)lunate ligament of Testut).

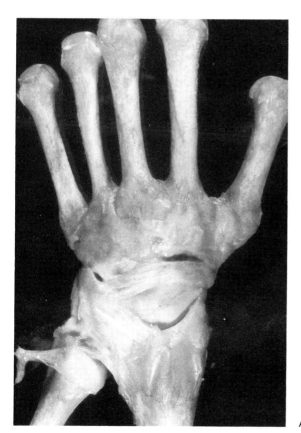

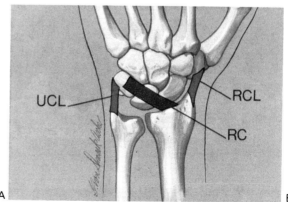

A B

Fig. 1.122   A. Dissection of the extrinsic ligaments of the dorsal aspect of the wrist. B. Diagram of the dorsum of the wrist. RC = dorsal radiocarpal ligament; RCL and UCL = the radial and ulnar collateral ligaments (of little importance). (Dissections by Dr Douglas Hanel; artwork by Grace von Drasek Ascher.)

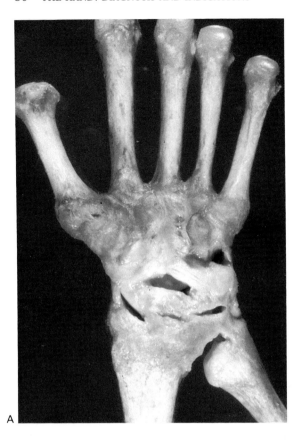

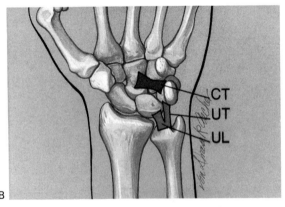

Fig. 1.123 A. Dissection of the palmar surface of the wrist following removal of the radioscaphocapitate and radiolunatotriquetral ligament. On the right, reading from proximally, lie the ulna, the triangular fibrocartilaginous complex, the triquetrum and the hamate. Passing from the triquetrum to the capitate is the triquetrohamatocapitate ligament. B. The palmar surface of the wrist showing the ulnolunate (UL) ligament and (UT) the ulnotriquetral ligament (together with the TFCC known also as the ulnocarpal complex (UCC)) and the capito (hamato) triquetral (CT) ligament. (Dissections by Dr Douglas Hanel; artwork by Grace von Drasek Ascher.)

A further ligament joins the carpal ends of these two:

(iii) The *triquetrohamatocapitate* (THC) (Fig. 1.123). This serves to prevent excessive dorsiflexion on the ulnar aspect of the wrist.

The triangle of carpus which lies bare between these three ligaments is the space of Poirier.

As the wrist extensors function to pull the complex of the metacarpus and distal carpal row dorsally, the last of these three ligaments pulls the proximal row into dorsiflexion on the ulnar aspect, complementing the stabilizing 'link' between the carpal rows on the radial aspect — the scaphoid. As the proximal row is arrested by the RLT transosseous ligament and the radio-scapholunate and ulnolunate interosseous ligaments, further extension occurs at the midcarpal joint placing under load both the scaphoid and two of the three transosseous ligaments — the RSC and the THC. By this mechanism, approximately 35% of extension occurs at the midcarpal joint, 65% at the radiocarpal. A similar mechanism drives the carpus in palmar flexion, 60% of the range being at the midcarpal joint, 40% at the radiocarpal.

The three transosseous, or extrinsic, palmar ligaments described above are paramount to the understanding of traumatic and attritional instabilities of the wrist. By contrast, the dorsal transosseous ligaments are of little significance in trauma simply because, as stated above, we fall onto the dorsiflexed hand. One of them is of importance, however, in the rheumatoid wrist (p. 367). There are two:

(iv) The dorsal *radiocarpal ligament* (DRC) which runs from the radius almost transversely in an ulnar direction to insert into the scaphoid, lunate and triquetrum.
(v) The *dorsal intercarpal ligament* (DIC) which binds the distal scaphoid to the capitate to the hamate.

The final element in the ligaments of the wrist, those around the distal radioulnar joint, are considered on page 220 (Ch. 2).

Blood supply of the carpus

The carpal bones are unique in that, to a varying degree, the major part of their surface is covered by the articular surfaces described above. Blood supply must enter through the often very limited non-articular surfaces remaining.

The extraosseous[336] arterial supply of the carpus consists of three dorsal and three palmar arches connected longitudinally at their borders by the ulnar and radial arteries. The distalmost of the palmar arches is the deep palmar arch. This shows two recurrent branches which anastomose with the terminal branches of the anterior interosseous artery.

The intraosseous blood supply[337] to the carpal bones divides them into three groups. Group I includes the scaphoid, the capitate[338] and 20% of the lunates in the series cited. Each has large areas of bone dependent upon a single intraosseous vessel. Group II includes the trapezoid and hamate which have two vessels but no anastomoses between them. Group III, the trapezium, triquetrum, pisiform and 80% of lunates has two vessels with consistent intraosseous anastomoses. Clearly, those carpal bones in Group I have a high risk of avascular necrosis of one fragment following fracture, a risk not shared by those in groups II and III.

All of the blood supply to the ligaments may derive from the synovium, as has been shown for the radioscaphocapitate ligament and the scapholunate interosseous ligament, which derive no flow from their bony attachments[339].

Mechanisms of injury
Direct blows to carpal bones, especially their prominences, may result in isolated fractures, such as those of the trapezial ridge, the hamulus or the pisiform[340] (see below). These do not interfere with the dynamics of the carpus as outlined above.

The vast majority of injuries to the carpus occur when the patient falls on the outstretched hand. With impact, the carpus extends, ulnar deviates and supinates relative to the forearm. Because the radial end of the carpus is relatively less mobile than the ulnar it is more prone to

injury in heavy falls. The force inflicted in such falls, which is dissipated at the ulnar end in many instances by midcarpal hyperextension, meets resistance in the radial column, which is levered at the waist of the scaphoid around the fulcrum of the dorsal lip of the radius. Three structures may yield: (i) the distal radius, as in the Colles fracture; (ii) the ligamentous tethers of the proximal pole of the scaphoid (of which more later); (iii) the scaphoid itself, fracturing across its waist as if to provide a more mobile midcarpal joint.

When the resultant vector is primarily one of extension, a scaphoid waist fracture results as described above. Where the vector is primarily one of ulnar deviation and intercarpal supination, ligamentous disruption and carpal dislocations result[341]. Pure ligamentous injuries pass around the lunate from radial to distal to ulnar, producing four stages of instability according to their extent:

I. Scapholunate failure which, by tearing the radioscapholunate ligament[342], releases the proximal pole of the scaphoid, resulting in *scapholunate instability* (see p. 218).

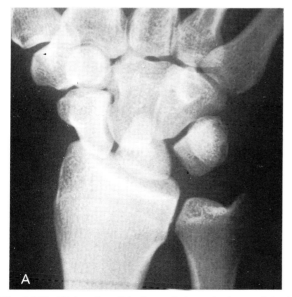

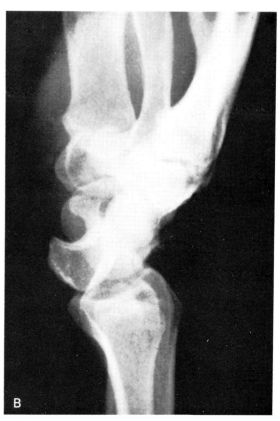

Fig. 1.124 Dislocation of the lunate is recognized on radiologic examination by its wedge-shaped appearance in the anteroposterior view (A) and in the lateral (B) by the fact that the capitate does not articulate with the 'cup' in the lunate.

II. Capitate-lunate failure, resulting in *dorsal subluxation of the capitate.*
III. Triquetrolunate failure; this may be accompanied by the presence of dorsal chip fractures of the triquetrum, which are thought to be due to impaction of a long ulnar styloid against the triquetrum in the extreme ulnar deviation of impact[343].
IV. Dorsal radiocarpal ligament failure, which permits anterior *lunate dislocation* (Fig. 1.124).

The lunate so displaced may produce acute carpal tunnel syndrome. (If the anteriorly located interosseous SL and TL ligaments are torn, again the lunate subluxes anteriorly due to its wedge shape, which is wider anteriorly. Dorsal lunate dislocations occur rarely (Fig. 1.125) and may cause extensor tendon rupture[344], as may palmar perilunar dislocation[345].)

Injuries which follow this perilunar pattern are said to occur in the *'lesser arc'* of the vulnerable zone for carpal fractures and dislocations[346]. The *'greater arc'* passes through the waist of the scaphoid, and the bodies of the capitate, hamate and triquetrum in turn. Extensions of the arc may occur, causing fractures of the radial and ulnar styloids. Combinations of lesser and greater arc injuries produce the apparently diverse and confusing variety of carpal fracture dislocations which are simply combinations and extensions of the two arcs: trans-scaphoid perilunate fracture dislocation (Fig. 1.126), scaphocapitate syndrome, indeed, any combination the reader creates from these arcs can and does occur.

When one considers the initial force which creates these lesser- and greater-arc injuries, it is evident that the skeleton distal to the line of injury is driven dorsally. It may remain there[347] (as in Fig. 1.126). More commonly the musculotendinous forces acting on the distal carpometacarpal complex return the distal skeleton to its original position with one of two consequences:

(i) That proximal portion of the carpus — often the lunate alone — which hung on grimly to its original anatomical position while the hurricane blew over its head, so to speak, may be knocked off its now insecure perch by the returning distal skeleton, coming to lie in an anterior dislocated position (see Fig. 1.124).
(ii) The carpus may assume a remarkably normal appearance — only detailed study will reveal the presence of injury.

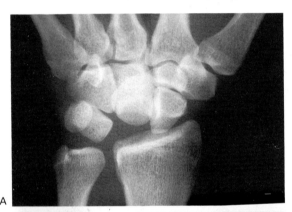

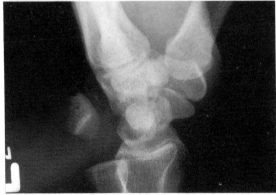

Fig. 1.125 Dorsal lunate dislocation A. In the posteroanterior view, the lunate is clearly displaced and there is a rotatory subluxation of the scaphoid. B. On the lateral, the lunate can be seen lying subcutaneously on top of the extensor retinaculum, where it was found at exploration.

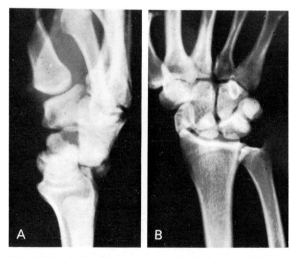

Fig. 1.126 A. It can be seen that only the lunate and the proximal pole of the scaphoid maintain their normal relationship with the radius and that the remainder of the carpus lies dorsal to these portions of the carpus. B. In the anteroposterior view there is wide separation of the two fragments of the scaphoid.

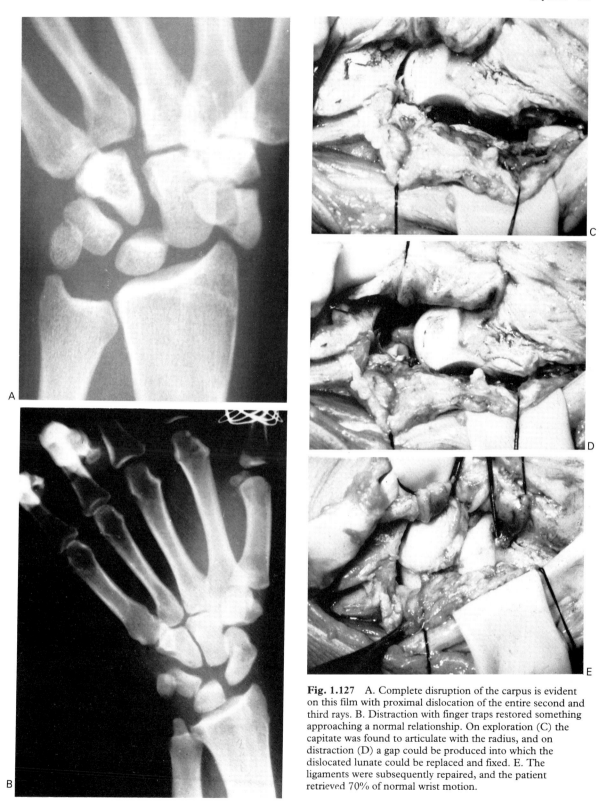

Fig. 1.127 A. Complete disruption of the carpus is evident on this film with proximal dislocation of the entire second and third rays. B. Distraction with finger traps restored something approaching a normal relationship. On exploration (C) the capitate was found to articulate with the radius, and on distraction (D) a gap could be produced into which the dislocated lunate could be replaced and fixed. E. The ligaments were subsequently repaired, and the patient retrieved 70% of normal wrist motion.

Midcarpal instability (p. 219) results from incompetence of the *triquetrohamatocapitate* ligament, which, by contrast with the radial column injuries described above, probably comes about through congenital laxity or chronic attenuation rather than acute injury[348]. As such it is considered in Chapter 2.

Presentation

Excluding those resulting from saw, axe, gun or similar agent, carpal injuries which are seen in the emergency room or casualty department can be classified into four groups:

1. Obvious, open disruptions due to massive trauma; these may be transverse[349], or axial[350,351] (Fig. 1.4B).
2. Closed fractures or dislocations which are *evident* on standard postero-anterior and lateral radiographs.
3. Closed fractures or dislocations which are associated with considerable pain, massive swelling, bruising and dysfunction of tendons, nerves and/or

vessels, but which are *not evident* on standard radiographs.
4. Closed fractures or dislocations which are not associated with major complaints, and are not evident on standard radiographs.

The hand surgeon will probably be consulted in the emergency room for the first three. The fourth group will commonly be diagnosed as *'sprains'* and treated without consultation by placing the patient in a wrist support splint. If so advised, the patient may present at an early juncture in the hand surgeon's office. If not, it may be many months before persistent symptoms, mainly pain and weakness of grip, bring him there (see under Reconstruction, p. 202).

Group 1 patients will require no additional clinical evaluation other than that for viability, skin cover, and integrity of tendon and nerve already detailed. Patients in groups 2 and 3 will be assessed for the common features of fractures and dislocations — locations of swelling, bruising and deformity, loss of motion, presence of

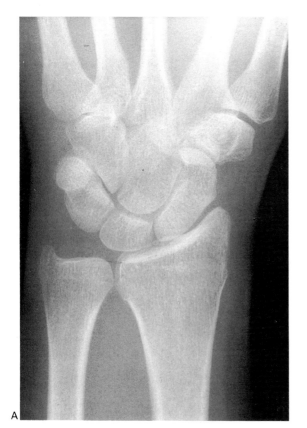
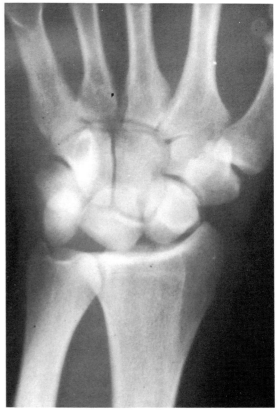

A   B

Fig. 1.128   Carpal arcs. A. The carpal arcs (see text) here are intact. B. The carpal arcs here (as in Fig. 1.130B) are disrupted due to a lunate dislocation.

abnormal motion, tenderness and the integrity of skin cover, nerve supply and arterial flow.

Radiologic examination

Further evaluation of patients in group 1 will be delayed until they are anaesthetized and prepared for surgery, when further views aided by suspension and traction (Fig. 1.127) will further clarify the injury.

Postero-anterior views of the wrist should be standardized by ensuring that the wrist is at the neutral position with respect to flexion and extension, ulnar-radial deviation and pronation–supination of the forearm. This is achieved by placing the palm flat on the table, with the elbow resting there also and with the shoulder level with the elbow. Apart from examining each carpal bone in turn for evidence of a fracture, four features, three of which are likely to reveal ligamentous disruption, should be studied[352]:

(i) The *carpal arcs* (Fig. 1.128) (these are also known as 'Gilula's lines' and are not to be confused with the arcs of injury mentioned above). Arc 1 is the proximal convex outline of the scaphoid, lunate and triquetrum; arc 2 the distal curve of the same bones; arc 3 the convex surfaces of the capitate and hamate. A break in any arc indicates disruption of ligamentous integrity.

(ii) The *width of the intercarpal joint spaces* — all should be equal.

(iii) The *shape* of the various *carpal bones*. The normal lunate shows four sides, but if displaced posteriorly or anteriorly, as in isolated dislocation or intercalated segment instability, it becomes triangular; whether the palmar or dorsal pole lies further distal can be determined by an algorithm[353], but it takes less time to look at the lateral view than to recall the algorithm!

(iv) *Ulnar variance*, which is the relationship of the distal outline of the ulnar head to that of the articular surface of the radius; this can be measured in three different ways with equal reliability. The technique of perpendiculars requires the examiner to draw, perpendicular to the axis of the radius, the line which passes through that point on the radiograph which marks the junction of the distal articular surface and the sigmoid notch of the radius; the variance is negative if the ulnar head fails to reach that line, positive if it projects beyond it, and neutral if it lies in the exact line.

The lateral view (Fig. 1.129) should be taken with the radius in the same line as the third metacarpal and avoiding radial or ulnar deviation. This can best be

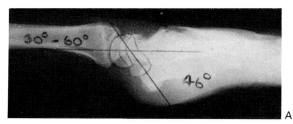

A

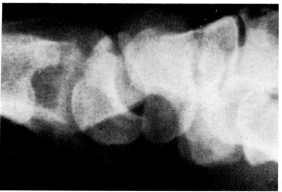

B

Fig. 1.129 True lateral of the wrist. A. The true lateral can be interpreted only if, as here, the third metacarpal is in direct line with the dorsal surface of the radius. The normal palmar tilt of the articular surface of a radius of 10° is seen here together with the colinearity of the radius, lunate and capitate and the normal scapholunate angle. This should normally lie between 30 and 60°, and it averages 47°. B. By contrast, here the colinearity of the radius, lunate and capitate has been lost. The lunate is dorsiflexed and the capitate is subluxed. The shadow of the scaphoid lies perpendicular to the axis of the radius creating a scapholunate angle of some 120°.

achieved by giving the patient a flat piece of plastic or wood, several of which are kept handy, and instructing the patient to insist that this be laid firmly along the back of the wrist while the view is taken. A good lateral is further ensured by having the wrist and the shoulder on the same level as above. Whether or not a true lateral has been achieved is determined by seeing that the scaphoid tubercle, and only its tubercle, protrudes anterior to the outline of the pisiform. In studying the lateral view, the lunate outline represents the proximal carpal row, the capitate the distal. Again, as in the antero-posterior view, four features should be observed:

(i) The *angle of the distal radius*; the normal palmar tilt of 10 to 15° may be reversed, usually after a Colles fracture.

(ii) The *colinearity* of the radius, lunate and capitate. The axes of the capitate and the radius are easily drawn; that of the lunate is a line perpendicular to a line drawn between its dorsal and ventral poles — in lunate dislocation[354], the capitate remains centred over the radius, whereas in perilunate dislocation, the lunate remains in line and the capitate is displaced.

(iii) The *angle of the lunate* relative to the axis of the radius; its axis may point dorsally, in which case it is dorsiflexed, and vice versa (it should be recalled that spurious dorsiflexion can be produced by ulnar deviation, palmar flexion by radial, hence the need for careful neutral positioning).

(iv) The *scapholunate angle* should be measured: a close approximation to the scaphoid axis can be obtained by drawing a line tangentially through the proximo-anterior outline of both the proximal and distal poles. The angle measured is that created by the *two axes extended distally*. The normal angle averages 47°, with a normal range from 30 to 60° [355]. Although, when using a standard goniometer, this may appear to be an inexact measure, it has been shown to be reproducible to within 7.4° [356]

Special additional views may be required to investigate suspicions established clinically or by study of the standard radiographs.

Scaphoid view, postero-anterior of the carpus in three positions: supinated by 45°, neutral and pronated by 45°; the majority of fractures will show in the latter two views [357]. Ulnar deviation (Fig. 1.130), by extending the scaphoid, will also assist in revealing fractures, although the reader should be aware that Russe [358] warned against undue distraction of the fragments. An occult fracture may not be revealed in any plain radiograph (Fig. 1.131), and a high level of clinical suspicion should be maintained.

Carpal tunnel view [359] (Fig. 1.132) may reveal fractures of the hook of the hamate and of the trapezial ridge [360] — the use of this view is sometimes made impossible by the inability to achieve the necessary extreme hyperextension of the wrist.

Hook of hamate view [361] (Fig. 1.133), with the hand

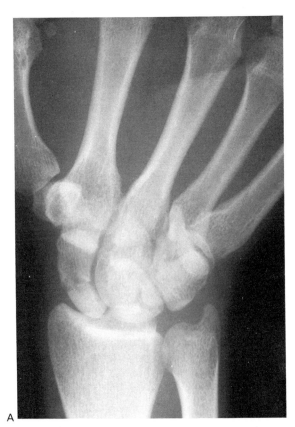 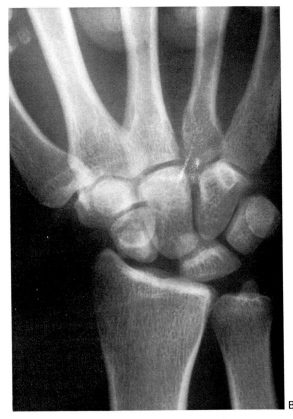

A   B

Fig. 1.130 The merits of wrist deviation in posteroanterior views of the wrist. This patient had an unusual combination. A. Ulnar deviation revealed a waist fracture of the scaphoid. B. Radial deviation with a clenched fist showed a coincidental scapholunate instability.

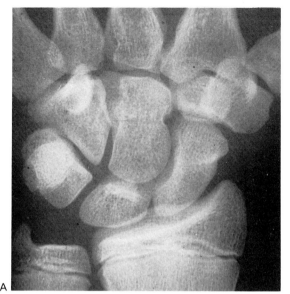

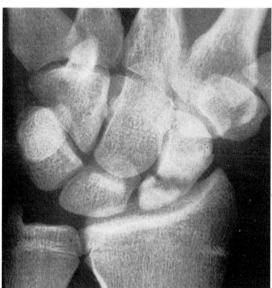

Fig. 1.131 This youth sustained a heavy fall but initial radiographs revealed no evidence of fracture. He presented some two years later complaining of wrist pain with no further injury. Radiograph (B) revealed an old scaphoid fracture. It was at that time that the original film shown in (A) was reviewed.

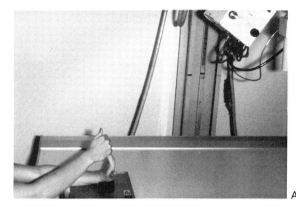

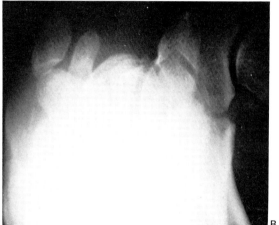

Fig. 1.132 Carpal tunnel view. A. Technique. B. Result.

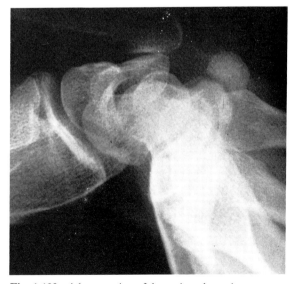

Fig. 1.133 A hamate view of the patient shown in Figs. 1.132 A and B. revealed the suspected fracture.

in midsupination and the wrist dorsiflexed; it is often necessary to repeat this study, varying the position slightly to reveal the hamulus.

The difficulties encountered in visualizing this fracture have led to the development of at least one other technique[362], in which a true lateral is taken, with the thumb in maximum abduction and the wrist in

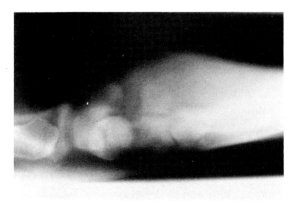

Fig. 1.134 Lateral tomography shows a fracture of the hook of the hamate.

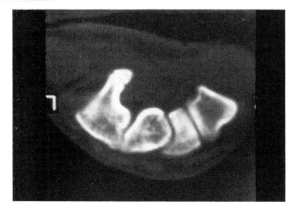

Fig. 1.135 CT scan also demonstrates the hamate well, here showing a non-union at an unusual site — the fracture is usually much closer to the body of the hamate. CT has been abandoned by the author as lateral tomography is less expensive in his institution.

full radial deviation. When clinical evidence is strong, but radiologic proof lacking after three attempts, lateral tomograms[363] (Fig. 1.134), or CT scan (Fig. 1.135)[364,365] should be employed.

Indications in closed carpal injuries

As a general rule, fractures or dislocations of the carpus which are *undisplaced and stable* are treated by immobilization in an anterior splint until swelling has subsided, when a cast is substituted. Qualifying comments to this generality are appropriate for certain fractures.

Scaphoid fractures, as is evident from the above discussion of mechanisms of injury, can occur in two quite distinct ways;

(i) The *isolated* scaphoid fracture which results from a pure extension vector will commonly be *undisplaced and stable*; while controversy exists on every aspect of immobilization, which is well reviewed by Taleisnik[366], suffice it to say that a longarm thumb spica circular cast with the wrist in radial deviation, slight palmar flexion and pronation for six weeks, followed by a similar shortarm for a further six, offers a high chance of union.

(ii) An apparently isolated, apparently undisplaced fracture may be the only evidence of a *reduced transcaphoid perilunate fracture dislocation*. This circumstance can be recognized by the presence of an offset between the fragments of more than 1 mm or by evidence of proximal row instability as seen by changes in the alignment of the lunate on the true lateral view. Such fractures should be opened, reduced and internally fixed with Kirschner wires[367,368] or with screws, including that designed by Herbert[369-375] (Fig. 1.136).

Fractures of the hook of hamate should be excised[376], despite isolated recommendations to fix the fracture[377]. Care should be taken to avoid injury to adjacent structures[378], especially the ulnar nerve. Fractures or dislocations which are *displaced* should be reduced[379]. Whether or not this is done as an emergency is determined by whether the carpal injury is complicated by vascular or neurological impairment. If it is not, there may be some merit and no loss in resting the limb in elevation for 72 hours. This will allow reduction of soft-tissue swelling which might otherwise complicate skin closure after any incisions which prove necessary. Reduction can be attempted closed, but should be carried out under sterile conditions, with finger trap traction and fluoroscopic control (Fig. 1.137). Some surgeons use the image intensifier as an operating table[380]. Repeat radiographs should be taken with *release of traction after* successful reduction, for frequently such views will demonstrate that the reduction has been lost or that a collapse pattern has ensued. In such circumstances, the surgeon should proceed with open reduction, internal fixation and ligamentous repair.

As emphasized previously, many significant carpal dislocations and instability patterns will be deemed to be sprains, and will be seen long after injury by the hand surgeon in his office. For this reason, these less evident injuries are discussed under Reconstruction (p. 202).

Much has been written on other fractures and dislocations of individual carpal bones. Diagnosis and indications follow the rules laid out above. The following

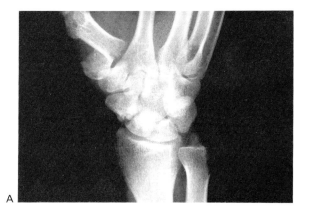

A

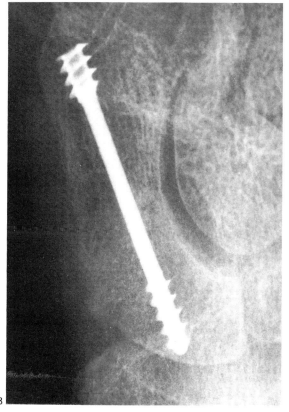

B

Fig. 1.136 A. Waist fracture of the scaphoid which was deemed to be unstable (coincident extra-articular fracture of the first metacarpal). B. Healing following Herbert screw fixation (case of Dr Charles J. Eaton).

is a selection of the literature relevant to each bone, and combination of bones:

trapezium[381-386]
scaphoid + lunate[387-391]
triquetrum[392-395]

pisiform[396]
hamate (body)[397-401]
hamate + pisiform[402]
trapezoid[403-408]
hamate (hook) + trapezium (ridge)[409,410]

See Green D P 1993 Operative Hand Surgery, 3rd edn. Churchill Livingstone, New York, pp. 807, 811, 846, 852, 883, 896, 901, 910 and 915.

In concluding consideration of the initial emergency-room examination, it is worth restating that, in the crush injuries which form an increasing proportion of the major hand injuries in an industrial society, the initial examination on arrival plays a small role. It is concerned mainly with sensibility and viability, a basic radiograph, and making sure that the patient is fit to go to the operating room. The pain is so severe, and the conclusions reached in such surroundings so limited, that full assessment is wisely postponed until formal exploration of the anaesthetized hand.

EXPLORATION

Although it has taken many pages to describe the history and initial examination, an experienced surgeon will complete the process in between five and fifteen minutes. As has become apparent, the first examination can confirm only some of the suspicions aroused by the history. The final diagnosis in other cases is only made at exploration, the second examination.

This is always conducted under completely aseptic conditions in the operating room after thorough preparation and sterile draping of the limb. It may or may not be felt necessary by the surgeon to have tourniquet control during exploration but it does facilitate thorough cleansing of the wound and identification of structures.

An inflated tourniquet is *essential* during radical debridement, otherwise bleeding from tissue which is viable will obscure the lack of it from that which is dead. Use of the tourniquet[411,412], both upper arm and digital[413, 414], is not without potential complications[415, 416]. Where a prolonged procedure is anticipated, a double cuff[417,418] may be used to extend the ischaemia time, which should be limited to two hours.

Massive wounds. It is here that the surgeon first encounters the massively injured extremity which he has elected not to examine in the emergency room, with the important exception of determining, if possible, whether or not nerve and blood supply to the hand remains intact. On that knowledge will depend, in certain limbs, the decision to amputate or reconstruct. That

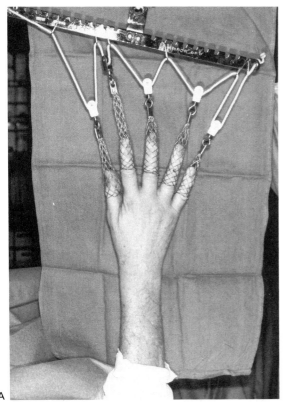

A

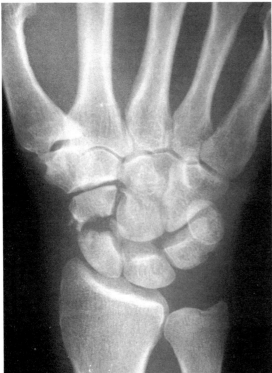

B

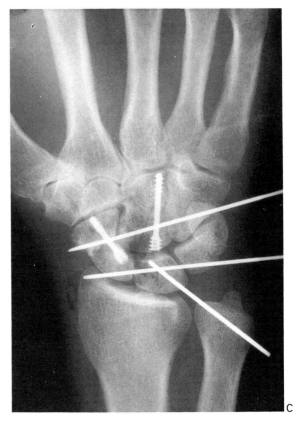

C

Fig. 1.137   A. Finger trap traction assists both in diagnosis and treatment. B. With such traction, a scaphocapitate fracture was demonstrated. C. Preliminary fixation was done with Kirschner wires. The fractures were then fixed with Herbert screws and a final radiograph taken, with no traction. The Kirschner wires were then removed. (Operation performed in conjunction with Dr D. A. Coleman)

specific knowledge aside, the decision regarding *amputation* is based on several questions:

1. Can we achieve primary healing? This depends on the following three questions concerned with the 'tripod' on which primary healing stands — tripod because, with failure of any one, the whole edifice of primary repair will collapse.
2. Can we ensure perfect *perfusion* to all tissues? This is achieved by *debridement* and *revascularization*.
3. Can we achieve *rigid fixation* of the skeleton?
4. Can we provide *skin cover* of guaranteed viability with *tension-free closure* of all wounds?
5. If we achieve all these goals, will the function of the hand be undoubtedly superior to that which would be achieved by amputation and, where necessary, prosthetic fitting?

The last question may be overlooked in the natural enthusiasm of the surgeon to preserve tissue and to exercise the marvellous armamentarium with which modern surgery has endowed him. It is of equal importance to the other questions, and if it cannot be answered in the affirmative, amputation should be performed primarily (Fig. 1.138). The soft tissue from the part may be used to provide cover for the stump[419], thereby preserving valuable length. In more unique circumstances, the amputation may yield a hand which is sufficiently uninjured to be able to be stored ectopically for later replantation[420].

Open fractures. In evaluating open tibial fractures, the classification of Gustilo[421] has proved of value in management and prognosis, and may be applied to fractures of the upper limb:

Type I   Associated clean wound of less than 1 cm
Type II   Laceration more than 1 cm but no extensive soft-tissue damage, flaps or avulsion

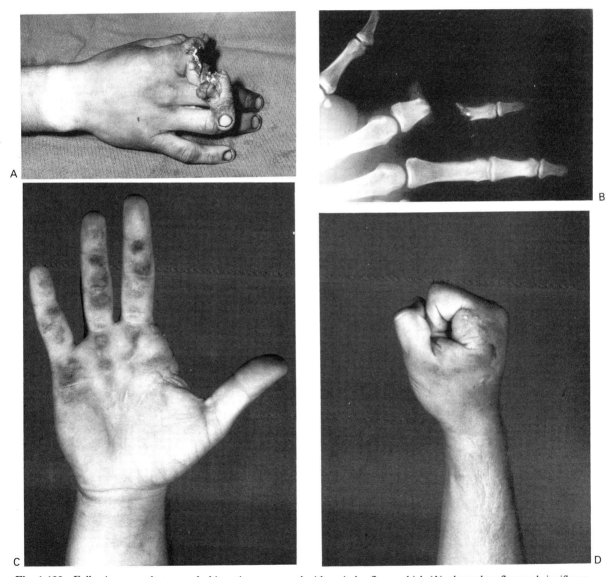

Fig. 1.138 Following a gunshot wound, this patient presented with an index finger which (A), showed no flow and significant soft-tissue loss and (B), on radiographic examination, loss of the proximal interphalangeal joint skeleton. Although reconstruction would have been possible, immediate amputation restored the patient early to work and function (C, D).

Type IIIA   Adequate soft-tissue coverage of the fracture despite extensive flaps *or* any injury from high-energy trauma
    IIIB   Extensive soft-tissue loss, periosteal stripping and heavy contamination
    IIIC   An arterial injury requiring repair.

Type IIIB wounds were found to have the highest sepsis rate, but early wound coverage lowered that rate — 'Delay of soft-tissue coverage enhances sepsis' (Gustilo[422]). The quality of local wound care is paramount in limiting infection[423].

Antibiotic therapy. While antibiotic cover appears to have no influence on the incidence of infection in the full spectrum of hand injuries, and therefore can be safely withheld[424], its use in open fractures is of definite merit[425]. It need only be a short course, one study having shown no difference between one and five days of cephalosporin therapy[426]. Certainly its efficacy is directly related to the *speed* with which it is given after injury. There appears to be no established need to continue therapy for more than 48 hours after definitive wound closure has been achieved[425]. It should be emphasized that no antibiotic can compensate for inadequate debridement (see below).

The first step in exploration, often time consuming, is to thoroughly cleanse the wound. This should be carried out using some form of pulsatile flow of normal saline or Ringer's lactate achieved by the use of a large chip syringe or the 'water-pick'. The addition of local antibiotics to the irrigating fluid has been shown to significantly reduce the bacterial contamination[427] of the wound, and a mixture of polymyxin B 50 mg/ml and bacitracin 50 u/ml[428] is a satisfactory choice. Cleansing of contaminated areas in the stream of saline is best done with the surgeon's glove finger. All interstices of the wounds must be sought out. The extent of a penetrating wound is often difficult to determine and partial division of tendons may be missed. In such a situation the presence of *blood staining of the tissue is a valuable guide* to the extent of the wound. Open joints should receive particularly careful scrutiny as foreign material may have been sucked into their far recesses.

The process should be continued patiently until all contamination has been cleaned out. The longer the delay between injury and surgery the more difficult this becomes. Where it proves impossible a choice must be made between:

1. *Sharp debridement of contaminated tissue.* This may be undesirable where it involves opening a joint, exposing bare bone or tendon or excising vital structures.
2. *Leaving soiled tissue.* This will inevitably lead to inflammation and result in an increase in early oedema and late fibrosis. It will predispose to infection.

INDICATIONS IN MASSIVE WOUNDS

With increasing use of immediate or early wound coverage with free tissue transfers[429–431], early decisions regarding the need and suitability of a wound for such transfers require to be made, for delay increases the risks of failure and infection dramatically[429]. As a general rule, massive wounds which are relatively clearly defined — those resulting from gunshot wounds and road traffic accidents are examples — can be best treated by *radical* techniques (Table 1.3, Fig. 1.139).

Table 1.3

	Conservative	Radical
Debridement	Obviously dead	'Pseudo' tumour resection[432]
Incisions	None additional	Through viable tissue
Longitudinal structures	Often not seen	Cleanse under the microscope
Bone fragments	Remove	Cleanse and fix
Irrigation	Copious	Less significant, after resection
Culture	Multiple swab	Quantitative biopsy post-debridement
Bone fixation	Percutaneous Kirschner wires	Open, plates, screws, external fixation
Primary repair (tendons, nerves)	Rarely	Customary
'Second look'	Necessary	Only if culture >10⁴/cc[433]
Disadvantages	Infection, scar (high incidence)	Flap failure, infection (low incidence, < 2% if <72 hours)
Operations	Multiple	Few
Hospital days	Many	Few
Final function	Poor to moderate	Superior

(Compare Figs 1.35 + 1.157, conservative, with Figs 1.139 + 1.178, radical <24 hours)

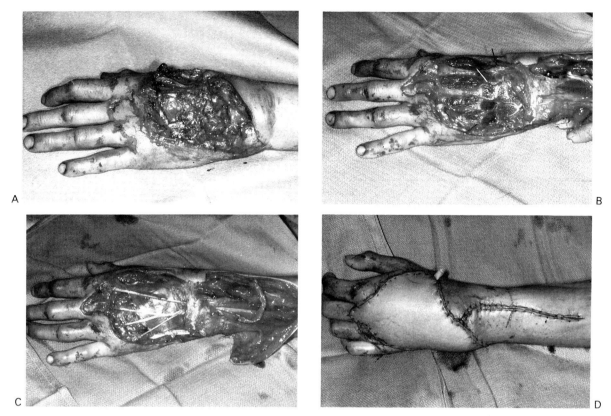

Fig. 1.139 Radical debridement. A. This patient presented after a rollover injury. B. Following radical debridement, which involved sharp excision of soft tissues and bone, internal fixation was employed in the form of a buttress plate on the radius and Kirschner wire fixation of the carpus. C. The dorsal capsule was reconstructed with fascia lata and extensor tendon grafts inserted. D. The whole reconstruction was covered with a tailored latissimus dorsi free flap. With one extensor tenolysis, the patient recovered full function. (From Lister, G. D. (1993) Free skin and composite flaps. In: Green, D. P. (ed) Operative hand surgery, 3rd edn. Churchill Livingstone, Edinburgh; further details of the technique are described therein.)

Crush or blast injuries — in which there are multiple fractures and dislocations, poor and patchy definition of probable survival of skin and soft tissue, and where digits are unexpectedly viable, but to which the source of arterial supply is unknown — are best approached with *conservative* methods (see Fig. 1.35).

Despite the evident advantage of radical surgery, it must be emphasized that is will succeed only where debridement is *absolute*, and that it can be absolute only in certain wounds.

Widely scattered fragments of metal, which are relatively non-reactive, such as occur in shotgun injuries or explosions, are commonly left but their pursuit may reveal unexpected injuries to deep structures. Leaving foreign bodies is not without hazard, for late complications may develop[434] including delayed nerve injury[135], tendon rupture[436], purulent tenosynovitis[437] and lead poisoning[438,439]. The removal of sea urchin spines,

often present in large numbers, can be facilitated by the use of soft-tissue radiographs[440]. If difficulty is encountered in locating radiolucent foreign bodies, *xeroradiography* may be of assistance[441,442].

Adequate exploration may require surgical extension of the skin wound. This practice has been criticised in the past but is completely justifiable provided cleansing as described has been meticulously performed. It may be essential to expose fractures for fixation and to identify structures where primary repair is intended. The line of the extending incision should be chosen with three factors in mind:

1. The viability of the skin flaps.
2. The avoidance of subsequent contracture. For example, on the flexor aspect of the digit, an appropriate modification of the midlateral or Bruner incisions should be used.

3. The history of injury, since the hand posture at that time indicates the probable site of tendon laceration in relation to the skin wound (p. 4).
4. The probable location of injured structures as suggested by the shape of the wound (p. 21).

In thoroughly cleansing all aspects of the wound the surgeon does more than that. He also compiles a list of injured structures, considers how they are to be repaired and establishes an order for the ensuing operation. The sequence of repair usually pursued will be followed in considering each specific structure.

See Green D P 1993 Operative Hand Surgery, 3rd edn. Churchill Livingstone, New York, p. 1108.

Bone and joint

FRACTURES

All fractures should be reduced and immobilized as the first step in the repair of the injured hand for only then, in certain instances, can an accurate assessment be made of damage to other structures. Such instances include flow in vessels, viability of tissues and the presence and extent of defects in skin, vessel, tendon and nerve.

In most compound injuries of the hand fractures can be dissected and visualized. Fragments entirely loose should be removed except in the circumstances outlined in Table 1.3; those retaining periosteal attachments should be kept. Periosteum should be carefully preserved, for its repair over a well reduced fracture will do much to prevent adhesion of overlying structures to the fracture site. Not uncommonly, periosteal repair will be the only practical means of holding the reduction of some of the fragments in a badly comminuted fracture.

Fractures, once exposed, should be inspected under loupe magnification with four objectives:

(i) Meticulous cleansing of all fragments without disturbing soft tissue attachments.
(ii) Removal of all interposed soft tissue.
(iii) Identification and matching of all fragments; this is best done by commencing with the most stable fragment, fixing it firmly with an appropriate instrument and then bringing the more mobile fragment to the stable one, seeking irregularities in the fracture line to 'key' together, thereby ensuring exact reduction. Where there are multiple fragments one moves progressively away from the original stable fragment; temporary fixation with fine Kirschner wires may be helpful in some

circumstances where they will not compromise the definitive fixation.
(iv) Selection of the technique of fixation to be used.

Clearly, in practice (iii) and (iv) are frequently done in direct sequence, the reduction being maintained by bone-holding instruments where possible, by the surgeon where not, while the assistant applies the fixation.

In crush and friction injuries, the viability of bone may be in question. This is most difficult to resolve at the time of primary exploration. Vessel refilling on release of the tourniquet, so helpful in assessing the skin, is of much less value in assessing blood supply to bone. In addition, periosteal flow is not essential to survival of the cortex if medullary blood supply is good. Resection of bone, except where done as part of the process of resecting non-viable soft tissues, is therefore not performed as a primary procedure in such injuries.

Particular attention should be given to obtaining an anatomically perfect reduction of fractures involving the articular surface[443] or, in children, the growing epiphysis (Fig. 1.140). In complex, open injuries this may require careful threading of various fragments on to interosseous wires in order to restore articular integrity (Fig. 1.141).

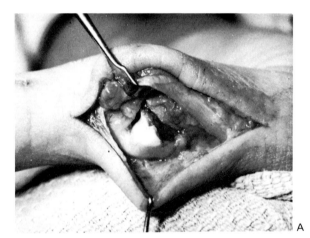

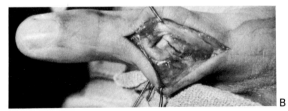

Fig. 1.140 A, B. Surgical exposure of an articular fracture permits accurate reduction and internal fixation to be performed.

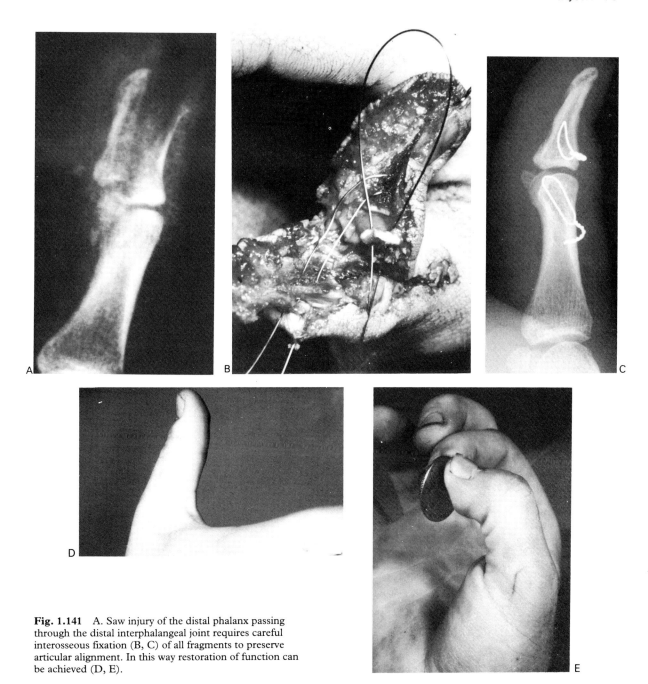

Fig. 1.141 A. Saw injury of the distal phalanx passing through the distal interphalangeal joint requires careful interosseous fixation (B, C) of all fragments to preserve articular alignment. In this way restoration of function can be achieved (D, E).

In all fractures of the digits and metacarpal bones, rotational mal-alignments must be excluded or malfunction will result (see Fig. 1.118). This is best achieved by visualization of the fracture during precise reduction and fixation. Where this is not possible, or

not applicable — as in comminution with bone loss — the relationship of the planes of the finger nails with the interphalangeal joints flexed should be compared with that on the uninjured hand. A better known fact, but one which cannot always be applied, is that all fingers when flexed at metacarpophalangeal and proximal interphalangeal joints point to the tubercle of scaphoid (Fig. 1.24). Repeated simultaneous flexion of injured and uninjured fingers to ensure that they are 'tracking' correctly is a further method of checking alignment. Appropriate fixation is selected.

Where there are significant defects in an exposed bone[444], correct alignment and rigid fixation of the remaining fragments is of equal, if not greater, importance. *Optimal skeletal length must be determined and maintained from the time of the initial surgery.* Once lost, wound contracture will prevent its recovery. Occasionally the object of alignment may be achieved by further bone resection to achieve good contact at the site of osteosynthesis, but this has the distinct disadvantage of relatively lengthening the tendons. This can be offset by equivalent shortening where they also are divided — this is common practice in the course of replantation and revascularization where shortening aids neuro-vascular repair.

Where shortening is not permissible the bone defect remains. If all tissues are clearly viable or can be made so, or if it is necessary to support a significant fragment such as an articular segment, then immediate cancellous bone grafting is indicated. In other circumstances, it can with benefit be left for 48 to 72 hours and should certainly be performed within 10 days. Results are good[445].

Where the skeletal defect is due to loss of a joint, length can be maintained by insertion either of a cortico cancellous bone graft to achieve fusion or of an immediate joint replacement. Although this sounds hazardous, the author has done it with success and with no complications in fifteen cases (Fig. 1.142). The need for adequate debridement and good skin cover is heightened in all such procedures.

In the operative management of all fractures, from the most simple to the most complex, peroperative radiography plays an essential role.

Indications in open fractures
Rigid fixation is desirable in all cases, provided that all tissues are viable and that reliable skin cover can be assured. In the fingers, whenever possible, the fixation should be applied without immobilizing the joints, thereby permitting early protected motion. Fixation may be achieved internally or externally. Where internal[446,447], the fixation is most commonly achieved by Kirschner wires, with or without intraosseous wiring[448], preferably on the tension surface[449], in the phalanges and by plates and screws[450] in the metacarpals. Intramedullary fixation, using accurately cut selected Steinmann pins, is an excellent method of managing a badly comminuted phalangeal fracture, especially in the

elderly, for it best maintains the soft-tissue attachments of the fragments[451] (Fig. 1.109). *External fixation* is most indicated in the presence of extensive comminution or bone defects which preclude rigid fixation by other means. Such bone destruction is usually associated with severe open injuries of the arm or hand[452,453]. External fixation is excellent preparation for delayed bone grafting and can be maintained in the upper limb until bone healing is attained[454]. Complications are few[455] if the apparatus is correctly applied and maintained[456]. External fixation may employ a sophisticated device such as the mini-Hoffman[457] or may be constructed by Kirschner wires 'spot-welded' by methyl methacrylate[458] (Fig. 1.143). Wherever possible the external fixation should be applied only to the bone which is fractured. This may, however, be inadequate and it may prove necessary to go to the next bone. When this is done, the intervening joint must be transfixed or fracture fixation will not be achieved and alignment will be lost.

Whenever, in applying either internal or external fixation, joints must be transgressed, then it is imperative to place them in the 'safe' position, that is, extension of the interphalangeal joints, flexion of the metacarpophalangeal.

See Green D P 1993 Operative Hand Surgery, 3rd edn. Churchill Livingstone, New York, pp. 695, 701, 708, 713, 721, 735, 760, 949.

DISLOCATIONS

The presence of dislocation should be confirmed, and where reduction does not restore to the joint its original range and stability, the periarticular structures should be inspected. In the absence of juxta-articular fractures, instability will be due to disruption of the collateral ligament or palmar plate. It is important to determine whether the disruption is in the substance of the ligament or is an avulsion of the ligament from the bone as the technique of repair may differ. Where the range of motion is decreased by reduction of the dislocation, or where reduction cannot be achieved, it is probable that a portion of the periarticular structures is trapped in that joint space and this should be sought. Quite frequently, the entrapped tissue proves to be the palmar plate, torn in a hyperextension injury, as in complex dislocation of the index metacarpal already described or the interposed extensor tendon[459,460]. Alternatively, the trapped tissue may be unrelated to the joint — a so-called *complicated dislocation*[461]. This is especially common in the elbow joint where the brachial artery, median[462], ulnar and radial nerves can all become caught in an elbow dislocation and retained there after reduction.

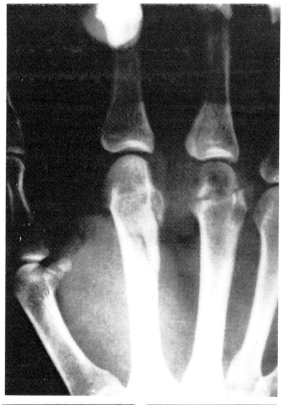

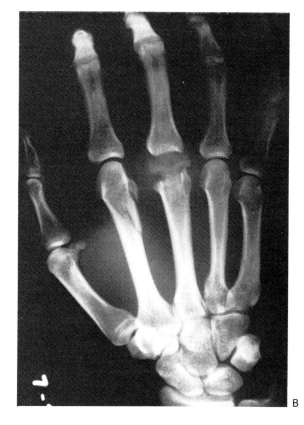

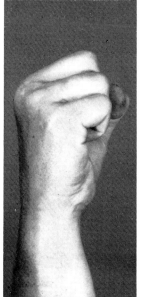

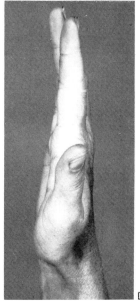

Fig. 1.142 A. This lady sustained an open, untidy injury when her hand was caught in a cement mixer. Exploration revealed that the metacarpal head of the middle phalanx was loose, and that the fracture of the second metacarpal was stable. B. Immediate joint replacement was undertaken, uneventful healing occurred, and she retrieved full function as seen three years later (C, D).

If a joint is lying open or is surgically explored, the articular surface should be examined directly for fractures and also to determine that no flakes of cartilage are lying free in the joint (Fig. 1.144).

Indications in open dislocations
As previously stated, absolutely precise reduction of avulsion fractures should be achieved. If there is no adequate 'key', then type B intraosseous wiring[463], screw fixation, or two Kirschner wires are required, for a condyle can rotate around a single pin. Ligamentous re-attachment can be attained with type B wiring. Both repair and re-attachment in the fingers should be achieved wherever possible without transfixing the joint, in order to permit early protected motion.

See Green D P 1993 Operative Hand Surgery, 3rd edn. Churchill Livingstone, New York, pp. 771, 783.

In *crush injuries of the carpus*, fractures and dislocations often coexist[464]. Displacement of the elements occurs either through the injuring force or because of the traction exerted by tendons at the time of the injury. Exploration should be aimed at determining the nature of any disorientation of these carpal bones and fragments. This is achieved by knowledge of the normal

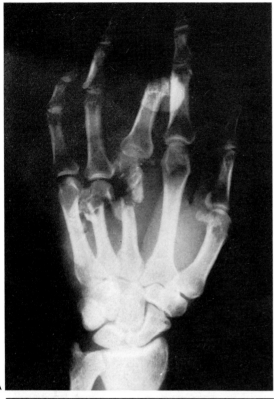

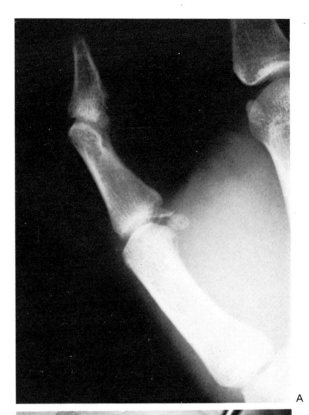

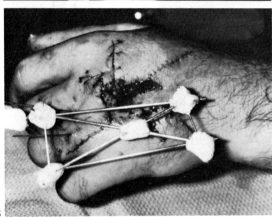

Fig. 1.143   A. Following a gunshot wound this patient had a significant segmental loss of the third and fourth rays. B. The length was maintained at the time of the initial debridement by the use of Kirschner wires 'spot welded' with methyl methacrylate.

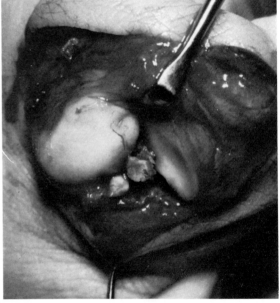

anatomy and by locating and matching the articular facets on each. Reduction is often facilitated by applying finger trap distraction and is further aided by repeated study of the radiographs (Figs 1.127, 1.137) (see p. 96).

Fig. 1.144   A. Radiographic examination of this patient, who sustained a game-keeper's thumb, revealed a suspicious fragment on the palmar aspect of the joint. B. Exploration of the joint revealed not only a fracture fragment from the anterior lip of the proximal phalanx, but also a depressed condylar fracture of the radial aspect of the metacarpal head.

Tendon and muscle

In the tidy hand injury, fairly firm conclusions will have been made about which tendons have been lacerated during the initial examination. These conclusions should be confirmed at exploration. The problems then remaining concern distinction of tendon from nerve, matching of tendon ends and exposure in the digit.

TENDON OR NERVE?

Locating the ends of divided structures for identification, matching and suture can be a frustrating exercise. Clearly, flexing the wrist and fingers fully will help to bring the ends towards the wound but then, even with retraction, the ends may be obscured by blood clot. Herein lies the solution. By dissecting where the clot is most dense and pure, the ends will be revealed as white gleams through the gore (Fig. 1.145). Working in this bloodstained synovium is like wading through quick-

sand. Rather it should be excised sharply, revealing the contained structures, which can be identified by:

Colour. Tendon: whitish yellow; nerve: whitish grey.
Texture of the surface. Tendon: smooth and firm; nerve: softer and somewhat more irregular due to the fascicular bundles appearing as longitudinal strands.
Median artery. If the structure believed to be the median nerve is inspected closely with magnification, an artery of differing diameter will almost always be found on its surface. Both nerve ends can be so identified. The artery also serves to ensure that the correct orientation of the nerve ends is selected for repair.
Retraction. Nerve ends retract much less than do divided tendons.
Nerve fascicles. After irrigation, if the nerve end is turned end-on and inspected with magnification, the fascicular bundles can be seen, shiny and hemispherical.
Passive movement. Selective flexion of the digital joints will identify individually the *distal* tendons ends. Once

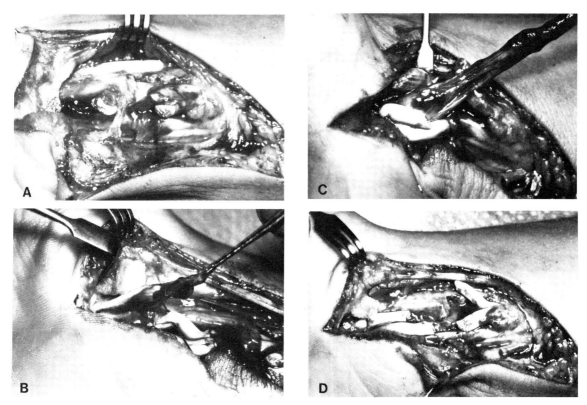

Fig. 1.145 A. This patient had sustained a clean laceration of the palmar aspect of the wrist. The proximal tendon ends had been retrieved with little difficulty, but even with full finger flexion the distal tendon ends were obscured in the dark blood clots seen at the proximal end of the carpal tunnel (on the left of the photograph). By dissecting where the blood clot was most dense (B, C), the distal tendon ends were revealed as a white gleam through the synovium. After transfixing the tendons with straight needles they were suitably approximated for subsequent primary tendon suture (D).

the *proximal* ends have been identified with a high degree of confidence, grasp them in turn by the cut end with fine toothed forceps and pull gently. A characteristic gliding motion will result and often the muscle belly will be revealed.

FLEXOR TENDON IDENTIFICATION AND PREPARATION

At the wrist: distal ends
In multiple flexor tendon injuries at the wrist, identification of the distal ends is straightforward after they have been located, profundus tendons flexing the distal interphalangeal joint, superficialis tendons the proximal interphalangeal joint. Traction on the distal end should be performed with the same care as on the proximal end by grasping the cut tendon end with fine toothed dissecting or mosquito forceps in order to avoid damage to the outer surface of the tendon (Fig. 1.146). Pulling on any finger flexor at the wrist, but especially a profundus tendon, will produce flexion to a varying degree in fingers adjacent to the finger to which the tendon goes, due to the interconnections between the tendons and due to the common synovial sheath. This spurious movement can be distinguished from that in the correct finger by gently resisting the pull with a finger on each digital pulp in turn. In the correct finger there is a precise transmission of pull from tendon to finger tip compared with the 'dampened' pull in the adjacent finger.

Proximal ends
The correct matching of the proximal ends at the wrist is rather more taxing as all pass through the space which occupies only 3 cm to the ulnar side of the median nerve. Four features aid in identification:

Anatomy. The finger flexor tendons lie in three layers:
    superficial: flexor digitorum superficialis to middle and ring (Fig. 1.147)

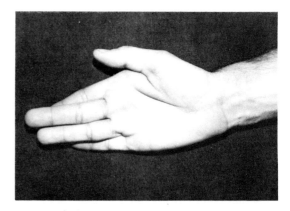

Fig. 1.147 In this posed photograph, the relationship of the superficialis tendons at the wrist is demonstrated. Those to the middle and ring fingers lie superficial to those to the small and index fingers.

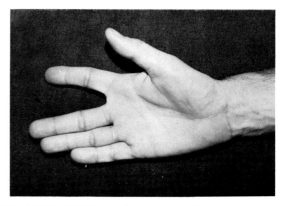

Fig. 1.148 All of the profundus tendons lie in the same plane. Those to the middle, ring and small fingers are, however, conjoined at the wrist, arising as they do from a common muscle belly while that to the index finger is quite separate.

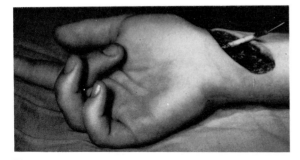

Fig. 1.146 Traction on the distal tendon end will effect flexion of either the proximal or the distal interphalangeal joint thereby revealing, as here, a flexor digitorum superficialis.

    middle: flexor digitorum superficialis to index and small
    deep: flexor digitorum profundus to all fingers; those to middle, ring and small are conjoined; that to index is separate (Fig. 1.148)
Cross-section. No two tendons have identical cross-section, either in diameter or shape.
Angle of cut. Despite the fact that all have been injured by the one blow it is surprising how the angle of the cut varies. This also affects the cross-sectional appearance.
Length. If the tendon ends are brought into exact apposition with no gap or overlap and held there, ready for suturing, by transfixion of the tendon ends with straight needles, the normal balanced posture of the

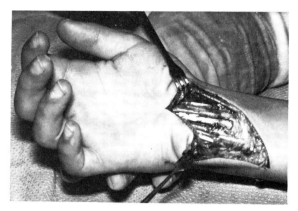

Fig. 1.149 The patient whose hand is illustrated in Fig. 1.145 had sustained an oblique laceration. After approximation and repair of the tendon ends it is evident that the correct proximal end was selected by the positioning of the fingers which lie in the normal cascade, the relationship of the fingers one to another being that which is seen in the uninjured hand.

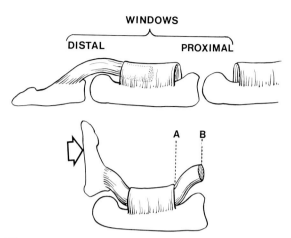

Fig. 1.150 Assessment for exposure during flexor tendon repair (see text).

finger should result (Fig. 1.149). Standard hypodermic needles should be used for this task for they are sharp and they inflict little damage; also, because of their hub, they cannot stray or be forgotten.

While describing retrieval of proximal tendon ends, an anatomical point should be made with regard to the flexor carpi radialis. It lies neither above the fascia nor below it but rather within it, in its own separate tunnel. If the surgeon remembers this he will retrieve it either by looking for the tunnel end-on, where it will be marked by tell-tale blood clot, or he will seek it from above or below the fascia where the tendon will shine through and can be released by incision.

In the digit

Having extended the incision as required to expose the distal end as dictated by the posture of the hand at the time of injury (p. 4) the flexor tendon sheath is exposed. Current theory and increasing practice dictate that the sheath should be preserved and repaired after flexor tendon repair[465,466]. Sheath repair is relatively easy in its retinacular or cruciate portions and rather difficult in the annular pulleys. The latter should therefore be preserved intact whenever possible. With this in mind the cut end of the distal tendon should be located by looking through the sheath while flexing the finger. It will be seen as a moving junction of white tendon and dark red blood. The length of this tendon, which can be seen in the retinacular portion of the sheath with full flexion, is then measured (Fig. 1.150):

AB	
1 cm or more	The entire tendon repair can be done by opening a 'window' in that retinacular portion of the sheath — a proximal window repair[467].
0.5 to 1 cm	The 'core' suture (Mason–Allen, modified Kessler etc.) cannot be placed in the distal tendon end through that window, so both it and the next window distally must be opened — a combined window repair.
less than 0.5 cm	Even the peripheral running suture cannot be inserted through that window so that the major part of the work must be done in the next window — a distal window repair.

If the superficialis is lacerated over the proximal phalanx where its two parts are wrapping around the profundus to reach their insertion, care should be taken to recognize the sinister effects of the *superficialis spiral*[468]. After complete laceration the spiral unwinds so that both ends move from their correct orientation which is in the sagittal plane to lie in the coronal plane of the finger. The problem arises because the two ends unwind in opposite directions. If repaired as they lie, where the flat ends, when approximated, look deceptively correct, the smooth tunnel they formerly created for the profundus will be grossly distorted.

EXTENSOR TENDONS

The *distal ends* can be identified by the action produced on traction, bearing in mind the effect of the intertendinous connections.

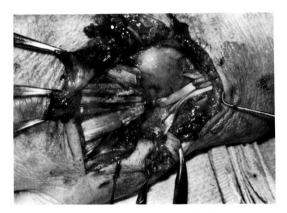

Fig. 1.151 In this clean-cut laceration of all the extensor tendons at the wrist, the variation in cross-sectional dimension, in angle of cut and in the length of the various tendons can be seen.

The *proximal ends* can be classified into groups if they remain in their compartment beneath the extensor retinaculum or if they can be replaced there with confidence by tracing them into the sheath from which they have retracted. Which tendons come through which compartment can be recalled by using Table 1.1 (p. 16). Further identification depends, as with the flexor tendons, on studying:

cross-section
angle of cut
length (Fig. 1.151).

PARTIAL DIVISION OF TENDONS

This may not have been revealed on examination (p. 30) but may subsequently result in tendon rupture if not repaired. Where some tendons have been totally divided this gives a strong clue as to the site of any partial divisions inflicted on others. Partial divisions of tendons should be sought by inspecting each tendon in the vicinity of the skin wound along as much of its length as can be delivered into the wound by full flexion of all joints with traction alternately directed both proximally and distally. The traction should be exerted by gripping the tendon with a gauze swab moistened with saline or by the use of a smooth sharp tendon hook. This process should be repeated at all wounds for all tendons regardless or whether or not they have already been found to be divided in one wound. Injuries at multiple levels do occur and may be missed, especially if the division is only partial at one of them. It is worthy of re-emphasis that all blood clot and bloodstaining should be thoroughly pursued and explored for this frequently reveals partial injuries.

ABRASION AND AVULSION OF TENDONS

Such injuries, especially of the extensors, are not uncommon in industrial and road traffic accidents. Much raw tendon is exposed to which adhesion can occur and the chance of successful function following primary repair is considerably less than it is in tidy lacerations.

Where the extensor tendon has been only partially abraded, the paratenon is lost and the blood supply of the tendon compromised. Gross contamination is the rule rather than the exception. These considerations apart, however, such unpromising material often does surprisingly well, although later tenolysis is very likely to be required. If satisfactory skin cover can be obtained, therefore, the tendon should be thoroughly cleansed, loose ends trimmed away and the tendon retained.

Tendons which have been avulsed are often found lying dangling from the wound in crush and roller injuries. However, their substance is often remarkably undamaged and if there is a chance that the part on which they act can be salvaged, they should be cleansed and sutured back in place, either from whence they came or to an adjacent motor better preserved, for they are difficult — and in some instances impossible — to replace.

MUSCLE

Muscle bellies are frequently injured in crush and avulsion injury. Dead muscle is an ideal medium for the growth of anaerobic organisms. At exploration the identification and excision of all non-viable muscle is therefore imperative. This is done using three criteria.

Appearance. Due to venous congestion and oedema, the muscle which is probably non-viable bulges from its fascial covering and has a dark plum-red colour contrasting with the brownish red of adjacent normal muscle.

Twitch. When normal muscle is grasped gently with toothed dissecting forceps, it twitches. Dead muscle does not. This test is valid regardless of the agents being used by the anaesthetist, but twitch decreases progressively with tourniquet ischaemia.

Perfusion. Especially in macroreplantation, it is important to know whether muscle in the amputated part will be perfused after vessel repair. Therefore, perfusion through the major artery is undertaken before replantation with heparinized Ringer's lactate. Any muscle which does not ooze lactate is excised. This practice has markedly increased survival and decreased infection. It is equally applicable in revascularization.

INDICATIONS

Primary repair of all injured tendons, regardless of the site, offers the best chance of speedy return of good function[469–471]. Contraindications are few. They include:

Loss of a segment of tendon — best judged by approximating the ends and assessing the resultant posture.
Joint injuries of such severity that they preclude early motion.
Fractures which cannot be accurately reduced and securely fixed.
Skin loss which requires distant flap coverage.

This is not the place to detail technique and postoperative management, only to stress that meticulous attention to these details is imperative if this philosophy is to prove successful.

Distal injuries of flexor digitorum profundus. Tendon advancement was commonly practiced in the past, with limits ranging from 0.75 to 2.5 cm. Attempting to resolve the issue, one cadaveric study determined that 1 cm was the maximum permissible shortening[472]. *Any* advancement risks the development of a *quadriga syndrome* (p. 174). Rather, direct repair should be undertaken in all cases. Repair of an *avulsion* of the profundus, which is often diagnosed long after injury, can be performed after various delays which depend upon the level at which the tendon has arrested proximally (p. 36). If repair has been left undone for too long, and the joint becomes unstable, fusion of the distal interphalangeal joint is indicated[473].

Although there is debate on the matter[474], partial tendon injuries should be repaired to avoid later triggering, entrapment or rupture[475] (Fig. 1.152).

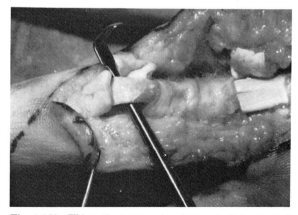

Fig. 1.152 This patient was explored secondarily because of lack of motion in a previously lacerated finger. He was found to have a partial laceration which was locking on the A2 pulley, preventing motion.

Muscle lacerations should be repaired with the expectation that useful, but not normal[476], function will be regained. Suture of muscle is sufficiently difficult in some instances that tendon grafts should be used to strengthen the repair[477].

See Green D P 1993 Operative Hand Surgery, 3rd edn. Churchill Livingstone, New York, pp. 1827, 1937.

Nerve

LACERATION

Where sensory and motor loss of characteristic distribution has been demonstrated on initial examination, exploration usually reveals a clear division of the nerve. Being softer and rather more adherent to adjacent soft tissue, nerve ends are somewhat less easy to locate than are the firmer tendon ends. The proximal end of the *ulnar nerve* divided at the wrist tends to adhere to the deep, radial surface of flexor carpi ulnaris and during exploration of the wound tends to be retracted with it. Likewise, the proximal end of the *median nerve* divided somewhat higher adheres to the deep surface of flexor digitorum superficialis. The ulnar nerve is further obscured by the more superficial and anterior ulnar artery with which it constitutes a neurovascular bundle invested by adipose tissue. Any difficulty encountered in locating nerve ends should be overcome by applying the rule which is absolute in *secondary* exploration — one must always dissect from normal tissue towards the injury. Thus in seeking out the end of a lacerated structure — and this is especially true in difficult exposures such as the upper forearm or the deep spaces of the hand — the incision should be extended adequately and the nerve, or vessel, displayed in uninjured tissue and traced from there. In applying this maxim to an injured nerve, there is clearly more hazard in dissecting the distal nerve end from distal proximally, for branches will be encountered and must be protected and incorporated in the nerve as the surgeon advances.

Once the ends have been located, correct orientation is essential in mixed nerves if the fullest recovery is to follow nerve suture. This is achieved, using magnifying loupes, by:

1. Matching blood vessels.
2. Drawing a fascicular plan (Fig. 1.153): gripping the epineurium with very fine forceps, the nerve endings are rotated so that they can be examined either through strong loupes or the operating microscope. The fascicular bundles are of different size and, if the microscope is being used, can be seen to consist of a differing number of fascicles. A plan should be drawn of each end in turn, either

PROXIMAL   DISTAL

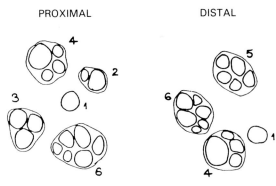

Fig. 1.153 This is a sketch of the fascicular bundles of the proximal and distal ends of a severed median nerve. It will be seen by comparing the size and number of fascicles contained in each bundle that accurate matching can be undertaken.

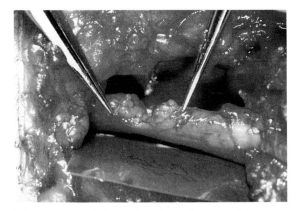

Fig. 1.154 Partial laceration of a median nerve injury. Primary repair is mandatory.

mentally or using a sterile pen and paper, and then the two ends matched.

3. Knowledge of the normal *internal anatomy* of the peripheral nerves[478–481] will allow one to predict the location of certain nerves, such as the motor branches of ulnar and median. If the similarity in size, shape and fascicular content is not recognized by the techniques in (2) above, this knowledge will help to orient the proximal end. The distal end can be mapped by tracing the relevant motor branch proximally from its actual take-off to the site of injury.

4. *Electrical stimulation* of the proximal stump[482,483] has not gained wide use as it involves a 'wake-up' general anaesthesia technique.

5. *Histochemical identification*[484,485] of motor and sensory fascicles is theoretically of most value where a nerve defect has to be grafted. While logical, there is no clinical evidence as yet that this is beneficial.

Indications
Primary or secondary repair of nerves has been the subject of some controversy. The ease of matching in the fresh injury, the impracticality of performing a delayed repair when tendons have been sutured primarily and the increased tension which results from the greater resection of nerve end necessary in secondary repair has made primary epineural suture[486,487], supplemented where necessary by fascicular aligning sutures, the method of choice for the author. There is also experimental evidence that the results are superior[488] following primary repair. Partial nerve lacerations (Fig. 1.154) must *always* be repaired primarily, for separating intact from divided fascicles secondarily is an inexact science.

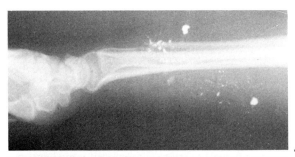

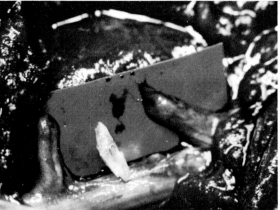

Fig. 1.155 A fracture of the ulna was inflicted on this child when she came between victim and assailant. The exploration revealed an injury of the ulnar nerve due to bone fragment. The nerve damage was sufficiently well localized as to justify primary nerve graft.

Where a defect exists in the nerve primary grafting should be performed only when the surgeon is confident that he is joining good nerve, that the skeleton is well stabilized, that the nerve graft has soft tissue cover which is well-vascularized and that healing will occur per primam (Fig. 1.155).

If *any* doubt exists as to the quality of nerve presenting for repair, it should be left and explored once the wounds are healed. An unsatisfactory suture does the patient a disservice because several months will pass before a decision will be taken to explore a nerve which is recorded as 'repaired' in the initial operation note. When it is elected to wait, there is some merit in attaching the nerve ends one to the other to prevent retraction and thereby shorten the gap.

Considerations of *splintage* following surgery clearly have no place in this text, concerned as it is with diagnosis and indications. However, the reader may perhaps excuse one observation. It is common practice to splint to protect a nerve repair, for example, wrist flexion following median nerve suture. This may be unwise, for scar will form to adjacent tissues which will then place traction on the nerve with wrist extension, and will limit the necessary longitudinal excursion present in all nerves with wrist motion[489]. It may be wiser perhaps to splint against the nerve repair to a degree which peroperative inspection shows that the repair can sustain. With the radial cutaneous nerve, so prone to painful neuroma formation, it is the author's practice to splint in full *ulnar* deviation provided the repair remains secure.

See Green D P 1993 Operative Hand Surgery, 3rd edn. Churchill Livingstone, New York, p. 1320.

AVULSION

Where a nerve has been avulsed the injury is inflicted at differing levels in different fascicles and traction damage occurs both proximal and distal to the obvious division. This is revealed by several observations:

The ends, both proximal and distal, are much thinner than expected or indeed than is the nerve itself when it is dissected out further away from the wound.
The ends frequently overlap.
When inspected with magnification the nerve can be seen to be the site of multiple sub-epineurial haemorrhages for some distance from its end.

Suture carries a greatly reduced hope of full function, although superior in children compared to adults[490].

INJURIES IN CONTINUITY

When characteristic sensory and motor loss have been found on examination, but, despite exhaustive exploration of all wounds, the nerve in question is found to be intact an *axonotmesis* or *neurapraxia* — Sunderland injuries types I and II — (p. 42 and p. 241) has been sustained. In order to facilitate possible secondary neurolysis, the exact site and extent of any bruising or swelling of the nerve should be recorded at exploration. If such swelling is significant, primary epineurotomy *may* reduce nerve damage and speed recovery.

Traction injury
A long section of the nerve is damaged in traction injuries; it is swollen throughout to a varying degree and considerable quantities of extravasated blood may be visible through the epineurium. If this is creating tension, evidenced by induration of the nerve on palpation, then it should be released by incising the epineurium.

Compression
Prolonged compression sufficient to produce lasting nerve disturbance is an unusual primary injury but may be found during exploration of an acute carpal tunnel or compartment syndrome. In the latter situation the nerve injury corresponds exactly to the extent of the forearm muscle bellies. The nerve is constricted, pale and avascular.

In all injuries in continuity, the significant point is whether or not the continuity of the axons themselves has been broken. The two possibilities have been given distinct names and the prognosis differs considerably (p. 241):

Neurapraxia. Axons intact; prognosis: early, full recovery.
Axonotmesis. Axons divided; prognosis: late, possibly incomplete, recovery.

It is not possible to distinguish between the two at the time of primary injury. Nerve conduction studies are of no value in making the distinction until some 48 hours to 8 days after injury, when conduction distal to the site of injury will remain only in the neurapraxia (the time until loss of distal conduction differs in various studies).

Vessel

Named arteries in the region of injury should be inspected, both under tourniquet control and after its release. Lacerations in large vessels should be occluded proximally and distally with bulldog clamps and in small vessels with microvascular clamps. In the large vessel it is also prudent to dissect out the next most proximal branch and place a soft sling around the main vessel just above to afford immediate control should a clamp slip. The tourniquet should then be released and the speed of arterial inflow through other vessels to the region served by the lacerated one assessed before the choice between vascular repair and ligation is made.

Viability should not be the only criterion of the need to perform a vascular repair as relative ischaemia may produce later disability. Radial or ulnar arteries at the wrist should be repaired if the division is clean and the injury otherwise suitable. Studies have shown that approximately half of the vessels repaired at the wrist will remain patent, that there is no absolute determinant of the need for repair, but that eventual patency will be more likely when the back pressure in the distal cut end is low and the hand is relatively ischaemic[491–494]. Most fingers have a dominant digital artery as evidenced by the calibre of the vessel. The larger vessel is usually on the ulnar border of the thumb, the index and middle fingers and on the radial border of the ring and small. Where only one has been divided it should be repaired if experience is available both to judge that it is of significant calibre and to perform the microvascular repair. When neither carries flow, the finger is likely to be non-viable and vascular reconstruction is essential.

Partial lacerations are especially likely to produce considerable blood loss as haemostasis cannot be effected by the usual means of vessel retraction (p. 45).

Torsion and compression of vessels may result in marked spasm and this may persist despite removal of the cause. The vessel should be observed until the spasm settles. This may be encouraged by the application of a stream of warm lignocaine 20%[495], or, as reported from one institution, phosphoenolpyruvate[496]. Where it does not resolve in vessels of consequence, flow should be restored by exploratory arteriotomy and replacement with a reversed vein graft where significant damage to the vessel is found.

Where vascular repair is to be performed, three major factors influence the outcome and these should be assessed during exploration.

1. *Proximal flow*. On release of the tourniquet it is probable that there will be no flow evident, due to vasospasm and a small terminal thrombus. These problems should be overcome by dilatation of the vessel after resection of its cut end. This should result in brisk, pulsatile bleeding of considerable force which does not reduce provided the vessel is held out to length (Fig. 1.156). As a simple guide to desired force, blood from a digital artery should reach the end of the hand table, from the radial or ulnar it should reach the near side of the nurse's table and from the brachial artery the far side!

2. *Uninjured vessel ends*. These should be inspected under magnification appropriate to the vessel size, seeking any evidence of intimal damage or

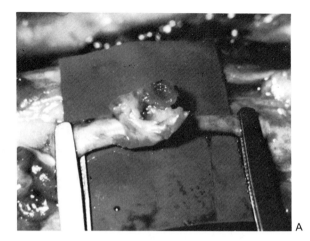

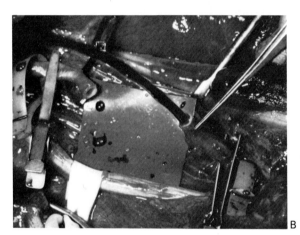

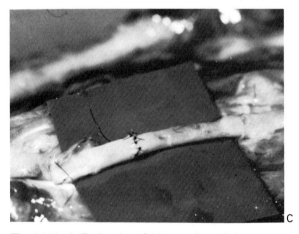

Fig. 1.156 A. Exploration of this wound revealed a traumatic aneurysm due to a partial laceration in the ulnar artery. B. After application of clamps and controlling slings, resection revealed good proximal flow. C. Direct anastomosis proved possible.

separation, of intramural or intraluminal thrombus or of vessel disease.

3. *Good run-off.* The amputated part of the limb distal to the vascular injury should be examined again for any evidence of injury likely to involve the distal vessel. The vessel distal to the injury should be exposed for a length which varies according to the degree of avulsion thought to be involved in the trauma. That vessel should be inspected for any evidence of damage, and in particular for:

(i) thrombus

(ii) avulsed branches — the repair should be performed *distal* to the first intact branch encountered

(iii) intimal tears, which can be seen through the wall as transverse areas of discoloration and which can be felt as irregularities with micro-forceps moved gently along the vessel lightly gripped.

(iv) the 'ribbon sign'[497] — this a series of curls in the course of a vessel normally straight, similar to those which can be produced in ribbons by pulling them firmly through a constriction. It is a sign of irreversible vessel damage.

Any damaged vessel must be resected and replaced by a suitable substitute, usually vein although arterial grafts[498] are superior in the following circumstances (Fig. 1.157):

1. Long defects, commonly encountered in revascularizations

2. Where the defect is between a large-calibre vessel and one or more of small calibre

3. In thumb replantation in which a long bypass from the radial artery improves exposure.

The arterial grafts are obtained from the posterior interosseous artery or the subscapular tree.

Skin

The possibility of deep damage underlying apparently innocuous puncture wounds has been emphasised. They must be explored to their full extent using a probe and the presence of blood staining as guides.

INJECTION INJURIES

The urgency required in handling similar small wounds due to *high compression injection*[499–502] cannot be stressed too strongly. Such injuries may inject any number of substances — paint[503–506], grease[507], hydraulic fluid, molten plastic[508] are only the most common. The distance injected is a function of the pressure in the

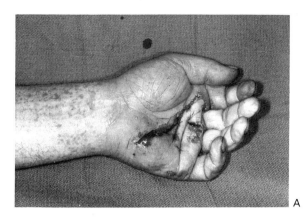

A

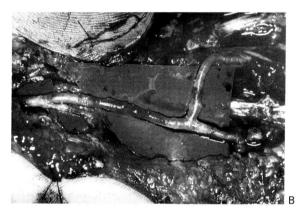

B

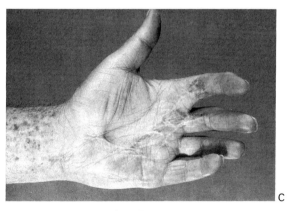

C

Fig. 1.157 Arterial graft. A. This patient presented with devascularization of the fingers following an untidy, ill-defined crush injury to the hand. Conservative management was undertaken with respect to the debridement and skin cover. B. A graft taken from the subscapular tree was used to revascularize the digits. The subscapular artery was anastomosed to the ulnar artery (left of the field), the circumflex scapular to the deep palmar arch and two branches of the thoracodorsal artery to the common digital arteries to the second and fourth spaces respectively. C. Satisfactory revascularization was achieved.

system[509] — hydraulic fluid has been reported in the chest wall following a fingertip puncture. The damage done to the tissues is a function of the nature of the material enhanced by the passage of time. In those instances where the material is radio-opaque, a radiograph will give some guidance as the extent of spread and, after debridement, the adequacy of removal[510].

Indications

Regardless of the extent of the necessary incisions, the absolute responsibility of the surgeon is to remove all of the foreign material, no matter how many hours that may take (Fig. 1.158). If this is not done, the immediate result may be infection, gangrene and amputation, and the long-term outcome fibrosis and discharging sinuses from granulomas which cripple the hand[511,512]. If the injected material is removed, the wounds sutured loosely and early motion begun, full function can be the reward (Fig. 1.159). The management of another potentially serious small wound — the human bite — is considered on page 331.

Total viable skin cover is of prime importance in the emergency management of hand injuries. Two facts have to be determined: *skin viability* and *skin loss*.

SKIN VIABILITY

While viability has been assessed during examination on the basis of colour, design of flaps and return of flow after finger tip expression, the final decision is made at exploration:

1. After all fractures have been reduced and immobilized
2. After all vessels subjected to torsion or compression have been seen to be free of spasm
3. After all appropriate vessels have been repaired and seen to transmit flow
4. After the tourniquet has been applied for a period in excess of 20 minutes and then released
5. After 10 minutes has been allowed to elapse following tourniquet release.

Fig. 1.158   A. This patient sustained a high-pressure injection injury with hydraulic fluid on the pulp of the left thumb. B. The fluid was traced into all compartments of the hand, through the carpal tunnel and up above the wrist. After evacuation of all foreign fluid and thorough irrigation (C) the wounds were closed lightly and irrigating catheters inserted. The patient healed slowly but satisfactorily (D).

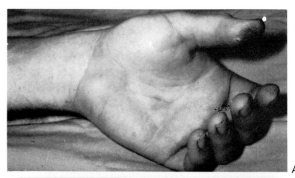

A

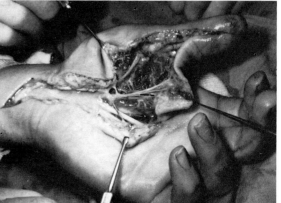

B

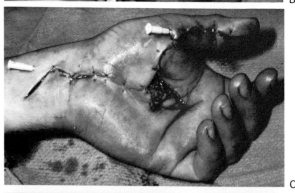

C

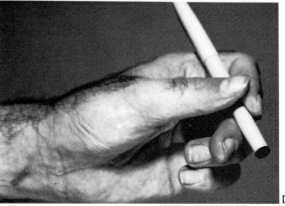

D

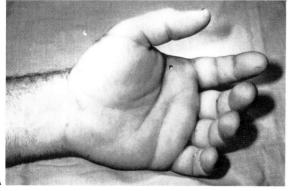

A

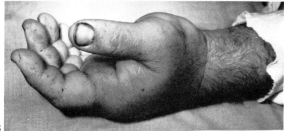

B

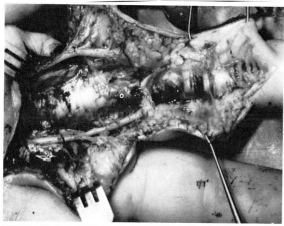

C

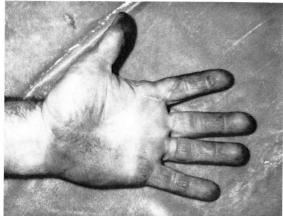

D

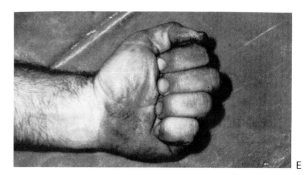

E

The release of the tourniquet will result in brisk oozing from the wounds in uncompromised cases. In more doubtful circumstances a very clear *line of demarcation* will appear between the region of *reactive hyperaemia* and the pallor of skin with no blood supply. This line should be marked with a skin pencil. If the decision were taken at this stage, however, too much would be sacrificed. Rather, the hand should be elevated for a period related to the length of tourniquet application, then lowered, haemostasis achieved and the wounds washed free of blood. If the skin flaps are then re-examined, the line of demarcation will be less evident, for the hyperaemia will have settled, but in most instances circulation will be clearly seen beyond the mark made with the skin pencil. Provided that no undue tension or distortion is subsequently applied to the flap, this second line can be selected for the excision. If, however, skin grafts or a flap are in any event to be applied and wider excision does not expose an unsatisfactory bed for the former, then the excision can be more radical, approaching the first demarcation line. The most unequivocal evidence of acceptable skin blood flow is brisk *dermal bleeding* on incision (Fig. 1.160). In extensive avulsion flaps these incisions are made parallel to the edge of the flap, proceeding further and further from the edge until viability is unequivocally demonstrated. This is the criterion applied in radical debridement (p. 92).

Fluorescein[513] has been advocated by some to demonstrate flow. This it certainly will do, but it has been shown to be consistently pessimistic, resulting in unnecessary sacrifice of skin (Fig. 1.161)

In extensive 'degloving' injuries of the limbs, immediate removal of the non-viable skin back to a bleeding margin is indicated, for valuable grafts can subsequently

Fig. 1.159 A. This patient presented with severe pain and oedema 24 hours after injection of car undersealant. B. The material was followed throughout the hand and all removed. C. Light suture and irrigation resulted in restoration of full function (D, E).

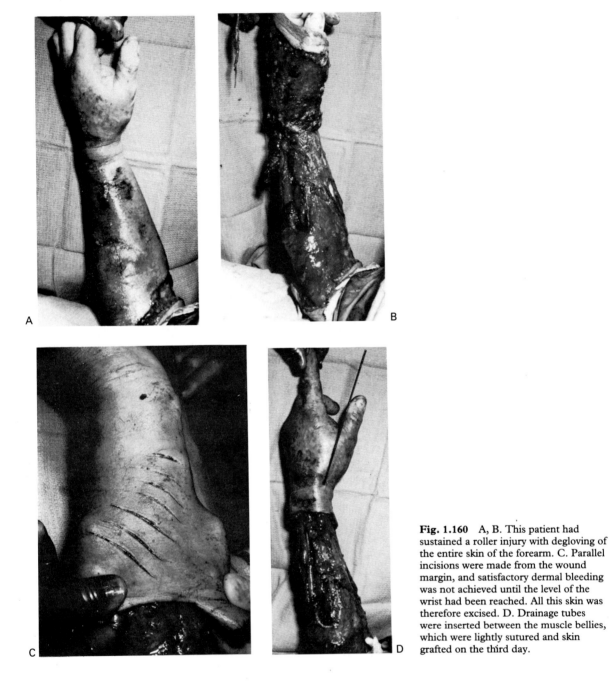

Fig. 1.160 A, B. This patient had sustained a roller injury with degloving of the entire skin of the forearm. C. Parallel incisions were made from the wound margin, and satisfactory dermal bleeding was not achieved until the level of the wrist had been reached. All this skin was therefore excised. D. Drainage tubes were inserted between the muscle bellies, which were lightly sutured and skin grafted on the third day.

be cut from the less damaged portions of the excised tissue.

Some argue that flaps should be sutured back provided that all deep non-viable tissue has been removed, since survival cannot be predicted with absolute accuracy. While the premise is true, the conclusion is not

acceptable since subsequent skin necrosis encourages sepsis and endangers repair performed deep to it. Marginally viable skin is probably worst of all because it multiplies the length of convalescence, delaying mobilization, promoting oedema and fibrosis in the hand and, if at length it survives, proving itself to be in-

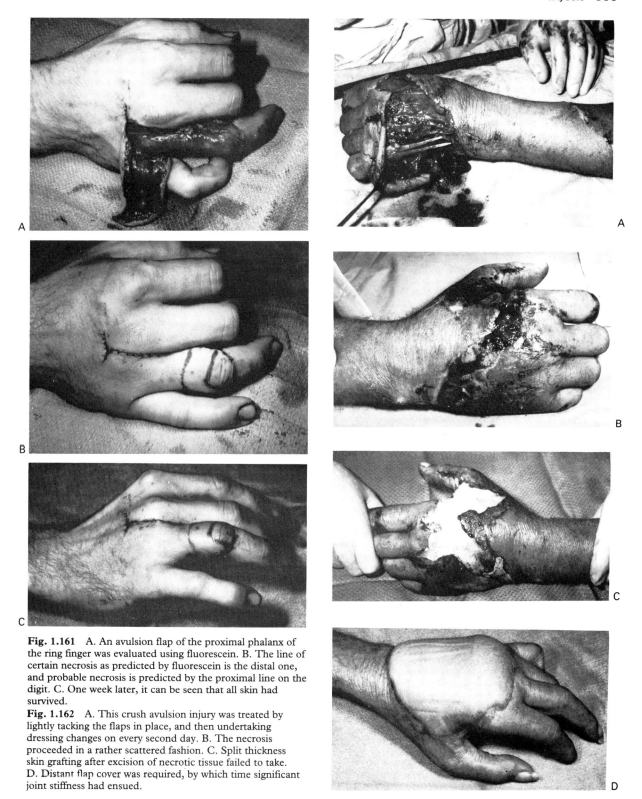

Fig. 1.161 A. An avulsion flap of the proximal phalanx of the ring finger was evaluated using fluorescein. B. The line of certain necrosis as predicted by fluorescein is the distal one, and probable necrosis is predicted by the proximal line on the digit. C. One week later, it can be seen that all skin had survived.

Fig. 1.162 A. This crush avulsion injury was treated by lightly tacking the flaps in place, and then undertaking dressing changes on every second day. B. The necrosis proceeded in a rather scattered fashion. C. Split thickness skin grafting after excision of necrotic tissue failed to take. D. Distant flap cover was required, by which time significant joint stiffness had ensued.

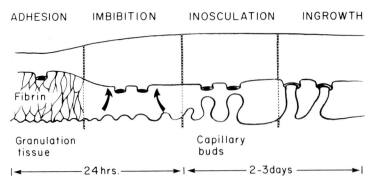

Fig. 1.163   A diagram of the normal process involved in skin graft take, proceeding from left to right (see text).

durated and adherent (Fig. 1.162). If despite these considerations, doubtfully viable flaps are placed into position this should be done without tension for they are more likely to survive than if they are stretched out to their original dimension[514].

SKIN LOSS

Especially in complex injuries, the wounds will gape apart and flaps of skin will retract markedly. *Landmarks* which correspond on either wound edge should be sought. Those available in the hand are the many unique *skin creases*, the *nail folds* and the margins of *hair-bearing skin* of the dorsum of forearm, hand and fingers. Once these points have been matched the surgeon can decide whether or not skin has been lost.

Dorsal skin is more mobile than palmar, but it is so to accommodate finger flexion. Closure should not be achieved by 'pulling the wound edges together'.

Where the nail bed has been injured it is particularly important to locate all parts of this specialized structure. Not uncommonly portions are to be found on flaps of digital pulp which have carried the nail bed well away from its dorsal origin. These should be replaced accurately to avoid late deformity of the nail which can be functionally disabling. (Fingertip injuries are considered below, p. 117.)

INDICATIONS

When skin has been lost, the replacement chosen should be the simplest compatible with the best and speediest functional recovery[515–518]. The simplest of skin cover is provided by the free skin graft. What is required by any skin graft is a bed which is vascular enough to produce capillary buds in sufficient quantity quickly enough to revitalize its dying cells (Fig. 1.163). The

periosteum of bone, paratenon and even cancellous bone are all capable of doing so, and therefore free split skin can be directly applied to them. Whether or not this is designed to produce the 'best and speediest functional recovery' is another matter entirely. For the very reason that they gain their blood supply by capillary budding from the bed, grafts in due course become firmly adherent to that bed. If movement of the bed is required through a greater range than that of the overlying skin — or vice versa, as in the movement of skin over bone — or if subsequent surgery such as tendon grafting will be required in the layer between skin and bed, then grafts are not suitable as a permanent cover. They may in complex injuries or in hands inexperienced in plastic surgical procedures be the correct *temporary* cover even in the situations described. If, however, the injury, the patient and the surgeon are fitted for immediate flap cover where it will eventually be undoubtedly required then an appreciable saving in time and money will be effected by the use of a primary flap.

Split skin is available in profusion and has the advantage that it takes readily. It can be meshed to cover large areas, conform with contour defects or permit drainage of secretions (Fig. 1.164). The disadvantages of split skin are that it is associated with considerable contracture[519], which may produce joint deformities, and that it is not as durable as full-thickness skin.

Full-thickness skin is in relatively short supply, takes less well than split, but does not contract and is of course thicker and therefore more durable (Fig. 1.165). As will be evident from what is said above, no skin graft takes on bare bone, tendon or ligament or over a cavity. Bringing with it an intrinsic blood supply, a flap[520,521] is necessary in such circumstances.

Local skin flaps[522] are of similar texture, they can be transferred in one procedure — this is the sole, somewhat artificial, distinction between local and regional

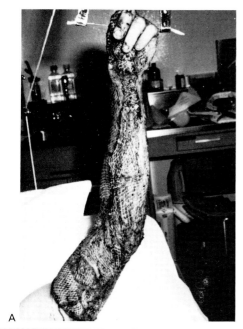

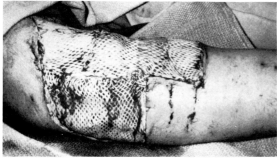

Fig. 1.164 Meshed skin grafts can be used to cover extensive areas as in this total degloving of the upper extremity (A) or to fit the contours of irregular defects and allow drainage of secretions (B).

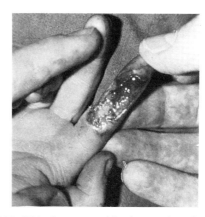

Fig. 1.165 This clean cut avulsion loss on the palmar aspect of the right index finger of a child exposed no significant deep structures. The bed showed a good blood supply, and because of its extent, situation, and vascularity was ideal for the use of a primary full-thickness graft.

axial flag and neurovascular island — they are considered in somewhat greater detail under finger-tip injuries. If the defect is too large to be covered by a local or regional flap, then distant tissue must be used.

The major disadvantages of local flaps have been their *limited availability*, their inability to fill *deep defects*, and the fact that their use inflicted an *additional injury* to an already injured extremity. With the recognition and description of the axial supply of many areas of skin, fascia and muscle[526] throughout the body, studies inspired in part by the increased use of free tissue transfer, the first two of these former disadvantages have been largely overcome. The third — that of adding further injury to a hand and arm already severely damaged — should be weighed carefully before employing these more recent local flaps (listed with references below), for the larger and deeper they have to be to reconstruct the primary defect, so too must be the secondary defect.

Cutaneous
Palmar digital vascular island[527]
First web[528]
Dorsal metacarpal[529,530]
  first dorsal metacarpal artery island[531]
  second dorsal metacarpal artery island[532]
  reversed or distally based[533,534]

Fasciocutaneous
Reversed radial forearm or 'Chinese'[535–542]
  with bone, tendon or 'outflow' addition[543–546]
(Fig. 1.169)
Reversed ulnar artery island[547–549]
Posterior interosseous artery island[550–552]
Medial septocutaneous of the arm[553]

flaps, the latter requiring a second stage for pedicle division — and they may bring with them some nerve supply. With this in mind, areas adjacent to the defect should be inspected to determine whether or not they can, without detriment, provide a transposition, advancement or rotation flap (Fig. 1.166). While the planning of such flaps is beyond the scope of this text, suffice it to say that the larger the flap constructed, the more likely is it to achieve the objective. Occasionally the skeleton of a viable digit is irreparably damaged. This can then serve as an incomparable source of local skin as a filletted finger flap[523,524] (Figs 1.167, 1.168).

If no local flap is available, then other sources of hand skin should be considered for construction of a *regional flap*[525]. Such regional flaps include cross-finger, thenar,

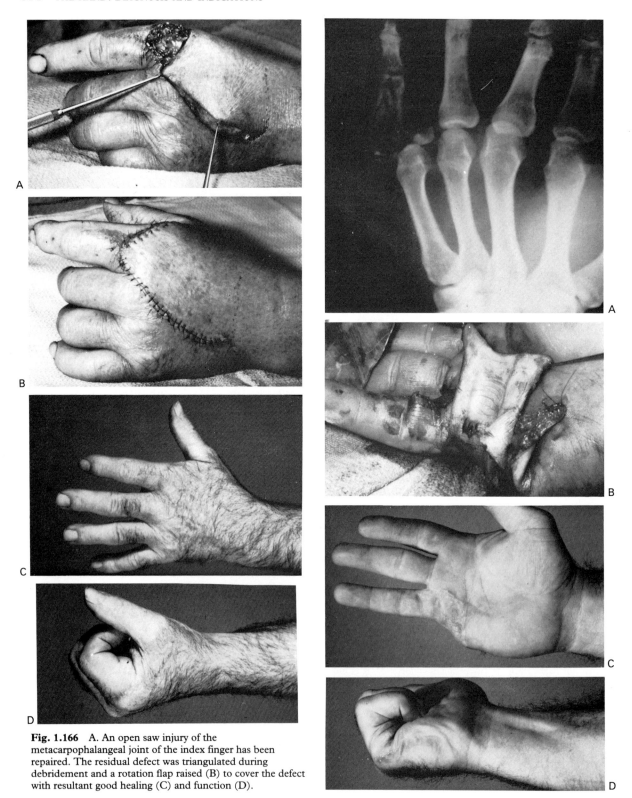

Fig. 1.166 A. An open saw injury of the metacarpophalangeal joint of the index finger has been repaired. The residual defect was triangulated during debridement and a rotation flap raised (B) to cover the defect with resultant good healing (C) and function (D).

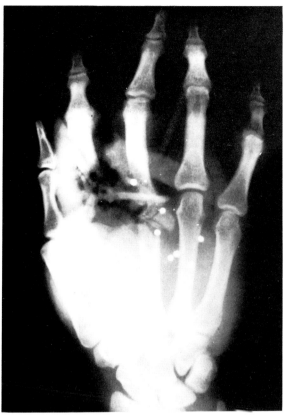

A

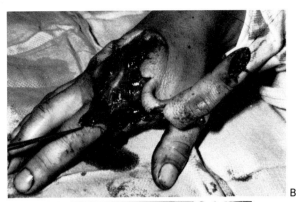

B

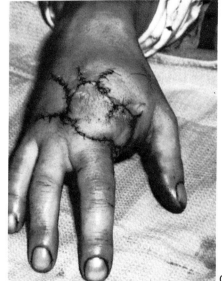

C

Fig. 1.168 Dorsal fillet flap. A. A shotgun injury to the metacarpophalangeal joint region of the index and middle fingers resulted in extensive skeletal damage to the index, such that it was sacrificed to produce a long fillet flap (B) which could be employed to cover the immediate joint replacement in the metacarpophalangeal joint of the middle finger with undoubtedly viable skin (C).

Musculocutaneous
The blood supply of muscles has been classified into five types[554]:

I   One vascular pedicle
II   One dominant plus other minor
III Two dominant
IV   Several, equal, segmental
V   One dominant plus peripheral

Fig. 1.167 (*Facing page, right*). Palmar fillet flap. A. The small finger was irrevocably injured by crushing, but the skin remained viable. B. A palmar fillet flap was therefore used to cover the reconstruction of the ring finger with resulting primary healing (C) and full range in the remaining digits (D).

In types I, II and V, one dominant pedicle[555] is capable of supporting the entire muscle if the others are ligated. Theoretically, therefore, any muscle in the upper extremity which belongs to one of these three types can be transposed on its pedicle. Several have been described:

latissimus dorsi to the upper arm[556-560] (Fig. 1.170)
deltoid to the shoulder[561]
brachioradialis[562] *extensor carpi radialis longus*[563] and *flexor carpi radialis*[564], all to the elbow
flexor digitorum superficialis to the antecubital fossa[565]
extensor carpi ulnaris and *flexor digitorum profundus* to the proximal ulna[566]
pronator quadratus[567] and *abductor digiti minimi*[568,569] to the wrist
the *first dorsal interosseous* to the first metacarpal and to the third metacarpal[570]

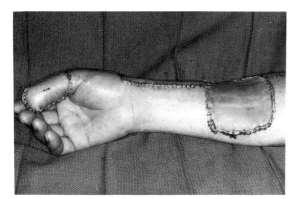

Fig. 1.169 Reversed radial forearm flap. Forty-eight hours following amputation and adverse exploratory assessment for replantation, thumb reconstruction was completed with a bone graft and reversed radial forearm flap.

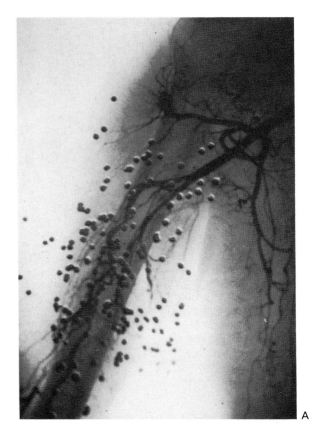

A

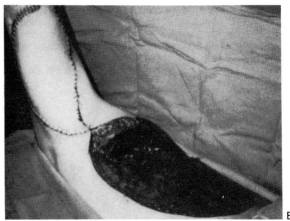

B

Fig. 1.170 A. A shotgun blast to the upper arm resulted in loss of flow in the brachial artery. An immediate vein graft was performed, and (B) the resultant skin defect closed with a pedicled latissimus dorsi musculocutaneous flap.

Distant flaps[571–573] may be of random blood supply, dependent upon the subdermal plexus, or axial[574] where a known vessel supplies the flap. *Random flaps* have the advantage of being thin and of potentially small dimension. Thus, *cross-arm flaps*[575–577] are ideal for resurfacing small, palmar defects, and *tubed acromiothoracic flaps* are ideal for cover of a thumb from which the skin has been avulsed. Both have the disadvantage, especially in the female, of creating cosmetically unsatisfactory defects. *Axial flaps* may be of skin alone, fasciocutaneous or musculocutaneous. They may be transferred on a pedicle or by microvascular techniques as a free flap. The *groin flap*[578–583] is the most widely used pedicle flap for the hand, almost to the exclusion of all others (Fig. 1.171). It provides predictably reliable skin cover of relatively good quality for large defects permitting immediate deep reconstruction where appropriate (Fig. 1.172). It can be split to a degree to cover two surfaces (Fig. 1.173) and on occasion has been used bilaterally to cover both hands simultaneously (Fig. 1.174). When even it cannot provide all the skin required it can be supplemented by free skin grafts (Fig. 1.175) or by the simultaneous use of a hypogastric[584, 585] or tensor fascia lata[586] flap. Increasingly, *emergency free flaps*[587,588] are being used in departments with sufficient experience and adequate staff. The advantages of providing skin cover which has a permanent blood supply are clear, especially in injuries where circumferential flap cover is required, where the defect is too proximal for a groin flap, where external fixation of the forearm has been required, where major primary reconstruction of deep structures takes precedence in dictating the postoperative posture of the limb, where nerve supply is also required, as in restoring a thumb pulp (Fig. 1.176) or where illness, such as un-

controlled epilepsy, makes immobilization a problem (Fig. 1.177). Many free flaps carry with them an excessive amount of tissue, and in circumstances requiring cover of a large area while avoiding bulk the use of a *free*

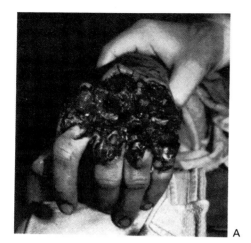

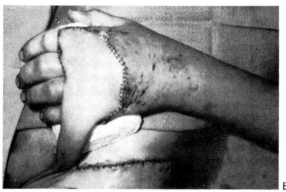

Fig. 1.171 A. This high-velocity gunshot wound of the metacarpophalangeal joint region required immediate bony stabilization and revascularization of one digit. B. Immediate viable skin cover was provided by a pedicle groin flap.

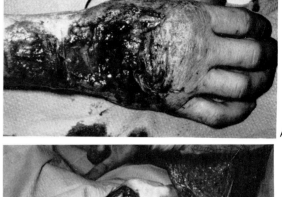

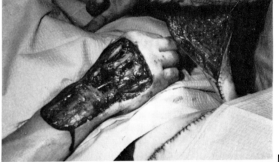

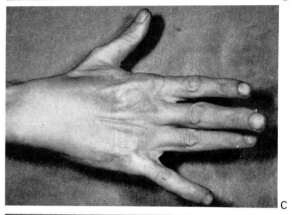

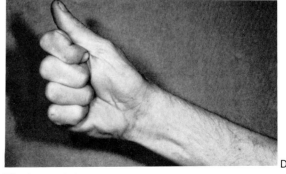

Fig. 1.172 A. This patient sustained a roll-over injury in a truck which removed all extensor tendons plus the dorsal surface of the metacarpals. B. Immediate groin flap cover permitted extensor tendon reconstruction and restoration of good function (C, D).

muscle flap with subsequent application of split skin grafts has decreased this problem (Fig. 1.178).

Many free tissue transfers have now been described for reconstruction of the hand[589,590]. Those most commonly used are: (i) the *tailored latissimus dorsi*[591]; (ii) the *rectus abdominis*[592]; (iii) the *serratus anterior*[593–595]; (iv) the *lateral arm*[596–598]; (v) the *radial forearm*[599–600] — although it has admitted complications[601–604]; (vi) the *dorsalis pedis*[605]; (vii) the *ulnar forearm*[606]; (viii) the *groin*[607–608], which has the great merit of its inconspicuous donor defect — which it shares with (ix) the *temporoparietal*[609–612].

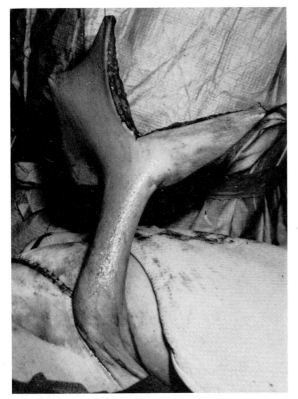

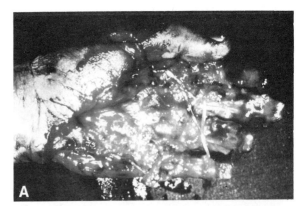

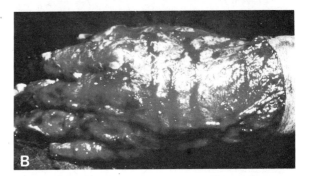

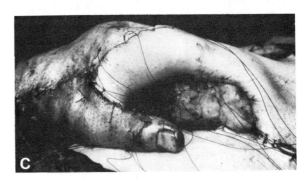

Fig. 1.173   Groin flap split to cover two surfaces.

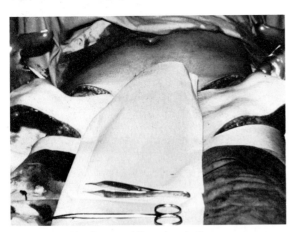

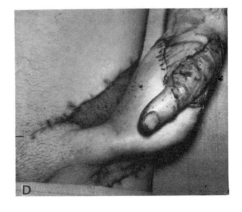

Fig. 1.174   Simultaneous bilateral groin flaps to cover bilateral electrical burns excised primarily.

Fig. 1.175   A, B. This patient suffered an avulsion injury while in his employment as a maintenance engineer, exposing both dorsal and palmar aspects of the hand. C. A primary groin flap was applied to cover the digits and palmar surface of the hand, split thickness skin grafts being used on the dorsum. D. On account of the tube pedicle, a primary groin flap allows adequate mobilization of the wrist and small joints of the hand while in place. (Further reconstruction on this patient is illustrated in Fig. 2.25.)

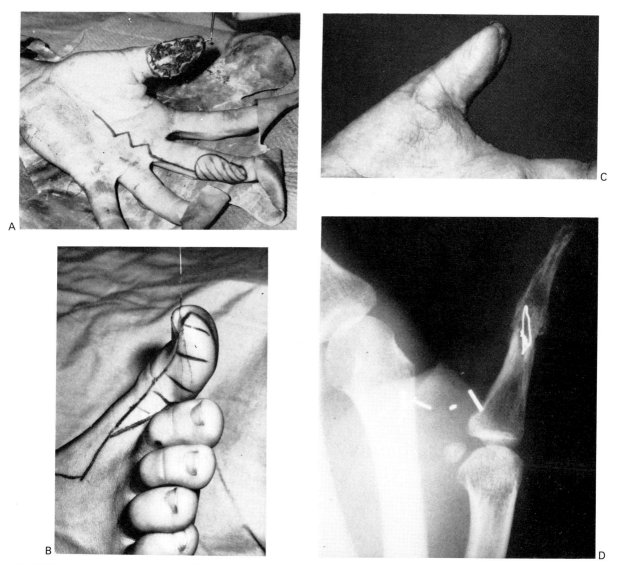

Fig. 1.176 A severe gouging injury of the pulp of the thumb required shortening of the skeleton with immediate arthrodesis of the distal interphalangeal joint. A. The choice lay between a pedicle neurovascular island from the hand or (B) a free neurovascular island from the pulp of the toe. After discussion with the patient the latter was selected. C. Satisfactory healing and return of sensation resulted with good bony union of the osteosynthesis (D).

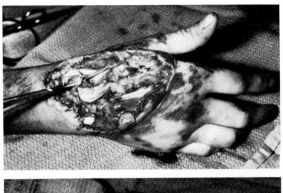

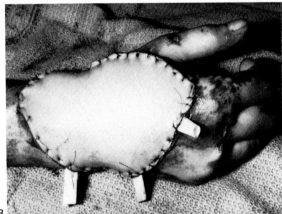

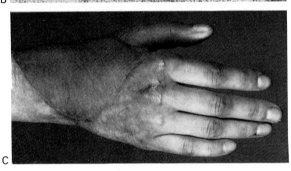

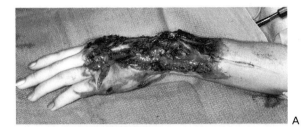

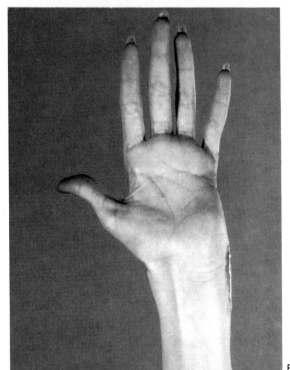

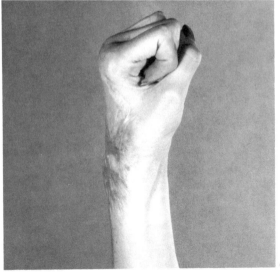

Fig. 1.177 This poorly-controlled epileptic sustained a deep road abrasion injury (A) which required stabilization of the wrist, reconstruction of the capsule and immediate tendon transfer. Application of a free groin flap (B) as an emergency permitted appropriate splintage, avoided problems during two subsequent seizures and showed trouble-free healing (C). Her hospital stay was for two days after injury.

Fig. 1.178 Free latissimus flap with skin graft. A. This patient suffered an injury similar to that shown in Figure 1.139. Following identical management with radical debridement, internal fixation and immediate extensor tendon grafts, a latissimus muscle flap was used with application of a split-thickness skin graft. Following an extensor tenolysis, the patient recovered good function (B, C). Of particular note is the almost total atrophy of the latissimus flap, giving a satisfactory contour to the hand.

Summarizing the indications for different types of skin cover discussed above:

1. Areas with good blood supply, no exposed bone, tendon or ligament:
   free skin graft
   (a) large areas on the dorsum or arm }
   (b) non-contact side of the digit }
       → *split skin*
       (i) irregular or discharging wounds
           → *meshed split skin*
   (c) small areas on flexion surface }
   (d) contact side of digit }
       → *full thickness skin*
2. Poor blood supply to bed, exposed structures, later surgery planned:
   flap
   (a) small defects; skin available
       → *local flap*
   (b) small defects; no local skin available
       → *regional flap*
       (i) thumb pulp
           → *neurovascular island flap*
   (c) small defects; no local or regional skin available }
   (d) total thumb skin avulsion }
       → *distant random flap*
           infraclavicular
           cross-arm
   (e) large defects
       → *distant axial flap*
       (i) circumferential, forearm, external fixation or splint
           → *free flap*
       (ii) thumb pulp
           → *free NVI flap from great toe.*

See Green D P 1993 Operative Hand Surgery, 3rd edn. Churchill Livingstone, New York, pp. 1103 and 1741.

FINGER-TIP INJURIES

The finger tip is an area in which examination of skin loss and the nature of the exposed tissue is unusually important in selecting the method of reconstruction and thereby influencing the outcome[613].

1. Pulp
Here, sensation, adequate padding and total freedom from discomfort are essential. The points to be noted are:

(a) *Whether or not bone is exposed.* If none is exposed, and the defect is smaller than 1 cm², remarkable results have been reported from merely dressing the wound[614-616] (Fig. 1.179). If the defect is larger than 1 cm² in an adult, a free skin graft is indicated. Split thickness skin is used for small defects, particularly on the ulnar side of the digit, for contraction will draw in normally sensible skin (Fig. 1.180). Full-thickness grafts are employed on larger areas of well-vascularized soft tissue, especially on the radial, contact, aspect of the finger.

   If bone is exposed, a graft may take but contraction would not occur and an adherent, tender scar would result. A flap is therefore required if length is to be maintained.

(b) *The angle at which tissue loss has occurred.* If more tissue has been lost from the dorsal than from the palmar aspect, then, if other factors make it appropriate, a local VY advancement flap is an excellent solution (Fig. 1.181)[617-620]. If the angulation is reversed, however, with more lost from the palmar than from the dorsal aspect, any attempt to use a local flap will be doomed to failure through undue tension, and another solution must be sought. In the thumb, distal to the interphalangeal joint, a palmar angled defect, if not too great, may be closed by a Moberg advancement flap[621-624] (Fig. 1.182) or by a dorsal neurovascular island flap from the thumb itself[625].

   Where bone is exposed and the angulation of the wound is unsuitable for local flap repair, the choice lies between:

(i) *Cross-finger flap*[626-629]; this is the most common solution, the main excluding factor being injury to the dorsum of the adjacent donor finger. The cross-finger flap to the thumb[630,631] can be taken from the proximal phalanx of the index finger or from the middle phalanx of either the middle or ring fingers. When taken from the index finger, the radial nerve can be blocked at the wrist and the area of resultant anaesthesia mapped out. If it includes the proximal phalanx, the radial nerve branches can be preserved in raising the flap (Fig. 1.183). The proximal course of the nerve is then transferred to the thumb at the second stage.

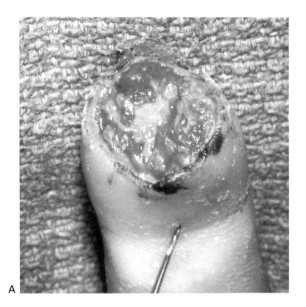

A

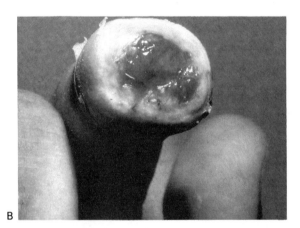

B

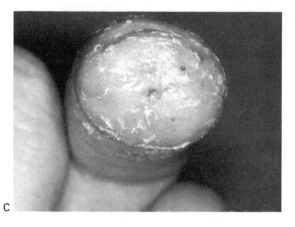

C

Alternatively the nerve can be transferred in one stage if a first dorsal metacarpal artery island flap[632] is used. A nerve supply to the thumb tip is thereby preserved[633-635]. A word of caution should be offered on the radial-nerve innervated cross-finger flap. It may, at some point after the division, show gradually decreasing sensation. This appears to be more common the longer the thumb and may be due to neurapraxia as the thumb is used in more and more abduction. It should probably therefore be reserved for thumbs amputated at the level of the interphalangeal joint, although division of the nerve and coaptation to a digital nerve stump can also serve.

Where more mobility is required, especially in cross-finger flaps from the dorsum of the proximal phalanx, the axial flag flap can provide it[636], so covering difficult defects on adjacent digits (Figs 1.184 and 1.185). Multiple cross-finger flaps are used for multiple fingertip amputations (Fig. 1.186).

(ii) *Thenar flap*[637]. Where a cross-finger flap cannot be employed, a flap from the metacarpophalangeal crease of the thumb is of use, but it should be restricted to patients 'biologically' under 40 or unacceptable proximal interphalangeal joint contracture may result (Fig. 1.187). "Biologic" age is inversely proportional to the hyperextensibility of the proximal interphalangeal joints. It is the flap of choice in younger women as it avoids an unsightly donor scar on the dorsum of a finger.

(iii) *Immediate neurovascular island*[638]— applicable only where the pulp lost is that of the thumb, only where it is the major injury, only where the surgeon is experienced in the technique and only where the wound is sufficiently recent and clean as to mimic a surgical excision. Care must be taken to check that flow exists in all relevant vessels (p. 174). Some disrepute has fallen on this procedure on account of poor sensation in the transferred pulp[639]. This does not occur if care is taken to avoid all tension on the neurovascular pedicle, both during dissection, and even more important after its application. At surgery, the

Fig. 1.179 Finger-tip dressing alone. A. This finger-tip injury was treated with dressings alone, resulting in: (B) granulation, epithelialization and finally complete healing. C. Desensitization was commenced at the stage shown in B.

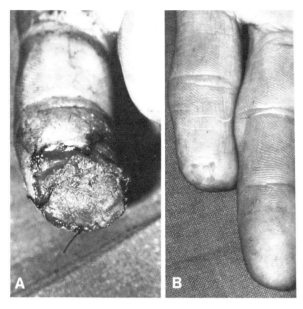

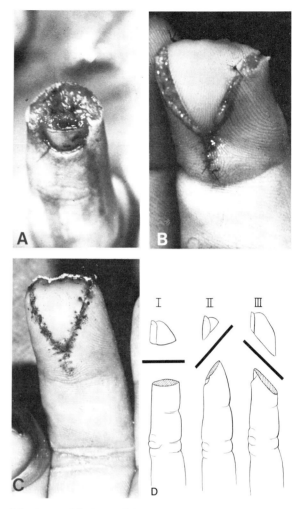

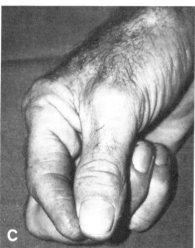

Fig. 1.180 A. This amputation of an index finger just distal to the distal interphalangeal joint was covered with a split thickness skin graft in a casualty department. When seen for review, the skin graft appeared to be of good appearance and was left undisturbed. Subsequent contraction of the graft drew normal digital skin over the amputation stump and the patient made good use of this simple repair (B, C).

Fig. 1.181 The bone of the distal phalanx was exposed in this amputation of a middle finger and therefore flap cover was required. Since the angle of amputation was transverse a V–Y advancement, (B) was appropriate and this resulted in satisfactory healing (C). D. The angle of amputation determines whether or not a local advancement flap can be used (not appropriate in type III).

pedicle must be seen to be loose with the flap in place on a fully abducted and extended thumb. Good results can then be expected[640–642] (Fig. 1.188).

(iv) *Revision of amputation.* Sacrifice of length is always a disturbing procedure, but, where other solutions have been rejected, it provides a sensitive well-healed stump. It is appropriate in isolated loss of a finger tip in older patients where a cross-finger flap is ruled out. It should not be employed on the thumb.

The questions which the examiner asks as he explores the finger tip injury under anaesthesia are:

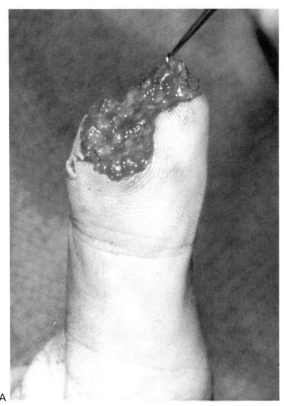

A

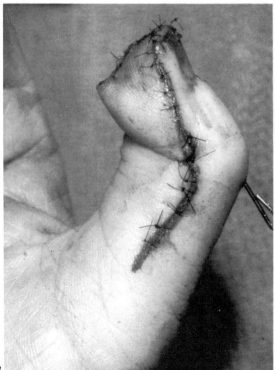

B

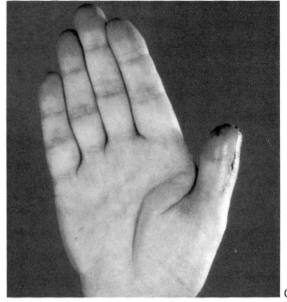

C

Fig. 1.182   Moberg advancement flap. A. Loss of the pulp; B the tip of the thumb was reconstructed with a Moberg advancement flap with closure of a 'dog-ear' and use of a Kirschner wire to maintain interphalangeal flexion. C. Satisfactory coverage was achieved and extension of the interphalangeal joint was restored, but healing was slow.

Q. Tissue loss or not?
    no tissue loss
        Q. Tidy or untidy?
            tidy → cleanse and repair
            untidy → debride → now significant tissue
                                  loss?
    tissue loss
Q. Bone exposed or not?
    not exposed → skin graft
        Q. Contact surface or not?
            contact → full-thickness skin graft
            non-contact → split thickness skin graft
    exposed
Q. Angle of tissue loss?
    more loss dorsally → local flap
        transverse → local flap
    more loss pulp
Q. Biological age?
    advanced → revise amputation
    not so → regional flap
        Q. Digit involved and area of loss?
            thumb and large loss → primary NVI flap
            finger or small loss → regional random flap
                Q. Sex?
                    female → thenar flap
                    male → cross-finger flap

These questions can be summarized in an algorithm:

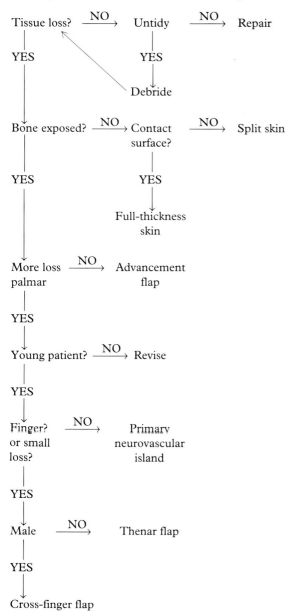

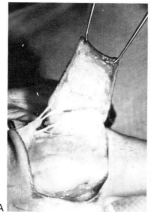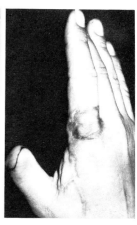

A   B

Fig. 1.183 Before raising a cross-finger flap for coverage of a thumb defect the distribution of the radial nerve was mapped out by blocking it at the level of the wrist. It was found to include the donor area for the flap. In the process of raising the flap from the dorsum of the proximal phalanx of the index finger the terminal branches of the radial nerve were carefully dissected out and preserved (A). On division and inset of the flap, the radial nerve branch to the index finger was dissected back on the dorsum of the first web space and then transferred to the ulnar aspect of the thumb through another incision. With this innervated cross-finger flap, the patient regained sensation on the tip of the amputated thumb (B).

2. Nail bed[643–648]

Here, adequate support for the nail and avoidance of any significant nail distortion are necessary if the nail is not to be functionally a nuisance and cosmetically an embarrassment. The injured nail bed should be inspected under magnification, using loupes or the operating microscope, with these points in mind. Adequate inspection may dictate removal of part or all of the nail.

(a) The distal half of the terminal phalanx should be present and, if fractured, stably reduced usually with the help of a fine Kirschner wire. The more phalanx is missing the greater is the likelihood of a curved nail and ablation should be considered. A curved nail can be avoided only if the nail bed is *supported by bone throughout its length.* (Fig. 1.189).

(b) Accurate localization and matching of both germinal and sterile nail bed should be made prior to careful repair. Otherwise, deformity will result.

(c) The eponychium should be similarly inspected. Any adhesion between it and the nail bed will result in a grooved or split nail. This is prevented by careful repair of all layers of the nail fold and insertion of a splint[649] to keep the cul-de-sac open during healing.

(d) If any nail bed is missing, it is best replaced with a split thickness graft of nail bed[650–652], taken either from the injured finger or from a toe (Fig. 1.190). These have been shown to be most effective on the sterile matrix, poor on the germinal[653]. Reversed dermal skin grafts are also useful substitutes but only on the sterile matrix in the acute phase[654].

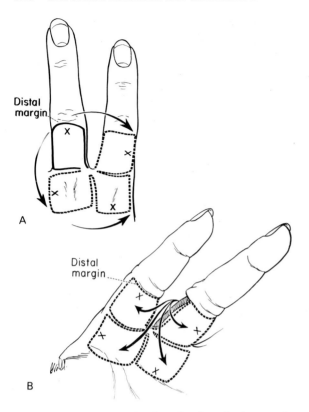

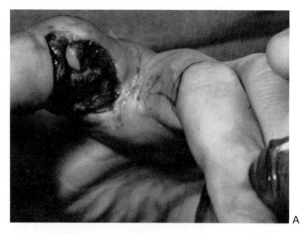

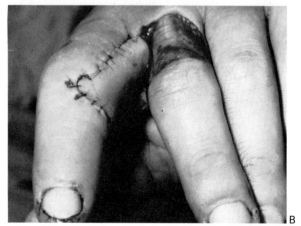

Fig. 1.184   A. The axial flag flap taken from the dorsum of the proximal phalanx can be rotated to cover any area within reach through 360°. B. A flap can also be brought through the web space to cover palmar defects.

(e) When the nail is completely destroyed but distal phalanx remains, length can be maintained by covering the soft-tissue defect with a reversed de-epithelialized cross-finger flap[655] (Fig. 1.191).

THERMAL INJURY

(For reasons of efficiency and convenience, the history, examination and indications in burns — thermal, electrical and chemical — and frostbite are considered here together).

Burns

HISTORY[656]

Thermal

The temperature of the source has to be very high if third- or fourth-degree burns are to be inflicted before the hand is withdrawn. This is especially true for burns

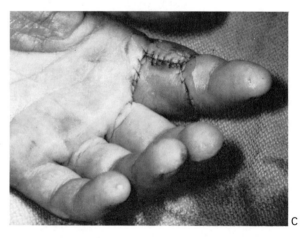

Fig. 1.185   A. This defect revealing an open joint is on both the ulnar and palmar aspects of the index finger. Employing an axial flag flap but with a 2 mm pedicle, well vascularized cover was achieved for the lateral and (C) palmar aspect of the wound. (From Lister, G. D. (1981) The theory of the transposition flap and its practical application in the hand. Clinics in Plastic Surgery 8: 115.)

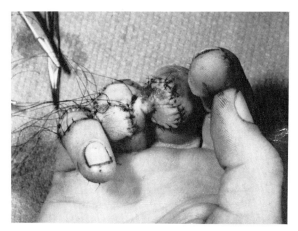

Fig. 1.186 Cross-finger flaps raised from adjacent fingers give very satisfactory cover for multiple fingertip amputations.

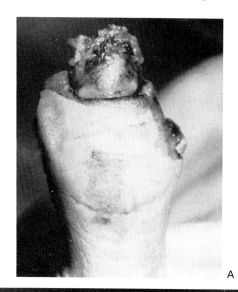

A

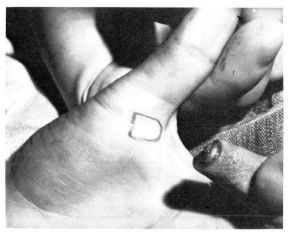

Fig. 1.187 A plan of the defect on the tip of this index finger of a twenty-two-year-old girl has been marked out over the metacarpophalangeal crease of the thumb. A thenar flap was subsequently raised somewhat larger than the plan. The secondary defect was closed directly, thereby eliminating the need for a skin graft.

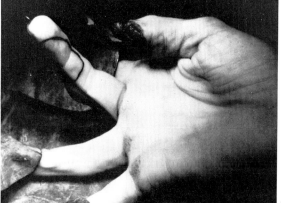

B

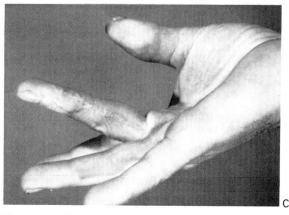

C

of the palm where the skin is thickest and sensitivity most acute. Thus, scalds, kitchen accidents and coal fire contact will all tend to produce first- or superficial second-degree burns.

By contrast, where the temperature is indeed very high or where the hand cannot be removed quickly in response to pain, third- and fourth-degree burns are probable. These circumstances apply in contact with electric fires, especially bar radiators, hot plates where the victim is impaired (see below) and in general body

Fig. 1.188 This patient sustained a crush avulsion of the entire pad of the dominant right thumb. A, B. An immediate neurovascular island flap was taken from the ulnar aspect of the middle finger with satisfactory restitution of the thumb pulp and good healing of the full-thickness graft on the secondary defect (C).

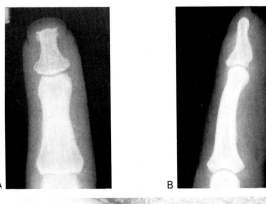

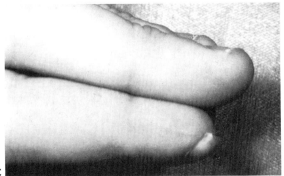

Fig. 1.189 A. The tip of the distal phalanx has been trimmed back, as shown on these radiographs, to a point where it offers inadequate support to the nailbed. B. This results in a curved nail, evident when it is compared with the normal finger on the opposite hand.

burns, as in nightdress accidents or when the patient is trapped in a house fire.

Electrical[657,658]

The electric fire burn[659,660] is usually a largely *thermal* injury unless the device is inadequately earthed or incorrectly wired or the conductive nature of the patient has been increased in some way, for example, by standing wet and barefoot on a stone floor.

True electrical injuries are classified in two ways:

1. *AC* (alternating current)
   (a) systemic effects: severe, with ventricular fibrillation, respiratory arrest and death
   (b) local burn: often minor
   DC (direct current)
   (a) systemic effects: moderate, not life-threatening
   (b) local burn: severe
2. *Low voltage*, i.e. less than 1000 volts
   (a) systemic effects: immediate if AC; none later

   (b) local burn: relatively minor full-thickness
   High voltage, i.e. > 1000 volts; often from *high-tension* lines carrying up to 350 000, averaging 14 000, volts[661]
   (a) systemic effects: severe and sustained, including marked hypovolaemia, cardiac arrythmias and renal failure
   (b) local burns:
      (i) entry wound(s) — full-thickness, charred (Fig. 1.192)
      (ii) exit wound(s) — explosive, often larger
      (iii) arc burns, across joints — 4th degree, wrist, elbow, shoulder
      (iv) thermal burns — due to clothing lit by arc burns

Chemical

More than 25 000 industrial chemicals can cause burns[662]. The majority are treated successfully with copious water lavage followed by routine burn care. The most commonly encountered which are so treated are:

alkyl mercuric agents[663]	gasoline, hydrocarbons[671-673]
ammonia[664]	hydrochloric (muriatic) acid[668]
asphalt/tar[665]	lithium[668,669]
chromic acid[666]	lye (including sodium, calcium
cantharide[663]	and potassium hydroxides)[674]
cement[667]	nitric acid[668]
creosote[668]	potassium permanganate[668]
dichromate salts[663,669]	propane[675]
formic acid[670]	sulphuric acid[668]
freon[668]	trichloracetic acid[668]

Five other common sources of chemical burn require more customized management:

Hydrofluoric acid[674,676-679]. Widely used in industry for glass and metal cleaning, rust removal, silicon chip and glass etching and the production of fluorocarbons and high-octane fuels, burns are characterized by (i) deep, severe pain which may be delayed in onset, (ii) no apparent lesion at that stage, (iii) progressive skin necrosis, often subungual, progressing to bony erosion. The fluoride ion must be bound, initially by the application of calcium gluconate gel or calcium carbonate mixture[677]. If pain persists this is followed progressively by local injection of 10% calcium gluconate[678] and by intra-arterial infusion[679]. Observation is essential. Admission is required if any patient meets the following criteria:

1. 1% body surface exposure to a solution of >50%
2. 5% body surface exposure to any solution
3. inhalation of a 60% solution.

Phenol[668, 680]. Patients should be observed closely for several hours after wide exposure, even after removal

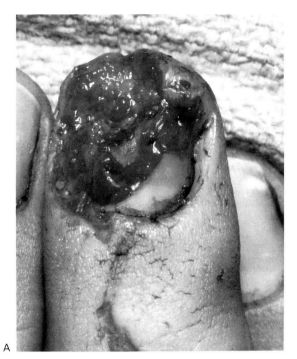

A

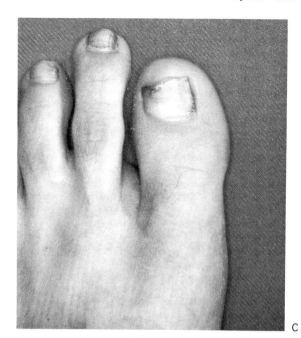

C

Fig. 1.190 Nailbed graft. A. The loss of nailbed shown was replaced with a split nailbed graft from the great toe with an acceptable result, both in the finger (B) and the toe (C).

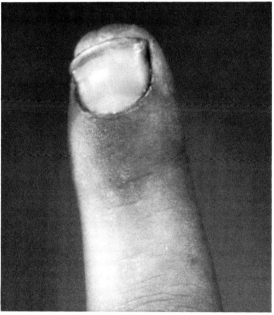

B

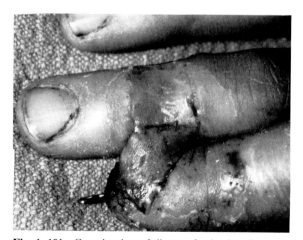

Fig. 1. 191 Complete loss of all cover for the dorsal aspect of distal phalanx can be treated with a de-epithelialized inverted cross-finger flap, subsequently split skin grafted.

by showering, as absorption may result in arrythmias, convulsions and collapse.

White phosphorus[681] ignites on exposure to air, which should be prevented by coating the involved area with mineral oil. The particles can be seen under a Wood's lamp and should be removed with that aid. (1% copper sulphate has been recommended, but absorption can result in haemolysis and renal failure — if used it should be washed off *immediately*.)

Elemental sodium and potassium[682] both *explode on contact with water.* The burns should be covered with mineral oil. The particles should then be removed, the

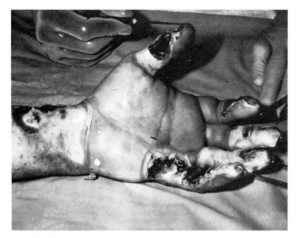

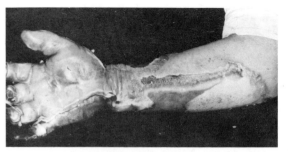

Fig. 1.193   This patient sustained a gross fourth-degree burn to his right hand from an open coal fire. He had no other burns and he proved to be an untreated epileptic who, at the time of injury, was also heavily intoxicated.

Fig. 1.192   The patient had sustained a high-voltage electrical burn, the point of entry being his non-dominant left hand. A fourth-degree injury has been sustained, the full-thickness loss evident at the wrist covering an area of destruction of superficial flexor tendons and the ulnar nerve and artery.

sodium placed in pure isopropyl alcohol, the potassium in tert-butyl alcohol.

Blast

Blast burns sustained in explosions commonly involve the face and hands. Although considerable oedema and crusting exudation ensue and can be alarming, these burns almost without exception are superficial second-degree. The significant aspect of blast injuries is the damage caused to the airway both internally and through the later development of neck oedema.

Epilepsy, intoxication and unconsciousness

A full-thickness localized burn may be sustained from a relatively low-temperature thermal source in the patient whose response to pain has been dulled or totally eliminated. This occurs in grand mal seizures, usually in undiagnosed or uncontrolled epileptics, in gross intoxication with alcohol or drugs and where injury or neuropathy has rendered the limb insensible (Fig. 1.193). More rarely such burns may occur where unconsciousness has arisen through other causes: head injury, cerebrovascular accident or circulatory collapse. As these patients require help in ways other than in the management of their burn, localized full-thickness thermal burns should always initiate more thorough investigation. If no systemic cause is present, then a local neurological deficit should be suspected and sought by examination.

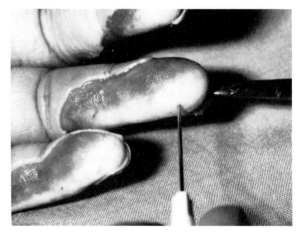

Fig. 1.194   A full-thickness third-degree burn does not bleed when stuck with a needle.

EXAMINATION

Degree

In all burns it has become the practice to classify the depth of skin destruction by degrees according to certain symptoms and signs. To some extent, this classification determines the line of treatment. These degrees are:

Degree	Appearance	Sensitivity	Graft
First *superficial*	Erythema	Hyperaesthetic	No
Second *partial-thickness*	Blistering	Hyperaesthetic	Sometimes (see below)
Third *full-thickness*	Hard, dry, waxy white	Anaesthetic	Yes

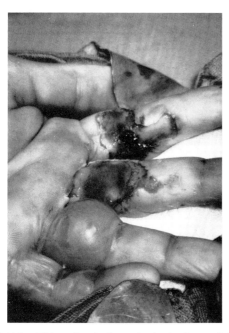

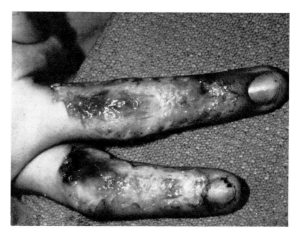

Fig. 1.196   An area of deep dermal burning treated by immediate excision and grafting.

Fig. 1.195   This patient had sustained mixed superficial second, deep dermal, and full-thickness burns. The blisters were debrided on the ring and small fingers and the burns on the index and middle excised and grafted.

The vascularity or otherwise of the skin can be demonstrated by the speed of capillary refilling after finger-tip pressure. In first- and second-degree burns, immediate refilling occurs, whereas in third-degree burns no change occurs either as a result of the pressure or of its release. Blood is present in the skin vessels of a third-degree burn which might cause some confusion on cursory examination, but this blood, like all the tissues of the skin in full-thickness burns, is coagulated and does not move with pressure. Neither does the finger bleed when stabbed with a needle (Fig. 1.194).

The classification laid out above is simple and fairly practical. However, like all simplifications it requires expansion.

1. *Second-degree burns.* It has become apparent that two distinct categories exist, having quite different implications as regards the eventual outcome (Fig. 1.195):
   (a) *Superficial partial-thickness.* Characterized by blistering and erythema, this burn is very sensitive to touch. Without complications, it will heal of its own accord leaving stable, mobile, non-hypertrophic and uncontracted skin.

(b) *Deep dermal.* Blistering is less marked and there may be some superficial coagulation and even loss of sensitivity (Fig. 1.196). Deep dermal burns are fairly pale. Pressure renders them even more pale over a wider area than in the superficial burn because of the tension already created by oedema. Sometimes a thin layer of redness persists due to very superficial intravascular coagulation. Although strictly partial-thickness, this burn has destroyed the major part of the skin and only the deep dermis and appendages remain alive. Healing will slowly ensue from these structures only provided that infection does not destroy them. Even then the resulting skin will be alternately thin and hypertrophic, relatively immobile and liable to crack and ulcerate and contract. While healing does occur, so that skin grafts are not essential, skin of such quality is quite unsuitable for satisfactory hand function. Early tangential excision and skin grafting are therefore desirable.

2. A category of *fourth-degree* has much to commend it to the hand surgeon. Since the three standard degrees of burn indicate only the depth of skin loss, and offer guidance only as to whether or not skin replacement will prove necessary, a fourth degree is helpful in distinguishing those cases in which structures of significance deep to the skin have been damaged by the burn injury.

By these criteria the distinction between superficial, partial-thickness, deep-dermal and full-thickness burns is more certainly made on the dorsum of the hand than

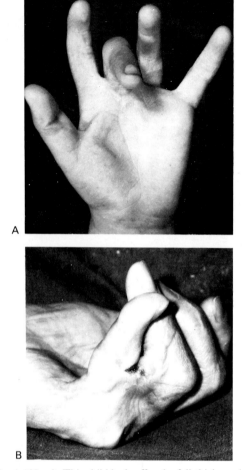

Fig. 1.197 A. This child had suffered a full-thickness burn of the palmar aspect of his middle finger which had been excised and covered with a split skin graft. At the time of examination, this was his maximum degree of extension. B. This patient sustained a full-thickness burn to the fourth web space.

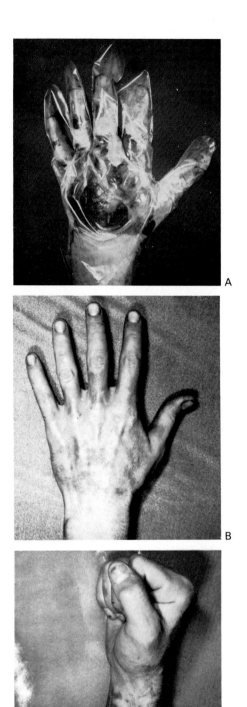

Fig. 1.198 A. The application of antibiotic ointment such as silver sulphadiazine, covered with plastic dressing gloves which can be bandaged at the wrist, permits full function while treating superficial second-degree burns. This results in rapid healing (B) with maintenance of full function (C).

it is on the palmar aspect. Splintage in correct posture (see below) and repeated examination are therefore more commonly employed than early surgery in burns of doubtful degree in the palm of the hand.

Extent
This should be carefully noted and can most efficiently be recorded on outline drawings of the hand. The area of burn should be broken up into the different regions with various degrees of burn depth, and this is usually done by distinctive cross-hatching on the diagram.

Posture

Oedema, inevitable in the burned hand, will be most apparent on the dorsum, but more significantly will also involve the periarticular structures. This results in the joints adopting the position in which the collateral ligaments are slack. Thus the metacarpophalangeal joints are straight and the interphalangeal joints flexed. Unless controlled by splintage and early motion, the ligaments will contract in this position causing fixed deformity.

In the fourth-degree burn of the distal palm due to electric bar radiator injuries, the metacarpophalangeal and proximal interphalangeal joints of all fingers are in equal fixed flexion of about 80°.

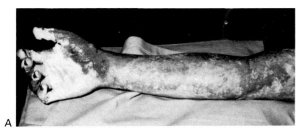

A

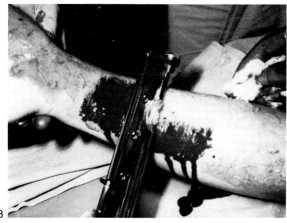

B

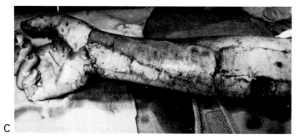

C

Fig. 1.199 Deep dermal burns (A) extending over a wide area should be tangentially excised (B) and immediately grafted with split-thickness skin (C).

Viability

The viability of digits distal to a burn should be checked by colour and circulatory return following expression of blood, especially useful in the nailbed. Doppler ultrasound may be required where skin is burned or macerated. The significance and timing of vascular impairment differs with the site and degree of the burn.

1. *Palm or digit, fourth-degree.* Immediate vascular embarrassment is not uncommon and indicates that both digital arteries have ceased to function. As the most *dorsal* of the vital structures on the *palmar* surface of the hand, this implies that both tendons and nerves have also been irretrievably destroyed. With this in mind, and considering that vascular repair would require the use of a vein graft beneath a flap, salvage of the digit is an impractical proposition.
2. *Forearm, third-degree.* Late vascular embarrassment in the hand may well occur, especially if the burn is circumferential. The mechanism and treatment is that of a compartment syndrome (p. 40). Oedema in the forearm beneath the unyielding eschar occludes the arterial inflow after a period of increasing venous congestion. The process can be arrested by slitting the eschar through its full thickness longitudinally until circulation is re-established. Every effort should be made to avoid exposing vital structures in the escharotomy wound as they are likely to become dessicated and die.

INDICATIONS

Will skin cover be required? If so, of what type? Skin cover is mandatory in all hand burns except first-degree and superficial second-degree, that is, the erythematous and the blistered burns. Split skin grafts will be used after early tangential excision of the deep dermal burn. In small areas of full-thickness loss split skin will probably subsequently contract to an unacceptable degree in regions of functional significance such as the palmar surface of the digits, and in the web spaces (Fig. 1.197). Full-thickness skin grafts are preferable but have a higher risk of poor 'take' when used acutely. Grafts will not take where bare tendons or bone are exposed by the burn. Primary skin flaps are then required, which can often be transposed from the lateral aspect of the same digit.

What deep structures are damaged? Electrical burns, the hook posture, skin charring, loss of digital viability, of sensation, and of movement all indicate injury to deep structures.

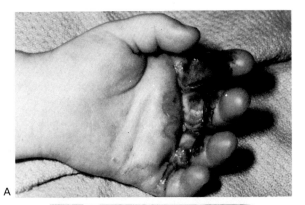

A

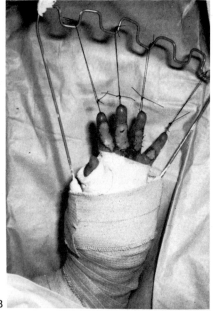

B

Fig. 1.200 Full-thickness electrical burns of the palmar aspect of the fingers in a child (A) should be excised immediately and grafted with full-thickness skin (B).

commence immediate motion. This is facilitated by applying antibiotic cream and then covering the hands with only a loose plastic disposable glove[683] (Fig. 1.198). Elevation and splintage is important between periods of exercise.

Spontaneous separation of dead tissue may take several weeks, and for this reason primary excision of

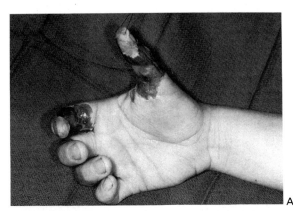

A

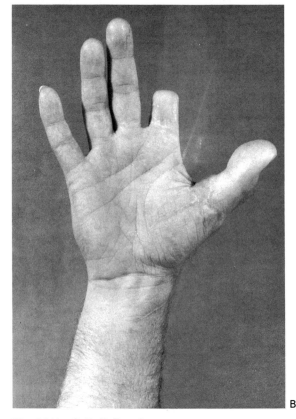

B

Fig. 1.201 C, D, E, F con't on next page.

What immediate treatment is appropriate? The best *posture* of the hand should be sought from the outset. That is, the wrist should be dorsiflexed, the metacarpophalangeal joints should be flexed as close to 90° as possible and the interphalangeal joints splinted in 20° of flexion. The collateral ligaments are so held taut and contraction is prevented. This position is very difficult to maintain in the burned hand. The use of Kirschner wires driven through the metacarpal head into the proximal phalanx has been found to hold the correct position most effectively without complication.

The alternative course, more applicable in more superficial and therefore less oedematous burns, is to

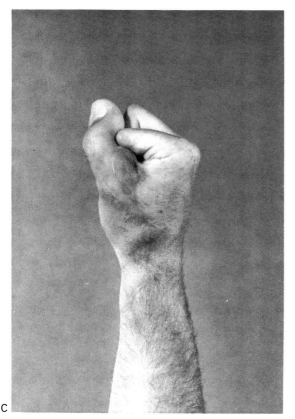

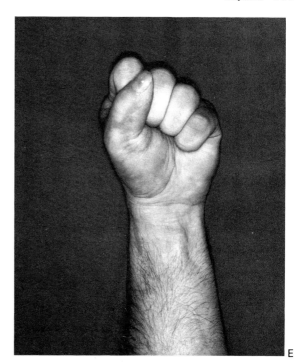

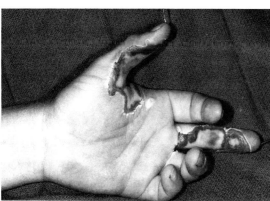

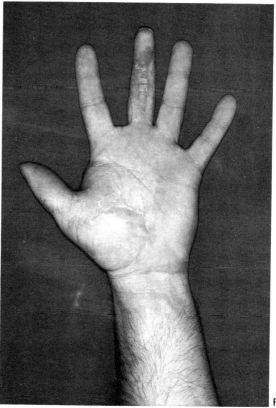

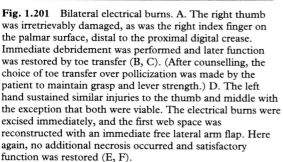

Fig. 1.201 Bilateral electrical burns. A. The right thumb was irretrievably damaged, as was the right index finger on the palmar surface, distal to the proximal digital crease. Immediate debridement was performed and later function was restored by toe transfer (B, C). (After counselling, the choice of toe transfer over pollicization was made by the patient to maintain grasp and lever strength.) D. The left hand sustained similar injuries to the thumb and middle with the exception that both were viable. The electrical burns were excised immediately, and the first web space was reconstructed with an immediate free lateral arm flap. Here again, no additional necrosis occurred and satisfactory function was restored (E, F).

hand burns is recommended. It is certainly indicated as follows:

(i) tangential excision of deep dermal burns of the dorsum with immediate grafting[684-687] (Fig. 1.199)
(ii) full-thickness excision of localized full-thickness burns with immediate or delayed grafting or flap cover (Fig. 1.200)
(iii) full-thickness excision of electrical burns, with preservation of intact tendons and nerves with immediate free flap application[688] (Fig. 1.201).

Electrical burns present similar problems to crush injuries, for tissues initially thought to be viable may subsequently die, resulting in loss of grafts applied to an apparently satisfactory bed. Repeated excision with trial homografts or heterografts has been recommended by some, and early flap cover has been recommended by others. The author has been impressed by the frustrations of the former and the relatively trouble-free healing obtained with early application of a flap (Fig. 1.201D, E, F).

In fourth-degree burns, nerves and tendons in continuity and apparently involved by burn should not be excised as they often, surprisingly, show later function.

Escharotomy[689-691] should be considered in all third- and fourth-degree burns. The burn need *not be* circumferential for it to produce hazardous compression, since oedema in association with a significant burn can produce a tourniquet effect. Any distal circulatory or sensory changes, or pain unrelieved by analgesics, should alert the surgeon to the need for decompression. As with fasciotomy — which should often be performed in conjunction with the escharotomy – if *any* indication exists, escharotomy should be undertaken.

See Green D P 1993 Operative Hand Surgery, 3rd edn. Churchill Livingstone, New York, p. 2007.

Frostbite[692,693]

Frostbite results from exposure to cold. The rapidity of onset and severity of injury are influenced by the intensity of the cold, wind velocity, the duration of exposure, wetness of the part, or immobility, which may result from sleep, inebriation or wounds. Any factors which reduce circulation will clearly increase the damage, including chronic cigarette smoking, vascular disease or constrictive clothing.

The pathological process involves extreme vasoconstriction with a rapid drop in temperature of the part even to the point of tissue freezing, with ice crystals forming in living tissues. This is the *first phase* of cold injury. Rewarming results in hyperaemia due to increased blood flow, but this is through vessels damaged

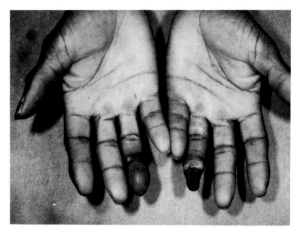

Fig. 1.202 Frosbite with some residual blister formation and frank necrosis.

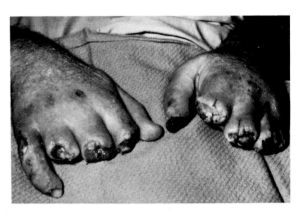

Fig. 1.203 Amputation some four weeks after frostbite injury to both upper extremities.

to a varied degree so that oedema, haemoconcentration, intravascular thrombosis and increased sympathetic tone produce vasoconstriction. This may cause loss of a part apparently well-perfused — the *second phase.*

Four degrees of frostbite have been described which correspond to the four degrees of burn:

1st — numbness, oedema, erythema
2nd — blistering
3rd — bluish-grey oedema (develops after the hyperaemic phase)
4th — cold, cyanotic, anaesthetic with *no* hyperaemic phase.

One of the major problems in frostbite is recognition of the various degrees. Another is that several, or all degrees may be present simultaneously in the same digit, being worse peripherally, improving the more proximal the part (Fig. 1.202). Loss of those portions of the digit with third- and fourth-degree changes is inevitable (Fig. 1.203). A simple classification has been proposed in which *superficial frostbite* implies skin damage only, and *deep* involves damage to deeper structures. The late effects of frostbite may be due to sympathetic overactivity and are similar to established sympathetic dystrophy — pain, discoloration, oedema and sweating. Children, even those apparently only mildly affected, may nonetheless show early epiphyseal closure[694].

INDICATIONS

Rapid rewarming in a whirlpool at 42°C is required, with appropriate analgesia for the often severe pain which will accompany this process. If hyperaemia does not result, intra-arterial reserpine, stellate ganglion block or immediate sympathectomy may reduce the area of tissue damage. Aspirin, urokinase[695] and low-molecular-weight dextran may reduce intra-vascular coagulation and improve flow. Control of treatment by use of the Doppler flowmeter and digital plethysmography (PVR)[696] and by analysis of blister fluid[697] may prove of value in the future. Conservation should be the theme with respect to the local injury which is too ill-defined for any other course, digits being left untouched for as long as two to three months. The late effects are greatly helped by sympathectomy.

See Green D P 1993 Operative Hand Surgery, 3rd edn. Churchill Livingstone, New York, p. 2033.

REFERENCES

1. Kelsey J L, Pastides H, Kreiger M, Harris C, Chernow R A 1980 Upper extremity disorders: a survey of their frequency and cost in the United States. C V Mosby, St Louis
2. Blair S J 1991 Prevention of occupational hand injuries. In: Kasdan M L (ed) Occupational hand and upper extremity injuries and diseases. Hanley & Belfus, Philadelphia
3. Committee on Injury Scaling. 1985 The abbreviated injury scale 1985 revision. American Association for Automotive Medicine, Morton Grove, IL
4. MacKenzie F J, Shapiro S, Siegel I 1988 The economic impact of traumatic injuries. JAMA 260: 3290–3296
5. Sanguinetti M V 1977 Reconstructive surgery of roller injuries of the hand. J Hand Surgery 2: 134–140
6. Strahan J, Crockett D J 1969 Wringer injury. Injury 1: 57
7. Justis E J, Moore S V, LaVelle D G 1987 Woodworking injuries: an epidemiologic survey of injuries sustained using woodworking machinery and hand tools. J Hand Surg (Am) 12: 890–895
8. Schwager R G, Smith J W, Goulian D 1975 Small deep forearm lacerations. Plastic Reconstr Surg 55: 190–194
9. Joseph K N, Kalus A M, Sutherland A B 1981 Glass injuries of the hand in children. Hand 13: 113–119
10. Sharrard W J W 1968 Injection injuries. J Bone Joint Surg 50B: 1
11. Elstrom J A, Pankovich A M, Egwele R 1978 Extra-articular low-velocity gunshot fractures of the radius and ulna. J Bone Joint Surg 60A: 335–341
12. Elton R C 1975 Gunshot and fragment wounds of the hand. Contemp Surg 7: 13–18
13. Luce E A, Griffen W 1978 Shotgun injuries of the upper extremity. J Trauma 18: 487–492
14. Marcus N A, Blair W F, Shuck J M, Omer G E 1980 Low-velocity gun-shot wounds to extremities. J Trauma 20: 1061–1064
15. Shepard G H 1980 High-energy, low-velocity, close-range shotgun wounds. J Trauma 20: 1065–1067
16. Robinson D W, Hardin C A 1955 Corn picker injuries. Am J Surg 89: 780–783
17. Campbell D C, Bryan R S, Cooney W P, Ilstrup D 1979 Mechanical cornpicker hand injuries. J Trauma 19: 678–681
18. Gorsche T S, Wood M B 1988 Mutilating corn-picker injuries of the hand. J Hand Surg (Am) 13: 423–427
19. Grogono B J S 1973 Auger injuries. Injury 4: 247–257
20. Beatty M E, Zook E G, Russell R C, Kinkead L R 1982 Grain auger injuries: The replacement of the corn picker injury? Plastic Reconstr Surg 69: 96–102
21. Jazheimer E C, Morain W D, Brown F E 1981 Woodsplitter injuries of the hand. Plastic Reconstr Surg 68: 83–88
22. Hellstrand P H 1989 Injuries caused by firewood splitting machines. Scand J Plastic Reconstr Surg Hand Surg 23: 51–54
23. Smith J R, Asturias J 1968 Card injury of the hand: its characteristics and treatment. J Bone Joint Surg 50A: 1161–1170
24. Barry T P, Linton P 1977 Biophysics of rotary mower and snowblower injuries of the hand: high vs. low velocity 'missile' injury. J Trauma 17: 214–221
25. Almdahl S M, Saebe-Larsen J, Due J Jr 1989 Injuries to the hand inflicted by rotary snowcutters. J Trauma 29: 227–228
26. Millea T P, Hansen R H 1989 Snowblower injuries to the hand. J Trauma 29: 229–233
27. Ross P M, Schwentker E P, Bryan H 1976 Mutilating lawnmower injuries in children. J Am Med Assoc 236: 408
28. Johnstone B R, Bennett C S 1989 Lawnmower injuries in children. Aust NZ J Surg 59: 713–718
29. McGregor I A, Jackson I T 1969 Sodium chlorate bomb injuries of the hand. Br J Plastic Surg 22: 16–29
30. Reid D A C 1973 Escalator injuries of the hand. Injury 5: 47
31. Charters A C, Davis J W 1978 The roll-bar hand. J Trauma 18: 601–604

32. Harris C, Wood V 1978 Rollover injuries of the upper extremity. J Trauma 18: 605–607
33. Mehrotra O N, Crabb D J M 1979 The pattern of hand injuries sustained in the overturning motor vehicle. Hand 11: 321–328
34. Heycock M H 1966 On the management of hand injuries caused by woodworking tools. Br J Plastic Surg 19: 58
35. Caldwell E H, McCormack R M 1980 Acute radiation injury of the hands: report on a case with a twenty-one year follow-up. J Hand Surg 5: 568–571
36. Ciano M, Burlin J R, Pardoe R, Mills R L, Hentz V R 1981 High-frequency electromagnetic radiation injury to the upper extremity: local and systemic effects. Ann Plastic Surg 7: 128–135
37. McCabe W P, Ditmars D M 1973 Soft tissue changes in the hands of drug addicts. Plastic Reconstr Surg 52: 538–540
38. McKay D, Pascarelli E F, Eaton R G 1973 Infections and sloughs in the hands in drug addicts. J Bone Joint Surg 55A: 741–746
39. Neviaser R J, Butterfield W C, Wiechi D R 1972 The puffy hand of drug addiction. A study of the pathogenesis. J Bone Joint Surg 54A: 629–633
40. Ryan J J, Hoopes J E, Jabaley M E 1974 Drug injection injuries of the hands and forearms in addicts. Plastic Reconstr Surg 53: 445–451
41. Snyder C C, Straight R, Glenn J 1972 The snakebitten hand. Plastic Reconstr Surg 49: 275–282
42. Marten E 1979 Hand deformities in patients with snakebite. Plastic Reconstr Surg 64: 554
43. Huang T T, Blackwell S J, Lewis S R 1978 Hand deformities in patients with snakebite. Plastic Reconstr Surg 62: 32–36
44. Grace T G, Omer G E 1980 The management of upper extremity pit viper wounds. J Hand Surg 5: 168–177
45. Rees R, Shack R B, Withers E, Madden J, Franklin J, Lynch J B 1981 Management of the brown recluse spider bite. Plastic Reconstr Surg 68: 768–773
46. Zeichner D M, Hoehn J G 1981 Karate-induced hand injuries. Orthopaedic Rev 10: 127–131
47. McLatchie G R, Davies J E, Caulley J H 1980 Injuries in karate — a case for medical control. J Trauma 20: 956–958
48. Nieman E A, Swann P G 1977 Karate injuries. Br Med J 223
49. Curtin J, Kay N R M 1976 Hand injuries due to soccer. Hand 8: 93–95
50. Al-Arabi K M, Sabet N A 1984 Severe mincer injuries of the hand in children in Saudi Arabia. J Hand Surg (Br) 9: 249–250
51. Viegas S F, O'Meara C 1986 Hand injuries from shrimp boat winches. J Trauma 26: 851–853
52. Kirwan L A, Scott F A 1988 Roping injuries in the hand: mechanism of injury and functional results. Plastic Reconstr Surg 81: 54–61
53. Morgan R F, Nichter L S, Friedman H I, McCue F C 3rd 1984 Rodeo roping thumb injuries. J Hand Surg (Am) 9: 178–180
54. Lesavoy M A, Meals R A 1984 Pay phone receiver cord injuries to the hand. J Hand Surg (Am) 9: 908–909
55. Dickason W L, Barutt J P 1984 Investigation of an acute microwave-oven hand injury. J Hand Surg (Am) 9A: 132–135
56. Green J, Harzinder K, Leon-Barth C A, Hamm A 1989 Microwave hand injury. Contemp Orthopaedics 19: 564–566
57. Nicholson C P, Grotting J C, Dimick A R 1987 Acute microwave injury to the hand. J Hand Surg (Am) 12: 446–449
58. Mitchell G M, Morrison W A, Papadopoulos A et al 1985 A study of the extent and pathology of experimental avulsion injury in rabbit arteries and veins. Br J Plastic Surg 38: 278
59. Chick L R, Lister G D 1991 Emergency management of thermal, electrical, and chemical burns. In: Kasdan M L (ed) Occupational hand and upper extremity injuries and diseases. Hanley & Belfus, Philadelphia
60. Chiu H Y, Chen M T 1984 Revascularization of digits after thirty-three hours of warm ischemia time: a case report. J Hand Surg (Am) 9A: 63–67
61. Frey M, Mandl H, Holle J 1980 Secondary operations after replantations. Chirurgia Plastica 5: 235–241
62. Gelberman R, Urbaniak J, Bright D, Levin L S 1978 Digital sensibility following replantation. J Hand Surg 3: 313–319
63. Kleinert H E, Jablon M, Tsai T 1980 An overview of replantation and results of 347 replants in 245 patients. J Trauma 20: 390–398
64. Morrison W, O'Brien B, MacLeod A 1978 Digital replantation and revascularization. A long-term review of one hundred cases. Hand 10: 125–134
65. Scott F A, Howar J W, Boswick J A 1981 Recovery of function following replantation and revascularization of amputated hand parts. J Trauma 21: 204–214
66. Blomgren I, Blomqvist G, Ejeskar A, Fogdestam I et al 1988 Hand function after replantation or revascularization of upper extremity injuries. A follow-up of 21 cases operated on 1979–1985 in Goteborg, Sweden. Scand J Plastic Reconstr Surg Hand Surg 22: 93–101
67. Koman L A, Nunley J A 1986 Thermoregulatory control after upper extremity replantation. J Hand Surg (Am) 11: 548–552
68. Yamauchi S, Nomura S, Yoshimura M, Ueno T et al 1983 A clinical study of the order and speed of sensory recovery after digital replantation. J Hand Surg (Am) 8: 545
69. Goldner R D, Fitch R D, Nunley J A, Aitken M S, Urbaniak J R 1987 Demographics and replantation. J Hand Surg (Am) 12: 961–965
70. Lister G D 1991 Replantation. In: Smith J W, Aston S J (eds) Grabb & Smith's plastic surgery, 4th edn. Little, Brown and Company, Boston, pp 1079–1112
71. Kaplan's functional and surgical anatomy of the hand. 3rd edn. 1984 Spinner M (ed). Lippincott, Philadelphia
72. Guyon F 1861 Note sur une disposition anatomique propre a la face anterieure de la region du poignet et non encore decrite. Bull Society Anat Paris 36: 184–186
73. Denman E E 1978 The anatomy of the space of Guyon. Hand 10: 69–76
74. McFarlane R M, Mayer J R, Hugill J V 1976 Further observations on the anatomy of the ulnar nerve at the wrist. Hand 8: 115–117
75. Lassa R, Shrewsbury M 1975 A variation in the path of the deep motor branch of the ulnar nerve at the wrist. J Bone Joint Surg 57A: 990–991

76. Engber W D, Gmeiner J G 1980 Palmar cutaneous branch of the ulnar nerve. J Hand Surg 5: 26–29

77. Coleman S S, Anson B J 1961 Arterial patterns in the hand based on a study of 650 specimens. Surg Gynecol Obstet 113: 409–424

78. Ikeda A, Ugawa A, Kazihara Y, Hamada N 1988 Arterial patterns in the hand based on a three-dimensional analysis of 220 cadaver hands. J Hand Surg (Am) 13: 501–509

79. Graham W P III 1973 Variations of the motor branch of the median nerve at the wrist. Plastic Reconstr Surg 51: 90–91

80. Lanz U 1977 Anatomical variations of the median nerve in the carpal tunnel. J Hand Surg 2: 44–53

81. Taleisnik J 1973 The palmar cutaneous branch of the median nerve and the approach to the carpal tunnel. J Bone Joint Surg 55A: 1212–1217

82. Hobbs R A, Magnussen P A, Tonkin M A 1990 Palmar cutaneous branch of the median nerve. J Hand Surg 15A: 38–43

83. Meals R A, Shaner M 1983 Variations in digital sensory patterns: a study of the ulnar nerve–median nerve palmar communicating branch. J Hand Surg (Am) 8: 411–414

84. Taleisnik J, Gelberman R H, Miller B W, Szabo R M 1984 The extensor retinaculum of the wrist. J Hand Surg (Am) 9: 495–501

85. Cusenz B J, Hallock G G 1986 Multiple anomalous tendons of the fourth dorsal compartment. J Hand Surg (Am) 11: 263–264

86. Leslie B M, Ericson W B Jr, Morehead J R 1990 Incidence of a septum within the first dorsal compartment of the wrist. J Hand Surg (Am) 15: 88–91

87. Patel M R, Desai S S 1988 Anomalous muscles of the first dorsal compartment of the wrist. J Hand Surg (Am) 13: 829–831

88. Steichen J B, Petersen D P 1984 Junctura tendinum between extensor digitorum communis and extensor pollicis longus. J Hand Surg (Am) 9: 674–676

89. Barfred T, Adamsen S 1986 Duplication of the extensor carpi ulnaris tendon. J Hand Surg (Am) 11: 423–425

90. McGregor I A, Glover L 1988 The E-flat hand. J Hand Surg (Am) 13: 692–693

91. Wood V E 1988 The extensor carpi radialis intermedius tendon. J Hand Surg (Am) 13: 242–245

92. Strauch B, de Moura W 1990 Arterial system of the fingers. J Hand Surg (Am) 15: 148–154

93. Brand P W, Cranor K C, Ellis J C 1975 Tendon and pulleys at the metacarpophalangeal joint of a finger. J Bone Joint Surg 57A: 779–783

94. Chuinard R G, Friermood T G, Lipscomb P R 1979 The 'suicide' wrist: epidemiologic study of the injury. Orthopaedics 2: 499–502

95. Argenta L C, Duus E C, Lane G A 1983 Carotid injury and cerebral infarction in a revascularization hand injury case. J Hand Surg (Am) 8: 935–937

96. Wei F C, Chuang C C, Chen H C, Tsai Y C, Noordhoff M S 1984 Ten-digit replantation. Plastic Reconstr Surg 74: 826–832

97. Van Alphen W A, Smith A R, ten Kate F J 1988 Maximum hypothermic ischemia in replants containing muscular tissue. J Hand Surg (Am) 13: 415–422

98. Goldner R D, Stevanovic M V, Nunley J A, Urbaniak J R 1989 Digital replantation at the level of the distal interphalangeal joint and the distal phalanx. J Hand Surg (Am) 14: 214–220

99. Yamano T 1985 Replantation of the amputated distal part of the fingers. J Hand Surg (Am) 10: 211–218

100. Nunley J A, Spiegl P V, Goldner R D, Urbaniak J R 1987 Longitudinal epiphyseal growth after replantation and transplantation in children. J Hand Surg (Am) 12: 274–279

101. Bieber E J, Wood M B, Cooney W P, Amadio P C 1987 Thumb avulsion: results of replantation/revascularization. J Hand Surg (Am) 12: 786–790

102. Carroll R 1974 Ring injuries in the hand. Clin Orthopaedics 104: 175–182

103. Urbaniak J R, Evans J P, Bright D S 1981 Microvascular management of ring avulsion injuries. J Hand Surg 6: 25–30

104. Nissenbaum M 1984 Class IIA ring avulsion injuries: an absolute indication for microvascular repair. J Hand Surg (Am) 9: 810–815

105. Weil D J, Wood V E, Frykman G K 1989 A new class of ring avulsion injuries. J Hand Surg (Am) 14: 662–664

106. Kay S, Werntz J, Wolff T W 1989 Ring avulsion injuries: classification and prognosis. J Hand Surg (Am) 14: 204–213

107. Tsai T M, Manstein C, DuBou R, Wolff T W et al 1984 Primary microsurgical repair of ring avulsion amputation injuries. J Hand Surg (Am) 9A: 68–72

108. Ferraiouli E B 1968 Repair of the disrupted flexor mechanism of the hand. Asoc Med Puerto Rico Bol 60: 11–16

109. Apley A G 1956 Test of the power of flexor digitorum sublimis. Br Med J 1: 25–26

110. Baker D S, Gaul S, Williams V K, Graves M 1981 The little finger superficialis — clinical investigation of its anatomic and functional shortcomings. J Hand Surg 6: 374–378

111. Austin G J, Leslie B M, Ruby L K 1989 Variations of the flexor digitorum superficialis of the small finger. J Hand Surg (Am) 14: 262–267

112. Kaplan E B 1969 Muscular and tendinous variations of the flexor superficialis of the fifth finger of the hand. Bull Hosp Joint Dis 30: 59

113. Kisner W H 1980 Double sublimis tendon to fifth finger with absence of profundus. Plastic Reconstr Surg 65: 229–230

114. Walker L G, Lesavoy M A 1990 Traumatic rupture of the profundus tendon proximal to the lumbrical origin. J Hand Surg (Am) 15: 484–486

115. Kumar S, James R 1985 Closed rupture of flexor profundus tendon in the palm. J Hand Surg (Br) 10: 193–194

116. Lillmars S A, Bush D C 1988 Flexor tendon rupture associated with an anomalous muscle. J Hand Surg (Am) 13: 115–119

117. Imbriglia J E, Goldstein S A 1987 Intratendinous ruptures of the flexor digitorum profundus tendon of the small finger. J Hand Surg (Am) 12: 985–991

118. Bynum D K Jr, Gilbert J A 1988 Avulsion of the flexor digitorum profundus: anatomic and biomechanical considerations. J Hand Surg (Am) 13: 222–227

119. Manske P R, Lesker P A 1978 Avulsion of the ring finger flexor digitorum profundus tendon. Hand 10: 52–55

120. Ogunro O 1983 Avulsion of flexor profundus, secondary to enchondroma of the distal phalanx. J Hand Surg (Am) 8: 315–316
121. Langa V, Posner M A 1986 Unusual rupture of a flexor profundus tendon. J Hand Surg (Am) 11: 227–229
122. Gordon L, Monsanto E H 1987 Acute vascular compromise after avulsion of the distal phalanx with the flexor digitorum profundus tendon. J Hand Surg (Am) 12: 259–261
123. Gibson C T, Manske P R 1987 Isolated avulsion of a flexor digitorum superficialis tendon insertion. J Hand Surg (Am) 12: 601–602
124. Chang W H J, Thoms O J, White W L 1972 Avulsion injury of the long flexor tendons. Plastic Reconstr Surg 50: 260–264
125. Leddy J P, Packer J W 1977 Avulsion of the profundus tendon insertion in athletes. J Hand Surg 2: 66–69
126. Stahl S, Wolff T W 1988 Delayed rupture of the extensor pollicis longus tendon after nonunion of a fracture of the dorsal radial tubercle. J Hand Surg (Am) 13: 338–341
127. Denman E 1979 Rupture of the extensor pollicis longus — a crush injury. Hand 11: 295–298
128. Simpson R G 1977 Delayed rupture of extensor pollicis longus tendon following closed injury. Hand 9: 160–161
129. Engkvist O, Lundborg U, Lundborg G 1979 Rupture of the extensor pollicis longus tendon after fracture of the lower end of the radius. A clinical and microangiographic study. Hand 11: 76–86
130. Mackay I, Simpson R G 1980 Closed rupture of extensor digitorum communis tendon following fracture of the radius. Hand 12: 214–216
131. Sadr B 1984 Sequential rupture of extensor tendons after a Colles fracture. J Hand Surg (Am) 9A: 144–145
132. Southmayd W W, Millender L H, Nalebuff E A 1975 Rupture of the flexor tendons of the index finger after Colles' fracture. J Bone Joint Surg 57A: 562–563
133. Younger C P, DeFiore J C 1977 Rupture of flexor tendons to the fingers after a Colles fracture. Case report. J Bone Joint Surg 59A: 828–829
134. Rosenfeld N, Rascoff J H 1980 Tendon ruptures of the hand associated with renal dialysis. Plastic Reconstr Surg 65: 77–79
135. Siegel D, Gebhardt M, Jupiter J B 1987 Spontaneous rupture of the extensor pollicis longus tendon. J Hand Surg (Am) 12: 1106–1109
136. Carducci A T 1981 Potential boutonniere deformity — its recognition and treatment. Orthopaedic Rev 10: 121–123
137. Furnas D, Spinner M 1978 The 'sign of horns' in the diagnosis of injury or disease of the extensor digitorum communis of the hand. Br J Plastic Surg 31: 263–265
138. Itoh Y, Horiuchi Y, Takahashi M, Uchinishi K, Yabe Y 1987 Extensor tendon involvement in Smith's and Galeazzi's fractures. J Hand Surg (Am) 12: 535–540
139. Kettelkamp D B, Flatt A E, Moulds R 1971 Traumatic dislocation of the long finger extensor tendon. A clinical anatomical and biomechanical study. J Bone Joint Surg 53A: 229–240
140. Albright J A, Linburg R M 1978 Common variations of the radial wrist extensors. J Hand Surg 3: 134–138
141. Lubahn J D 1989 Mallet finger fractures: a comparison of open and closed technique. Hand Surg (Am) 14: 394–396
142. Crawford G P 1984 The molded polythene splint for mallet finger deformities. J Hand Surg (Am) 9: 231–237
143. Miura T, Nakamura R, Torii S 1986 Conservative treatment for a ruptured extensor tendon on the dorsum of the proximal phalanges of the thumb (mallet thumb). J Hand Surg (Am) 11: 229–233
144. Patel M R, Lipson L B, Desai SS 1986 Conservative treatment of mallet thumb. J Hand Surg (Am) 11: 45–47
145. Rayan G M, Mullins P T 1987 Skin necrosis complicating mallet finger splinting and vascularity of the distal interphalangeal joint overlying skin. J Hand Surg (Am) 12: 548–552
146. Stern P J, Kastrup J J 1988 Complications and prognosis of treatment of mallet finger. J Hand Surg (Am) 13: 329–334
147. Ritts G D, Wood M B, Engber W D 1985 Nonoperative treatment of traumatic dislocations of the extensor digitorum tendons in patients without rheumatoid disorders. J Hand Surg (Am) 10: 714–716
148. Carroll C 4th, Moore J R, Weiland A J 1987 Posttraumatic ulnar subluxation of the extensor tendons: a reconstructive technique. J Hand Surg (Am) 12: 227–231
149. Saldana M J, McGuire R A 1986 Chronic painful subluxation of the metacarpal phalangeal joint extensor tendons. J Hand Surg (Am) 11: 420–423
150. Magnell T D, Pochron M D, Condit D P 1988 The intercalated tendon graft for treatment of extensor pollicis longus tendon rupture. J Hand Surg (Am) 13: 105–109
151. Matsen F A 1980 Compartmental syndromes. Grune & Stratton, New York
152. Volkmann R 1967 Die ischaemischen muskellahmugen und-kontrakturen. Centrabl F Chir (translation by Edgar Bick). Clin Orthopedics 50: 5–6
153. Sarokhan A J, Eaton R G 1983 Volkmann's ischemia. J Hand Surg (Am) 8: 806–809
154. Garfin S R, Mubarak S J, Evans K L, Hargens A R, Akeson W H 1981 Quantification of intracompartmental pressure and volume under plaster casts. J Bone Joint Surg 63A: 449–453
155. Zweifach S S, Hargens A R, Evans K L, Smith R K, Mubarak S J, Akeson W H 1980 Skeletal muscle necrosis in pressurized compartments associated with haemorrhagic hypotension. J Trauma 20: 941–947
156. O'Neil D, Sheppard J E 1989 Transient compartment syndrome of the forearm resulting from venous congestion from a tourniquet. J Hand Surg (Am) 14: 894–896
157. Hastings H 2nd, Misamore G 1987 Compartment syndrome resulting from intravenous regional anesthesia. J Hand Surg (Am) 12: 559–562
158. Trumble T 1987 Forearm compartment syndrome secondary to leukemic infiltrates. J Hand Surg (Am) 12: 563–565
159. Joseph F R, Posner M A, Terzakis J A 1984 Compartment syndrome caused by a traumatized vascular hamartoma. J Hand Surg (Am) 9: 904–907
160. Hung L K, Kinninmonth A W, Woo M L 1988 Vibrio vulnificus necrotizing fasciitis presenting with

compartmental syndrome of the hand. J Hand Surg (Br) 13: 337–339

161. Imbriglia J E, Boland D M 1984 An exercise-induced compartment syndrome of the dorsal forearm — a case report. J Hand Surg (Am) 9A: 142–143

162. Halpern A, Mochizuki R M 1980 Compartment syndrome of the interosseous muscles of the hand. Orthopaedic Rev 9: 121–127

163. Spinner M, Aiache A, Silver L, Barsky A S 1973 Impending ischemic contracture of the hand. Plastic Reconstr Surg 50: 341–349

164. Matsen F A, Winquist R A, Krugmire R B 1980 Diagnosis and management of compartmental syndromes. J Bone Joint Surg 62A: 286–291

165. Mubarak S J, Owen C A, Hargens A R, Garetto L P, Enneking W F 1978 Acute compartment syndromes. Diagnosis and treatment with the aid of the wick catheter. J Bone Joint Surg 60A: 1091–1099

166. Bingold A C 1979 On splitting plasters. J Bone Joint Surg 61B: 294–295

167. Wolfort F G, Cochran T C, Filtzer H 1973 Immediate interossei decompression following crush injury of the hand. Arch Surg 106: 826–828

168. Holden C E A 1979 The pathology and prevention of Volkmann's ischaemic contracture. J Bone Joint Surg 61B: 296–300

169. Sunderland S 1978 Nerves and nerve injuries, 2nd edn. Churchill Livingstone, Edinburgh

170. Seddon Sir H J 1972 Surgical disorders of peripheral nerves. Williams & Wilkins, Baltimore

171. Dellon A L 1978 The moving two-point discrimination test: clinical evaluation of the quickly adapting fiber/receptor system. J Hand Surg 3: 474–481

172. Weber E H 1835 Ueber den Tastsinn. Arch Anat Physiol Wissenischs Med 3: 152–160

173. Moberg E 1964 Evaluation and management of nerve injuries in the hand. Surg Clin North Am 44: 1019

174. Mackinnon S E, Dellon A L 1985 Two-point discrimination tester. J Hand Surg (Am) 10: 906–907

175. Dellon A L, Mackinnon S E, Crosby P M 1987 Reliability of two-point discrimination measurements. J Hand Surg (Am) 12: 693–696

176. Louis D S, Greene T L, Jacobson K E, Rasmussen C et al 1984 Evaluation of normal values for stationary and moving two-point discrimination in the hand. J Hand Surg (Am) 9: 552–555

177. Learmonth J R 1919 A variation in the distribution of the radial branch of the musculo-spiral nerve. J Anat Physiol 53: 371–372

178. Mackinnon S E, Dellon A L 1985 The overlap pattern of the lateral antebrachial cutaneous nerve and the superficial branch of the radial nerve. J Hand Surg (Am) 10: 522–526

179. Gwathmey F W, House J H 1984 Clinical manifestations of congenital insensitivity of the hand and classification of syndromes. J Hand Surg (Am) 9: 863–869

180. Parker R D, Froimson A I 1986 Neurogenic arthropathy of the hand and wrist. J Hand Surg (Am) 11: 706–710

181. Earle A S, Vlastou C 1980 Crossed fingers and other tests of ulnar nerve motor function. J Hand Surg 5: 560–565

182. Martin D F, Tolo V T, Sellers D S, Weiland A J 1989 Radial nerve laceration and retraction associated with a supracondylar fracture of the humerus. J Hand Surg (Am) 14: 542–545

183. Gelberman T H, Menon J, Fronek A 1980 The peripheral pulse following arterial injury. J Trauma 20: 948–950

184. Adar R, Schramek A, Khodadadi J, Zweig A, Golcman L, Romanoff H 1980 Arterial combat injuries of the upper extremity. J Trauma 20: 297–302

185. Lord R S A, Irani C N 1974 Assessment of arterial injury in limb trauma. J Trauma 14: 1042–1053

186. Linson M A 1980 Axillary artery thrombosis after fracture of the humerus. J Bone Joint Surg 62A: 1214–1215

187. Broudy A S, Jupiter J, May J W 1979 Management of supracondylar fracture with brachial artery thrombosis in a child. J Trauma 19: 540–544

188. Tse D H W, Slabaugh P B, Carlson P A 1980 Injury to the axillary artery by a closed fracture of the clavicle. J Bone Joint Surg 62A: 1372–1376

189. Sturn J T, Rothenberger D A, Strate R 1978 Brachial artery disruption following closed elbow dislocation. J Trauma 18: 364–366

190. Lev–El A, Adar R, Rubinstein Z 1981 Axillary artery injury in erect dislocation of the shoulder. J Trauma 21: 323–325

191. Shuck J M, Omer G E, Lewis C E 1972 Arterial obstruction due to intimal disruption in extremity fractures. J Trauma 12: 481–489

192. Robbs J, Baker L 1978 Major arterial trauma: review of experience with 267 injuries. Br J Surg 65: 532–538

193. Raju S, Carner D V 1981 Brachial plexus compression: complication of delayed recognition of arterial injuries of the shoulder girdle. Arch Surg 116: 175–178

194. Ashbell T S, Kleinert H E, Kutz J E 1967 Vascular injuries about the elbow. Clin Orthopaedics 50: 107–127

195. Scherr D D, Lichti E L, Lambert K L 1973 Tissue viability assessment with Doppler ultrasonic flowmeter in acute injuries of extremities. J Bone Joint Surg 55A: 157–161

196. Yao S, Gourmos C, Papathanasiou K, Irvine W 1972 A method for assessing ischemia of the hand and fingers. Surg Obstet Gynecol 135: 373–378

197. McCormick T M, Burch B H 1979 Routine angiographic evaluation of neck and extremity injuries. J Trauma 19: 384–387

198. May J W Jr, Atkinson R, Rosen H 1984 Traumatic arteriovenous fistula of the thumb after blunt trauma: a case report. J Hand Surg (Am) 9: 253–255

199. Samson R, Pasternak B M 1980 Traumatic arterial spasm — rarity or nonentity. J Trauma 20: 607–609

200. Koman L A, Nunley J A, Wilkinson R H Jr, Urbaniak J R, Coleman R E 1983 Dynamic radionuclide imaging as a means of evaluating vascular perfusion of the upper extremity: a preliminary report. J Hand Surg (Am) 8: 424–434

201. Taweepoke P, Frame J D 1990 Acute ischaemia of the hand following accidental radial artery infusion of Depo-Medrone. J Hand Surg (Br) 15: 118–120

202. Zingaro E A, Kilgore E S 1988 Partial hand amputation following radial artery cannulation. Contemp Orthopaedics 16: 46–47

203. Grossland S G, Nevisser R 1977 Complications of radial artery catheterization. Hand 9: 287–290

204. Mandel M, Dauchot P 1977 Radial artery cannulation in 1000 patients: precautions and complications. J Hand Surg 2: 482–485

205. Serafin D, Puckett C L, McCarty G 1976 Successful treatment of acute vascular insufficiency in a hand by intra-arterial fibrinolysin, heparin and reserpine. Plastic Reconstr Surg 58: 506–509

206. Neviaser R J, Adams J, May G 1976 Complications of arterial puncture in anticoagulated patients. J Bone Joint Surg 58A: 218–220

207. Schmidt P E, Hewitt R L 1980 Severe upper limb ischemia. Arch Surg 115: 1188–1191

208. Aulicino P L, Klavans S M, DuPuy T E 1984 Digital ischemia secondary to thrombosis of a persistent median artery. J Hand Surg (Am) 9: 820–823

209. Richards R R, Urbaniak J R 1984 Spontaneous retrocarpal radial artery thrombosis: a report of two cases. J Hand Surg (Am) 9: 823–827

210. Baur G, Porter J, Bardana E, Wesche D, Rosch J 1977 Rapid onset of hand ischemia of unknown etiology. Ann Surg 186: 184–189

211. Roberts B 1976 The acutely ischemic limb. Heart Lung 5: 273–276

212. Saveyev V, Zarevakhin I, Stepanov N 1977 Artery embolism of the upper limbs. Surgery 81: 367–375

213. Adams J T, McEvoy R K, DeWeese J A 1965 Primary deep venous thrombosis of upper extremity. Arch Surgery 91: 29–42

214. Paletta F X 1981 Venous gangrene of the hand. Plastic Reconstr Surg 67: 67–69

215. Stain S C, Yellin A E, Weaver F A, Pentecost M J 1989 Selective management of nonocclusive arterial injuries. Arch Surg 124: 1136–1141

216. Sachagello C R, Ernst C B, Griffen W O 1974 The acutely ischemic upper extremity: selective management. Surgery 76: 1002–1009

217. Caffee H H, Master N T 1984 Atherosclerosis of the forearm and hand. J Hand Surg (Am) 9: 193–196

218. Godina M 1986 Arterial autografts in microvascular surgery. Plastic Reconstr Surg 78: 293–294

219. Conklin W T, Dabb R W, Danyo J J 1981 Microvascular salvage of the embolized hand. Orthopaedic Rev 10: 169–171

220. Kartchner M M, Wilcox W C 1976 Thrombolysis of palmar and digital arterial thrombosis by intra-arterial thrombolysin. J Hand Surg 1: 67–74

221. Jelalian C, Mehrohof A, Cohen IK, Richardson J, Merritt W H 1985 Streptokinase in the treatment of acute arterial occlusion of the hand. J Hand Surg (Am) 10: 534–538

222. Cooney W P 3rd, Wilson M R, Wood M B 1983 Intravascular fibrinolysis of small-vessel thrombosis. J Hand Surg (Am) 8: 131–138

223. Dacey L J, Dow R W, McDaniel M D, Walsh D B, Zwolak R M, Cronenwett JL 1988 Cost-effectiveness of intra-arterial thrombolytic therapy. Arch Surg 123: 1218–1223

224. Pasch A R, Bishara R A, Schuler J J, Lim L T, Meyer J P, Merlotti G, Barrett J A, Flanigan P 1986 Results of venous reconstruction after civilian vascular trauma. Arch Surg 121: 607–611

225. Miller A, Campbell D R, Gibbons G W, Pomposelli F B, Freeman D V, Jepsen S J, Lees R S, Isaacsohn J L, Purcell D, Bolduc M, LeGerfo F W 1989 Routine intraoperative angioscopy in lower extremity revascularization. Arch Surg 124: 604–608

226. Sahdev P, Jacobs L, Ellison L 1989 Extremity vascular injury from blunt trauma. Contemp Surg 35: 20–25

227. Inoue G, Maeda N 1987 Irreducible palmar dislocation of the distal interphalangeal joint of the finger. J Hand Surg (Am) 12: 1077–1079

228. Crick J C, Conners J J, Franco R S 1990 Irreducible palmar dislocation of the proximal interphalangeal joint with bilateral avulsion fractures. J Hand Surg (Am) 15: 460–463

229. Jones N F, Jupiter J B 1985 Irreducible palmar dislocation of the proximal interphalangeal joint associated with an epiphyseal fracture of the middle phalanx. J Hand Surg (Am) 10: 261–264

230. Green S M, Posner M A 1985 Irreducible dorsal dislocations of the proximal interphalangeal joint. J Hand Surg (Am) 10: 85–87

231. Boyes J H 1980 The measuring of motions. J Hand Surg 5: 89–90

232. Salter R B, Harris W R 1963 Injuries involving the epiphyseal plate. J Bone Joint Surg 45A: 587–622

233. Barton N J 1979 Fractures of the phalanges of the hand in children. Hand 11: 134–143

234. Schneider L H 1988 Fractures of the distal phalanx. Hand Clin 4: 537–547

235. Shrewsburry M M, Johnson R K 1983 Form, function, and evolution of the distal phalanx. J Hand Surg (Am) 8: 475–479

236. Thayer D T 1988 Distal interphalangeal joint injuries. Hand Clin 4: 1–4

237. Vicar A J 1988 Proximal interphalangeal joint dislocations without fractures. Hand Clin 4: 5–13

238. Eaton R G, Littler J W 1976 Joint injuries and their sequelae. Clin Plastic Surg 3: 85–98

239. Bogumill G P 1983 A morphologic study of the relationship of collateral ligaments to growth plates in the digits. J Hand Surg (Am) 8: 74–79

240. Hankin F M, Janda D H 1989 Tendon and ligament attachments in relationship to growth plates in a child's hand. J Hand Surg (Br) 14: 315–318

241. Bowers W H, Wolf J W, Nehil J L, Bittinger S 1980 The proximal interphalangeal joint volar plate. I. An anatomical and biomechanical study. J Hand Surg 5: 79–88

242. Bowers W H 1981 The proximal interphalangeal joint volar plate. A clinical study of hyperextension injury. J Hand Surg 6: 77–81

243. Lubahn J D 1988 Dorsal fracture dislocations of the proximal interphalangeal joint. Hand Clin 4: 15–24

244. Stern P J, Lee A F 1985 Open dorsal dislocations of the proximal interphalangeal joint. J Hand Surg (Am) 10: 364–370

245. Peimer C A, Sullivan D J, Wild D R 1984 Palmar dislocation of the proximal interphalangeal joint. J Hand Surg (Am) 9A: 39–48

246. Posner M A, Kapila D 1986 Chonic palmar dislocation of proximal interphalangeal joints. J Hand Surg (Am) 11: 253–258

247. Margles S W 1988 Intra-articular fractures of the metacarpophalangeal and proximal interphalangeal joints. Hand Clin 4: 67–74

248. Hastings H 2nd, Carroll C 4th 1988 Treatment of closed articular fractures of the metacarpophalangeal and proximal interphalangeal joints. Hand Clin 4: 503–527

249. Kiefhaber T R, Stern P J, Grood E S 1986 Lateral stability of the proximal interphalangeal joint. J Hand Surg (Am) 11: 661–669

250. Smith R J 1977 Post-traumatic instability of the metacarpophalangeal joint of the thumb. J Bone Joint Surg 59A: 14–21

251. Mogensen B A, Mattsson H S 1980 Post-traumatic instability of the metacarpophalangeal joint of the thumb. Hand 12: 85–90

252. Minami A, An K N, Cooney W P 3rd, Linscheid R L, Chao E Y 1985 Ligament stability of the metacarpophalangeal joint: a biomechanical study. J Hand Surg (Am) 10: 255–260

253. Miller R J 1988 Dislocations and fracture dislocations of the metacarpophalangeal joint of the thumb. Hand Clin 4: 45–65

254. Hooper G J 1987 An unusual variety of skier's thumb. J Hand Surg (Am) 12: 627–629

255. White G M 1986 Ligamentous avulsion of the ulnar collateral ligament of the thumb of a child. J Hand Surg (Am) 11: 669–672

256. Browne E Z Jr, Dunn H K, Snyder C C 1976 Ski pole thumb injury. Plastic Reconstr Surg 58: 19–23

257. Smith M A 1980 The mechanism of acute ulnar instability of the metacarpophalangeal joint of the thumb. Hand 12: 225–230

258. Redler I, Williams J T 1967 Rupture of a collateral ligament of the proximal interphalangeal joint of the finger. J Bone Joint Surg 49A: 322–326

259. Stener B 1962 Displacement of the ruptured ulnar collateral ligament of the MCP joint of the thumb. J Bone Joint Surg 44B: 869–879

260. Stern P J 1981 Stener lesion after lateral dislocation of the proximal interphalangeal joint — indication for open reduction. J Hand Surg 6: 602–604

261. Light T R 1981 Buttress pinning techniques. Orthopaedic Rev 10: 49–55

262. Burkhalter W E 1989 Closed treatment of hand fractures. J Hand Surg (Am) 14: 390–393

263. Belsky M R, Eaton R G, Lane L B 1984 Closed reduction and internal fixation of proximal phalangeal fractures. J Hand Surg (Am) 9: 725–729

264. Widgerow A, Edinburg M, Biddulph S L 1987 An analysis of proximal phalangeal fractures. J Hand Surg (Am) 12: 134–139

265. Black D M, Mann R J, Constine R M, Daniels A U 1986 The stability of internal fixation in the proximal phalanx. J Hand Surg (Am) 11: 672–677

266. Vanik R K, Weber R C, Matloub H S, Sanger J R, Gingrass RP 1984 The comparative strengths of internal fixation techniques. J Hand Surg (Am) 9: 216–221

267. Lister G 1978 Intraosseous wiring of the digital skeleton. J Hand Surg 3: 427–435

268. Greene T L, Noellert R C, Belsole R J, Simpson L A 1989 Composite wiring of metacarpal and phalangeal fractures. J Hand Surg (Am) 14: 665–669

269. Barton N 1989 Conservative treatment of articular fractures in the hand. J Hand Surg (Am) 14: 386–390

270. O'Rourke S K, Gaur S, Barton N 1989 Long-term outcome of articular fractures of the phalanges: an eleven year follow up. J Hand Surg (Br) 14B: 183–193

271. Schenck R R 1986 Dynamic traction and early passive movement for fractures of the proximal interphalangeal joint. J Hand Surg (Am) 11: 850–858

272. Eaton R G, Malerich M M 1980 Volar plate arthroplasty of the proximal interphalangeal joint: a review of ten years' experience. J Hand Surg 5: 260–268

273. Incavo S J, Mogan J V, Hilfrank B C 1989 Extension splinting of palmar plate avulsion injuries of the proximal interphalangeal joint. J Hand Surg (Am) 14: 659–661

274. Abrahamsson S O, Sollerman C, Lundborg G, Larsson J, Egund N 1990 Diagnosis of displaced ulnar collateral ligament of the metacarpophalangeal joint of the thumb. J Hand Surg (Am) 15: 457–460

275. Louis D S, Buckwalter K A 1989 Magnetic resonance imaging of the collateral ligaments of the thumb. J Hand Surg (Am) 14: 739–741

276. Pichora D R, McMurtry R Y, Bell M J 1989 Gamekeepers thumb: a prospective study of functional bracing. J Hand Surg (Am) 14: 567–573

277. Hansen C A, Peterson T H 1987 Fracture of the thumb sesamoid bones. J Hand Surg (Am) 12: 269–270

278. Ishizuki M 1988 Injury to collateral ligament of the metacarpophalangeal joint of a finger. J Hand Surg (Am) 13: 444–448

279. Hubbard L F 1988 Metacarpophalangeal dislocations. Hand Clin 4: 39–44

280. Ramirez Ruiz G, Combalia Aleu A, Valer Tito A, Bordas Sales J L, Rofes Capo S 1985 Simultaneous subluxation of the metacarpophalangeal joints of all four fingers: a case report. J Hand Surg (Am) 10: 78–80

281. Hall R F Jr, Gleason T F, Kasa R F 1985 Simultaneous closed dislocations of the metacarpophalangeal joints of the index, long, and ring fingers: a case report. J Hand Surg (Am) 10: 81–85

282. Araki S, Ohtani I, Tanaka T 1987 Open dorsal metacarpophalangeal dislocations of the index, long, and ring fingers. J Hand Surg (Am) 12A: 458–460

283. Kaplan E B 1957 Dorsal dislocation of the metacarpophalangeal joint of the index finger. J Bone Joint Surg 39A: 1081–1086

284. Green D P, Terry G C 1973 Complex dislocation of the metacarpophalangeal joint. J Bone Joint Surg 55A: 1480–1486

285. Nussbaum R, Sadler A H 1986 An isolated, closed, complex dislocation of the metacarpophalangeal joint of the long finger: a unique case. J Hand Surg (Am) 11: 558–561

286. Lineaweaver W, Mathes S J 1988 Distal avulsion of the palmar plate of the interphalangeal joint of the thumb. J Hand Surg (Am) 13: 453–455

287. Posner M A, Ambrose L 1989 Boxer's knuckle — dorsal capsular rupture of the metacarpophalangeal joint of a finger. J Hand Surg (Am) 14: 229–236

288. Koniuch M P, Peimer C A, VanGorder T, Moncada A 1987 Closed crush injury of the metacarpophalangeal joint. J Hand Surg (Am) 12: 750–757

289. Lane C S 1977 Detecting occult fractures of the metacarpal head: the Brewerton view. J Hand Surg 2: 131–133

290. Light T R, Ogden J A 1987 Metacarpal epiphyseal fractures. J Hand Surg (Am) 12: 460–464

291. McElfresh E C, Dobyns J H 1983 Intra-articular metacarpal head fractures. J Hand Surg (Am) 8: 383–393

292. Breen T F, Gelberman R H, Jupiter J B 1988 Intra-articular fractures of the basilar joint of the thumb. Hand Clin 4: 491–501

293. Pellegrini V D Jr 1988 Fractures at the base of the thumb. Hand Clin 4: 87–102

294. Bennett E H 1886 On fracture of the metacarpal bone of the thumb. Br Med J 2: 12–13

295. Walker L G 1989 Bennett's fracture. Surg Rounds Orthopaedics 3: 79–80

296. Peterson P, Sacks S 1986 Fracture-dislocation of the base of the fifth metacarpal associated with injury to the deep motor branch of the ulnar nerve: a case report. J Hand Surg (Am) 11: 525–528

297. Rolando S 1910 Fracture de la base du premier metacarpien: et principalement sur une variete non encore decrite. Presse Medicale 33: 303

298. Cain J E Jr, Shepler T R, Wilson M R 1987 Hamatometacarpal fracture–dislocation: classification and treatment. J Hand Surg (Am) 12: 762–767

299. Marck K W, Klasen H J 1986 Fracture-dislocation of the hamatometacarpal joint: a case report. J Hand Surg (Am) 11: 128–130

300. Bergfield T G, DuPuy T E, Aulicino P L 1985 Fracture-dislocations of all five carpometacarpal joints: a case report. J Hand Surg (Am) 10: 76–78

301. Gunther S F, Bruno P D 1985 Divergent dislocation of the carpometacarpal joints: a case report. J Hand Surg (Am) 10: 197–201

302. Laforgia R, Specchiulli F, Mariani A 1990 Dorsal dislocation of the fifth carpometacarpal joint. J Hand Surg (Am) 15: 463–465

303. Mueller J J 1986 Carpometacarpal dislocations: report of five cases and review of the literature. J Hand Surg (Am) 11: 184–188

304. Rawles J G Jr 1988 Dislocations and fracture-dislocations at the carpometacarpal joints of the fingers. Hand Clin 4: 103–112

305. Stevanovic M V, Stark H H 1984 Dorsal dislocation of the fourth and fifth carpometacarpal joints and simultaneous dislocation of the metacarpophalangeal joint of the small finger: a case report. J Hand Surg (Am) 9: 714–716

306. Weiland A J, Lister G D, Villarreal-Rios A 1976 Volar fracture dislocations of the second and third carpometacarpal joints associated with acute carpal tunnel syndrome. J Trauma 16: 672–675

307. Ho P K, Choban S J, Eshman S J, Dupuy T E 1987 Complex dorsal dislocation of the second carpometacarpal joint. J Hand Surg (Am) 12: 1074–1076

308. Carroll R E, Carlson E 1989 Diagnosis and treatment of injury to the second and third carpometacarpal joints. J Hand Surg (Am) 14: 102–107

309. Henderson J J, Arafa M A 1987 Carpometacarpal dislocation. An easily missed diagnosis. J Bone Joint Surg 69B: 212–214

310. Robert P 1936 Radiographie de l'articulation trapezometacarpienne. Les athroses de cette jointure. Bulletins et memoires de la Societe de Radiologie medicale de France 24: 687–690

311. Bowers W H, Hurst L C 1977 Gamekeeper's thumb.

Evaluation by arthrography and stress roentgenography. J Bone Joint Surg 59A: 519–524

312. McElfresh E C, Dobyns J H 1983 Intra-articular metacarpal head fractures. J Hand Surg (Am) 8: 383–393

313. Hunter J M, Cowen N J 1970 Fifth metacarpal fractures in a compensation clinic population. A report on one hundred and thirty-three cases. J Bone Joint Surg (Am) 52: 1159–1165

314. Barton N J 1984 Fractures of the hand. J Bone Joint Surg (Br) 66: 159–167

315. Smith R J, Peimer C A 1977 Injuries to the metacarpal bones and joints. Adv Surg 11: 341–374

316. Flatt A E 1966 Closed and open fractures of the hand. Fundamentals of management. Postgrad Med 39: 17–26

317. Pritsch M, Engel J, Farin I 1981 Manipulation and external fixation of metacarpal fractures. J Bone Joint Surg 63A: 1289–1291

318. Workman C E 1964 Metacarpal fracture. Missouri Med 61: 687–690

319. Gropper P T, Bowen V 1984 Cerclage wiring of metacarpal fractures. Clin Orthop 188: 203–207

320. Butt W D 1962 Fractures of the hand. I. Description. Can Med Assoc J 86: 731–735

321. Griffiths J C 1964 Fractures at the base of the first metacarpal bone. J Bone Joint Surg 46B: 712

322. Pollen A G 1968 The conservative treatment of Bennett's fracture-subluxation of the thumb metacarpal. J Bone Joint Surg (Br) 50: 91–101

323. Gedda K O 1954 Studies on Bennett's fracture: anatomy, roentgenology, and therapy. Acta Chir Scand (suppl): 193: 5–108

324. Flatt A E 1972 Care of minor hand injuries, 3rd edn. CV Mosby, St Louis

325. Heim U, Pfeiffer KM 1988 Internal fixation of small fractures, 3rd edn. Springer Verlag, Heidelburg

326. Walker L G 1989 Bennett's fracture. Surg Rounds Orth 3: 79–80

327. Dabezies E J, Schutte J P 1986 Fixation of metacarpal and phalangeal fractures with miniature plates and screws. J Hand Surg (Am) 11: 283–288

328. Jabaley M E, Freeland A E 1986 Rigid internal fixation in the hand: 104 cases. Plastic Reconstr Surg 77: 288–298

329. Burgess R C 1990 Anatomic variations of the midcarpal joint. J Hand Surg (Am) 15: 129–131

330. Ruby L K, Cooney W P 3rd, An K N, Linscheid R L, Chao E Y 1988 Relative motion of selected carpal bones: a kinematic analysis of the normal wrist. J Hand Surg (Am) 13: 1–10

331. Seradge H, Sterbank P T, Seradge E, Owens W 1990 Segmental motion of the proximal carpal row: their global effect on wrist motion. J Hand Surg (Am) 15: 236–239

332. Drewniany J J, Palmer A K, Flatt A E 1985 The scaphotrapezial ligament complex: an anatomic and biomechanical study. J Hand Surg (Am) 10: 492–498

333. Anderson W J, Bowers W H 1985 Congenital absence of the triquetrum: a case report. J Hand Surg (Am) 10: 620–622

334. Simmons B P, McKenzie W D 1985 Symptomatic carpal coalition. J Hand Surg (Am) 10: 190–193

335. Palmer A K, Werner F W, Murphy D, Glisson R 1985

Functional wrist motion; a biomechanical study. J Hand Surg (Am) 10: 39–46

336. Gelberman R H, Panagis J S, Taleisnik J, Baumgaertner M 1983 The arterial anatomy of the human carpus. Part I. The extraosseous vascularity. J Hand Surg (Am) 8: 367–375

337. Panagis J S, Gelberman R H, Taleisnik J, Baumgaertner M 1983 The arterial anatomy of the human carpus. Part II. The intraosseous vascularity. J Hand Surg (Am) 8: 375–382

338. Vander Grend R, Dell P C, Glowczewskie F, Leslie B, Ruby L K 1984 Intraosseous blood supply of the capitate and its correlation with aseptic necrosis. J Hand Surg (Am) 9: 677–683

339. Hixson M L, Stewart C 1990 Microvascular anatomy of the radioscapholunate ligament of the wrist. J Hand Surg (Am) 15: 279–282

340. Failla J M, Amadio P C 1988 Recognition and treatment of uncommon carpal fractures. Hand Clin 4: 469–476

341. Mayfield J K, Johnson R P, Kilcoyne R K 1980 Carpal dislocations: pathomechanics and progressive perilunar instability. J Hand Surg 5: 226–241

342. Ruby L K, An K N, Linscheid R L, Cooney W P 3rd, Chao E Y 1987 The effect of scapholunate ligament section on scapholunate motion. J Hand Surg (Am) 12: 767–771

343. Garcia-Elias M 1987 Dorsal fractures of the triquetrum-avulsion or compression fractures? J Hand Surg (Am) 12: 266–268

344. Schwartz M G, Green S M, Coville F A 1990 Dorsal dislocation of the lunate with multiple extensor tendon ruptures. J Hand Surg (Am) 15: 132–133

345. Minami A, Ogino T, Hamada M 1989 Rupture of extensor tendons associated with a palmar perilunar dislocation. J Hand Surg (Am) 14: 843–847

346. Johnson R P 1980 The acutely injured wrist and its residuals. Clin Orthop 149: 33

347. Jasmine M S, Packer J W, Edwards G S Jr 1988 Irreducible trans-scaphoid perilunate dislocation. J Hand Surg (Am) 13: 212–215

348. Lichtman D M, Schneider J R, Swafford A R et al 1981 Ulnar midcarpal instability. Clinical and laboratory analysis. J Hand Surg 6: 515–523

349. Nyquist S R, Stern P J 1984 Open radiocarpal fracture-dislocations. J Hand Surg (Am) 9: 707–710

350. Garcia-Elias M, Dobyns J H, Cooney W P 3rd, Linscheid R L 1989 Traumatic axial dislocations of the carpus. J Hand Surg (Am) 14: 446–457

351. Norbeck D E Jr, Larson B, Blair S J, Demos T C 1987 Traumatic longitudinal disruption of the carpus. J Hand Surg (Am) 12: 509–514

352. Gilula L A 1979 Carpal injuries: analytic approach and case exercises. Am J Roentgenol 133: 509

353. Cantor R M, Braunstein E M 1988 Diagnosis of dorsal and palmar rotation of the lunate on a frontal radiograph. J Hand Surg (Am) 13: 187–193

354. Campbell R D, Lance E M, Chin Bor Yeoh 1964 Lunate and perilunar dislocations. J Bone Joint Surg 46B: 55–72

355. Linscheid R L, Dobyns J H, Beabout J W, Bryan R S 1972 Traumatic instability of the wrist. J Bone Joint Surg 54A: 1612–1632

356. Garcia-Elias M, An K N, Amadio P C, Cooney W P,

357. Linscheid RL 1989 Reliability of carpal angle determinations. J Hand Surg (Am) 14: 1017–1021

358. Leslie I J, Dickson R A 1981 The fractured carpal scaphoid. J Bone Joint Surg 63B: 225–230

359. Russe O 1960 Fracture of the carpal navicular. Diagnosis, nonoperative treatment and operative treatment. J Bone Joint Surg (Am) 42: 759

360. Hart V L, Gaynor V 1941 Roentgenographic study of the carpal canal. J Bone Joint Surg 23: 382–383

361. Palmer A K 1981 Trapezial ridge fractures. J Hand Surg 6: 561–564

362. Andress M R, Peckar V G 1970 Fracture of the hook of the hamate. Br J Radiol 93: 141–143

363. Papilion J D, DuPuy T E, Aulicino P L, Bergfield T G, Gwathmey F W 1988 Radiographic evaluation of the hook of the hamate: a new technique. J Hand Surg (Am) 13: 437–439

364. Bishop A T, Beckenbaugh R D 1988 Fracture of the hamate hook. J Hand Surg (Am) 13: 135–139

365. Egawa M, Asai T 1983 Fracture of the hook of the hamate: report of six cases and the suitability of computerized tomography. J Hand Surg (Am) 8: 393–398

366. Polivy K D, Millender L H, Newberg A, Philips C A 1985 Fractures of the hook of the hamate — a failure of clinical diagnosis. J Hand Surg (Am) 10: 101–104

367. Taleisnik, Julio 1985 The wrist. Churchill Livingstone, New York, Edinburgh, London, Melbourne

368. Moneim M S 1988 Management of greater arc carpal fractures. Hand Clin 4: 457–467

369. Nathan R, Lester B, Melone C P Jr 1987 The acutely injured wrist — an anatomic basis for operative treatment. Orthopaedic Rev 16: 80–95

370. Herbert T J 1989 Internal fixation of the carpus with the Herbert bone screw system. J Hand Surg (Am) 14: 397–400

371. Adams B D, Blair W F, Reagan D S, Grundberg A B 1988 Technical factors related to Herbert screw fixation. J Hand Surg (Am) 13: 893–899

372. Viegas S F, Bean J W, Schram R A 1987 Transscaphoid fracture/dislocations treated with open reduction and Herbert screw internal fixation. J Hand Surg (Am) 12: 992–999

373. Duncan G J, Walker L G 1990 Herbert screw fixation of scaphoid fractures: indications and technique. Contemp Orthopedics 21: 384–388

374. Sprague H H, Howard F M 1988 The Herbert screw for treatment of the scaphoid fracture. Contemp Orthopaedics 16: 19–25

375. Botte M J, Gelberman R H 1987 Modified technique for Herbert screw insertion in fractures of the scaphoid. J Hand Surg (Am) 12: 149–150

376. Botte M J, Mortensen W W, Gelberman R H, Rhoades C E, Gellman H 1988 Internal vascularity of the scaphoid in cadavers after insertion of the Herbert screw J Hand Surg (Am) 13: 216–220

377. Stark H H, Chao E K, Zemel N P, Rickard T A, Ashworth C R 1989 Fracture of the hook of the hamate. J Bone Joint Surg (Am) 71: 1202–1207

378. Watson H K, Rogers W D 1989 Nonunion of the hook of the hamate: an argument for bone grafting the nonunion. J Hand Surg (Am) 14: 486–490

379. Smith P 3rd, Wright T W, Wallace P F, Dell P C 1988 Excision of the hook of the hamate: a retrospective

survey and review of the literature. J Hand Surg (Am) 13: 612–615

379. Campbell R D, Thompson C, Lance E M, Adler J B 1965 Indications for open reduction of lunate and perilunate dislocations of the carpal bones. J Bone Joint Surg 47A: 915–937

380. Hanel D P, Robson D B 1987 The image intensifier as an operating table. J Hand Surg (Am) 12: 322–323

381. Goldberg I, Amit S, Bahar A, Seelenfreund M 1981 Complete dislocation of the trapezium (multangulum majus). J Hand Surg 6: 193–195

382. Seimon L P 1972 Compound dislocation of the trapezium. J Bone Joint Surg 54A: 1297–1300

383. Sherlock D A 1987 Traumatic dorsoradial dislocation of the trapezium. J Hand Surg (Am) 12: 262–265

384. Freeland A E, Finley J S 1984 Displaced vertical fracture of the trapezium treated with a small cancellous lag screw. J Hand Surg (Am) 9: 843–845

385. Jones J A, Pellegrini V D Jr 1989 Transverse fracture-dislocation of the trapezium. J Hand Surg (Am) 14: 481–485

386. Griffin A C, Gilula L A, Young V L, Strecker W B, Weeks P M 1988 Fracture of the dorsoulnar tubercle of the trapezium. J Hand Surg (Am) 13: 622–626

387. Gordon S L 1972 Scaphoid and lunate dislocation. J Bone Joint Surg 54A: 1769–1772

388. Brown R H L, Muddu B N 1981 Scaphoid and lunate dislocation. Hand 13: 303–307

389. Coll G A 1987 Palmar dislocation of the scaphoid and lunate. J Hand Surg (Am) 12: 476–480

390. Sarrafian S K, Breihan J H 1990 Palmar dislocation of scaphoid and lunate as a unit. J Hand Surg (Am) 15: 134–139

391. Kupfer K 1986 Palmar dislocation of scaphoid and lunate as a unit: case report with special reference to carpal instability and treatment. J Hand Surg (Am) 11: 130–134

392. Fryktman E 1980 Dislocation of the triquetrum. Scand J Plastic Reconstr Surg 14: 205–207

393. Soucatos P N, Hartofilakidis-Gsrofalidis G C 1981 Dislocation of the triangular bone: report of a case. J Bone Joint Surg 63A: 1012–1014

394. Bieber E J, Weiland A J 1984 Traumatic dorsal dislocation of the triquetrum: a case report. J Hand Surg (Am) 9: 840–842

395. Goldberg B, Heller A P 1987 Dorsal dislocation of the triquetrum with rotary subluxation of the scaphoid. J Hand Surg (Am) 12: 119–122

396. Minami M, Yamazaki J, Ishii S 1984 Isolated dislocation of the pisiform: a case report and review of the literature. J Hand Surg (Am) 9A: 125–127

397. Freeland A E, Finley J S 1986 Displaced dorsal oblique fracture of the hamate treated with a cortical mini lag screw. J Hand Surg (Am) 11: 656–658

398. Ogunro O 1983 Fracture of the body of the hamate bone. J Hand Surg (Am) 8: 353–355

399. Loth T S, McMillan M D 1988 Coronal dorsal hamate fractures. J Hand Surg (Am) 13: 616–618

400. Kimura H, Kamura S, Akai M, Ohno T 1988 An unusual coronal fracture of the body of the hamate bone. J Hand Surg (Am) 13: 743–745

401. Roth J H, de Lorenzi C 1988 Displaced intra-articular coronal fracture of the body of the hamate treated with a Herbert screw. J Hand Surg (Am) 13: 619–621

402. Gainor B J 1985 Simultaneous dislocation of the hamate and pisiform: a case report. J Hand Surg (Am) 10: 88–90

403. Meyn M A, Roth A M 1980 Isolated dislocation of the trapezoid bone. J Hand Surg 5: 602–604

404. Bendre D V, Baxi V K 1981 Dislocation of trapezoid. J Trauma 21: 899–900

405. Kopp J R 1985 Isolated palmar dislocation of the trapezoid. J Hand Surg (Am) 10: 91–93

406. Goodman M L, Shankman G B 1984 Update: palmar dislocation of the trapezoid — a case report. J Hand Surg (Am) 9A: 127–131

407. Goodman M L, Shankman G B 1983 Palmar dislocation of the trapezoid — a case report. J Hand Surg (Am) 8: 606–609

408. Rhoades C E, Reckling F W 1983 Palmar dislocation of the trapezoid — case report. J Hand Surg (Am) 8: 85–88

409. Jensen B V, Christensen C 1990 An unusual combination of simultaneous fracture of the tuberosity of the trapezium and the hook of the hamate. J Hand Surg (Am) 15: 285–287

410. Ohshio I, Ogino T, Miyake A 1986 Dislocation of the hamate associated with fracture of the trapezial ridge. J Hand Surg (Am) 11: 658–660

411. Tajima T 1983 Considerations on the use of the tourniquet in surgery of the hand. J Hand Surg (Am) 8: 799–802

412. Moore M R, Garfin S R, Hargens A R 1987 Wide tourniquets eliminate blood flow at low inflation pressures. J Hand Surg (Am) 12: 1006–1011

413. Lubahn J D, Koeneman J, Kosar K 1985 The digital tourniquet: how safe is it? J Hand Surg (Am) 10: 664–669

414. Hixson F P, Shafiroff B B, Werner F W, Palmer A K 1986 Digital tourniquets: a pressure study with clinical relevance. J Hand Surg (Am) 11: 865–868

415. Palmer A K 1986 Complications from tourniquet use. Hand Clin 2: 301–305

416. Nitz A J, Dobner J J 1989 Upper extremity tourniquet effects in carpal tunnel release. J Hand Surg (Am) 14: 499–504

417. Neimkin R J, Smith R J 1983 Double tourniquet with linked mercury manometers for hand surgery. J Hand Surg (Am) 8: 938–941

418. Dreyfuss U Y, Smith R J 1988 Sensory changes with prolonged double-cuff tourniquet time in hand surgery. J Hand Surg (Am) 13: 736–740

419. Rees M J, de Geus J J 1988 Immediate amputation stump coverage with forearm free flaps from the same limb. J Hand Surg (Am) 13: 287–292

420. Godina M, Bajec J, Baraga A 1986 Salvage of the mutilated upper extremity with temporary ectopic implantation of the undamaged part. Plastic Reconstr Surg 78: 295–299

421. Gustilo R B, Anderson J T 1976 Prevention of infection in the treatment of one thousand and twenty-five open fractures of long bones. Retrospective and prospective analysis. J Bone Joint Surg 58A: 453–458

422. Gustilo R B, Gruninger R P, Davis T 1987 Classification of Type III (severe) open fractures relative to treatment and results. Orthopedics 10: 1781–1788

423. Dellinger E P, Miller S D, Wertz M J, Grypma M,

Droppert B, Anderson P A 1988 Risk of infection after open fracture of the arm or leg. Arch Surg 123: 1320–1327

424. Peacock K C, Hanna D P, Kirkpatrick K, Breidenbach W C et al 1988 Efficacy of perioperative cefamandole with postoperative cephalexin in the primary outpatient treatment of open wounds of the hand. J Hand Surg (Am) 13: 960–964

425. Antrum R M, Solomkin J S 1987 A review of antibiotic prophylaxis for open fractures. Orthopaedic Rev 16: 81–89

426. Dellinger E P, Caplan E S, Leaver L D et al 1988 Duration of preventive antibiotic administration for open extremity fractures. Arch Surg 123: 333–339

427. Scherr D D, Dodd T A 1976 In vitro bacteriological evaluation of the effectiveness of antimicrobial irrigating solution. J Bone Joint Surg 58A: 119–122

428. Scherr D D, Dodd T A, Buckingham W W 1972 Prophylactic use of topical antibiotic irrigation in uninfected surgical wounds. A microbiological evaluation. J Bone Joint Surg 54A: 634–640

429. Godina M 1986 Early microsurgical reconstruction of complex trauma of the extremities. Plastic Reconstr Surg 78: 285–292

430. Lister G D 1988 Emergency free flaps. In: Green D P (ed) Operative hand surgery, 2nd edn. Churchill Livingstone, Edinburgh

431. Lister G, Scheker L 1988 Emergency free flaps to the upper extremity. J Hand Surg (Am) 13(1): 22–28

432. Guttman L 1956 The problem of treatment of pressure sores in spinal paraplegics. Br J Plastic Surg 8: 196–213

433. Breidenbach W C 3rd 1989 Emergency free tissue transfer for reconstruction of acute upper extremity wounds. Clin Plastic Surg 16: 505–514

434. Morgan W J, Leopold T, Evans R 1984 Foreign bodies in the hand. J Hand Surg (Br) 9: 194–196

435. Browett J P, Fiddian N J 1985 Delayed median nerve injury due to retained glass fragments. A report of two cases. J Bone Joint Surg (Br) 67: 382–384

436. Jablon M, Rabin S I 1988 Late flexor pollicis longus tendon rupture due to retained glass fragments. J Hand Surg (Am) 13: 713–716

437. Jozsa L, Reffy A, Demel S, Balint J B 1989 Foreign bodies in tendons. J Hand Surg (Br) 14: 84–85

438. Viegas S F, Calhoun J H 1986 Lead poisoning from a gunshot wound to the hand. J Hand Surg (Am) 11: 729–732

439. Watson N, Songcharoen G P 1985 Lead synovitis in the hand: a case report. J Hand Surg (Br) 10: 423–424

440. Newmeyer W L 3rd 1988 Management of sea urchin spines in the hand. J Hand Surg (Am) 13: 455–457

441. Carneiro R S, Okunski W J, Hefernan A H 1977 Detection of a relatively radiolucent foreign body in the hand by xerography. Plastic Reconstr Surg 59: 862–863

442. Boxers D G, Lynch J B 1977 Xeroradiography for nonmetallic foreign bodies. Plastic Reconstr Surg 60: 470–471

443. Lee M H 1963 Intra-articular and peri-articular fractures of the phalanges. J Bone Joint Surg 45B: 103–109

444. Peitner C A, Smith R J, Leffert R D 1981 Distraction in the primary treatment of metacarpal bone loss. J Hand Surg 6: 111–124

445 Freeland A E, Jabaley M E, Burkhalter W E, Chaves

A M 1984 Delayed primary bone grafting in the hand and wrist after traumatic bone loss. J Hand Surg (Am) 9A: 22–28

446. Barton N 1989 Internal fixation of hand fractures [editorial]. J Hand Surg (Br) 14: 139–142

447. Meals R A, Meuli H C 1985 Carpenter's nails, phonograph needles, piano wires, and safety pins: the history of operative fixation of metacarpal and phalangeal fractures. J Hand Surg (Am) 10: 144–150

448. Lister G 1978 Intraosseous wiring of the digital skeleton. J Hand Surg 3: 427–435

449. Rayhack J M, Belsole R J, Skelton W H Jr 1984 A strain recording model: analysis of transverse osteotomy fixation in small bones. J Hand Surg (Am) 9: 383–387

450. Segmuller G 1973 Surgical stabilization of the skeleton of the hand. Williams & Wilkins, Baltimore

451. Grundberg A B 1981 Intramedullary fixation for fractures of the hand. J Hand Surg 6: 568–573

452. Riggs S A Jr, Cooney W P 3rd 1983 External fixation of complex hand and wrist fractures. J Trauma 23: 332–336

453. Fernandez D L, Ghillani R 1987 External fixation of complex carpal dislocations: a preliminary report. J Hand Surg (Am) 12: 335–347

454. Stein H, Horer D, Horesh Z 1984 The use of external fixators in the treatment and rehabilitation of compound limb injuries. Orthopedics 7: 707–714

455. Seitz W H Jr, Gomez W, Putnam M D, Rosenwasser M P 1987 Management of severe hand trauma with a mini external fixateur. Orthopedics 10: 601–610

456. Stuchin S A, Kummer F J 1984 Stiffness of small-bone external fixation methods: an experimental study. J Hand Surg (Am) 9: 718–724

457. Bilos J, Eskestrand T 1979 External fixator use in comminuted gunshot fractures of the proximal phalanx. J Hand Surg 4: 357–359

458. Scott M M, Mulligan P J 1980 Stabilizing severe phalangeal fractures. Hand 12: 44–50

459. Inoue G, Maeda N 1987 Irreducible palmar dislocation of the distal interphalangeal joint of the finger. J Hand Surg (Am) 12: 1077–1079

460. De Smet L, Vercauteren M 1984 Palmar dislocation of the proximal interphalangeal joint requiring open reduction: a case report. J Hand Surg (Am) 9: 717–718

461. Fernandez D L 1981 Irreducible radiocarpal fracture dislocation and radioulnar dissociation with entrapment of the ulnar nerve, artery and flexor profundus II–V — case report. J Hand Surg 6: 456–461

462. Matev I 1976 A radiological sign of entrapment of the median nerve in the elbow joint after posterior dislocation. J Bone Joint Surg 58B: 353–355

463. Lister G 1978 Intraosseous wiring of the digital skeleton. J Hand Surg 3: 427–435

464. Green D P, O'Brien E T 1978 Open reduction of carpal dislocations: indications and operative techniques. J Hand Surg 3: 250–265

465. Eiken O, Hagberg L, Lundborg G 1981 Evolving biologic concepts as applied to tendon surgery. Clin Plastic Surg 8: 1–12

466. Lister G 1985 Indications and techniques for repair of the flexor tendon sheath. Hand Clin 1: 85–95

467. Lister G D 1983 Incision and closure of the flexor sheath during primary tendon repair. Hand 15: 123–135

468. Lister G D 1985 Pitfalls and complications of flexor tendon surgery. Hand Clin 1: 133–146

469. Lister G D, Kleinert H E, Kutz J E, Atasoy E 1977 Primary flexor tendon repair followed by immediate controlled mobilization. J Hand Surg 2: 441–455

470. Strickland J W 1985 Flexor tendon repair. Hand Clin 1: 55–68

471. Urbaniak J R 1985 Repair of the flexor pollicis longus. Hand Clin 1: 69–76

472. Malerich M M, Baird R A, McMaster W, Erickson J M 1987 Permissible limits of flexor digitorum profundus tendon advancement — an anatomic study. J Hand Surg (Am) 12: 30–33

473. Leddy J P 1985 Avulsions of the flexor digitorum profundus. Hand Clin (1): 77–83

474. Weeks P M 1981 Invited comment on three complications of untreated partial laceration of flexor tendons — entrapment, rupture and triggering. J Hand Surg 6: 396–398

475. Schlenker J D, Lister G D, Kleinert H E 1981 Three complications of untreated partial laceration of flexor tendons — entrapment, rupture and triggering. J Hand Surg 6: 392–396

476. Garrett W E Jr, Seaber A V, Boswick J, Urbaniak J R, Goldner J L 1984 Recovery of skeletal muscle after laceration and repair. J Hand Surg (Am) 9: 683–692

477. Botte M J, Gelberman R H, Smith D G, Silver M A, Gellman H 1987 Repair of severe muscle belly lacerations using a tendon graft. J Hand Surg (Am) 12: 406–412

478. Sunderland S 1978 Nerves and nerve injuries, 2nd edn. Churchill Livingstone, Edinburgh

479. Williams H B, Jabaley M E 1986 The importance of internal anatomy of the peripheral nerves to nerve repair in the forearm and hand. Hand Clin 2: 689–707

480. Chow J A, Van Beek A L, Meyer D L, Johnson M C 1985 Surgical significance of the motor fascicular group of the ulnar nerve in the forearm. J Hand Surg (Am) 10: 867–872

481. Bonnel F 1985 Histologic structure of the ulnar nerve in the hand. J Hand Surg (Am) 10: 264–269

482. Gaul J S Jr 1983 Electrical fascicle identification as an adjunct to nerve repair. J Hand Surg (Am) 8: 289–296

483. Gaul J S Jr 1986 Electrical fascicle identification as an adjunct to nerve repair. Hand Clin 2: 709–722

484. Ganel A, Engel J, Luboshitz S, Melamed R, Rimon S 1981 Choline acetyltransferase nerve identification method in early and late nerve repair. Ann Plastic Surg 6: 228–230

485. Riley D A, Lang D H 1984 Carbonic anhydrase activity of human peripheral nerves: a possible histochemical aid to nerve repair. J Hand Surg (Am) 9A: 112–120

486. Bowers W H, Carlson E C, Wenner S M, Doyle J R 1989 Nerve suture and grafting. Hand Clin 5: 445–453

487. Omer G E Jr 1986 Acute management of peripheral nerve injuries. Hand Clin 2: 193–206

488. Bolesta M J, Garrett W E Jr, Ribbeck B M, Glisson R R et al 1988 Immediate and delayed neurorrhaphy in a rabbit model: a functional, histologic, and biochemical comparison. J Hand Surg (Am) 13: 352–357

489. Wilgis E F, Murphy R 1986 The significance of longitudinal excursion in peripheral nerves. Hand Clin 2: 761–766

490. Stevenson J H, Zuker R M 1986 Upper limb motor and sensory recovery after multiple proximal nerve injury in children: a long term review in five patients. Br J Plastic Surg 39: 109–113

491. Gelberman R H, Nunley J A, Koman L A, Gould J S et al 1982 The results of radial and ulnar arterial repair in the forearm. Experience in three medical centers. J Bone Joint Surg (Am) 64: 383–387

492. Gelberman R H, Gould R N, Hargens A R, Vande Berg J S 1983 Lacerations of the ulnar artery: hemodynamic, ultrastructural, and compliance changes in the dog. J Hand Surg (Am) 8: 306–309

493. Trumble T, Seaber A V, Urbaniak J R 1987 Patency after repair of forearm arterial injuries in animal models. J Hand Surg (Am) 12: 47–53

494. Nunley J A, Goldner R D, Koman L A, Gelberman R, Urbaniak J R 1987 Arterial stump pressure: a determinant of arterial patency? J Hand Surg (Am) 12: 245–249

495. Puckett C L, Winters R R, Geter R K, Goelel D 1985 Studies of pathologic vasoconstriction (vasospasm) in microvascular surgery. J Hand Surg (Am) 10: 343–349

496. Bruch H P, Lanz U, Horl M, Wolter J 1985 Rigor of small human vessels. J Hand Surg (Am) 10: 985–988

497. Van Beek A L, Kutz J E, Zook E 1978 Importance of the ribbon sign, indicating unsuitability of the vessel, in replanting a finger. Plastic Reconstr Surg 61: 32–35

498. Godina M 1986 Arterial autografts in microvascular surgery. Plastic Reconstr Surg 78: 293–294

499. O'Reilly R J, Blatt G 1975 High-pressure injection injury. J Am Med Assoc 233: 533–534

500. Gelberman R, Posch J L, Jurist J M 1975 High-pressure injection injuries of the hand. J Bone Joint Surg 57A: 935–937

501. Schoo M J, Scott F A, Boswick J A 1980 High pressure injection injuries of the hand. J Trauma 20: 229–238

502. Harter B T Jr, Harter K C 1986 High-pressure injection injuries. Hand Clin 2: 547–552

503. Scher C, Schun F D, Harvin J S 1973 High pressure paint gun injuries of the hand. Br J Plastic Surg 26: 167–171

504. Waters W R, Penn I, Ross H M 1967 Airless paint gun injuries of the hand. 39: 613–618

505. Stark H H, Ashworth C R, Boyes J H 1967 Paint gun injuries of the hand. J Bone Joint Surg 49A: 637–647

506. Thakore HK 1985 Hand injury with paint–gun. J Hand Surg (Br) 10: 124–126

507. Stark H H, Ashworth C R, Boyes J H 1961 Grease gun injuries of the hand. J Bone Joint Surg 43A: 485–491

508. Flint M H 1966 Plastic injection moulding injury. Br J Plastic Surg 19: 70–78

509. Geller E R, Gursel E 1986 A unique case of high-pressure injection injury of the hand. J Trauma 26: 483–485

510. Crabb D J M 1981 The value of plain radiographs in treating greasegun injuries. Hand 13: 39–42

511. Ramos H, Posch J L, Lie K K 1970 High-pressure injection injuries of the hand. Plastic Reconstr Surg 45: 221–226

512. Kaufman H D 1968 High-pressure injection injuries. Br J Surg 55: 214–218

513. Dibbell D, Hedberg J, McGraw J, Rankin J, Souther S A 1979 Quantitative examination of the use of

fluorescein in predicting viability of skin flaps. Ann Plastic Surg 3: 101–105

514. Elliott R, Hoehn J, Stayman J W 1979 Management of the viable soft tissue cover in degloving injuries. Hand 11: 69–71

515. London P S 1961 Simplicity of approach to treatment of the injured hand. J Bone Joint Surg 43B: 454–464

516. Beasley R W 1983 Principles of soft tissue replacement for the hand. J Hand Surg (Am) 8: 781–784

517. Ketchum L D 1985 Symposium on skin and soft tissue coverage of the upper extremity. Hand Clin 1: 597–776

518. Chase R A 1985 Historical review of skin and soft tissue coverage of the upper extremity. Hand Clin 1: 599–608

519. Ross R 1979 Inhibition of myofibroblasts by skin grafts. Plastic Reconstr Surg 63: 473–481

520. Horn J J 1951 The use of full thickness hand skin flaps in the reconstruction of injured fingers. Plastic Reconstr Surg 7: 463–481

521. Lister G D 1993 Skin flaps. In: Green D P (ed) Operative Hand Surgery, 3rd edn. Churchill Livingstone, New York, pp 1741–1822

522. Lister G 1985 Local flaps to the hand. Hand Clin 1: 621–640

523. Lanier V C 1981 The fillet flap principle. Orthopaedic Rev 10: 63–66

524. Chase R A 1968 The damaged index digit — a source of components to restore the crippled hand. J Bone Joint Surg 50A: 1152–1160

525. Russell R C, Van Beek A L, Wavak P, Zook E G 1981 Alternative hand flaps for amputations and digital defects. J Hand Surg 6: 399–405

526. Him F P, Casanova R, Vasconez L O 1985 Myocutaneous and fasciocutaneous flaps in the upper limb. Hand Clin 1: 759–768

527. Rose E H 1983 Local arterialized island flap coverage of difficult hand defects preserving donor digit sensibility. Plastic Reconstr Surg 72: 848–858

528. Earley M J 1989 The first web hand flap. J Hand Surg 14B: 65–69

529. Earley M J, Milner R H 1987 Dorsal metacarpal flaps. Br J Plastic Surg 40: 333–341

530. Healy C, Mercer N S, Earley M J, Woodcock J 1990 Focusable Doppler ultrasound in mapping dorsal hand flaps. Br J Plastic Surg 43: 296–299

531. Small J O, Brennen M D 1990 The first dorsal metacarpal artery neurovascular island flap. Br J Plastic Surg 43: 17–23

532. Earley M J 1989 The second dorsal metacarpal artery neurovascular island flap. J Hand Surg (Br) 14: 434–440

533. Maruyama Y 1990 The reverse dorsal metacarpal flap. Br J Plastic Surg 43: 24–27

534. Quaba A A, Davison P M 1990 The distally-based dorsal hand flap. Br J Plastic Surg 43: 28–39

535. Muhlbauer W, Herndl E, Stock W 1982 The forearm flap. Plastic Reconstr Surg 70: 336–342

536. Song R, Gao Y, Song Y, Yu Y, Song Y 1982 The forearm flap. Clin Plastic Surg 9: 21

537. Yang G et al 1981 Forearm free skin flap transplantation. Natl Med J China 61: 139

538. Soutar D S, Tanner N S 1984 The radial forearm flap

539. Meland N B, Lincenberg L S M, Cooney W P III, Wood M B, Hentz V R 1989 Experience with the island radial forearm flap in local hand coverage. J Trauma 29: 489–493

540. Reyes F A, Burkhalter W E 1988 The fascial radial flap. J Hand Surg (Am) 13: 432–437

541. Naasan A, Quaba A A 1990 Successful transfer of two reverse forearm flaps despite disruption of both palmar arches. Br J Plastic Surg 43: 476–479

542. Lin S D, Lai C S, Chiu C C 1984 Venous drainage in the reverse forearm flap. Plastic Reconstr Surg 74: 508–512

543. Matev I 1985 The osteocutaneous pedicle forearm flap. J Hand Surg (Br) 10: 179–182

544. Reid C D, Moss L H 1983 One-stage repair with vascularised tendon grafts in a dorsal hand injury using the 'Chinese' forearm flap. Br J Plastic Surg 36: 473–479

545. Foucher G, van Genechten F, Merle N, Michon J 1984 A compound radial artery forearm flap in hand surgery: an original modification of the Chinese forearm flap. Br J Plastic Surg 37: 139–148

546. Mahoney J, Naiberg J 1987 Toe transfer to the vessels of the reversed forearm flap. J Hand Surg (Am) 12: 62–65

547. Guimberteau J C, Goin J L, Panconi B, Schuhmacher B 1988 The reverse ulnar artery forearm island flap in hand surgery: 54 cases. Plastic Reconstr Surg 81: 925–932

548. Glasson D W, Lovie M J 1988 The ulnar island flap in hand and forearm reconstruction. Br J Plastic Surg 41: 349–353

549. Li Z T, Liu K, Cao Y D 1989 The reverse flow ulnar artery island flap: 42 clinical cases. Br J Plastic Surg 42: 256–259

550. Zancolli E A, Angrigiani C 1988 Posterior interosseous island forearm flap. J Hand Surg (Br) 13: 130–135

551. Bayon P, Pho R W 1988 Anatomical basis of dorsal forearm flap based on posterior interosseous vessels. J Hand Surg (Br) 13: 435–439

552. Costa H, Soutar D S 1988 The distally based island posterior interosseous flap. Br J Plastic Surg 41: 221–227

553. Carriquiry C E 1990 Versatile fasciocutaneous flaps based on the medial septocutaneous vessels of the arm. Plastic Reconstr Surg 86: 103–109

554. Mathes S J, Nahai F 1981 Classification of the vascular anatomy of muscles: experimental and clinical correlation. Plastic Reconstr Surg 67: 177–187

555. McCraw J B, Dibbell D G, Carraway J H 1977 Clinical definition of independent myocutaneous vascular territories. Plastic Reconstr Surg 60: 341–352

556. Brones M F, Wheeler E S, Lesavoy M A 1982 Restoration of elbow flexion and arm contour with the latissimus dorsi myocutaneous flap. Plastic Reconstr Surg 69: 329–332

557. Landra A P 1979 The latissimus dorsi musculocutaneous flap used to resurface a defect on the upper arm and restore extension to the elbow. Br J Plastic Surg 32: 275–277

558. Stern P J, Neale H W, Gregory R O, Kreilein J G 1982

Latissimus dorsi musculocutaneous flap for elbow flexion. J Hand Surg 7: 25–30

559. Abu Jamra F N L, Akel S R, Shamma A R 1981 Repair of major defect of the upper extremity with a latissimus dorsi myocutaneous flap: a case report. Br J Plastic Surg 34: 121–123

560. Silverton J S, Nahai F, Jurkiewicz M J 1978 The latissimus dorsi myocutaneous flap to replace a defect of the upper arm. Br J Plastic Surg 31: 29–31

561. Handle N, Winspur I, Hoehn R 1979 Coverage of a shoulder wound with a deltoid muscle flap. Ann Plastic Surg 3: 277–279

562. Lai M F, Krishna B V, Pelly A D 1981 The brachioradialis myocutaneous flap. Br J Plastic Surg 34: 431–434

563. Ohtsuka H, Imagawa S 1985 Reconstruction of a posterior defect of the elbow joint using an extensor carpi radialis longus myocutaneous flap: case report. Br J Plastic Surg 38: 238–240

564. Kenney J G, Morgan R F, McLaughlin R, Edgerton M T 1983 The 'fold-back' flexor ulnaris muscle flap for repair of soft tissue losses about the elbow. Contemp Orthop 7: 63–66

565. Hodgkinson D J, Shepard G H 1983 Muscle musculocutaneous and fasciocutaneous flaps in forearm reconstruction. Ann Plastic Surg 10: 400–407

566. Cohen B E 1982 Local muscle flap coverage of the proximal ulna without functional loss. Plastic Reconstr Surg 70: 745–748

567. Dellon A L, Mackinnon S E 1984 The pronator quadratus muscle flap. J Hand Surg (Am) 9: 423–427

568. Reisman N R, Dellon A L 1983 The abductor digiti minimi muscle flap: a salvage technique for palmar wrist pain. Plastic Reconstr Surg 72: 859–863

569. Mathes S J, Vasconez L O, Jurkiewicz M J 1977 Extension and further applications of the muscle flap transposition. Plastic Reconstr Surg 60: 6–13

570. Lubahn J D, Carlier A, Lister G D 1985 The denervated first dorsal interosseous muscle flap: a case report. J Hand Surg (Am) 10: 684–686

571. Russell R C, van Beek A L, Wavak P, Zook E G 1981 Alternative hand flaps for amputations and digital defects. J Hand Surg 6: 399–405

572. Winspur I 1985 Distant flaps. Hand Clin 1: 729–739

573. Lister G D 1993 Skin flaps. In: Green D P (ed) Operative Hand Surgery, 3rd edn. Churchill Livingstone, New York, pp 1741–1822

574. McGregor I A, Morgan G 1973 Axial and random pattern flaps. Br J Plastic Surg 26: 202–213

575. Yeschua R, Wexler M R, Neuman Z 1977 Cross-arm triangular flaps for correction of adduction contracture of the web space in the hand. Plastic Reconstr Surg 59: 859–861

576. Holevich J 1965 Early skin grafting in the treatment of traumatic avulsion injuries of the hand and fingers. J Bone Joint Surg 47A: 944–957

577. Jarev A, Hirshowitz B 1978 A two stage cross arm flap for severe multiple degloving injury of the hand. Hand 10: 276–278

578. Lister G D, McGregor I A, Jackson I T 1973 Groin flap in hand injuries. Br J Accident Surg 4: 229–239

579. May J W, Bartlett S P 1981 Staged groin flap in reconstruction of the pediatric hand. J Hand Surg 6: 163–171

580. Schlenker J D, Averill R M 1980 The iliofemoral (groin) flap for hand and forearm coverage. Orthopaedic Rev 9: 57–63

581. Schlenker J D 1980 Important considerations in the design and construction of groin flaps. Ann Plastic Surg 5: 353–357

582. Freedlander E, Dickson W A, McGrouther D A 1986 The present role of the groin flap in hand trauma in the light of a long-term review. J Hand Surg (Br) 11: 187–190

583. Reinisch J F, Winters R, Puckett C L 1984 The use of the osteocutaneous groin flap in gunshot wounds of the hand. J Hand Surg (Am) 9A: 12–17

584. Schlenker J D, Atasoy E, Lyon J 1980 The abdominohypogastric flap — axial pattern flap for forearm coverage. Hand 12: 248–252

585. Shaw D T 1980 Tubed pedicle construction: the single pedicle abdominal tube and the acromiopectoral flap. Ann Plastic Surg 4: 219–223

586. Watson A C, McGregor J C 1981 The simultaneous use of a groin flap and a tensor fascia latae myocutaneous flap to provide tissue cover for a completely degloved hand. Br J Plastic Surg 34: 349–352

587. Lister G, Scheker L 1988 Emergency free flaps to the upper extremity. J Hand Surg (Am) 13: 22–28

588. Lister G D 1993 Free skin and composite flaps. In: Green DP (ed) Operative Hand Surgery, 3rd edn. Churchill Livingstone, New York, pp 1103–1158

589. Hing D N, Buncke H J, Alpert B S, Gordon L 1985 Free flap coverage of the hand. Hand Clin 1: 741–758

590. Ikuta Y 1985 Vascularized free flap transfer in the upper limb. Hand Clin 1: 297–309

591. Godina M 1991 A thesis. Presernova Druzba, Ljubljana

592. Press B H, Chiu D T, Cunninghan B L 1990 The rectus abdominis muscle in difficult problems of hand soft tissue reconstruction. Br J Plastic Surg 43: 419–425

593. Logan S E, Alpert B S, Buncke H J 1988 Free serratus anterior muscle transplantation for hand reconstruction. Br J Plastic Surg 41: 639–643

594. Brody G A, Buncke H J, Alpert B S, Hing D N 1990 Serratus anterior muscle transplantation for treatment of soft tissue defects in the hand. J Hand Surg (Am) 15: 322–327

595. Whitney T M, Buncke H J, Alpert B S, Buncke G M, Lineaweaver WC 1990 The serratus anterior free muscle flap: experience with 100 consecutive cases. Plastic Reconstr Surg 86: 481–490

596. Katsaros J, Schusterman M, Beppu M, Banis J C Jr, Acland R D 1984 The lateral upper arm flap: anatomy and clinical applications. Ann Plastic Surg 12: 489–500

597. Lister G, Scheker L 1988 Emergency free flaps to the upper extremity. J Hand Surg (Am) 13: 22–28

598. Scheker L R, Kleinert H E, Hanel D P 1987 Lateral arm composite tissue transfer to ipsilateral hand defects. J Hand Surg (Am) 12: 665–672

599. Mahaffey P J, Tanner N S, Evans H B, McGrouther D A 1985 The degloved hand: immediate complete restoration of skin cover with contralateral forearm free flap. Br J Plastic Surg 38: 101–106

600. Swanson E, Boyd J, Manktelow R T 1990 The radial forearm flap; reconstructive applications and donor site defects in 35 consecutive patients. Plastic Reconstr Surg 85: 258–266

601. Jones B M, O'Brien C J 1985 Acute ischaemia of the hand resulting from elevation of a radial forearm flap. Br J Plastic Surg 38: 396–397

602. Timmons M J, Missotten F E, Poole M D, Davies D M 1986 Complications of radial forearm flap donor sites. Br J Plastic Surg 39: 176–178

603. Bardsley A F, Soutar D S, Elliot D, Batchelor A G 1990 Reducing morbidity in the radial forearm flap donor site. Plastic Reconstr Surg 86: 287–292

604. McGregor A D 1987 The free radial forearm flap — the management of the secondary defect. Br J Plastic Surg 40: 83–85

605. Zuker R M, Manktelow R T 1986 The dorsalis pedis free flap; technique of elevation, foot closure, and flap application. Plastic Reconstr Surg 77: 93–104

606. Lovie M J, Duncan G M, Glasson D W 1984 The Ulnar artery forearm free flap. Br J Plastic Surg 37: 486–492

607. Salibian A H, Anzel S H, Mallerich M M, Tesoro V E 1984 Microvascular reconstruction for close-range gunshot injuries to the distal forearm. J Hand Surg (Am) 9: 799–804

608. Swartz W M 1984 Immediate reconstruction of the wrist and dorsum of the hand with a free osteocutaneous groin flap. J Hand Surg (Am) 9A: 18–21

609. Upton J, Rogers C, Durham-Smith G, Swartz W M 1986 Clinical applications of free temporoparietal flaps in hand reconstruction. J Hand Surg (Am) 11: 475–483

610. Brent B, Upton J, Acland R D, Shaw W W et al 1985 Experience with the temporoparietal fascial free flap. Plastic Reconstr Surg 76: 177–188

611. Rose E H, Norris M S 1990 The versatile temporoparietal fascial flap; adaptability to a variety of composite defects. Plastic Reconstr Surg 85: 224–232

612. Hing D N, Buncke H J, Alpert B S 1988 Use of the temporoparietal free fascial flap in the upper extremity. Plastic Reconstr Surg 81: 534–544

613. Grad J B, Beasley R W 1985 Fingertip reconstruction. Hand Clin 1: 667–676

614. Louis D S, Palmer A K, Burney R E 1980 Open treatment of digital tip injuries. J Am Med Assoc 244: 697–698

615. Allen M J 1980 Conservative management of fingertip injuries in adults. Hand 12: 257–265

616. DeBoer P, Collinson P O 1981 The use of silver sulphadiazine occlusive dressings for fingertip injuries. J Bone Joint Surg 4: 545–547

617. Tranquilli-Leali E 1935 Ricostruzione dell'apice delle falangi ungueali mediante autoplastica volare peduncolata per scorrimento. Infort Traum Lavoro 1: 186–193

618. Atasoy E, Ioakimidis E, Kasdan M, Kutz J E, Kleinert H E 1970 Reconstruction of the amputated fingertip with a triangular volar flap. J Bone Joint Surg 52A: 921–926

619. Snow J W 1985 Volar advancement skin flap to the fingertip. Hand Clin 1: 685–688

620. Shepard G H 1983 The use of lateral V–Y advancement flaps for fingertip reconstruction. J Hand Surg (Am) 8: 254–259

621. Macht S D, Watson H K 1980 The Moberg volar advancement flap for digital reconstruction. J Hand Surg 5: 372–376

622. Posner M A, Smith R J 1971 The advancement pedicle flap for thumb injuries. J Bone Joint Surg 53A: 1618–1621

623. Arons M S 1985 Fingertip reconstruction with a palmar advancement flap and free dermal graft: a report of six cases. J Hand Surg (Am) 10: 230–232

624. Dellon A L 1983 The extended palmar advancement flap. J Hand Surg (Am) 8: 190–194

625. Pho R W H 1979 Local composite neurovascular island flap for skin cover in pulp loss of the thumb. J Hand Surg 4: 11–16

626. Cronin T D 1951 The cross-finger flap — a new method of repair. Ann Surg 17: 419–425

627. Curtis R M 1957 Cross-finger pedicle flap in hand surgery. Ann Surg 145: 650

628. Hoskin H D 1960 The versatile cross-finger flap. J Bone Joint Surg 42A: 261–277

629. Kappel D A, Burech J G 1985 The cross-finger flap. An established reconstructive procedure. Hand Clin 1: 677–683

630. Vlastou C, Earle A S, Blanchard J M 1985 A palmar cross-finger flap for coverage of thumb defects. J Hand Surg (Am) 10: 566–569

631. Gaul J S Jr 1987 A palmar-hinged flap for reconstruction of traumatic thumb defects. J Hand Surg (Am) 12: 415–421

632. Small J O, Brennen M D 1988 The first dorsal metacarpal artery neurovascular island flap. J Hand Surg (Br) 13: 136–145

633. Adamson J E, Horton C E, Crawford H H 1967 Sensory rehabilitation of the injured thumb. Plastic Reconstr Surg 40: 53–57

634. Gaul J S 1969 Radial innervated cross-finger flap from index to provide sensory pulp to injured thumbs. J Bone Joint Surg 51A: 1257–1263

635. Walker M A, Hurley C B, May J W Jr 1986 Radial nerve cross-finger flap differential nerve contribution in thumb reconstruction. J Hand Surg (Am) 11: 881–887

636. Lister G D 1981 The theory of the transposition flap and its practical application in the hand. Clin Plastic Surg 8: 115–128

637. Flatt A E 1957 The thenar flap. J Bone Joint Surg 39B: 80–85

638. Markley J M Jr 1985 Island flaps of the hand. Hand Clin 1: 689–699

639. Krag C, Rasmussen B 1975 The neurovascular island flap for defective sensibility of the thumb. J Bone Joint Surg 57B: 495–499

640. Henderson H P, Reid D A C 1980 Long term follow up of neurovascular island flaps. Hand 12: 113–122

641. Markley J M 1977 The preservation of close two-point discrimination in the interdigital transfer of neurovascular island flaps. Plastic Reconstr Surg 59: 812–816

642. Tubiana R, DuParc J 1961 Restoration of sensibility in the hand by neurovascular skin island transfer. J Bone Joint Surg 43B: 474–480

643. Zook E G, Guy R J, Russell R C 1984 A study of nail bed injuries: causes, treatment, and prognosis. J Hand Surg (Am) 9: 247–252

644. Zook E G 1985 Nail bed injuries. Hand Clin 1: 701–716

645. Zook E G 1990 Anatomy and physiology of the perionychium. Hand Clin 6: 1–7

646. Guy R J 1990 The etiologies and mechanisms of nail bed injuries. Hand Clin 6: 9–19
647. Van Beek A L, Kassan M A, Adson M H, Dale V 1990 Management of acute fingernail injuries. Hand Clin 6: 23–35
648. Shepard G H 1990 Management of acute nail bed avulsions. Hand Clin 6: 39–56
649. Seckel B R 1986 Self-advancing silicone rubber splint for repair of split nail deformity. J Hand Surg (Am) 11: 143–144
650. Shepard G H 1983 Treatment of nail bed avulsions with split-thickness nail bed grafts. J Hand Surg (Am) 8: 49–54
651. Saito H, Suzuki Y, Fujino K, Tajima T 1983 Free nail bed graft for treatment of nail bed injuries of the hand. J Hand Surg (Am) 8: 171–178
652. Shepard G H 1990 Nail grafts for reconstruction. Hand Clin 6: 79–102
653. Pessa J E, Tsai T M, Li Y, Kleinert H E 1990 The repair of nail deformities with the nonvascularized nail bed graft: indications and results. J Hand Surg (Am) 15: 466–470
654. Clayburgh R H, Wood M B, Cooney W P 3rd 1983 Nail bed repair and reconstruction by reverse dermal grafts. J Hand Surg (Am) 8: 594–598
655. Atasoy E 1982 Reversed cross-finger subcutaneous flap. J Hand Surg 7: 481–483
656. Magierski M, Sakiel S, Buczak B, Koisar J, Kepny A, Ciembroniewicz W 1979 Analysis of reasons and locations of burns on hands. Scand J Plastic Reconstr Surg 13: 141–142
657. Salisbury R E, Hunt J L, Warden G D, Pruitt B A 1973 Management of electrical burns of the upper extremity. Plastic Reconstr Surg 51: 648–652
658. Sullivan W G, Scott F A, Boswick J A 1981 Rehabilitation following electrical injury to the upper extremity. Ann Plastic Surg 7: 347–353
659. Gunn A 1967 Electric fire burn. Br Med J 3: 764–766
660. Stone P A 1973 Hand burns caused by electric fires. Injury 4: 240–246
661. Luce E A, Gottlieb S E 1984 'True' high-tension electrical injuries. Ann Plastic Surg 12: 321–326
662. Curreri P W, Asch M J, Pruitt B A 1970 The treatment of chemical burns. J Trauma 10: 634
663. Jelenko C 1974 Chemicals that burn. J Trauma 14: 65–72
664. Edelman P A 1987 Chemical and electrical burns. In: Achauer B M (ed) Management of the burned patient. Appleton & Lange, Norwalk, C T, pp 183–202
665. Hill M B, Achauer B M, Martinez S 1984 Tar and asphalt burns. J Burn Care Rehabil 5: 271–274
666. Saydjari R, Abston S, Desai M H, Herndon D N 1986 Chemical burns. J Burn Care Rehabil 7: 404–408
667. Pike J, Patterson A, Arons MS 1988 Chemistry of cement burns: pathogenesis and treatment. J Burn Care Rehabil 9: 258–260
668. Ellenhorn M J, Barceloux D G 1988 Medical toxicology: diagnosis and treatment of human poisoning. Elsevier, New York
669. Leonard LG 1982 Chemical burns: effect of prompt first aid. J Trauma 22: 420–422
670. Sigurdsson J, Bjornsson A, Gudmundsson ST 1983 Formic acid burn — local and systemic effects. Burns 9: 358–361
671. Hansbrough J F, Zapata-Sirvent R, Dominic W et al 1985 Hydrocarbon contact injuries. J Trauma 25: 250–252
672. Hunter G A 1968 Chemical burns of the skin after contact with petrol. Br J Plastic Surg 21: 337–341
673. Simpson L A, Cruse C W 1981 Gasoline immersion injury. Plastic Reconstr Surg 67: 54–57
674. Greco R J, Hartford C E, Haith L R et al 1988 Hydrofluoric acid-induced hypocalcemia. J Trauma 28: 1593–1596
675. Hicks L M, Hunt J L, Baxter C R 1979 Liquid propane cold injury: a clinicopathologic and experimental study. J Trauma 19: 701–703
676. Brown T D 1974 The treatment of hydrofluoric acid burns. J Soc Occup Med 24: 80–89
677. Kohnlein H E, Achinger R 1982 A new method of treatment of hydrofluoric acid burns of the extremities. Chir Plast 6: 297–305
678. Chick L R, Borah G B 1992 Treatment of hydrofluoric acid burns of the hand. Plastic Reconstr Surg (in press)
679. Dibell D G, Iverson R E et al 1970 Hydrofluoric acid burns of the hand. J Bone Joint Surg 52A: 931–936
680. Pardoe R, Minami R T, Sato R M, Schlesinger S L 1977 Phenol burns. Burns 3: 29–41
681. Monzingo DW, Smith AA, McManus WF et al 1988 Chemical burns. J Trauma 28: 642–647
682. Clare RA, Krenzelok EP 1988 Chemical burns secondary to elemental metal exposure. Am J Emerg Med 6: 355–357
683. James J H, Morris A M 1977 The use of hand bags compared with a conventional dressing in the treatment of superficial burns of the hand. Chirurgia Plastica 4: 67–72
684. Chait L A 1975 The treatment of burns by early tangential excision and skin grafting. South African Med J 49: 1375–1379
685. Wexler M R, Yeschua R, Neuman Z 1975 Early treatment of burns of the hand by tangential excision and grafting. Plastic Reconstr Surg 54: 268–273
686. Levein B A, Sirinek K R, Peterson H D, Pruitt B A 1979 Efficacy of tangential excision and immediate autografting of deep second-degree burns of the hand. J Trauma 19: 670–673
687. Malfeyt G A M 1976 Burns of the dorsum of the hand treated by tangential excision. Br J Plastic Surg 29: 78–81
688. Chick L R, Lister G D, Souder L 1992 Early free flaps in the management of electrical burns. Plastic Reconstr Surg 89: 1013–1019
689. Salisbury R E, Pruitt B A 1976 Burns of the upper extremity. Saunders W B, Philadelphia
690. Salisbury R, McKeel D 1974 Ischemic necrosis of the intrinsic muscles of the hand after thermal injuries. J Bone Joint Surg 56A: 1701–1707
691. Salisbury R E, Taylor J W, Levine N S 1976 Evaluation of digital escharotomy in burned hands. Plastic Reconstr Surg 58: 440–443
692. Schumacker H B 1982 Frostbite. In: Flynn J E (ed) Hand surgery, 3rd edn. Williams & Wilkins, Baltimore, p 591
693. Mills W J, Whaley R, Fish W 1960 Frostbite: experience with rapid rewarming and ultrasonic therapy. Alaska Med 2: 1–3, 114–122
694. Nakazato T, Ogino T 1986 Epiphyseal destruction of

children's hands after frostbite: a report of two cases. J Hand Surg 11A: 289–292

695. Zdeblick T A, Field GA, Shaffer J W 1988 Treatment of experimental frostbite with urokinase. J Hand Surg (Am) 13: 948–953

696. Rakower S, Shahgoli S, Wong S 1978 Doppler ultrasound and digital plethysmography to determine the need for sympathetic blockage after frostbite. J Trauma 18: 713–718

697. Robson M C, Heggers J P 1981 Evaluation of hand frostbite blister fluid as a clue to pathogenesis. J Hand Surg 6: 43–47

2. Reconstruction

Before considering reconstruction of the previously injured hand the surgeon must not only possess a thorough knowledge of the deficiencies in structure and function in the affected limb; he must also understand the demands that the patient places on the limb both in his occupation and in his recreation. Knowing that nothing he does will prove successful without the active participation of the patient after surgery, he must in addition assess the patient's attitude and motivation.

Time may be on the patient's side, or against him. While nerve function is slow to return, and time should be allowed for it to do so, joint contracture for whatever reason will become fixed and the joint itself increasingly damaged if intervention is unduly delayed. To choose the stage at which to operate is therefore a subtle art. One rule which proves helpful is never to operate while the patient shows steady improvement. This can be called 'plateau surgery' since it is undertaken when the patient ceases to progress in the climb to recovery. This necessitates regular repeated examination. Such repeated assessment is the key to management of patients likely to require reconstructive surgery of the hand. It not only permits close observation of slowly recovering function, but also gives the opportunity to adjust or change splints or physical therapy, to get to know the patient and his problems and to encourage him to take a positive, aggressive attitude, which will prove invaluable when operation is thought appropriate.

HISTORY

Original injury

Nature of injury. The injuring agent must be ascertained — especially the presence of crush, heat or electrical damage.

Closed injuries, in particular, present problems. It is important to obtain details of the occurrence in order to clarify the mechanism, which may help in deducing the anatomical location and pathology. Whether or not the patient was able to continue work is some guide to the severity of the injury.

Date and time of injury. The circumstances under which an accident occurred may be of relevance. Whether or not it happened at work is of great moment in some societies. The work, or compensation, injury offers the patient a cushion, in that he receives disability payment while off work, his medical bills are settled, and he may receive lump-sum compensation for any permanent partial disability. This cushion is good in that it reduces the financial concerns of the injured. It may also have bad effects, leading to erroneous statements regarding the original circumstances, lack of effort in rehabilitation, reluctance to return to work and exaggeration of residual complaints.

Primary treatment. Details of primary treatment are often best obtained from the primary treating physician. In this time of litigation, questions regarding the original care may easily be misinterpreted as criticism. One must even be careful of emphasis and inflection in asking the simple question, 'Who was your original doctor?' The way in which the answer is phrased can also be enlightening with regard to the patient's attitude, which may strongly influence the outcome of the later treatment.

Subsequent progress and therapy.

Previous injury to the part. Previous injuries may materially influence both the presenting injury and the required treatment. This often requires prompting from the examiner which may reveal forgotten childhood falls, automobile wrecks and several sports injuries! The surgeon is then left at first medically, and later legally, to untangle the knot.

Occupation

Details of the patient's occupation are relevant to the surgeon's planning of treatment and rehabilitation. They also give him some early insight into financial, social and domestic problems on which he may legitimately be asked to advise.

Did this injury happen at work?
How exactly did it occur?
Did you quit right away? (Clearly this is not asked of those severely and obviously injured.)
Did you report it right away?
What exactly do you do?
How long have you been doing that kind of work?
With your current employer?
Are they holding your job?

And later, once you have come to know the patient and his companions better:

Do you hope to go back to the same job?
How many are there at home?
Anyone else working?

While this chapter is concerned primarily with reconstruction following a single identifiable injury, it will become apparent, especially in considering wrist disability (p. 202), that it is not always possible to identify a solitary incident which was responsible for the patient's complaints. It may transpire that the problem is due to repeated stress placed on the upper extremity by the need to perform single or multiple manual activities repetitively throughout the day, within time limits[1] strictly applied by the needs of automated production. Such problems have come to be called cumulative trauma disorders.

Cumulative trauma disorders[2] (CTD). While these are due in most instances to nerve compression or to musculotendinous disorders, and as such will be considered in the following two chapters, they may well complicate the management of the presenting injury and the return of the patient to the workplace. They are associated with identified risk factors: repetitiveness, forcefulness, certain postures, mechanical stresses, and exposure to vibration and to low temperatures[3,4]. The prevalence of such disorders has been found to be sufficiently high as to (i) result in a high incidence of worker transfer to positions with less risk factors[5], (ii) require repeated evaluation[6,7] and (iii) initiate programmes to eliminate the causative factors[8,9]. Tool redesign prompted by these efforts will have the secondary benefit of reducing other work-related injuries[10-12].

The mental and economic well-being of the patient depends largely on his ability to return to his original employment. Ideally the surgeon would observe the man at work but this is not practical. The second alternative would require the patient to return to his place of work for trial employment. Many patients, and even more employers, are reluctant to participate in such a trial, and this is frequently made more difficult by the attitude of insurance companies or government departments. Wherever possible it should be arranged, especially where doubt exists as to whether or not further treatment is required. If, after return to work, the patient volunteers that he is fully capable of carrying out his original employment, then no matter how much loss of function in individual structures the surgeon may elicit on subsequent examination, he must be very guarded in suggesting any further surgical treatment.

Where he cannot do his job, the patient's explanation and demonstration of his difficulty should be carefully observed and analysed.

In the common circumstance mentioned above, where the patient cannot return for a trial period of employment, or where he refuses to do so with the often valid fear that his return may prompt his discharge simply because he *is* unable to perform efficiently, the third alternative is to commit the patient to a formal return-to-work programme. A complete programme has eight components[13,14]:

(i)   Physical evaluation[15,16]; this demands the use of several hand assessment techniques of proven reliability[17], which neither time nor space permit in the surgeon's examining room.
(ii)   Psychological assessment of the subjective effects of the injury (see p. 163).
(iii) Biomechanical job analysis.
(iv)   Work simulation.
(v)   Re-evaluation.
(vi)   Labour market survey.
(vii) Vocational re-education[18].
(viii) On-the-job training.

The skills required in such a programme are those possessed by physical and occupational therapists, rehabilitation nurses and counsellors, job analysis experts, claims examiners and consulting attorneys. Many programmes have been developed throughout the United States under various titles. Many offer all of the above services, many do not. The hand surgeon is wise if he investigates, better instigates, the programme he employs for his patients. In the sequence, detailed above, the surgeon is likely to play his most significant role[19] at the stage of re-evaluation, when he will be required to decide whether or not he can surgically correct those deficiencies which have been shown to be preventing the patient's return to his original employment.

This goal-oriented approach should start soon after a wage-earner has been injured, whether on or off the job, for it maintains his place in the community. It also serves to direct his attention from his damaged extremity to matters which are probably causing him great concern and in the solution of which he is required to play an active role in a programme such as that detailed above. Goal orientation can be further enhanced by the surgeon and the patient, in the presence of their contact with the return-to-work programme, agreeing on a firm date for being back on the job. When this is done with the patient's full commitment, it can then be communicated to all interested parties, to assist in their planning, with the confidence that it will not alienate the patient.

Current complaints

How can I help you? With appropriate reference to self-evident problems, such as an amputation or an open wound, the question allows the patient to expand on his needs as he sees them, and often reveals hidden difficulties. It may also inform the surgeon that his role has already been defined and is limited to rendering a disability evaluation or a second opinion. While this knowledge should make his examination no less thorough, in the first circumstance he can legitimately limit his records to those details salient to his calculations[20], while in the second he should be cautious in rendering an opinion regarding the surgery indicated. He must also, as always, be non-committal in his responses regarding any colleague. If, on conclusion of the consultation, the patient should ask whether the consultant would assume his care, he should always be returned to his referring doctor with the knowledge that a full report will be sent. If the referring doctor elects, in writing, to send the patient for treatment, only then may the consultant assume that patient's care. Neither one's practice, nor the respect of one's colleagues, is augmented by suborning patients. In our competitive society, the second surgeon will be *thought* to have done so often enough, without actually having to commit that breach in ethical behaviour.

Complaints will be expressed in one or more phrases from a brief list: *pain*, *loss of strength*, *inability to achieve certain hand positions*, which may wholly, or in part, be due to *loss of motion* in a specific joint or joints, and *numbness*. All of these may cause noticeable *clumsiness* and *loss of speed and dexterity*, difficulties heightened by the presence of an impaired and therefore *unused part*.

PAIN[21]

The nature and location of pain and of factors which initiate it should be determined.

Where is your pain?
Does it radiate elsewhere?
The patient should be encouraged to indicate the site and radiation with one finger. This should later be correlated with tenderness on palpation or pain on ma-

nipulation. As a general rule, the more diffuse the pain, the greater is the problem diagnostically for the surgeon and the longer and more taxing will be his relationship with the patient.

How bad is it?
It is impossible to quantify pain. Some estimate can be obtained by asking them to indicate a number on a scale from 0 to 10, where 0 represents no pain and 10 constant, unremitting pain preventing sleep despite narcotics and making the patient feel suicidal.

Is it there all the time?
Does it keep you awake at night?
Constant pain which keeps the patient awake at night is more commonly of a neurological origin with or without some psychological overlay, than of a musculo-skeletal origin.

What makes it worse?
What makes it better?
Rest helps most musculo-skeletal pain, activity makes it worse. This question may well elicit the demonstration by the patient of particular movements or postures which elicit pain. Once again, these should be noted and correlated with later examination.

Pain secondary to injury is usually one of three types:

Musculo-skeletal — due to distortion and stretch of injured or inadequate muscle, tendon, ligament or bone and is usually associated with activity.
Neuro-cutaneous — due to contact with neuromata, either at the macroscopic level of a neuroma (p. 234) or at the nerve endings in hypersensitive or unsuitable skin (p. 167). This is usually associated with contact.
Post-traumatic sympathetic dystrophy.

POST-TRAUMATIC SYMPATHETIC DYSTROPHY (= reflex sympathetic dystrophy = algodystrophy = causalgia)[21-24]

The following syndrome may arise after injury or surgery and consists of:

Pain inappropriate for the injury or operation; it is elicited by even the slightest contact or movement, and the examiner is impressed by the *protected immobility* of the affected limb.
Swelling — again, more severe than would be anticipated.
Stiffness affecting all joints of the hand.
Discoloration which, though commonly purplish in character, differs from case to case and time to time; the hand is often mottled in appearance, and it always differs from the contralateral limb.
Hyperhidrosis.

Increased hair growth as time progresses, the hair being thicker and darker than that on the opposite hand.
Shiny skin due, at least in part, to the swelling.
Osteoporosis, commonly described in the later stages, has been seen by the author as early as two weeks after the provoking event.

Factors which predispose to the development of dystrophy are:

An *initiating painful event*, which may be relatively minor.
A predisposing *diathesis* involving both a tendency to increased sympathetic tone and a specific psychological make-up[25].
Abnormally high *sympathetic activity*.

It has also been shown in one series to be more common in smokers[26]. In the author's experience dystrophy occurs most commonly when a tight dressing has been left in place, the pain relieved by increasing doses of analgesic. This may well account for the high incidence following closed reduction of Colles' fracture[27,28] and immobilization with a plaster cylinder cast, which the orthopaedist is reluctant to remove lest the reduction be lost. The practice of *always* splitting hand dressings to skin before giving pain medication yields a very low incidence of dystrophy.

Three stages are described classically[29], but they are related less to management than the following modification:

I   *Immediate*: inappropriate pain in the first 48 hours following injury or surgery, (children are not immune[30], and, when the diagnosis is suspected, should receive the same management detailed below).
II   *Early*: characterized by all or most of the features described above, commencing within one week and lasting for about three months.
III *Late* (Sudeck's atrophy[31,32]): the hand now demonstrates little or no evidence of sympathetic overactivity, for it is dry, painful, stiff and atrophic, often accompanied by limitation of shoulder motion — the *shoulder–hand syndrome*.

Diagnosis should be made at stage I, at which point the syndrome may be averted. If seen in stage II, the suspicions aroused by the clinical appearance can be confirmed by:

Radiographic examination of both hands on one film which permits ease of comparison and will show osteoporosis early (see Fig. 2.11) in the periarticular region and in the carpus — dystrophy may occasionally be confined to one digit[33].

Three-phase radionuclide bone scan has been said to be highly specific in phase III, showing diffuse increased uptake[34], although just how specific it is has been questioned[35].
Response to sympathetic blockade is felt by some to be necessary for a firm diagnosis[29].

Indications

Stage I   Immediate splitting of all circumferential dressings down to skin on two sides; vigorous therapy; frequent consultations for strong encouragement
Stage II   'Stress loading' programme[36] (the author's preference), stellate ganglion block, intermittent or continuous[37] intravenous steroids and/or guanethidine followed by manipulation[38,39]
Stage III As for stage II with sympathectomy

In both stages II and III, a thorough search should be made for *underlying pathology*, such as carpal tunnel syndrome. Any such source of continuing noxious afferent stimuli should be eliminated, despite concerns about operating on a dystrophic limb. Major factors in management are *honesty* and *indoctrination*. Patients must be told that however hard they work, which they must, it will be at least one year before they are well. They must be indoctrinated as follows:

'*Your hand is lying to you.* It will tell you very persuasively that, if you will only let it rest, it promises to get well. *It is lying* and if you heed it and leave it alone, it will become very much worse.'
'*You must be in charge of your hand*, not your hand in charge of you, which is the state of affairs at the moment. Let it know that however much it kicks and screams, you are going to ignore it and keep on using it as much as *you* wish.'

See these patients often, for they need your support and encouragement. Most important of all, keep their numbers few by being vigilant in the first 48 hours following injury or elective surgery.
See Green D P 1993 Operative Hand Surgery, 3rd edn. Churchill Livingstone, New York, p. 642.

LOSS OF POSITION AND POWER

Eight basic positions of the hand make up most manoeuvres, and the ability of the hand to adopt these positions and to exert force while in them should be determined.

1. *Precision pinch* (*nail pinch*). The tips of finger nails of the index finger and thumb are brought together as

in lifting a pin from a flat surface (Fig. 2.1).

2. *Pulp pinch.* The pulps of index and thumb are opposed with the distal interphalangeal joints extended as in gripping a sheet of paper (Fig. 2.2). The resistance to the thumb flexor can be increased by placing the middle finger on top of the index. The power exerted can be measured with a pinch dynamometer. Normal 5–10 pounds.

3. *Key pinch.* The pulp of the thumb is opposed to the radial side of the middle phalanx of the index finger, as in turning a key. The resistance exerted against the thumb is increased by 'stacking up' the other fingers behind the index using the interossei. The power can be measured again with a pinch dynamometer. Normal 13–20 pounds (Fig. 2.3).

4. *Chuck grip.* The digital pulps of index and middle fingers are brought into contact with the pulp of the thumb as in exerting longitudinal traction on a pencil. The index finger pronates and the middle finger supinates so that the three digits come to resemble the chuck of a power drill (Fig. 2.4).

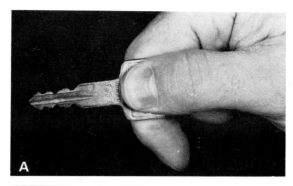

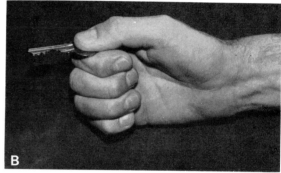

Fig. 2.3 A. Key pinch. B. The power exerted in key pinch can be increased by strong flexion of the thumb. The resistance offered by the index finger is supplemented by the 'stacking up' of the other fingers behind it.

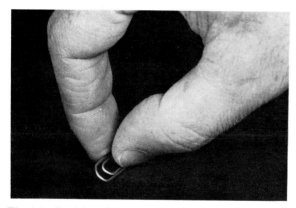

Fig. 2.1 Precision pinch.

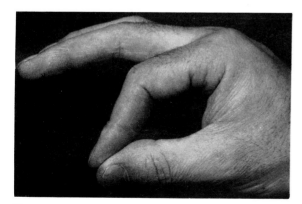

Fig. 2.2 Pulp pinch.

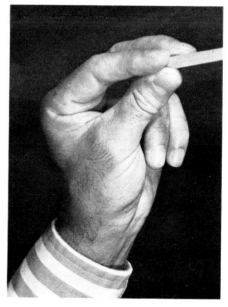

Fig. 2.4 Chuck grip, in which the thumb, index finger and middle finger come together round a narrow cylindrical object as does the chuck of a drill.

5. *Hook grip.* The fingers are all flexed at the interphalangeal joints and extended at the metacarpophalangeal joints as in carrying a suitcase (Fig. 2.5).

6. *Span grasp.* From the hook grip the interphalangeal joints are extended to approximately 30° and the thumb is abducted fully as in lifting a large glass or bottle (Fig. 2.6). Span is measured as the maximum distance attainable actively between the distal digital creases of thumb and index finger and of thumb and small finger. Alternatively, it can be assessed by the ability to lift cylinders of differing circumference.

7. *Power grasp.* The fingers are flexed fully and the opposed thumb is flexed over the fingers to increase the power as in using a hammer (Fig. 2.7). The force generated can be measured with a grip dynamometer[40] (normal 90–100 pounds). The grip is compared with that in the other hand. The

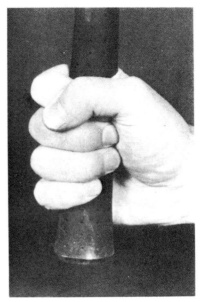

Fig. 2.7 Power grasp.

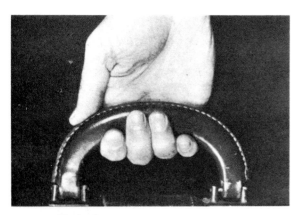

Fig. 2.5 Hook grip.

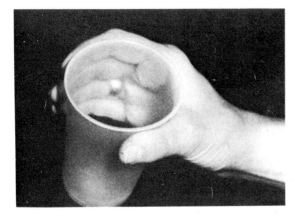

Fig. 2.6 Span grasp.

normal variation between hands is some 10% but, rather surprisingly, the dominant is not always the stronger. Both the grip and pinch dynamometer have been shown to be reliable and reproducible[41], with two provisos: (i) the elbow should be flexed during all tests[42] and (ii) the average of several tests should be taken, as variations are as high as 23.7% in grip and 17.6% in pinch[43]. By using a work simulator, normal data can be accumulated to act as a goal, and the patient's progress can be documented[44]. When a grip dynamometer is not available a useful substitute is a pneumatic tourniquet cuff rolled up and bound with tape and inflated to 30 mm of mercury. The average male can grasp this with sufficient force to push the mercury off the usual scale, that is, 300 mm of mercury. Here, comparison with the normal hand is even more important.

8. *Flat hand.* All fingers and the thumb are extended at all joints and the thumb is adducted to lie in the same plane as the hand, as in pushing against a flat surface, or inserting the hand between closely approximated surfaces (Fig. 2.8).

It will be appreciated that the radial side of the hand plays the major role in fine movements, and this is one reason why loss of median nerve sensation is much more significant than of the ulnar nerve distribution. The ulnar side of the hand is more significant in powerful manipulations. The thumb is of prime importance in

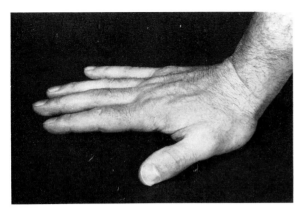

Fig. 2.8 The flat hand as used in pushing against a flat surface. It should be noted that in this posture the wrist requires to be in marked dorsiflexion.

all except the hook grip and the flat hand and even the flat hand posture can be impeded by an immobile thumb fixed in palmar abduction.

The posture and movement of the wrist and forearm are very significant in most of these positions. Full dorsiflexion of the wrist is essential in pushing with either the flat hand or in applying full power grasp. Wrist flexion with power grasp is necessary in a pronated position in many reaching and lifting manoeuvres. Pronation and supination of the forearm are required in all powerful turning activities performed by the hand. Torque is applied to smaller objects by rolling movements of the digits engaged in a chuck grip — impossible without ulnar innervated intrinsics, difficult without median sensation.

Often a patient may lack several of the postures of the hand, but commonly one is of paramount significance in preventing him from resuming employment. This must be identified and then analysed during examination and return-to-work evaluation (see above) into specific structural and dynamic deficiencies. Thereafter, by correcting these deficiencies, treatment can be directly aimed at achieving occupational function.

LOSS OF SENSATION

The nature and distribution of sensory loss will be elicited during subsequent examination.

UNUSED PARTS

The presence of unused parts may inhibit the patient's ability to adopt one of the eight basic positions of the hand or to exert power in that position. This should be noted, for where the part cannot be rendered useful,

judicious amputation may greatly enhance function. The stiff or painful index finger can often be disregarded, for all of the above positions can be assumed simply by using the middle and ring fingers as if they were index and middle (Fig. 2.9). The patient has, in effect, amputated his own index finger.

Personality, intelligence and reliability

It is not necessary to take a formal psychiatric history to gain an assessment of the patient's personality. Several simple guides can be offered in determining whether the patient is likely to respond well to further treatment, cooperate in rehabilitation and indeed whether or not he wishes to achieve full recovery.

Attendance
While most patients are genuinely unable to keep one appointment for unexpected reasons, the one whose record is repeatedly marked with failure to attend must be suspected of lacking interest.

Meeting the surgeon's gaze
A hypnotic stare lasting seconds is *not* implied, but even shy patients meet the surgeon's eye when he is explaining something or asking a question and failure to do so should raise fears of future problems. Failure of the surgeon to meet the patient's gaze is probably equally significant but is outwith the scope of this text.

Response to instructions
It is inevitable that some patients will be encountered who have insufficient intelligence to cooperate in their care. These should be recognized by their inability to perform with their normal hand simple movements carefully and repeatedly explained and demonstrated.

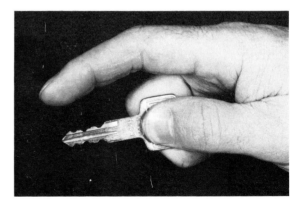

Fig. 2.9 The middle finger is substituted, often subconsciously, for the injured index.

Honesty

Patients indicate to some degree their reliability in subsequent management by the honesty with which they answer questions. Some will, for example, claim to have used a splint continuously or left a dressing undisturbed when even cursory inspection shows this to be untrue.

Inappropriate affect

Patients who complain vehemently but with apparent relish of disability and especially pain, often ill-defined, but who show little other evidence of distress when the pain is elicited constitute a group little understood, difficult to manage and invariably unchanged by surgical intervention.

Liability

When a patient returns often to the matter of liability for his original injury, he must be suspected of wishing to extract maximum compensation. While such an attitude is understandable and often justified, it is not compatible with a single-minded effort to achieve full recovery.

Malingering

A patient may malinger for financial gain, to avoid work, to inspire sympathy, possibly for other reasons. Whatever the cause, the surgeon must attempt to detect the fact for a number of reasons. Several manoeuvres are helpful.

Glove hypaesthesia. Sensory loss following injury exists in recognizable anatomic dermatomes (see p. 228), with some fluctuation due to variation and overlap. Few patients know these dermatomes — although an increasing number know the features of carpal tunnel syndrome — and pinwheel testing of the entire upper extremity, marking the point of change from normal to hypaesthetic with each sweep of the device, may show the alleged hypaesthesia to have a 'glove distribution'. The proximal margin may be at any level from the wrist to the neck, but never in an anatomical distribution.

Repeated 1, decreasing 2PD. If a patient claims total absence of sensation, it is relatively easy to disprove in that he shows a normal sweat or wrinkle pattern (pp. 230 and 233) or occasionally he can be misled — 'Tell me each time you *do not* feel me touch you'. More subtle and difficult is the patient who attempts to deceive on testing of two-point discrimination, knowing that to be some measure of sensory return. Initial testing may reveal a 2 PD of 15 mm in an area the examiner suspects to be normal. He should then apply a stream of 30 to 40 applications of 1 point alone, to the stage that the patient begins to doubt his own sensibility. This can be accompanied by occasional expressions of disbelief

— 'Are you sure?' — and by the narrowing of the gap. The two points are at last applied, the patient in relief exclaims 'Two!' and the examiner has a 2 PD reading of 5 mm — and some information about the patient's veracity.

The flat curve. Using the grip strength dynamometer, the patient's grip strength should be measured at all five settings from narrow to wide span grasp. However badly injured a hand may be the plot of the resulting strengths should always be a curve as in the normal hand (see below), skewed to right or left depending upon the injury. A flat curve, that is, the same strength at every setting, should raise suspicions. They can largely be confirmed by:

Rapid exchange grip strength. When he has time to concentrate, the malingerer can produce less than maximal strength repeatedly. If he is encouraged to alternate rapidly from one hand to the other, strongly gripping the dynamometer set at the central position, this control disappears. Normally with rapid exchange, grip strength falls slightly, but rises often dramatically in the patient who is malingering[45]. Thus a suspicious recording might read as follows:

Hand	\multicolumn{5}{c}{Dynamometer setting}	Rapid exchange
	1	2	3	4	5	
Injured	20	20	20	25	20	90
Normal	85	100	110	140	120	120

Breakaway. When testing muscle strength, if the examiner initially encounters resistance but, without his applying extra force, the offered resistance suddenly gives way and cannot be reproduced, this is evidence of an attempt to deceive.

Distracted function. The movement which the patient claims is impossible is reproduced passively by the examiner. While maintaining the position he then asks the patient to perform a new, and relatively complex, manoeuvre with his other hand. After the patient has attempted this for some moments, the examiner helps him, thereby releasing the passive hold on the limb in question. If the posture is maintained, active function exists and deception is proved.

Such deception may have complex causes, and the physician should remember that his first responsibility is to his patient, without ever being dishonest. As an example, take the high-achievement young violinist, an only child. Her expenses to audition for a prestigious school of music are being paid by a subscription raised by her township. Suddenly, without injury, she is unable to flex her small finger on her left hand. The *distracted function test* reveals her deception, but only to her physician. By informing her parents, he would disgrace and discredit her, when all she needs is some relief from the load of expectations and responsibility. Qualified reassurance is given, 'She will certainly recover, but may not be at her best for a while'. The load is removed, self-respect maintained, function returns, the audition is successful.

It may be seen from this example that the boundary between conscious malingering on the one hand and factitious injury (see p. 164) and hysteria on the other is grey indeed.

From all or any of these criteria the surgeon must form an opinion of a patient's desire and ability to cooperate in any further surgery. While the benefits of any doubt should be given to the patient, where the surgeon has serious fears on this score, he should not undertake surgery. Much can often be gained by sharing these reservations with the patient. You may lose him, but this will only confirm your decision not to treat him.

Increasing knowledge carries both assets and liabilities. *Because* we have now recognized the prevalence of *cumulative trauma disorders* we can, through the actions of return-to-work programmes and more enlightened employers, strive to prevent the vicious cycle to which many workers were subjected, by which their cure was followed by their return to the initiating activity which led inevitably to their recurrent impairment[2]. On the other side of the balance sheet, workers have learned the symptoms associated with CTD, symptoms which, in many cases, have no objective means for confirmation or denial. In some locations, such as Australia, where CTD is known as RSD — *repetitive stress disorder* — this knowledge created havoc in the workers' health care and compensation field, requiring legislative action.

The psychological stress undoubtedly inflicted on the severely injured worker has been recognized, analysed and successfully managed notably by one group in Milwaukee[46-48]. *Post-traumatic stress disorder* PTSD (note the potential confusion for the abbreviations PTSD and RSD) is characterized by *avoidance reactions*. Study of the flashbacks which are experienced by all patients injured on the job revealed three types: (i) *replay flashbacks* which involve incidents up to the injury, (ii) *appraisal flashbacks* which give an image of the hand after trauma, and (iii) *projected flashbacks* in which the hand is perceived as worse than was actually so. The first group (replay) showed a 95.2% return to work with minimal psychotherapy, while of those experiencing the second two sets of images a mere 10.3% returned, despite prolonged psychological counselling. Early return to the work site, graded work exposure and on-site job evaluations were all shown to increase the rate and speed of return to work.

With this increasing body of knowledge, it is clear that the hand surgeon needs information from many specialized individuals in making a final assessment of the injured worker. It is honest to indicate, in those who have been shown to be malingering by the methods detailed above, that it is not possible to give a rating 'as no anatomical basis can be found for some of the complaints'. Such a statement will never be disputed by the third party carrier, the employer or even the patient's own attorney, for all can abandon him with a clear conscience. But the patient, who is our primary concern, *has* been abandoned, even by his physician, by the promulgation of such a report. It is humane and professional in such cases to explain the situation to him and try to obtain his cooperation in consulting others in the large team now necessary. If, as indicated above sometimes happens, he walks out, then the report should be softened by the strong recommendation that the patient be seen by these other consultants.

Past medical history

Social history

Systematic enquiry

Quickly done, these questions frequently reveal fascinating and highly relevant information which the experienced examiner knows to pursue: the mastectomy five years previously in the patient with radiating pain; the 60 pack-years of smoking in the patient with a painful bony swelling; the polyuria and polydypsia in the patient whose wounds will not heal.

EXAMINATION AND INDICATIONS

Observation

Much can be learned by observing the hand at rest and in use before formal examination is begun.

Posture or balance
Any disturbance in the posture will quickly be detected. This may be due to disorders of bones, joints, tendons or nerves and will be discussed under each heading.

Protection
The posture adopted may not be due to joint or tendon problems but rather due to the desire to avoid pain. This is also a common cause of complete failure to use a hand which has sustained only a local injury. Examples of such protective postures include:

(a) The flexed wrist held across the abdomen indicative of a median nerve neuroma at the wrist

(b) The finger excluded from pick-up movements due to digital nerve neuroma, a poorly healed nail bed or an adherent amputation stump

(c) The immobile hand cradled in the other arm, suggestive of early dystrophy.

The hand at rest is never truly so, for the fit hand constantly moves in gesticulation, nervousness and personal mannerisms.

Cleanliness

That the hand which may be used in the consulting room is *not* used anywhere else is suggested by the extreme cleanliness of the palms, digital pulps and nails in contrast to the other hand. Cleanliness of one area of the hand may indicate lack of use. It may, however, be due to absence of sweating and because the skin ridges or 'finger-prints' are less pronounced, both a result of incomplete return of sensation.

The contrary is also true. Work staining on a hand or digit which is 'too painful to use' belies that claim.

Swelling

Oedema is always more evident on the dorsum of the hand. In the healed but little used hand it may not be striking but when that hand is compared with the dorsum of the other, swelling can be seen to have obliterated any intertendinous depression, making the extensor tendons more difficult to see. Variation in the amount of oedema can be recorded by volumetric displacement, immersing the hand to a precise landmark so that repeated tests may give comparable results (Fig. 2.10A). Oedema in the fingers can be most easily recorded by using a set of jeweller's sizing rings (Fig. 2.10B, C).

Oedema from disuse arises in a somewhat passive fashion. More 'active' oedema results from infection, injury or venous or lymphatic obstruction and these are discussed elsewhere. Where the oedema is a major problem of obscure origin, the possibility of repeated infection, injury or obstruction inflicted by the patient must be considered.

Factitious injury[49]

Factitious lymphoedema[50]. Most factitious lymphoedema is caused by the surreptitious use of a tourniquet, the minority by repeated blows — often evidenced by recurrent bruising — or by self-injection[51] which may result in recurrent low-grade infection. The diagnosis is suggested by transverse marking at the proximal edge of the oedema (Fig. 2.11). It is often necessary to admit the patient to hospital where the diagnosis is confirmed by:

radiological exclusion of other causes; includes venography and lymphangiography

laboratory confirmation of normal chemistry

irregularly timed nursing staff visits which may reveal the use of a tourniquet — it is usually obscured by clothing

bulky or occlusive dressings preventing access, and which cause resolution.

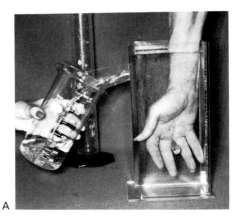

A

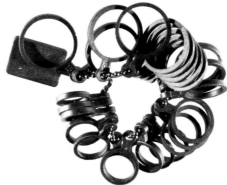

B

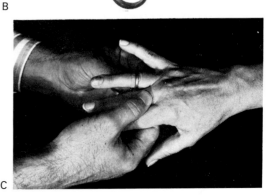

C

Fig. 2.10 A. Volumetric displacement to measure oedema. B, C. The progression of oedema of the fingers can be best and quickly recorded by the use of a set of jeweller's sizing rings.

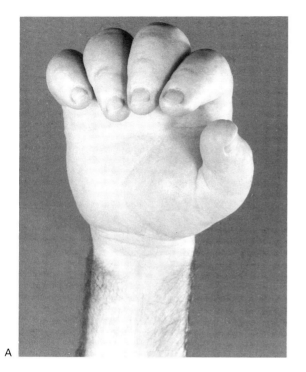

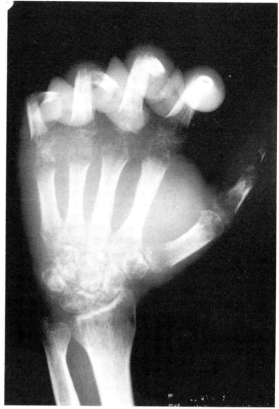

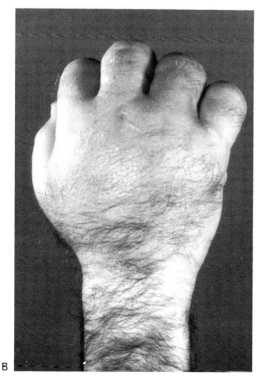

Fig. 2.11 Factitious lymphoedema. After a minor injury to the dorsum of the hand, this patient developed total disuse of his dominant right hand. A, B. Marked lymphoedema with some erythema confined entirely to the hand. The wrist is normal, and a strip of skin was noted to be much paler than the hand distally or the forearm proximally. C. Advanced periarticular and carpal osteoporosis typical of both disuse and post-traumatic sympathetic dystrophy.

Secretan's disease[52,53] is a hard oedema of the dorsum of the hand which results in peritendinous fibrosis. It is now believed by most[54] to be factitious in nature and surgery is no longer recommended[55].

Factitious ulceration[56] is another manifestation of self-inflicted injury (Figs 2.12, 2.13; see also Figs. 1.32 and 6.9). It should be suspected if a wound fails to heal as expected, and becomes virtually certain if evidence of interference appears such as fresh bleeding (Fig. 2.14) or excoriation, and can be confirmed by the application of tetracycline dressings beneath an easily removable window in a cast. The patient is instructed not to touch the dressing. Subsequent fluorescence of the opposite

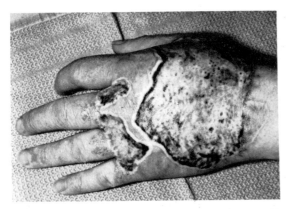

Fig. 2.12 Infrequently, a patient with a self-inflicted wound will present as an emergency. The full-thickness burn shown here, the patient claimed, was caused by chemicals found in the toilet of a bus. Histology showed it to be thermal in nature, while enquiry revealed that the victim was known in psychiatric units throughout the state.

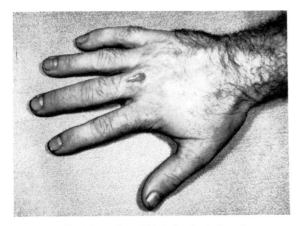

Fig. 2.13 Factitious ulcer. This lesion healed on three successive occasions when completely occluded in a cast only to recur on removal of that cast.

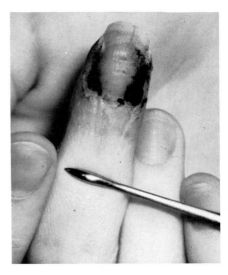

Fig. 2.14 This patient was treated for a variety of diagnoses for a painful finger. Only when fresh blood was seen around the base of the nail was the diagnosis made. On psychiatric consultation the patient admitted that her injury was self-inflicted.

hand under ultra-violet light gives the confirmatory[57] evidence. Healing will result with application of an occlusive cast.

Factitious contracture of the elbow has been reported[58].

The diagnosis of factitious injury is made more difficult both by the fact that most cases commence with a definite, though minor, injury to the area and also by the friendly, relaxed, gentle, cooperative, but unconcerned, affect of the patient. This contrasts with the behaviour of patients with similar complaints:

(a) dystrophy — usually over-anxious
(b) clenched-fist syndrome[59] — characterized by immovable digital flexion which is released by anaesthesia; these patients have poor defenses and may show great anger
(c) SHAFT syndrome[60]: Sad, Hostile, Anxious, Frustrating, Tenacious.

'Malingering is feigning illness for secondary gain. Patients with factitious lymphoedema are not *feigning* illness: they are *causing* illness' (Smith, 1975)[50]. All require psychotherapy. Confrontation of the patient with your suspicions will cause a dramatic change in his demeanour, to one hostile in all respects. Not only for this reason but also for the patient's own good, confrontation is contraindicated[49].

Systematic examination
Examination of the limb should first be directed at significant regions remote from the site of injury lest they be subsequently omitted.

Neck

The neck should be put through a full range of guided active motion — extension, flexion, lateral flexion and rotation. Any limitation or pain on these movements must be fully investigated for they may seriously affect function in the hand and may even be the origin of all residual symptoms. Investigations include:

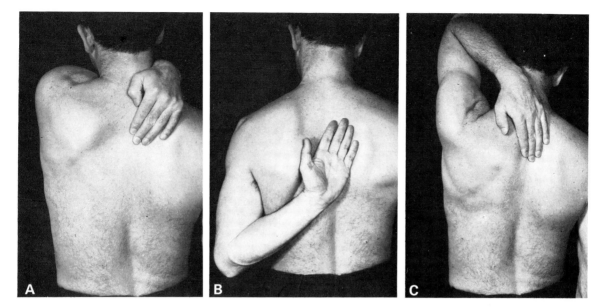

Fig. 2.15 The motion of the shoulder can be quickly checked by asking the patient to touch between the shoulder blades (A) over the contralateral shoulder which is performed by flexion and adduction (B) under the homolateral axilla, which demonstrates extension and internal rotation, and (C) over the homolateral shoulder, which demonstrates abduction and external rotation.

neurological examination of the trunk and lower limbs; radiographic examination of cervical spine: AP, lateral — in flexion and extension, oblique; myelogram where indicated.

Shoulder

The shoulder may have been injured in the same incident as was the hand, may be incapacitated by the same root injury or may be the seat of intrinsic derangement which contributes to the patient's disability. The joint should be put through a full range of guided active movement. This can quickly and reliably be effected by asking the patient to touch the interscapular region by three different routes:

1. Over the contralateral shoulder: *flexion, adduction* (Fig. 2.15A)
2. Under the ipsilateral axilla: *extension, internal rotation* (Fig. 2.15B)
3. Over the ipsilateral shoulder by carrying the arm directly out from the side: *abduction, external rotation* (Fig. 2.15).

If difficulty is encountered in any of these actions then each component movement should be checked in turn and radiographs obtained.

More distal examination of the upper limb secondary to injury will be considered structure by structure rather than on a regional basis, with the exception of the thumb (p. 176).

Skin

Ideally the skin should provide an unbroken, mobile cover for the hand which can accommodate to any position adopted by the underlying joints, while being capable of withstanding certain forces, both direct and tangential. It must be fully sensible but not painful. The initial injury, or subsequent surgery, may have left several skin features which may or may not require correction: scars, burn deformities, ulceration, skin grafts or flaps. These are considered in turn.

SCARS

These should be inspected for any evidence of incomplete healing, hypertrophy or contracture (Fig. 2.16). They should be palpated for adhesion to the underlying tissues, inelasticity or points of tenderness. When tenderness is located, the precise position and extent of the hypersensitivity or of a Tinel's sign (p. 227) should be mapped out with a blunt-pointed instrument such as a probe and any area of associated numbness with a pinwheel (p. 230). These should be marked with a skin

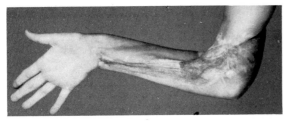

Fig. 2.16 Extensive scarring from the upper arm to the wrist has produced an immobile contracture of the elbow and less so of the wrist.

pencil and photographed or drawn in the patient's record.

BURN DEFORMITIES[61]

In the case of burn scars, hypertrophy, inelasticity, contracture and fragility may follow on the spontaneous healing of a deep dermal burn. While the primary structure damaged in the burn is the skin, correction of the resultant deformities often requires surgery on more structures than the skin alone. A classification of burned hand deformities[62] is used below to also suggest the indications.

Deformity	Probable indicated procedures
Claw	Release and skin graft
	Arthrodesis PIP joints
Palmar contracture	Full-thickness graft
Web space contracture	Release and local flaps[63,64]
	Release adductor pollicis and 1st dorsal interosseous
Hypertrophic scars and isolated bands	Release and skin graft
Amputations	First web release
	Rotational osteotomies
	Digital transposition[65]
	Toe-to-hand transfer
Wrist and elbow contractures	Release and local muscle, fasciocutaneous[66] or free flap

Personal experience has taught that, whereas the delay between injury and reconstruction following trauma should be at least six months, that delay in burned patients should be one year, for many months were consumed initially in achieving complete healing. If free flaps are to be used, the surgeon must be very aware of the lack of elasticity in grafted and in donor areas. Flap design therefore requires to be more precise, with a generous margin for error, and should include skin to cover the entire length of the pedicle and beyond if the recipient vessel lies beneath an area previously grafted.

ULCERATION

Persistent or recurrent ulceration in the hand is caused by one of the following:

1. *Loss of sensation* — discussed later; (p. 227).
2. *Vascular insufficiency* — discussed later; (p. 258).
3. *Unstable scars* — most commonly encountered following burns, they arise through repeated trauma to fragile or adherent skin or through the intermittent ischaemia produced by the raised tension created in extending or flexing a joint against a skin contrature.
4. *Retained 'foreign body'* — this may be retained since the injury and may truly be a foreign body, including non-absorbable surgical material, or may be necrotic tissue in the form of slough or sequestrated bone.
5. *Factitious wounding* — suggested by the bizarre nature of the wound and the affect of the patient; (see p. 164).
6. *Malignant change* — a Marjolin's ulcer; (see p. 427).

SKIN GRAFTS

Not all grafts applied at the time of emergency surgery are employed because they provide the ideal solution. Frequently considerations of infection, coincident injuries, early mobilization or the experience of the surgeon may have dictated the use of the simplest and most sure means of achieving immediate skin cover. Grafts should be regarded as rather specialized scars, attention being paid to hypertrophy, contracture, adherence, inelasticity, fragility and ulceration, points of tenderness and differences in pigmentation. Plans to operate on structures beneath the graft (for example, the insertion of tendon grafts) should be considered, as should any likely increase in trauma to the area with return to work.

Indications

Increasingly, with the much larger selection of flaps available — especially in the form of free tissue transfers — modern practice dictates total *excision* of scar remaining from the initial injury. Recognizing that scar is relatively avascular and immobile, and therefore likely to impair the desired result, complete scar removal has become mandatory when reparative surgery on skeletal and neurovascular structures is planned. Thus, complex reconstruction commences with radical debridement which differs little from that described in the management of selected massive injuries (p. 92). 'Pseudotumour' resection is performed by incision only through entirely normal tissue, confident that whatever defect is created can be filled with a well vascularized flap. That said, there remains a clear place, where no deep reconstruction is intended, for simple *incision* of scarred skin where its release alone will achieve the required improvement in function.

Revision, release or replacement of scars or grafts is one of the most rewarding forms of reconstruction. Particular attention should be paid to the *thumb–index web space*, where release of contracture in the adductor pollicis and first dorsal interosseous allied with introduction of better skin cover may convert a crippled hand to a functional one (p. 178).

Several techniques of scar revision or replacement are available:

Split skin grafts have a role in covering well vascularized defects in which contracture is unlikely to occur or can be prevented. They have been found by some to be as acceptable as full-thickness following release of burn contractures[67].

Full-thickness grafts. These may be used after release of a scar contracture but they require a smooth, perfectly vascularized bed and therefore cannot be used where that is not available. They are therefore rarely applicable to the web spaces.

Where the floor of the defect created by incision or excision of scar is deemed unsuitable for a skin graft, either because it would be unlikely to take or because deep reconstruction has been performed, then a flap should be used, local, regional or distant; if distant, random or axial; if axial, pedicled or free[68]. A review of the flaps available has been made on p. 113.

Z-plasty (Fig. 2.17)[69]. In this procedure the skin to

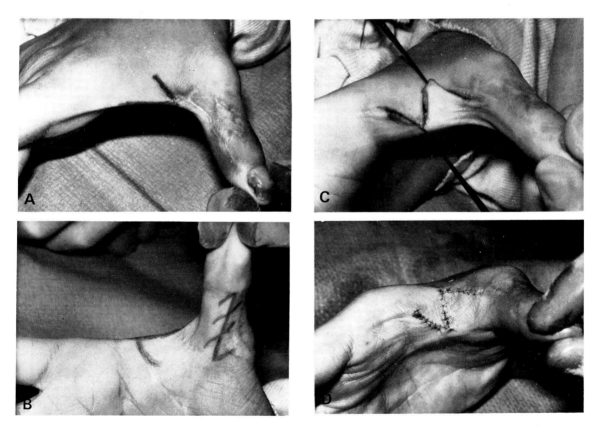

Fig. 2.17 As a result of a crush injury to the thumb, this patient had sustained a scar contracture on its ulnar aspect. This produced a limitation of span grasp by shortening of the web which was composed of good-quality skin on both dorsal and palmar aspects. A Z-plasty was constructed, (A, B), and after exposure of the web space and release of some fascial contracture the flaps were transposed (C) and sutured into position (D), providing increase in the depth of the first web space and also in the length of span grasp.

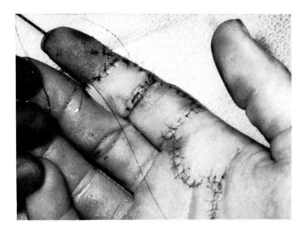

Fig. 2.18 The index finger was the seat of a severe contracture. Release required the insertion of a silastic rod and nerve graft, with excision of the scarred skin. Cover was achieved with a cross-finger flap.

release the contracture is gained from the transverse dimension, so the skin on either side of the scar should be inspected to see that it is of good quality and available in sufficient quantity. In effect, two transposition flaps of adjacent skin are interposed into the central limb which is the line of the contracture. If the entire Z-plasty is constructed within scar tissue the single contracture or bridle scar may become two, one to each side of the Z-plasty.

Local flaps. Transposition flaps, such as that from the dorsum of the index finger to the first web space described by Brand[70], are valuable in deepening a web space. The defect created when a flexion contracture of a digit is released can frequently be covered with a flap from the side of the same digit[71] — the flap where possible should include the dorsal digital arteries and nerves[72]. The planning and application of all such transposition flaps requires knowledge of the theory underlying their design[63,73]. Local flaps for larger defects are available in profusion, and are summarized on p. 113.

Regional flaps, usually in the form of a cross-finger flap, provide appropriate cover when release of a flexion contracture requires tendon and nerve surgery as well as scar excision (Fig. 2.18).

Distant flaps. These are necessary where inadequate local or regional skin is available and full-thickness grafts are not applicable or appropriate, for example prior to tendon grafting (Fig. 2.19). While on the dorsal aspect a pedicled axial groin flap can be used for scar replacement, in smaller defects or on the palm, thinner, random pattern flaps give superior results. These can come from the thorax (Fig. 2.20) or, better still, from

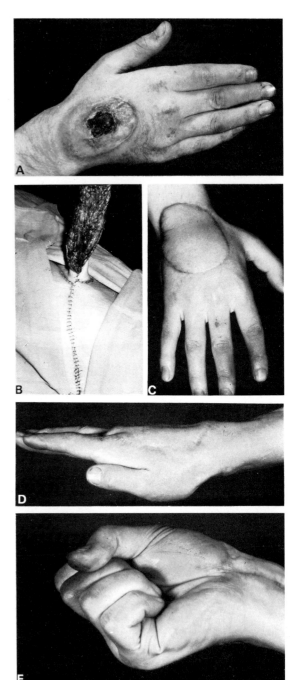

Fig. 2.19 A. This patient had sustained a full-thickness fourth-degree burn of the hand with destruction of the extensor tendons and contracture of the metacarpophalangeal joints in extension. B. A groin flap was raised and applied to the area following excision of the graft producing satisfactory cover (C) through which extensor tendon grafting was performed after release of the metacarpophalangeal joints. The outcome was full extension (D) and powerful flexion (E).

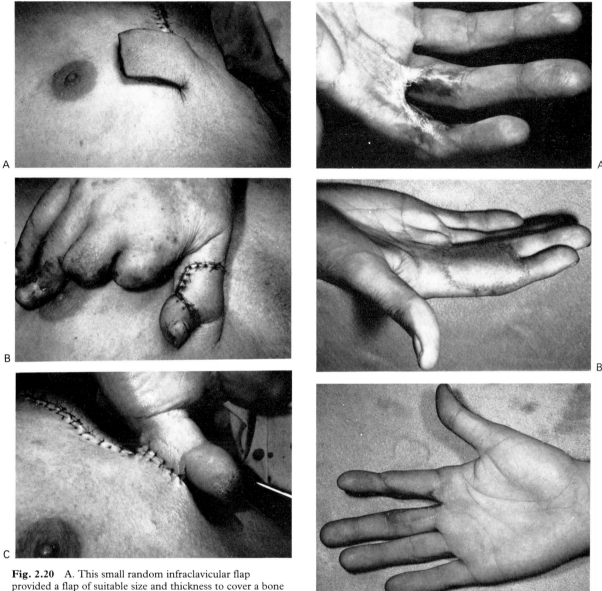

Fig. 2.20 A. This small random infraclavicular flap provided a flap of suitable size and thickness to cover a bone graft in this mutilated hand (B). C. The attachment is made secure by raising a small flap on the *recipient* site to suture to the free margin of the donor defect thereby elimininating raw areas and facilitating healing by primary intention.

Fig. 2.21 A. This small area of dense palmar scarring required excision both for comfort and also for access to the index finger for tendon and nerve grafting. This was achieved (B) with a cross-arm flap which was subsequently divided (C) to provide good skin cover.

the other arm[74] (Fig. 2.21). Forearm defects require either a random pattern flap from the abdomen (Fig. 2.22) or a free flap (Fig. 2.23).

The selection of free flaps is virtually unlimited in area, depth and quality (p. 115). Their merits are now widely recognized: (i) a permanent pedicle, (ii) a single operative procedure, (iii) a completely closed wound,

(iv) total operating time and hospital stay which are now less than with conventional pedicle flaps, (v) freedom to perform complex reconstruction on the underlying structure and thereafter to position and elevate the limb as the needs of the reconstruction dictate.

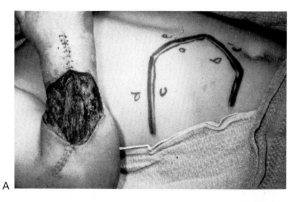

A

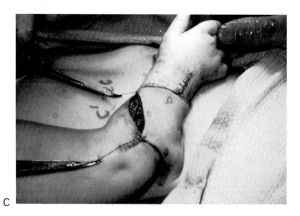

B

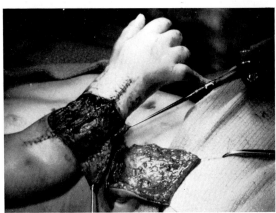

C

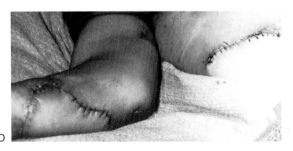

D

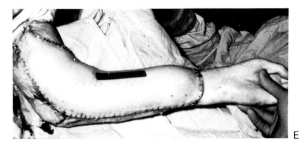

E

Fig. 2.23 After excision of extensive scarring of the arm and forearm, the only flap capable of providing sufficient cover was a latissimus dorsi musculocutaneous free flap.

An even more recent addition to the armamentarium is the technique of soft-tissue expansion. It has been recommended for use in the upper extremity[75,76], but has not gained wide acceptance. The author has no experience with the method.

Selecting which flap to employ to cover defects in different areas of the hand can be difficult. The reader is referred to a personal review by the author in Green's *Operative Hand Surgery*[68].

A note of caution should be sounded regarding scar or graft excision solely for treatment of points of tenderness. Sensory re-education by exposure to a high frequency of different stimuli should be first employed. If surgery is later performed, such re-education should certainly be practised postoperatively at a very early stage.

See Green D P 1993 Operative Hand Surgery, 3rd edn. Churchill Livingstone, New York, pp. 1103 and 1741.

FLAPS

Local flaps in the hand used at the time of injury, provided they were well-designed, are the least likely of all skin cover to require further attention. However, faults in design may result in any or even all of the problems referred to above in relation to scars in the hand.

Any secondary defects from which a flap was harvested and which were covered with skin grafts should be carefully examined for possible revision.

Fig. 2.22 A. This congenital skin defect on the dorsal aspect of the forearm was too proximal for an axial groin flap. A random flap was therefore raised (B) and a secondary flap similar to that referred to in Fig. 2.20 can be seen here raised from the forearm. The flap was applied (C) and divided three weeks later (D).

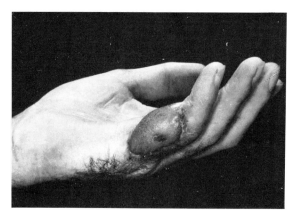

Fig. 2.24 A cross-arm flap had been applied to the palmar aspect of the left small finger in this patient following an avulsion injury which exposed both tendons and neurovascular bundle. The bulk of this flap limited flexion of the small finger and revision was required before full function could be restored.

Distant flaps invariably present unsatisfactory features at secondary assessment:

Bulk. In the majority of distant flaps an excess of both skin and fat is introduced initially, mainly in the interest of preserving the blood supply of the flap. This bulk may limit motion purely by its presence (Fig. 2.24). Needless excision of skin should be avoided, however, for frequently none need be discarded. It should rather be redistributed by the use of Z-plasties in the marginal wound, since contracture along the line of that wound is responsible for the bulky 'pin-cushion' appearance.

Insensitivity. Sensation is always poor in distant flaps. This will improve with time and with thinning but rarely provides more than protective sensation. Usually little can be done to improve this situation, but occasionally fine sensation may be imported to critical areas of a large flap, using a neurovascular island flap (Fig. 2.25).

PULP INJURIES AND DIGITAL AMPUTATIONS

Indications

The digital pulp is a region where length should be preserved in the emergency situation and where split skin grafts are often employed both with this in mind and also in order to ensure primary healing. In other cases distant flaps may have been used ill-advisedly and will then require thinning, reduction and even replacement. The requirements in the digital pulp are freedom from pain, good sensation and stable padding which is adequate, but not excessive. Free graft reconstruction of the fingertip may give an excellent result with good

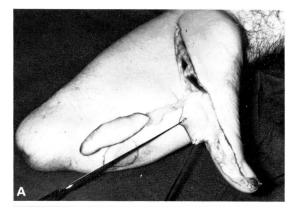

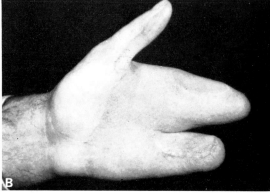

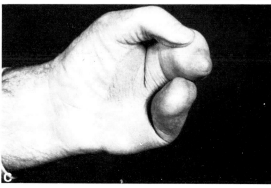

Fig. 2.25 A. This patient who had sustained a gross avulsion injury of the left hand was treated primarily with a groin flap (Fig. 1.175, p. 119). Sensation was provided to the flap together with some augmentation of its blood supply by a neurovascular island taken from the non-contact, radial aspect of the thumb. The improved blood supply permitted a later conversion of the mitten hand to one of three digits (B) with adequate flexion and key pinch between two areas with sensation. C. The patient has since returned to his occupation as a maintenance engineer.

tactile gnosis[77]. As a general rule, it seems that the thicker the donor skin the better the functional result, the smaller the area the better the sensibility[78]. If the graft has retracted markedly, as it will do if not adherent to bone, sufficient pulp may have been drawn in to make the result satisfactory or alternatively to permit the use of a secondary local flap. The local flap employed may be of an advancement type, such as those described by Kutler[79], Moberg, and the V-Y advancement flap apparently originally designed by Tranquilli-Leali and introduced into the English literature by Atasoy and others (p. 119). (A recent translation[80] indicates that Tranquilli–Leali divided the neurovascular pedicles!) Joshi[81] has reported a transposition flap containing the dorsal digital nerve. All local flap procedures have the major merit of restoring sensation. If local flaps are not possible then the choice lies between re-amputation more proximally, cross-finger flap, thenar flap, and neurovascular island flap.

The neurovascular island flap (p. 122) is justifiable only in the thumb and in a finger having unique occupational significance. Before undertaking a neurovascular island flap care should be taken to ensure that there is flow not only in the vessel which will supply the flap but also in the other digital artery of that finger and in the *contralateral* vessel of the finger immediately adjacent (Fig. 2.26) — otherwise severe cold intolerance or even necrosis may result.

A free neurovascular island transfer from the fibular aspect of the great toe offers the advantages of correctly oriented sensation and no surgery on another digit in the hand. It is the *only* available technique when donor fingers are absent or injured. The result are good[82] (Fig. 1.176).

The choice between the remaining solutions should be made after explaining the time factor involved to the patient and discussing the choice with him in the light of his occupation.

Cross-finger and *thenar flaps* on the pulp have two major disadvantages: insensitivity, which improves with time[83,84], and stiffness in the involved digits, which is more common, more prolonged and therefore more significant in the older patient. They do, however, provide satisfactory pain-free padding in the great majority of cases. If taken from the metacarpophalangeal crease of the thumb, which can be closed directly, thenar flaps have the advantage that they create no cosmetically undesirable secondary defect, but the serious disadvantage of prolonged proximal interphalangeal joint flexion in the recipient finger[85]. They should therefore be reserved for young patients in whom the appearance of the hand is unusually important. Even then, the need for vigorous physical therapy after division must be made clear to the patient before a thenar flap is used.

Re-amputation more proximally is apparently a simple solution to the problem of tender pulp scars. It may have serious disadvantages of which the surgeon should be fully aware before embarking on this course:

1. The hazard of a tender scar remains, however careful the amputation technique, and to this must be added the possibility of the formation of a neuroma on either or both digital nerves (p. 234).
2. A surprising amount of skeleton has to be resected if tension-free closure with good skin is to be achieved.
3. If the eventual amputation is through the middle phalanx, flexion of the proximal interphalangeal joint may be limited by the detached flexor digitorum profundus acting as an extensor via the lumbrical. This 'lumbrical plus' (p. 254) can be offset by suturing the tendon of profundus to the flexor sheath in the relaxed position.
4. *Quadriga syndrome*[86]. The practice of suturing the flexor to the extensor tendon over the end of an amputation of middle, ring or small finger seriously impairs the motion in the uninjured fingers due to the common origins of the flexors and of the extensors. This may even occur when the tendons have not been so tethered and is due simply to scarring. This is predominantly of the flexor tendon and the patient complains of weakness of grip. Examination reveals a flexion deficit in the uninjured digits which have a normal passive range.

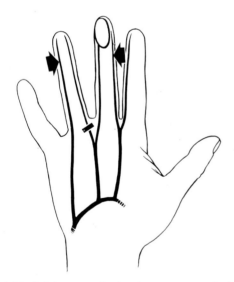

Fig. 2.26 It is important in planning a neurovascular island flap that not only is flow in the vessel to the flap and in the remaining vessel to that digit confirmed, but also flow to the contralateral digital artery of the adjacent finger. This will provide the only flow to that digit, since the artery to its other side will be divided in the course of dissection.

It will be noted that the stump of the amputated digit is more strongly flexed than the others. Verdan[87] termed this the quadriga syndrome after the Roman chariot in which the reins of all four horses were controlled in unison. Release of the flexor tendon remnant, done under local anaesthesia to ensure effectiveness, restores full power (Fig. 2.27). (It should be noted that the quadriga effect is present to reduce grip strength in all circumstances which prevent full excursion of one profundus tendon — ankylosis or arthrodesis of interphalangeal joints and adhesion after flexor repair are two examples).

It will be evident that management of the profundus is important in amputation, especially distal to the

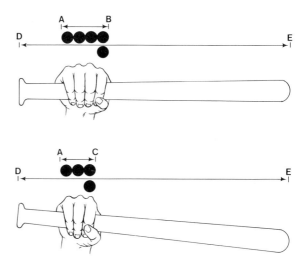

Fig. 2.28 This diagram illustrates how leverage is lost with removal of the index metacarpal ray. The length of the lever arm being reduced by one quarter has been shown to reduce leverage by almost 50%.

proximal interphalangeal joint: if left loose, lumbrical plus may result; if sutured under too much tension, a quadriga.

Ray amputation of a mutilated finger may prove beneficial. The disadvantage of the procedure is that, by removing one of the metacarpals, the leverage which the hand can apply is significantly reduced (Fig. 2.28). This adversely affects the use of a hammer, a spade, even a fishing rod. It is therefore indicated for:

stumps which impair function — for example, the stiff flexed index stump which reduces thumb–finger span grasp, or the painful small finger stump which is repeatedly struck

painful stumps — with the reservations expressed in 1 to 4 opposite

restoring competence in the respect that otherwise water or coins drop through a space created by proximal digital amputation (Fig. 2.29)

reasons of appearance — in salespersons, those engaged in communications and those concerned with cosmesis.

Ray amputation of the middle or ring should be accompanied by transposition of the index or small[88] which will yield predictably good results[89]. If not, 'scissoring' may occur (Fig. 2.30) or the remaining space will adversely affect the competence of the hand for containing liquids or small objects. If transposition is not performed, dorsal dermadesis and reconstruction of the deep transverse metacarpal ligament has been shown to give good results in 12 of 13 patients in one series[90].

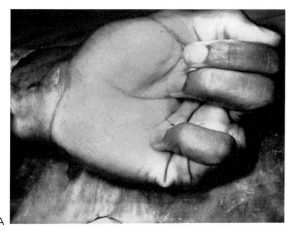

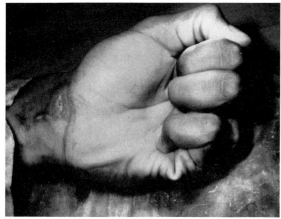

Fig. 2.27 Operative procedure under wrist block — quadriga syndrome. A. This patient is unable to fully flex his three remaining digits because the long flexor tendon is tethered out to length at the amputation stump. B. By division of the flexor digitorum profundus to the ring finger in the palm, full flexion was achieved.

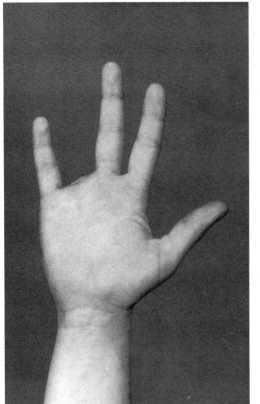
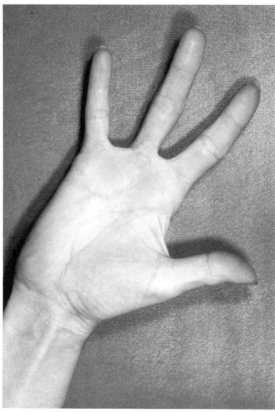

A   B

Fig. 2.29   Post-amputation competence. A. This patient, who had undergone proximal amputation without transposition following a ring avulsion injury, had problems with water and coins spilling from the palm of her hand through the defect. B. By contrast, this patient who had sustained the same injury underwent re-amputation and transposition of the fifth onto the fourth metacarpal rendering her hand competent.

See Green D P 1993 Operative Hand Surgery, 3rd edn. Churchill Livingstone, New York, pp. 62, 1766, 1773.

Thumb reconstruction[91,92]

The best method of restoring the critical loss of a thumb is to undertake replantation. Where this has not proved possible or where the injury has been of a more complex nature than clean amputation, the requirements for a functional thumb must be understood during examination and reconstructive planning.

Position is the first requirement, for if the thumb cannot be opposed to the fingers it cannot serve its normal function. This can often be achieved by release of an adduction contracture and transfer of necessary motors.

Stability can be of two varieties, fixed and mobile. The latter is preferable and is fully achieved by restoring ligamentous integrity and by transfers appropriate to restore the movements normally produced by the nine muscles of the thumb. This may be impossible, in which case joints can be maintained in good position by tenodesis or arthrodesis. Wherever possible, the basal carpometacarpal joint is kept mobile.

Strength sufficient to resist the forces of the fingers is provided, as is stability, by judicious fusions, tendon grafts and transfers.

Motion for the thumb comes as a consequence of restoring mobile stability and strength. In order of importance, efforts should be directed at (i) restoring opposition and abduction in the carpometacarpal joint, (ii) extension and flexion in the carpometacarpal and interphalangeal joints, (iii) adduction and finally (iv) metacarpophalangeal joint motion.

Sensation and *vascularity* of the terminal portion of the thumb are essential for its normal manipulative activity and are usually considered in conjunction with the final requirement, namely:

Length. The necessary length of a thumb depends

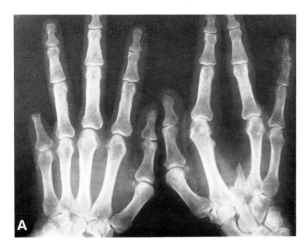

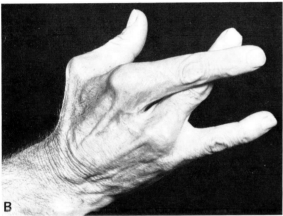

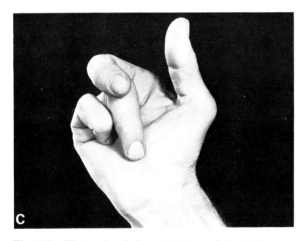

Fig. 2.30 This patient had sustained a mutilating injury to his middle finger which was treated by ray amputation. This resulted in severe functional incapacity as evidenced by scissoring in flexion and loss of the competence of the open hand. The situation was improved for the patient by transposition of the index finger on to the residual base of the middle finger metacarpal.

firstly, upon the *presence, length* and *mobility* of the fingers, for contact with force must be achieved, and, secondly, upon the occupational and social demands the patient will place upon it. Often the final decision may be made after a period of trial, both of occupation and recreations. Fitting the available procedures to the needs of the patient is a complex and individual process and the following is intended to act only as a guide.

INDICATIONS

Acceptable length — poor covering
Better skin and sensation can be obtained from a *palmar advancement* or *innervated cross-finger flap*[93,94] (pp. 69, 121–2, 174). Where improved blood supply, sensation and a better pulp is required only a *neurovascular island flap*, pedicle or free transfer can provide it.

Subtotal amputations
Subtotal amputations which have good skin cover and *nearly* acceptable length — which usually means an amputation at some point between the metacarpophalangeal and interphalangeal joints — can be restored by *phalangization*[95] (Fig. 2.31) or *metacarpal lengthening*[96,97] or *local flap and bone graft*[98]. This level of amputation, especially close to the metacarpophalangeal joint, is the perfect indication for *toe-to-hand transfer*. It demands only two motors, flexor and extensor, which are the only functions readily transferred with the toe.

Total amputation
Those in which there is no satisfactory function whatsoever can be reconstructed by *osteoplastic reconstruction*[99,100] (Fig. 2.32), *pollicization*[101–103] (Fig. 2.33), *toe-to-hand transfer*[104–106] (Fig. 2.34) or, rarely, by microvascular transfer of other parts electively amputated[107–108]. In making the choice the surgeon must pay heed to five factors:

1. *Occupation.* Manual workers may lose essential leverage across the palm of the hand by sacrificing the one metacarpal necessary in pollicization[109]; athletes will be ill-advised to surrender a toe despite the fact that foot problems after toe-to-hand transfer have been shown to be few[110].
2. *Sex.* Women will be understandably dissatisfied by the cosmetic appearance of an osteoplastic thumb reconstruction and also with the donor scar of the tube pedicle.
3. *Available digit.* If the patient is not prepared to surrender a toe, and no finger can be sacrificed —

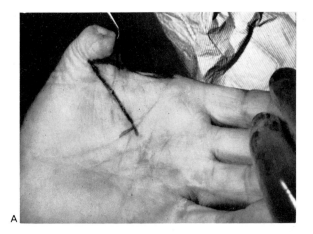

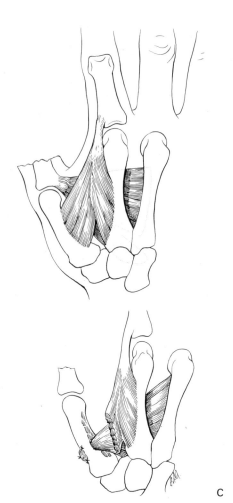

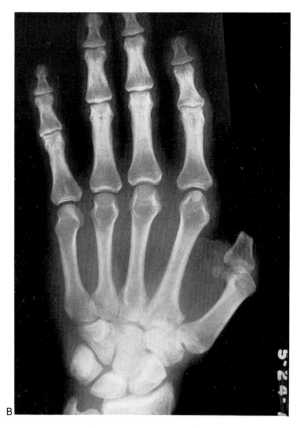

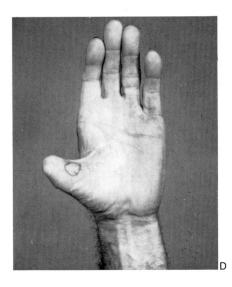

Fig. 2.31 A, B. This patient had suffered a thumb amputation at the midpoint of the proximal phalanx. As a result, he had no first web space with which to effect span grasp. The release of the muscles was performed as shown in (C), the first dorsal interosseous being detached from the first metacarpal, and the adductor pollicis being reinserted low on the metacarpal. A Z-plasty was also performed resulting in the acceptable space shown in (D).

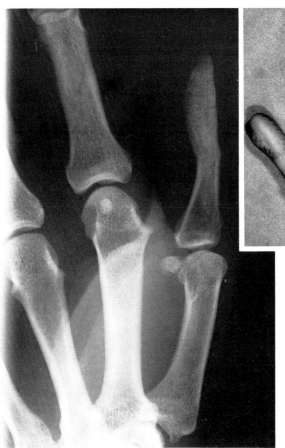

A

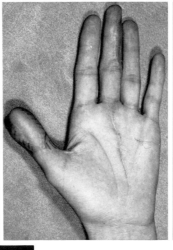

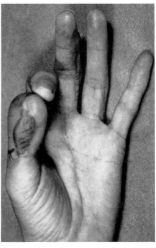

B   C

Fig. 2.32 Osteoplastic reconstruction. A. This patient had sustained amputation at the mid-point of the proximal phalanx with degloving of soft tissue to a more proximal level while water skiing. An immediate bone graft was inserted, and subsequently incorporated satisfactorily. The bone graft was covered with a tube pedicle and a later neurovascular island was applied. In (B) and (C) it can be seen that the thumb is bulky and that the neurovascular island pedicle is somewhat unstable despite attempts to attach it to the bone graft.

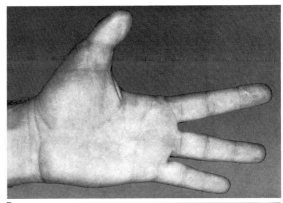

B

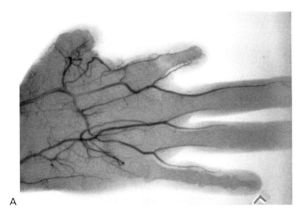

A

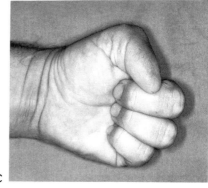

C

Fig. 2.33 Post-traumatic pollicization. Pollicization is indicated in two circumstances following traumatic loss of the thumb. First (A), where amputation of the thumb at the level of the metacarpophalangeal joint is accompanied by amputation of another digit — here the index finger — at a level which makes it functionally of no value; (B) and (C) show the result.

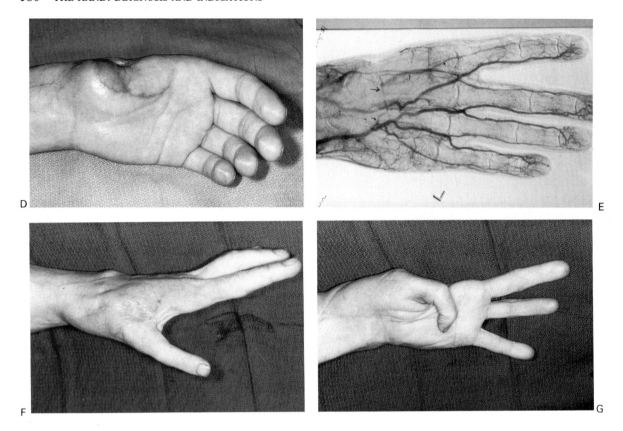

Fig. 2.33(*continued*)   Secondly (D,E), pollicization is indicated where the basal joint and intrinsic muscles of the thumb have been eliminated by proximal amputation. This patient also had a significant amount of scarring around the base and therefore pollicization was undertaken with simultaneous transfer of a free lateral arm flap. The result is shown in (F) and (G).

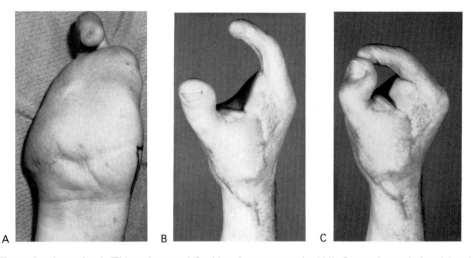

Fig. 2.34   Toe-to-hand transfer. A. This patient was left with only a contracted middle finger after an industrial accident. The palmar defect had previously been covered with a groin flap. B. By fusing the proximal interphalangeal joint of the middle at a satisfactory position and undertaking toe-to-hand transfer, a crude span grasp was achieved, and (C) some pinch was restored which gave him a good assist hand.

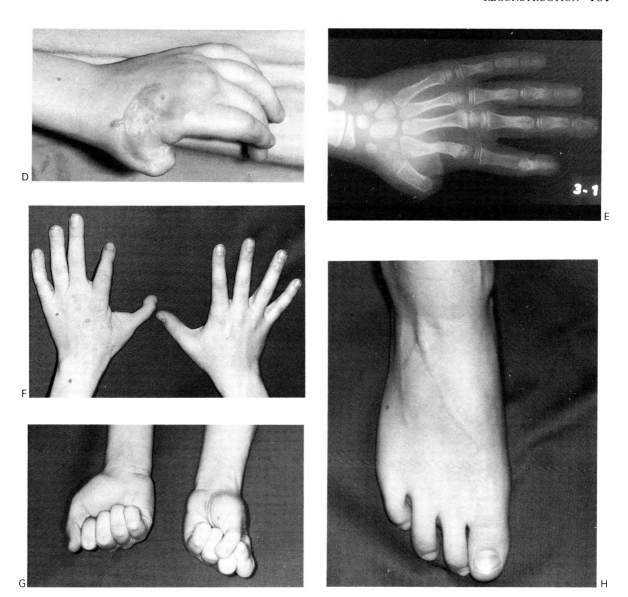

Fig. 2.34(*continued*)   D, E. Amputation in this child was at the level of the metacarpophalangeal joint of the thumb. Although the index finger was damaged, it was still functionally valuable. Second toe-to-hand transfer was performed and demonstrates (F) the inferior appearance of the new thumb, but (F, G) its satisfactory function and (H) the superior result in the foot.

either because they are absent or essential — only one of the three options remains.

4. *Basal joint.* Of the three procedures only pollicization adequately restores a basal joint to the thumb.
5. *Palmar and digital vessels.* When injury or disease has damaged the neurovascular structures of the fingers no pedicle is available either for pollicization or for conventional osteoplastic reconstruction, which requires a neurovascular island flap.
6. *Level of amputation.* The closer the amputation is to the basal joint, the less of the thumb motion detailed above can be restored by any procedure other than pollicization; if the base of the metacarpal is absent, pollicization, if a digit is available, is almost mandatory.

The influence of these six factors on the choice of procedure is shown in admittedly oversimplified form in Fig. 2.35. Other algorithms have been designed[111]. It will be evident from the above that angiography (p. 261) plays an important role in selection of the procedure most likely to succeed.

Toe-to-hand transfer offers unique advantages in digital reconstruction. The most commonly practiced, that of the great toe to replace the *thumb*[112,113], gives excellent results[114,115] (Fig. 2.34 A–C). Modifications to the original technique have been described[116–118], including the '*wrap-around*' method, intended to preserve some semblance of a toe[119,120]. The use of the *second toe* is preferred to the great toe by some in some cases[121–123], for reasons of appearance, commonly available footwear and — particularly — in children where the secondary defect is inconspicuous and the hope exists for adapta-

tion of the new thumb with growth[124] (Fig. 2.34 D–G).

Multiple digit loss can also be reconstructed by free tissue transfer[125–127], commonly using multiple toes[128–134].

Evaluation for toe-to-hand transfer requires:

(i) Assessment of:
Skin requirements. Ideally the foot should be closed with local skin, and the toe will therefore require additional skin cover when placed on the hand; further, the neurovascular pedicle should not be placed beneath skin grafts. Prior or simultaneous skin transfer may be necessary.
Skeletal reconstruction. Bone contact must ensure primary union and adequate length; measurement on the radiograph will be the basis of the plan.
Vascular anatomy, mainly by *Doppler studies* but supplemented by *angiography* of both hand and foot[135].

(ii) Thorough and repeated consultation with the patient and their family, emphasizing duration of procedure, possible failure, postoperative disappointment with appearance, donor foot function, delay in sensory recovery and chances for motion: photographs should be shared, and whenever possible a candidate for toe transfer should meet a graduate.

Prosthetic devices, both functional[136–139] and cosmetic[140,141], are becoming increasingly sophisticated. While not within the terms of this text, the surgeon must at least know of their availability and where to refer the patient for expert counselling.

See Green D P 1993 Operative Hand Surgery, 3rd edn. Churchill Livingstone, New York, p. 2073.

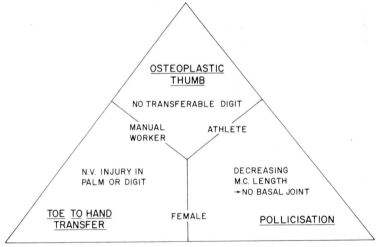

Fig. 2.35 This diagram summarizes the factors influencing the choice between pollicization, osteoplastic thumb reconstruction, and toe-to-hand transfer (see text).

Nail bed[142,143]

Following nail-bed injuries four distinct problems may be found.

Remnants of nail

Where an unsuccessful attempt has been made to excise totally the germinal matrix small spicules of the nail persist, growing in irregular manner through the skin. These cause pain and annoyance. Formal ablation should be recommended.

Split nail

An injury of the nail bed in which the eponychium has been allowed to heal to the germinal matrix causes a longitudinal split in the nail (Fig. 2.36). This should be revised by excision and resuture under magnification.

Non-adherent nail

Where loss of sterile matrix has been replaced with a graft the nail which subsequently grows over it may not adhere, resulting in painful packing of dirt under the nail. The area of nail bed which is failing in its function should be defined under magnification and shaved down to a bleeding bed to which a split thickness nail bed graft should be applied.

Before undertaking any revisionary surgery of the nail bed, the surgeon is well-advised to warn the patient of the unpredictability of the procedure.

Hook nail

This deformity results from failure to maintain a length of distal phalanx equal to the remaining nail bed at the

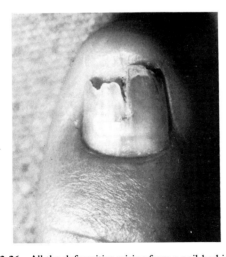

Fig. 2.36 All the deformities arising from a nail-bed injury are shown in this nail which is split, non-adherent, and the source of recurrent discomfort and infection.

time of the original injury. (p. 125) If ablation is declined, reconstruction can be performed. It will require addition of skin using a regional flap and usually a bone graft into the distal phalanx, although supporting the nail bed with Kirschner wires has been reported to give good results[144].

In rare circumstances, an unsatisfactory or absent nail can be replaced by microvascular transfer of an entire nail from the foot[145-147]. Prosthetic nails are a less expensive alternative[148].

(Reconstruction of bone and joint are considered separately, except in the wrist, where they are discussed together in a section devoted to that region and which follows.)

Bone

Three problems may arise following fractures of the hand: non-union, osteitis and malunion.

NON-UNION

Non-union comes about through *lack of adequate contact* between the bone ends or through *avascularity*. Lack of adequate sustained contact may be due to:

Too large a gap. This may be due to:
(i) Appropriate debridement of damaged bone, say after a gunshot wound, but failure to insert a bone graft
(ii) The interposition of soft parts such as a tendon or palmar plate (Fig. 2.37)
(iii) The presence between the viable ends of pieces of dead bone
(iv) The interposition of tumour as in a pathological fracture
(v) Excessive traction applied in attempting to immobilize the part
(vi) Internal fixation, poorly applied, which holds the fragments apart rather than together.

Excessive motion between the ends. Certain fractures are unstable and can be judged to be so at the time they are incurred (p. 52). If it has been decided nonetheless to manage them closed with cast immobilization, the joints at either end of the bone should *never* be moved until union is assured by the absence of tenderness at the fracture site; if the preferable treatment of internal or external fixation has been adopted but has failed to achieve *immobility* between the fragments[149], the same rules apply as if no fixation had been attempted — the joints cannot be moved. If attempts *are* made to move those joints in the presence of an unstable or poorly

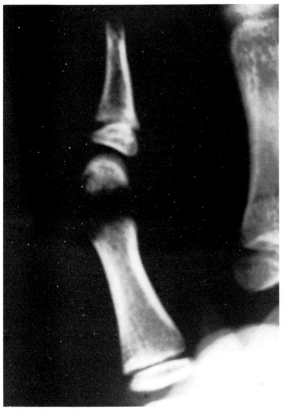

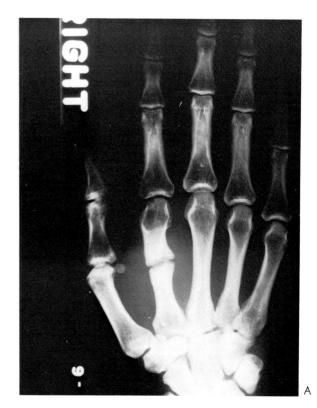

A

Fig. 2.37 This child presented with a persistently painful thumb after injury. Radiographic examination revealed the presence of a wide gap, and exploration showed that this gap contained the long flexor tendon, preventing union.

fixed fracture, motion is more likely at the fracture site than at the — by now — oedematous joint, which, with time, becomes increasingly immobile, even ankylosed, throwing progressively more movement on the fracture site — a pseudarthrosis (Fig. 2.38). The *rest and protection* splint allied to early protected motion (p. 66) must be reserved for the management of inherently stable fractures, or in rare cases where one makes a reasoned decision to accept the lesser evil of non-union in the interests of achieving soft-tissue healing while maintaining as much joint motion as possible.

Avascularity may arise in the long bones of the hand as a consequence of crush injuries with resultant comminuted or segmental fractures, the fragments of which

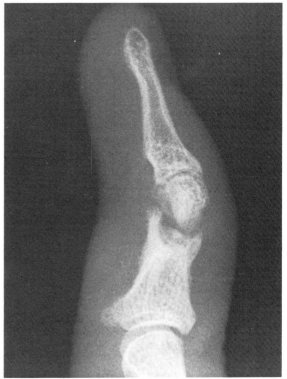

B

Fig. 2.38 The elements of pseudoarthrosis. A. Sclerosis in the bone ends. B. Ankylosis of an adjacent joint frequently plays a part in the development of motion at a nonunion.

are deprived of their blood supply. Such injuries also cause scarring and poor perfusion of surrounding soft tissues. The effect, when established, is that the bone ends become sclerotic and the scar tissue forms a *fibrous union* (Fig. 2.38).

On examination, the patient frequently has remarkably little pain and relatively good function. The presence of non-union may be detected by *tenderness on direct pressure*, by the presence of *motion*, either clinically or demonstrated on *stress films* or *cineradiography* or on lateral tomogram (Fig. 2.39).

Indications
Treatment of non-union in the long bones requires removal of the cause, excision of scarred and poorly vascularized soft tissue, debridement of the bone ends, rigid fixation[149], cancellous bone grafting and provision of well-vascularized skin cover. In many instances the lack of bone was recognized at the time of the injury and insertion of bone, either conventional[150] or vascularized[151], performed as a delayed procedure. Defects treated at a later stage are grafted with cancellous or corticocancellous autograft[152], allograft[153] or vascularized autograft[154,155]. The choice of graft is still subject to debate. However, all are agreed upon the absolute need for perfect soft-tissue cover, and the provision of such in the form of free tissue transfer is an essential part of the management of bony defects with associated soft-tissue injury. Whether thereafter 6, 8, 10 or 12 centimetres of bone gap is the upper limit beyond which a *vascularized* bone graft is required is a matter of personal preference and experience — fibula (Fig. 2.10E,F), iliac crest, scapular margin, radius and rib being the choices of vascularized bone in order of decreasing popularity.

See Green D P 1993 Operative Hand Surgery, 3rd edn. Churchill Livingstone, New York, pp. 717, 742, 961.

OSTEITIS (see Chapter 4, p. 330)

Osteitis is uncommon in association with fractures of the upper extremity and is always due to avascularity, as outlined above. The findings are those of osteitis elsewhere: a chronically discharging wound surrounded by inflamed, indurated skin. The radiograph will show a non-union, often with sequestration and sclerosis of bone fragments. Many organisms may be cultured, but they are merely opportunistic. They will disappear with adequate surgical treatment. The diagnosis of osteitis *unrelated* to fractures may be much more difficult and is considered in Chapter 4 (p. 330). That treatment is as for non-union — radical debridement of all avascular bone and soft tissue, adequate fixation, provision of well vascularized soft-tissue cover and cancellous bone graft, either simultaneously or some six weeks later when it is seen that all infection has settled (Fig. 2.40). In some instances of infected forearm non-unions, vascularized bone grafts may be indicated[156], often with microvascular soft-tissue cover[157] (Fig. 2.40).

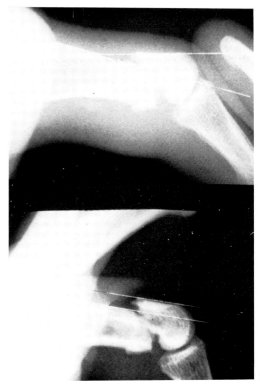

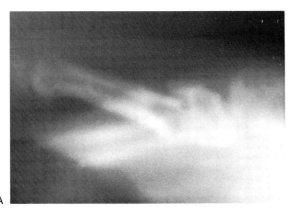

Fig. 2.39 A. Lateral (or sagittal) tomogram with apex palmar angulation. It was painless, and the patient presented for tenolysis. B. Hyperextension stress applied to this delayed union of a proximal phalanx reveals motion.

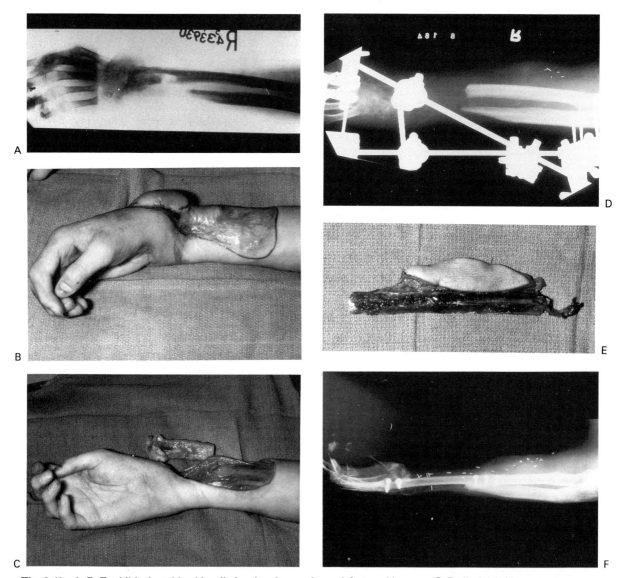

Fig. 2.40 A, B. Established osteitis with a discharging sinus and unsatisfactory skin cover. C. Radical debridement was performed (see p. 92) and (D) an external fixator and a combined serratus anterior and latissimus dorsi flap applied. Six weeks later there was no evidence of residual sepsis and therefore a vascularized fibula (E) was harvested and placed to establish a stable skeleton with simultaneous conversion to a one-bone forearm (F). (In part form Lister, G. D. (1993) Free Skin and Composite flaps In: Green D. P. (ed) Operative Hand Surgery, 3rd edn. Churchill Livingstone, New York.)

MALUNION

Malunion is due to shortening or incorrect alignment at the time of management of the original fracture (p. 52). Malalignment may be *rotational* or *angulatory*, the angulation being antero-posterior or lateral. The functional effects of malunion may be minor, as with that following a boxer's fracture of the fifth metacarpal, or significant.

Scissoring, in which fingers do not run on parallel tracks, but cross one another or diverge, results most commonly from rotation, usually in an oblique or spiral fracture of the metacarpal, sometimes of a phalanx (Fig. 2.30, p. 177).

Reduced motion may be due to adhesions, or to relative lengthening of the tendons, as in the Z deformity (like that in rheumatoid, p. 359) seen after an anteriorly

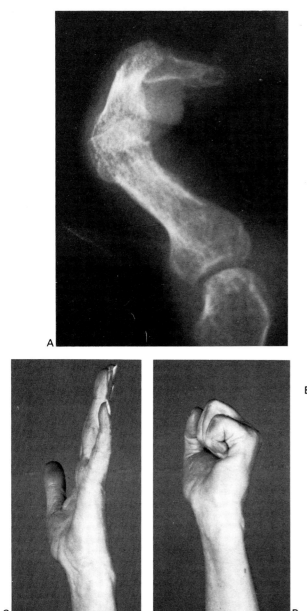

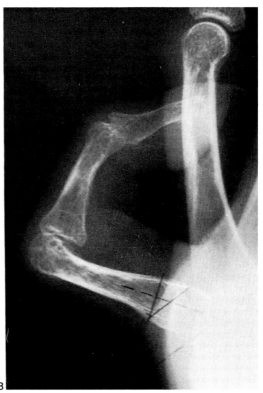

Fig. 2.41 This patient had gross malalignment of the proximal phalanx following a fracture at the junction of the proximal and middle thirds. In the anteroposterior view shown in (A) the malalignment can be partly appreciated. B. In the lateral, as always, the metacarpophalangeal joint is obscured, but is indicated by the dotted line which bisects the line marking the axis of the proximal phalanx. The appropriate wedge for closing osteotomy is marked out on this radiograph. C, D. With this correction of malalignment full range of motion was restored to the small finger.

angulated transverse fracture of the diaphysis of the proximal phalanx. Passive motion of the proximal interphalangeal joint may remain, or a flexion contracture may have developed. (Fig. 2.41).

Interference with normal function may arise as in (i) lateral angulation of a border digit which may catch on sliding the hand into a narrow space or (ii) apex dorsal angulation of a second or third metacarpal which may produce a painful mass in the palm — the metacarpal head — or (iii) apex dorsal angulation of the first metacarpal which reduces span grasp (Fig. 2.42).

Cosmetic considerations may be significant and valid. The precise amount of lateral angulation in the phalanges can be deduced from study of true anteroposterior radiographs in which the articular surfaces should be parallel. Determination from standard lateral

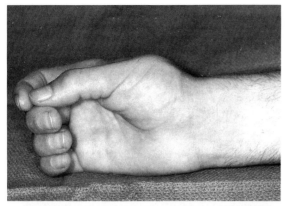

A

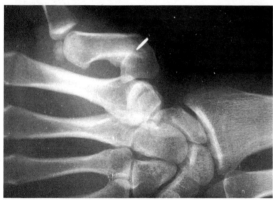

B

Fig. 2.42   A, B. Apex dorsal malunion of the first metacarpal resulting in significant loss of span grasp, thumb extension and radial abduction. The mark on the radiograph in (B) is a segment of pin placed during reversed wedge osteotomy to correct the malunion.

radiographs of the degree of antero-posterior angulation becomes progressively more difficult as the malunion lies more proximal to the diaphysis of the proximal phalanx. This is due to the superimposition of adjacent phalanges and metacarpals. *Sagittal tomograms* (see Fig. 2.39A) are required and are sometimes difficult to obtain. The exact amount of rotational malunion cannot be calculated preoperatively.

Indications[158]
Significant malunion requires surgical correction. Rotational malalignment in any bone in a digital ray is best achieved by osteotomy at the proximal metaphysis of the metacarpal, but its effectiveness in correcting phalangeal rotation is limited by the deep transverse metacarpal ligament to 20° in the index, middle and ring fingers, 30° in the small[159]. *Apex palmar or dorsal* malunions are best corrected by recalling that the dorsal surface of all long bones in the hand, excepting the

distal phalanges, is virtually flat. Osteotomies, usually closing wedge, designed to achieve that flat dorsal surface are indicated, combined with rigid fixation. The correction of *laterally* deviated malunions, in contrast with those above, can be planned on the true antero-posterior radiographs taken preoperatively. On such radiographs the exact amount of bone to be removed in a closing wedge, or inserted in an opening wedge osteotomy can be calculated (Fig. 2.43). Where corrective osteotomy[160] is not along the original fracture line, solid union of that fracture *must* be assured before surgery if the catastrophe is to be avoided of refracture during surgery yielding multiple unmanageable fragments. Usually a delay of six months after clinical and radiological union is a wise course to pursue.

See Green D P 1993 Operative Hand Surgery, 3rd edn. Churchill Livingstone, New York, pp. 715, 739, 961.

Joints

The patient should be asked to carry all joints in both upper extremities through a full range of active motion. In practice many of these are performed simultaneously with testing of the muscles which produce the motion.

Elbow:	flex and extend (biceps, brachialis and brachioradialis; triceps)
Forearm:	pronation and supination (pronators teres and quadratus; supinator and biceps)
Wrist:	dorsiflexion and palmar flexion (ECU, ECRL, ECRB; FCR and FCU)
	radial and ulnar deviation (ECRL and APL; FCU and ECU)
Fingers:	close and open hand (FDP and FDS; ED, EI, and EDM)
	adduct and abduct (Palmar interossei 'PAD' (Palmar ADduct) Dorsal interossei 'DAB' (Dorsal ABduct) and ADM)
Thumb:	touch tip of small finger and flex down to the palm = opposition and flexion (APB; FPL and FPB); extend (EPL, EPB, APL); adduct to the index finger (AP)

RANGE OF MOTION

Disregarding the position of the shoulder, *all joints are at zero degrees* when the upper limb is in the extended 'anatomical position' with the forearm midway between pronation and supination. '*Extension*' is the term used to describe movement from the flexed position towards neutral. It can also be used to describe motion beyond neutral, where that movement is normal, as at the wrist. However, the use of 'dorsiflexion' for that movement frees 'extension' of any ambiguity. '*Hyperextension*' is the term used when such motion beyond neutral is

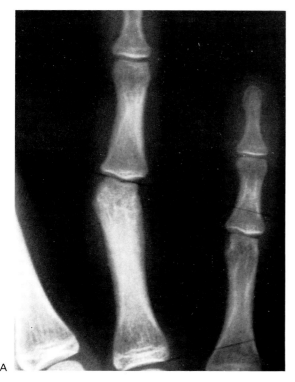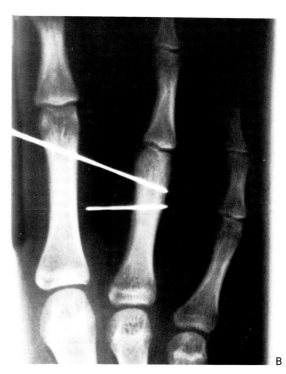

A   B

Fig. 2.43 A. The lateral angulation in the proximal phalanx of this ring finger can be seen by drawing lines touching the condyles at the base and at the head (B). Correction is achieved by osteotomy after placing Kirschner wires in position parallel to the joint surfaces. The holes so drilled later accommodate the intraosseous wire.

common but unnecessary for function, as at the IP joint of the thumb or the MP joints of the fingers or where it is unnatural, as at the proximal interphalangeal joints in *recurvatum* and *swan-neck* deformities. Hypermobility occurs in Ehlers–Danlos syndrome which may result in joint problems in the hand and wrist[161].

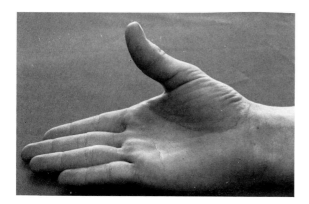

Fig. 2.44 Palmar abduction.

Abduction and *adduction* of the fingers are those motions, respectively, away from and towards the line of the middle finger.

Movements of the thumb
Palmar abduction. With the hand flat on the table with the dorsum down, palmar abduction is vertical motion away from the index finger and is measured as the maximum angle attainable between index finger and thumb (Fig. 2.44). A simple method of measuring this angle, using wooden blocks of different angles has been described[162].

Radial abduction. Movement of the thumb away from the index finger in the plane of the flat hand (Fig. 2.45).

Adduction. Approximation of the thumb to the index finger with both in extension (Fig. 2.46).

Flexion. The motion produced on flexing interphalangeal, metacarpophalangeal and carpometacarpal joints (Fig. 2.47).

Extension. The opposite movement to flexion, it brings the thumb to a point mid-way through the arc from radial to palmar abduction.

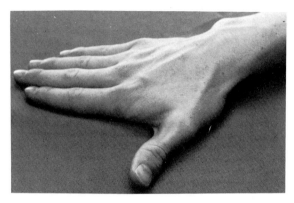

Fig. 2.45 Radial abduction.

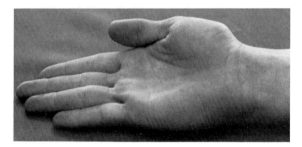

Fig. 2.46 Adduction.

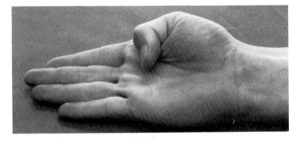

Fig. 2.47 Flexion.

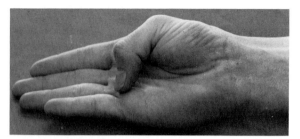

Fig. 2.48 Opposition.

Opposition. A composite movement of abduction, rotation and flexion of the thumb, this is recorded as the minimum attainable distance in centimetres between the tip of the thumb and the proximal digital crease of the small finger (Fig. 2.48). The carpometacarpal joint at which this action mainly occurs has several planes of motion which permit and guide this composite movement[163]. Measurement is therefore difficult and may require radiologic analysis[164].

The normal range for any joint is best taken as that of the uninjured opposite extremity. Where that has also been injured, or is absent, an average range has been prepared by the American Academy of Orthopaedic Surgeons. For ease of memory, these figures have been modified and rounded off to the nearest five degrees in Table 2.1.

The aggregate range of motion in the metacarpophalangeal and interphalangeal joints of the thumb varies very widely in normal individuals from 120° to over 300°[165].

Composite records are used to note the flexion and extension deficits in the fingers. These are defined as:

Extension deficit. With active extension, the aggregate *minimum* flexion in degrees for the metacarpal, proximal interphalangeal, and distal interphalangeal joints; expressed differently, this is the minimum angle obtainable between the axes of the metacarpal and the distal phalanx (Fig. 2.49).

Flexion deficit. With active flexion, the minimum attainable distance in centimetres between the plane of the finger nail and the palmar crease (Fig. 2.50).

Total active motion (TAM). This is a simple addition of the ranges of motion available in the metacarpophalangeal, proximal and distal interphalangeal joints in any one digit. The normal is therefore 270°. While

Table 2.1   Normal ranges of motion

Elbow	flexion		145°
	extension		0°
Forearm	pronation		70°
	supination		85°
Wrist	dorsiflexion		70°
	palmar flexion		75°
	ulnar deviation		35°
	radial deviation		20°
Thumb	abduction		60°
	flexion	IP	80°
		MP	55°
		CM	45°
	(hyper)extension	IP	15°
		MP	10°
Fingers	Flexion	(Hyper)extension	
DIP	80°	0	
PIP	100°	0	
MP	90°	0–45	

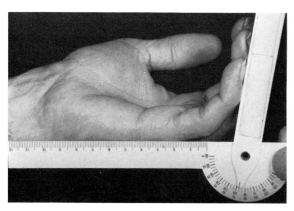

Fig. 2.49 Extension deficit. This is measured as the composite lack of extension for all three finger joints and is represented as the minimum angle which can be obtained between the axes of the metacarpal and the distal phalanx.

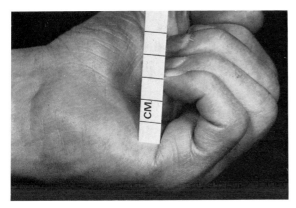

Fig. 2.50 Flexion deficit. This is measured as the distance between the distal palmar crease and, because of variations in the point formerly chosen on the digital pulp, the plane of the nail of the involved finger.

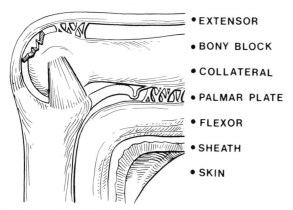

- • EXTENSOR
- • BONY BLOCK
- • COLLATERAL
- • PALMAR PLATE
- • FLEXOR
- • SHEATH
- • SKIN

Fig. 2.51 This diagram lists all of the factors which may cause flexion contracture.

useful, caution should be exercised in interpreting results so expressed. For example, 210° suggests fairly useful motion, but if the lost 60° is all from the proximal interphalangeal joint, the finger is severely disabled.

For this reason, the composite records outlined above should be used only for loss of motion due entirely to tendon injuries and even then TAM for the interphalangeal joints alone is a more valid criterion. Where joints are also damaged, individual ranges must be recorded.

Once the patient has gone through normal active motion in joints in the upper limbs, the examiner can concentrate his attention on those evidently disabled.

LIMITATION OF NORMAL MOTION[166]

As will be emphasized below, limitation of extension or of flexion may be of both active and passive, or of active alone. Only when both are impaired does a *contracture* exist.

Flexion contracture (Fig. 2.51)
Disregarding camptodactyly[167] (p. 477), which is a congenital flexion deformity, flexion contracture may be due to tightness in one or more of the structures on the palmar aspect of the joint.

Skin — scar contracture, especially following palmar burns[168] (Fig. 2.52).

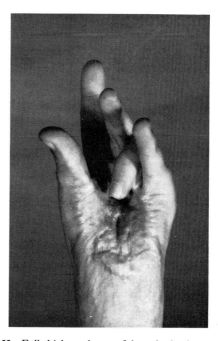

Fig. 2.52 Full-thickness burns of the palm inadequately treated inevitably result in gross flexion contracture.

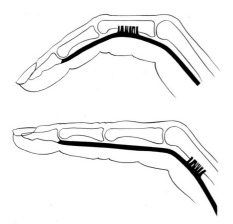

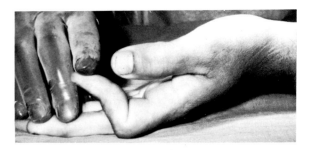

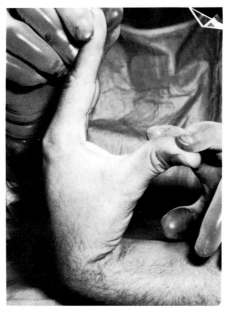

Fig. 2.53 Adjustment of the joints proximal to that which appears to be the seat of contracture may reveal the primary source of that deformity. In this diagram the flexion contracture is at the proximal interphalangeal joint. Flexion of the metacarpophalangeal joint in the presence of an adhesion over the proximal phalanx (upper figure) has no effect on the flexion contracture of the proximal interphalangeal joint. If, however, the adhesion of the flexor tendons lies proximal to the metacarpophalangeal joint, flexion of that joint will result in correction of the contracture apparently present in the proximal interphalangeal joint (lower figure).

Palmar fascia — as in Dupuytren's contracture (see below).

Flexor tendon sheath.

Flexor tendon (see p. 253). If adjustment of the position of the joints proximal to an apparently contracted joint results in its full extension then the limitation is due either to tendon shortening or to tendon adhesions proximal to the joints adjusted. For example, if firm flexion of the metacarpophalangeal joints permits full extension of an apparently limited proximal interphalangeal joint, then the flexor tendon is either short or adherent proximal to the metacarpophalangeal joint (Fig. 2.53). In the presence of Volkmann's contracture of the flexors in the forearm, the passive extension of the digital joints is limited in wrist extension, not so if the wrist is flexed (Fig. 2.54). It follows that the full passive range of a joint can be recorded only after the range has been checked with more proximal joints in differing positions. Alternatively, if a flexor tendon functions on joints more proximal but not on the one being tested it may be assumed that one factor at least in the flexion contracture of that joint is adhesion of the tendon to the bone immediately proximal to the joint. In this circumstance, assuming the extensor tendon is healthy, passive flexion will exceed active flexion and may well be normal, while the extension deficit will be the same both actively and passively.

Fig. 2.54 A. With the wrist fully extended the proximal interphalangeal joint here shows a 90° flexion contracture. B. With full flexion of the wrist the index finger fully extends. From this it can be deduced that the long flexor tendon is adherent proximal to the wrist joint, and this proved to be the case on exploration.

Capsular structures (collateral ligament, accessory collateral ligament, palmar plate) may be the sole cause of limited extension, usually by shortening of the palmar plate or adhesions of the collateral ligament. As the collateral ligament at the proximal interphalangeal joint is taut in all positions of the joint, and as the metacarpophalangeal joint is *normally* taut in flexion, it follows that collateral ligament *shortening* can never produce or be part of a flexion contracture. Even where other structures are the primary cause of a flexion contracture in an *interphalangeal* joint the palmar plate becomes contracted at an early stage.

In the great majority of cases flexion contractures are due to tightness of structures on the flexor aspect. Occasionally, however, the joint may be *prevented from extending* by incongruity of the articular surfaces, or adhesion of the dorsal capsule or of the extensor tendon to the articular surface of the head of the proximal bone.

Where dorsal adhesions are the cause, not only will there be a flexion contracture but there will also be marked limitation of flexion.

Locking of a joint implies that it is *temporarily* fixed in a particular posture, but can be released by some manipulation of the joint, usually painful. This usually occurs in flexion and may, by progression of the process, result in fixed flexion contracture. Trigger finger (p. 345) is by far the most common cause, producing proximal interphalangeal joint flexion. Locking, usually at the metacarpophalangeal joint, may also be due to intracapsular tumours or more commonly to loose bodies, osteophytes, capsular tears or distortion of the articular surfaces[171-174] (Fig. 2.55).

Dupuytren's[175] *disease*[176-178]

Since micro-trauma[179,180] to the palmar fascia followed by myofibroblast contracture[181-183] is now blamed by many for the development of this disorder, the point may be stretched to include it at this juncture. A familial disorder, the patient when pressed can usually recall some member of his family, often distant, who has suffered from this complaint. It has also been reported to be more common in diabetics[184] and cigarette smokers[185]. It normally commences with the development of a nodule in the palm which is frequently painful. This may or may not proceed to the next stage, which is the development of bands of Dupuytren's contracture[186]. The bands develop in specific relationships to the flexor tendon sheath and neurovascular

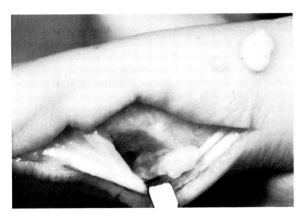

Fig. 2.55 This joint was subject to intermittent locking and periods of painful swelling. Radiographic examination revealed nothing of note, but exploration of the proximal interphalangeal joint yielded the loose body shown in the photograph.

bundles of the finger[187] and affect, in order of frequency, the ring, small, middle, and rarely, the thumb and index fingers[188]. A close relationship with the tendon of abductor digiti minimi exists[189,190].

The examiner may attempt to predict the presence of a significant displacement of the neurovascular bundle by the method described by Watson[191] — in which there is a 'soft, pulpy mass' between the palmar crease and the proximal digital crease overlying a spirally located nerve — or by the Doppler ultrasound examination[192]. Finally, he should ensure that no other areas are afflicted, for Dupuytren's-like fibromatosis can occur in the foot[193] and on the penis[194].

Indications. If the fascial bands are not causing contracture then no surgery is required and the patient is advised to return when contracture commences. If contracture has occurred then surgery should be scheduled. A variety of procedures have been recommended, including:

(i) *Palmar fasciotomy*, best reserved for the elderly patient, or one with skin maceration, or mainly MP involvement[195]
(ii) *Limited fasciectomy*
(iii) *Radical fasciectomy*
(iv) *Dermofasciectomy and skin graft*[196]

Some, including the author, favour (ii), leaving transverse wounds open[197,198]; others combine fasciotomy with skin graft[199]. For the reasons outlined previously, full extension is more likely to be achieved after release of a metacarpophalangeal than of an interphalangeal contracture where 53% improvement has been reported after removal of an isolated digital cord[200]. Such a cord, by traction on the transverse retinacular ligament, may produce a boutonniere deformity[201] (Fig. 2.56). Other factors reported to have an adverse effect on the result are: early age of onset, being of the fair sex[202], the presence of Garrod's[203] knuckle pads[204], the number of rays involved[205] and the patient being an epileptic or an alcoholic — there is a higher incidence of coexistence with these conditions than would be expected randomly[206].

Following severe recurrence of over 70° PIP contracture, amputation by disarticulation at that joint, or arthrodesis at a better angle[207] will ameliorate a considerable hindrance.

See Green D P 1993 Operative Hand Surgery, 3rd edn. Churchill Livingstone, New York, p. 569.

Limitation of flexion (extension contracture) (Fig. 2.57)
This may be due to one or more of all the structures on the dorsal aspect of the joint.

Skin — scar contracture.

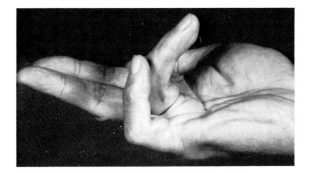

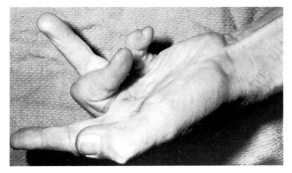

Fig. 2.56 A, B. Dupuytren's contracture. Of the joints contracted, the metacarpophalangeal joint of the ring finger will be most readily released. The proximal interphalangeal joint contractures and the interphalangeal joint contracture of the thumb in (B) will prove most difficult to release.

Long extensor. Again, adjustment of the adjacent joints may yield a diagnosis of tendon shortening or of adhesion proximal to that adjusted joint. Limited flexion caused by long extensor adhesion is most commonly seen in the proximal interphalangeal joint, the

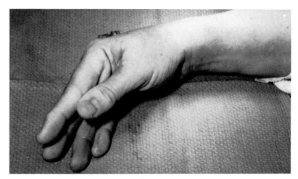

Fig. 2.58 This hand is in the extreme intrinsic plus position with metacarpophalangeal joint flexion and interphalangeal extension.

adhesion being to the proximal phalanx consequent upon either a fracture or severe crush injury of the finger. Active extension of the joint will be severely limited or absent. Commonly it falls markedly short of passive extension.

Intrinsics. Contracture of one or more intrinsics may follow ischaemia and muscle fibrosis (p. 251) or may occur for non-ischaemic reasons[208] (p. 385). If very marked this may be apparent from the 'intrinsic plus' posture of the hand in which the fingers are flexed at the metacarpophalangeal joints and extended at the interphalangeal joints (Fig. 2.58). In less evident contracture, its presence is detected by attempting to flex the proximal interphalangeal joint while passively extending the corresponding metacarpophalangeal joint. In intrinsic tightness this movement is restricted (Fig. 2.59). The restriction can be differentiated from that caused by extensor tendon adhesion or capsular ligament dis-

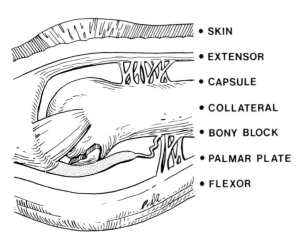

- • SKIN
- • EXTENSOR
- • CAPSULE
- • COLLATERAL
- • BONY BLOCK
- • PALMAR PLATE
- • FLEXOR

Fig 2.57 This diagram shows all of the factors which may be involved in loss of flexion (extension contracture).

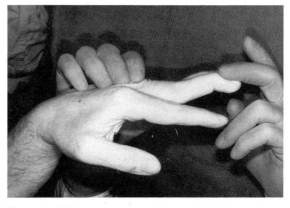

Fig. 2.59 With the metacarpophalangeal joint extended, attempts to flex the proximal interphalangeal joint in this patient with intrinsic tightness met with resistance while still in hyperextension.

order by thereafter allowing the metacarpophalangeal joint to flex. In other disorders the inability to fully flex the proximal interphalangeal joint will persist whereas in pure intrinsic tightness the proximal interphalangeal joint will increasingly flex as the metacarpophalangeal joint also flexes (Fig. 2.60). The intrinsic tightness present is recorded by noting the passive flexion which is possible at the proximal interphalangeal joint (a) when the metacarpophalangeal joint is extended and (b) when that joint is flexed. As an example, the record of the patient in Figures 2.59 and 2.60 read '0/0–80 (intrinsic tightness)'. A *'saddle deformity'* has been reported[209] in which adhesions between the lumbrical and interosseous result in painful impingement on the deep transverse metacarpal ligament with intrinsic contraction, the ligament being the 'saddle', the two muscles the 'legs of the rider'.

Capsular structures (dorsal capsule, collateral ligament, accessory collateral ligament, palmar plate). These structures alone may limit flexion by adhesion of any one of them to the head of the proximal bone of the joint. If other structures are primarily responsible, the capsular structures are likely to become involved in addition. In contrast to flexion contracture, which is more common in the interphalangeal joints and particularly the proximal, stiffness in extension due to collateral ligament shortening is much more likely in the metacarpophalangeal joint. This is because that ligament is normally slack in extension and tight in flexion. Loss of flexion at the metacarpophalangeal joints can come about simply by immobilization in the incorrect, extended position. In addition to a shortened collateral

ligament, metacarpophalangeal flexion may be prevented by adhesion of the palmar plate to the palmar surface of the metacarpal head. It is possible to distinguish between palmar plate adhesion and collateral ligament tightness as the cause of metacarpophalangeal joint fixation in extension. If the collateral ligaments are the cause then abduction and adduction of the fingers, normally at least 45° combined in this extended position, will be virtually eliminated. In the less likely situation in which the palmar plate is the major or sole culprit, attempted passive flexion will produce an opening of the dorsal aspect of the joint. This comes about as the anterior lip of the base of the proximal phalanx jams against the adherent plate and the unaffected and therefore still loose collateral ligament permits the flexion force to rock the dorsal lip away from the metacarpal head. This is subtle, is felt as a recess dorsally between head and base and may be best appreciated under anaesthesia and should always be sought after tight collateral ligaments have been released (Fig. 2.61).

Postburn claw contractures (p. 168) involve fixed extension of the metacarpophalangeal joints. They have been classified in such a way as to guide treatment and indicate prognosis[210], as shown in Table 2.2.

Apart from factors on the extensor aspect and in the joint capsule limiting flexion, it may be blocked by palmar structures:

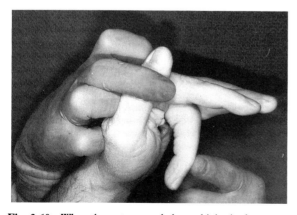

Fig. 2.60 When the metacarpophalangeal joint in the patient illustrated in Figure 2.59 was allowed to flex, significant increase in the flexion in the proximal interphalangeal joint resulted, demonstrating that the limitation of motion at that joint was due to intrinsic tightness.

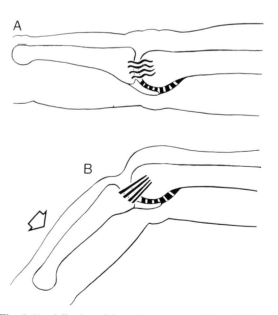

Fig. 2.61 Adhesion of the palmar plate to the head of the metacarpal with no involvement of the collateral ligament results in rubbery resistance to flexion and causes an opening of the dorsal aspect of the joint.

Table 2.2

Type	Examination	Structures involved	Improvement (%)
I	>30° Flexion with wrist extended	Skin	95
II	<30° Flexion with wrist extended	Skin; extensor apparatus; dorsal capsule	73
III	>30° hyperextension	Skin; extensor apparatus; dorsal capsule; joint (subluxed)	47

Flexor tendon: a flexor tendon adherent within the sheath may be sufficiently bulky as to block full flexion of an interphalangeal joint.

Bone: this may take the form of a true block (Fig. 2.62) or may be the result of articular incongruity or destruction (Fig. 2.63).

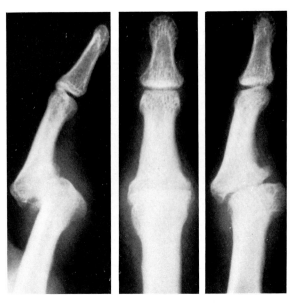

Fig. 2.63 This patient had previously sustained fracture-dislocation of the proximal interphalangeal joint which was not adequately reduced. This has gone on to post-traumatic osteoarthritis.

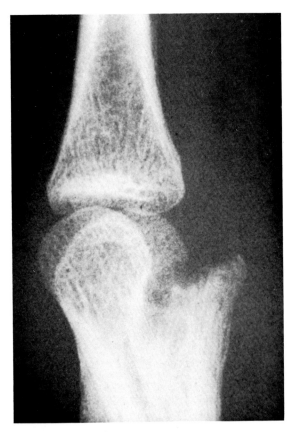

Fig. 2.62 A bony block clearly limiting flexion.

Chondral fractures may present a diagnostic problem. The patient complains of a persistently painful joint which remains swollen, although the swelling tends to wax and wane, limiting flexion to a varying degree. Radiographic examination reveals nothing. This condition most frequently affects the metacarpophalangeal joint, and questioning may cause the patient to recall an injury, usually minor, but one which involved a direct blow to the metacarpal head or a twist which could have caused the proximal phalangeal base to impinge on the head. Exploration may reveal the chondral fracture and often a consequent loose body in the joint cavity (Fig. 2.64).

The severely injured hand becomes very oedematous. Unless prevented from doing so the joints assume the posture in which their ligaments are most relaxed. Ligamentous contracture and fibrosis causes the joints to become virtually immobile in this position, which is characteristically:

Wrist	— flexion
Thumb	— adduction
Metacarpophalangeal	— extension
Proximal interphalangeal	— flexion (Fig. 2.65)

The first procedure the surgeon may have to undertake in such a neglected or mismanaged hand is to release the contractures.

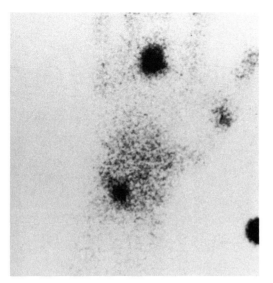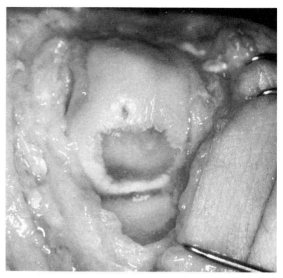

Fig. 2.64 Chondral fracture. Following a localized, closed injury this patient presented with recurrent swelling, discomfort and limitation of function in the metacarpophalangeal joint of the middle finger. A. Bone scan revealed that this joint was hot indeed, although a normal radiograph showed no abnormality. B. Exploration revealed the presence of chondromalacia.

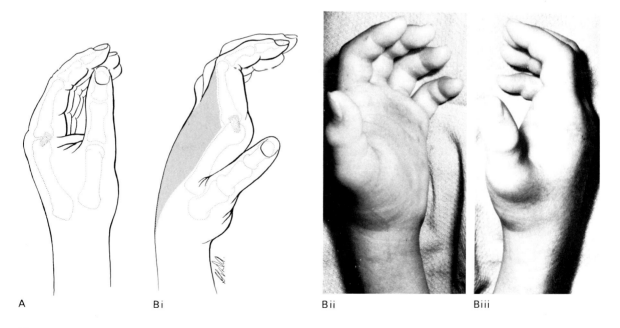

A   B i   B ii   B iii

Fig. 2.65 A. Diagrammatic representation of the posture of the relaxed uninjured hand. B. With injury, oedema accumulates in the available space on the dorsal aspect of the hand. This drives the wrist into flexion, the metacarpophalangeal joints into hyperextension, the proximal interphalangeal joints into flexion and the thumb into adduction. In this position the collateral ligament of the metacarpophalangeal joint, the palmar plate of the proximal interphalangeal joint and the tissues of the first web space will shorten and scar.

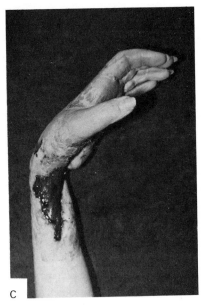

C

Fig. 2.65(*continued*)   C. If this development is not controlled by external or internal splintage in the severely injured hand, these developments will result in severe fixed contractures.

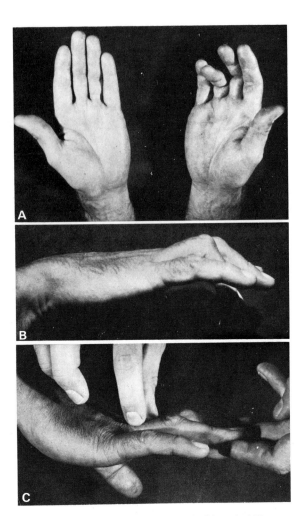

Fig. 2.66   A, B. This patient presented with an inability to extend the proximal interphalangeal joints of both ring and middle fingers. His active range of motion in the ring finger was recorded as 60–90°. C. His passive range was, however, 10–90°, indicating that the cause of his loss of extension lay in the tendon and not in the proximal interphalangeal joint itself.

Recording range of motion

As each joint is carried by the examiner to its full *passive* range, and this is recorded, the patient should be invited to 'keep it there'. The *active* range can then be recorded also. It is common practice to record active range only. This can be misleading as it is not a true reflection of the capabilities of that joint but rather of the limitations of the muscles acting upon it. Paralysis or tendon adhesions, for example, will cause the active range to fall far short of the passive and only the two can accurately pinpoint the problem (Fig. 2.66)

The active range should be recorded as recommended by Koch and Mason, adding the passive range in brackets:

$$\frac{\text{maximum extension}}{\text{maximum flexion}} \quad \text{e.g.} \quad \frac{(10)\ 60}{90} \quad \begin{array}{l}\text{in the patient shown}\\\text{in Figure 2.66}\end{array}$$

All recordings should be made with a goniometer applied to the dorsal aspect of the joint. Only in this way can accurate measure be taken, especially by different observers, of improvement or deterioration between visits.

ABNORMAL MOTION

Having recorded the passive and active range of *normal* movement of the joints, the surgeon should test for the presence of *abnormal* movements. Chronic *hyperextension* or *recurrent dorsal dislocation*[211,213] may follow an untreated tear of the palmar plate or fracture-dislocation of the proximal, or more rarely distal, interphalangeal joint. This may present openly or masked as a swollen, 'weak' joint. Clinically it can be revealed by passive stress with or without anaesthesia.

The collateral ligaments of each joint should be stressed by placing the examiner's thumb or index finger on the opposite side of the joint to act as a stable fulcrum while holding the joint in extension and stressing the collateral ligament using the distal part of the limb or digit as a lever arm to exert force. This may reveal frank laxity and sublux the joint. More commonly the patient withdraws his hand, complaining of pain over the collateral ligament under test. The precise point of tenderness on the collateral ligament should be sought by pressure with the digital pulp. Lateral stress radiographs should be taken. If pain is severe, this should be performed under appropriate nerve block. Care should be taken to avoid rotation, and therefore spurious lateral movement, of the proximal interphalangeal joint which has a flexion contracture, by testing for lateral instability in that joint with the metacarpophalangeal joint locked in full flexion. That flexed posture is also the one in which lateral stability of the metacarpophalangeal joint should be tested since it tightens the collateral ligament.

Recording abnormal motion is done by placing skin marks over the mid-point of the lax joint and also of the joints immediately adjacent. The angle produced by stress between these joints can then be measured with varying degrees of difficulty and therefore inaccuracy (Fig. 2.67).

Greater ease and accuracy can be achieved by measuring on stress radiographs.

Injuries to the ulnar collateral ligament of the metacarpophalangeal joint of the thumb (gamekeeper's, ski-pole) are frequently ignored by the patient or splinted by his physician. When he presents later the patient will have painful weakness of his thumb[214] and will show radial instability and some palmar subluxation on examination. The palmar plate offers some stability with the joint in extension, so with lesser degrees of instability stress should be applied with the joint in flexion[215]. As mentioned previously, care should be taken to prevent rotation of the proximal bone when applying lateral stress to a flexed joint, lest an incorrect diagnosis of instability be made. In the future, arthrography may become a routine part of the investigation, helping to predict the pathology more accurately[216]. Depending on the state of the joint surfaces the choice lies between reconstruction and arthrodesis (Fig. 2.68).

RADIOLOGICAL EXAMINATION

Interphalangeal joints — true anteroposterior, lateral and obliques (best taken on dental film laid alongside the joint)

Metacarpophalangeal joints — anteroposterior, Brewerton (p. 394) and two *angled laterals*
— 30° pronation for index and middle
— 30° supination for ring and small

Study of these radiographs will reveal *incongruity* due to a healed intra-articular fracture, a bony block, or chronic dislocation, or evidence of *traumatic arthritis* in the form of loss of joint space, eburnation — sclerosis — of the bone ends, cyst formation and osteophytic spurs. The findings may dictate what line of treatment can be pursued.

INDICATIONS[217]

Significant *abnormal* motion is a definite indication for exploration and reconstruction or stabilization. Except where radiological examination has shown definite incongruity or advanced degeneration, *limited normal motion in a stable joint* should always be treated initially by dynamic splintage, only to be abandoned when no further gain can be achieved as evidenced by unchanging measurements on successive visits.

If active range does not equal passive, there is no benefit whatsoever to be gained from operation on the joint alone. Rather should the cause of the loss of active motion be located and remedied whereafter passive range should be reassessed during surgery and cap-

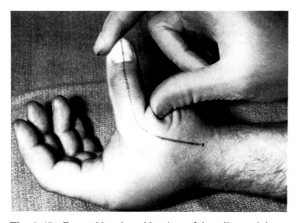

Fig. 2.67 By marking the mid-points of the adjacent joints, angulation can be appreciated on stress, even when it is of a much less significant degree than in this tear of the ulnar collateral ligament.

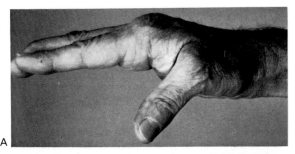

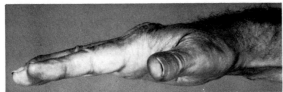

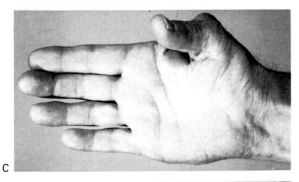

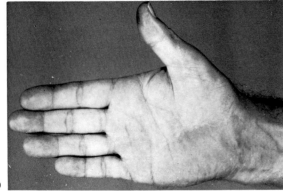

Fig. 2.68 Restoration of function by arthrodesis for chronic instability of the metacarpophalangeal joint. A, B. Restoration of alignment in extension. C, D. Restoration of radial abduction.

sulectomy performed if necessary. Thereafter the excursion of the joint may improve appreciably through exercise of the muscles, now released, which normally produce the full range. Conversely, no substitution surgery, either tendon graft or tendon transfer, will have

sufficient power to improve the passive range of motion in a joint. Thus, for example, it is fruitless to recommend a flexor tendon graft to a patient with stiff digital joints or, as happens more commonly, to perform an opponensplasty on a patient with limited passive abduction of the thumb.

Since active range cannot *exceed* passive range, there is no way in which the surgeon can determine at examination whether or not the tendon acting on a joint can take advantage of any improvement he may achieve by operating to relieve a limited passive range. Thus it is most important at surgery to check, for example, that the flexor tendon is capable of actively achieving the new-found flexion attained passively, either by working under local anaesthetic and enlisting the patient's help or by exposing the tendon away from the joint and pulling on it. Otherwise a puzzling discrepancy will exist postoperatively between the active function present then and the passive range achieved at operation.

If it has been determined that the contracture is in the joint and periarticular structures, and if the articular surfaces are good, soft tissue release may well restore motion[218,219]. The procedure in most cases will involve a dorsal approach and exploration of all possible causes of contracture — extensor tendon, dorsal capsule, true collateral, accessory collateral, palmar plate[220], flexor sheath and flexor tendon in that sequence. After each is released, motion should be checked, and for this and other reasons local anaesthesia is most helpful, for the patient can provide the power to move the joint (Fig. 2.69). In addition, his active function obviates the need, otherwise essential, to check through separate incisions that the motor tendons of the joint are free to function. Further, the range achieved can be demonstrated to the patient, potent reinforcement during immediate postoperative therapy. Hyperextension of the joint can be corrected by palmar plate repair, advancement or reconstruction[221].

If the articular surface is destroyed, soft tissue release will not suffice. The choice lies between *arthroplasty* and *arthrodesis*. *Perichondrial arthroplasty*, by which it is hoped to restore cartilage cover to the bone ends[222-227], may be of value in young patients following trauma[228,229], but it has not gained wide acceptance.

Resection arthroplasty is a good procedure in the basal joint of the thumb (p. 336), but results in too much laxity in digital joints, especially the interphalangeal. *Resection with insertion of a silicone spacer* was an effective procedure, although with gradually reducing motion and an admittedly limited term, but the problems reported with silicone (p. 338) dictate that any surgeon would be ill-advised to use such implants, especially in the young, post-traumatic joint. No satisfactory *total*

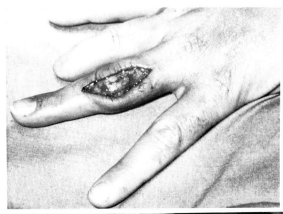

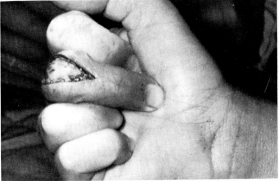

Fig. 2.69 Local anaesthesia in capsulectomy (see text).

joint replacement for the digital joints is currently available. *Interpositional arthroplasty*, using local tissue, such as the palmar plate or the extensor apparatus, gives only limited motion. However, studies conducted during 11 activities of daily living have shown that a surprisingly small range is actually required — the *maximum* employed was 60° at each of the metacarpophalangeal and proximal interphalangeal joints and 39° at the distal[230]. It may be that improved technique in interpositional arthroplasty may yield such ranges, and this is the current choice in the metacarpophalangeal joint for non-rheumatoid patients in whom perichondrial arthroplasty is contraindicated.

One surface of a joint, especially the head of the metacarpal, can be restored by non-vascularized metatarsal transfer[231] (see Fig. 6.19). *Vascularized joint transfer* has been practiced for as long as many of the currently popular other free tissue transfers. It has, however, failed to gain wide acceptance, despite isolated reports of its use[232,233]. This is probably because the resultant range of motion is poor[234] and it requires sacrifice of a toe. It should be reserved for isolated digital joint injuries in children, for the joint transfer

carries with it the epiphysis and therefore the chance of growth. From all that has been said, it follows that in most interphalangeal joints irreversibly damaged and symptomatic, arthrodesis[235-237] should be strongly recommended. A wide range of techniques is available[238-245]. Selection of the angle of arthrodesis must be considered at the time of examination. The metacarpophalangeal joint and interphalangeal joint of the thumb should be fused in 20° of flexion, and the *distal* interphalangeal joint of the fingers at 10, 20, 30 and 40° of flexion, reading from index to small. These figures are adjusted to individual functional needs but less so than in the *proximal* interphalangeal joints where other considerations apply, as follows. In the index finger, the position should be such as brings the pulp of the finger in firm contact with that of the thumb (Fig. 2.70). In the ulnar three fingers, a position should be chosen which brings the finger down into power grasp, while avoiding undue malalignment of the pulp of the digit with the other fingers when the hand is extended. The latter depends entirely on the ability of the metacarpophalangeal joint to hyperextend (Fig. 2.71). Fortunately, this tends to increase from the radial to the ulnar side of the hand, as does the need for proximal interphalangeal joint flexion to give powerful grasp. Thus, as a general rule, the angles chosen for arthrodesis are index 20°, middle 30°, ring 40°, and small 50°.

The carpometacarpal joints may be symptomatic following injury. Fusion of the second and third is the only treatment. Fusion[246] or resection arthroplasty[247] may be used on the fourth and fifth. The first will be considered in Chapter 4, since arthritis following trauma in that joint is far exceeded by idiopathic degenerative disease.

See Green D P 1993 Operative Hand Surgery, 3rd edn. Churchill Livingstone, New York, pp. 99, 144, 1201.

ADDUCTION DEFORMITY OR CONTRACTURE OF THE THUMB

This crippling loss of thumb function can come about as a result of one or any combination of a number of disorders:

skin contracture
adductor fibrosis
basal joint disease (p. 336)
loss of active palmar abduction (Fig. 2.72).

It is imperative that all factors be dealt with in such a way as to avoid swift recurrence. For example, adductor release without provision of mobile adequate skin would be valueless. Release with provision of skin will fail to give maximum benefit if the patient has no means to hold the thumb out in abduction, either static, in the form of a carpometacarpal arthrodesis or a temporary

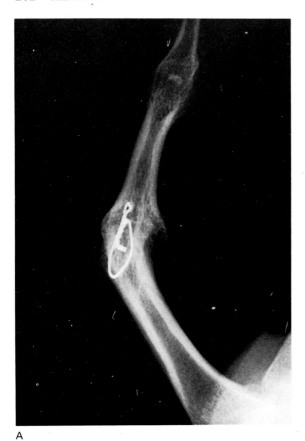

A

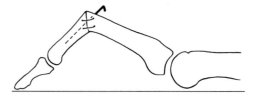

Fig. 2.71 The angle at which the proximal interphalangeal joint should be fused is determined by the available hyperextension of the metacarpophalangeal joint which permits the tip of the flexed digit to remain in the plane of the palm.

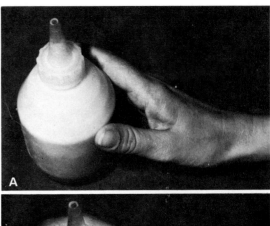

A

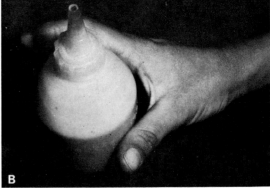

B

Fig. 2.72 This patient had sustained a high median nerve injury with resultant loss of opposition. Her attempts to grasp objects of large diameter are impeded by her inability to abduct the thumb. In this case, she has compensated to some extent by hyperextension of the metacarpophalangeal joint of the index finger. Span grasp in a hand with normal abduction is shown for comparison.

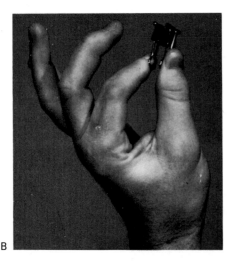

B

Fig. 2.70 A. The angulation is chosen for arthrodesis of the proximal interphalangeal joint of the index finger that approximates the pulp of that digit to that of the thumb. B. This is particularly important in this patient who has previously undergone fusion of the distal interphalangeal joint.

internal splint, or better dynamic, by provision of a strong opponensplasty at the time of release (p. 242).

Wrist[248,249]

The anatomy and mechanics of the carpus have been discussed on pp. 15 and 75.

HISTORY

While some patients present with a firm diagnosis which requires only confirmation, the majority of those with wrist problems come with no diagnosis but with one or more of the following complaints: (i) *pain*, (ii) *weakness*, (iii) *loss of motion* or, less commonly, (iv) *instability* which may be accompanied by a '*clunk*' which they feel, rather than hear.

On questioning, there may be clear recall of a specific injury, and, indeed, they may have presented to the emergency room or casualty department and, after examination and radiographic examination, may have been diagnosed as having a 'sprain' (group 4 on p. 84). If a specific injury is known, then the *mechanism* should be determined, for a direct fall or a twisting motion offer clues to the pathology. *Symptoms* and *provoking and alleviating factors*, both immediately after the injury and at present, should be ascertained:

How did you fall on your hand, in which direction and from what height?
Can you show me how that twist happened?
Did you experience pain immediately?
If not, when did it commence?
Did you stop what you were doing?
Was there a definite 'snap' or 'pop' when it occurred?
Did you see a doctor right away?
Do you have (can you get) the radiographs taken at that time?
How was the hand that night? And the next day?
Was there any bruising, and if so, where exactly?
Has the problem gone away only to come back? How often?
Have you been able to return to work?
Anything in particular that makes the pain better? Or worse?
Can you point to the spot or area where the pain is located?
Is the loss of motion due to pain, or does the movement just stop?
Show me the movement which gives you pain. And that which feels unstable.
What treatment have you had so far?
Have you had any previous injuries to this hand or arm?

EXAMINATION

Examination of the wrist, as always, should follow a set pattern to avoid omission. A full examination of the remainder of the extremity should also be performed.

Palpation

The patient is asked to rest his elbow on a firm surface. The forearm is pronated and the wrist flexed. Cradling the wrist in both hands, each bone and joint space on the dorsal surface is palpated firmly, in turn, with either thumb. A definite sequence is followed: radial styloid, taking care to palpate the first dorsal compartment, the dorsal lip of the radius, moving from there proximally just radial to the radial tubercle to the point at which the abductor pollicis longus 'intersects' with the radial wrist extensors, where lies the mysterious abductor bursa thence moving on to the radioulnar joint, ulnar head, ulnar styloid, triquetrum, lunatotriquetral joint, lunate, scapholunate joint — remembering that it is directly distal to the radial tubercle in the neutral wrist — scaphotrapezoidal joint, scaphocapitate joint, capitate, capitatelunate joint, capitatehamate joint, hamate, hamatotriquetral joint and all four of the ulnar carpometacarpal joints — all can be palpated from the dorsal aspect. Moving the wrist to neutral both in pronation and in flexion–extension, ulnar deviate the wrist. Now, on the radial side of the wrist, palpate the anatomical snuffbox, its boundaries and its contents, the radial styloid, the scaphoid, the trapezium and the base of the first metacarpal. By adducting the thumb, the first metacarpal is moved anteriorly giving evidence of the exact location of the basal joint of the thumb. It also should be palpated and a torque test applied — more of that later (p. 336). By flexing the elbow fully and carrying the wrist into radial deviation, present the ulnar aspect of the wrist for palpation of the base of the fifth metacarpal, the extensor carpi ulnaris tendon, the hamate, hamatotriquetral joint, triquetrum, TFCC and ulnar head. Other areas we appear to have overlooked will be picked up during the dynamic tests below. During palpation of all these points, so laboriously listed on the dorsum and lateral aspects of the wrist, *tenderness* is sought, together with any other less likely findings such as *abnormal motion*, *crepitus* and *swellings*, *cystic* or *hard*. If found, points of tenderness should be marked with a skin pencil. Of equal importance, they should be compared with the identical point on the opposite wrist, for the tenderness elicited may be bilateral and therefore probably physiologic.

Dynamic or manipulative tests

In these tests the examiner moves the wrist in particular ways to elicit *pain* and *instability*. We were palpating the ulnar border of the wrist, the ulnar head to be exact. Moving anteriorly and distally, each by 2 cm, palpate the pisiform lying beneath the distal wrist crease at its ulnar extreme. Push it firmly in a radial direction, thereby moving the pisotriquetral joint (Fig. 2.73). Pain suggests arthritis therein (p. 340). Moving the palpating thumb 2 cm further in the same direction, now distally and radialwards, firm pressure will meet the hamulus,

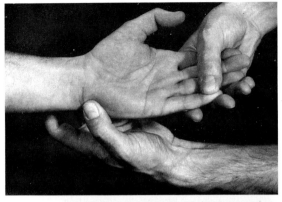

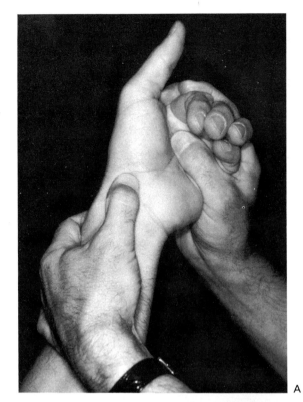

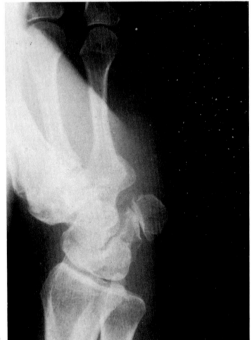

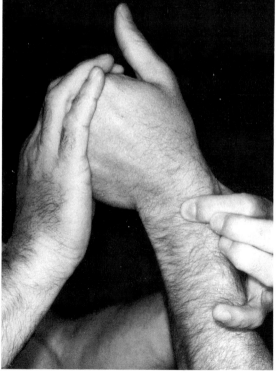

Fig. 2.73   A. The pisiform is palpated at the ulnar end of the distal wrist crease. If moving the pisiform produces pain, it is probable that pisotriquetral arthritis is present. B. Radiographic findings. Excision of the pisiform will cure the problem.

which is always tender, for the deep motor branch of the ulnar nerve crosses it. But compare.

At the point at which the thenar crease loses its emphasis just before reaching the wrist crease, palpate the obvious bony prominence, the distal pole of the scaphoid (Fig. 2.74A). With the patient's wrist in ulnar deviation, place the examining thumb firmly on the prominence, the index finger of the same hand on the radial tubercle dorsally. Maintaining firm pressure with

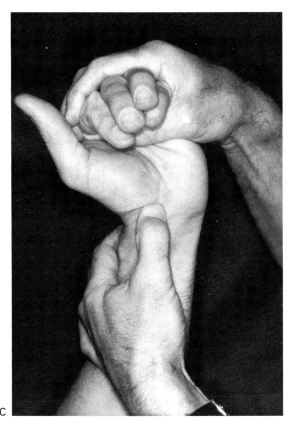

C

Fig. 2.74 The scaphoid shift test. A. With the wrist in ulnar deviation, the thumb is placed on the distal pole of the scaphoid and (B) the index finger on the radial styloid dorsally. C. The wrist is then moved firmly into radial deviation, maintaining firm pressure on the distal pole of the scaphoid. In scapholunate instability, the pressure on the distal pole will cause the proximal pole to sublux dorsally where it hits the examining index finger.

the thumb, with the other hand push the wrist strongly into radial deviation. In radial deviation, the scaphoid flexes. If all ligamentous attachments are intact, direct transmission of force will occur, and the radially deviating hand will easily overcome the resisting thumb. If however, the ligaments of the proximal pole of the scaphoid are lax or torn, the resisting thumb will prevent the forward motion of the bowing scaphoid, whose 'feet' — the proximal pole — 'will slip out from under him'. The proximal pole will jump over the dorsal lip of the radius with a 'clunk', felt most convincingly by the waiting index finger. This is the *scaphoid shift test* of Watson[50], suggestive if positive of scapholunate instability. It is, however, positive in some normal wrists, especially those of young ladies, and should therefore be repeated on the opposite hand before gathering the

crowd. Just distal to the prominence lies the scapho-trapezial joint and now is the most opportune time to palpate for tenderness.

Return the wrist to the original position, pronation and palmar flexion. Radially deviate the wrist and observe the prominence of the triquetrum 2 cm distal to the ulnar head. Ulnar deviate the wrist (Fig. 2.75) and it should disappear as it rides distally and forward on its helicoid joint with the hamate. If it initially becomes more prominent and then vanishes with a palpable 'clunk' the *Lichtman test* for ulnar midcarpal instability is positive, suggesting attrition of the triquetro-hamatocapitate ligament. This also may be spuriously positive, so the opposite wrist should be tested and, even if it is negative, no firm conclusions should be drawn.

Take the triquetrum just observed between the finger and thumb of one hand, the lunate between those of the other. Attempt to move them in opposite directions on one another in an anteroposterior plane. This is the *LT ballottement test* which is positive for lunatotriquetral strain or rupture if the movement produces undue motion, pain or crepitus.

With the patient's elbow still resting on the table, stand and, with your elbow pointing to the ceiling, take his hand as if to shake it in greeting. With the other hand, grip his forearm firmly at the junction of middle and distal thirds such as to compress the distal radioulnar joint. Now with the first hand, successively pronate and supinate his forearm, while maintaining compression. Pain referred to the ulnar head will suggest chondromalacia thereon.

Range of motion

The forearm and wrist should now be carried through all motions permitted by its three degrees of freedom. Release the forearm compression, sliding that hand distally to gently encircle the wrist, but not restrict its free movement. With the other hand, first pronate and then supinate the forearm, giving a 'tweak' at each extreme to stress the inferior radioulnar joint. Pain in extreme pronation will suggest either chondromalacia of the head or damage to the anterior radioulnar ligament (p. 220), in extreme supination either chondromalacia or damage to the dorsal ligament. Other movements of the wrist should also be carried to their extreme and then modest load applied. Throughout these manoeuvres, pain should be noted, as should any irregularity in motion or 'clicks'[251] detected by the 'listening' hand lightly holding the wrist.

Ulnar deviation is especially significant, for when carried to the extreme it may produce pain on either side of the wrist. On the ulnar side it will suggest *ulnar*

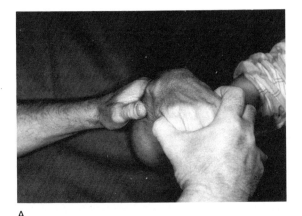

A

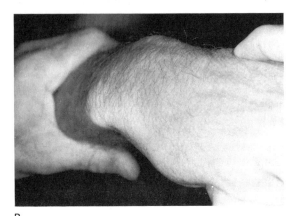

B

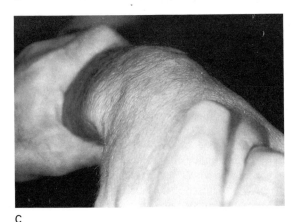

C

Fig. 2.75   Ulnar mid-carpal instability. A. The wrist is held in flexion with the forearm pronated. B. Radial deviation of the wrist produces a prominence of the triquetrum just distal to the ulnar head. C. Ulnar deviation should produce smooth dorsiflexion of the triquetrum causing its dorsal surface to move anteriorly, creating a hollow on the ulnar side of the wrist. If this prominence becomes more pronounced and then disappears with a 'clunk', ulnar mid-carpal instability is probable.

impingement (or impaction or abutment) syndrome. If the pain is on the radial side, it should be repeated with the thumb of the patient clasped in his palm — the *Finkelstein test* for *de Quervain's tenosynovitis* (p. 343). If the Finkelstein test is no more positive than simple ulnar deviation, the radial cutaneous nerve should be percussed for a Tinel sign (p. 227) and its dermatome examined for hypaesthesia — neuritis, sometimes caused by entrapment of that nerve as it emerges beneath the tendon of brachioradialis (p. 313), may cause wrist pain, as of course may more common nerve entrapments.

A brisk movement similar to that employed in the Finkelstein test should also be used into extreme dorsiflexion for it may reveal *flexor carpi radialis tendinitis* (p. 346).

The range of motion in the wrist can be measured somewhat inaccurately with a large goniometer, its fulcrum placed over the radiocarpal joint. Flexion and extension are best measured from the ulnar aspect, the line of the hand being the dorsal aspect of the third metacarpal, that of the forearm, the subcutaneous border of the ulna. Another guide to loss of motion is gained by comparison with the opposite wrist. More precise measurement can await a full set of radiographs.

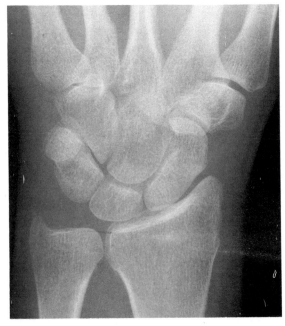

A

Fig. 2.76   Carpal arcs. A. The carpal arcs (see text) here are intact. B. The carpal arcs here (as in Fig. 1.128B) are disrupted due to a lunate dislocation. C. The strongly positive ulnar variance is associated in this patient with ulnar impaction syndrome.

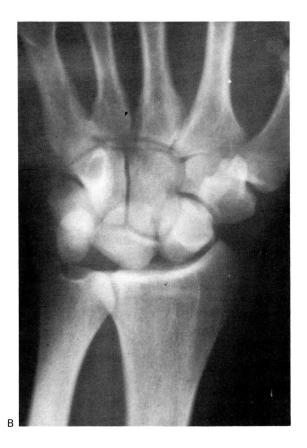

B

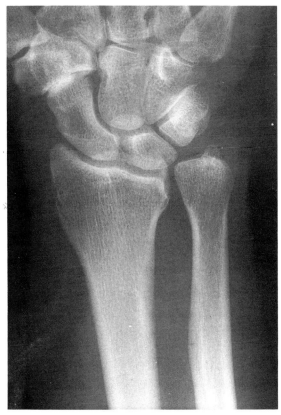

C

Grip strength measurement

The grip strength is measured with the Jamar dynamometer, taking care to place the elbow in flexion. Repeated measurements are taken and averaged in each of the five positions of the instrument. The significance of the readings, and those on rapid exchange, in revealing the malingerer have already been detailed (p. 162). Any significant reduction when compared with the opposite hand, if felt to be an honest reading, is indicative of wrist pathology provided all other possible causes for weakness have been eliminated. Conversely, and perhaps of greater economic significance, an equal grip strength to the other hand carries a high probability that there is no significant injury[252]. If standard radiographs (see below) are normal and the patient is content with reassurance, a programme involving (i) no further studies, (ii) a therapy programme including work hardening, and (iii) further full examination in six weeks may well yield an asymptomatic patient who has incurred minimal expense. If his problems persist six weeks later, more detailed examination is then pursued.

Local anaesthesia

If a site of precise tenderness has been found during examination and it can accurately and without exception be reproduced, and if the grip strength is equal and the radiographic examination clear, infiltration of the point with local anaesthetic containing adrenaline (epinephrine), mixed with a soluble steroid, should be performed and the examination repeated. Any new sites of reproducible tenderness which then appear should be similarly injected. If, by such injection, all pain and tenderness is eliminated and, then again, after inspection of normal standard radiographs, nothing further should be done. The exact location of the injection in the carpus, not on the skin, should be known and noted by the examiner, the patient should be encouraged to exercise gently and should be seen again in two weeks. The purpose of including steroid in the injectate is that, if the problem is local inflammation and the elimination of pain by the local anaesthetic indicates that the correct point has been injected, no further treatment may be required.

INVESTIGATION

Standard posteroanterior and lateral views (described in full on page 85) should be requested, taking care that the limb is positioned correctly[253].

Each carpal bone should be examined in turn for evidence of pathology in the form of fractures, cysts and increased radiodensity, possibly indicative of avascular necrosis.

On the *postero-anterior view* (Fig. 2.76), four features should be examined:

(i)   The *carpal arcs* — a break in any of the three suggests ligamentous disruption.

(ii) The *width and colinearity of the intercarpal joint spaces.*

(iii) The *shape* of the individual *carpal bones.*

(iv) *Ulnar variance,* which is the relationship of the distal outline of the ulnar head to that of the articular surface of the radius; this can be measured in three different ways with equal reliability[254]. The technique of *perpendiculars* requires the examiner to draw, perpendicular to the axis of the radius, that line which passes through the junction of the distal articular surface and the sigmoid notch of the radius — the variance is *negative* if the ulnar head fails to reach that line, *positive* if it projects beyond it, and *neutral* if it lies in the exact line.

Positive ulnar variance (Fig. 2.76C) is associated with a *thinner TFCC*[255] and with a higher incidence of ulnar column disorders, especially *ulnar impaction syndrome* (p. 220). Negative ulnar variance accompanies a higher incidence of *Kienbock's disease* and possibly also radial column pathology, especially *scapholunate dissociation*[256].

The *lateral view* (Fig. 2.77) should be exposed and examined as described in Chapter 1 and reprinted here for convenience:

The *lateral* view should be taken with the radius in the same line as the third metacarpal. This can best be achieved by giving the patient a flat piece of plastic or wood, several of which are kept handy, and instructing the patient to insist that this be laid firmly along the back of the wrist while the view is taken. A good lateral is further ensured by having the wrist and the shoulder on the same level as above. Whether or not a true lateral has been achieved is determined by seeing that the scaphoid tubercle, and only its tubercle, protrudes anterior to the outline of the pisiform. In studying the lateral view, the lunate outline represents the proximal carpal row, the capitate the distal. Again, as in the anteroposterior view, four features should be observed:

(i) The *angle of the distal radius*; the normal palmar tilt of 10° to 15° may be reversed, usually after a Colles fracture (Fig. 2.79A).

(ii) The *colinearity* of the radius, lunate and capitate. The axes of the capitate and the radius are easily

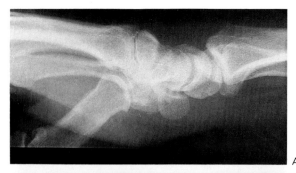

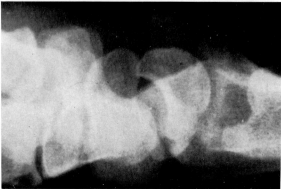

Fig. 2.77 True lateral of the wrist. A. The true lateral can be interpreted only if, as here, the third metacarpal is in direct line with the dorsal surface of the radius. The normal palmar tilt of the articular surface of a radius of 10° is seen here together with the colinearity of the radius, lunate and capitate and the normal scapholunate angle. This should normally lie between 30° and 60° and it averages 46°. B. By contrast, here the colinearity of the radius, lunate and capitate has been lost. The lunate is dorsiflexed and the capitate is subluxed. The scaphoid lies perpendicular to the axis of the radius creating a scapholunate angle of some 120°.

drawn; that of the lunate is a line perpendicular to a line drawn between its dorsal and ventral poles — in lunate dislocation[257], the capitate remains centred over the radius, whereas in perilunate dislocation, the lunate remains in line and the capitate is displaced.

(iii) The *angle of the lunate* relative to the axis of the radius; its axis may point dorsally, in which case it is dorsiflexed, and vice versa (it should be recalled that spurious dorsiflexion of the lunate can be produced by ulnar deviation, palmar flexion by radial, hence the need for careful neutral positioning).

(iv) The *scapholunate angle* should be measured: a close approximation to the scaphoid axis can be obtained by drawing a line through the proximo-anterior outline of the proximal and distal poles.

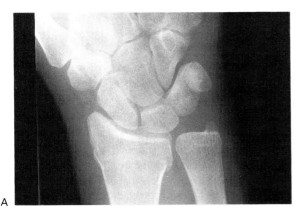

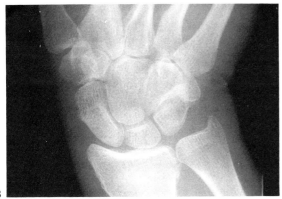

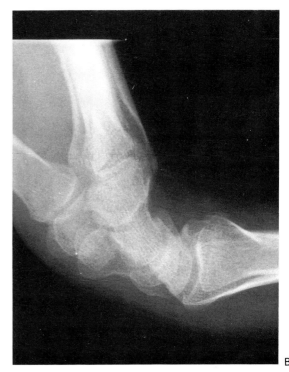

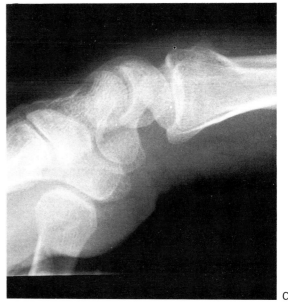

Fig. 2.78 A. Radial deviation. This causes the scaphoid to flex and is likely to reveal scapholunate disassociation. Note the clear joint space between the hamate and triquetrum. B. Ulnar deviation. This causes the scaphoid to extent and is a good view in which to see a scaphoid fracture (see Fig. 1.130A). In addition one can see the overriding of the hamate and the triquetrum. This contact causes the helicoid joint between these bones to engage and produces dorsiflexion of the proximal row, evidenced by the overlap of the lunate and capitate (see pp. 15 and 76).

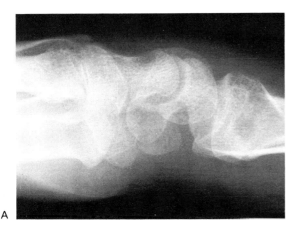

Fig. 2.79 A. This lateral view shows the reversal of palmar tilt of the radius associated with a Colles fracture, together with the carpal instability pattern non-dissociative (CIND) characteristic of this post-Colles deformity. B. Demonstrates good dorsiflexion in the same patient with much of the motion occuring at the midcarpal joint. C. Demonstrates poor palmar flexion with, again, much of the motion occuring at the midcarpal joint — although here there is a little more radiocarpal activitiy than in dorsiflexion.

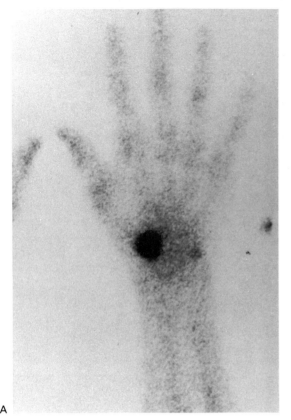

A

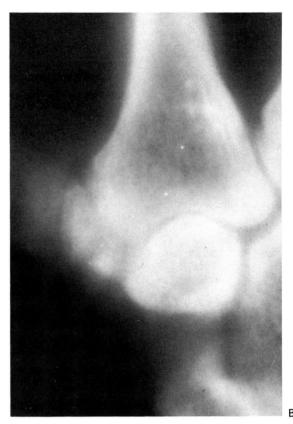

B

Fig. 2.80 A. Bone scan of this patient who had obscure wrist pain revealed significant uptake in the region of the basal joint of the index metacarpal. B. Subsequent polytomography revealed an occult fracture of the radial beak of the base of the second metacarpal.

The angle measured is that created by the *two axes extended distally*. The normal angle averages 47°, with a normal range from 30 to 60°[258]. Although when using a standard goniometer this may appear to be an inexact measure, it has been shown to be reproducible to within 7.4°[259].

In a standard posteroanterior view centred on the carpometacarpal joint and including the full length of the metacarpus, the *carpal height* should be calculated by measuring the distance from the base of the third metacarpal to the distal radial articular surface. The *carpal height ratio* is that measurement divided by the length of the third metacarpal. In normal hands this is a very constant figure of 0.54 ± 0.03[260]. Reduction in this ratio is evidence of *carpal collapse*.

If no pathology is found, additional views should be ordered:

1, 2 Posteroanterior in *radial and ulnar deviation* (Fig. 2.78); the former will emphasize any tendency to scapholunate instability (SLI), the latter better reveal an occult scaphoid fracture.

3, 4 Posteroanterior and lateral with a *clenched fist*; the former may drive the capitate between the scaphoid and lunate in SLI, the latter may reveal a collapse pattern of the carpus, most often encountered following malunion of a Colles fracture[261] (Fig. 2.79).

5, 6 Lateral views in *extension and flexion*, especially in the presence of limitation of these movements, will reveal the relative motion occurring in the radiocarpal and midcarpal joints (Fig. 2.79B and C).

Cysts within any of the carpal bones may be seen on a radiograph. They are the cause of pain only if they have *sclerotic margins* or they *communicate* with the joint space (page 341).

If by this stage a diagnosis has not been made, it may safely be concluded that the patient has *obscure wrist pain*!

Special studies
Any of the following studies may be indicated and have been shown to be of value in further evaluating obscure wrist pain:

Radionuclide imaging (bone scan)[262,263] is of particular value in localizing a disease process in the wrist, where that is poorly defined (Fig. 2.80); imaging is 95% accurate[264] in demonstrating fractures or complete ligamentous tears and 96% accurate in negative reading, that is, giving a cold scan when no pathology could be demonstrated by any other technique. Bone scans give false-negative readings in partial ligamentous tears.

Cineradiography (fluoroscopy) should be conducted in the presence of the hand surgeon to ensure that the correct manoeuvres are performed. The study is especially useful when a 'clunk' can be reliably reproduced on examination for it may well demonstrate a dynamic instability[265], that is, one which occurs only with motion; it can, with benefit, be done in conjunction with arthrography[266].

Arthrography[267] is perhaps best performed by the hand surgeon, certainly in his presence; if that is not possible, video imaging should be retained for him to study. Arthrography is most valuable in delineating tears, often partial and therefore 'cold' on bone scan, in the scapholunate ligament, the lunotriquetral ligament and the TFCC[268], the last of which has a complex arthrographic anatomy[269,270]. Triple injections — radiocarpal, midcarpal and inferior radioulnar joints — have been recommended for maximum yield[271]; the author finds that these give much more post-study discomfort and therefore reserves them for cases in whom the single radiocarpal injection has been negative. Digital subtraction techniques have been found by some to facilitate interpretation[272]; the author believes that distraction during arthrography may offer some evaluation of the thickness of cartilage — though only in the single plane viewed — it being represented by the dark line between bone and dye (Fig. 2.81).

Polytomography (trispiral[273] or ellipsoid) (Fig. 2.82) offers the opportunity to study the carpal bones in greater detail; it may yield evidence of occult fractures and erosive lesions. It is of value in assessing union of both fractures and intercarpal arthrodeses. The plane — sagittal, coronal or transverse — should be indicated by the surgeon; in an example from another location, only sagittal tomograms give a useful view of proximal phalangeal malunion (see Fig. 2.39A). Its use in conjunction with arthrography may yield evidence regarding ligamentous tears otherwise not available[274].

Computerised tomography (CT scan) gives information which is somewhat more refined than that obtainable with polytomography (Fig. 2.83), and it is particularly valuable in evaluating the distal radioulnar joint[275,276] (Fig. 2.84). Views in neutral, pronation and supination will demonstrate subluxation with more certainty than even the most accurately positioned lateral radiograph.

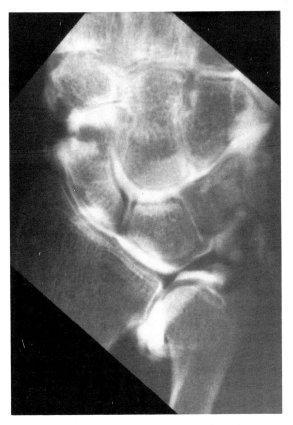

Fig. 2.81 A triple arthrogram has been performed. Distraction is applied, and the dark line between the dye and the subchondral bone is clearly displayed. This represents articular cartilage.

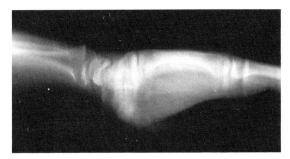

Fig. 2.82 Lateral polytomography. In another case of obscure wrist pain, lateral polytomography was performed and this revealed a midcarpal instability pattern as the only positive finding.

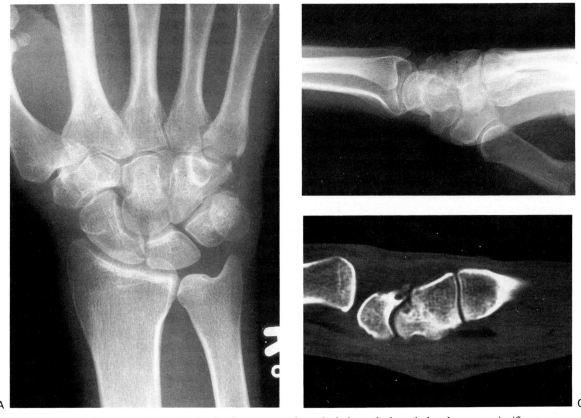

Fig. 2.83 Lateral CT scan. A, B. Standard wrist views suggested, particularly on the lateral, that there were significant problems in the midcarpal region of this patient who, approximately one year after a fall from a height had been classified as a malingerer. C. Lateral CT scan clearly showed a malunion of the capitate with significant interference with midcarpal joint function.

Whether or not the lack of a joint space indicates loss of cartilage, as the author suspects, has not yet been confirmed to the best of his knowledge. Three-dimensional images can be constructed[277,278] but they have no clinical application at this stage.

Arthroscopy[279-287] (Fig. 2.85) is the only method of ascertaining the presence of damage to the cartilaginous surface, but clumsily performed it can produce it — it should therefore be performed only after full training on the cadaveric model and clinical practice on those already scheduled for wrist arthrodesis; even then it should be reserved, in the opinion of those most expert[288], for patients still undiagnosed three months after the onset of wrist pain. With increased use of arthroscopy, the author has been impressed with how frequently it shows more than one pathological process, thereby improving quality of care. Combined with wrist manipulation it may demonstrate non-dissociative carpal instability[289].

Digital angiography[290] may occasionally be required to show bone tumours in the carpus, of which wrist pain is the only symptom.

It is evident that the armamentarium available is both rich and expensive. It is also important to recognize that surgery based on one observation alone may be entirely erroneous[272]. The thorough history and examination remains the cornerstone on which a sound diagnostic programme is constructed: a 'clunk' may be clarified by cineradiography alone, DRUJ dislocation diagnosed by a single CT scan. In patients in whom truly no clues exist an algorithm of diagnosis may assist both in reaching a valid conclusion and in limiting costs.

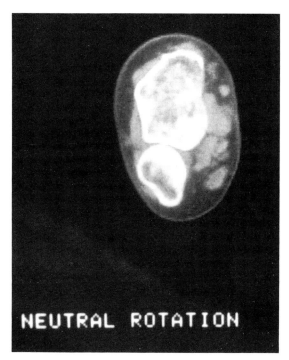

Fig. 2.84 Computerized tomography is the only satisfactory way of studying the inferior radio-ulnar joint.

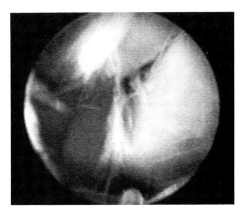

Fig. 2.85 Arthroscopy. This reveals a total scapholunate tear. The lunate is in the right side of the field and the proximal pole of the scaphoid, which is subluxed dorsally and therefore creates a 'step off', is in the top of the field. At between 9 and 10 o'clock, a white shadow is seen which is the edge of a significant defect in the articular cartilage. Because of this wear, which could be satisfactorily detected only by arthroscopy, a stabilization of the subluxation of this scaphoid was deemed to be an inadequate procedure.

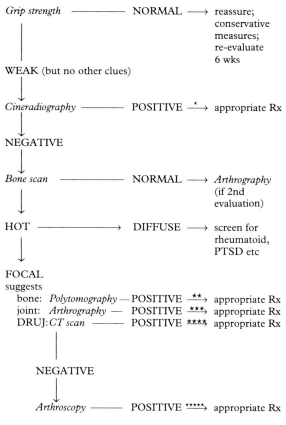

Grip strength ——————— NORMAL ⟶ reassure; conservative measures; re-evaluate 6 wks

WEAK (but no other clues)

Cineradiography ——————— POSITIVE —[*]→ appropriate Rx

NEGATIVE

Bone scan ——————— NORMAL ⟶ *Arthrography* (if 2nd evaluation)

HOT ——————————————⟶ DIFFUSE ⟶ screen for rheumatoid, PTSD etc

FOCAL
suggests
  bone: *Polytomography* — POSITIVE —[**]→ appropriate Rx
  joint: *Arthrography* — POSITIVE —[***]→ appropriate Rx
  DRUJ: *CT scan* ——————— POSITIVE —[****]→ appropriate Rx

NEGATIVE

Arthroscopy ——————— POSITIVE —[*****]→ appropriate Rx

[*]   carpal instability
[**]   occult fracture, erosion or tumour
[***]   partial ligamentous tear
[****] DRUJ disorder
[*****] cartilage damage, loose body

Magnetic resonance imaging (MRI) (Fig. 2.86) offers exciting potential in assessing patients with wrist pain[291]. While on first consideration the current cost of $750 to $1000 appears prohibitive, if it were to replace more than one of the studies outlined above, it would prove economical. MRI offers several advantages in imaging the wrist[292]:

(i)   The ability to study wrist anatomy in multiple positions and planes
(ii) Clear visualization of soft tissues, including ligament, nerve and tendon
(iii) High sensitivity in detecting occult fractures and tumours
(iv) Inspection of articular cartilage.

Ultrasound transmission imaging[293] may also prove to be part of the new wave.

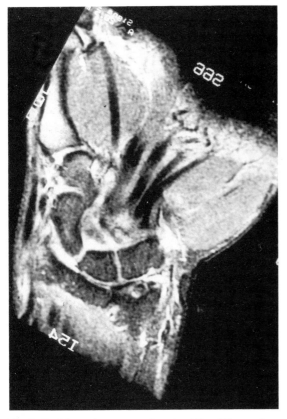

Fig. 2.86 Magnetic resonance imaging. The difference in alignment and intercarpal joint space is seen between the lunatotriquetral joint and the scapholunate joint. The patient had a partial tear of the scapholunate ligament which caused pain, but no instability.

NON-UNION

While other carpal bones may be the seat of non-union, notably the capitate[294,295], the incidence is miniscule when compared to that of the scaphoid[296]. All three factors previously stated to cause non-union (p. 183) — *avascularity of the fragments, separation of the bone ends* and *undue motion at the fracture site* — play a potent role in the high incidence of scaphoid non-union. Avascularity of the proximal pole (Fig. 2.87) results from the distal entry of the sole blood supply[297]. Separation of the fragments is more likely to occur when the apparently isolated fracture in fact represents the only bony injury in a major fracture dislocation of the carpus (pp. 82 and 88). Motion between the fragments is a consequence of the fracture line becoming the natural extension of the mid-carpal joint (Fig. 2.88). That this occurs, resulting in decreased motion of the proximal row and increased motion of the distal, has been shown in cadaveric studies[298]. The same study showed that the proximal row tended to become more extended (DISI) and the distal more flexed. The effect is to produce a more flexed scaphoid — the *humpback deformity* — which can be detected on lateral views of the wrist, but is best visualized on tomograms[299] or CT scans[300] in the axis of the bone. Even if the scaphoid heals in this position, there is a loss of wrist extension proportional to the scaphoid flexion[301] and a significantly poorer clinical outcome[302]. If non-union persists, arthritis occurs in the majority and in a definite sequence: (i) the scaphoid and radial styloid, (ii) the radio-scaphoid joint as far as the fracture line, and (iii) the capitolunate joint. This has been termed *scapholunate advanced collapse* or the *SLAC wrist*[303,304] (Fig. 2.89).

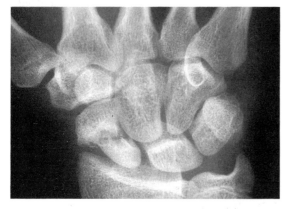

Fig. 2.87 Probable avascular necrosis of the proximal pole of the scaphoid in a non-union. In addition, there is more than 1 mm shift between the two scaphoid fragments, and the carpal arcs are disrupted by the lunate, which is dorsiflexed.

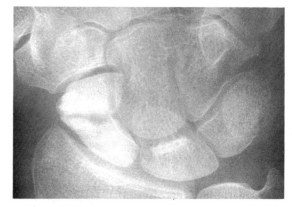

Fig. 2.88 Scaphoid non-union. The sclerosis between the fragments indicates that non-union is established. The abnormal outline of the lunate testifies to the established DISI pattern.

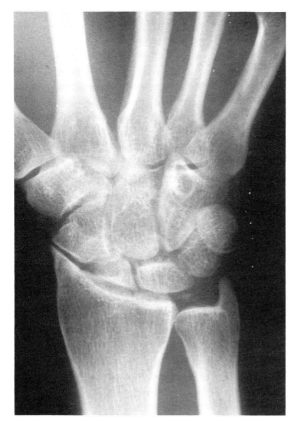

Fig. 2.89 SLAC wrist. In an established scaphoid non-union with a dorsal collapse pattern of the proximal row, arthritis has commenced between the radial styloid and the distal scaphoid. Of note is the lack of arthritis between the proximal pole and the remainder of the scaphoid fossa. The collapse between the capitate and the lunate presages development of arthritis at that joint.

Indications

No avascular necrosis, no arthritis. It is evident that scaphoid non-union, indeed scaphoid malunion, is to be avoided. If there is no evidence of shift of the fragments one or the other of more than 1 mm, and there is no DISI deformity on the lateral view, then immobilization is indicated (p. 88). In all other circumstances more active steps are required, but which? Recommended procedures include electrical stimulation[305], percutaneous pin fixation[306], screw fixation, including that designed by Herbert[307-311], bone graft alone from both dorsal and palmar approaches[312], from sources including the radius, ulnar and iliac crest[313] (Fig. 2.90), soft-tissue arthroplasty[313,314], anterior bone graft and correction of the humpback deformity with Herbert[315,316] or AO[317] screw or staple[318] fixation. The author's preference is for the modification of the Russe

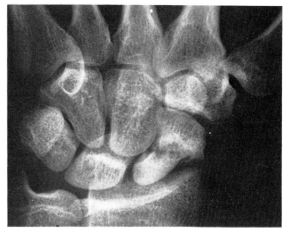

A

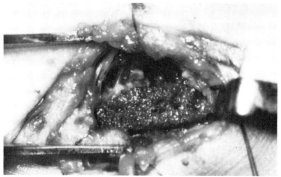

B

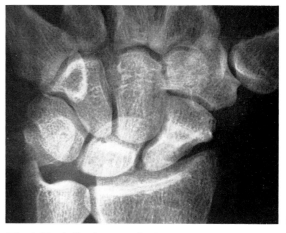

C

Fig. 2.90 A. Persistent cystic change in this scaphoid was allied to motion evident on cineradiography but no clear evidence of aseptic necrosis or arthritis. B. A cancellous bone graft was inserted resulting in (C) satisfactory late union.

technique described by Green[319] (Fig. 2.91), for the corticocancellous graft from the radius, when wedged into the anterior trough created in the scaphoid with the wrist in dorsiflexion, both corrects the humpback de

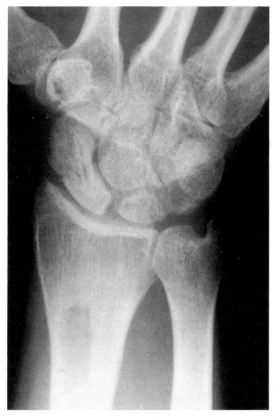

Fig. 2.91   Scaphoid bone graft. Healing has been achieved using cortico-cancellous bone grafts taken from the anterior cortex of the radius through the same incision (see text).

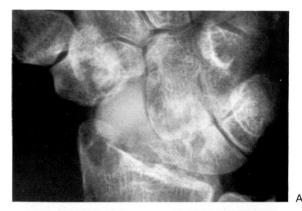

A

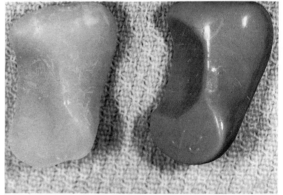

B

Fig. 2.92   Silicone synovitis. A. This patient shows both subluxation of the scaphoid implant and also cystic changes in the adjacent radius, lunate, capitate and trapezium. Note the capitolunate arthritis, the untreated element of the SLAC wrist. B. On removal of the implant, significant wear is to be seen. The implant is to the left, a sizer to the right for comparative purposes.

formity and is subjected to compression in so doing. Some concern has been expressed that the anterior approach, by dividing the major wrist ligaments, produces carpal collapse[320]. Care should be taken in their repair.

Avascular necrosis, no arthritis. As Green has emphasized[319], avascular necrosis, although suspected on the radiograph, can only be diagnosed at surgery. If in any doubt, I would graft as above. If definitely avascular and unmanageable, the proximal pole should be removed. Some would have inserted silicone[321] before the recognition of problems with instability, wear and silicone synovitis (see under trapezial implant, Chapter 4, p. 338) (Fig. 2.92), others a rolled tendon graft or fascia[332]. The prognosis is guarded.

Arthritis confined to the scaphoid. If only with the styloid, radial styloidectomy will give relief of unpredicted degree and duration. If throughout the radioscaphoid joint, the choices are radioscaphoid fusion, proximal row carpectomy[323-326], and resection with capitolunatehamatotriquetral arthrodesis (a 'four-corner'

fusion) to prevent collapse. Wrist denervation[327] offers relief in two-thirds of cases, but is more popular East of the Atlantic than West.

SLAC wrist. Total wrist arthrodesis[328-332].

See Green D P 1993 Operative Hand Surgery, 3rd edn. Churchill Livingstone, New York, p. 809.

AVASCULAR NECROSIS

While this occurrence, apparently without prior injury, has been reported in the scaphoid — *Preiser's disease*[333] — and in the pisiform, it is by far most commonly encountered in the lunate, where it is termed lunatomalacia or *Kienbock's disease*[334-337]. It may well result from micro-fractures of the lunate impairing its blood supply. It is more common in patients with *negative ulnar variance*[338]. There are four stages:

I   Tender lunate; no changes on routine radiographic examination; increased uptake on *bone scan*; dark low-signal-intensity on T1-weighted MRI[339]

II   Increased *radiodensity but no collapse* (except a little on the radial aspect in later cases in this stage)

III   *Lunate collapse*, confirmed by a *reduced carpal height* (p. 210) (Fig. 2.93A)

IV   *Carpal arthritis*

Indications

Stage I   Immobilization.

II   Several procedures have been recommended to revascularize the lunate or to 'unload' it, including various intercarpal fusions[340], lengthening of the ulna and shortening of the capitate or of the radius; studies have shown[341] that operations on the forearm are most efficacious and least injurious; radial shortening by 4 mm, or by the amount required to restore neutral ulnar variance,

whichever is the greater, is the easier procedure (Fig. 2.93B).

III   Radial shortening ± Lunate resection[342] — the lunate was formerly replaced with a silicone spacer with good results[343,344], but fear of the now well-established complications[345] of silicone implants make this unacceptable; the space may be left, or filled with tendon; proximal migration of the capitate may occur and procedures to prevent this have been described but have no proven advantage.

IV   Proximal row carpectomy or wrist fusion.

See Green D P 1993 Operative Hand Surgery, 3rd edn. Churchill Livingstone, New York, p. 839.

INSTABILITY

Instability disorders of the wrist[346,347] result from tearing or stretching of the ligaments of the carpus (p. 81). Complete tears result in gaps which can be seen on rou-

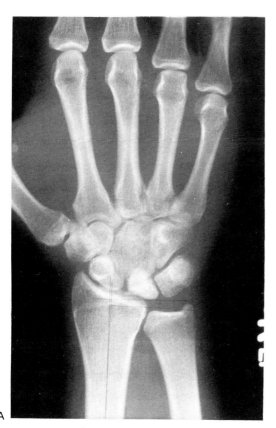

A

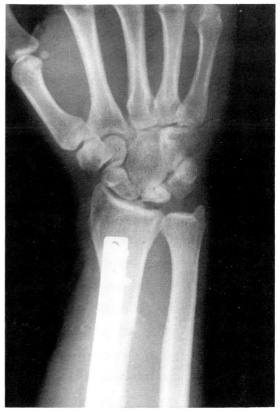

B

Fig. 2.93 Kienbock's disease. A. Stage three disease is confirmed by the increased opacity and reduction in size of the lunate. The carpal height is reduced to 0.45 (normal 0.54 +/− 0.03). Negative ulnar variance is evident. B. The lunate has been unloaded by radial shortening which significantly alleviated the patient's discomfort.

tine radiographs, and may therefore be called *static*. Stretching is more subtle, causing problems which are not seen on standard films but are produced with movement and loading of the wrist. These can be termed dynamic. Scapholunate instability is the most common of the static group, ulnar midcarpal instability of the *dynamic*. A further classification[348] separates instability between bones of the same row, usually the proximal — *dissociated carpal instability* (CID) — from those of the radiocarpal and midcarpal joints which lie between rows — *non-dissociative instability* (CIND). The latter is most common following the reversal of tilt associated with Colles fracture (Fig. 2.79).

Scapholunate instability (= scapholunate dissociation = rotatory subluxation of the scaphoid[349])
This most commonly occurs as a result of a fall on the outstretched hand in which the primary vector is ulnar deviation and intercarpal supination. It represents stage I of Mayfield's four stages[350] of perilunar injury (p. 81). It may also result from an anatomical predisposition[351], a fall on the elbow[352] or excision of a dorsal ganglion cyst[353]. The diagnostic features other than the pain and loss of grip strength characteristic of all wrist disorders are:

(i) A positive *Watson scaphoid shift* test (p. 204).
(ii) Increased space between the scaphoid and lunate on the posteroanterior radiograph (Figs 2.94, 2.95); dubbed the *Terry Thomas sign*[354] after the English actor who had a wide space between his front teeth (wider gaps have been called the Leon Spinks sign after the American boxer who had *no* front teeth). If questionable, this is exaggerated by *radial deviation* and by the *clenched fist* view (*not* named after Spinks).
(iii) The *signet ring sign* (Fig. 2.94A) is seen on the posteroanterior view and is due to the flexed posture of the scaphoid, which is seen more end-on than is normal — the distal pole forms the 'ring', the proximal pole its 'stone'.
(iv) An *increase in the scapholunate angle* on the lateral view above the upper limit of normal of 60° (p. 86) (Fig. 2.94B).
(v) A *dorsal intercalated segment instability (DISI)* pattern (pp. 76 and 85) (Fig. 2. 94C).

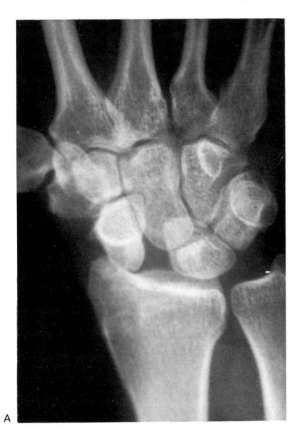

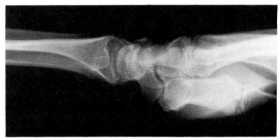

Fig. 2.94 A. Terry Thomas sign, signet ring sign, and evident overriding of the lunate on the capitate. B. Modest change in the scapholunate angle at 75° (normal 30–60°). C. More pronounced DISI pattern with loss of colinearity of the radius, lunate and capitate (demonstrated by the lines) and a scapholunate angle of 90°.

A

B

C

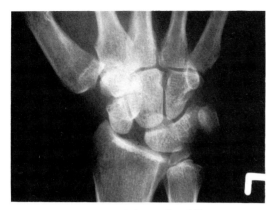

Fig. 2.95 Established scapholunate instability.

Quite apart from the problems caused by the instability itself, the dramatic reduction in the load-bearing contact area between scaphoid and radius brought about by the scaphoid rotation[355,356] causes the early development of radioscaphoid and later pancarpal *arthritis*.

Indications. Clearly this problem should be corrected. Equally clearly, there is no general agreement upon what should be done. If encountered early, with an understanding of the mechanism, there is clear merit in attempting direct repair of the ligaments. Unfortunately, most patients present long after the injury when repair is no longer possible. *Triscaphe or STT fusion* (Fig. 2.96), in which the scaphoid, trapezoid and trapezium are fused, has had wide popularity[357-361] with good results on follow-up for an average of 56 months[362]. However, there have been complications, both in the short term[363] and the long term, the latter largely due to the altered wrist mechanics[364,365], such that an original proponent of the procedure now recommends routine partial radial

styloidectomy as part of the triscaphe fusion[366]. The alternatives are few, including ligamentous re-attachment[367] and capsulodesis[368]. Before any reconstructive procedure is selected it is prudent to inspect the cartilaginous surfaces of the radius, scaphoid, capitate and lunate for evidence of wear which would presage the development of a SLAC wrist and also would be very likely to cause continued symptoms if surgery addressed only the instability. Such inspection is best done through the arthroscope so that the final options can be discussed with the patient.

See Green D P 1993 Operative Hand Surgery, 3rd edn. Churchill Livingstone, New York, p. 883.

Ulnar midcarpal instability[369]
Laxity of the triquetrohamatocapitate ligament, which most commonly arises from chronic attrition, permits the proximal row of the carpus to tilt in a palmar direction, a *volar intercalated segment instability (VISI)* pattern. Disruption or attrition of the lunatotriquetral ligament — ulnar perilunate instability as opposed to the radial perilunate instability which produces scapholunate dissociation — may also produce a VISI pattern. Taken together, the two may be considered as constituting the full pattern of ulnar midcarpal instability[370-372]. However, the concept is complicated by the fact that isolated lunotriquetral injuries occur, apparently resulting from hyperextension and twisting of the wrist, and made more probable if there is a positive ulnar variance[373]. The diagnoses are made as follows:

1. Ulnar midcarpal instability:
   (i) A positive *Lichtman test* (p. 205)
   (ii) A *decrease in the scapholunate angle* (Fig. 2.97) to less than the lower limit of normal 30°

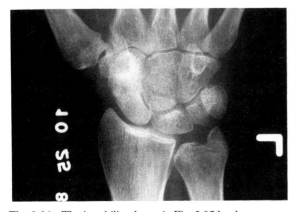

Fig. 2.96 The instability shown in Fig. 2.95 has been corrected by triscaphe fusion.

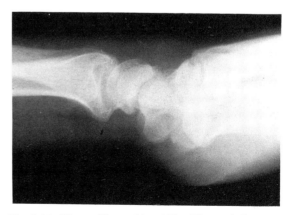

Fig. 2.97 Ulnar mid-carpal instability. The scapholunate angle is at the lower limits of normal at 30° (normal range 30–60°), as a result of a VISI pattern of the proximal carpal row.

(iii) A *VISI pattern* on the lateral radiograph
(iv) A demonstrable snap from VISI to DISI with ulnar deviation on the *lateral cineradiogram*
2. Lunotriquetral strain[374,375]
   (i) A positive *ballottement test* (p. 205)
   (ii) An LT leak demonstrated on *arthrogram*

Indications. Stabilization of the lunatotriquetral joint can be achieved by fusion of that joint alone, but a relatively high failure rate, shared by the author, has been reported[373–375], greater success being achieved by 'four-corner' fusion of *hamate–triquetrum–lunate–capitate*, which is, in any event, indicated in full ulnar midcarpal instability. If the problem exists in the presence of a positive ulnar variance, simultaneous *ulnar shortening* should be done.

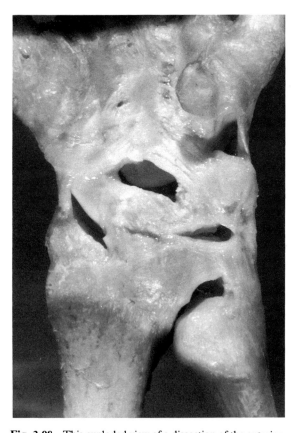

Fig. 2.98 This exploded view of a dissection of the anterior surface of the left wrist demonstrates on the right from lower to upper, the head of the ulna, the triangular fibrocartilaginous complex (TFCC) the triquetrum and the hamate with its hook in evidence. The anterior ligaments have been removed with the exception of the triquetrocapitate ligament. The attachment of the TFCC from the ulnar styloid to the sigmoid notch on the radius is seen. (Dissection by Dr Douglas Hanel.)

See Green D P 1993 Operative Hand Surgery, 3rd edn. Churchill Livingstone, New York, p. 896.

THE DISTAL RADIO-ULNAR JOINT (DRUJ)[376–378] (Fig. 2.98)

The cylindrical head of the ulna articulates with the sigmoid notch of the radius. In order to achieve the normal range of pronation and supination (p. 190), 270° of the circumference of the head is covered with cartilage, as also is a portion of its distal end. Between that portion of the distal head and the ulnar styloid is a recess, termed the fovea. The triangular fibrocartilaginous complex (TFCC) connects the ulna at the fovea to the radius at the ulnar aspect of the lunate fossa (which corresponds to the distal margin of the sigmoid notch). The anterior and posterior margins of this triangular portion of the TFCC are thickened to form the anterior and dorsal radio-ulnar ligaments respectively. The TFCC also incorporates the ulnar collateral ligament, the sheath of extensor carpi ulnaris, the strong, anteriorly located ulnotriquetral ligament and the relatively weak anterior ulnolunate ligament. Together with the meniscus homologue, the whole constitutes the ulnocarpal complex. As the forearm pronates, the ulna moves distally and dorsally relative to the radial sigmoid notch, tightening the anterior radioulnar ligament. As supination occurs, so do the converse movements and the posterior ligament comes under tension. Perforations of the TFCC — causing free communication from the distal radio-ulnar joint to the radiocarpal joint — are absent in childhood, but become progressively more common until they are present in the majority over the age of 50.

Pathology
Painful conditions around the ulnar head include:

(i) DRUJ chondromalacia or arthritis — diagnosed by compression–rotation (p. 205), bone scan and CT (Fig. 2.99)
(ii) Subluxation of the ECU tendon[379–382]
(iii) TFCC afflictions[383]
   (a) acute, including dislocation of the DRUJ[384]
   (b) chronic, including ulnar impaction syndrome.

Acute TFCC injuries involve avulsion of the ligament, usually from its radial attachment. Those which are complete result in dislocation of the distal radio-ulnar joint, which can be diagnosed by examination, a true lateral radiograph and confirmed by CT scan. Those which are incomplete leave either or both of the radio-ulnar ligaments intact, creating an acute perforation, which is relatively rare. The diagnosis is made by arthrography or arthroscopy, though great caution must

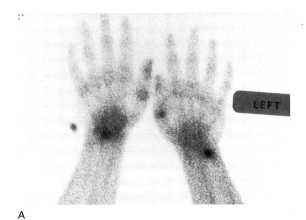

A

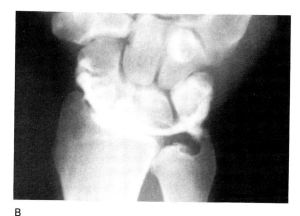

B

C

Fig. 2.99 Chondromalacia of the distal radio-ulnar joint. A. In this bone scan for a patient with obscure wrist pain, increased uptake was seen in the region of the distal radio-ulnar joint. B. An arthrogram failed to reveal any leak from the radiocarpal joint into the distal radio-ulnar joint. C. CT scan appears to show some subluxation of the ulnar head with contact between radius and ulnar head and probably chondromalacia. Exploration showed this to be the case and relief was obtained by a matched osteotomy of the ulnar head.

be exercised in declaring that the tear is the source of ulnar-sided wrist pain[385].

Chronic TFCC problems are invariably associated with a *positive ulnar variance* (Fig. 2.100). They develop with the passage of time in four phases:

1. Pain and swelling — ulnar variance is the only clue
2. TFCC perforation — demonstrable on *arthrography*
3. Ulnolunate abutment — positive *bone scan*, erosions on *polytomography*, changes seen at *arthroscopy*
4. LT strain — see above

In addition to the abutment of the overlong ulnar head against the lunate, the ulnar styloid may strike the triquetrum, another manifestation of the ulnar impaction or impingement syndrome. Again the *bone scan* will be positive and *polytomography* will show erosions, this time in the triquetrum.

Indications

DRUJ arthritis is treated in a manner similar to arthritis in other joints of the hand, by resection arthroplasty — a Darrach procedure or a matched osteotomy of the ulnar head — or by fusion of the distal radio-ulnar joint[386], preserving forearm rotation by a proximal osteotomy.

Dislocation is treated by immobilization in a long-arm splint in full supination for six weeks. If that proves unsuccessful, a fusion of the radio-ulnar joint with proximal osteotomy[386] is required.

Incomplete TFCC tears, if they are central and are felt to be the cause of symptoms, are managed by arthroscopic excision of the central portion of the TFCC where it overlies the distal part of the ulnar head[387,388]. *Peripheral* tears can be repaired successfully, as the blood supply there is superior to that present centrally[389].

Ulnar impaction, impingement or abutment are relieved by ulnar shortening[390–392].

A number of these procedures — proximal row carpectomy, ulnar head hemiresection and, most commonly, excision of partial TFCC tears — have been done through the arthroscope[393–395].

See Green D P 1993 Operative Hand Surgery, 3rd edn. Churchill Livingstone, New York, p. 991.

Nerve

In assessing the effect of nerve injury, which may have been complete or partial, single or multiple, accurately repaired or not, after a period of recovery which may still be progressing, the assessment can be of value only if the same tests are repeated at regular intervals of six weeks, wherever possible by the same examiner. The tests selected should be as objective as can be devised.

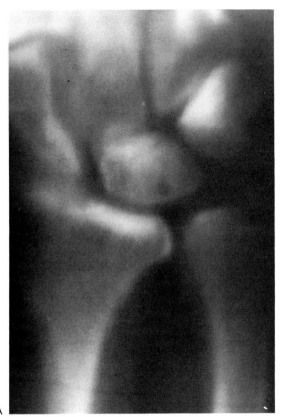
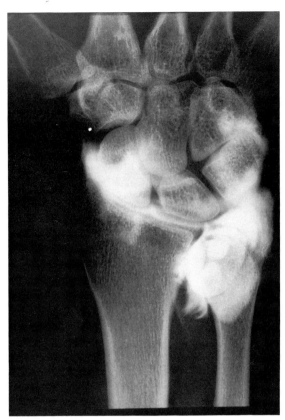

A   B

Fig. 2.100   A. This patient with ulnar-sided pain, on polytomography showed a positive ulnar variance and also cystic changes in the lunate. B. An arthrogram revealed a leak in the TFCC, but no escape through the lunatotriquetral interosseous ligament. At exploration chondromalacia of the lunate was found corresponding to the cyst. Ulnar shortening gave the patient relief.

In observing the hand of a patient known or believed to have a nerve injury, clues to the location of the injury may be seen.

Skin changes
(a) *Site of scar*. The site of scars in the arm allied to a knowledge of the surface markings of the major structures at risk, leads the surgeon to suspect which nerves may by involved.
(b) *Ulcers*. Areas with no protective sensation are injured inadvertently — these are most commonly on the finger tips. This is the deformity most prevalent in patients suffering from Hansen's disease (leprosy)[396].
(c) *Smoothness, dryness and cleanliness of skin*. The skin ridges in areas of sensory loss become less pronounced. This smoothness and loss of sweating minimizes dirt retention. Allied to reduced use this results in the area being much cleaner than those adjacent.

(d) *Absence of calluses*. The hands of workmen show thickening of the palmar skin. In areas of sensory loss the skin becomes softer and calluses disappear.
(e) *Circulatory and colour changes*. Due to absence of sympathetic control the colour of adjacent innervated and denervated areas often differs markedly, the denervated area being most frequently red and shiny.
(f) *Temperature changes*. For the first few weeks after nerve injury the denervated digits are warm, as their vessels have been freed from sympathetic control. Thereafter the fingers become cold to the touch when compared with adjacent, innervated areas.

Alteration of contour
   Muscle wasting. Paralysed muscles become increasingly atrophic. Those muscles in the hand which do so most noticeably are:

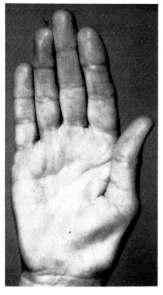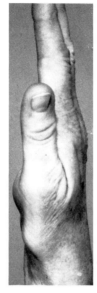

Fig. 2.101 A, B. Atrophy of the abductor pollicis brevis in median nerve injury.

abductor pollicis brevis — median nerve (Fig. 2.101)
abductor digiti minimi $\left.\right\}$ ulnar nerve (Fig. 2.102)
1st dorsal interosseous

The wasting is most easily appreciated if the injured hand is compared with the uninjured one. The deformity has two components — depression due to loss of muscle bulk and prominence of bones normally masked by muscle. In more proximal injuries, the arm and forearm lose bulk and this should be recorded as a difference in circumference from the unaffected arm at a measured distance above and below the olecranon.

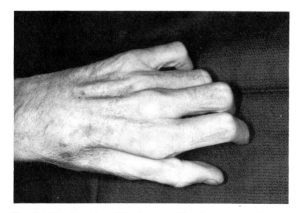

Fig. 2.102 Atrophy of the interossei in ulnar nerve palsy.

Spindling of the fingers. The bulk of subcutaneous tissue becomes reduced in most fingers deprived of their sensory supply and this results in a noticeable tapering of the distal portion of the affected digits.

Pathognomonic postures

Changes in posture due to nerve injury may be very evident at rest or may only be observed or become more pronounced when the patient is asked to perform certain functions. As a general rule, the higher the lesion, the more likely is the postural change to be seen immediately. With the passage of time also, a postural *deformity*, which is passively correctable, becomes a *contracture*, which is not. This is due to joint changes, and one of the major responsibilities of those following a patient with a nerve injury is to prevent contracture by correct splinting. Such splinting often serves to improve function also.

Cerebral palsy (p. 247). This differs from all other nerve lesions commonly affecting the upper extremity — apart from a cerebrovascular accident, which resembles it in many ways — in that the lesion is of an upper motor neuron rather than a lower one and there is therefore usually a marked degree of *spasticity*. There are two groups of postural change:

extrinsic — flexion contracture of elbow, wrist and fingers
pronation contracture of the forearm
adduction ± flexion contracture of the thumb
intrinsic — intrinsic-plus deformity of the fingers, that is, flexion of the metacarpophalangeal joints and extension, often swan-neck, of the interphalangeal joints.

Upper roots of the brachial plexus — 'Erb's palsy'[397] (Fig. 2.103) (p. 243). Originally described in relation to birth injuries this nerve lesion may be produced by any powerful blow to the shoulder with associated contralateral flexion of the cervical spine. This is not uncommon in motorcyclists wearing a crash helmet, which skids on landing — throwing the force on to the angle of the neck and shoulder. The roots are disrupted from above in turn.

C5 and C6. Due to loss of shoulder abduction (deltoid) and external rotation (spinati), of elbow flexion (biceps, brachialis, brachioradialis) and forearm supination (biceps, supinator) the arm hangs by the patient's side internally rotated, extended at the elbow and pronated.

C7. The additional loss of elbow extension (triceps) increases the limpness of the posture while the loss of wrist extension (extensor carpi radialis longus et brevis

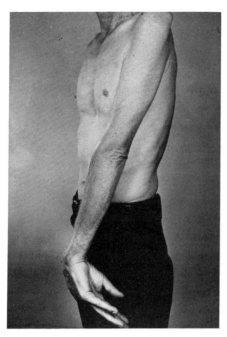

Fig. 2.103 Erb's palsy. The patient sustained a brachial plexus gunshot injury. He shows shoulder adduction, elbow extension, forearm pronation and wrist flexion — the 'porter's tip' position.

and ulnaris) results in some wrist flexion. In its full form this turns the palm of the hand upwards to the rear at the level of the mid-thigh, a posture adopted for the surreptitious receipt of money — 'porter's tip' position.

Radial nerve above the elbow. Due to loss of the wrist and finger extensors, a 'drop wrist' posture results (Fig. 2.104). The fingers may appear to extend remarkably well but this is due to (i) the tenodesis effect of wrist flexion in extending the metacarpophalangeal

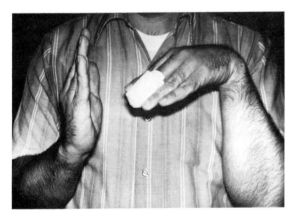

Fig. 2.104 This patient had sustained a spontaneous radial palsy and demonstrates the characteristic 'drop wrist' posture.

joints and (ii) active intrinsic ulnar-innervated extension of the interphalangeal joints.

Ulnar nerve at the wrist — 'claw hand' (Fig. 2.105)[398]. The characteristic posture of hyperextension of the metacarpophalangeal joints and flexion of the interphalangeal joints is adopted by the ring and small fingers only in pure ulnar nerve loss at the wrist. Paralysis of the flexor digiti minimi and the lumbrical muscles of these fingers disturbs the balance of the metacarpophalangeal joints of which these muscles are the prime flexors. If the joints are sufficiently mobile, the long extensors hyperextend them and in young hands this it may do by as much as 60°. The long extensors thus lose and the long flexors gain mechanical advantage at the interphalangeal joints, which therefore adopt a flexed posture.

'Ulnar clawing' does not result in all ulnar nerve lesions. This can be for any one of the following reasons:

1. *The ulnar nerve does not serve the lumbricals.* The lumbricals exercise control over the metacarpophalangeal joints, as is evidenced by the absence of clawing in the middle and index fingers in ulnar nerve injuries, when all intrinsics to these fingers other than the lumbricals are paralysed. The innervation of the lumbricals varies and hence, so will the presence of clawing. High ulnar nerve injuries, above an existing Martin–Gruber anastomosis — in which ulnar intrinsic fibres travel with the median nerve to the forearm before crossing to join the ulnar nerve (p. 235) — will also show no clawing.

2. *The metacarpophalangeal joint is not hyperextensible, through age, disease, injury, or inherent stiffness.* This fact can be demonstrated in the recently acquired ulnar claw hand. By blocking the hyperextension of the metacarpophalangeal joint, clawing no longer occurs with extension — the Bouvier manoeuvre

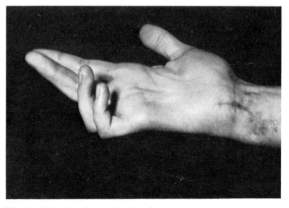

Fig. 2.105 An ulnar claw hand.

(see below). Prevention of metacarpophalangeal hyperextension is the basis of many operative procedures for ulnar claw hand.

3. *Either the long flexors or the long extensors are not functioning*:
   (a) If the ulnar nerve injury is above the motor branch to the flexor digitorum profundus of the ring and small fingers, clawing does not occur. As the nerve recovers proximal to distal, the long flexors will recover first, and temporary clawing may then be seen.
   (b) In the unusual event of an associated radial nerve injury above the branch to extensor digitorum or division of the tendon itself.

The *Bouvier manoeuver*[399] is important in assessing the claw hand. Hyperextension of the metacarpophalangeal joint is prevented as described above, and the patient is asked to extend the finger. One of three circumstances will result:

1. *Bouvier-positive* (Fig. 2.106) — the finger extends at the interphalangeal joints; only an anticlaw procedure will be required.
2. *Bouvier-negative* — the finger does not extend at the interphalangeal joints, and is either

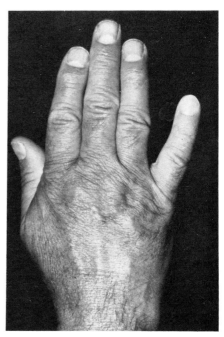

Fig. 2.107 An ulnar abducted finger in ulnar palsy. This occurs in patients in whom the metacarpophalangeal joint cannot hyperextend and thus the long extrinsic extensors abduct the finger, no resistance being offered by the paralysed third palmar interosseous.

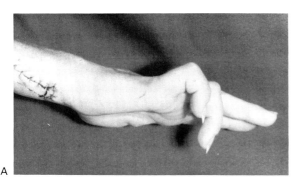

A

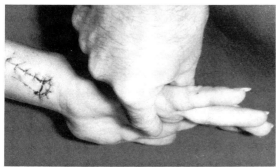

B

Fig. 2.106 A, B. Bouvier manoeuvre. This patient is Bouvier-positive.

   (a) *Passive-positive* — the examiner is able to extend the interphalangeal joints passively, indicating that the extensor apparatus is incompetent at that joint, due to dysfunction, probably on account of distension.
   (b) *Passive-negative* — even passively the finger is fixed in flexion as a result of skin shortening, flexor adhesions, palmar plate contracture or the other causes discussed on p. 191.

Ulnar abducted finger[400] (Fig. 2.107). If the metacarpophalangeal joint cannot hyperextend, the finger does not claw. In some of these patients, the loss of the third palmar interosseous causes the small finger to abduct markedly in extension. This is often an impediment when sliding the hand into narrow spaces, such as into a trouser pocket.

Froment's sign[401] (Fig. 2.108). The patient is asked to pull on a sheet of paper with index finger and thumb while the examiner withdraws it strongly. The normal patient maintains maximum contact of his digital pulp with the paper by extending the interphalangeal joint of the thumb. In ulnar palsy, for the reasons explained on page 37, the flexor pollicis longus is too powerful for

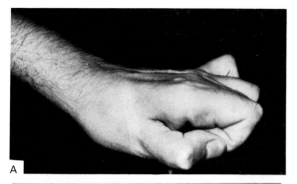

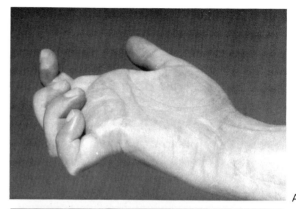

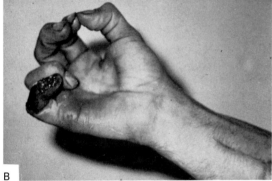

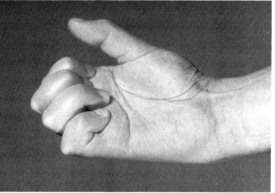

Fig. 2.108 Froment's sign. A. In attempting to exert powerful key pinch in which the interphalangeal joint of the thumb is normally extended that joint flexes. Note the clawing of the small and ring fingers and also the wasting of the first dorsal interosseous. B. This patient shows all the deficits of an ulnar nerve injury — the Froment posture, clawing and sensory deficit as evidenced by the full-thickness burn of the small finger which was sustained when it was inadvertently immersed in hot oil.

Fig. 2.109 Combined median and ulnar nerve lesion. A. The characteristic claw posture of all four fingers is demonstrated. B. On attempting to make a fist, the typical roll up of the fingers is noted, preventing a wide span grasp. (The intact thenar musculature suggests anomalous innervation.)

the combined interphalangeal joint extensors weakened by the loss of the contribution from adductor pollicis. In addition, the control of the metacarpophalangeal joint is lost through the paralysis of adductor pollicis and the deep head of flexor pollicis brevis. It collapses into hyperextension, balance is lost and the interphalangeal joint flexes. Many other active postural tests have been described to confirm ulnar nerve paralysis[402].

Median nerve. The radial half of the hand becomes flattened. This is partly because of thenar muscle wasting but also because the loss of abductor pollicis brevis results in an adducted posture of the thumb. This is for two reasons:

(a) Adductor pollicis is unopposed
(b) Extensor pollicis longus, always an adductor of the adducted thumb, becomes more strongly so due to shift of the dorsal expansion under the action of the unopposed adductor pollicis.

Combined median and ulnar nerve at the wrist[403] — 'simian hand' (Fig. 2.109). A full claw hand *plus* thenar and hypothenar flattening *plus* thumb adduction and flexion results. The thumb hyperextends at the basal joint and is more flexed than usual at the metacarpophalangeal and interphalangeal joints[404]. This posture is very characteristic and has been called the 'simian hand' because of its similarity to the hand of the ape. Apart from combined ulnar and median nerve injuries, this posture is also seen in:

Charcot–Marie–Tooth disease. An inherited disorder, this is characterized by palsy commencing peripherally, firstly in the lower limb. It affects primarily median and ulnar innervated intrinsics, sparing the radial nerve and usually leaving sensation intact (Fig. 2.110).

Lower roots of the brachial plexus: 'Klumpke paralysis'[405], *C8 and T1*. This results from violent upward traction on the upper limb such as can occur obstetrically in management of breech or arm presentation. The roots

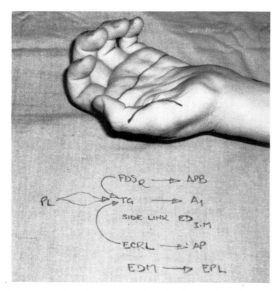

Fig. 2.110 The characteristic flat claw hand of median and ulnar nerve motor loss is seen here in a patient with Charcot–Marie–Tooth disease. The planned transfers and tenodeses are written out on the sterile sheet.

are disrupted from below. Loss of all intrinsic muscles of the hand produces flattening and marked wasting but there may be less dramatic change in posture due to weakness or absence of function in the long flexors.

Tinel's sign[406,407]

If the ends of growing axons are tapped, tingling paraesthesiae are felt in the area of sensory distribution of the nerve to which these axons belong. It should be understood that the Tinel's sign gives no indication whatsoever of:

1. *The quality of eventual recovery*, which may be anything from mere paraesthesiae to acceptable two-point discrimination
2. *The quantity of eventual recovery*, for the sign can be evoked from a very small percentage of the total nerve axon population.

The test is performed by lightly tapping as in percussing the chest, commencing distally and proceeding proximally along the line of the nerve. The Tinel's sign is elicited over a varying length of the nerve. The most proximal and distal points of the Tinel's sign are localized by measuring their distance from chosen fixed bony points. These should be recorded for further comparison as progression of the sign indicates continued axon growth. The rate of growth varies from 1 to 4 mm per day; the speed is directly related to the size of the

axons involved and inversely to the age of the patient and the distance from the injury to the hand. Henderson, in exhaustive studies on prisoners of war[408], found the Tinel's sign most useful for drawing conclusions as follows:

Strong Tinel at injury + none distally = no chance of recovery

Reducing Tinel at injury + advancing distally = good chance of useful recovery

Strong Tinel at injury + advancing distally = poor chance of useful recovery.

SENSORY ASSESSMENT (Table 2.3, Figs 2.111, 2.112)

The areas of the upper limb served by its several nerves are to be found illustrated in most textbooks of anatomy and general surgery. The diagrams do not correspond exactly, which is understandable, since there is significant overlap. Clinically, this overlap results in a patient under examination reporting a large area of 'different' sensation and a small area of *absolute sensory loss*. Precise boundaries are therefore neither present nor necessary to the examiner. Rather should he be aware of areas of different sensation significant in localizing the site of a nerve injury. Further confusion is sometimes caused by the failure to distinguish between diagrams of *dermatomes*, which strictly are areas served by one spinal nerve, and diagrams of areas of *cutaneous nerve distribution*, which differ because most cutaneous nerves communicate with more than one spinal nerve via the brachial plexus.

There are several reasons for the difficulties encountered in assessing areas of sensory loss:

(a) *Shrinkage* of the area of reduced sensation will occur, quickly in the first few days, and slowly thereafter.
(b) *Joint sense* is rarely completely lost, and therefore movement of the region may be misinterpreted as cutaneous sensation.
(c) Any test of sensation which requires patient responses cannot be objective and will be unreliable in the young, the mentally unfit and in patients intent upon obtaining maximum compensation for injury. (See p. 162.)
(d) Even in total recent nerve division, the area of *absolute sensory loss* is small compared with the total area of reduced loss. Absolute sensory loss is most commonly limited to the following areas, which have been called *autonomous zones* (cross-hatched in Figs 2.111 and 2.112):

ulnar nerve	palmar aspect of small finger
median nerve	palmar aspect of index finger
radial nerve	small area on the dorsum of the MP joint of the thumb
root C5	over the belly of the deltoid
C6	the thenar eminence
C7	NIL
C8	ulnar border of the hand
T1	ulnar border of the elbow
T2	inner aspect of upper arm

Sweating

Sympathetic denervation following peripheral nerve injury results in loss of sweating. This loss is complete in the autonomous zone of the divided nerve. In the *intermediate zone* surrounding the autonomous, sweating is greatly diminished.

The presence of beads of sweat on innervated skin can be detected using the + 20 dioptre lens of an ophthalmoscope. Loss of sweating is of functional importance, for the lack of the adhesion which sweat provides

Table 2.3   Dermatomes and cutaneous nerve distribution

	Dermatomes (Figs 2.111, 2.112)			
	On top of the shoulder	C4	Ulnar aspect forearm and hand	C8
	Outer aspect upper arm	C5	Inner aspect elbow	T1
	Radial aspect forearm and hand	C6	Inner aspect upper arm	T2
	Hand (*overlapped by adjacent dermatomes*)	C7		

Abbreviation in figure	*Nerve*	*Cutaneous nerve distribution* (Figs 2.111, 2.112)
	Supraclavicular nerves (C3, 4)	On top of shoulder and anterior chest
A	Axillary nerve (C5, 6)	Proximal lateral aspect of upper arm
LIC	Lateral inferior cutaneous nerve of arm (C5, 6, a branch of the radial nerve)	Distal lateral aspect of upper arm
LCF	Lateral cutaneous nerve of the forearm (C5, 6, the termination of the musculocutaneous nerve)	Radial aspect of forearm
R	Superficial radial nerve (C6, 7)	Radial dorsum of the hand to the PIP joints[1]
M	Median nerve (C6, 7, 8)	Thumb, index, middle and radial side of ring finger
PCM	Palmar cutaneous branch of the median nerve (C6, 7, 8)	Palmar triangle[2]
U	Ulnar nerve (C8, T1)	Small, ulnar side of ring finger, hypothenar eminence
DSU	Dorsal sensory branch of the ulnar nerve (C8, T1)	Ulnar dorsum of the hand to the PIP joints[3]
MCF	Medial cutaneous nerve of the forearm (C8, T1, from the medial cord)	Ulnar border of forearm
MCA	Medial cutaneous nerve of the arm (C8, T1, from the medial cord)	Inner aspect of the upper arm (distal)
ICB	Intercostobrachial nerve (T2)	Inner aspect of the upper arm (proximal)
PCF	Posterior cutaneous nerve of the forearm (C5–8, from the radial nerve)	Dorsum of forearm

[1] The dorsal innervation of the fingers distal to the proximal interphalangeal joints is from the digital nerves via constant dorsal digital branches.
[2] The 'palmar triangle' is that small area defined by the distal palmar crease and the thenar and hypothenar creases. Sensory change there is significant since the palmar cutaneous nerve arises some centimetres above the wrist and does not pass through the carpal tunnel. The nerve may in addition supply palmar skin more distal, as far as the PIP joints.
[3] Sensory change in dorsal sensory territory has similar significance in ulnar nerve disorders as palmar cutaneous loss in median nerve problems — it localizes the lesion proximal to the wrist.

Figs 2.111 and 2.112   In these figures, the regions served by cutaneous nerves are outlined and lettered according to the abbreviations given in the table. Due to overlap these are not absolute territories of innervation, with the result that hypaesthesia, not anaesthesia, is the outcome of cutaneous nerve division. Areas of absolute sensory supply of the nerve roots and of the radial (R), median (M) and ulnar (U) nerves are indicated by cross-hatching.

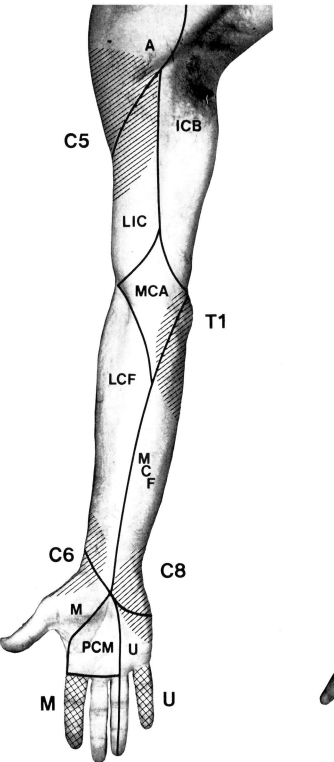

Fig. 2.111 Anterior aspect of upper limb.

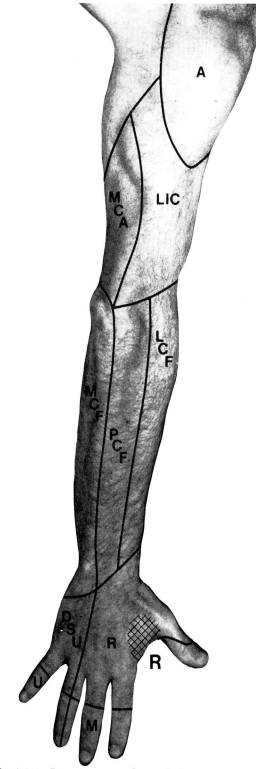

Fig. 2.112 Posterior aspect of upper limb.

seriously interferes with span grasp of smooth cylindrical objects and with finger manipulations in precision or chuck grip. The latter problem can readily be appreciated by recalling the difficulty of manipulating small objects with cold hands.

Smoothness is largely due to the absence of sweat, the lack of which reduces the friction between the skin and objects moved across it. While this can be detected by the examiner's finger if his hands are cold, clearly any sweat on his hands will substitute for that of the patient and the distinction may not be clear.

The *tactile adherence test*[409] (p. 42). The friction on normal and denervated fingers is best tested with a smooth plastic object such as the barrel of a pen. In the denervated areas the plastic glides smoothly and compares with the definite resistance felt on areas of normal innervation.

In the unusual situation where sweating is absent from even sensible areas, it has been stimulated for the purpose of testing by several means:

(a) *Pneumatic tourniquet.* If applied to the upper arm at above-systolic pressure for ten to fifteen minutes, the reactive hyperaemia consequent on release is accompanied by sweating in normally innervated areas.
(b) *Wrapping in hot blankets* is especially appropriate for children.
(c) *Hot room, heated bed cradle* or specially designed 'hot box'.
(d) *Exercise.*

One of the above methods is most often employed before conducting formal sweat pattern tests.

Sweat pattern tests have been designed, most of which depend on staining techniques and some on the fact that dry skin has a much higher resistance than moist to the passage of an electrical current[410].

Staining techniques
Iodine–starch. Iodine is painted on the area to be assessed. Starch powder is then dusted over the iodine. Sweating areas become dark.

Ninhydrin printing test[411–413]. The digits are pressed in turn on to a strip of paper. This is then developed in acidified 1% ninhydrin in acetone, dried and heated. The sweat pattern of black dots which emerges can then be fixed in acidified copper nitrate in acetone.

Bromophenol blue[414]. In this test the paper has been previously immersed in 5% bromophenol blue in acetone. The sweat pattern appears as blue dots on a yellow background.

Cobalt chloride. A solution of 25% cobalt chloride in 99% alcohol is painted on the injured hand; perspiration changes the solution from blue to pink.

Quinizarin. Quinizarin powder, sodium carbonate and rice starch are dusted firmly on to the patient's extremity before stimulating sweating, which produces a deep violet colour.

All of these tests have the disadvantage of being time-consuming, while some are messy. Seddon, who employed the quinizarin test for ten years, stated that the regular employment of one of these tests is unnecessary. They are of use where meticulous visual records are required.

Return of sweating to an area of sensory loss is one of the last cutaneous functions to return during nerve regeneration and closely parallels the return of two-point discrimination. There are three exceptions to this useful rule:

1. Sweating is *not* lost in lesions of the roots of the brachial plexus proximal to the entry of the postganglionic sympathetic fibres — important in examination of patients who have suffered a brachial plexus injury (p. 243).
2. Sweating returns to distant flaps applied to the hand, even if two-point discrimination does *not* return to the flap, probably due to sudomotor fibres accompanying ingrowing vessels since the sweating disappears with brachial block.
3. Patients who have undergone cervical sympathectomy.

With these rare exceptions, examination of sweating is a useful immediate guide to the patient's sensory recovery. If present, the examiner should proceed to qualitative evaluation of the static two-point discrimination. If absent, then first pin-prick and then awareness of moving and constant touch should be assessed.

Pinprick
If absence of sweating suggests dense sensory loss then the distribution of loss should be mapped out. This can be swiftly and accurately done using a pin wheel (Fig. 2.113), moving from areas of normal to abnormal sensation, marking the points of change on the skin. These should then be transferred to an outline of the hand in the patient's record. Pain perception is involved in the use of the pin wheel and the area of analgesia does not quite correspond with that of anaesthesia, being somewhat smaller. Once pinprick is present, the patient has entered the stage of 'protective sensation'.

Touch — moving and constant[415]
If pinprick is present throughout, then moving and constant touch should be applied to the area under examination. By using his own finger the examiner can be certain that contact has been made. Some precautions should be taken to avoid misleading responses.

1. What the examiner intends to do should be shown to the patient before he is asked to look away.

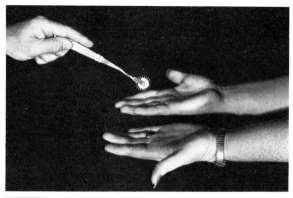

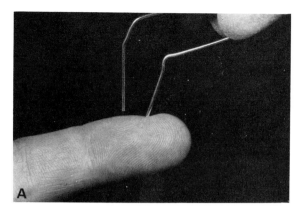

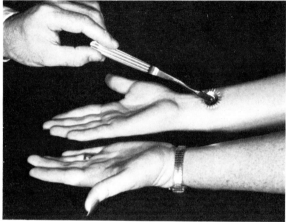

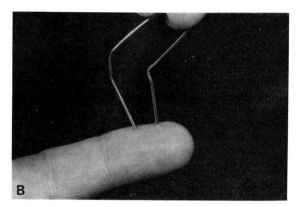

Fig. 2.113 The pinwheel provides a swift and adequate method of mapping out an area of sensory change.

2. Comparison should always be made with areas known to be normal on either the same or the other hand.
3. Occasional mock motions should be made without making contact to ensure that the patient is responding to touch and not simply to the examiner's movements.
4. Care should be taken to test known 'significant areas' such as the areas of absolute loss.

Fig. 2.114 A, B. Two-point discrimination is determined by alternately applying one or two points to the area under examination. A very satisfactory tool for this test can be produced by twisting a paper clip. C. Little force should be applied in testing for two points. If too much force is applied, (D), the sensory receptors between the two points will be stimulated and, even in the presence of two-point discrimination, the patient will feel the application of only one.

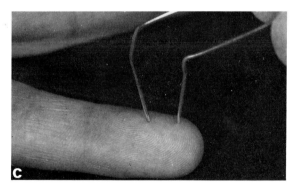

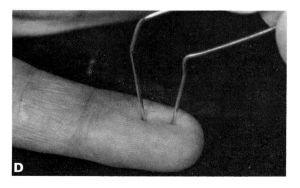

Moving touch will be appreciated before static, and the presence of either is the signal to move to their quantitative equivalent, moving or static two-point discrimination.

Two-point discrimination (2PD) (Fig. 2.114)
This test is performed either with a calibrated caliper or, more simply, with a paper clip twisted into shape. The test should first be explained to the patient and a quick test done on the opposite hand, for rare cases of congenital absence of two-point discrimination have been reported. The points of the caliper are set at 15 mm at first and progressively brought together as accurate responses are obtained.

As the minimum distance apart at which the patient can discriminate is approached, errors will be made. At this stage the following discipline should be adopted.

1. An interval of 3–4 seconds should be allowed between applications of the caliper to the skin.
2. The caliper should be applied with only slight force, just less than that required to cause blanching of the skin around each point (Fig. 2.114, C and D).
3. When two points are being applied they must make contact simultaneously and should be in the line of the digit.
4. The test should commence at the finger tips and should proceed across all finger tips before being carried out more proximally.

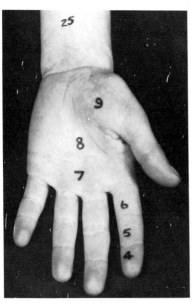

Fig. 2.115 The values for normal two-point discrimination differ significantly in various areas of the hand and are shown here in millimetres.

5. The same marking system should be used in all tests.
Omer[416] — two correct out of three applications is a 'pass'.
Moberg[417] — 10 applications of two points and 10 applications of one point are made randomly[418]. The total of *incorrect* one-point applications is subtracted from the total of *correct* two-point applications. An answer of five or more is considered a 'pass'.

The values for normal two-point discrimination differ from one area of the hand to another[419] (Fig. 2.115). It is necessary for the surgeon to be aware of this to recognize complete recovery and to avoid wasting time using settings too close for even the normal hand.

distal phalanx	3–5 mm
middle phalanx	3–6 mm
proximal phalanx	4–7 mm
palm	
distal to distal palmar crease	5–8 mm
centre of palm	6–9 mm
thenar and hypothenar	7–10 mm
dorsum	7–10 mm
forearm	20–50 mm
arm	65–70 mm

The results of two-point discrimination are seriously compromised if the hand is oedematous or callused.

This is a meticulous and time-consuming test. If the results on separate occasions, often by different observers, are to assess regeneration accurately, this care and time is necessary.

Moving[420] and static (constant)[421]. Moving two-point discrimination depends for its presence on the quickly adapting nerve fibres which return more quickly and in greater density than the slowly adapting fibres on which constant touch depends. Thus, moving 2PD returns earlier, by some 6 months, and has a value generally 8–10 mm smaller, or better, than constant 2PD. It is a measure of the capability of the hand to feel objects provided hand motion is possible, which is the normal circumstance. Constant 2PD indicates the capacity of the hand to be aware of objects held quite still which usually returns when constant 2PD is less than 15 mm. From the above it will be realized that a hand with 10 mm of moving 2PD will be able to detect and identify objects unseen, but that once that object is lifted and held immobile, the patient will not know whether or not he still has it in his grasp.

Semmes–Weinstein monofilaments[422]
A measure of constant touch, the monofilament test, is

highly reproducible but time-consuming. It gives an excellent graphic record of sensory status.

Programme of sensory evaluation and care after nerve repair

To perform the complete battery of tests outlined above is both unnecessary and illogical. Rather should the patient progress through a series of stages. During the time normally expected for axon growth, the presence of an advancing Tinel is sufficient confirmation of progress and skin and joint care fulfil the patient's needs. Once advance and time has proceeded, pinprick and touch perception should be assessed. When moving touch returns, moving 2PD can serve as the sole criterion for recovery and the patient commences an intensive course of daily 'sensory re-education',[423,424]. Once moving 2PD falls below 10 mm the surgeon should seek the constant 2PD which, once found, can serve as the monitor of the final stages.

Grading sensory recovery

Based upon the tests of light touch, pain and two-point discrimination, sensory recovery can be graded according to the scale adopted by the British Medical Research Council:

S0   No sensation
S1   Pain sensation
S2   Pain and some touch sensation
S3   Pain and touch with no over-reaction
S3+   Some two-point discrimination
S4   Complete recovery

All assessments are based on recovery of sensory faculties in the autonomous areas of the injured nerve.

This system will still be encountered in some reports and is included for that reason, but should now be superseded by a system based on a statement of the stage that a patient has reached, thus:

anaesthetic
  → pin-prick (protective)
    → moving touch
      → moving 2PD of X mm
        → static 2PD of Y mm

Other clinical sensory tests

The important aspects of clinical testing are that it should advise of progress or arrest of reinnervation and that it should be as objective as possible. Quite apart from the methods of assessment detailed above, many other clinical tests have been used and are still used by different clinicians. These will not all be described here because space does not allow it, because it would pos-

sibly cause confusion, because some have been found to be of questionable accuracy[425] and because the author does not use them. With one exception.

In infants

Wrinkling (Fig. 2.116)[426]. In very young children it may be difficult to perform even simple sweat tests although tactile adherence is usually detectable. If the normal hand is immersed in warm water for five minutes the digital pulps become wrinkled. It has been noted that this wrinkling occurs only in skin with some sensory innervation, remaining smooth in denervated areas. The exact stage of sensory return after injury at which wrinkling appears has not been established.

PAIN

Pain may also be elicited in the course of examination. It falls under four broad headings.

Neuroma — painful paraesthesiae as described below are caused by palpating a neuroma.

Burning pain — this is sometimes present over the nerve distal to Tinel's sign.

Over-reaction (hyperpathia) — return of sensation to an area is often accompanied by hypersensitivity, which causes the patient to back away from the examining hand. Protection and disuse may result. This must be recognized and firmly discouraged for the patient has reached an important juncture. If allowed to continue protection, an established pattern of hypersensitivity and disuse will be created. If, on the other hand, the

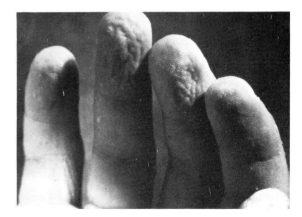

Fig. 2.116 This patient who is recovering from division and primary repair of her radial digital nerve to the index finger, shown on the right of the picture, has had the hand immersed in warm water for a period of five minutes. The very characteristic wrinkling which is produced in normal skin is seen on the small, ring, and middle fingers and is starting to reappear on the index finger.

patient is exhorted to engage in 'sensory rehabilitation', recovery and full function can be anticipated. Rehabilitation requires the patient to make more contact with the previously denervated digit than with others, and with as wide a variety of surfaces as possible.

Reflex sympathetic dystrophy (p. 157), of which *causalgia*[427] is a particularly intractable form resulting from nerve injury.

Neuroma

If, on palpating the scar, the patient withdraws or complains of pain of a tingling nature, this is strong evidence of a neuroma adjacent to the scar. A large neuroma may be visible or its margins palpable. The exact location of a smaller neuroma can be defined by repeating the palpation with a bluntly pointed instrument. More than one neuroma may be present when a cutaneous nerve has been divided. Probing should therefore be performed around all margins of the scar marking each neuroma with a skin pencil (Fig. 2.117). A persistently tender neuroma may respond to sensory re-education and/or transcutaneous nerve stimulation but, if not, is an indication for nerve exploration, as the patient will be understandably reluctant to use the hand normally.

Bowler's thumb[428,429]. In ten-pin bowling, the edge of the thumb-hold presses firmly against the palmar aspect of the proximal phalanx of the thumb. At the point of pressure, both digital nerves to the thumb lie close together over the sheath of flexor pollicis longus and are therefore compressed against an unyielding structure. Minor injury to the nerve or nerves results but is rarely sufficient to cause the player to give up the game. The trauma is therefore repeated and a neuroma in continuity forms.

Symptoms. The patient complains of pain on the palmar aspect of the thumb which may be associated with numbness on one or other or both aspects of the thumb pulp.

Examination. Palpation reveals a nodule, which, if the examiner is not familiar with the diagnosis, may be mistaken for a ganglion. It is more mobile than a flexor sheath ganglion in a transverse plane but not along the axis of the thumb. Firm pressure on the swelling may produce paraesthesiae in the digital nerve distribution (Fig. 2.118).

Indications

If the neuroma is in the substance of a major nerve, then its presence alone is an indication for resection and grafting (p. 242). The choice of surgical procedure for relief of neuroma problems in non-essential nerves or in amputation stump attests to the lack of universal success with any[430–441]. Certainly, whichever is chosen, immediate postoperative sensory re-education contributes greatly to success. There *was* only one cure for bowler's thumb — to stop bowling. However, transfer of the ulnar digital nerve to the dorsal aspect of the adductor pollicis has been described[442].

See Green D P 1993 Operative Hand Surgery, 3rd edn. Churchill Livingstone, New York, p. 1390.

MOTOR ASSESSMENT (see Appendix, p. 513)

All major muscles in the injured limb are tested. Selective testing is not acceptable for a number of reasons:

1. Nerve injury may be partial only.
2. Recovery after repair may be only partial.

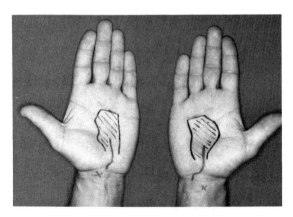

Fig. 2.117 Following bilateral carpal tunnel release this patient had significant dysaesthesia. This has been marked out using a pin wheel. The locations of the neuromata are marked with crosses.

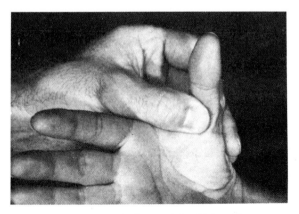

Fig. 2.118 Palpation of a firm nodule which produces paraesthesiae in the thumb. The nodule, being mobile transversely but not longitudinally, is diagnostic of a 'bowler's thumb'.

3. In multiple penetrative lacerations, such as are inflicted by shattered glass, branches of main nerves may have been divided, either alone or in combination with division of the main trunk.

4. In traction or compression injuries, the motor loss may be of an unpredictable distribution.

5. Loss of function in isolated muscles may not be appreciated by the patient or recognized by the surgeon unless a full systematic examination is performed and yet it may reduce the patient's power or manipulative ability.

6. Innervation may be anomalous. In a small minority of patients cross-links exist between the three main nerves of the upper limb. The *Martin–Gruber anastomosis*[443–445] is an anomaly in which motor fibres, normally carried in the ulnar nerve throughout its course, join it from the median nerve only in the forearm. The anastomosis may be from the median nerve proper or from the anterior interosseous nerve. The clinical significance is in high injuries above the link. In a complete anastomosis, the consequence will be:

high ulnar nerve   no motor loss
high median nerve   total motor loss in the hand

In the first instance, a high median nerve block will distinguish the anomaly from a partial ulnar nerve lesion. In the latter, selective nerve stimulation studies will clarify the situation if they are done within the first few days after injury. In later cases, exploration will reveal an intact ulnar nerve.

In the course of motor examination, it is necessary that the patient understands what is required of him. Several approaches may be employed.

'*Bend it like this.*' The patient is invited to copy with his injured limb a movement demonstrated by the examiner. While satisfactory with coarse movement such as bending the elbow, the examiner cannot be certain whether or not the patient has understood.

'*Do this with your good hand and then with the bad*' (Fig. 2.119). A better approach, this shows that the patient understands and also demonstrates his normal range in the uninjured hand as the criterion against which his injured hand is to be judged. However, it presupposes the presence of a 'good' hand and bilateral injuries are not uncommon. Further, it is often the case that patients 'forget' how to perform some movement with the injured hand and the wrong conclusion may be drawn.

'*Hold your hand like that, keep it there, don't let me move it*' (Fig. 2.120). The examiner places the hand or digit in the position which the muscle under test would normally produce and assesses the power it can generate. This method is the best, for the patient is not required to interpret a movement made by the examiner, it can be used in bilateral injuries and it places the limb in the required posture, reinforcing the patient's memory of how to achieve it. It also speeds the process of examination, because the examiner can record the passive range of joints while achieving each posture.

The examiner should palpate the relevant muscle belly and tendon while the patient is performing this

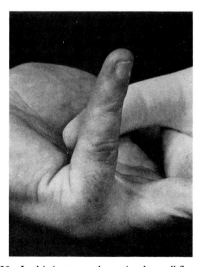

Fig. 2.120 In this instance, the patient's small finger has been placed in the position which flexor digiti minimi produces and the patient has then been instructed to keep it in that position and resist the attempts of the examiner to move it. This demonstrates the presence of an active flexor digiti minimi.

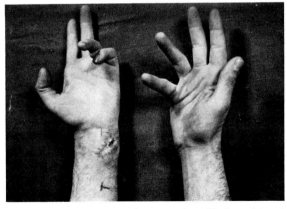

Fig. 2.119 This patient is demonstrating with the uninjured right hand that he is able to flex the metacarpophalangeal joint of his small finger with flexor digiti minimi but is unable to do so with the injured hand.

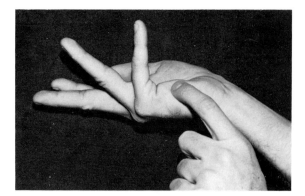

Fig. 2.121 The muscle belly under examination should be palpated as this test is performed.

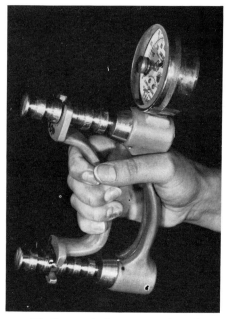

Fig. 2.122 The Jamar grip dynamometer is used to record the strength of power grasp.

manoeuvre (Fig. 2.121). In this way muscular activity can be detected which is not strong enough to maintain the joint position and when the joint on which the muscle acts has little or no range of motion due to injury or disease.

In assessing motor function, the examiner should remember that muscles act synergistically with, and are dependent for their power in part upon, muscles elsewhere often having a different nerve supply. For example, grip strength (ulnar and median) fell by 77% in one study[446] in the absence of radial nerve function.

In conducting the muscle test it is important to determine the power which the muscle is capable of generating. This is significant not only in charting the patient's improvement but is necessary in planning a beneficial programme of tendon transfers where appropriate. The scale of power employed is:

0 *Total paralysis* — no contraction detactable on palpation
1 *Flicker* — no movement, but contraction palpable
2 *Movement with gravity eliminated* — this is achieved by placing the line of action of the muscle in a horizontal plane; this is not possible with all muscles
3 *Movement against gravity*
4 *Movement against gravity and resistance*
5 *Full power*

While universally in use, this scale has serious limitations, for all weakly active muscles are graded power 4. Wherever possible a quantitative assessment should be employed comparing with the opposite hand, if normal. Those most used are:

Jamar grip dynamometer — this records grip power in pounds per square inch. It is important that the slot

in which the adjustable bar is placed is noted (Fig. 2.122) (p. 162)
Pinch dynamometer (Fig. 2.123)

Clearly a large number of quantitative recording devices could be designed but it would be impractical to employ them all. In the case of certain muscles, the examiner may pit his own against that of the patient's, both normal and injured, thereby gauging the difference between them. This can be done, for example, with abductor digiti minimi, the first dorsal interosseous, the superficialis tendons and pronator teres. The reader can undoubtedly make the list more comprehensive, and

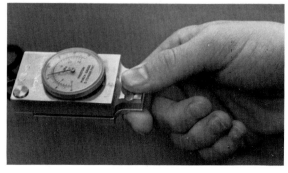

Fig. 2.123 The pinch dynamometer is employed to record pinch strength.

Table 2.4 Reflexes

Muscle	Action	Percussion point	Level of reflex arc
Biceps (Fig. 2.124)	Elbow flexion	Biceps tendon	C5 (6)
Brachioradialis (Fig. 2.125)	Elbow flexion in neutral pronation–supination	Radial styloid	C(5) 6
Triceps (Fig. 2.126)	Elbow extension	Triceps tendon	C7
Extensor carpi ulnaris (Fig. 2.127)	Wrist extension and ulnar deviation	Base of 5th metacarpal	C7

the examiner's day more exhausting! This is not quantitative, however useful, and it remains that no widely applicable technique of categorizing grade 4 has been devised.

Although using similar digits the scale above has certain differences from that of the British Medical Research Council, and the examiner should be aware of it also to avoid confusion as it may be encountered in some reports:

M0 No contraction
M1 Perceptible contraction in proximal muscles
M2 Perceptible contraction in both proximal and distal muscles
M3 All important muscles able to work against resistance
M4 All synergic and independent movements possible
M5 Complete recovery

This classification is more applicable in proximal nerve lesions and, like the MRC sensory grading, has probably outlived its usefulness.

The muscles tested, their action, and the nerve or root injury in which they are paralysed are detailed in the Appendix (p. 513).

Reflexes (see Table 2.4; Figs 2.124–2.127)
Using a tendon hammer, reflexes should be tested with the relevant muscle contracted against moderate resistance.

Reflexes will be *absent* if the arc is interrupted, that is, in lower motor neuron disorders such as division of a peripheral nerve. They will be *exaggerated* if higher control has been eliminated, as in upper motor neuron injury and at certain levels in some cases of cord transection.

Having now accumulated all the necessary evidence, the precise level of a nerve lesion can be deduced in the majority of cases (see Table 2.5).

ELECTROMYOGRAPHY[447–449] AND NERVE CONDUCTION STUDIES

There are two basic groups of investigation in common use for study of muscle function following denervation and during regeneration and recovery. In the first the stimulus is applied directly to the muscle or to its nerve at the end plate and the differing response to different strengths of stimulus applied for different durations is an indication of the condition of the muscle. This group

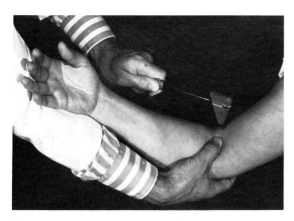

Fig. 2.124 Biceps tendon reflex. While palpating the tendon of biceps, the examiner's thumb nail is percussed with a tendon hammer.

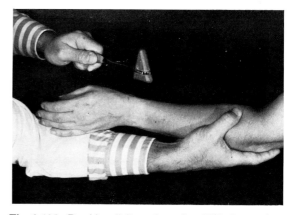

Fig. 2.125 Brachioradialis tendon reflex. With the arm in mid-pronation–supination, and while palpating the belly of the brachioradialis, the partially flexed forearm is percussed firmly with a tendon hammer proximal to the radial styloid.

Table 2.5   Sensory, motor and reflex loss in differing levels of nerve injury
Abbreviations employed in table:
1. T = thumb, I = index, M = middle, R = ring, S = small
2. Muscles as in full muscle test chart (p. 513)

Nerve	Level	Loss		
		Sensory	*Motor*	*Reflex*
Median	wrist	palmar aspect TIM ½R	APB OP FPB (supf. head) lumbricals I + M	—
	above wrist	*add* 'palmar triangle'		
	elbow or above		*add* FCR PT FDS FDP (I and M) FPL PQ	
Ant. interosseous	forearm	nil	FPL FDP (I and M) PQ	
Ulnar	palm (deep branch)	nil	IO AP FPB (deep head)	
	wrist	palmar ½RS	*add* ADM FDM ODM lumbricals R + S	
	above wrist	*add* ulnar aspect of dorsum		
	elbow or above		*add* FCU FDP (R and S)	
Radial	wrist	dorsum 1st web	—	—
Posterior interosseous	forearm	nil	ECU ED EDM EPL EI APL EPB	ECU
Radial	elbow	dorsum 1st web	*add* S	
	spiral groove	*add* dorsum of forearm	*add* ECRL ECRB BR	*add* BR
	axilla	*add* distal lateral aspect of upper arm	*add* T	*add* T
Medial cord	axilla	ulnar aspect of arm of forearm and of hand	*all* finger flexors *all* small hand muscles	nil
	subclavicular		*add* sternocostal head of PM	nil
Lateral cord	axilla	radial aspect of forearm and of hand	elbow flexion forearm pronation wrist flexion (FCR)	BB
	subclavicular		*add* clavicular head of PM	BB
Posterior cord	axilla	over deltoid posterior aspect upper arm dorsum of forearm dorsum 1st web	abduction of shoulder all upper limb extensors + BR	T BR ECU
	subclavicular		*add* LD	T BR ECU
Roots			*motor loss of varying degree in isolated root lesions; increased in multiple.*	
C5	posterior triangle	over deltoid	ext. rotation and abduction of shoulder	

Table 2.5 Cont'd

Nerve	Level	Loss		
		Sensory	*Motor*	*Reflex*
C6	posterior triangle	thenar eminence	int. rotation and adduction of shoulder elbow flexion forearm supination	BR + BB
C7	posterior triangle	nil	elbow, wrist and finger extension forearm pronation	T ECU
C8	posterior triangle	ulnar border forearm	wrist, finger and thumb flexion	
T1	posterior triangle	inner aspect elbow	intrinsic movements	—

includes studies of the rheobase and chronaxie response to galvanic and faradic stimulation, strength duration curves and galvanic–tetanus ratios. The second group of tests are all based on electromyographic observation with and without stimulation of the relevant motor nerve. While both groups can provide useful information, the latter has certain advantages over the first.

1. By adjusting the recording needle electrode the activity in any part of the muscle under investigation can be observed, whereas direct muscle stimulation studies only the most superficial fibres.
2. The technique can be used for studying other causes of muscle weakness or paralysis such as neuropathies and compression syndromes.
3. Using the same basic equipment studies of sensory nerve activity can be performed.

For these reasons, and in order to present a single, comprehensive means of investigating innervation electrically, only the second group will be considered here.

Electromyography. The electrical activity in a muscle is recorded by inserting a sterile needle electrode into the appropriate muscle belly. Apart from insertion this should normally not be painful. If the discomfort persists it is possible that the needle has been inserted into the motor point — the point at which the neuro-muscular end plates are situated. In this circumstance, the needle should be removed and reinserted. This should be done in any case on three or four occasions to each muscle, noting the electrical activity for each successive insertion.

The activity recorded by the needle electrode is fed into an oscilloscope and it can then be both heard and seen. Analysis of the wave form on the oscilloscope can

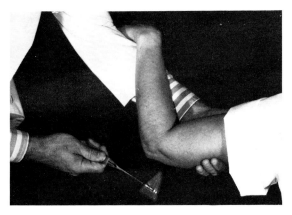

Fig. 2.126 Triceps tendon reflex. With the elbow flexed and relaxed over the examiner's arm, the triceps tendon is struck with the tendon hammer behind the elbow while palpating the belly of the muscle in the upper arm.

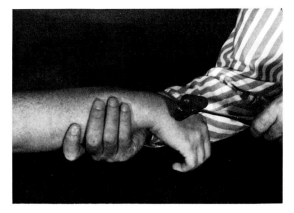

Fig. 2.127 Extensor carpi ulnaris tendon reflex. With the arm in pronation and the tendon of the extensor carpi ulnaris being palpated, the base of the fifth metacarpal is struck with a tendon hammer.

be greatly eased by use of a storage monitor which retains each wave on a calibrated screen until it is cleared by the operator. Basically, five wave forms will be encountered (Table 2.6).

Nerve conduction studies are superimposed on this study by applying stimulating electrodes over the course of the motor nerve proximally and recording the muscle activity. The stimulating current is gradually increased until a maximum action potential is attained. Using the storage monitor this is easily recognized and is usually achieved with a voltage of 400 mV. A stimulus 20% supramaximal is used thereafter. The time between the stimulus and the action potential can then be read off the calibrated scale and is referred to as *distal latency*. In studying the median and ulnar nerves the electrode is inserted in abductor pollicis brevis and flexor digiti minimi respectively and the nerve stimulated at the wrist.

Normal distal motor latency
Median 2.99 millisecs + 0.004 × age (SD ± 0.39)
Ulnar 2.21 millisecs + 0.01 × age (SD ± 0.34)

In normal hands the distal latency of the ulnar nerve is two-thirds that of the median nerve. Latency can be affected by cold, compression and neuropathy. The test should therefore be conducted in comfortably warm surroundings and the latency should be checked in the normal limb to exclude generalized neuropathy.

If, despite adjusting the position of the stimulating electrode no action potential is recorded, then the nerve has been divided. This inability to transmit current develops distally from the site of injury and therefore false positives may be obtained until 48 hours after injury. In nerve contusion, compression and traction it is possible to differentiate between

Axonotmesis   No distal nerve conduction after 48 hours (the lapse may be longer, see p. 105)

Neurapraxia   Distal nerve conduction remains normal

This distinction cannot be made at surgical exploration except with nerve stimulation.

After nerve injury, with or without repair, distal latency will only return once the ingrowing axons have reached the neuromuscular junction but thereafter recovery action potentials will be evident some time before motor activity is evident clinically.

No estimate of the number of motor axons present can be made from the amplitude of the action potential.

Having marked the skin at the point where the nerve was stimulated at the wrist, the stimulus is re-applied at the elbow. Care should be taken that a matching wave form is obtained, indicating that the same fibres have been stimulated, and this is best achieved by leaving the action potential obtained at the wrist on the storage monitor. This also facilitates measurement of the difference in time taken for the potentials to appear after stimulus at the wrist and at the elbow. By also measuring the distance between the points of stimulation the conduction velocity can be calculated in metres per second.

$$\frac{\text{distance between points (cm)}}{100} \times \frac{1000}{\text{time difference (msec)}} = \text{conduction velocity (m/sec)}$$

$$\text{e.g} \quad \frac{13}{100} \times \frac{1000}{3.25} = 40 \text{ m/sec}$$

The minimum normal conduction velocity in nerves of the upper limb is 50–60 metres per second. Thus the example above could indicate a compression neuropathy between elbow and wrist.

After recovery of a nerve division conduction velocity across the lesion and distal to it is reduced. This improves gradually until about 18 months after repair.

Table 2.6 Electromyographic features

Wave	Interpretation	Audio	Voltage
Straight line	Normal muscle at rest	Nil	Isoelectric
Motor-unit action potential	Contraction of normal muscle	Thump	10 mV
Fibrillation potential	Appears 2–3 weeks after injury Denervated muscle at rest Contraction — no effect	High-pitched clicks	1 mV
Recovery action potential	Contraction of reinnervated muscle during recovery	Thump	10 mV
Recovered motor unit action potential	Recovered muscle hypertrophy of motor unit	Thump	20 mV

Sensory studies
Sensory nerves can be stimulated *antidromically*, that is, against the normal direction of impulses, by placing recording electrodes around each finger in turn and stimulating at the wrist as before but with a current of 50 mV. This produces a large potential but considerable interference may occur due to motor activity. Therefore *orthodromic* stimulation is favoured. Two finger stimulating electrodes are placed over the digital nerve under study and the recording electrodes are strapped to the wrist. Stimulation is applied with a current of 50 mV. Unlike the motor action potential, the sensory action potential is quantitative, the minimum normal amplitude being 10 microvolts.

Normal distal sensory latency
Median 3.07 millisecs + 0.01 × age (SD ± 0.94)
Ulnar 1.78 millisecs + 0.03 × age (SD ± 0.96)

Until regrowth has occurred, of course, no sensory potentials will be detected, and in one study of nerve lacerations of the wrist this was found never to occur before 10 months[450]. Thereafter amplitude of orthodromic action potential indicates the percentage of functioning sensory fibres and in the same study this never exceeded 40%. Using similar techniques of distal stimulation and proximal recording at the elbow, it is possible by moving the stimulus proximal along the course of the nerve to determine the site of a nerve division, no action potentials being transmitted from below the lesion to above.

In summary, what can electromyography offer to the clinician carrying out a secondary assessment of an injured limb?

1. After 48 hours neurapraxia can be differentiated from axonotmesis and complete division by the presence or absence of action potentials on stimulation of the nerve distal to the lesion.
2. After three weeks, denervation can be confirmed by the presence of fibrillation potentials on electromyography.
3. A division can be localized in some cases using orthodromic sensory stimulation.
4. In brachial plexus lesions, the persistence of sensory conduction from an anaesthetic area indicates that the lesion is medial or proximal to that dorsal root ganglion and therefore not available to be grafted.
5. Re-innervation can be detected prior to clinical evidence of motor return.
6. Compression neuropathies can be detected and localized.
7. In the very difficult re-exploration of the partially functioning nerve repair, evoked action potential

studies during surgery may identify the transmitting, and therefore intact, fascicles[448].

Electromyographic interpretation clearly requires experience, and, clearly, experienced advice is desirable. However, it is important that the hand surgeon understands the basic principles of such a useful tool and can go some way towards interpreting the results it yields.

GRADES OR NERVE DAMAGE (see also p. 42)

Especially in closed injuries, or as a result of gunshot wounds, nerves may suffer less than complete transection. In 1942 Seddon[451] introduced the following classification of nerve injury.

Neurotmesis and axonotmesis
In both of these the integrity of the nerve fibres is interrupted, but in axonotmesis the *anatomical* continuity of the nerve is preserved as the Schwann cells which form the sheath are uninterrupted. The clinical and electrical findings are identical and it is therefore impossible to distinguish them clinically. Exploration is therefore required. If anatomical continuity is found, surgical repair is not necessary, as recovery, although proceeding at the same rate of 1–2 mm per day as a neurotmesis after repair, may eventually be good.

Neurapraxia
This is due to selective demyelinization of larger fibres in the nerve: no axonal degeneration occurs. The essential features which distinguish neurapraxia from the two more severe degrees of injury are:

1. Sensation and sympathetic activity may be intact.
2. Muscle atrophy rarely occurs although motor paralysis is complete.
3. Electrically there is:
   (a) no reaction of degeneration, and
   (b) nerve conduction distal to the lesion is preserved, although voluntary action potentials disappear.
4. Recovery occurs after an unpredictable interval and in no set order, that is, muscle action does not return from proximal to distal as in the other two forms.

Thus, neurapraxia can often be diagnosed without surgery. If it is, conservative measures can be adopted with confident reassurance of the patient.

The delay before recovery from the different grades of nerve damage varies so greatly that only a very wide approximation can be offered to the patient. A neurapraxia should show full recovery, regardless of the level, in 1 to 4 months. Return of function from an axonotmesis depends on the level of injury and may take from 4 to 18 months. Traction injuries require significantly longer for recovery than other forms of axonotmesis.

INDICATIONS

The decision to intervene following nerve injury can be one of the more difficult which the hand surgeon has to make. Nerves which have sustained neurapraxia do not require exploration. Nerves which are known from operation reports to have been divided and not repaired should be explored.

Between these relatively clear extremes lies the area of difficult decision. Problems include:

The unknown lesion
The unknown repair, both whether and how
The nerve which appears to have been divided partially (anomalous innervation should be excluded by selective nerve block)
The nerve divided completely, repaired and showing only partial recovery.

The decision to explore such injuries should be made on the basis of repeated examination conducted at maximum intervals of 6 weeks. Indications for exploration are:

1. A static Tinel's sign at the presumed site of injury (the converse is *not* true — since growth of a very small proportion of the axons can produce an advancing Tinel, such an advance is not in itself a contraindication to exploration, see p. 227).
2. Absence of recovery action potentials on electromyography or, somewhat later, of clinical evidence of motor activity in the most proximal paralysed muscle by the time at which it would be expected to occur. This time can be calculated from Seddon's composite figure for rate of return in which one day is allowed for each millimetre of nerve distal to the supposed site of injury.
3. Failure to recover sensation in the median nerve distribution.
4. Painful neuroma formation.

The introduction of the *operating microscope* has made fascicular dissection of major nerves a practical proposition, permitting complete internal as well as external neurolysis in instances of partial nerve injury. The experimental and limited operative use of microelectrical evaluation of individual fascicular conductivity in partial nerve injuries promises much for the future in these very difficult injuries[448, 452].

Elimination of crippling neuromata and provision of sensation in median nerve distribution are the only absolute indications for exploration of partially divided or previously repaired nerves in isolated major nerve injuries. This is because good motor function can be provided by selected tendon transfers. Indeed, since full motor recovery cannot be anticipated, especially in adults, appropriate transfers may be performed before motor power could be expected to return[453]. This is the more justifiable the more proximal the lesion. Resection of neuromata with or without grafting offers no guarantee that pain will be eliminated[454].

Nerve grafts
The placement of interfascicular grafts has now become the accepted surgical technique for overcoming a gap between nerve ends, eliminating suture under tension, re-routing, exaggerated joint flexion and other erstwhile mechanisms of effecting end-to-end repair[455]. *Matching of proximal and distal corresponding fascicular groups* by *visual techniques*, knowledge of the *internal anatomy*[456-459], *electrical stimulation*[460,461] and *histochemical identification*[462,463] has been discussed on p. 103. For reconstruction of larger nerves, the *sural nerve* is that most commonly employed[464] as a graft. To replace the digital nerve, both the *lateral*[465,466], and *medial antebrachial cutaneous nerve*[467] have their proponents. My preference is for the medial, or more recently, for the posterior interosseous nerve at the wrist, since the lateral antebrachial cutaneous may supersede the function of the radial cutaneous nerve (p. 43). Prosthetic tubes[468] and vascularized pseudosheaths[469] are currently being investigated as alternatives to autogenous nerve grafts. *Sensory nerve transfer* of dorsal cutaneous nerves to more significant areas has been performed with success[470,471], although on a limited scale. Where long defects exist in more than one peripheral nerve, a pedicled graft of one less significant may be used to replace another — the St Clair Strange procedure[472,473]. Although *vascularized nerve grafts*[474,475] have been shown experimentally[476] to have no advantage in a well-perfused soft-tissue bed, they may have merit where the grafts must be placed in scar.

See Green D P 1993 Operative Hand Surgery, 3rd edn. Churchill Livingstone, New York, p. 1325.

Tendon transfers[477-479].
Armed with the results of the full muscle test, the examiner can select suitable motor units for transfer. While consideration of specific transfers is outwith the scope of this text, certain basic rules can be stated.

1. All joints on which the transfer is to act should have a full passive range of motion.

2. Transfer of a muscle must not cause the loss of an essential function.

3. Any transferred muscle loses at least 1 grade on the power scale — thus only grade 5 muscles are really satisfactory motors, although grade 4 will suffice for certain transfers.

4. The amplitude of movement produced by the muscle for transfer should approximate to that which it is replacing. It should be remembered that the amplitude of any tendon which crosses the wrist is increased by 2–3 cm by full motion in that joint. This is invaluable in tetraplegics especially, and contraindicates wrist fusion. The selection of a transfer has been greatly refined by the analysis of the amplitude and mass fraction of all upper extremity muscles (Brand)[480,481].

5. The effectiveness of certain transfers which retain their original function after transfer depends on the activity of the antagonist to that original function, which must therefore be tested. For example, brachioradialis is an effective dorsiflexor transfer to the wrist only if triceps is strong enough to resist its normal elbow flexor action[482].

6. Any acute angulation in the course of a transferred tendon should be avoided.

7. The correct biomechanics of insertion are usually achieved by attaching the transfer to the tendon of the paralysed muscle. Where nerve repair carries some hope of recovery in that muscle, the attachment should be done in an end-to-side manner.

The knowledge and practice of available transfers for median[483,484], ulnar, radial[487] and multiple[488] nerve lesions permits the surgeon to offer early assistance to the patient awaiting nerve recovery, and the only chance of improved function for one who has no hope of such recovery because either the nerve or the muscle it supplied have been irretrievably damaged. Such plans for transfer commonly include judicious use of selected tenodeses to provide passive control of certain functions[489]. In some massive injuries, insufficient transfers are available. In such cases, *free muscle transplantation*[490] can provide invaluable function, attainable by no other means.

While keeping a patient under review pending possible surgery, the examiner is of course responsible for keeping deterioration to a minimum by preventing deformity and joint stiffness with appropriate static and dynamic splints and by insturcting the patient in basic physical therapy. Muscle bulk *may rarely* be maintained with the use of a portable galvanic muscle stimulator. Although formerly sceptical of the value of such treatment, a few obsessive patients have convinced the author of the value of regular use. However, these patients applied the stimulus hourly— such enthusiasm gives startling results after precise primary fascicular repair, but is difficult to communicate to those less devoted to their recovery.

See Green D P 1993 Operative Hand Surgery, 3rd edn. Churchill Livingstone, New York, pp. 1407, 1419, 1451.

BRACHIAL PLEXUS INJURIES

Plexus dysfunction may result from open wounds, closed traction or follow anaesthesia (types I, II and III of Leffert[491]).

It will be appreciated that, while C5 and T1 may each be injured independently by avulsion, isolated *root* lesions of C6–8 are very unlikely. The *trunks* of the brachial plexus lie in the posterior triangle where, apart from the more common traction injuries, they are also vulnerable to stab or gunshot wounds. The defects resulting from injury of the trunks are identical to the corresponding root lesions:

Upper trunk	C5 and C6
Middle trunk	C7
Lower trunk	C8 and T1

If follows that it is not possible to differentiate between injuries of roots and of the trunk which they form except when the roots are damaged proximal to the posterior primary rami, the sympathetic rami communicantes or the motor nerves arising directly from the roots. This occurs most often in traction injuries of the plexus. In those instances it is important to attempt to determine at what level the root is divided, since injuries outside the spinal canal can be grafted with some hope for recovery of function. Millesi[492] has classified plexus injuries according to level:

I	Supraganglionic
II	Infraganglionic
III	Trunk
IV	Cord

More detailed information should be sought for levels I and II root injuries.

Level of root injury (considered from distal to proximal)
The levels of root injury and the corresponding clinical signs are given in Table 2.7, see also Figure 2.128.

Tinel sign[495]
By percussion in the posterior triangle and distal to the clavicle, a Tinel sign should be sought. By identifying the dermatome(s) in which the patient describes paraesthesia in the presence of anaesthesia the surgeon will know which root neuromas are sufficiently intact to produce cortical awareness.

Table 2.7

Lesion	Clinical sign
Just proximal to the trunks	Rhomboids active (C5), serratus anterior active (C5, 6, 7) (may require EMG to detect innervation)
Proximal to white ramus communicantes of T1 (C8)	*Horner's syndrome*: lid lag, pupillary constriction, conjunctival hyperaemia, loss of sweating in head and neck. (Note: Horner's syndrome will also result from *disruption of the sympathetic chain* at any level above C8 T1.) (Fig. 2.128)
Proximal to grey rami communicantes	Sweating will persist in limb in areas that are anaesthetic
Proximal to dorsal ramus	Paralysis of paravertebral muscles — may be shown by posterior cervical electromyography[493]

Proximal to the dorsal nerve root ganglion	(i) Axon reflexes[494] will remain intact:
	    (a) *Histamine response.* The flare of the 'triple response' to 1% histamine is lost in peripheral lesions but preserved when the injury is proximal to the sensory spinal ganglion
	    (b) *Cold vasodilation.* The rise in skin temperature which occurs 5–10 minutes after cold immersion in the normal digit, but is lost in peripheral nerve injury, is maintained in preganglionic lesions
	(ii) Sensory conduction distally will be normal despite anaesthesia in the relevant dermatome

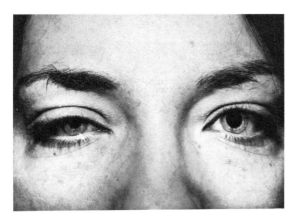

Fig. 2.128 Horner's syndrome with constriction of the pupil, conjunctival injection and ptosis of the upper lid.

Imaging
Fractures of the clavicle, transverse processes of the cervical spine and neck of the first rib give some indication of the level and severity of the original injury.

Radiographic examination of the chest may reveal evidence of damage to the phrenic nerve in the form of diaphragmatic paralysis.

Myelography may be performed in brachial plexus traction injuries. Certainly the presence of a meningocele at the level of injury strongly suggests a hopeless prognosis (Fig. 2.129). However, a number of cases have now been reported where a root suitable for grafting, showing intraoperative evoked potentials[496], has been found at the level known to have shown a pseudomyelomeningocele. For this reason, the author has abandoned routine myelography.

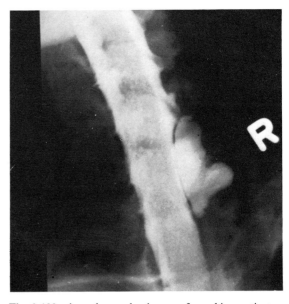

Fig. 2.129 A myelogram has been performed in a patient who had sustained a traction injury of the brachial plexus. A meningocele is demonstrated at three levels, indicating avulsion of the roots from the cord.

High resolution CT myelography and *magnetic resonance imaging* both give excellent visualization of the nerve roots within the dural sheath, but poor resolution outside the spinal canal.

Partial plexus injuries
Detailed records of sensory and motor function by the techniques detailed above, must be made in such cases:

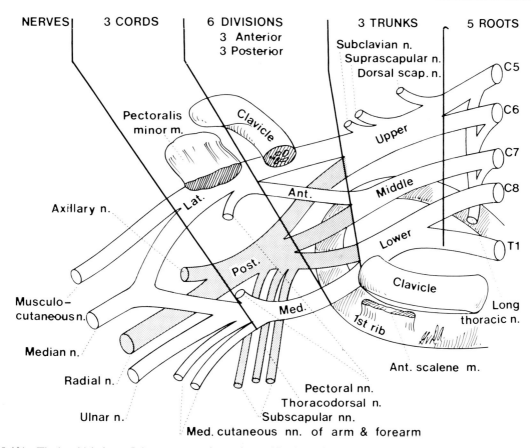

NERVES | 3 CORDS | 6 DIVISIONS | 3 TRUNKS | 5 ROOTS
3 Anterior
3 Posterior

Subclavian n.
Suprascapular n.
Dorsal scap. n.

C5
C6
C7
C8
T1

Pectoralis minor m.
Clavicle
Upper
Middle
Lower
Clavicle
1st rib
Ant. scalene m.

Axillary n.
Lat.
Ant.
Post.
Med.

Musculo-cutaneous n.
Median n.
Radial n.
Ulnar n.

Long thoracic n.

Pectoral nn.
Thoracodorsal n.
Subscapular nn.
Med. cutaneous nn. of arm & forearm

Fig. 2.130 The brachial plexus. It is necessary to know the ramifications of the plexus in order to deduce the location of lesions from observed peripheral loss. In addition, the relationship to the bony skeleton can provide information if fractures are evident on radiographic examination.

1. To determine whether selected arthrodeses and transfers could restore acceptable function
2. To locate precisely in the plexus where the lesion lies, and to avoid injury to intact nerves during exploration (Fig. 2.130).
3. To monitor improvement.

Pain

Pain of a neuralgic nature may be a major complaint of the patient. This is especially true if the plexus palsy is consequent upon irradiation for carcinoma[497], usually of the breast. If this pain is becoming more severe after a long period of quiescence, one must suspect the presence of recurrent carcinoma in the plexus. In either case, patients must be made aware that pain is usually a poor prognostic sign[498].

Birth palsies

It is very difficult to test muscles in children and while

the following should be tried, any or all may be fruitless on any particular visit.

1. *Observation.* Careful study of the child while at play, concentrating attention on one movement at a time, may reveal postural changes indicating a deficit (Fig. 2.131) or, conversely, may enable the surgeon to demonstrate convincingly to the mother motion that even she had not noticed; two-handed toys are a necessary tool.
2. *Maintenance of position.* If the limb is placed in the position produced by a particular muscle, it may be held there momentarily after release.
3. *Stretch-induced contraction.* Conversely, if a muscle is put on full stretch and palpated, contraction may be felt or, alternatively, may occur on release after some thirty seconds of stretch.

An optimistic prognosis is justified as 80%[499] make a full recovery. Muscles which will recover will all be evident by 15 months of age[500].

A

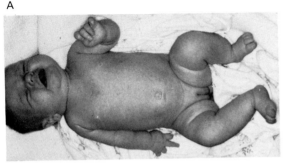

B

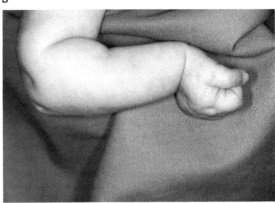

Fig. 2.131 Observation of these newborn children reveals (A) characteristic Erb's posture of the right upper extremity (C5, 6 (7)) suggestive of dystocia in a vertex delivery. B. Characteristic Klumpke posture, (C(7) 8, 1) suggestive of difficulties during breech delivery.

Indications[501,502]

Obstetric palsy. While, as stated above, most babies with obstetric palsy do recover, early identification and exploration are worthy objectives in the minority who will not do so. Electromyography and nerve conduction studies will assist in the identification of those with complete lesions[503]. If such studies are not available, or are equivocal, it is appropriate to explore if there is *no return of biceps function by 3 months*[504].

Open injuries. These patients are usually explored by the vascular service, who should be encouraged to call the hand surgeon to be present during the procedure. The indications for nerve repair or delayed graft are those given on pp. 45 and 104.

Closed traction injuries. The principles of repeated examination, both clinical and electromyographic, laid out in the first paragraph of this section on nerves apply (p. 221). When a plateau of improvement is reached, or there is uneqivocal EMG evidence of a total lesion, the decision must be made whether to proceed with *exploration and graft*, or *tendon and muscle transfers*, or both. At exploration, much time will be gained and no benefit lost if the surgeon adheres strictly to the rule of exploration that one should proceed from normal to scarred tissue, stopping when scar is encountered. *Neurolysis, nerve graft or neurotization*, or any combination thereof, may be required and may offer a 50% chance of improvement[505]. If roots are found, *intraoperative evoked cortical potentials* are invaluable to ensure that grafts are not wasted on roots with no central connection. If more than one root is found to which grafts can be placed, the first should be joined to the lateral cord or the musculo-cutaneous nerve (depending on the level, free from scar, at which the distal end of the nerve is located), the sec-

ond to the posterior cord or radial nerve, the third — a very rare situation — to the medial cord or median nerve. Sural nerve grafts are used, but they are often insufficient. The ulnar nerve, it will be seen from above, is last in priority and can be used as a graft if paralysed, preferably vascularized as it is of large diameter. If no roots are found, grafts may be run from the *intercostal* nerves[506,507], the *spinal accessory*[508] or, if it has been spared, the *thoracodorsal*[509]. If a nerve, such as the musculocutaneous, is found to have been avulsed directly from muscle, Brunelli[510] has reported good results following direct implantation, *neurotization. Tendon and muscle transfers* can assist in both obstetric[511] and adult[512,513] palsies by restoring function to the shoulder[514–516], the *elbow*[517–521] and in partial lesions, to wrist and fingers (see p. 242).

Postirradiation lesions of the plexus offer a more gloomy prognosis for the reasons detailed above. If grafting is performed the grafts should be wrapped and covered with a pedicled or free soft-tissue transfer in an attempt to improve the vascularity of the heavily scarred region. *Omentum* is a common choice of transfer[522].

The majority of patients who sustain brachial plexus injuries are young and otherwise healthy. If therefore there is *any* evidence of a proximal nerve root which could be grafted, then exploration is worthwhile if only to give the patient and his family the small comfort of possessing absolute information regarding the nature of the injury and of having tried all.

All patients, both before and after surgery, successful or otherwise, should be considered for orthotics and assisted with rehabilitation[523].

See Green D P 1993 Operative Hand Surgery, 3rd edn. Churchill Livingstone, New York, p. 1494.

CEREBRAL PALSY

Only a small percentage of children with cerebral palsy can be helped by surgery. The surgeon must spend the necessary time to evaluate those factors which serve to select those children. This requires several visits, because the findings often change as the patient becomes less nervous, during which the surgeon can make the point to the parents that even if surgery seems indicated the aim is to provide a better 'assist hand'.

Intelligence is often severely impaired. The simple use of an arbitrary figure of Intelligence Quotient will probably result in exclusion of some who would benefit and the inclusion of some who would not. Rather should the following qualities be sought with the advice and help of parents and therapist:

interpretation attention
collaboration perception — both visual and auditory
motivation emotional stability

All of these qualities are required in some measure if the child is to benefit from surgery.

Spontaneous use of the limb should be observed. If none whatsoever is seen it is unlikely that a tendon transfer will make the child aware of the hand.

Examination

If the child has not been disqualified on either of the above scores, examination should be directed at sensory and motor function.

Sensation may vary from absence to normality. In the former instance the patient is unlikely to benefit from surgery for he has no afferent input and probably displays no spontaneous use of the limb. Patients can be arbitrarily divided into three groups:

1. No sensation, even to pinprick — no spontaneous use
— no surgery
2. Some touch and pain; no proprioception; no 2PD
— reluctant spontaneous use when encouraged
— qualified prognosis
3. Proprioception, 2PD — spontaneous use
— good prognosis following surgery

Motor function. The nature of the disorder should be observed, for only spastic children can be helped by surgery. Significant degrees of *athetosis, tremor, ataxia* or *rigidity* therefore eliminate any potential benefit to be derived from surgical assistance. Spasticity itself is of varying degrees which change according to emotions, which differ from day to day. The spasticity can be classified by its response to *stretch*[542]:

severe — strong reflex which halts initial motion
moderate — visible response
minimum — palpable response

The more severe the stretch response, the more that tendon requires tenotomy, and the less predictable will be its activity and antagonism if it is transferred.

The majority of patients will show the extrinsic type of spastic hand with the typical flexion–pronation deformity. The system of selection for surgery proposed by Zancolli is recommended[525]. This is based largely on the ability to extend the fingers and the wrist:

Group 1 finger extension *full* with wrist *neutral*
Group 2 finger extension *full* with wrist *flexed*
(a) wrist extension with fingers flexed
(b) *no* wrist extension even with fingers flexed
Group 3 finger extension *nil* even with wrist *flexed*

Thumb contractures (Fig. 2.132) are simply classified:

Grade I contracture of basal joint (1st dorsal interosseous and adductor)
Grade II + metacarpophalangeal joint (+ FPB)
Grade III + interphalangeal joint (+ FPL)

Voluntary control of possible motors for transfer should be assessed. EMG studies are useful, for muscles which are active in attempts at both grasp and release are not good potential transfers.

Indications[526–529]

Zancolli Group 1 patients require no surgery apart from correction of any thumb deformity, which is probably mild. Group 3 shows very poor results with surgery. They may, like those disqualified on the grounds of intelligence or spontaneous use, benefit from surgery purely for cosmetic and toilet reasons[530,531]. Group 2 are good surgical candidates. Surgery for spasticity has two distinct elements: *release*, by myotomy, tenotomy, neurectomy or tendon lengthening of spastic muscles and *tendon transfer*, in some cases to supplement the weak antagonists of the spastic muscles. Both sub-groups 2 (a) and (b) require release of the ventral muscles at the upper part of the forearm[532] and correction of the thumb deformities by release and tenodesis or transfer[533,534]. Group 2(a) requires simple tenotomy of flexor carpi ulnaris, while 2(b) requires transfer to restore wrist extension[535,536]. The best age at which to perform this evaluation and undertake the surgery is between 6 and 10.

See Green D P 1993 Operative Hand Surgery, 3rd edn. Churchill Livingstone, New York, p. 217.

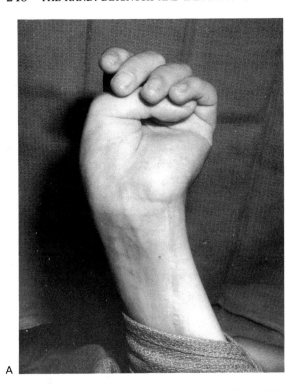

A

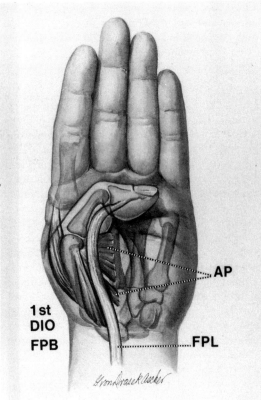

1st
DIO
FPB

AP

FPL

B

ADULT ACQUIRED SPASTIC HEMIPLEGIA

This arises most commonly as a result of head trauma or a cerebrovascular accident, a stroke. This produces a clinical picture which resembles cerebral palsy, but which differs in the important respects that it occurs in patients more likely to have other significant health problems, and less likely to be able to adapt, either to the catastrophe which has befallen them, or to the changes in function of specific muscles which tendon transfer would demand. Assessment needs to be even more guarded and recommendations even more guaranteed than in the spastic child. Systematic evaluation[537] includes assessment, in turn, of:

1. *Cognitive capacity*
2. *Motivation*
3. *Awareness of body image*
4. *Hand placement* — shoulder and elbow control play a major role
5. *Proprioception*
6. *Sensibility*
7. *Volitional motor control*

Using the above criteria, Pinzur[537] developed a functional capacity rating from 1 to 7 used for both selection and postoperative evaluation. He was able to report improvement by two functional levels in 73% of patients selected for surgery. A team approach, involving neurologists, psychologists, occupational therapists and others is necessary for such detailed and essential evaluation[538]. In determining volitional control, greater accuracy can be achieved with the use of dynamic electromyography[539]. Selective nerve blocks, especially of the high median nerve, give information on the likely efficacy of release of spastic motors.

Indications
Percutaneous phenol blocks are used to control spasticity of the *pectoralis major*[540], the *elbow flexors*[541] and the *intrinsics*[542]. Surgery is directed, as in the child with cerebral palsy, at release of spastic motors and tendon transfer to weak antagonists of spastic muscles. This may require, for:

Elbow spasticity, lengthening of biceps and brachialis, release of the lacertus fibrosus

---

Fig. 2.132 Cerebral palsy. A. This thumb-in-palm deformity is grade III. B. Diagrammatic representation of the spastic muscles — first dorsal interosseous and adductor pollicis (grade I), flexor pollicis brevis (grade II), flexor pollicis longus (grade III).

Wrist flexor spasticity, lengthening or release of FCU and FCR

Spastic wrist and finger flexors, fractional lengthening[543] or superficialis-to-profundus transfer[544,545]

Absent wrist extension, transfer or tenodesis[537]

Absent finger extension, brachioradialis to extensor digitorum transfer[546]

Thumb-in-palm deformity, Z-plasty of the web skin, lengthening or recession of intrinsics and/or arthrodesis of the interphalangeal joint[547].

See Green D P 1993 Operative Hand Surgery, 3rd edn. Churchill Livingstone, New York, p. 227.

NEURALGIC AMYOTROPHY[548,549] (= shoulder girdle syndrome = Parsonage–Turner syndrome = paralytic brachial neuritis)

This condition is of unknown aetiology, but commonly follows on an injection of some kind. It is characterized by *pain* followed by *paralysis*. The pain is sudden in onset and is usually a constant severe ache across the

Table 2.8 Clinical classification of the quadriplegic upper limbs and possible function obtained by surgery[1]

Group	Lowest functioning cord segments	Remaining motor function	Subgroups		Function regained by surgery
1 Flexor of the elbow 13%	5–6	Biceps, brachialis	A	Without brachioradialis (1– A)	–
			B	With brachioradialis (1 – B)	Elbow extension and weak lateral grip and grasping
2 Extensor of the wrist 74%	6–7	Extensor carpi radialis longus and brevis	A	Weak and complete wrist extension (2–A)	
			B	Strong wrist extension (2–B) 82%	I Without pronator teres, flexor carpi radialis, and triceps (2–B: I) 76%	Elbow extension Good lateral grip and grasping
					II Without flexor radialis and triceps; and with pronator teres (2–B: II) 16%	
					III With pronator teres, flexor carpi radialis, and triceps (2–B: III) 8%	Good lateral grip and better grasping than 2–B: I and 2–B: II
3 Extrinsic extensor of the finger 6.8%	7–8	Ext. digit. communis Ext. digit. quinti Ext. carpi ulnaris	A	Complete extension of ulnar fingers and paralysis of radial fingers and thumb (3–A)	Good lateral and pulp grips and excellent grasping (better in subgroup 3–B)
			B	Complete extension of all fingers and weak thumb extension (3-B)	
4 Extrinsic flexor of the fingers and extensor of the thumb 6.2%	8–1	Flexor digit. prof. Ext. indicis proprius Ext. pollicis longus Flexor carpi ulnaris	A	Complete flexion of ulnar fingers and paralysis or weakness of flexion of the radial fingers and thumb. Complete thumb extension (4–A)	Excellent lateral and pulp grips and grasping (better in subgroup 4–B: II)
			B	Complete flexion of the fingers and thumb, with total intrinsic paralysis (4–B)	I Without flexor superficialis (4–B: I)	
					II With flexor superficialis (4–B: II)	

[1]Reproduced from Zancolli, E. A. 1979 Structural and dynamic bases of hand surgery, 2nd edn. Lippincott, Philadelphia. p. 230, with kind permission of the author and publisher.

Table 2.9   Classifications of quadriplegia

	Freehafer	Moberg	Zancolli
Elbow flexion — no BR	Ib	O:0	1A
— + BR		O:1	1B
Weak wrist extension	II		2A
Strong BR and ECRL	III	OCu: 2	
+ ECRB		OCu: 3	2B I
+ PT		OCu: 4	2B II
+ triceps, FCR	IV	OCu: 5	2B III
Finger extension			
— ulnar digits		OCu: 6	3A
— all, including thumb		OCu: 7	3B
Finger flexion			
— ulnar digits		OCu: 8	4A
— all — no FDS			4B I
— + FDS	V	OCu:9	4B II
Exceptions		OCu: X	

shoulder girdle and down into the arm. It may persist for hours to weeks but it improves markedly with the onset of paralysis. The paralysis is of a *lower motor neuron type*, with flaccidity, rapid wasting, but no fasciculations. The palsy may afflict peripheral nerves individually or in combination, nerve roots or the spinal cord itself. It may be unilateral or bilateral. The peripheral nerves most commonly involved are the long thoracic, the axillary, the radial, the anterior interosseous, the suprascapular and the musculo-cutaneous nerves, in that order. The upper roots of the plexus C5–7 are those affected in root loss. Sensation is normally not markedly reduced. The prognosis is for recovery in the majority of cases, but that may take several years.

CERVICAL CORD TRANSECTION = QUADRIPLEGIA = TETRAPLEGIA[550,551]

Patients should always be evaluated by a hand surgeon for function can be improved in the majority of patients. Formerly, these injuries were classified according either to the level of cord or of bony lesion. More recently, emphasis has been laid on residual function, both motor and sensory, which need not coincide with respect to cervical level. Freehafer[552], Lamb[553] and Zancolli[554] have introduced motor classifications which correspond except in minor detail. Zancolli has linked classification to potential surgical gain (Table 2.8) in a most practical way. Study of Table 2.8 reveals that, in his series, the majority of patients fell into the group with strong wrist extension — the so-called 'strong C6' — a group who can be helped greatly by surgery. Moberg[555],

whose classification was modified at the International Conference in Giens, France, in 1984, has emphasized the importance of sensibility in tetraplegia. He has classified patients as Cu = Cutaneous, being patients with useful sensory afferents from the hands and as O = Ocular, where all information available to the patient is visual. In the latter group he recommends reconstruction in only one hand since only one at a time can be controlled by visual input. Unfortunately, any attempt to rationalize the three main classifications currently in vogue (Table 2.9) reveals that there is but a poor fit. Communication therefore requires either a knowledge of all classifications, an arbitrary adoption of one or a detailed description of the individual patient.

After taking a history which determines efficiency in activities of daily living, examination is conducted as follows:

1. Test sensation, using moving 2PD — in the majority, C6 will be intact and therefore sensibility will be present in thumb and index.
2. Check joint range of motion — note contractures — hyperextensibility of MP joints. The latter, if present, may require control by tenodesis or transfer, active or passive.
3. Determine presence, spasticity and strength of muscle activity. Remember that almost all muscles are innervated from more than one root (Table 2.10) and therefore strength will increase the lower is the cervical lesion. Only power 4 and 5 muscles should be transferred.

Indications[556–562]

Table 2.11 serves only as a guide to potential substitutes. For more detailed guidance and for transfers to restore intrinsic function the reader should consult Zancolli's classic text[554]. The aim of surgery should be to achieve independent transfer as from bed to chair and, in the majority, 'strong C6' group, to restore strong grasp and lateral pinch[563,564]. The recent use of implantable functional neuromuscular stimulators[565–567] promises an enhanced capability to assist tetraplegic patients.

The timing of reconstruction for tetraplegia should be late enough for all motors to have returned to maximum strength and for the patient to have had time to understand fully his limitations. Conversely, it should be early enough for the patient not to have completely adjusted to his life style to a degree that the time lost by surgery becomes an intrusion. In practical terms, this usually means surgery about 1 year after the cervical injury[568].

See Green D P 1993 Operative Hand Surgery, 3rd edn. Churchill Livingstone, New York, p. 1519.

Table 2.10 The root values of muscles (after Zancolli)

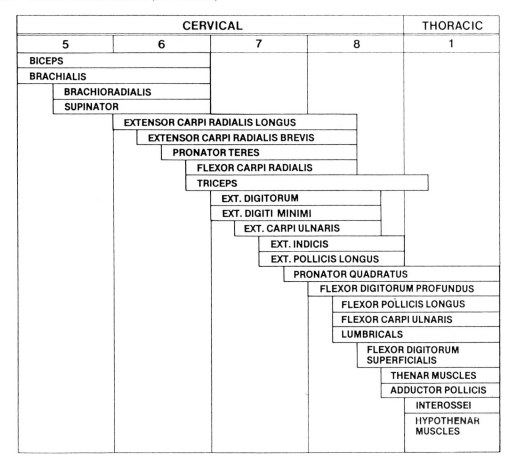

	CERVICAL				THORACIC
	5	**6**	**7**	**8**	**1**

BICEPS

BRACHIALIS

BRACHIORADIALIS

SUPINATOR

EXTENSOR CARPI RADIALIS LONGUS

EXTENSOR CARPI RADIALIS BREVIS

PRONATOR TERES

FLEXOR CARPI RADIALIS

TRICEPS

EXT. DIGITORUM

EXT. DIGITI MINIMI

EXT. CARPI ULNARIS

EXT. INDICIS

EXT. POLLICIS LONGUS

PRONATOR QUADRATUS

FLEXOR DIGITORUM PROFUNDUS

FLEXOR POLLICIS LONGUS

FLEXOR CARPI ULNARIS

LUMBRICALS

FLEXOR DIGITORUM SUPERFICIALIS

THENAR MUSCLES

ADDUCTOR POLLICIS

INTEROSSEI

HYPOTHENAR MUSCLES

Muscle and tendon

Much of the assessment of muscle and tendon injury has been made in performing the full muscle test and examining the joints. It is necessary now to consider factors over and above the presence or absence of muscle function. Active motion may be absent or diminished because of (i) division, (ii) rupture, (iii) contracture in the muscle, (iv) adhesions, (v) bowstringing, (vi) lumbrical plus, (vii) recurvatum deformity, or (viii) the quadriga syndrome[580].

FLEXOR

Division, rupture or paralysis?
The full muscle test may have revealed total lack of function in one or more muscles. It is usually apparent whether this is due to tendon division or to nerve injury from the site of the wound, the presence of muscle

Table 2.11 Tendon transfers and tenodeses in quadriplegia

		Normal motor	Potential substitute
(i)	Elbow flexion	Biceps	–
		Brachialis	
		Brachioradialis	
(ii)	Elbow extension[569,570]	Triceps	Post. deltoid, biceps
(iii)	Wrist extension	ECRL	Brachioradialis[571]
		ECRB	
(iv)	Pronation	Pronator teres	Biceps (Zancolli 2A)
(v)	Wrist flexion	FCR	–
(vi)	Finger and thumb extension	ED	Brachioradialis or
		EPL	tenodesis
(vii)	Thumb flexion[572–577]	FPL	Brachioradialis or tenodesis
(viii)	Finger flexion	FDP	Brachioradialis
		FDS	pronator teres[578] or ECRL[579]

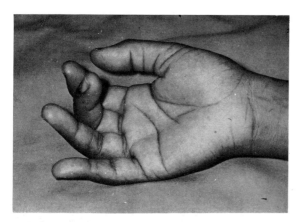

Fig. 2.133 This patient shows an abnormal posture of the ring and small fingers suggestive of adhesions or rupture of both flexor tendons to the small finger and of the entire profundus and possibly a portion of the superficialis to the ring finger. This deduction was subsequently confirmed at surgical exploration.

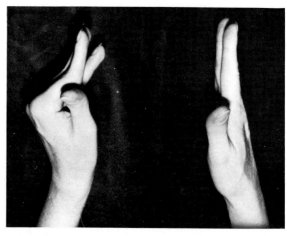

Fig. 2.134 This patient is attempting to extend both hands. In the left she shows severe advanced intrinsic contracture with metacarpophalangeal flexion contracture and hyperextension deformities of the proximal interphalangeal joints.

wasting, the pattern of motor loss and the associated sensory disturbance, but this may not be entirely clear or may require confirmation.

Posture. The posture produced by division of various tendons has been detailed on p. 30. Nerve injury may eliminate active function but would not result in the posture typical of tendon injury. In the case of the long flexor tendon, for example, denervation would not produce the characteristically extended finger of a complete tendon laceration (Fig. 2.133). By altering the position of the wrist more can be learned about tendon integrity from the resulting changes in posture due to the tenodesis effect.

Defect. Palpation may detect the absence of a tendon from its sheath when compared with an uninjured finger or may reveal a defect in the wrist distal to the bulge of the muscle belly, which can be emphasized by attempted contraction.

Passive motion. This test is valuable in checking the integrity of long flexor tendons (p. 32). Firm pressure exerted over the junction of middle and distal thirds of the forearm produces distinct flexion of the fingers in the presence of intact long flexor tendons. Similar pressure over the radius a little further distally flexes the thumb via an intact pollicis longus.

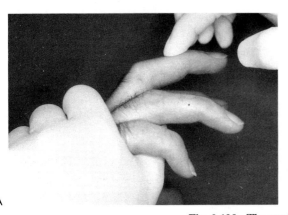

A

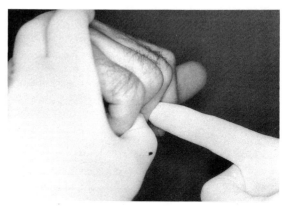

B

Fig. 2.135 The test for intrinsic tightness.

Contracture

Contracture occurs most commonly in the muscle bellies of the intrinsics and of the finger flexors of the forearm as a result of a compartment syndrome (p. 40) which was not recognized or was treated too late to avoid muscle death and fibrosis. The tenodesis effect on the joints crossed by the tendons of contracted muscles has been detailed on p. 192.

Flexion contracture (Volkmann's). Attempt to extend all the fingers while also extending the forearm and hand. In the presence of a contracture the fingers will resist the attempt, remaining flexed. Flexion of the wrist will, however, allow the fingers to extend, confirming the presence of shortening, or adhesion, of the muscles above the wrist.

Intrinsic tightness (contracture) (Fig. 2.134). With the metacarpophalangeal joint passively hyperextended, attempt to flex the proximal interphalangeal joint (Fig. 2.135). In the presence of intrinsic tightness, this will meet with rubbery resistance which will decrease if the metacarpophalangeal joint is now allowed to flex. If it is suspected that one or other of the radial or ulnar intrinsics is responsible for the tightness, the finger should be deviated at the metacarpophalangeal joint each way in turn. If tightness is more marked in radial deviation of the finger, the ulnar intrinsic is responsible, and vice versa.

Adhesions

The most common cause of inadequate range of motion in tendons, in the presence of a palpable powerful muscle belly contraction and an adequate range of passive joint motions is adhesion of the tendon, usually most firm at the site of injury which may have been to the tendon itself or to adjacent structures, most commonly bone.

By limiting tendon movement, adhesions produce active deficits in joint motion which exceed the passive but are also responsible for a passive deficit in the opposite movement. For example, assuming the absence of other contractures, if the flexor pollicis longus is adherent to the proximal phalanx there will be a flexion and often an extension deficit in the interphalangeal joint of the thumb. The active and the passive extension deficit will be equal because the adherent tendon acts as a check on both. However, in flexion the passive range will exceed the active since the examiner can exert more power on the joint than can the adherent tendon (Fig. 2.136).

Site of adhesion. The primary adhesion will be at the location of the original injury and repair, but in most cases will have spread to involve much of the length of the tendon. Adhesion of muscle or tendon to the skin of

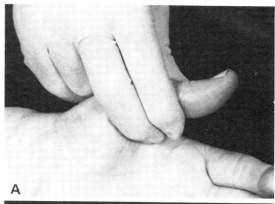

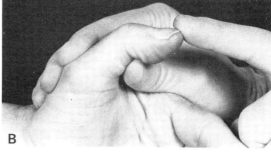

Fig. 2.136 This patient had sustained a laceration of flexor pollicis longus which at exploration subsequent to this illustration proved adherent at the site of repair. A. The patient is attempting active flexion but is achieving none. B. The passive range of motion can be seen to considerably exceed that achieved actively.

the forearm is easily appreciated, for each muscle contraction produces puckering of the skin. Adhesion to other tendons is indicated by mass action of normally independent tendons when the patient attempts to flex only one.

The location of an adhesion can occasionally be accurately determined by adjusting the position of the joints. Considering the proximal interphalangeal joint with a flexion deficit, if full flexion of the metacarpophalangeal joint permits the proximal interphalangeal joint to extend, the adhesion must be proximal to the metacarpophalangeal joint. If it does not, the flexor tendon is adherent to the proximal phalanx (Fig. 2.137).

Bowstringing

Doyle and Blythe[581] have shown that both the A2 and A4 pulleys — those at the proximal and middle phalanx respectively (Fig. 2.138C) — are required for full flexion to be possible. If either is divided, the flexor tendon stands out from the digital skeleton like the string on a bow. This increases the moment arm on whichever joint is further removed from the tendon than is customary. A flexor deformity, later a contracture, will

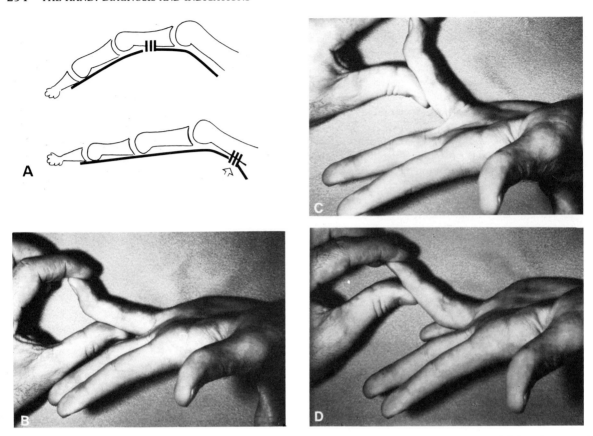

Fig. 2.137   A. Adjustment of the joints proximal to that which appears to be the seat of contracture may reveal the primary source of that deformity. In this diagram the flexion contracture is at the proximal interphalangeal joint. Flexion of the metacarpophalangeal joint in the presence of adhesion over the proximal phalanx (upper figure) has no effect on the flexion contracture of the proximal interphalangeal joint. If, however, the adhesion of the flexor tendons lies proximal to the metacarpophalangeal joint, flexion of that will result in correction of the contracture apparently present in the proximal interphalangeal joint. B. This patient has a flexion contracture of the distal interphalangeal joint present when both metacarpophalangeal and proximal interphalangeal joints are extended. C. Flexion of the metacarpophalangeal joint has little or no effect on the flexion contracture of the distal interphalangeal joint. D. However, when the proximal interphalangeal is flexed, the distal interphalangeal joint can be fully extended. It can therefore be concluded that the flexion contracture is due to limitation of flexor tendon motion and further that the tendon is adherent in the region of the proximal phalanx.

occur at that joint, poorer flexion at others. This not only decreases the mechanical efficiency of the tendon but also increases the likelihood of tendon adhesion to the soft tissue. Bowstringing can be detected both on inspection (Fig. 2.138) and on palpating the tendon while asking the patient to flex the finger.

Lumbrical plus[582]
This disability occurs whenever the flexor digitorum profundus is released distally to a degree which causes its contraction to act through the lumbrical, causing extension of the interphalangeal joints instead of flexion. This may occur following laceration of the tendon, amputation through the finger distal to the

proximal interphalangeal joint, insertion of an overlong tendon graft or the development of adhesions distal to the lumbrical. It is recognized by the occurrence of paradoxical extension on strong flexion of the fingers (Fig. 2.139).

Recurvatum (Fig. 2.140)
This hyperextension of the proximal interphalangeal joint occurs in supple patients after excision of the superficialis tendon during primary repair or tendon graft and is akin to *swan-neck deformity* encountered in rheumatoid disease (p. 389). Initially slight, it may increase to the degree where it produces a 'slow finger', flexion occurring later than in adjacent fingers. Indeed,

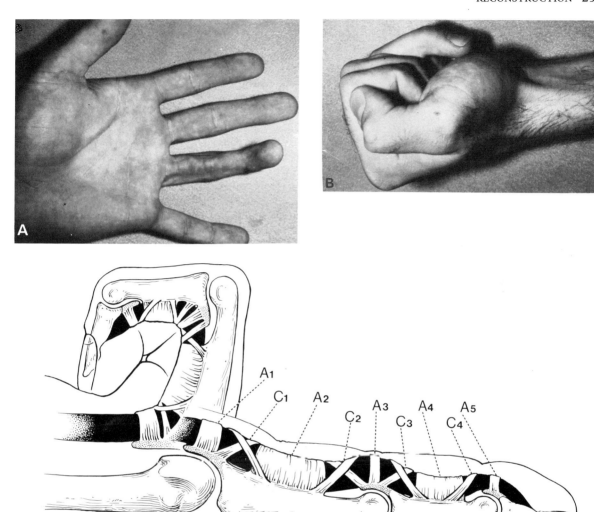

Fig. 2.138 A. This patient can clearly be seen to have no pulleys over the flexor tendon to the ring finger, the tendon standing out through the skin. B. The flexor tendon, although pulling through, is mechanically inefficient on account of the lack of pulleys. C. This diagram shows the placement and nomenclature of the normal pulley mechanism, although other namings of the C pulleys are common (the most frequent is to omit C1 shown here renaming 2, 3 and 4 as C1 2 and 3).

the patient may have to help the finger around the head of the proximal phalanx with the adjacent digit before flexion can ensue. It can be avoided by not excising that portion of the superficialis distal to its chiasm.

Quadriga syndrome (see p. 174).

Indications[583]
If neither finger flexor is functioning, and no tendon repair was performed primarily, then a *tendon graft*[584,585] should be planned and the sources of the graft checked

during examination. In order of preference these are palmaris longus from either arm, one of the two tendons of extensor digiti minimi or one of the tendons of extensor digitorum longus from either the second, third or fourth toes. Many surgeons use the divided flexor digitorum superficialis or the plantaris[586]. The author finds the first too thick and worries about its nutrition; the second he finds too thin and is concerned about its strength.

If flexor digitorum superficialis is intact and functioning, the choice lies between tendon graft and fixing the distal

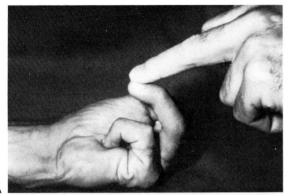

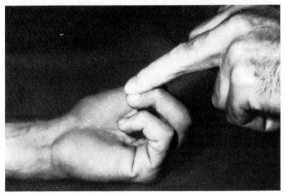

Fig. 2.139 Lumbrical plus. In (A) the patient is lightly flexing the hand without power. The examiner's finger is resting lightly on the distal phalanx of the ring finger. B. With powerful grasp the small finger comes down into full flexion, but the ring finger paradoxically *extends* against the resisting finger.

interphalangeal joint, preferably by *tenodesis* or *capsulodesis*. Littler has shown what a small proportion of the sweep of finger flexion is represented by motion of the distal interphalangeal joint and to hazard all for this

small gain is indicated in only a small proportion of well-motivated patients with specialized occupations. For the great majority who have not had the benefit of a primary repair of profundus, tenodesis of the distal interphalangeal joint is the procedure of choice. If tendon graft is selected the choice must be made between sacrificing the superficialis and grafting past it. The former has been done successfully but no report exists of its consistent reliability and the latter technique certainly has a higher chance of maintaining proximal interphalangeal joint function.

The choice of motor for a tendon graft is made finally during surgery, but a preliminary selection can be undertaken at the time of examination. The surgeon should determine that the muscle can be felt contracting in the forearm and that there is prima facie evidence that the tendon crosses at least one joint. Experience has shown that this assures that the motor has adequate power and amplitude.

If primary repair or tendon graft has been performed and rupture has occurred, immediate re-operation is indicated[587]. If the same procedures have resulted in adhesions, then *tenolysis*[588, 589] should be proposed, preferably commencing under wrist block (Fig 2.141). In doing so, the surgeon must always warn the patient of the possibility that exploration may reveal a totally unsatisfactory tendon, and graft or silicone rod insertion[590–593] may be necessary.

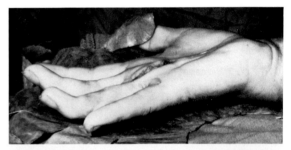

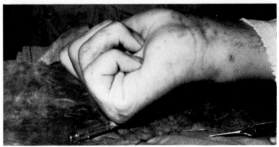

Fig. 2.141 Tendolysis under wrist block permits the patient to participate in the procedure. The intravenous cannula seen in (B) is to permit the administration of intravenous anaesthesia should forearm exploration prove necessary.

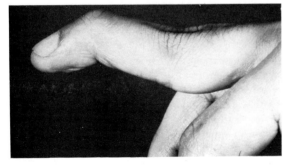

Fig. 2.140 This very supple 18-year-old patient had achieved an excellent result following flexor tendon graft to his middle finger but subsequently developed a progressive recurvatum deformity of the proximal interphalangeal joint.

A *silicone rod* is indicated in the following circumstances:

Unsatisfactory skin coverage, where, for example, a cross-finger flap must be done at the same procedure

Absence of pulleys, in which situation pulley reconstruction must always be performed

Limitation of passive joint motion, where capsulectomy and early motion with or without dynamic splintage is required

A generally unsatisfactory bed, with extensive scarring and exposure of bare bone.

As previously emphasized, no tendon graft can possibly increase the range of motion in a contracted joint, and this must be corrected by splintage or surgery before grafting is considered. Where secondary tendon surgery is being considered and, in particular, where there is a significant flexion contracture, care must be taken to evaluate the skeletal structures, skin and, sometimes overlooked, the blood supply to the digit involved. This can be done by use of the *digital Allen test* or, more precisely, by employing a Doppler flow meter or colour duplex ultrasonography (p. 47). If flow is absent in both vessels, surgery should probably be reconsidered. If flow is present in one or even both, the patient should still be warned that release of the contracture, however meticulous, may result in no flow to the pulp, necessitating return of the finger to the flexed position. As opposed to immediate replacement, late reconstruction of digital arteries is less successful due largely to poor run-off, although lengthening of shortened arteries which are carrying flow has been performed using arterial or reversed vein grafts.

In the ultimate situation — several operations, a flexion contracture, joint damage and an insensate digit with no detectable blood flow — a simple operation may be preferable. Depending upon several factors — occupation, recreation, the condition of the other digits and the patient's preference — *arthrodesis*, tenodesis or *amputation* may be selected.

In some circumstances, notably in replacing flexor pollicis longus[594,595], *tendon transfer*, usually of the superficialis of the ring finger will be selected in preference to a tendon graft. *Bowstringing* is corrected by *pulley reconstruction*, for which there are several techniques. My preference is for a combination of extensor retinaculum to replace the A2 and A4[596], and palmar plate[597] to replace A3, the latter, of course, only in circumstances where a graft or rod are being inserted.

Lumbrical plus deformities may be eliminated by the tendon surgery planned. If the finger functions well otherwise, simple division of the lumbrical under local anaesthetic will cure the problem. If the patient

scheduled for simple division has hyperextensible metacarpophalangeal joints, he should be warned that there is the possibility that he may develop a claw deformity.

Recurvatum is corrected by capsulodesis, or by tenodesis of the proximal interphalangeal joint, if tendon remains, or by transfer from the lateral band as in correcting swan-neck deformity (p. 389).

It will be evident that, in obtaining informed consent to operate on a digit showing flexion contracture following tendon repair, the surgeon may need to offer a daunting list of options, depending in part on the findings at surgery: tenolysis, possible tendon graft, possible tendon transfer, possible pulley reconstruction, possible rod placement, possible capsulectomy, possible vein graft, possible cross-finger flap, possible arthrodesis, possible amputation. The patient should also be warned that graft or two-stage reconstruction alike may require further tenolysis, and so on.

However daunting for the patient, he should be cheered by the fact that, if he persists through whatever is required and works hard, the great majority of digits come to work well[598]. Parents should be encouraged to commit their children to a reconstructive programme, for an immobile digit grows less well[599].

See Green D P 1993 Operative Hand Surgery, 3rd edn. Churchill Livingstone, New York, p. 1859.

EXTENSOR

Of the eight ills which afflict the patient with a previous flexor injury (p. 250), only rupture and adhesions plague the extensor tendons. However, the extensor apparatus over the dorsum of the finger is of such complex structure that rupture of a repair, or, more commonly, failure to recognize the injury initially, results in postural changes difficult to correct — the mallet finger and the boutonniere deformity. They are easy to recognize and have been described previously (p. 38). The examiner need only ensure that the underlying bone is not the seat of non-union or malunion and that the joints are not subluxed or the seat of arthritis, or both.

Injuries of the extensors more proximally are usually due to lacerations. The extensor pollicis longus is frequently subject to rupture (p. 37) which may go unnoticed for long periods. The patient may complain of clumsiness, or it may be found in the course of routine examination for another complaint. It is detected by weakness of interphalangeal flexion and the inability of the patient to raise the thumb when the hand is placed flat on the table.

Indications

Mallet finger should be treated initially by prolonged

splintage[600]. If the patient will persist, it rarely fails. If the deformity persists and the patient will not, reconstruction can be performed by graft or transfer[601], the joint can be fused, or the entire apparatus encouraged to migrate proximally by doing a tenotomy of the central slip at the proximal joint[602].

Chronic boutonniere[603] should be managed initially by restoring full joint motion and, as with the mallet, prolonged splintage. This is a more difficult splint to wear, and the patient who discards it more worthy of sympathy. Reconstruction has been performed by innumerable techniques, some staged[604]. Fractional advancement of the central slip and raising of the lateral bands by folding over and suturing the transverse retinacular ligaments from either side of the finger, performed under *local anaesthesia* so that balance can be ensured, followed by six weeks of Kirschner wire immobilization has proved most successful for the author. ('Most' is here used in its comparative form, not its superlative.)

Loss of extensors further proximally may not require reconstruction[605]. However, most are replaced by transfers[606], described in more detail on p. 242.

See Green D P 1993 Operative Hand Surgery, 3rd edn. Churchill Livingstone, New York, p. 1961.

Vessel

(Vascular occlusion may occur dramatically, in which circumstance the patient will present in the emergency room. Such cases have been discussed under 'non-traumatic vascular emergencies' on p. 48).

The symptoms of obliterative arterial disease tend to indicate the level of obstruction[607].

Group I   proximal subclavian — steal syndrome
Group II distal subclavian, axillary or brachial — intermittent claudication
Group III distal disease and distal symptoms

It will be evident that higher occlusions may masquerade as ones more distal, whereas the reverse cannot occur.

HISTORY

Inadequate circulation to a limb or digit, according to its degree, will declare itself by one or more of the following symptoms.

Subclavian steal syndrome[608]
In this syndrome there is an occlusion of the proximal subclavian or innominate artery. The name is derived from its most dramatic symptom which is fainting during vigorous exercise of the limb. The demand in the arm causes reversal of flow in the vertebral artery, which arises from the first part of the subclavian, thereby stealing blood from the cerebral circulation. The syndrome may present with upper extremity symptoms alone, of pain, weakness, easy fatigue and numbness. The pulse is diminished, the blood pressure is lower than in the other arm, and the diagnosis is confirmed by arch angiography. 'Shunt steal' which arises in dialysis patients is considered on page 443.

Intermittent claudication
Much less common in the upper than in the lower limb, this is characterized by increasing pain with continued exercise which forces rest (not strictly 'claudication'; L. *claudicare* = to limp). Most often encountered in the forearm muscles, this is due to an obstruction of the brachial artery.

Frank necrosis
The dead part will be black or mottled brown, hard and cold (Fig. 2.142). The part may be firmly adherent and the surgeon should not dislodge it until he has planned the closure of the wound and indeed prepared the patient for admission. In some cases, mostly in young children, often following attempted replacement of a fingertip with or without vascular repair, it may be best to leave the part to separate spontaneously, which will take several months but may leave a well-healed non-tender amputation stump. This approach is also adopted where surgery is contraindicated by severe ischaemia, or in polyarteritis, scleroderma and frostbite (see p. 136).

Persistent ulceration
When a wound on a digit fails to heal, or minor trauma results in skin breakdown which fails to heal, the sur-

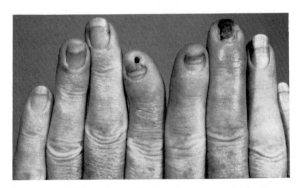

Fig. 2.142 This patient with thromboangitis obliterans demonstrates frank and incipient necrosis in several digits.

geon should suspect an inadequate blood supply, provided the other causes of ulceration (p. 168) have been eliminated (Fig. 2.143).

Cold intolerance

The patient who complains that any fall in ambient temperature results in pain and pallor in one or more digits has some obstruction of his vascular tree, temporary or permanent, localized or diffuse.

Colour change

The finger appears deep red with a bluish tinge. The patient may report that the finger becomes absolutely white in cold weather, and this can often be demonstrated by immersion in ice water.

Stiffness of the joints

The finger or part will be less used by the patient, resulting in both oedema and stiffness, both active and passive.

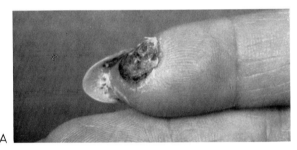

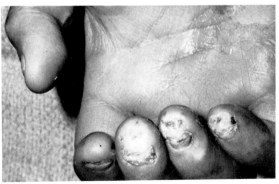

Fig. 2.143 A. This patient had ulnar artery thrombosis resulting in poor flow to the index finger. B. Persistent ulceration in this patient's fingertips was thought to be due to nerve injuries in the forearm. However, investigation of the vascular tree and reconstruction with reversed vein grafts resulted in satisfactory healing of the fingertips before sensation improved.

EXAMINATION

Examination may reveal any of the following signs of vascular impairment.

Skin temperature

A difference in temperature between the affected hand or digit and its normal counterpart can be detected simply by touch, and is a most helpful clinical tool. By advancing the examiner's hands up both extremities of the patient, a definite level of temperature change may be detected. A more exact record can be made by the use of a portable thermocouple with digital read-out. This allows improvement to be charted and demonstrated to the patient — the basis of biofeedback techniques.

Slow refill after expression

This can be detected by comparing the nail bed with that of a normal finger or by applying a digital Allen test.

Absent pulses

Only the radial pulse can be palpated with sufficient confidence to declare it absent. The ulnar artery and digital arteries can frequently be felt pulsating if the hand is warm, but failure to do so is not evidence of absent flow.

Blood pressure

Recordings taken in *both arms* may reveal a significant difference due to a proximal block.

Allen test[609]

The patency of the ulnar and radial arteries at the wrist and of the two digital arteries at the base of a finger can be determined clinically by this technique (although its validity has been challenged[610]). Both arteries at the wrist are occluded by the examiner's middle and index fingers of both hands (Fig. 2.144). The patient is then asked to close the hand firmly while the occlusion is maintained, thereby expelling much of the blood. With the hand then relaxed and occlusion continued, the palm appears pale. Occasionally, despite continued occlusion of both arteries, the palm will refill. This is due to a *persistent median* or other anomalous artery. Failure to observe this may lead the examiner to draw false reassurance regarding radial or ulnar artery patency, or both. It is therefore important to confirm the *persistence* of palmar pallor before proceeding with the test. Removal of the occlusion from *one* of the vessels in the presence of a block in that vessel will result in no immediate change. By contrast, if the vessel is patent a

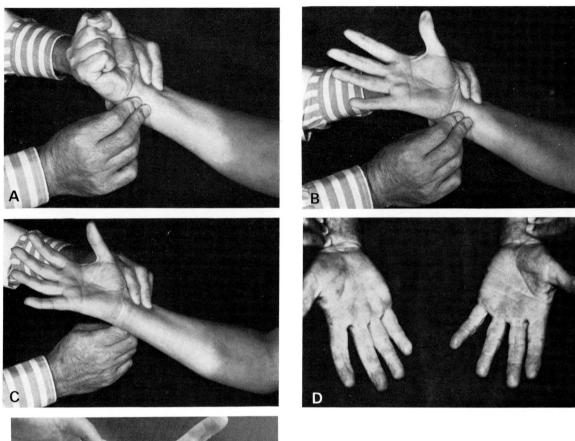

Fig. 2.144 The Allen test. Both radial and ulnar arteries are occluded at the wrist by the examiner. The patient is asked to firmly flex all fingers and the thumb thereby expelling blood from the hand (A). B. The patient is then asked to open the hand in a relatively relaxed posture and the pallor of the palm can be appreciated. C. Release of the compression on one or other of the arteries under test will, if that vessel is patent, result in rapid return of normal colour to the palm of the hand. D. If, as in this patient, one ulnar artery is thrombosed then the pallor persists when compared with the normal hand. E. On release of this patient's ulnar artery, only the small, ring, and half of the middle finger filled. This illustrates absence of any significant palmar arches.

pink blush spreads rapidly across the palm. In the event of obstruction being present the occlusion on the other vessel should be released and the response again noted. When the first vessel tested was patent the examination should be repeated for the other vessel. The Allen test has been quantified both by timing refill[611] and measuring digital systolic pressure[612].

The *digital Allen test* is performed in similar manner except that the examiner should first exsanguinate the

digit by brisk proximal massage before occluding the digital arteries against the proximal phalanx (Fig. 2.145).

If either test is equivocal, warming the hand in hot water before repeating the test will eliminate doubt.

Doppler flowmeter[613]
Flow can be detected with ease in all significant arteries in the upper extremity using ultrasound. Because of

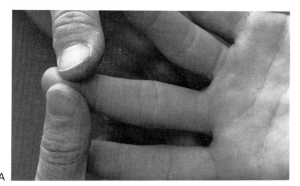

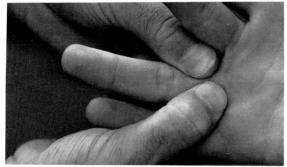

Fig. 2.145 The digital Allen test. A. The thumbs of the examiner are placed on either side of the anterior surface of the digit, and (B) are swept firmly and proximally to exsanguinate the digit, coming to rest over the digital arteries on the proximal phalanx, thereby occluding inflow. As with the Allen test, release of one or other thumb will reveal the presence or absence of flow through that vessel.

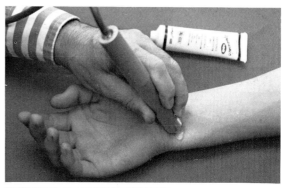

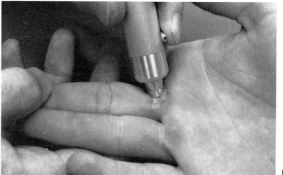

Fig. 2.146 The use of the Doppler flow meter for (A) ulnar and (B) digital arteries.

the presence of significant arches in the hand and the fingers it is important to determine the direction of flow, either by using a meter which indicates this or, more simply, by occluding any potential source of backflow while listening. Thus, while checking flow in the ulnar artery, proper or digital, the radial equivalent should be occluded, and vice versa (Fig. 2.146).

A diagnosis can be arrived at in most patients with the relatively simple office techniques which are detailed. To confirm or quantify this diagnosis or to investigate the more obscure cases, the more sophisticated techniques available in a *vascular laboratory*[614,615] may be employed:

temperature	— thermography, infra-red radiometry
	— cold stress testing[616], before and after digital nerve block
perfusion	— plethysmography[617,618] or pulse volume record (PVR)
	— transcutaneous oxygen monitor[619]

stenosis or occlusion	— Doppler wave-form analysis[620], velocity/time, pulsatility index
	— high-resolution ultrasound, duplex scanner[621,622]

In many cases, these studies will provide all necessary information and the more invasive methods will not be required.

Digital subtraction angiography (DSA) is now the technique of choice in most instances for visualization of the vessels as it may not require cannulation of the arterial tree.

IMAGING

Arteriography of the conventional kind is required to confirm, or sometimes make, a diagnosis; to determine the location and distribution of pathologic changes; to ensure the presence of other, apparently unaffected, vessels, to gain an impression of the state of health of the vascular tree; and to assist in the planning of surgical procedures.

Maximum vasodilatation is desirable in these studies. By comparisons performed in the course of studying patients with bilateral disease, we have determined that

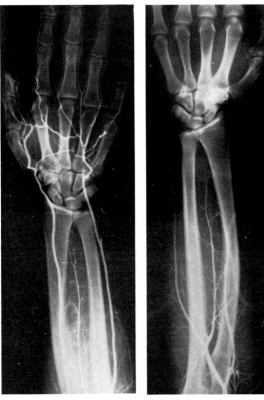

Fig. 2.147 Simultaneous arteriography performed (R) without regional block, and (L) with regional block. The patient had bilateral symptoms which were more severe in (L) than in (R). As can be seen, he had an ulnar artery thrombosis in the superficial branch of the left side, but no diagnosis could be made in the arteriogram of the right, which was performed without anaesthesia.

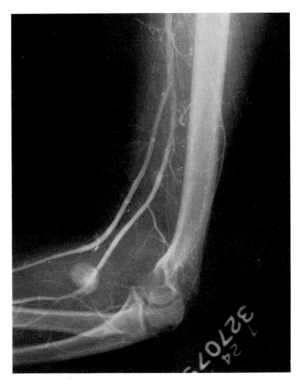

Fig. 2.148 Arteriography shows a traumatic aneurysm in the antecubital fossa. There is also a high bifurcation of the brachial artery. If the dye had been introduced below the level of the bifurcation, a faulty conclusion may have been reached regarding the circulation to this extremity.

this is achieved to a greater and more reliable degree after *regional nerve block* than with general anaesthesia, intra-arterial vasodilators, stellate ganglion block, sedation or with no preparation whatsoever (Fig. 2.147). Introduction of the dye is preferably made through a catheter in the femoral artery at the groin, passing retrograde through the aorta thence to the subclavian and axillary arteries. This not only permits study of the proximal portions of the vascular tree to the upper extremity where unsuspected anomalies or pathology may lie but also avoids inflicting iatrogenic insult to an arterial system already in trouble (Fig. 2.148)

Subtraction films made from the angiograms highlight the vessels in a useful way (Fig. 2.152). *Magnification angiography* permits easier study of detail in the vessels but its greater cost probably outweighs any diagnostic benefit.

These various studies may reveal one of the following vascular disorders:

Localized arterial occlusion (proximal occlusions have been considered on p. 49)

This is most common in the ulnar artery at the region of the canal of Guyon[623–627] (Fig. 2.149). Because thrombosis at this point probably results from the use of the butt of the hand as a blunt instrument, the condition is referred to as the 'hypothenar hammer syndrome'[628] (Fig. 2.150). A few cases of non-thrombotic occlusion have been reported[629,630]. It is usually associated with cold intolerance, pain and sometimes ulceration, most often of the ring finger.

Aneurysm (p. 443)

Generalized arterial disorders

These conditions affect many or all of the vessels in the limb and are therefore much less amenable to surgical

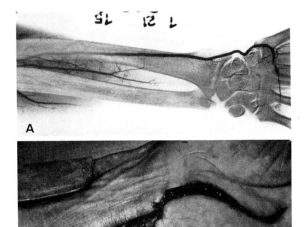

Fig. 2.149 A. A thrombosed ulnar artery is demonstrated on arteriogram in which the radial artery is seen to provide the only blood supply to the hand. The thrombosed segment of the ulnar artery is displayed after resection (B).

correction than the localized lesions. They can be classified:

degenerative organic disease	— atherosclerosis
vasospastic organic disease	— e.g. thromboangiitis obliterans[631], (Fig. 2.151)
vasospastic functional disease	— Raynaud's — erythromelalgia

Raynaud's disease[632]. Due to small vessel spasm of unknown cause, this disorder is characterized by cyclical colour and temperature changes in the digits. The sudden onset of extreme pallor progressing to a cold, pale cyanosis, which is followed after a varying period by painful reactive hyperaemia, is diagnostic of the condition. The idiopathic disease is invariably symmetrical and bilateral and usually found in females between fifteen and forty-five.

Raynaud's phenomenon presents in the same manner but has some underlying associated disorder[633]. Thus, the phenomenon is encountered in the following conditions: scleroderma[634], polyarteritis nodosa, systemic

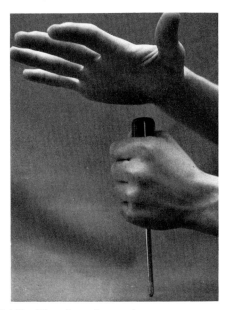

Fig. 2.150 'Hypothenar hammer'.

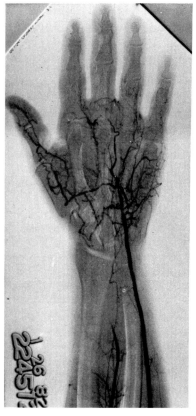

Fig. 2.151 This patient shows extensive vasospastic disease in the digital arteries with absent flow in the radial artery. (Arteriograms by courtesy of C. S. Wheeler.)

lupus erythematosus, mixed connective tissue disease, rheumatoid arthritis, cervical rib, thromboangiitis obliterans, cryoglobulinaemia, the use of vibratory tools[635,636] and others. Investigations should be instituted to exclude such underlying disease.

In both the phenomenon and the disease, a minority of cases become progressively worse, with later development of trophic changes in the affected digits, recurrent infection and even focal gangrene.

Vibration syndrome (= dead hand syndrome[637] = white finger disease[638] = occupational Raynaud's disease[639]). This syndrome occurs in those who use vibratory tools, especially if those tools are worn and are used in a cold workplace. It is characterized by changes in both the nerves[640,641] and the vessels of the digits. The cold immersion test is used to evaluate the severity of the condition, and a 'squeeze test' has been described[642] in which the patient squeezes a grip dynamometer for 5 seconds. If positive, clear demarcation results between the perfused and non-perfused portions of the digits and persists for more than 60 seconds.

Cumulative trauma disorders (CTD) (p. 156) may be associated with reduction in radial and ulnar arterial blood flow[643].

INDICATIONS

The first service that the physician can perform for any patient with vessel disease is to persuade him to *stop smoking*[644]. Indeed, the deleterious effects of smoking on flow are such as to compromise any proposed surgical procedure, and the surgeon is justified in refusing to perform that surgery until the patient has abstained for six weeks. Sometimes drawing a parallel between what is happening in the digital vessels with what may be going on in the coronary and cerebral circulation serves to drive home the point.

Proximal occlusions should be explored, excised and repaired; this usually requires a vein graft. The *in situ* technique, now commonly used in the lower extremity, has been employed in the upper[645].

Ulnar artery thrombosis is cured in most patients by resection of the thrombosed segment. In itself, resection is surprisingly effective, probably by removing any vasospastic effects of the thrombus and also by effecting a local sympathectomy[646]. In this, as in other major vessel resections, replacement with a reversed vein graft increases the chances of a successful outcome. The difficulty in performing such a graft lies in finding a point in the vascular tree for the distal anastomosis with sufficient run-off to prevent graft failure, while not interfering appreciably with existing circulation. Such a vein graft is not itself without potential complications

(Fig. 2.152). *Microangioscopy*[647] is of value in inspecting vessels distal to occlusions of the ulnar artery and also of vessels more distally. With microvascular techniques, exploration of digital occlusions is well justified.

Where no localized occlusion is encountered, and no systemic cause can be found, or when treated, leaves persistent generalized peripheral vascular problems, biofeedback techniques should first be tried[648]. If these fail, *sympathectomy* may be of value. In those cases in whom the results of the cold immersion test were markedly improved by digital nerve block, digital sympathectomy[649–652] has been shown to be of value. In occasional patients improvement in the cold immersion test may be poor after digital nerve block, better after stellate ganglion block. In such circumstances, cervical sympathectomy[653,654] may give relief. Patients should be warned that the gain may prove to be only temporary. The changes seen in CTD are better managed by exercise than by rest[643].

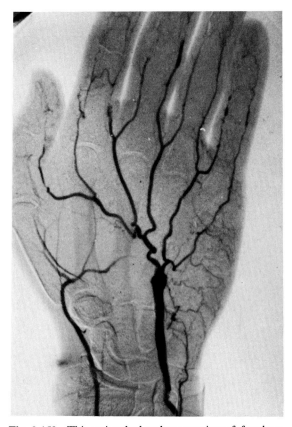

Fig. 2.152 This patient had undergone vein graft for ulnar artery thrombosis. It can be seen in this subtraction angiogram that multiple emboli are present throughout the digital arterial tree, probably arising from mural thrombi in the vein graft.

See Green D P 1993 Operative Hand Surgery, 3rd edn. Churchill Livingstone, New York, p. 2262.

Surgical planning

On completion of examination, the surgeon knows which of the eight basic hand functions are impaired and, of those, which are most required by the patient in pursuit of his occupation and recreation. He has also determined as fully as possible what contribution each anatomical structure makes to the impairment of hand function. Assuming that the patient is at a 'plateau' in his recovery and that all conservative aids offered by physical therapy and splintage have been exhausted, it remains for him to plan a surgical programme designed to restore the maximum hand function attainable. In doing so, efforts should be directed primarily at the functions which by their impairment prevent the patient from doing his regular job. For example, after severe injury, a hand may show loss of five of the eight basic functions (p. 158). However, of those only one, let us say power grasp in the non-dominant hand, may be essential. Having analysed the anatomical deficits, the surgeon may realize that, while they are multiple, only absence of flexion in the proximal interphalangeal joints of the badly injured ring and small fingers is preventing power grasp. Damage to both extensors and flexors may make the achievement of active motion unlikely but arthrodesis in a carefully selected position would result in a functional hand despite the other disabilities. In short, the reconstruction should be tailored to the individual needs of the patient. This approach is not only the most pragmatic but also serves to simplify for the surgeon what may be a bewildering complexity of structural and dynamic disturbance.

Certain general rules should assist the surgeon in reconstruction. Adequate *blood supply* must be present to ensure healing of wounds by primary intention. The *skeleton* is the structure on which all reconstruction is built. Non-union and malunion of fractures should therefore be corrected by bone graft and osteotomy allied with internal or external fixation. *Skin cover* must be stable and sufficiently robust as to permit whatever procedures on deep structures may be necessary. These are the three basic prerequisites. If they are unsound, steps should be taken to restore them. Sensation must be restored to a degree which is at the least protective. *Joint motion* must be secured before tendons can be expected to function. This may require not only capsulectomy in its various forms but also tenolysis and release of contractures in muscle and skin, as in adduction deformities of the thumb. Only after all these preliminaries have been completed successfully can the ultimate goal of restoration of motion be approached by appropriate *tendon grafts* or *transfers*.

Every attempt should be made to reduce the number of surgical procedures, for each is an assault, however elegant technically, from which the hand must recover. Grouping of procedures is one of the intellectual pleasures of reconstructive surgery of the hand. Release of an adduction contracture of the thumb can well be combined with an opponensplasty, for nought will be lost to the former by the immobilization required for the success of the transfer. If, however, the release reveals a lack of skin cover sufficient to require a distant pedicle flap, then the transfer must be postponed and the release maintained by static means. The passive motion necessary in the proximal interphalangeal joint for a tendon graft to function may require extensive work on the capsular structures, the benefit of which may be maintained only by early motion with appropriate dynamic splintage. The tendon graft must clearly wait. Many more hypothetical situations could be put forward to illustrate the point, some simple, some sufficiently problematical as to have several correct solutions — or none at all. The essence of the matter is that as many steps should be taken as possible in one procedure while being confident that the benefits of none are lost in the process.

REFERENCES

1. Arndt R 1987 Work pace, stress, and cumulative trauma disorders. J Hand Surg (Am) 12: 866–869
2. Louis D S 1987 Cumulative trauma disorders. J Hand Surg (Am) 12: 823–825
3. Punnett L 1987 Upper extremity musculoskeletal disorders in hospital workers. J Hand Surg (Am) 12: 858–862
4. Armstrong T J 1986 Ergonomics and cumulative trauma disorders. Hand Clin 2: 553–565
5. Silverstein B, Fine L, Stetson D 1987 Hand-wrist disorders among investment casting plant workers. J Hand Surg (Am) 12: 838–844
6. Buckle P 1987 Musculoskeletal disorders of the upper extremities: the use of epidemiologic approaches in industrial setting. J Hand Surg (Am) 12: 885–889
7. Muffly-Elsey D, Flinn-Wagner S 1987 Proposed screening tool for the detection of cumulative trauma disorders of the upper extremity. J Hand Surg (Am) 12: 931–935
8. Lutz G, Hansford T 1987 Cumulative trauma disorder controls: the ergonomics program at Ethicon, Inc. J Hand Surg (Am) 12: 863–866

9. Blair S J, Bear-Lehman J 1987 Prevention of upper extremity occupational disorders. J Hand Surg (Am) 12: 821–822
10. Smith B L 1987 An inside look: hand injury-prevention program. J Hand Surg (Am) 12: 940–943
11. Meagher S W 1987 Tool design for prevention of hand and wrist injuries. J Hand Surg (Am) 12: 855–857
12. Blair S J, McCormick E 1985 Prevention of trauma: cooperation toward a better working environment. J Hand Surg (Am) 10: 953–958
13. Schultz-Johnson K 1987 Assessment of upper extremity — injured persons' return to work potential. J Hand Surg (Am) 12: 950–957
14. Benner C L, Schilling A D, Klein L 1987 Coordinated teamwork in California industrial rehabilitation. J Hand Surg (Am) 12: 936–939
15. Jones L A 1989 The assessment of hand function: a critical review of techniques. J Hand Surg (Am) 14: 221–228
16. Herbin M L 1987 Work capacity evaluation for occupational hand injuries. J Hand Surg (Am) 12: 958–961
17. Fess E E 1986 The need for reliability and validity in hand assessment instruments. J Hand Surg (Am) 11: 621–623
18. Blumenthal S M 1987 Vocational rehabilitation with the industrially injured worker. J Hand Surg (Am) 12: 926–930
19. Dobyns J H 1987 Role of the physician in workers' compensation injuries. J Hand Surg (Am) 12: 826–829
20. Guides to evaluation of permanent impairment, 3rd edn. 1990 American Medical Association, Chicago, IL
21. Goldner J L 1983 Pain: general review and selected problems affecting the upper extremity. J Hand Surg (Am) 8: 740–745
22. Kleinert H E, Cole N M, Wayne L, Harvey R, Kutz J E, Atasoy E 1973 Post-traumatic sympathetic dystrophy. Orth Clin North Am 4: 917–927
23. Kozin F, McCarty D J, Genant H 1976 The reflex sympathetic dystrophy syndrome I. Clinical and histologic studies: evidence for bilaterality, response to corticosteroids and articular involvement. Am J Med 60: 321–331
24. Kozin F, Genant C, Bekerman C, McCarty D J 1976 The reflex sympathetic dystrophy syndrome II. Roentgenographic and scintigraphic evidence of bilaterality and of periarticular accentuation. Am J Med 60: 332–338
25. Pak T J, Martin G M, Magness J L, Kavanaugh G L 1970 Reflex sympathetic dystrophy, review of 140 cases. Minn Med 53: 507–512
26. An H S, Hawthorne K B, Jackson W T 1988 Reflex sympathetic dystrophy and cigarette smoking. J Hand Surg (Am) 13: 458–460
27. Colles A 1814 On fracture of the carpal extremity of the radius. Edin Med Surg J 10: 181 (reprinted in Clin Orth Rel Res (1972) 83: 3–5)
28. Atkins R M, Duckworth T, Kanis J A 1990 Features of algodystrophy after Colles' fracture. J Bone Joint Surg (Br) 72: 105–110
29. Lankford L L 1993 Reflex sympathetic dystrophy. In: Green D P (ed) Operative hand surgery. Churchill Livingstone, New York, pp 627–660
30. Forster R S, Fu F H 1985 Reflex sympathetic dystrophy in children: a case report and review of literature. Orthopedics 8: 475–476
31. Sudeck P 1900 Uber die akute entzundliche Knochenatropie. Arch Klin Chir 11: 147
32. Rohrich R J, Stevenson T R, Piepgrass W 1987 End-stage reflex sympathetic dystrophy. Plastic Reconstr Surg 79: 625–626
33. Lagier R, Chamay A 1984 Localized Sudeck's dystrophy and distal interphalangeal osteoarthritis of a finger: anatomicoradiologic study. J Hand Surg (Am) 9: 328–332
34. Mackinnon S E, Holder L E 1984 The use of three-phase radionuclide bone scanning in the diagnosis of reflex sympathetic dystrophy. J Hand Surg (Am) 9: 556–563
35. Werner R, Davidoff G, Jackson M D, Cremer S et al 1989 Factors affecting the sensitivity and specificity of the three-phase technetium bone scan in the diagnosis of reflex sympathetic dystrophy syndrome in the upper extremity. J Hand Surg (Am) 14: 520–523
36. Watson H K, Carlson L 1987 Treatment of reflex sympathetic dystrophy of the hand with an active 'stress loading' program. J Hand Surg (Am) 12: 779–785
37. Linson M A, Leffert R, Todd D P 1983 The treatment of upper extremity reflex sympathetic dystrophy with prolonged continuous stellate ganglion blockade. J Hand Surg (Am) 8: 153–159
38. Poplawski Z J, Wiley A M, Murray J F 1983 Post-traumatic dystrophy of the extremities. A clinical review and trial of treatment. J Bone Joint Surg 65A: 642–655
39. McKain C W, Urban B J, Goldner J L 1983 The effects of intravenous regional guanethidine and reserpine — a controlled study. J Bone Joint Surg (Am) 65: 808–811
40. Bechtol C O 1954 Grip test: use of dynamometer with adjustable handle spacings. J Bone Joint Surg 36A: 820–824
41. Mathiowetz V, Weber K, Volland G, Kashman N 1984 Reliability and validity of grip and pinch strength. J Hand Surg (Am) 9: 222–226
42. Mathiowetz V, Rennells C, Donahoe L 1985 Effect of elbow position on grip and key pinch strength. J Hand Surg (Am) 10: 694–697
43. Young V L, Pin P, Kraemer B A, Gould R B et al 1989 Fluctuation in grip and pinch strength among normal subjects. J Hand Surg (Am) 14: 125–129
44. Anderson P A, Chanoski C E, Devan D L, McMahon B L, Whelan E P 1990 Normative study of grip and wrist flexion strength employing a BTE Work Simulator. J Hand Surg (Am) 15: 420–425
45. Hildreth D H, Breidenbach W C, Lister G D, Hodges A D 1989 Detection of submaximal effort by use of the rapid exchange grip. J Hand Surg (Am) 14: 742–745
46. Grunert B K, Devine C A, Matloub H S, Sanger J R, Yousif N J 1988 Flashback after traumatic hand injuries: prognostic indicators. J Hand Surg (Am) 13: 125–127
47. Grunert B K, Devine C A, McCallum-Burke S, Matloub H S et al 1989 On-site work evaluations: desensitisation for avoidance reactions following severe hand injuries. J Hand Surg (Br) 14: 239–241
48. Grunert B K, Matloub H S, Sanger J R, Yousif N J 1990 Treatment of posttraumatic stress disorder after work-related hand trauma. J Hand Surg (Am) 15: 511–515

49. Louis D S, Lamp M K, Greene T L 1985 The upper extremity and psychiatric illness. J Hand Surg (Am) 10: 687–693
50. Smith R J 1975 Factitious lymphedema of the hand. J Bone Joint Surg 57A: 89–94
51. Kusumi R K, Plouffe J F 1981 Gas in soft tissue of forearm in an 18-year-old emotionally disturbed diabetic. J Am Med Assoc 246: 679–680
52. Secretan H 1901 Hard edema and traumatic hyperplasia of the dorsum of the metacarpus. Rev Med Suisse Rom 21: 409
53. Romm S 1986 Henri-Francois Secretan. Hand Clin 2: 453–456
54. Reading G 1980 Secretan's syndrome: hard edema of the dorsum of the hand. Plastic Reconstr Surg 65: 182–187
55. Saferin E H, Posch J L 1976 Secretan's disease. Posttraumatic hard edema of the dorsum of the hand. Plastic Reconstr Surg 58: 703–707
56. Agris J, Simmons C 1978 Factitious (self-inflicted) skin wounds. Plastic Reconstr Surg 62: 686–692
57. Phelps D B, Buchler U, Boswick J A 1977 The diagnosis of factitious ulcer of the hand: a case report. J Hand Surg 2: 105–108
58. Vetter W L, Weiland A J, Arnett F C 1983 Factitious extension contracture of the elbow: case report. J Hand Surg (Am) 8: 277–279
59. Simmons B P, Vasile R 1980 The clenched fist syndrome. J Hand Surg 5: 420–427
60. Wallace P, Fitzmorris C 1978 The S-H-A-F-T syndrome in the upper extremity. J Hand Surg 3: 492–494
61. Salisbury R E, Dingeldein G P 1988 The burned hand and upper extremity. In: Green D P (ed) Operative hand surgery, 2nd edn. Churchill Livingstone, Edinburgh
62. Achauer B M, Brody G S, Wilson-Mackby L 1979 A classification of burned hand deformities. Orthopaedic Rev, 8: 71–77
63. Lister G D 1985 Local flaps to the hand. Hand Clin 1: 621–640
64. Matthews R N, Morgan B D 1987 Multiple seagull flaps for digital contractures in electrical burns. Br J Plastic Surg 40: 47–51
65. May J W Jr, Donelan M B, Toth B A, Wall J 1984 Thumb reconstruction in the burned hand by advancement pollicization of the second ray remnant. J Hand Surg (Am) 9: 484–489
66. Cherup L L, Zachary L S, Gottlieb L J, Petti C A 1990 The radial forearm skin graft-fascial flap. Plastic Reconstr Surg 85: 898–902
67. Pensler J M, Steward R, Lewis S R, Herndon D N 1988 Reconstruction of the burned palm: full thickness versus split-thickness skin grafts — long-term follow-up. Plastic Reconstr Surg 81: 46–49
68. Lister G D 1993 Skin Flaps. In: Green D P (ed) Operative hand surgery. Churchill Livingstone, New York, pp 1741–1822
69. Furnas D W 1985 Z-plasties and related procedures for the hand and upper limb. Hand Clin 1: 649–665
70. Spinner M 1969 Fashioned transpositional flap for soft tissue adduction contracture of the thumb. Plastic Reconstr Surg 44: 345–348
71. Green D P, Dominguez O J 1979 A transpositional skin flap for release of volar contractures of a finger at the MP joint. Plastic Reconstr Surg 64: 516–520
72. Joshi B B 1972 Dorsolateral flap from same finger to relieve flexion contracture. Plastic Reconstr Surg 49: 186–189
73. Lister G D 1981 The theory of the transposition flap and its practical application in the hand. Clin Plastic Surg 8: 115–128
74. McCash C R 1956 Cross-arm bridge flaps in the repair of flexion contractures of the finger. Br Plastic Surg 9: 25–33
75. Mackinnon S E, Gruss J S 1985 Soft tissue expanders in upper limb surgery. J Hand Surg (Am) 10: 749–754
76. Morgan R F, Edgerton M T 1985 Tissue expansion in reconstructive hand surgery: case report. J Hand Surg (Am) 10: 754–757
77. Matev I B 1980 Tactile gnosis in free skin grafts in the hand. Br J Plastic Surg 33: 434–439
78. Porter R W 1968 Functional assessment of transplanted skin in volar defects of the digits. J Bone Joint Surg 50A: 955–963
79. Freiburg A, Manktelow R 1972 The Kutler repair for fingertip amputations. Plastic Reconstr Surg 50: 371–375
80. Lister GD 1991 The VY advancement flap. In: Foucher G (ed) Fingertip and nailbed injuries. Churchill Livingstone, Edinburgh, pp 52–61
81. Joshi B B 1974 A local dorsolateral island flap for restoration of sensation after avulsion injury of fingertip pulp. Plastic Reconstr Surg 54: 175–182
82. Kato H, Ogino T, Minami A, Usui M 1989 Restoration of sensibility in fingers repaired with free sensory flaps from the toe. J Hand Surg (Am) 14: 49–54
83. Nicolai J P A, Hentenaar G 1981 Sensation in cross-finger flaps. Hand 13: 12–16
84. Kleinert H E, McAlister C G, MacDonald C J, Kutz J E 1974 A critical evaluation of cross-finger flaps. J Trauma 14: 756–763
85. Flatt A E 1957 The thenar flap. J Bone Joint Surg 39B: 80–85
86. Neu B R, Murray J F, MacKenzie J K 1985 Profundus tendon blockage: quadriga in finger amputations. J Hand Surg (Am) 10: 878–883
87. Verdan C 1960 Syndrome of the quadriga. Surg Clin North Am 40: 425–426
88. Posner M 1979 Ray transposition for central digital loss. J Hand Surg 4: 242–257
89. Colen L, Bunkis J, Gordon L, Walton R 1985 Functional assessment of ray transfer for central digital loss. J Hand Surg (Am) 10: 232–237
90. Steichen J B, Idler R S 1986 Results of central ray resection without bony transposition. J Hand Surg (Am) 11: 466–474
91. Littler J W 1976 On making a thumb: one hundred years of surgical effort. J Hand Surg 1: 35–51
92. Verdan C 1968 The reconstruction of the thumb. Surg Clin North Am 48: 1033–1061
93. Miura T 1973 Thumb reconstruction using radial innervated cross-finger pedicle graft. J Bone Joint Surg 55A: 563–569
94. Rybka F J, Pratt F E 1979 Thumb reconstruction with a sensory flap from the dorsum of the index finger. Plastic Reconstr Surg 64: 141–144
95. Bunnell S 1931 Physiologic reconstruction of the thumb after total loss. Surg Obstet Gynecol 52: 245–248

96. Matev I B 1980 Thumb reconstruction through metacarpal bone lengthening. J Hand Surg 5: 482–487

97. Matev I B 1989 The bone-lengthening method in hand reconstruction: twenty years' experience. J Hand Surg (Am) 14: 376–378

98. Reid D A C 1980 The Gillies thumb lengthening operation. Hand 12: 123–129

99. Chase R A 1973 Atlas of hand surgery. W B Sanders Co, Philadelphia

100. Morgan L R, Stein F 1972 Method for a rapid and good thumb reconstruction. Plastic Reconstr Surg 50: 131–133

101. Buck-Gramcko D 1971 Pollicisation of the index finger. J Bone Joint Surg 53A: 1605–1617

102. Buck-Gramcko D 1977 Thumb reconstruction by digital transposition. Orthopedic Clin North Am 8: 329–342

103. Ward J W, Pensler J M, Parry S W 1985 Pollicization for thumb reconstruction in severe pediatric hand burns. Plastic Reconstr Surg 76: 927–932

104. Lister G D, Kalisman M, Tsai T M 1983 Reconstruction of the hand with free microneurovascular toe-to-hand transfer: experience with 54 toe transfers. Plastic Reconstr Surg 71: 372–386

105. Yoshimura M 1980 Toe-to-hand transfer. Plastic Reconstr Surg 66: 74–83

106. Lister G D 1988 Microsurgical transfer of the second toe for congenital deficiency of the thumb. Plastic Reconstr Surg 82: 658–665

107. Bourne M H, Wood M B, Cooney W P 1988 Reconstruction by free-tissue transfer of electively amputated parts. Surg Rounds Ortho 56–61

108. May J W Jr, Rothkopf D M, Savage R C, Atkinson R 1989 Elective cross-hand transfer: a case report with a five year follow-up. J Hand Surg (Am) 14: 28–34

109. Murray J F, Carman W, MacKenzie J K 1977 Transmetacarpal amputation of the index finger: a clinical assessment of hand strength and complications. J Hand Surg 2: 471–481

110. Lipton H A, May J W Jr, Simon S R 1987 Preoperative and postoperative gait analyses of patients undergoing great toe-to-thumb transfer. J Hand Surg (Am) 12: 66–69

111. Koman L A, Poehling G G, Price J L 1986 Thumb reconstruction — an algorithm. Ortho 9: 873–878

112. May J W Jr, Bartlett S P 1985 Great toe-to-hand free tissue transfer for thumb reconstruction. Hand Clin 1: 271–284

113. Lister G D, Kalisman M, Tsai TM 1983 Reconstruction of the hand with free microneurovascular toe-to-hand transfer: experience with 54 toe transfers. Plastic Reconstr Surg 71: 372–386

114. Frykman G K, O'Brien B M, Morrison W A, MacLeod A M 1986 Functional evaluation of the hand and foot after one-stage toe-to-hand transfer. J Hand Surg (Am) 11: 9–17

115. Poppen N K, Norris T R, Buncke H J Jr 1983 Evaluation of sensibility and function with microsurgical free tissue transfer of the great toe to the hand for thumb reconstruction. J Hand Surg (Am) 8: 516–531

116. Wilson C S, Buncke H J, Alpert B S, Gordon L 1984 Composite metacarpophalangeal joint reconstruction in great toe-to-hand free tissue transfers. J Hand Surg (Am) 9: 645–649

117. Wei F C, Chen H C, Chuang C C, Noordhoff M S 1988 Reconstruction of the thumb with a trimmed-toe transfer technique. Plastic Reconstr Surg 82: 506–515

118. Koman L A, Weiland A J, Moore J R 1985 Toe-to-hand transfer based on the medial plantar artery. J Hand Surg (Am) 10: 561–566

119. Morrison W A, O'Brien B M, MacLeod A M 1980 Thumb reconstruction with a free neurovascular wrap-around flap from the big toe. J Hand Surg 5: 575

120. Urbaniak J R 1985 Wrap-around procedure for thumb reconstruction. Hand Clin 1: 259–269

121. Leung P C 1980 Transplantation of the second toe to the hand. A preliminary report of sixteen cases. J Bone Joint Surg (Am) 62: 990–996

122. Wang W 1983 Keys to successful second toe-to-hand transfer: a review of 30 cases. J Hand Surg (Am) 8: 902–906

123. Leung P C 1985 Thumb reconstruction using second-toe transfer. Hand Clin 1: 285–295

124. Lister G D 1988 Microsurgical transfer of the second toe for congenital deficiency of the thumb. Plastic Reconstr Surg 82: 658–665

125. Singer D I, O'Brien B M, Angel M F, Gumley G J 1989 Digital distraction lengthening followed by free vascularized epiphyseal joint transfer. J Hand Surg (Am) 14: 508–512

126. Furnas D W, Achauer B M 1983 Microsurgical transfer of the great toe to the radius to provide prehension after partial avulsion of the hand. J Hand Surg (Am) 8: 453–460

127. Morrison W A, O'Brien B M, MacLeod A M 1984 Ring finger transfer in reconstruction of transmetacarpal amputations. J Hand Surg (Am) 9A: 4–11

128. Yu Z J 1987 Reconstruction of a digitless hand. J Hand Surg (Am) 12: 722–726

129. Krylov V S, Milanov N O, Borovikov A M, Trofimaov E I, Shiriaev A A 1985 Functional reconstruction of both hands by free transfer of combined second and third toes from both feet. Plastic Reconstr Surg 75: 584–589

130. Wei F C, Chen H C, Chuang C C, Noordhoff M S 1988 Simultaneous multiple toe transfers in hand reconstruction. Plastic Reconstr Surg 81: 366–377

131. Wei F C, Colony L H, Chen H C, Chuang C C, Noordhoff M S 1989 Combined second and third toe transfer. Plastic Reconstr Surg 84: 651–661

132. Rose E H 1984 Reconstruction of central metacarpal ray defects of the hand with a free vascularized double metatarsal and metatarsophalangeal joint transfer. J Hand Surg (Am) 9A: 28–31

133. Gordon L, Leitner D W, Buncke H J, Alpert B S 1985 Hand reconstruction for multiple amputations by double microsurgical toe transplantation. J Hand Surg (Am) 10: 218–225

134. Wei F C, Chen H C, Chuang C C, Noordhoff M S 1986 Reconstruction of a hand, amputated at the metacarpophalangeal level, by means of combined second and third toes from each foot: a case report. J Hand Surg (Am) 11: 340–344

135. Greenberg B M, May J W Jr 1988 Great toe-to-hand transfer: role of the preoperative lateral arteriogram of foot. J Hand Surg (Am) 13: 411–414

136. Lamb D W 1983 Prosthetics in the upper extremity. J Hand Surg (Am) 8: 774–777

137. Northmore-Ball, Heger H, Hunter G A 1980 The below-elbow myo-electric prosthesis with the hook and functional hand. J Bone Surg (Br) 62: 363–367

138. Dick T, Lamb D W, Douglas W B 1984 A wrist-powered hand prosthesis. J Bone Joint Surg (Br) 66: 742–744

139. Lamb D W, Dick T D, Douglas W B 1988 A new prosthesis for the upper limb. J Bone Joint Surg (Br) 70: 140–144

140. Pillet J 1983 Esthetic hand prostheses. J Hand Surg (Am) 8: 778–781

141. Beasley R W 1987 Hand and finger prostheses. J Hand Surg (Am) 12: 144–147

142. Kleinert H E, Putcha S M, Ashbell T S, Kutz J E 1967 The deformed fingernail, a frequent result of failure to repair nailbed injuries. J Trauma 7: 176–190

143. Zook E G, Russell R C 1990 Reconstruction of a functional and esthetic nail. Hand Clin 6: 59–68

144. Atasoy E, Godfrey A, Kalisman M 1983 The antenna: procedure for the 'hook-nail' deformity. J Hand Surg (Am) 8: 55–58

145. Lister G D 1990 Microvascular free transfer of the nail. In: Strauch B, Vasconez L O, Hall-Findlay E J (eds) Grabb's Encyclopedia of flaps. Little Brown & Co, Boston, pp 898–901

146. Morrison W A 1990 Microvascular nail transfer. Hand Clin 6: 69–76

147. Koshima I, Soeda S, Takase T, Yamasaki M 1988 Free vascularized nail grafts. J Hand Surg (Am) 13: 29–32

148. Beasley R W, de Beze G M 1990 Prosthetic substitution for fingernails. Hand Clin 6: 105–110

149. Jupiter J B, Koniuch M P, Smith R J 1985 The management of delayed union and nonunion of the metacarpals and phalanges. J Hand Surg (Am) 10: 457–466

150. Calkins M S, Burkhalter W, Reyes F 1987 Traumatic segmental bone defects in the upper extremity. J Bone Joint Surg (Am) 69: 19–27

151. Gordon L, Buncke H J, Alpert B S, Wilson C, Kock R A 1985 Free vascularized osteocutaneous transplants from the groin for delayed primary closure in the management of loss of soft-tissue and bone in the hand and wrist. Report of two cases. J Bone Joint Surg (Am) 67: 958–964

152. Rinaldi E 1987 Autografts in the treatment of osseous defects in the forearm and hand. J Hand Surg (Am) 12: 282–286

153. Smith R J, Brushart T M 1985 Allograft bone for metacarpal reconstruction. J Hand Surg (Am) 10: 325–334

154. Wood M B 1987 Upper extremity reconstruction by vascularized bone transfers: results and complications. J Hand Surg (Am) 12: 422–427

155. Kumar V P, Satku K, Helm R, Pho R W 1988 Radial reconstruction in segmental defects of both forearm bones. J Bone Joint Surg (Br) 70: 815–817

156. Dell P C, Sheppard J E 1984 Vascularized bone grafts in the treatment of infected forearm nonunions. J Hand Surg (Am) 9: 653–658

157. Lister G D 1993 Free skin and composite flaps. In: Green D P (ed) Operative hand surgery, 3rd edn. Churchill Livingstone, New York, pp 1103–1158

158. Seitz W H Jr, Froimson A I 1988 Management of malunited fractures of the metacarpal and phalangeal shafts. Hand Clin 4: 529–538

159. Gross M S, Gelberman R H 1985 Metacarpal rotational osteotomy. J Hand Surg (Am) 10: 105–108

160. Froimson A I 1981 Osteotomy for digital deformity. J Hand Surg 6: 585–589

161. Kornberg M, Aulicino P L 1985 Hand and wrist joint problems in patients with Ehlers–Danlos syndrome. J Hand Surg (Am) 10: 193–196

162. Srinivasan H 1981 A simple method for assessing abduction of the thumb. J Hand Surg 6: 583–584

163. Kuczynski K 1974 Carpometacarpal joint of the human thumb. J Anat 118: 119–126

164. Cooney W P, III Lucca M J, Chao E Y S, Linscheid R L 1981 The kinesiology of the thumb trapeziometacarpal joint. J Bone Joint Surg 63A: 1371–1381

165. Harris H, Joseph J 1949 Variation in the extension of the metacarpophalangeal and interphalangeal joints of the thumb. J Bone Joint Surg 31B: 547–559

166. Wilson R L, Liechty B W 1986 Complications following small joint injuries. Hand Clin 2: 329–345

167. Smith R J, Kaplan E B 1968 Camptodactyly and similar atraumatic flexion deformities of the proximal interphalangeal joints of the fingers. J Bone Joint Surg 50A: 1187–1203

168. Stern P J, Neale H W, Graham T J, Warden G D 1987 Classification and treatment of postburn proximal interphalangeal joint flexion contractures in children. J Hand Surg (Am) 12: 450–457

169. Fernandez G N 1988 Locking of a metacarpophalangeal joint caused by a haemangioma of the volar plate. J Hand Surg (Br) 13: 323–324

170. Alldred A 1954 A locked index finger. J Bone Joint Surg 36B: 102–103

171. Aston J N 1960 Locked middle finger. J Bone Joint Surg 42B: 75–79

172. Rankin E A, Uwagie-Ero S 1986 Locking of the metacarpophalangeal joint. J Hand Surg (Am) 11: 868–871

173. Posner M A, Langa V, Green S M 1986 The locked metacarpophalangeal joint: diagnosis and treatment. J Hand Surg (Am) 11: 249–253

174. Ostrowski D M 1990 Locking of the metacarpophalangeal joint: a case report and literature review. Cont Ortho 21: 265–269

175. Dupuytren G 1834 Permanent retraction of the fingers produced by an affliction of the palmar fascia. Lancet 2: 222

176. McFarlane R M 1983 The current status of Dupuytren's disease. J Hand Surg (Am) 8: 703–708

177. Hill N A, Hurst L C 1989 Dupuytren's contracture. Hand Clin 5: 349–357

178. Boswick J A, Burkhalter W E, Gonzalez R, Kilgore E S, Watson H K 1988 Symposium: Dupuytren's contracture. Cont Ortho 16: 71–110

179. Larsen R D, Takagishi N, Posch J L 1960 The pathogenesis of Dupuytren's contracture. J Bone Joint Surg 42A: 993–1007

180. Skoog T 1963 The pathogenesis and etiology of Dupuytren's contracture. Plastic Reconstr Surg 31: 258–267

181. Gabbiani G, Majho G 1972 Dupuytren's contracture:

fibroblast contraction? Am J Pathol 66: 131–138

182. Guber S, Rudolph R 1978 The myofibroblast. Surg Obstet Gynecol 146: 641–649

183. Badalamente M A, Stern L, Hurst L C 1983 The pathogenesis of Dupuytren's contracture: contractile mechanisms of the myofibroblasts. J Hand Surg (Am) 8: 235–243

184. Noble J, Heathcote J G, Cohen H 1984 Diabetes mellitus in the aetiology of Dupuytren's disease. J Bone Joint Surg (Br) 66: 322–325

185. An H S, Southworth S R, Jackson W T, Russ B 1988 Cigarette smoking and Dupuytren's contracture of the hand. J Hand Surg (Am) 13: 872–874

186. Luck J U 1959 Dupuytren's contracture. J Bone Joint Surg 41A: 635–664

187. McFarlane R M 1974 Patterns of diseased fascia in the fingers in Dupuytren's contracture. Plastic Reconstr Surg 54: 31–44

188. Mikkelsen O A 1976 Dupuytren's disease — a study of the pattern of distribution and stage of contracture in the hand. Hand 8: 265–271

189. White S 1984 Anatomy of the palmar fascia on the ulnar border of the hand. J Hand Surg (Br) 9: 50–56

190. Barton N J 1984 Dupuytren's's disease arising from the abductor digiti minimi. J Hand Surg (Br) 9: 265–270

191. Short W H, Watson H K 1982 Prediction of the spiral nerve in Dupuytren's contracture. J Hand Surg 7: 84–86

192. Elsahy N I 1976 Doppler ultrasound detection of displaced neurovascular bundles in Dupuytren's contracture. Plastic Reconstr Surg 57: 104–105

193. Gordon S 1964 Dupuytren's contracture, plantar involvement. Br J Plastic Surg 17: 421–423

194. Williams J L, Thomas C G 1968 Natural history of Peyronie's disease. Proc Roy Soc Med 61: 876–877

195. Bryan A S, Ghorbal M S 1988 The long-term results of closed palmar fasciotomy in the management of Dupuytren's contracture. J Hand Surg (Br) 13: 254–256

196. Ketchum L D, Hixson F P 1987 Dermofasciectomy and full-thickness grafts in the treatment of Dupuytren's contracture. J Hand Surg (Am) 12: 659–664

197. Lubahn J D, Lister G D, Wolfe T 1984 Fasciectomy and Dupuytren's disease: a comparison between the open-palm technique and wound closure. J Hand Surg (Am) 9A: 53–58

198. Schneider L H, Hankin F M, Eisenberg T 1986 Surgery of Dupuytren's disease: a review of the open palm method. J Hand Surg (Am) 11: 23–27

199. Gonzalez R I 1985 The use of skin grafts in the treatment of Dupuytren's contracture. Hand Clin 1: 641–647

200. Strickland J W, Bassett R L 1985 The isolated digital cord in Dupuytren's contracture: anatomy and clinical significance. J Hand Surg (Am) 10: 118–124

201. Kuhlmann J N, Boabighi A, Guero S, Mimoun M, Baux S 1988 Boutonniere deformity in Dupuytren's disease. J Hand Surg (Br) 13: 379–382

202. Zemel N P, Balcomb T V, Stark H H, Ashworth C R et al 1987 Dupuytren's disease in women: evaluation of long-term results after operation. J Hand Surg (Am) 12: 1012–1016

203. Garrod A E 1875 Concerning pads upon the finger

204. Mikkelsen O A 1977 Knuckle pads in Dupuytren's disease. Hand 9: 301–305

205. Legge J H, McFarlane R M 1980 Prediction of results of treatment of Dupuytren's disease. J Hand Surg 5: 608–616

206. Wolfe S J, Summerskill W H J, Davidson C S 1956 Thickening and contraction of the palmar fascia (Dupuytren's contracture) associated with alcoholism and hepatic cirrhosis. New Eng J Med 255: 559–563

207. Watson H K, Lovallo J L 1987 Salvage of severe recurrent Dupuytren's contracture of the ring and small fingers. J Hand Surg (Am) 12: 287–289

208. Smith R J 1971 Non-ischemic contractures of the intrinsic muscles of the hand. J Bone Joint Surg 53A: 1313–1331

209. Chicarilli Z N, Watson H K, Linberg R, Sasaki G 1986 Saddle deformity. Posttraumatic interosseous-lumbrical adhesions: review of eighty-seven cases. J Hand Surg (Am) 11: 210–218

210. Graham T J, Stern P J, True M S 1990 Classification and treatment of postburn metacarpophalangeal joint extension contractures in children. J Hand Surg (Am) 15: 450–456

211. Donaldson W R, Millender L W 1978 Chronic fracture subluxation of the proximal interphalangeal joint. J Hand Surg 3: 149–153

212. Kleinert H E, Kasdan M L 1965 Reconstruction of chronically subluxated proximal interphalangeal finger joint. J Bone Joint Surg 47A: 958–964

213. Palmer A K, Linscheid R L 1978 Chronic recurrent dislocation of the proximal interphalangeal joint of the finger. J Hand Surg 3: 95–97

214. Helm R H 1987 Hand function after injuries to the collateral ligaments of the metacarpophalangeal joint of the thumb. J Hand Surg (Br) 12: 252–255

215. Palmer A, Louis D 1978 Assessing ulnar instability of the metacarpophalangeal joint of the thumb. J Hand Surg 3: 542–546

216. Stothard J, Caird D M 1981 Experience with arthrography of the first metacarpophalangeal joint. Hand 13: 257–266

217. Tajima T 1988 Treatment of post-traumatic contracture of the hand. J Hand Surg (Br) 13: 118–129

218. Harrison D H 1977 The stiff proximal interphalangeal joint. Hand 9: 102–108

219. McCue F C, Honner R, Johnson M C, Gieck J H 1970 Athletic injuries of the proximal interphalangeal joint requiring surgical treatment. J Bone Joint Surg 52A: 937–956

220. Watson H K, Light T R, Johnson T R 1979 Checkrein resection for flexion contracture of the middle joint. J Hand Surg 4: 67–72

221. Eaton R G, Malerich M M 1980 Volar plate arthroplasty of the proximal interphalangeal joint: a review of ten years' experience. J Hand Surg 5: 260–268

222. Engkvist O, Johansson S H 1980 Perichondrial arthroplasty. Scand J Plastic Reconstr Surg 14: 71–87

223. Engkvist O, Ohlsen L N 1979 Reconstruction of articular cartilage with free autologous perichondrial grafts: an experimental study in rabbits. Scand J Plastic Reconstr Surg 13: 269–274

224. Engkvist O, Skoog V, Pastacaldi P, Yormuk E, Juhlin R 1979 The cartilaginous potential of the perichondrium

joints and their clinical relationships. Br Med J 1: 665

in rabbit ear and rib: a comparative study in vivo and vitro. Scand J Plastic Reconstr Surg 13: 275–280

225. Ohlsen L 1978 Cartilage regeneration from perichondrium. Experimental studies and clinical applications. Plastic Reconstr Surg 62: 507–513

226. Skoog T, Johansson S H 1976 The formation of articular cartilage from free perichondrial grafts. Plastic Reconstr Surg 57: 1–6

227. Upton J, Sohn S A, Glowacki J 1981 Neocartilage derived from transplanted perichondrium: what is it? Plastic Reconstr Surg 68: 166–172

228. Wu G, Johnson D E 1983 Perichondrial arthroplasty in the hand: a case report. J Hand Surg (Am) 8: 446–453

229. Seradge H, Kutz J A, Kleinert H E, Lister G D et al 1984 Perichondrial resurfacing arthroplasty in the hand. J Hand Surg (Am) 9: 880–886

230. Hume M C, Gellman H, McKellop H, Brumfield R H Jr 1990 functional range of motion of the joints of the hand. J Hand Surg (Am) 15: 240–244

231. Menon J 1983 Reconstruction of the metacarpophalangeal joint with autogenous metatarsal. J Hand Surg (Am) 8: 443–446

232. Tsai T M, Singer R 1984 Elective free vascularized double transfer of toe joint from second toe to proximal interphalangeal joint of index finger: a case report. J Hand Surg (Am) 9: 816–820

233. O'Brien B, Gould J S, Morrison W A, Russell R C et al 1984 Free vascularized small joint transfer to the hand. J Hand Surg (Am) 9: 634–641

234. Foucher G, Sammut D, Citron N 1990 Free vascularized toe-joint transfer in hand reconstruction: a series of 25 patients. Recon Microsurg 6: 201–208

235. Carroll R E, Hill N A 1969 Small joint arthrodesis in hand reconstruction. J Bone Joint Surg 51A: 1219–1221

236. Moberg E 1960 Arthrodesis of finger joints. Surg Clin North Am 40: 465–470

237. Robertson D C 1964 The fusion of interphalangeal joints. Can J Surg 7: 433–437

238. Ferlic D C, Turner B D, Clayton M L 1983 Compression arthrodesis of the thumb. J Hand Surg (Am) 8: 207–210

239. Ayres J R, Goldstrohm G L, Miller G J, Dell P C 1988 Proximal interphalangeal joint arthrodesis with the Herbert screw. J Hand Surg (Am) 13: 600–603

240. McGlynn J T, Smith R A, Bogumill G P 1988 Arthrodesis of small joints of the hand: a rapid and effective technique. J Hand Surg (Am) 13: 595–599

241. Buchler U, Aiken M A 1988 Arthrodesis of the proximal interphalangeal joint by solid bone grafting and plate fixation in extensive injuries to the dorsal aspect of the finger. J Hand Surg (Am) 13: 589–594

242. Lewis R C, Nordyke M D, Tenny J R 1986 The tenon method of small joint arthrodesis in the hand. J Hand Surg (Am) 11: 567–569

243. Khuri S M 1986 Tension band arthrodesis in the hand. J Hand Surg (Am) 11: 41–45

244. Braun R M, Rhoades C E 1985 Dynamic compression for small bone arthrodesis. J Hand Surg (Am) 10: 340–343

245. Wright C S, McMurtry R Y 1983 AO arthrodesis in the hand. J Hand Surg (Am) 8: 932–935

246. Clendenin M B, Smith R J 1984 Fifth metacarpal/hamate arthrodesis for posttraumatic osteoarthritis. J Hand Surg (Am) 9: 374–378

247. Black D M, Watson H K, Vender M I 1987 Arthroplasty of the ulnar carpometacarpal joints. J Hand Surg (Am) 12: 1071–1074

248. Taleisnik, Julio 1985 The wrist. Churchill Livingstone, New York

249. Lichtman D M 1988 The wrist and its disorders. WB Saunders, Philadelphia

250. Watson H K, Ashmead D 4th, Makhlouf M V 1988 Examination of the scaphoid. J Hand Surg (Am) 13: 657–660

251. Jackson W T, Protas J M 1981 Snapping scapholunate subluxation. J Hand Surg 6: 590–594

252. Czitrom A A, Lister G D 1988 Measurement of grip strength in the diagnosis of wrist pain. J Hand Surg (Am) 13: 16–19

253. Hardy D C, Totty W G, Reinus W R, Gilula L A 1987 Posteroanterior wrist radiography: importance of arm positioning. J Hand Surg (Am) 12: 504–508

254. Steyers C M, Blair W F 1989 Measuring ulnar variance: a comparison of techniques. J Hand Surg (Am) 14: 607–612

255. Palmer A K, Glisson R R, Werner F W 1984 Relationship between ulnar variance and triangular fibrocartilage complex thickness. J Hand Surg (Am) 9: 681–682

256. Czitrom A A, Dobyns J H, Linscheid R L 1987 Ulnar variance in carpal instability. J Hand Surg (Am) 12: 205–208

257. Campbell R D, Lance E M, Chin Bor Yeoh 1964 Lunate and perilunar dislocations. J Bone Joint Surg 46B: 55–72

258. Linscheid R L, Dobyns J H, Beabout J W, Bryan R S 1972 Traumatic instability of the wrist. J Bone Joint Surg 54A: 1612–1632

259. Garcia-Elias M, An K N, Amadio P C, Cooney W P, Linscheid RL 1989 Reliability of carpal angle determinations. J Hand Surg (Am) 14: 1017–1021

260. Youm Y, Flatt A 1980 Kinematics of the wrist. Clin Orthop 149: 21–32

261. Taleisnik J, Watson H K 1984 Midcarpal instability caused by malunited fractures of the distal radius. J Hand Surg (Am) 9: 350–357

262. Belsole R J, Eikman A, Muroff L R 1981 Bone scintigraphy in trauma of the hand and wrist. J Trauma 21: 163–166

263. Batillas J, Vasilas A, Pizzi W, Gokcebay T 1981 Bone scanning in the detection of occult fractures. J Trauma 21: 564–569

264. Pin P G, Semenkovich J W, Young V L, Bartell T et al 1988 Role of radionuclide imaging in the evaluation of wrist pain. J Hand Surg (Am) 13: 810–814

265. Nielsen P T, Hedeboe J 1984 Posttraumatic scapholunate dissociation detected by wrist cineradiography. J Hand Surg (Am) 9A: 135–138

266. Hankin F M, White S J, Braunstein E M, Louis D S 1986 Dynamic radiography evaluation of obscure wrist pain in the teenage patient. J Hand Surg (Am) 11: 805–809

267. Shigematsu S, Abe M, Onomura T, Kinoshita M, Inoue T 1989 Arthrography of the normal and posttraumatic wrist. J Hand Surg (Am) 14: 410–412

268. Palmer A K, Levinsohn E M, Kuzma G R 1983 Arthrography of the wrist. J Hand Surg (Am) 8: 15–23

269. Hardy D C, Totty W G, Carnes K M, Kyriakos M et al

1988 Arthrographic surface anatomy of the carpal triangular fibrocartilage complex. J Hand Surg (Am) 13: 823–829

270. Reinus W R, Hardy D C, Totty W G, Gilula L A 1987 Arthrographic evaluation of the carpal triangular fibrocartilage complex. J Hand Surg (Am) 12: 495–503

271. Zinberg E M, Palmer A K, Coren A B, Levinsohn E M 1988 The triple-injection wrist arthrogram. J Hand Surg (Am) 13: 803–809

272. Belsole R J, Quinn S F, Greene T L, Beatty M E, Rayhack J M 1990 Digital subtraction arthrography of the wrist. J Bone Joint Surg (Am) 72: 846–851

273. Posner M A, Greenspan A 1988 Trispiral tomography for the evaluation of wrist problems. J Hand Surg (Am) 13: 175–181

274. Blair W F, Berger R A, el-Khoury G Y 1985 Arthrotomography of the wrist: an experimental and preliminary clinical study. J Hand Surg (Am) 10: 350–359

275. Mino D E, Palmer A K, Levinsohn E M 1983 The role of radiography and computerized tomography in the diagnosis of subluxation and dislocation of the distal radioulnar joint. J Hand Surg (Am) 8: 23–31

276. King G J, McMurtry R Y, Rubenstein J D, Ogston N G 1986 Computerized tomography of the distal radioulnar joint: correlation with ligamentous pathology in a cadaveric model. J Hand Surg (Am) 11: 711–717

277. Weeks P M, Vannier M W, Stevens W G, Gayou D, Gilula L A 1985 Three-dimensional imaging of the wrist. J Hand Surg (Am) 10: 32–39

278. Engel J, Salai M, Yaffe B, Tadmor R 1987 The role of three dimension computerized imaging in hand surgery. J Hand Surg (Br) 12: 349–352

279. Kelly E P, Stanley J K 1990 Arthroscopy of the wrist. J Hand Surg (Br) 15: 236–242

280. North E R, Thomas S 1988 An anatomic guide for arthroscopic visualization of the wrist capsular ligaments. J Hand Surg (Am) 13: 815–822

281. Botte M J, Cooney W P, Linscheid R L 1989 Arthroscopy of the wrist: anatomy and technique. J Hand Surg (Am) 14: 313–316

282. Bora F W Jr 1985 Wrist arthroscope. J Hand Surg (Am) 10: 308

283. North E R, Thomas S 1988 An anatomic guide for arthroscopic visualization of the wrist capsular ligaments. J Hand Surg (Am) 13: 815–822

284. Kaempffe F, Peimer C A 1990 Distraction for wrist arthroscopy. J Hand Surg (Am) 15: 520–521

285. Whipple T L 1990 Precautions for arthroscopy of the wrist. Arthroscopy 6: 3–4

286. Toby E B, Poehling G G, Koman A L 1989 Midcarpal arthroscopy. Surg Rounds Ortho: 23–27

287. Koman L A, Poehling G G, Toby E B, Kammire G 1990 Chronic wrist pain: indications for wrist arthroscopy. Arthroscopy 6: 116–119

288. Cooney W P, Dobyns J H, Linscheid R L 1990 Arthroscopy of the wrist: anatomy and classification of carpal instability. Arthroscopy 6: 133–140

289. Fitzpatrick D 1989 Arthroscopic surgery of the wrist. Can Oper Room Nurs J 7: 4, 6, 8–9

290. Marshall J H, Sonsire J M, Nielsen P E, Nigogosyan G, Terzian J 1987 Digital angiography and osteoblastoma of the triquetrum. J Hand Surg (Am) 12: 256–258

291. Zlatkin M B, Chao P C, Osterman A L, Schnall M D et al 1989 Chronic wrist pain: evaluation with high resolution MR imaging. Radiology 173: 723–729

292. Reicher M A, Kellerhouse LE 1990 MRI of the wrist and hand. Raven Press, New York

293. Hentz V R, Marich K W, Dev P 1984 Preliminary study of the upper limb with the use of ultrasound transmission imaging. J Hand Surg (Am) 9: 188–193

294. Minami M, Yamazaki J, Chisaka N, Kato S et al 1987 Nonunion of the capitate. J Hand Surg (Am) 12: 1089–1091

295. Freeman B H, Hay E L 1985 Nonunion of the capitate: a case report. J Hand Surg (Am) 10: 187–190

296. Osterman A L, Mikulics M 1988 Scaphoid nonunion. Hand Clin 4: 437–455

297. Panagis J S, Gelberman R H, Taleisnik J, Baumgaertner M 1983 The arterial anatomy of the human carpus. Part II: The intraosseous vascularity. J Hand Surg (Am) 8: 375–382

298. Smith D K, Cooney W P 3rd, An K N, Linscheid R L, Chao E Y 1989 The effects of simulated unstable scaphoid fractures on carpal motion. J Hand Surg (Am) 14: 283–291

299. Engdahl D E, Schacherer T G 1989 A new method of evaluating angulation of scaphoid nonunions. J Hand Surg (Am) 14: 1033–1034

300. Sanders W E 1988 Evaluation of the humpback scaphoid by computed tomography in the longitudinal axial plane of the scaphoid. J Hand Surg (Am) 13: 182–187

301. Burgess R C 1987 The effect of a simulated scaphoid malunion on wrist motion. J Hand Surg (Am) 12: 774–776

302. Amadio P C, Berquist T H, Smith D K, Ilstrup D M et al 1989 Scaphoid malunion. J Hand Surg (Am) 14: 679–687

303. Vender M I, Watson H K, Wiener B D, Black D M 1987 Degenerative change in symptomatic scaphoid nonunion. J Hand Surg (Am) 12: 514–519

304. Watson H K, Ballet F L 1984 The SLAC wrist: scapholunate advanced collapse pattern of degenerative arthritis. J Hand Surg (Am) 9: 358–365

305. Frykman G K, Taleisnik J, Peters G, Kaufman R et al 1986 Treatment of nonunited scaphoid fractures by pulsed electromagnetic field and cast. J Hand Surg (Am) 11: 344–349

306. Cosio M Q, Camp R A 1986 Percutaneous pinning of symptomatic scaphoid nonunions. J Hand Surg (Am) 11: 350–355

307. Herbert J 1989 Internal fixation of the carpus with the Herbert bone screw system. J Hand Surg (Am) 14: 397–400

308. Adams B D, Blair W F, Reagan D S, Grundberg A B 1988 Technical factors related to Herbert screw fixation. J Hand Surg (Am) 13: 893–899

309. Viegas S F, Bean J W, Schram R A 1987 Transscaphoid fracture dislocations treated with open reduction and Herbert screw fixation. J Hand Surg (Am) 12: 992–999

310. Botte M J, Gelberman R H 1987 Modified technique for Herbert screw insertion in fractures of the scaphoid. J Hand Surg (Am) 12: 149–150

311. Botte M J, Mortensen W W, Gelberman R H, Rhoades C E, Gellman H 1988 Internal vascularity of the scaphoid in cadavers after insertion of the Herbert screw. J Hand Surg (Am) 13(2): 216–220

312. Fernandez D L 1984 A technique for anterior wedge-shaped grafts for scaphoid nonunions with carpal instability. J Hand Surg (Am) 9: 733–737

313. Boeckstyns M E, Busch P 1984 Surgical treatment of scaphoid pseudarthrosis: evaluation of the results after soft tissue arthroplasty and inlay bone grafting. J Hand Surg (Am) 9: 378–382

314. Boeckstyns M E, Kjaer L, Busch P, Holst-Nielsen F 1985 Soft tissue interposition arthroplasty for scaphoid nonunion. J Hand Surg (Am) 10: 109–114

315. Cooney W P, Linscheid R L, Dobyns J H, Wood M B 1988 Scaphoid nonunion: role of anterior interpositional bone grafts. J Hand Surg (Am) 13: 635–650

316. Nakamura R, Hori M, Horii E, Miura T 1987 Reduction of the scaphoid fracture with DISI alignment. J Hand Surg (Am) 12: 1000–1005

317. Fernandez D L 1990 Anterior bone grafting and conventional lag screw fixation to treat scaphoid nonunions. J Hand Surg (Am) 15: 140–147

318. Korkala O L, Antti-Poika I U 1989 Late treatment of scaphoid fractures by bone grafting and compression staple osteosynthesis. J Hand Surg (Am) 14: 491–495

319. Green D P 1985 The effect of avascular necrosis on Russe bone grafting for scaphoid nonunion. J Hand Surg 10A: 597–605

320. Garcia-Elias M, Vall A, Salo J M, Lluch A L 1988 Carpal alignment after different surgical approaches to the scaphoid: a comparative study. J Hand Surg (Am) 13: 604–612

321. Zemel N P, Start K K, Ashworth C R, Rickard T A, Anderson DR 1984 Treatment of selected patients with an ununited fracture of the proximal part of the scaphoid by excision of the fragment and insertion of a carved silicone-rubber spacer. J Bone Joint Surg (Am) 66: 510–517

322. Eaton R G, Akelman E, Eaton B H 1989 Fascial implant arthroplasty for treatment of radioscaphoid degenerative disease. J Hand Surg (Am) 14: 766–774

323. Green D P 1987 Proximal row carpectomy. Hand Clin 3: 163–168

324. Inglis A E, Jones E C 1977 Proximal row carpectomy for diseases of the proximal row. J Bone Joint Surg 59A: 460–463

325. Neviaser R J 1983 Proximal row carpectomy for posttraumatic disorders of the carpus. J Hand Surg (Am) 8: 301–305

326. Imbriglia J E, Broudy A S, Hagberg W C, McKernan D 1990 Proximal row carpectomy: clinical evaluation. J Hand Surg (Am) 15: 426–430

327. Buck-Gramcko D 1977 Denervation of the wrist joint. J Bone Joint Surg 59A: 54–61

328. Viegas S F, Rimoldi R, Patterson R 1989 Modified technique of intramedullary fixation for wrist arthrodesis. J Hand Surg (Am) 14: 618–623

329. Louis D S, Hankin F M 1986 Arthrodesis of the wrist: past and present. J Hand Surg (Am) 11: 787–789

330. Benkeddache Y, Gottesman H, Fourrier P 1984 Multiple stapling for wrist arthrodesis in the nonrheumatoid patient. J Hand Surg (Am) 9: 256–260

331. Wood M B 1987 Wrist arthrodesis using dorsal radial bone graft. J Hand Surg (Am) 12: 208–212

332. Rayan G M 1986 Wrist arthrodesis. J Hand Surg (Am) 11: 356–364

333. Ferlic C D, Morin P 1989 Indiopathic avascular necrosis of the scaphoid: Preiser's disease? J Hand Surg 14A: 13–16

334. Linscheid R L 1985 Kienbock's disease. J Hand Surg 10A: 1–3

335. Kienbock R 1910 Uber traumatische malacie des mondbeins und ihre folgezustande: entartungsformen und kompressionfrakturen. Fortschr Geb Rontgenstrahlen 16: 78

336. Kienbock R 1910 Concerning traumatic malacia of the lunate and its consequences: degeneration and compression fractures (reprinted in Clin Orth Rel Res 149: 4–8, 1980)

337. Almquist E E 1987 Kienbock's disease. Hand Clin 3: 141–148

338. Gelberman R H, Bauman T, Menon J, Akeson W 1975 Ulnar variance in Kienbock's disease. J Bone Joint Surg 57A: 674–676

339. Sowa D T, Holder L E, Patt P G, Weiland A J 1989 Application of magnetic resonance imaging to ischemic necrosis of the lunate J Hand Surg 14A: 1008–1016

340. Watson H K, Ryu J, DiBella A 1985 An approach to Kienbock's disease: triscaphe arthrodesis. J Hand Surg 10A: 179–187

341. Horii E, Garcia-Elias M, Bishop A T, Cooney W P et al 1990 Effect on force transmission across the carpus in procedures used to treat Kienbock's disease. J Hand Surg (Am) 15: 393–400

342. Blanco R H 1985 Excision of the lunate in Kienbock's disease: long-term results. J Hand Surg (Am) 10: 1008–1013

343. Swanson A B, Maupin B K, de Groot Swanson G, Ganzhorn R W, Moss S H 1985 Lunate implant resection arthroplasty: long-term results. J Hand Surg (Am) 10: 1013–1024

344. Alexander A H, Turner M A, Alexander C E, Lichtman D M 1990 Lunate silicone replacement arthroplasty in Kienbock's disease: a long-term follow-up. J Hand Surg (Am) 15: 401–407

345. Kleinert J M, Lister G D 1986 Silicone implants. Hand Clin 2: 271–290

346. Linscheid R L, Dobyns J H, Beckenbaugh R D, Cooney W P 3rd, Wood M B 1983 Instability patterns of the wrist. J Hand Surg (Am) 8: 682–686

347. Cooney W P, Garcia-Elias M, Dobyns J H, Linscheid R L 1989 Anatomy and mechanics of carpal instability. Surg Rounds Ortho: 15–24

348. Cooney W P, Dobyns J H, Linscheid R L 1990 Arthroscopy of the wrist: anatomy and classification of carpal instability. Arthroscopy 6: 133–140

349. Howard F, Thomas F, Wojeie E 1974 Rotatory subluxation of the navicular. Clin Ortho Rel Res 104: 134

350. Mayfield J K, Johnson R P, Kilcoyne R K 1980 Carpal dislocations: pathomechanics and progressive perilunar instability. J Hand Surg 5: 226–241

351. Schuhl J F, Leroy B, Comtet J J 1985 Biodynamics of the wrist: radiologic approach to scapholunate instability. J Hand Surg (Am) 10: 1006–1008

352. Morgan W, Groves RJ 1984 Scapholunate dissociation from a fall on the elbow. J Hand Surg (Am) 9: 845–847

353. Crawford G P, Taleisnik J 1983 Rotatory subluxation of the scaphoid after excision of dorsal carpal ganglion and wrist manipulation — a case report. J Hand Surg (Am) 8: 921–925

354. Frankel V H 1977 The Terry-Thomas sign. Clin Ortho 129: 321

355. Burgess R C 1987 The effect of rotatory subluxation of the scaphoid on radio-scaphoid contact. J Hand Surg (Am) 12: 771–774

356. Blevens A D, Light T R, Jablonsky W S, Smith D G et al 1989 Radiocarpal articular contact characteristics with scaphoid instability. J Hand Surg (Am) 14: 781–790

357. Kleinman W B 1987 Management of chronic rotary subluxation of the scaphoid by scapho-trapezio-trapezoid arthrodesis. Rationale for the technique, postoperative changes in biomechanics, and results. Hand Clin 3: 113–133

358. Eckenrode J F, Louis D S, Greene T L 1986 Scaphoid-trapezium-trapezoid fusion in the treatment of chronic scapholunate instability. J Hand Surg (Am) 11: 497–502

359. Hastings D E, Silver R L 1984 Intercarpal arthrodesis in the management of chronic carpal instability after trauma. J Hand Surg (Am) 9: 834–840

360. Watson H K, Ryu J, Akelman E 1986 Limited triscaphoid intercarpal arthrodesis for rotatory subluxation of the scaphoid. J Bone Joint Surg (Am) 68: 345–349

361. Viegas S F, Patterson R M, Peterson P D, Pogue D J et al 1990 Evaluation of the biomechanical efficacy of limited intercarpal fusions for the treatment of scapho-lunate dissociation. J Hand Surg (Am) 15: 120–128

362. Kleinman W B 1989 Long-term study of chronic scapho-lunate instability treated by scapho-trapezio-trapezoid arthrodesis. J Hand Surg (Am) 14: 429–445

363. Frykman E B, Af Ekenstam F, Wadin K 1988 Triscaphoid arthrodesis and its complications. J Hand Surg (Am) 13: 844–849

364. Kleinman W B, Carroll C 4th 1990 Scapho-trapezio-trapezoid arthrodesis for treatment of chronic static and dynamic scapho-lunate instability: a 10-year perspective on pitfalls and complications. J Hand Surg (Am) 15: 408–414

365. Garcia-Elias M, Cooney W P, An K N, Linscheid R L, Chao EY 1989 Wrist kinematics after limited intercarpal arthrodesis. J Hand Surg (Am) 14: 791–799

366. Rogers W D, Watson H K 1989 Radial styloid impingement after triscaphe arthrodesis. J Hand Surg (Am) 14: 297–301

367. Taleisnik J 1985 The wrist. Churchill Livingstone, Edinburgh

368. Blatt G 1987 Capsulodesis in reconstructive hand surgery. Dorsal capsulodesis for the unstable scaphoid and volar capsulodesis following excision of the distal ulna. Hand Clin 3: 81–102

369. Brown D E, Lichtman D M 1987 Midcarpal instability. Hand Clinics 3: 135–140

370. Trumble T E, Bour C J, Smith R J, Glisson R R 1990 Kinematics of the ulnar carpus related to the volar intercalated segment instability pattern. J Hand Surg (Am) 15: 384–392

371. Trumble T, Bour C J, Smith R J, Edwards G S 1988 Intercarpal arthrodesis for static and dynamic volar intercalated segment instability. J Hand Surg (Am) 13: 384–390

372. Viegas S F, Patterson R M, Peterson P D, Pogue D J 1990 Ulnar-sided perilunate instability: an anatomic and biomechanic study. J Hand Surg (Am) 15: 268–278

373. Pin P G, Young V L, Gilula L A, Weeks P M 1989 Management of chronic lunotriquetral ligament tears. J Hand Surg (Am) 14: 77–83

374. Lichtman D M, Noble W H, Alexander C E 1984 Dynamic triquetrolunate instability. J Hand Surg 9: 185–189

375. Reagan D S, Linscheid R L, Dobyns J H 1984 Lunotriquetral sprains. J Hand Surg (Am) 9: 502–512

376. Palmer A K 1987 The distal radioulnar joint. Anatomy, biomechanics, and triangular fibrocartilage complex abnormalities. Hand Clin 3: 31–40

377. Hagert C G 1987 The distal radioulnar joint. Hand Clin 3: 41–50

378. King G J, McMurtry R Y, Rubenstein J D, Gertzbein S D 1986 Kinematics of the distal radioulnar joint. J Hand Surg (Am) 11: 798–804

379. Eckhardt W A, Palmer A K 1981 Recurrent dislocation of extensor carpi ulnaris tendon. J Hand Surg 6: 629–631

380. Burkhart S S, Wood M B, Linscheid R L 1982 Posttraumatic recurrent subluxation of the extensor carpi ulnaris tendon. J Hand Surg 7: 1–3

381. Chun S, Palmer A K 1987 Chronic ulnar wrist pain secondary to partial rupture of the extensor carpi ulnaris tendon. J Hand Surg (Am) 12: 1032–1035

382. Rowland S A 1986 Acute traumatic subluxation of the extensor carpi ulnaris tendon at the wrist. J Hand Surg (Am) 11: 809–811

383. Palmer A K 1989 Triangular fibrocartilage complex lesions: a classification. J Hand Surg (Am) 14: 594–606

384. Buterbaugh G A, Palmer A K 1988 Fractures and dislocations of the distal radioulnar joint. Hand Clin 4: 361–375

385. Taleisnik J 1988 Clinical and technologic evaluation of ulnar wrist pain (editorial). J Hand Surg (Am) 13: 801–802

386. Dell P C 1987 Distal radioulnar joint dysfunction. Hand Clin 3: 563–583

387. Menon J, Wood V E, Schoene H R, Frykman G K et al 1984 Isolated tears of the triangular fibrocartilage of the wrist: results of partial excision. J Hand Surg (Am) 9: 527–530

388. Palmer A K, Werner F W, Glisson R R, Murphy D J 1988 Partial excision of the triangular fibrocartilage complex. J Hand Surg (Am) 13: 391–394

389. Thiru R G, Ferlic D C, Clayton M L, McClure D C 1986 Arterial anatomy of the triangular fibrocartilage of the wrist and its surgical significance. J Hand Surg (Am) 11: 258–263

390. Darrow J C Jr, Linscheid R L, Dobyns J H, Mann J M 3rd et al 1985 Distal ulnar recession for disorders of the distal radioulnar joint. J Hand Surg (Am) 10: 482–491

391. Boulas H J, Milek M A 1990 Ulnar shortening for tears of the triangular fibrocartilaginous complex. J Hand Surg (Am) 15: 415–420

392. Linscheid R L 1987 Ulnar lengthening and shortening. Hand Clin 3: 69–79

393. Roth J H, Poehling G G 1990 Arthroscopic "-ectomy": surgery of the wrist. Arthroscopy 6: 141–147

394. Osterman A L 1990 Arthroscopic debridement of triangular fibrocartilage complex tears. Arthroscopy 6: 120–124

395. Roth J H, Poehling G G, Whipple T L 1988

Arthroscopic surgery of the wrist. Instr Course Lect 37: 183–194

396. Brunel W, Schecter W P, Schecter G 1988 Hand deformity and sensory loss due to Hansen's disease in American Samoa. J Hand Surg (Am) 13: 279–283

397. Erb W H 1874 Uber eine eigenthumliche Localisation von Lahemengen im Plexus brachialis. Verhandl d. Naturhist. Medical (Heidelberg) 2: 130

398. Brand P W 1958 Paralytic claw hand. J Bone Joint Surg 40B: 618–632

399. Bouvier M 1851–2 Note sur une paralysie partielle des muscles de la main. Bull Acad Nat Med 18: 125–139 (cited in Zancolli, reference 525)

400. Blacker G J, Lister G D, Kleinert H E 1976 The abducted little finger in low ulnar nerve palsy. J Hand Surg 1:190–196

401. Froment M J 1915 La paralysie de l'adducteur du pouce et le signe de la prehension. Rev Neurol 28: 1236–1240

402. Mannerfelt L 1966 Studies on the hand in ulnar nerve paralysis. A clinical and experimental investigation in normal and anomalous innervation. Acta Ortho Scand (suppl) 87

403. Zancolli E A 1957 Clawhand caused by paralysis of the intrinsic muscles. J Bone Joint Surg 39A: 1076–1081

404. Srinivasan H 1983 Postural changes in thenar paralysis and their significance. J Hand Surg (Am) 8: 194–196

405. Klumpke A 1885 Contribution a' l'etude des paralysies radiculaires du plexus brachial. Rev Med 5: 591–596

406. Tinel J 1915 Le signe du 'Fourrnillement' dans les lesion des Neufs Peripheriques. Press Med 47: 388–389

407. Tinel J 1917 Nerve Wounds. Bailliere Tindal and Cox, London

408. Henderson W R 1948 Clinical assessment of peripheral nerve injuries. Lancet i: 801–805

409. Harrison S H 1974 The tactile adherence test estimating loss of sensation after nerve injury. Hand 6: 148–149

410. Egyed B, Eory A, Veres T, Manninger J 1980 Measurement of electrical resistance after nerve injuries of the hand. Hand 12: 275–281

411. Aschan W, Moberg E 1962 The Ninhydrin finger printing test used to map out partial lesions to hand nerves. Acta Chir Scand 123: 365–370

412. Moberg E 1958 Objective methods for determining the functional value of sensibility in the hand. J Bone Joint Surg 40B: 454–476

413. Moberg E 1960 Examination of sensory loss by the ninhydrin printing test in Volkmann's contracture. Bull Hosp Joint Dis 21: 296–303

414. Sakurai M 1986 Use of bromphenol blue printing method for detecting sweat on the palm. J Hand Surg (Br) 11: 125–130

415. Dellon A L 1984 Touch sensibility in the hand. J Hand Surg (Br) 9: 11–13

416. Omer G E Jr 1968 Evaluation and reconstruction of the forearm and hand after acute traumatic peripheral nerve injuries. J Bone Joint Surg 50A: 1454–1478

417. Moberg E 1964 Evaluation and management of nerve injuries in the hand. Surg Clin North Am 44: 1019

418. Onne L 1962 Recovery of sensibility and sudo-motor activity in the hand after nerve suture. Acta Chir Scand (suppl) 300: 1–69

419. Gellis M, Pool R 1977 Two-point discrimination

420. Dellon A L 1981 Evaluation of sensibility and reeducation of sensation in the hand. Williams & Wilkins, Baltimore

421. Dellon A L, Kallman C H 1983 Evaluation of functional sensation in the hand. J Hand Surg (Am) 8: 865–870

422. Bell-Krotoski J, Tomancik E 1987 The repeatability of testing with Semmes–Weinstein monofilaments. J Hand Surg (Am) 12: 155–161

423. Dellon A L, Curtis R M, Edgerton M T 1974 Reeducation of sensation in the hand after nerve injury and repair. Plastic Reconstr Surg 53: 297–305

424. Parry C B, Salter M 1976 Sensory re-education after median nerve lesions. Hand 8: 250–257

425. Levin S, Pearsall G, Ruderman R J 1978 Von Frey's method of measuring pressure sensibility in the hand: an engineering analysis of Weinstein–Semmes pressure aesthesiometer. J Hand Surg 3: 211–216

426. O'Riain S 1973 New and simple test of nerve function in hand. Br Med J 3: 615–616

427. Mitchell S W 1872 Injuries of nerves and their consequences. Lippincott, Philadelphia

428. Bodyns J H, O'Brien E T, Linscheid R L, Farrow G M 1972 Bowler's thumb: diagnosis and treatment. J Bone Joint Surg 54A: 751–755

429. Kisner W H 1976 Thumb neuroma: a hazard of ten pin bowling. Br J Plastic Surg 29: 225–226

430. Herndon J, Eaton R, Littler J W 1976 Management of painful neuromas in the hand. J Bone Joint Surg 58A: 369–373

431. Tupper J W, Booth D M 1976 Treatment of painful neuromas of nerves in the hand: a comparison of traditional and newer methods. J Hand Surg 1: 144–151

432. Swanson A B, Boeve N R, Lumsden R M 1977 The prevention and treatment of amputation neuromata by silicone capping. J Hand Surg 2: 70–78

433. Wood V E, Mudge M K 1987 Treatment of neuromas about a major amputation stump. J Hand Surg (Am) 12: 302–306

434. Karev A, Stahl S 1986 Treatment of painful nerve lesions in the palm by 'rerouting' of the digital nerve. J Hand Surg (Am) 11: 539–542

435. Goldstein S A, Sturim H S 1985 Intraosseous nerve transposition for treatment of painful neuromas. J Hand Surg (Am) 10: 270–274

436. Robbins T H 1986 Nerve capping in the treatment of troublesome terminal neuromata. Br J Plastic Surg 39: 239–240

437. Brandner M D, Buncke H J, Campagna-Pinto D 1989 Experimental treatment of neuromas in the rat by retrograde axoplasmic transport of ricin with selective destruction of ganglion cells. J Hand Surg (Am) 14: 710–714

438. Hurst L C, Badalamente M A, Blum D 1984 Carbon dioxide laser transection of rat peripheral nerves. J Hand Surg (Am) 9: 428–433

439. Gorkisch K, Boese-Landgraf J, Vaubel E 1984 Treatment and prevention of amputation neuromas in hand surgery. Plastic Reconstr Surg 73: 293–299

440. Dellon A L, Mackinnon S E 1986 Treatment of the painful neuroma by neuroma resection and muscle implantation. Plastic Reconstr Surg 77: 427–438

441. Mass D P, Ciano M C, Tortosa R, Newmeyer W L, Kilgore E S Jr 1984 Treatment of painful hand neuromas by their transfer into bone. Plastic Reconstr Surg 74: 182–185

442. Belsky M R, Millender L H 1980 Bowler's thumb in a baseball player: a case report. Orthopedics 3: 122–123

443. Martin R 1763 Tal om Nervers allmanna Egenskaper i Manniskans kroop. L Salvius, Stockholm

444. Gruber W 1870 Uber die Verbundung des Nervus medianus mit dem Nervus ulnaris am unterarme des Meuchen und der Saugethiere. Arch Anat Physiol Med Leipzig 37: 501–522

445. Brandsma J W, Birke J A, Sims D S Jr 1986 The Martin-Gruber innervated hand. J Hand Surg (Am) 11: 536–539

446. Labosky D A, Waggy C A 1986 Apparent weakness of median and ulnar motors in radial nerve palsy. J Hand Surg (Am) 11: 528–533

447. Clippinger F W, Goldner J L, Roberts J M 1962 Use of the electromyogram in evaluating upper-extremity peripheral nerve lesions. J Bone Joint Surg 44A: 1047–1060

448. Van Beek A L 1986 Electrodiagnostic evaluation of peripheral nerve injuries. Hand Clin 2: 747–760

449. Stewart J D 1986 Electrodiagnostic techniques in the evaluation of nerve compressions and injuries in the upper limb. Hand Clin 2: 677–687

450. Ballantyne J P, Campbell M J 1973 Electrophysiological study after surgical repair of sectioned human peripheral nerves. J Neurol Neurosurg Psych 36: 797–805

451. Seddon Sir H J 1972 Surgical disorders of peripheral nerves. Williams & Wilkins, Baltimore

452. Terzis J K, Dykes R E, Hakstian R W 1976 Electrophysiological recordings in peripheral nerve surgery: a review. J Hand Surg 1: 52–66

453. Omer G E 1988 Timing of tendon transfers in peripheral nerve injury. Hand Clin 4: 317–322

454. Dellon A L, Mackinnon S E 1986 Pain after radial sensory nerve grafting. J Hand Surg (Br) 11: 341–346

455. Millesi H 1986 The nerve gap. Theory and clinical practice. Hand Clin 2: 651–663

456. Sunderland S 1978 Nerves and nerve injuries, 2nd edn. Churchill Livingstone, Edinburgh

457. Williams H B, Jabaley M E 1986 The importance of internal anatomy of the peripheral nerves to nerve repair in the forearm and hand. Hand Clin 2: 689–707

458. Chow J A, Van Beek A L, Meyer D L, Johnson M C 1985 Surgical significance of the motor fascicular group of the ulnar nerve in the forearm. J Hand Surg (Am) 10: 867–872

459. Bonnel F 1985 Histologic structure of the ulnar nerve in the hand. J Hand Surg (Am) 10: 264–269

460. Gaul J S Jr 1983 Electrical fascicle identification as an adjunct to nerve repair. J Hand Surg (Am) 8: 289–296

461. Gaul J S Jr 1986 Electrical fascicle indentification as an adjunct to nerve repair. Hand Clin 2: 709–722

462. Ganel A, Engel J, Luboshitz S, Melamed R, Rimon S 1981 Choline acetyltransferase nerve identification method in early and late nerve repair. Ann Plast Surg 6: 228–230

463. Riley D A, Lang D H 1984 Carbonic anhydrase activity of human peripheral nerves: a possible histochemical aid to nerve repair. J Hand Surg (Am) 9A: 112–120

464. Ortiguela M E, Wood M B, Cahill D R 1987 Anatomy of the sural nerve complex. J Hand Surg (Am) 12: 1119–1123

465. Tank M S, Lewis R C Jr, Coates P W 1983 The lateral antebrachial cutaneous nerve as a highly suitable autograft donor for the digital nerve. J Hand Surg (Am) 8: 942–945

466. Bourne M H, Wood M B, Carmichael S W 1987 Locating the lateral antebrachial cutaneous nerve. J Hand Surg (Am) 12: 697–699

467. Masear V R, Meyer R D, Pichora D R 1989 Surgical anatomy of the medial antebrachial cutaneous nerve. J Hand Surg (Am) 14: 267–271

468. Bora F W Jr, Bednar J M, Osterman A L, Brown M J, Sumner A J 1987 Prosthetic nerve grafts: a resorbable tube as an alternative to autogenous nerve grafting. J Hand Surg (Am) 12: 685–692

469. Mackinnon S E, Dellon A L 1988 A comparison of nerve regeneration across a sural nerve graft and a vascularized pseudosheath. J Hand Surg (Am) 13: 935–942

470. Bedeschi P, Celli L, Balli A 1984 Transfer of sensory nerves in hand surgery. J Hand Surg (Br) 9: 46–49

471. Matloubi R 1988 Transfer of sensory branches of radial nerve in hand surgery. J Hand Surg (Br) 13: 92–95

472. Louis D S, Eckenrode J F 1986 Autogenous nerve pedicle graft in the forearm. J Hand Surg (Am) 11: 703–706

473. Greenberg B M, Cuadros C L, Panda M, May J W Jr 1988 St Clair Strange procedure: indications, technique, and long-term evaluation. J Hand Surg (Am) 13: 928–935

474. Rose E H, Kowalski T A 1985 Restoration of sensibility to anesthetic scarred digits with free vascularized nerve grafts from the dorsum of the foot. J Hand Surg (Am) 10: 514–521

475. Doi K, Kuwata N, Sakai K, Tamaru K, Kawai S 1987 A reliable technique of free vascularized sural nerve grafting and preliminary results of clinical applications. J Hand Surg (Am) 12: 677–684

476. Shibata M, Tsai T M, Firrell J, Breidenbach W C 1988 Experimental comparison of vascularized and nonvascularized nerve grafting. J Hand Surg (Am) 13: 358–365

477. Smith R J 1986 Indications for tendon transfers to the hand. Hand Clin 2: 235–237

478. Riordan D C 1983 Tendon transfers in hand surgery. J Hand Surg (Am) 8: 748–753

479. Schneider L 1988 Tendon transfers in muscle and tendon loss. Hand Clin 4: 267–272

480. Brand P W 1988 Biomechanics of tendon transfers. Hand Clin 4: 137–154

481. Brand P W, Thompson D E 1982 Relative tension and potential excursion of muscles in the forearm and hand. J Hand Surg 6: 209–219

482. Brys D, Waters R L 1987 Effect of triceps function on the brachioradialis transfer in quadriplegia. J Hand Surg (Am) 12: 237–239

483. Cooney W P 1988 Tendon transfer for median nerve palsy. Hand Clin 4: 155–165

484. Cooney W P, Linscheid R L, An K N 1984 Opposition of the thumb: an anatomic and biomechanical study of tendon transfers. J Hand Surg (Am) 9: 777–786

485. Hastings H 2nd, Davidson S 1988 Tendon transfers for

ulnar nerve palsy. Evaluation of results and practical treatment considerations. Hand Clin 4: 167–178

486. Smith R J 1983 Extensor carpi radialis brevis tendon transfer for thumb adduction — a study of power pinch. J Hand Surg 8: 4–15

487. Reid R L 1988 Radial nerve palsy. Hand Clin 4: 179–185

488. Eversmann W W 1988 Tendon transfers for combined nerve injuries. Hand Clin 4: 187–199

489. Revol M P, Servant J M 1987 Classification of the main tenodesis technique used in hand surgery. Plastic Reconstr Surg 79: 237–242

490. Manktelow R T 1988 Functioning microsurgical muscle transfer. Hand Clin 4: 289–296

491. Leffert R D 1974 Brachial plexus injuries. New Engl J Med 291: 1059–1067

492. Millesi H 1977 Surgical management of brachial plexus injuries. J Hand Surg 2: 367–379

493. Bufalini C, Pescatori G 1969 Posterior cervical electromyography in the diagnosis and prognosis of brachial plexus injuries. J Bone Joint Surg 51B: 627–631

494. Bonney G 1954 The value of axon responses in determining the site of lesion in traction injuries of the brachial plexus. Brain 77: 588–609

495. Landi A, Copeland S 1979 Value of the Tinel sign in brachial plexus lesions. Ann Roy Coll Surg Engl 61: 470–471

496. Landi A, Copeland S A, Wynn, Parry C B, Jones S J 1980 The role of somatosensory evoked potentials and nerve conduction studies on the surgical management of brachial plexus injuries. J Bone Joint Surg 62B: 492–496

497. Match R M 1975 Radiation-induced brachial plexus paralysis. Arch Surg 110: 384–386

498. Rorabeck C H, Harris W R 1981 Factors affecting the prognosis of brachial plexus injuries. J Bone Joint Surg 63B: 404–407

499. Hardy A E 1981 Birth injuries of the brachial plexus. J Bone Joint Surg 63B: 98–101

500. Hoffer M M, Braun R, Hsu J, Mitani M, Temes K 1981 Functional recovery and orthopaedic management of brachial plexus palsies. J Am Med Assoc 246: 2467–2470

501. Millesi H 1984 Brachial plexus injuries. Clin Plastic Surg 2: 115–120

502. Narakas A 1981 Brachial plexus surgery. Orthop Clin North Am 12: 303–323

503. Terzis J K, Liberson W T, Levine R 1986 Obstetric brachial plexus palsy. Hand Clin 2: 773–786

504. Boome R S, Kaye J C 1988 Obstetric traction injuries of the brachial plexus. J Bone Joint Surg (Br) 70: 571–576

505. Kanaya F, Gonzalez M, Park C M, Kutz J E et al 1990 Improvement in motor function after brachial plexus surgery. J Hand Surg (Am) 15: 30–36

506. Nagano A, Tsuyama N, Ochiai N, Hara T, Takahashi M 1989 Direct nerve crossing with the intercostal nerve to treat avulsion injuries of the brachial plexus. J Hand Surg 14: 980–985

507. Minami M, Ishii S 1987 Satisfactory elbow flexion in complete (preganglionic) brachial plexus injuries; produced by suture of the third and fourth intercostal nerves to musculocutaneous nerve. J Hand Surg 12: 1114–1118

508. Allieu Y, Cenac P 1988 Is surgical intervention justifiable for total paralysis secondary to multiple avulsion injuries of the brachial plexus? Hand Clin 4: 609–618

509. Dai S Y, Lin D X, Han Z, Zhoug SZ 1990 Transference of thoracodorsal nerve to musculocutaneous nerve or axillary nerve in old traumatic injury. J Hand Surg 15: 36–37

510. Brunelli G, Monini L 1985 Direct muscular neurotization. J Hand Surg (Am) 10: 993–997

511. Zancolli E A, Zancolli E R Jr 1988 Palliative surgical procedures in sequelae of obstetric palsy. Hand Clin 4: 643–669

512. Leffert R D, Pess G M 1988 Tendon transfers for brachial plexus injury. Hand Clin 4: 273–288

513. Merle M, Foucher G, Dap F, Bour C 1989 Tendon transfers for treatment of the paralyzed hand following brachial plexus injury. Hand Clin 5: 33–41

514. Narakas A O 1988 Paralytic disorders of the shoulder girdle. Hand Clin 4: 619–632

515. Comtet J J, Herzberg G, Naasan I A 1989 Biomechanical basis of transfers for shoulder paralysis. Hand Clin 5: 1–14

516. Gilbert A, Romana C, Ayatti R 1988 Tendon transfers for shoulder paralysis in children. Hand Clin 4: 633–642

517. Alnot J Y 1989 Elbow flexion palsy after traumatic lesions of the brachial plexus in adults. Hand Clin 5: 15–22

518. Hoang P H, Mills C, Burke F D 1989 Triceps to biceps transfer for established brachial plexus palsy. J Bone Joint Surg (Br) 71: 268–271

519. Tsai T M, Kalisman M, Burns J, Kleinert H E 1983 Restoration of elbow flexion by pectoralis major and pectoralis minor transfer. J Hand Surg (Am) 8: 186–190

520. Stern P J, Caudle R J 1988 Tendon transfers for elbow flexion. Hand Clin 4: 297–307

521. Moneim M S, Omer G E 1986 Latissimus dorsi muscle transfer for restoration of elbow flexion after brachial plexus disruption. J Hand Surg (Am) 11: 135–139

522. LeQuang C 1989 Postirradiation lesions of the brachial plexus. Results of surgical treatment. Hand Clin 5: 23–32

523. Wynn Parry C B 1989 Orthotics and rehabilitation after extensive upper limb paralysis. Hand Clin 5: 97–105

524. Braun R M, Hoffer M M, Mooney V, McKeever J, Roper B 1973 Phenol nerve block in the treatment of acquired spastic hemiplegia in the upper limb. J Bone Joint Surg 55A: 580–585

525. Zancolli E A 1979 Structural and dynamic bases of hand surgery, 2nd edn. Lippincott, Philadelphia

526. Zancolli E A, Goldner L J, Swanson A B 1983 Surgery of the spastic hand in cerebral palsy: report of the Committee on Spastic Hand Evaluation (International Federation of Societies for Surgery of the Hand). J Hand Surg (Am) 8: 766–772

527. Goldner J L 1988 Surgical reconstruction of the upper extremity in cerebral palsy. Hand Clin 4: 223–265

528. Szabo R M, Gelberman R H 1985 Operative treatment of cerebral palsy. Hand Clin 1: 525–543

529. Hoffer M M, Lehman M, Mitani M 1989 Surgical indications in children with cerebral palsy. Hand Clin 5: 69–74

530. Suso S, Vicente P, Angles F 1985 Surgical treatment of

the non-functional spastic hand. J Hand Surg (Br)
10: 54–56

531. Hoffer M M, Zeitzew S 1988 Wrist fusion in cerebral
palsy. J Hand Surg (Am) 13: 667–670

532. Strecker W B, Emanuel J P, Dailey L, Manske P R
1988 Comparison of pronator tenotomy and pronator
rerouting in children with spastic cerebral palsy. J Hand
Surg (Am) 13: 540–543

533. House J H, Gwathmey F W, Fidler M O 1981
A dynamic approach to the thumb-in-palm deformity
in cerebral palsy. Evaluation and results in fifty-six
patients. J Bone Joint Surg 63A: 216–225

534. Manske P R 1985 Redirection of extensor pollicis
longus in the treatment of spastic thumb-in-palm
deformity. J Hand Surg (Am) 10: 553–560

535. Wenner S M, Johnson K A 1988 Transfer of the flexor
carpi ulnaris to the radial wrist extensors in cerebral
palsy. J Hand Surg (Am) 13: 231–233

536. Hoffer M M, Lehman M, Mitani M 1986 Long-term
follow-up on tendon transfers to the extensors of the
wrist and fingers in patients with cerebral palsy. J Hand
Surg (Am) 11: 836–840

537. Pinzur M S 1985 Surgery to achieve dynamic motor
balance in adult acquired spastic hemiplegia: a
preliminary report. J Hand Surg (Am) 10: 547–553

538. Swanson A B, de Groot Swanson G 1989 Evaluation
and treatment of the upper extremity in the stroke
patient. Hand Clin 5: 75–96

539. Keenan M A, Romanelli R R, Lunsford B R 1989 The
use of dynamic electromyography to evaluate motor
control in the hands of adults who have spasticity
caused by brain injury. J Bone Joint Surg (Am)
71: 120–126

540. Botte M J, Keenan M A 1988 Percutaneous phenol
blocks of the pectoralis major muscle to treat spastic
deformities. J Hand Surg (Am) 13: 147–149

541. Keenan M A, Tomas E S, Stone L, Gersten L M 1990
Percutaneous phenol block of the musculocutaneous
nerve to control elbow flexor spasticity. J Hand Surg
(Am) 15: 340–346

542. Keenan M A, Todderud E P, Henderson R, Botte M
1987 Management of intrinsic spasticity in the hand
with phenol injection or neurectomy of the motor
branch of the ulnar nerve. J Hand Surg (Am)
12: 734–739

543. Keenan M A, Abrams R A, Garland D E, Waters R L
1987 Results of fractional lengthening of the finger
flexors in adults with upper extremity spasticity. J Hand
Surg (Am) 12: 575–581

544. Keenan M A, Korchek J I, Botte M J, Smith C W,
Garland D E 1987 Results of transfer of the flexor
digitorum superficialis tendons to the flexor digitorum
profundus tendons in adults with acquired spasticity of
the hand. J Bone Joint Surg (Am) 69: 1127–1132

545. Botte M J, Keenan M A, Korchek J I, Waters R L 1987
Modified technique for the superficialis-to-profundus
transfer in the treatment of adults with spastic clenched
fist deformity. J Hand Surg (Am) 12: 639–640

546. Pinzur M S, Wehner J, Kett N, Trilla M 1988
Brachioradialis to finger extensor tendon transfer to
achieve hand opening in acquired spasticity. J Hand
Surg (Am) 13: 549–552

547. Botte M J, Keenan M A, Gellman H, Garland D E,
Waters R L 1989 Surgical management of spastic

thumb-in-palm deformity in adults with brain injury.
J Hand Surg (Am) 14: 174–182

548. Turner J W A, Parsonage M J 1957 Neuralgic
amyotrophy (paralytic brachial neuritis) with special
reference to prognosis. Lancet ii: 209–212

549. Parsonage M J, Turner J W A 1948 Neuralgic
amyotrophy: The shoulder-girdle syndrome. Lancet
i: 973–978

550. McDowell C L, Rago T A, Gonzalez S M 1989
Tetraplegia. Hand Clin 5: 343–349

551. Bedbrook G M 1979 Spinal injuries with tetraplegia
and paraplegia. J Bone Joint Surg 61B: 267–284

552. Freehafer A A, Vonhaam E, Allen V 1974 Tendon
transfers to improve grasp after injuries of the cervical
spinal cord. J Bone Joint Surg 56A: 951–959

553. Lamb D W, Lamdry R M 1972 The hand in
quadriplegia. Paraplegia 9: 204–212

554. Zancolli E A 1979 Structural and dynamic bases of
hand surgery, 2nd edn. J B Lippincott Co, Philadelphia

555. McDowell C L, Moberg E A, House J H 1986 The
second international conference on surgical
rehabilitation of the upper limb in tetraplegia. J Hand
Surg 11A: 604–608

556. Murphy C P, Chuinard R G 1988 Management of the
upper extremity in traumatic tetraplegia. Hand Clin
4: 201–209

557. Hentz V R, Brown M, Keoshian L A 1983 Upper limb
reconstruction in quadriplegia: functional assessment
and proposed treatment modifications. J Hand Surg
(Am) 8: 119–131

558. Lamb D W, Chan K M 1983 Surgical reconstruction of
the upper limb in traumatic tetraplegia. A review of 41
patients. J Bone Joint Surg (Br) 65: 291–298

559. Ejeskar A 1988 Upper limb surgical rehabilitation in
high-level tetraplegia. Hand Clin 4: 585–599

560. Hentz V R, Hamlin C, Keoshian L A 1988 Surgical
reconstruction in tetraplegia. Hand Clin 4: 601–607

561. Freehafer A A, Kelly C M, Peckham P H 1984 Tendon
transfer for the restoration of upper limb function after
a cervical spinal cord injury. J Hand Surg (Am)
9: 887–893

562. Kelly C M, Freehafer A A, Peckham P H, Stroh K 1985
Postoperative results of opponensplasty and flexor
tendon transfer in patients with spinal cord injuries.
J Hand Surg (Am) 10: 890–894

563. House J H, Gwathmey F W, Lundsgaard D K 1976
Restoration of strong grasp and lateral pinch in
tetraplegia due to cervical spinal cord injury. J Hand
Surg 1: 152–159

564. Colyer R A, Kappelman B 1981 Flexor pollicis longus
tenodesis in tetraplegia at the sixth cervical level — a
prospective evaluation of functional gain. J Bone Joint
Surg 63A: 376–379

565. Keith M W, Peckham P H, Thrope G B, Stroh K C
et al 1989 Implantable functional neuromuscular
stimulation in the tetraplegic hand. J Hand Surg (Am)
14: 524–530

566. Peckham P H, Keith M W, Freehafer A A 1988
Restoration of functional control by electrical
stimulation in the upper extremity of the quadriplegic
patient. J Bone Joint Surg (Am) 70: 144–148

567. Freehafer A A, Peckham P H, Keith M W 1988 New
concepts on treatment of the upper limb in the
tetraplegic. Surgical restoration and functional

neuromuscular stimulation. Hand Clin 4: 563–574

568. McDowell C, Moberg E A, Smith A G 1979 International conference on surgical rehabilitation of the upper limb in tetraplegia. J Hand Surg 4: 387–390

569. Lacey S H, Wilber R G, Peckham P H, Freehafer A A 1986 The posterior deltoid to triceps transfer: a clinical and biomechanical assessment. J Hand Surg (Am) 11: 542–547

570. Falconer D P 1988 Tendon transfers about the shoulder and elbow in the spinal cord injured patient. Hand Clin 4: 211–221

571. Freehafer A A, Peckham P H, Keith M W, Mendelson L S 1988 The brachioradialis: anatomy, properties, and value for tendon transfer in the tetraplegic. J Hand Surg (Am) 13: 99–104

572. House J H, Shannon M A 1985 Restoration of strong grasp and lateral pinch in tetraplegia: a comparison of two methods of thumb control in each patient. J Hand Surg (Am) 10: 22–29

573. Rieser T V, Waters R L 1986 Long-term follow-up of the Moberg key grip procedure. J Hand Surg (Am) 11: 724–728

574. Waters R, Moore K R, Graboff S R, Paris K 1985 Brachioradialis to flexor pollicis longus tendon transfer for active lateral pinch in the tetraplegic. J Hand Surg (Am) 10: 385–391

575. Waters R L, Stark L Z, Gubernick I, Bellman H, Barnes G 1990 Electromyographic analysis of brachioradialis to flexor pollicis longus tendon transfer in quadriplegia. J Hand Surg (Am) 15: 335–339

576. Hiersche D L, Waters R L 1985 Interphalangeal fixation of the thumb in Moberg's key grip procedure. J Hand Surg (Am) 10: 30–32

577. Colyer R A, Kappelman B 1981 Flexor pollicis longus tenodesis in tetraplegia at the sixth cervical level. A prospective evaluation of functional gain. J Bone Joint Surg (Am) 63: 376–379

578. Gansel J, Waters R, Gellman H 1990 Transfer of the pronator teres tendon to the tendons of the flexor digitorum profundus in tetraplegia. J Bone Joint Surg (Am) 72: 427–432

579. Mendelson L S, Peckham P H, Freehafer A A, Keith M W 1988 Intraoperative assessment of wrist extensor muscle force. J Hand Surg (Am) 13: 832–836

580. Lister G 1985 Pitfalls and complications of flexor tendon surgery. Hand Clin 1: 133–146

581. Doyle J R, Blythe W 1975 The finger flexor tendon sheath and pulleys: anatomy and reconstruction. Symposium on tendon surgery in the hand. AAOS. Mosby, St Louis

582. Parkes A 1971 The 'lumbrical plus' finger. J Bone Joint Surg 53B: 236–239

583. Lister G D 1990 Flexor tendon. In: McCarthy J G (ed) Plastic surgery. WB Saunders, Philadelphia, pp 4516–4564

584. Strickland J W 1989 Flexor tendon surgery. Part 2: Free tendon grafts and tenolysis. J Hand Surg (Br) 14: 368–382

585. Wilson R L 1985 Flexor tendon grafting. Hand Clin 1: 97–107

586. Harvey F J, Chu G, Harvey P M 1983 Surgical availability of the plantaris tendon J Hand Surg (Am) 8: 243–247

587. Allen B N, Frykman G K, Unsell R S, Wood V E 1987 Ruptured flexor tendon tenorrhaphies in zone II: repair and rehabilitation. J Hand Surg (Am) 12: 18–21

588. Strickland J W 1985 Flexor tenolysis. Hand Clin 1: 121–132

589. Jupiter J B, Pess G M, Bour C J 1989 Results of flexor tendon tenolysis after replantation in the hand. J Hand Surg (Am) 14: 35–44

590. LaSalle W B, Strickland J W 1983 An evaluation of the two-stage flexor tendon reconstruction technique. J Hand Surg (Am) 8: 263–267

591. Hunter J M, Jaeger S H, Matsui T, Miyaji N 1983 The pseudosynovial sheath — its characteristics in a primate model. J Hand Surg (Am) 8: 461–470

592. Hunter J M 1983 Staged flexor tendon reconstruction. J Hand Surg (Am) 8: 789–793

593. Hunter J M 1985 Tendon salvage and the active tendon implant: a perspective. Hand Clin 1: 181–186

594. Schneider L H, Wiltshire D 1983 Restoration of flexor pollicis longus function by flexor digitorum superficialis transfer. J Hand Surg (Am) 8: 98–101

595. Posner M A 1983 Flexor superficialis tendon transfers to the thumb — an alternative to the free tendon graft for treatment of chronic injuries within the digital sheath. J Hand Surg (Am) 8: 876–881

596. Lister G D 1979 Reconstruction of pulleys employing extensor retinaculum. J Hand Surg 4: 461–464

597. Karev A 1984 The 'belt loop' technique for the reconstruction of the pulleys in the first stage of flexor tendon grafting. J Hand Surg 9A: 923–924

598. Strickland J W 1985 Results of flexor tendon surgery in zone II. Hand Clin 1: 167–179

599. Cunningham M W, Yousif N J, Matloub H S, Sanger J R et al 1985 Retardation of finger growth after injury to the flexor tendons. J Hand Surg (Am) 10: 115–117

600. Patel M R, Desai S S, Bassini-Lipson L 1986 Conservative management of chronic mallet finger. J Hand Surg (Am) 11: 570–573

601. Kleinman W B, Petersen D P 1984 Oblique retinacular ligament reconstruction for chronic mallet finger deformity. J Hand Surg (Am) 9: 399–404

602. Grundberg A B, Reagan D S 1987 Central slip tenotomy for chronic mallet finger deformity. J Hand Surg (Am) 12: 545–547

603. Froehlich J A, Akelman E, Herndon J H 1988 Extensor tendon injuries at the proximal interphalangeal joint. Hand Clin 4: 25–37

604. Curtis R M, Reid R L, Provost J M 1983 A staged technique for the repair of the traumatic boutonniere deformity. J Hand Surg (Am) 8: 167–171

605. Quaba A A, Elliot D, Sommerlad B C 1988 Long term hand function without long finger extensors: a clinical study. J Hand Surg (Br) 13: 66–71

606. Schneider L H, Rosenstein R G 1983 Restoration of extensor pollicis longus function by tendon transfer. Plastic Reconstr Surg 71: 533–537

607. Welling R E, Cranley J J, Krause R J, Hafner C D 1981 Obliterative arterial disease of the upper extremity. Arch Surg 116: 1593–1596

608. Heath R D 1972 The subclavian steal syndrome. Cause of symptoms in the arm. J Bone Joint Surg 54A: 1033–1039

609. Allen E V 1929 Thromboangitis obliterans: methods of diagnosis of chronic occlusive arterial lesions distal to the wrist with illustrative cases. Am J Med Sci 178: 237–244

610. McGregor A D 1987 The Allen test — an investigation of its accuracy by fluorescein angiography. J Hand Surg (Br) 12: 82–85

611. Gelberman R H, Blasingame J P 1981 The timed Allen test. J Trauma 21: 477–479

612. Scavenius M, Fauner M, Walther-Larsen S, Buchwald C, Nielsen S L 1981 A quantitative Allen's test. Hand 13: 318–320

613. DeBenedetto M R, Nappi J F, Ruff M E, Lubbers L M 1989 Doppler mapping in hypothenar syndrome: an alternative to angiography. J Hand Surg (Am) 14: 244–246

614. Ernst D, Hurlow R, Strachan C, Chandler S 1978 The assessment of digital vessel disease by dynamic hand scanning. Hand 10: 217–225

615. Wilgis E, Jezic D, Stonesifer G, Classen J, Sekercan K 1974 The evaluation of small-vessel flow. J Bone Joint Surg 56A: 1199–1206

616. Koman L A, Nunley J A, Goldner J L, Seaber A V, Urbaniak J R 1984 Isolated cold stress testing in the assessment of symptoms in the upper extremity: preliminary communication. J Hand Surg (Am) 9: 305–313

617. Bendick P J, Mayer J R, Glover J L, Park H M 1979 A photoplethysmographic technique for detecting vascular compromise. J Trauma 19: 398–402

618. Smith D J Jr, Bendick P J, Madison S A 1984 Evaluation of vascular compromise in the injured extremity: a photoplethysmographic technique. J Hand Surg (Am) 9: 314–319

619. Dowd G S E 1986 Predicting stump healing following amputation for peripheral vascular disease using the transcutaneous oxygen monitor. Ann Roy Coll Surg 68: 31–35

620. Gross W, Louis D 1978 Doppler hemodynamic assessment of obscure symptomatology in the upper extremity. J Hand Surg 3: 467–473

621. Dooley T W, Welsh C F, Puckett C L 1989 Noninvasive assessment of microvessels with the duplex scanner. J Hand Surg (Am) 14: 670–673

622. Koman L A, Bond M G, Carter R E, Poehling G G 1985 Evaluation of upper extremity vasculature with high-resolution ultrasound. J Hand Surg (Am) 10: 249–255

623. Koman L A, Urbaniak J R 1985 Ulnar artery thrombosis. Hand Clin 1: 311–325

624. Kleinert H E, Volanitis G J 1965 Thrombosis of the palmar arterial arch and its tributaries: etiology and newer concepts in treatment. J Trauma 5: 446–457

625. Koman L A, Urbaniak J R 1981 Ulnar artery insufficiency: a guide to treatment. J Hand Surg 6: 16–24

626. Millender L, Nalebuff E, Dasdan E 1972 Aneurysms and thromboses of the ulnar artery in the hand. Arch Surg 105: 686–690

627. Eguro H, Goldner J L 1973 Bilateral thrombosis of the ulnar arteries in the hands. Plastic Reconstr Surg 52: 573–578

628. Coon J, Bergan J, Bell J 1970 Hypothenar hammer syndrome: Post-traumatic digital ischemia. Surgery 68: 1122–1128

629. Carneirio R S, Mann R J 1979 Occlusion of the ulnar artery associated with an anomalous muscle: a case report. J Hand Surg 4: 412–414

630. Cho K 1978 Entrapment occlusion of the ulnar artery in the hand. J Bone Joint Surg 60A: 841–843

631. Hirai M, Shinoya S 1979 Arterial obstruction of the upper limb in Buerger's disease: its incidence and primary lesion. Br J Surg 66: 124–129

632. Raynaud A G M 1862 De l'asphyxie locale et de la gangrene symetrique des extremites. Rignoux, Paris

633. Balas P, Tripolitis A J, Kaklamanis P, Mandalaki T, Paracharalampous N 1979 Raynaud's Phenomenon. Primary and secondary causes. Arch Surg 114: 1174–1177

634. Farmer R, Gifford R, Hines E 1961 Raynaud's disease with sclerodactylia. A follow-up study of seventy-one patients. Circulation 23: 13–15

635. Welsh C L 1980 The effect of vibration on digital blood flow. Br J Surg 67: 708–710

636. Teisinger J 1972 Vascular disease disorders resulting from vibrating tools. J Med 14: 129–133

637. Telford L E D, McCann M B, MacCormack D H 1949 Dead hand in users of vibrating tools. Lancet i: 359

638. Taylor W, Pelmear P L 1975 Vibration white finger in industry. Academic Press Inc, San Diego, CA pp 21–30

639. Blunt R J, Porter J M 1981 Raynaud syndrome. Semin Arthrit Rheum 10: 282–308

640. Lundborg G, Dahlin L B, Hansson H A, Kanje M, Necking L E 1990 Vibration exposure and peripheral nerve fiber damage. J Hand Surg (Am) 15: 346–351

641. Brammer A J, Piercy J E, Auger P L, Nohara S 1987 Tactile perception in hands occupationally exposed to vibration. J Hand Surg (Am) 12: 870–875

642. Pike J, Arons M S 1990 Vibration Syndrome: a new test and rating system for disability compensation. Con Ortho 20: 303–308

643. Hansford T, Bood H, Kent B, Lutz G 1986 Blood flow changes at the wrist in manual workers after preventive interventions. J Hand Surg (Am) 11: 503–508

644. Mosely L H, Finseth F 1977 Cigarette smoking: impairment of digital blood flow and wound healing in the hand. Hand 9: 97–100

645. Guzman-Stein G, Schubert W, Najarian D W, Press B H, Cunningham B L 1989 Composite in situ vein bypass for upper extremity revascularization. Plastic Reconstr Surg 83: 533–536

646. Given K S, Puckett C L, Kleinert H E 1978 Ulnar artery thrombosis. Plastic Reconstr Surg 61: 405–411

647. Rottler P D, Meystrik R, Puckett CL 1990 Microvascular angioscopy. Plastic Reconstr Surg 85: 397–403

648. Brown F E, Jobe J B, Hamlet M, Rubright A 1986 Induced vasodilation in the treatment of posttraumatic digital cold intolerance. J Hand Surg (Am) 11: 382–387

649. Wilgis E F 1985 Digital sympathectomy for vascular insufficiency. Hand Clin 1: 361–367

650. Flatt A E 1980 Digital artery sympathectomy. J Hand Surg 5: 550–556

651. Morgan R F, Reisman N R, Wilgis E F 1983 Anatomic localization of sympathetic nerves in the hand. J Hand Surg (Am) 8: 283–288

652. Morgan R F, Wilgis E F 1986 Thermal changes in a rabbit ear model after sympathectomy. J Hand Surg (Am) 11: 120–124

653. Arnulf G 1976 Physiological basis of sympathetic surgery for the upper limb in Raynaud's diseases. J Cardiovasc Surg 17: 354–357

654. Kirtley J A, Riddell D H, Stoney W S, Wright J K 1967 Cervicothoracic sympathectomy in neurovascular abnormalities of the upper extremity. Ann Surg 165: 869–879

3. Compression

The pathogenesis of peripheral nerve compression is varied:

Anatomical. In certain areas, nerves pass through unyielding surroundings, as in the carpal tunnel and beneath the arcade of Frohse.

Postural. Many occupations or recreations require repetitive motions[1-4]. If these are made in a posture which increases peripheral nerve compressions, symptoms may develop. Examples of such positions are:

(a) The flexed wrist which increases carpal tunnel compression, especially if weight is lifted in this posture
(b) Pronation of the forearm with an extended elbow and flexed wrist motion which compresses the radial nerve in its 'tunnel' at the elbow.

Developmental. Anomalous structures may overfill a tight compartment or may place a nerve on stretch, as occurs in the presence of a cervical rib or its fibrous anlage.

Inflammatory. Synovitis is the most common cause of nerve compression in the carpal tunnel. Usually non-specific, the increased bulk of inflamed synovium cannot be accommodated by the inexpansible tunnel and compression of the median nerve results. The specific synovitis of rheumatoid disease causes a higher incidence of nerve compression amongst those so afflicted than occurs in the general population.

Traumatic. Acute carpal tunnel syndrome, requiring urgent release, may complicate any hand injury in which significant oedema occurs. Delayed nerve compression may result from trauma as in the tardy ulnar palsy following on supracondylar fractures of the humerus.

Metabolic. Alterations in fluid distribution may well precipitate or exacerbate nerve compression. This is especially common in carpal tunnel syndrome, in which the characteristic night numbness is due in part to the increased peripheral circulation which occurs during sleep, largely as a means of temperature regulation. The syndrome is more prevalent in women and is often more troublesome in the premenstrual phase and during pregnancy when water retention occurs. Certain endocrine disorders, by disturbing fluid balance, show an increased incidence of nerve compression syndromes. Thus carpal tunnel syndrome in particular is more common in myxoedema[5] and diabetes[6].

Swellings, by taking up already overcrowded space, may produce compression syndromes.

Iatrogenic. Acute compression may be inflicted on nerves during surgical procedures. Such injury occurs most commonly to the radial nerve, travelling, as it does, for most of its course close to bone. It is therefore very vulnerable during internal fixation of fractures of the humerus and radius. The surgeon must identify and preserve it zealously when applying bone plates. Compression of peripheral nerves may also occur through poor positioning of the anaesthetized patient. Once again the radial nerve in the spiral groove is most at risk, although the axillary nerve and ulnar nerve above the elbow[7,8] have been injured by this means.

When subjected to constant compression a nerve becomes narrowed. This is commonly observed in the course of relieving a carpal tunnel syndrome (Fig. 3.1). If narrowing has been present for some time, fibrosis occurs in the epineurium and between the fascicles themselves[9]. In such circumstances, compression by fibrosis may persist even after release of the original compressing force. Curtis has demonstrated the value of splitting the epineurium in improving the results of carpal tunnel release[10]. Although he also recommended internal neurolysis, this is now deemed to be of no value[11].

If the compressive force is applied intermittently, as in the radial tunnel syndrome, a constriction in the nerve itself is much less likely. Thus confirmation of the diagnosis at the time of surgery is less convincing and there is rarely any need to perform an internal neurolysis.

'Double crush' syndrome[12] arises when a nerve is

283

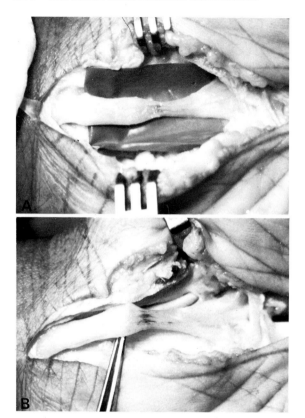

Fig. 3.1 A,B. This median nerve has been subjected to compression in the carpal tunnel and shows both narrowing of the nerve and hyperaemia of the narrow section.

compressed at more than one level. Second or subsequent compressions of the nerve occur more readily[13], and release of one without the other understandably is less likely to give relief [6,13].

HISTORY

When a patient presents with pain or dysaesthesia he should be questioned, in respect of each, regarding location, radiation, duration, fluctuation and periodicity, nature and time of onset and factors which provoke or relieve the symptoms. He may be unable to give precise replies. It is then useful to ask him to record the details during an attack and report them at his next visit. For example, patients may state that numbness involves all of their digits, but advised observation reveals that only those supplied by the median nerve are affected.

Other symptoms should be recorded and a general medical history and description of occupation obtained. Particular attention should be paid to any family history of diabetes, to symptoms suggestive of other endocrine

disorders, and to repetitive occupational postures or manoeuvres. If a full physical examination has been performed in the recent past, a report should be obtained.

SYMPTOMS AND SIGNS

Compression of peripheral nerves produces predictably one or more of four effects: pain, sensory disturbance, motor loss, electrophysiological change.

The *pain* of nerve compression may be located at the site of compression, but commonly radiates distally and proximally. Distal radiation is easily understood and knowledge of the distribution of, for example, a cervical root is necessary to localize the site of compression. Proximal radiation is more difficult to understand and may represent a generalized neuritis resulting from distal compression or referred pain to an area having a common cervical root origin with the compressed nerve. Pain occurs in compression of purely motor nerves, as in the *radial tunnel syndrome*. This is probably due to the fact that the nerve is not entirely efferent in flow, having afferent fibres from both muscles and joints.

Sensory disturbance in compression syndromes initially takes the form of intermittent *numbness* and *tingling* or *paraesthesia*. These are invariably within the exact sensory distribution of the compressed nerve, although not necessarily throughout it. Any indisputable extension beyond the boundaries of that distribution should make the examiner beware. He may be dealing with anomalous distribution, compression of more than one nerve, or, most probably, compression located more proximally than initially suspected.

While at first present only periodically, numbness soon becomes constant. Depending upon the nerve involved, this may be a nuisance or a distinct disability. Loss of sensation in median nerve distribution causes clumsiness in fine manipulation and this may be the patient's sole or major complaint.

Examination at all stages reveals some change in sensation. This is by no means total anaesthesia or analgesia. Two-point discrimination, sweating and even tactile gnosis are commonly all intact. The patient simply declares that on light touch or pinwheel testing 'it feels different' from other normal areas — this has been termed *dysaesthesia*. It follows that the area under examination must be repeatedly compared with other areas of normally similar sensibility in the same and the other hand. The boundaries of dysaesthesia should be marked out. Special attention should be paid to key areas, such as the 'palmar triangle' in median and the dorsum of the hand in ulnar nerve compression.

A Tinel's sign is often elicited at the site of compression or a little proximal to it, producing paraesthesia radiating into the sensory distribution of the nerve.

Tenderness may be present over the course of the nerve expecially when pain is the major symptom. This may be revealed by direct palpation or by the indirect compression produced by putting muscles on tension or by so positioning joints as to increase the pressure on the nerve.

Motor loss in nerve compression, unlike that following nerve section, is an insidiously progressive disability, of which the patient may be unaware. *Muscle wasting* may be far advanced but unnoticed by the patient's untrained eye. *Postural changes*, such as the development of a claw hand or abducted small finger in ulnar nerve compression, may be the first feature which commands his attention or it may be *weakness and clumsiness* in certain acts. The weakness is often slight and detectable only by careful comparison with the other, supposedly normal, hand. In certain instances it is possible to pit one muscle directly against its counterpart, as with the abductor pollicis brevis of each hand (Fig. 3.2).

Electrical activity may be altered in nerve compression syndromes, with a reduction in nerve conduction velocity across the area of compression. This is exemplified by the increase in distal motor or sensory latency often found in carpal tunnel syndrome. However, only a positive finding of slowing of nerve conduction is of value. Uninterrupted conduction in but a small percentage of fibres will give normal speeds of conduction for the whole nerve. Also, in those syndromes in which compression is intermittent, as in the radial tunnel, nerve conduction times are often normal. Thus a normal electrical study does not rule out a compression syndrome, while an abnormal study confirms the clinical findings. Such studies are often of greatest value in localizing the site of compression.

MEDIAN NERVE

Carpal tunnel syndrome

The carpal tunnel is a bony canal of which the margins can be palpated (Fig. 3.3).

The *scaphoid tubercle* is the bony prominence at the base of the thenar eminence just distal to the distal wrist crease. The tendon of flexor carpi radialis appears to attach to that prominence when rendered palpable by flexing the wrist against resistance — it in fact passes over the tubercle and into a groove beneath the *ridge of the trapezium*, which lies immediately adjacent distally. These two bones form the radial boundary of the carpal tunnel.

The *pisiform* is easily palpable at the ulnar end of the narrow area between the two wrist creases. Flexor carpi ulnaris attaches to the pisiform, gaining additional purchase through the piso-hamate and piso-metacarpal ligaments which insert into the hook of the hamate and the base of the fifth metacarpal respectively.

The *hook of the hamate*, with the pisiform, forms the ulnar margin of the tunnel. More difficult to palpate, the hook of the hamate lies two centimetres distal and slightly radial to the pisiform beneath the broken skin crease which demarcates the hypothenar eminence.

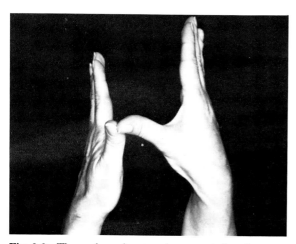

Fig. 3.2 The weakness in a muscle can sometimes be demonstrated by pitting it against its normal counterpart in the other hand. Here weakness of the abductor pollicis brevis in carpal tunnel syndrome is clearly demonstrated when the patient attempts to maintain both thumbs in palmar abduction while pushing one against the other.

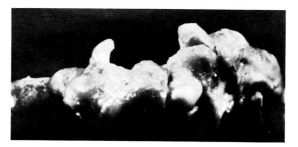

Fig. 3.3 The carpal tunnel view in relief in a dissection of the skeleton. The pisiform has been removed on the left of the photograph revealing the hook of the hamate which forms the ulnar border, while on the right of the photograph the tubercle of the scaphoid and the ridge of the trapezium are seen clearly forming the radial border. (Reproduced from Johnson M K and Cohen M J 1975, The Hand Atlas. Thomas, Springfield, with kind permission of the authors and publisher.)

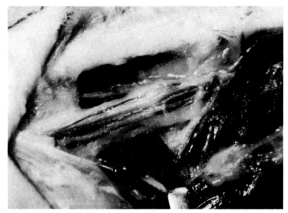

Fig. 3.4 Here a persistent median artery is seen on the surface of the median nerve. Flow has been diminished by the compression against the retinaculum.

Over the hook the motor branch of the ulnar nerve can be rolled by the examining finger.

The *flexor retinaculum* which roofs over the tunnel is a thick, rigid, fibrous sheet which attaches to its bony boundaries. A less substantial part of the retinaculum passes superficially to blend with the hypothenar fascia. Sometimes referred to as the *volar carpal ligament*, this is the roof of *Guyon's canal*, through which the ulnar nerve and artery pass, radial to the pisiform but ulnar to the hook of the hamate.

Ten structures pass through the carpal tunnel — the median nerve, flexor pollicis longus and the eight flexor tendons to the four fingers. Many variations in the anatomy and course of the median nerve, especially its motor branch, have been reported[14-18], although the

reported incidence of such variations differs widely[19]. The tendons are enveloped by the synovium of the radial and ulnar bursae. Any volumetric increase of this synovium will compress the median nerve[20].

Other less common causes of median nerve compression in the carpal tunnel include:

developmental — persistent median artery[21,22] (Fig. 3.4)
— unusually extensive lumbrical[23-27] or superficialis[28] muscle bellies (Fig. 3.5)
— anomalous muscles[29] of which the *reversed palmaris*[30-33] and *palmaris profundus*[34-36] are the most common

trauma[37] — the effects of trauma may be direct, as in carpal bone fractures or carpometacarpal dislocation (Fig. 3.6), or indirect due to the swelling resulting from an extensive hand injury or burn[38]

swellings — ganglion[39], fibroma[40], aneurysm of the median artery[41] or lipoma

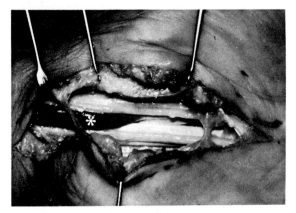

Fig. 3.5 The belly of the superficialis to the middle finger is unduly long and has produced compression in the carpal tunnel.

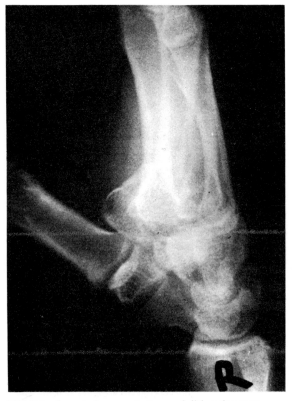

Fig. 3.6 An anterior carpometacarpal dislocation may produce pressure in the carpal tunnel resulting in acute median nerve compression.

inflammatory — rheumatoid disease, gout, tuberculosis[42-44], gonorrhoea[45], scleroderma[46] and amyloidosis[47]

metabolic — pyridoxine deficiency[48] and other
endocrine imbalance, the most com-
mon of which is pregnancy, peripheral neuropathy[49]

SYMPTOMS

Numbness is the most frequent complaint. Located in
the median nerve distribution, the digits most often
involved are the middle and index. Initially, the numbness is intermittent. The time of onset is characteristically in the early hours of the morning, induced by the
acute wrist flexion of the 'fetal' sleeping position, by
altered fluid distribution in the lying position and by
increased blood flow to the limb for thermoregulation.
For reasons which are obscure, symptoms are often
relieved by hanging the limb dependent. Carpal tunnel
syndrome may be provoked by working with the wrist
flexed, while driving or reading a newspaper.

Pain in the upper limb may be due to median nerve
compression in the carpal tunnel. This cause may be
overlooked, particularly if the pain is in the arm above
the tunnel. Discomfort due to carpal tunnel syndrome
may be present *as far proximal as the shoulder*[50].

Clumsiness may be due to sensory loss or to weakness
in the thenar musculature.

EXAMINATION

Muscle wasting is best detected by comparison with the
other hand, while viewing the thenar eminence in pro-
file (Fig. 3.7). It may rarely affect only part of the
abductor pollicis brevis, in which case it may be less
pronounced.

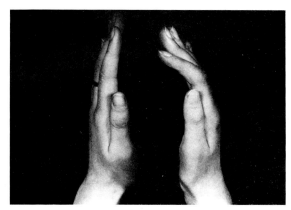

Fig. 3.7 Thenar wasting may be demonstrated best by
comparing it with the opposite normal hand.

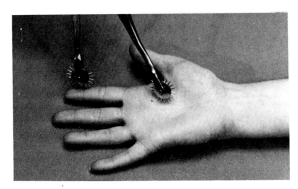

Fig. 3.8 As the pinwheel is passed from the index finger
into the palm, it moves from the area of absolute innervation
by the median nerve into that supplied by the palmar
cutaneous. In carpal tunnel syndrome, therefore, a change
will occur at some point between these two areas.

Sensory disturbance is mapped out using light touch
or, more expeditiously, by using a pin-wheel (Fig. 3.8).
Loss of sensation is not commonly so advanced as to
cause a detectable difference in two-point discrimination[51]. It follows that sweating is often present, in which
event those sensory tests based on its absence are
not applicable. In perfoming the examination, repeated
comparison should be made with ulnar innervated digits and with those on the other hand. The dysaesthesia
does not often involve the entire median nerve distribution and this does not cast doubt on the diagnosis.
However, particular attention should be paid to the
'palmar triangle' (p. 14). If sensation is diminished in
that area innervated by the palmar cutaneous nerve, a
diagnosis of carpal tunnel compression should be made
with reservations and with the knowledge that it is only
tenable if:

1. The 'palmar triangle' is not served by the palmar
cutaneous nerve, or
2. The palmar cutaneous nerve does not arise some
6 cm proximal to the retinaculum and pass
superficial to it as is normally the case, but
originates, as has been described, deep to it,
piercing the retinaculum to serve the palmar
triangle (Fig. 3.9).

The distribution of the palmar cutaneous nerve is not
limited strictly to the palmar triangle, as Erik Moberg
was quick to point out to the author after the first edition of this book. Using the pinwheel from the median
autonomous zone on the index finger and running
towards the palm, change may occur as far distal as the
middle digital crease. This *may* be due to thicker skin
on the digit, and the change should be compared with
that on the opposite hand.

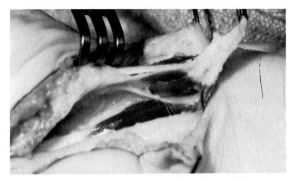

Fig. 3.9 The palmar cutaneous branch of the median nerve can be seen in this case arising just proximal to the carpal tunnel and passing through the retinaculum. This particular patient showed evidence of sensory loss in the distribution of the palmar cutaneous nerve.

A

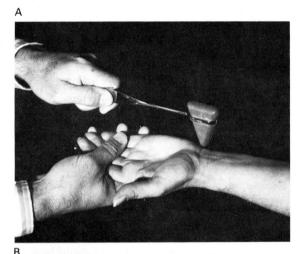

B

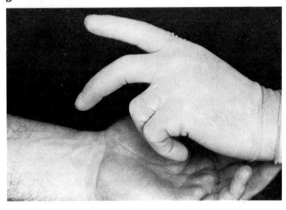

Fig. 3.10 A Tinel's sign is very frequently elicited in carpal tunnel syndrome just proximal to the tunnel. The percussion may be performed either with a tendon hammer or with the flexed middle finger as in percussing the chest.

Changes may also be detected in the ulnar nerve distribution in as many as one-third of cases of carpal tunnel syndrome[52].

A *Tinel's sign* is detected in the majority of patients with carpal tunnel syndrome. Tapping with the flexed finger or with a tendon hammer over the course of the nerve at the retinaculum, or more commonly just proximal to it, produces paraesthesiae radiating into the median nerve distribution (Fig. 3.10).

The *Phalen test*[53-55] increases the compression on the median nerve by placing the wrist in acute flexion, especially in patients with carpal tunnel syndrome[56]. This is achieved by putting the dorsum of one hand against that of the other with the fingers dependent and lowering the elbows as far as possible while maintaining that contact. By doing both hands at one time the normal acts as a control for the affected hand. However, both hands may be involved either with the patient's knowledge or subclinically. Therefore a timed Phalen test is of more value, any onset of numbness in less than one minute being considered diagnostic of carpal tunnel compression (Fig. 3.11). The patient may avoid flexing the wrist fully (as seen with the left hand in Fig. 3.11A), knowing from experience that it is uncomfortable. For this reason, the Phalen test can probably be performed more efficiently by the examiner. The wrist is fully flexed with the forearm supinated and then maintained in that position by holding the palmar abducted thumb towards the wrist. In patients in whom the wrist cannot be flexed, pressure over the median nerve immediately above the carpal tunnel will prove equally effective in diagnosis[57].

The *reversed Phalen test* is performed by placing the palms of the hands together and raising the elbows as high as possible. Occasionally, when the Phalen test is negative, the reverse test is positive, producing numbness and tingling in the median nerve distribution by placing the nerve on stretch (Fig. 3.12).

Abductor pollicis brevis should be tested. With the hand flat on the table, palm upwards, the patient should be asked to touch with his thumb the examiner's finger held above the hand. Strength is tested by having the patient resist downward pressure.

The diagnosis of carpal syndrome in the majority of cases will be made with confidence on the basis of the above examination. In those where doubt remains *electromyography* should be undertaken. Prolongation of the distal motor latency beyond 4 ms will confirm the presence of median nerve compression. Such an increase in distal motor latency is found in approximately two-thirds of patients with subsequently confirmed median nerve entrapment[58]. A normal result does not therefore rule out the diagnosis[59,60]. It has been reported

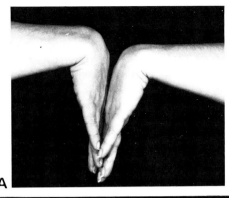

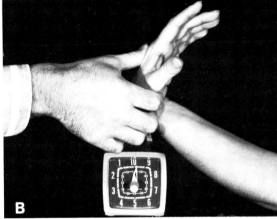

Fig. 3.11   A. The Phalen test is performed by having the patient place the backs of the hands against one another and flex the wrists fully. The development of paraesthesiae in the median nerve distribution is evidence of compression of the median nerve in the carpal tunnel. B. The test can also be performed by the examiner flexing the patient's wrist into the position shown in A. The test should be timed since the more rapid the onset of paraesthesiae the more definite the diagnosis.

that orthodromic sensory nerve conduction studies are a more sensitive index of compression, 85 to 95% of surgically confirmed cases showing prolongation of the distal sensory latency beyond 3.5 ms, which is the upper limit of normal (p. 241).

All patients with carpal tunnel syndrome should have the most likely systemic causes eliminated by basic laboratory work:

sedimentation rate — if elevated this should be followed with more sophisticated tests for rheumatoid disease and collagen disorders
two-hour postprandial blood sugar, serum uric acid, T3 resin uptake and T4 and T7 estimations.

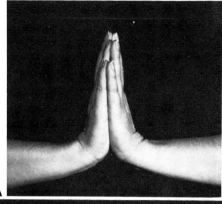

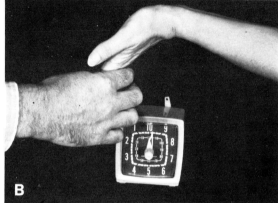

Fig. 3.12   Occasionally the reversed position with the palms together and the wrist dorsiflexed may produce paraesthesiae when the orthodox Phalen test has failed to do so.

RADIOLOGIC EXAMINATION

Standard and special views of the hand should be taken for they may reveal an unsuspected radio-opaque lesion producing pressure in the carpal tunnel. The specialized carpal tunnel view is most useful in this respect (Fig. 3.13)[61].

INDICATIONS

Conservative management is indicated in all patients who have only intermittent problems. While diuretics, pyridoxine[62] or anti-inflammatory agents may be of help, this usually consists of injection and splintage[63]. The tunnel is injected with 0.5 ml of local anaesthetic and 0.5 ml of soluble steroid at a point midway between the pisiform and the scaphoid tubercle and 1 cm distal, using a short 27 gauge needle with the bevel parallel to the nerve (Fig. 3.14). Care should be taken to ensure that the median nerve has not been impaled by asking

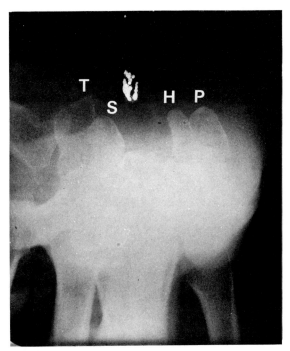

Fig. 3.13 A carpal tunnel radiologic view. The scaphoid, pisiform, trapezium, and hamate are marked with initial letters. This view is of value in demonstrating the presence of abnormal radio-opaque structures within the carpal tunnel.

the patient whether paraesthesiae have resulted from introduction of the needle. If they do, it should be re-inserted. The onset of *paraesthesiae during injection* tends to confirm the diagnosis since the addition of 1 ml of fluid should not cause significant compression of a normal nerve. The splint is worn to hold the wrist in slight dorsiflexion. Injection has been shown to cure 22–54%[63–65] of patients with appropriate symptoms. It is especially indicated in pregnant patients in whom the compression can be expected to abate with delivery.

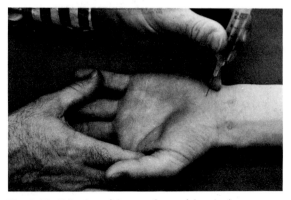

Fig. 3.14 Injection of the carpal tunnel (see text).

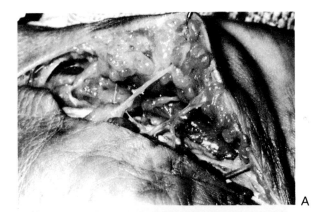

A

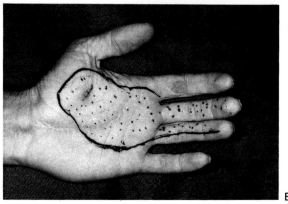

B

Fig. 3.15 A. The terminal branches of the palmar cutaneous nerve may be encountered in the process of making the incision for release of the carpal tunnel. B. This patient presented after carpal tunnel release with hypaesthesia and dysaesthesia in the extensive area marked out by the pen. He also had a fairly painful neuroma at the proximal end of the incision.

Surgical release of the flexor retinaculum[66] is indicated after failed conservative management or as the first line of treatment in those patients showing *constant numbness*, evident *motor weakness* or *increased distal latency*. These are also the cases in whom epineurotomy is required since Curtis has shown that scarring of the epineurium and around the fascicles can entirely negate the value of simple decompression. If the synovium around the flexor tendons is thickened and hypertrophied, some surgeons undertake synovectomy. Great care must be taken to protect the palmar cutaneous branches in making the incision (Fig. 3.15)[67]. The superficial palmar arch is also at risk during release of the carpal tunnel as is the motor branch of the median nerve[68] (Fig. 3.16). The nerve may be clearly constricted as in Figure 3.1, the site of the local blood flow reduction[69] (Fig. 3.4) or markedly hyperaemic (Fig. 3.17).

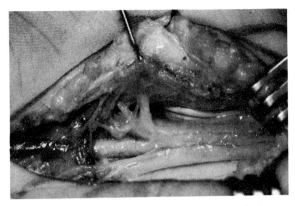

Fig. 3.16 The median nerve is seen passing beneath the superficial palmar arch which lies with one of its branches to the left end of the incision. Just proximal to the point at which it passes beneath the arch, the median nerve gives off its motor branch. Here there are two.

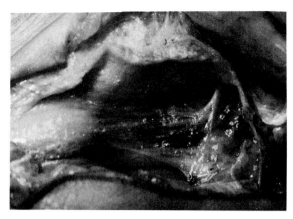

Fig. 3.17 Hyperaemia of the median nerve consequent upon compression.

The side effects of carpal tunnel release, their cause and rate of resolution are the source of disagreement in the literature. That the volume of the tunnel is increased is generally agreed[70]. That the grip strength decreases is also agreed, but its speed of recovery varies widely, from 3 months[71] to 9 months[72]. Whether or not the arch widens is disputed[70,73], as is the importance of that widening[73,74]. Suffice it to say that sensation improves rapidly[72] following simple release, even in those cases in which the ulnar nerve distribution was involved[52].

See Green D P 1993 Operative Hand Surgery, 3rd edn. Churchill Livingstone, New York, p. 1349.

Pronator syndrome[75]

On entering the forearm, the median nerve passes beneath the edge of the lacertus fibrosus of the biceps, between the two heads of pronator teres and then beneath the bridge or arch formed by the proximal edge of the flexor digitorum superficialis. The median nerve may be subjected to compression by any of these structures[76,77] or by anterior displacement of the radial head at this level. In less than one-tenth of patients, the nerve may pass through the humeral head or beneath both heads of pronator teres which increases the probability of compression. The significance of the pronator syndrome is that it may easily be mistaken for carpal tunnel compression and the wrong treatment undertaken.

Points of similarity to carpal tunnel syndrome
Numbness and paraesthesia in median innervated digits
Weakness of the thenar muscles
Pain in the wrist and forearm.

Points of contrast with carpal tunnel syndrome
No nocturnal complaints
No Tinel sign at the wrist
Nerve conduction may be delayed, but not at the wrist
Dysaesthesia in the 'palmar triangle'.

It might be expected that the Phalen test would be negative. However, it was positive in 50% of patients diagnosed as having pronator syndrome at the Mayo Clinic[78].

The patient with pronator syndrome complains primarily of pain[79] in the forearm, usually following activity, with associated dysaesthesia in the median nerve distribution and possible thenar weakness.

The *Tinel sign* is found over the median nerve either where it passes beneath the pronator teres at the junction of upper or middle thirds of the forearm or proximal to that in the antecubital fossa (Fig. 3.18).

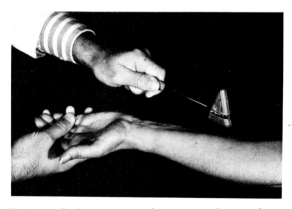

Fig. 3.18 In the pronator syndrome, percussion over the median nerve where it passes between the heads of pronator teres produces pain and paraesthesiae passing down into the median nerve distribution.

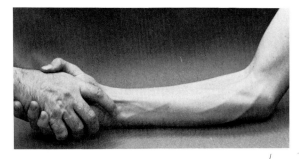

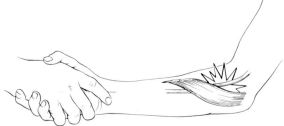

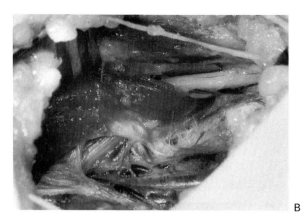

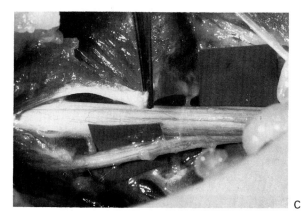

Fig. 3.19 Pronator syndrome. A. Testing pronator teres compression. B. Looking from the ulnar aspect with the hand to left side of the photograph, the median nerve can be seen passing between the superficial and deep heads of the pronator. The deep head has been retracted in a radial direction away from the examiner to demonstrate this relationship. C. After division of the deep head, the median nerve, which is hyperaemic, is released. The anterior interosseous nerve in the lower part of the photograph here has a rather low take-off from the median nerve.

Pain and paraesthesiae in the median nerve distribution are evoked by placing stress on the three likely compressing structures:

pronator teres	— resisted pronation of the *extended* forearm (Fig. 3.19)
lacertus fibrosus[80]	— resisted flexion of the elbow and supination of the forearm (Figs 3.21 and 3.23B)
arch of flexor digitorum superficialis	— resisted flexion of the proximal interphalangeal joint of the middle finger (Fig. 3.22)

Resisted pronation with the elbow flexed does not produce pain (Fig. 3.20), for only the ulnar head of pronator teres is rendered tense in this position, and the nerve is therefore not compressed.

Nerve conduction studies[78,81], both motor and sensory, may show no change in conduction as the compression exerted by the pronator teres or superficialis is intermittent, depending upon position and muscle contraction. If, however, there is slowing it will be located in the forearm. Electromyographic studies of the muscles served by the median nerve should also be performed.

INDICATIONS

Splintage in pronation and slight wrist flexion, with or without elbow flexion, allied with a change in occupational use of the arm if possible, may relieve the symptoms. If not, exploration is indicated with decompression of the median nerve by release of one head of pronator teres, the superficialis bridge and any associated compressing structures.

See Green D P 1993 Operative Hand Surgery, 3rd edn. Churchill Livingstone, New York, p. 1343.

Anterior interosseous syndrome

The anterior interosseous nerve arises from the median nerve some 4–6 cm below the elbow. It is an entirely motor nerve, serving flexor pollicis longus, flexor digitorum profundus to the index and middle fingers and pronator quadratus.

Compression of the anterior interosseous nerve was first described by Tinel in 1918. Spinner[82], in his monograph on nerve disorders in the forearm, lists the structures which may compress the nerve:

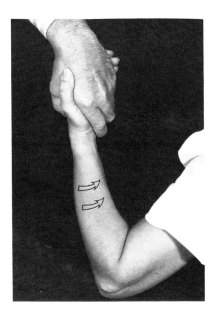

Fig. 3.20 When the resisted pronation is attempted with the elbow flexed, the patient has significantly less discomfort. In this position the humeral head of pronator teres plays little part in pronation of the forearm and therefore compression of the median nerve is not so marked.

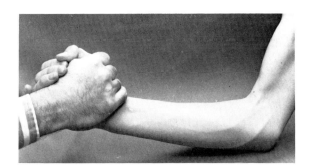

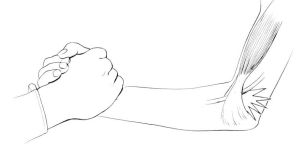

Fig. 3.21 Pronator syndrome. Testing for lacertus fibrosus compression.

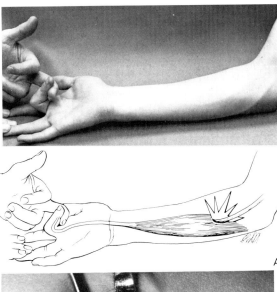

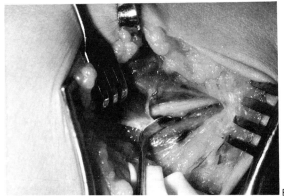

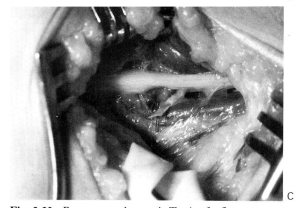

Fig. 3.22 Pronator syndrome. A. Testing for flexor digitorum superficialis compression. B. (The hand is to the left of this photograph. The incision is transverse.) The right angled retractor is lifting one head of the flexor digitorum superficialis beneath which the median nerve passes. C. After release of this head, the proximal hyperaemia, constriction at the point of compression and distal pseudoneuroma are all evident. These intraneural changes are by no means common in this dynamic compression (see text).

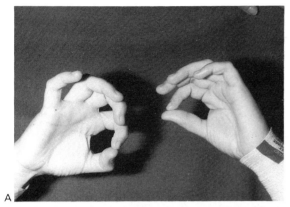

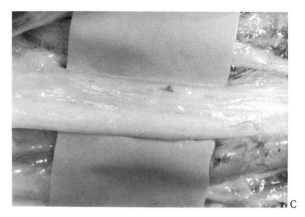

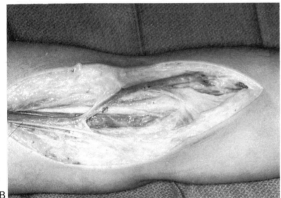

Fig. 3.23 Anterior interosseous palsy. A. Here, immediately following surgery, the patient is requested to make a circle with his thumb and index finger as he does on the left of this photograph. On the right, his lack of interphalangeal flexion in the thumb and weakness of distal interphalangeal flexion in the index produces the characteristic posture of anterior interosseous palsy. B. (The hand is to the right of the photograph.) Here the lacertus fibrosus is seen crossing the median nerve from proximal – radial to distal – ulnar. C. The different appearance of the two components of the median nerve can be seen on close inspection.

This patient presented with anterior interosseous syndrome. The upper part is the anterior interosseous component, the lower the median nerve proper. This occurred after a heavy work-out by this 20-year-old athlete. It was postulated that the longer course, with no branches, of the median nerve permitted it to fall away from the compressing lacertus in a manner the shorter anterior interosseous component could not do.

tendinous bands	— in the deep head of pronator teres
	— in the origin of flexor digitorum superficialis of the middle finger
	— in the origin of a palmaris profundus
accessory muscles	— from superficialis to profundus muscles
	— Gantzer's muscle (an accessory head to flexor pollicis longus)
vascular	— thrombosis of ulnar collateral vessels
	— aberrant radial artery
other	— an enlarged bicipital bursa

SYMPTOMS

Pain in the forearm is very commonly the presenting symptom. Pain is thus common to the three compression neuropathies of the median nerve. It occurs in this purely motor nerve for reasons discussed previously (p. 284).

Weakness of pinch occurs primarily through the loss of flexor pollicis longus. The fine pinch manoeuvre, which requires nail-to-nail contact as in lifting a pin from a flat surface, is lost due to paralysis of both flexor pollicis longus and flexor digitorum profundus to the index finger.

EXAMINATION

The fine pinch posture is abnormal. The pulp of the index finger, which is extended at the distal interphalangeal joint makes contact with the pulp of the thumb just distal to its hyperextended interphalangeal joint (Fig. 3.23).

Muscle testing reveals:

Flexor pollicis longus — absent or weak interphalangeal flexion of the thumb

Flexor digitorum profundus — absent or weak distal interphalangeal flexion of the index and, less commonly, the middle finger

Pronator quadratus — when compared with the normal limb pronation of the forearm with the elbow flexed (to reduce the power of pronator teres) is weaker.

Variations — differing distribution of the anterior interosseous nerve may result in variations of this clinical picture:

Only flexor pollicis longus or flexor digitorum profundus of the index may be affected[83,84], or

In addition to flexor pollicis longus, pronator quadratus and profundus to the index and middle fingers:

(i) parts of superficialis may be affected

(ii) in certain instances of the Martin–Gruber anastomosis, a varying number of intrinsics normally innervated by the ulnar nerve may be affected.

INDICATIONS

Observation should be pursued for 6–12 weeks for spontaneous recovery may occur[84]. Decompression should then be performed. If unsuccessful, it can be followed by appropriate tendon transfers some 3 to 6 months later.

See Green D P 1993 Operative Hand Surgery, 3rd edn. Churchill Livingstone, New York, p. 1345.

OTHER REPORTED CAUSES OF MEDIAN NERVE COMPRESSION

The reported causes of median nerve compression form an impressive list. The following is an incomplete guide to the literature.

Developmental
Aberrant and anomalous lumbricals[85-87]
Anomalous superficialis[88]
Persistent median artery[89-91]
Vessel perforating nerve[92]
Supracondylar process[93]

Traumatic
'Greenstick' fracture[94-96]
Colles[97]
Hook of hamate[98]
Cut superficialis[99]
Fracture–dislocation carpo-metacarpal[100]
Elbow dislocation[101-103]
Insect sting[104]

Metabolic
Amyloid[105]
Mucopolysaccharidoses[106]

Tumours — intraneural
Lipofibroma[107-108]
Haemangioma[109]

Degenerative
Osteophyte[110]
Cyst[111]
Bursa[112]
Ganglion[113]

Iatrogenic
Opponensplasty[114]
Dialysis[115-20]
Silicone rod[121]

ULNAR NERVE

Symptoms due to compression of the median nerve are most probably due to entrapment at the wrist or in the forearm. By contrast, similar problems in ulnar nerve distribution are more often due to involvement of the nerve at the elbow or of its roots in the neck.

Guyon's canal — ulnar tunnel syndrome[122,123]

The volar carpal ligament which roofs over the canal of Guyon is a structure less substantial than the flexor retinaculum which encloses the carpal tunnel (p. 13). Fewer structures, only the ulnar nerve and artery, pass through the canal, and it contains no synovium. For these reasons, compression of the ulnar nerve is much less common than median nerve entrapment at the wrist; when it does occur, it is more frequently associated with trauma or with the presence in the canal of an abnormal structure. The configuration of the hypothenar muscle origin is probably significant[124].

Trauma
Ulnar nerve involvement may follow on one heavy blow to the base of the hypothenar eminence but is more frequently due to repetitive occupational trauma of the type which is also responsible for thrombosis of the ulnar artery in this situation — 'hypothenar hammer syndrome' (p. 262). It may also result from the oedema following injury[125].

Abnormal structures
Swellings. A ganglion[126] is by far the most common cause of ulnar nerve palsy in Guyon's canal; indeed, four out of the first five explored by Seddon proved to be due to a ganglion (Fig. 3.24)[127,128].

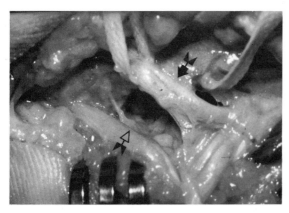

Fig. 3.24 This patient presented with loss of ulnar nerve function distal to Guyon's canal. Exploration revealed a ganglion compressing the deep branch (seen here immediately after the ganglion was opened).

Anomalous muscles[129–134]:
— reversed or accessory palmaris longus passing through the tunnel (Fig. 3.25);
— duplication of hypothenar muscles
— abnormal origin for the hypothenar muscles in the forearm
— aberrant flexor carpi ulnaris[135,136]

SYMPTOMS

Patients will present with *pain* which may be in the hand or forearm[137], and with varying combinations of *weakness, paraesthesia* and *hypaesthesia*, for six separate patterns of involvement have been described[138]:

1. Pure sensory deficit
2. Pure motor deficit involving:
   (a) all ulnar-innervated intrinsic muscles
   (b) all the above, except the hypothenar muscles
   (c) as in (a) but excepting the abductor digiti minimi
3. Mixed motor and sensory deficit, involving:
   (a) all ulnar-innervated intrinsic muscles
   (b) all the above, except the hypothenar muscles

EXAMINATION

Posture may be altered as for an ulnar nerve lesion (p. 224) (Fig. 3.26).

Sensory disturbance
The expected sensory loss will be, as in compression of the ulnar nerve at any level, of the palmar surface of the small finger and the ulnar half of the ring. However, the most significant part of the clinical examination is directed at the distribution of the *dorsal sensory branch*. If this shows hypaesthesia on pinwheel testing, the compression *cannot* be in Guyon's canal. If the test is normal, it *may* be or may not.

Motor loss
    Deep motor[139]: All the interossei and adductor pollicis are weak or paralysed, and this is evidenced by muscle wasting particularly noticeable in the first dorsal interosseous.
    Complete ulnar. In addition to the above, the hypothenar muscles are weak or paralysed. Again, this is demonstrated by wasting and on active testing.

Electromyography
Nerve conduction velocities will often be slowed from the wrist to the first dorsal interosseous.

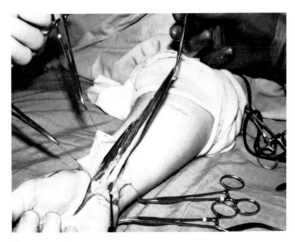

Fig. 3.25 Guyon's canal compression. An anomalous muscle arose from a reversed palmaris longus to pass into the canal, causing compression.

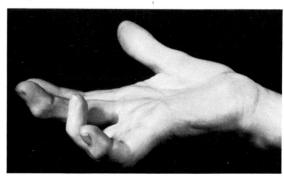

Fig. 3.26 The ulnar claw hand.

INDICATIONS

Ulnar nerve entrapment at Guyon's canal more frequently results in motor loss than median nerve compression in the carpal tunnel. In all cases with such loss, exploration should be performed.

See Green D P 1993 Operative Hand Surgery, 3rd edn. Churchill Livingstone, New York, p. 1366.

At the elbow — cubital tunnel syndrome[140]

Traumatic ulnar neuritis, tardy ulnar palsy or cubital tunnel syndrome at the elbow was the first chronic disorder of a peripheral nerve to be described. While there is an element of compression, friction plays a greater role here than in any other of the 'compression neuropathies'. Either or both may be due to one of several causes.

Anatomical. The aponeurosis between the two heads of flexor carpi ulnaris may be unusually tight.

Trauma — direct: any blow to the flexed elbow may injure the nerve. The exposed situation of the nerve is shown by the frequency with which the 'funny (or crazy) bone' is struck. If severe, such a blow may lead to a chronic neuritis.

Trauma — indirect: injuries to the bones of the elbow joint, especially in childhood, may result in 'tardy ulnar palsy' at a much later date.

fractures of lateral condyle
dislocation of radial head } → cubitus valgus
fractures of medial condyle → irregular ulnar groove

The latter has its effect by direct impingement on the nerve, the former by placing the nerve on undue stretch.

Recurrent dislocation of the nerve. Normally firmly seated in the ulnar groove, or cubital tunnel as it is also named, the ulnar nerve in some instances dislocates over the medial epicondyle on flexion. This movement in itself is sufficient to produce neuritis and also further exposes the nerve to trauma. It is important to remember that recurrent dislocation of the nerve was found in 16.2% of one series of entirely asymptomatic volunteers[141].

Arthritis. Osteoarthritis or rheumatoid disease of the humero-ulnar joint may result in cysts[142] or bone spurs (Fig. 3.27). These bone spurs may impinge upon the ulnar nerve.

Swellings. The ubiquitous ganglion is again the swelling most likely to embarrass the nerve.

Abnormal muscle. Anconeus epitrochlearis[143-145] passes from the medial border of the olecranon to the medial epicondyle and may compress the ulnar nerve.

Posture. The pressure in the cubital tunnel rises

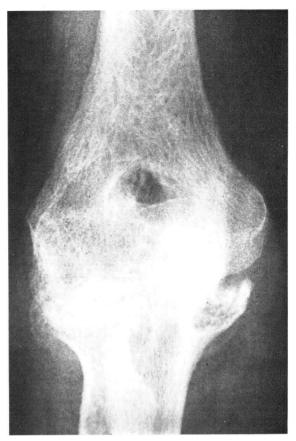

Fig. 3.27 Spurs around the elbow joint in association with rheumatoid arthritis may produce compression of the ulnar nerve in the cubital tunnel.

significantly with elbow flexion and with shoulder abduction. This is a major cause of nocturnal symptoms.

SYMPTOMS

Pain in the upper extremity, often of an ill-defined nature, may be the major complaint.

Paraesthesiae and numbness involving the ulnar innervated digits are usually present. The numbness and tingling may be similar to that of carpal tunnel compression, initially nocturnal and infrequent, later more constant. Elbow flexion makes the pain and paraesthesiae more troublesome, and commonly occurs while sleeping.

Weakness in the ulnar innervated musculature in the hand is common. The muscles in which weakness is most noticed by the patient are the adductor pollicis and the first dorsal interosseous, due to reduction in pinch strength and the *wasting* in the first web space which accompanies it.

EXAMINATION

Distinction between cubital tunnel neuritis and involvement of the ulnar nerve in Guyon's canal or more proximal compression of cervical roots C8 and T1 at the neck is, of course, mandatory if surgical relief is to be obtained. This distinction is not easily made.

Sensory disturbance

As in carpal tunnel syndrome, this is not always sufficiently severe to reduce two-point discrimination or sweating.

Dysaesthesia is more likely, involving the small and ring fingers, hypothenar eminence and the ulnar half of the dorsum of the hand. The last is of great diagnostic significance in eliminating Guyon's canal compression as the cause of the patient's complaints.

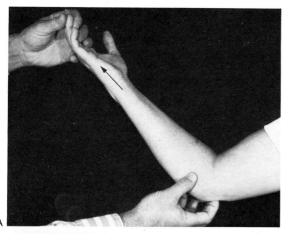

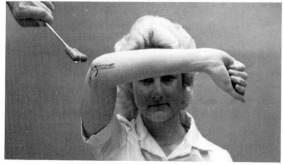

Fig. 3.28   A. Palpation of the ulnar nerve in the cubital tunnel will produce paraesthesiae radiating down to the small finger in the presence of ulnar neuropathy at the elbow. It is important to compare this with the unaffected limb as the ulnar nerve frequently shows a positive Tinel's sign in this position. B. Percussion of the ulnar nerve at the cubital tunnel can be more easily undertaken with the shoulder flexed and internally rotated, bringing the arm in front of the head.

Tinel's sign is invariably positive over the ulnar nerve in the cubital tunnel, producing tingling radiating into the ulnar two fingers (Fig. 3.28). However, the normal ulnar nerve often 'Tinel's' in this situation and therefore only a difference from the unaffected side is significant.

Flexion of the elbow produces pain and paraesthesiae in the ulnar nerve distribution and is virtually diagnostic of cubital tunnel syndrome (Fig. 3.29). It is something akin to the Phalen test in carpal tunnel syndrome, and, like that, can be timed to give some measure of severity.

Motor loss

Weakness or *paralysis* and *wasting* of the ulnar innervated muscles in the hand occurs in established ulnar neuropathy at the elbow. Active testing should be performed on all the intrinsic muscles. Froment's sign may be present (p. 225) as may clawing, affecting only the ring and small fingers.

The nerve supply to flexor digitorum profundus of the ring and small fingers comes from the ulnar nerve five or six centimetres distal to the cubital tunnel. Paralysis of these muscles may therefore be encountered in ulnar nerve compression at the elbow but is surprisingly rare. So also is palsy of flexor carpi ulnaris and this may be for the same reason, namely, that the fascicles to these muscles are located on the deep surface of the nerve in the cubital tunnel. Active testing will reveal this loss. If flexor digitorum profundus is affected it will have two consequences:

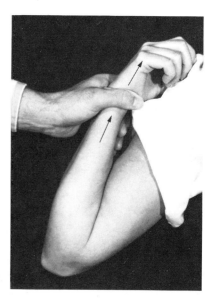

Fig. 3.29   If the paraesthesiae and pain are produced by forceful flexion of the elbow, this is virtually diagnostic of an ulnar neuropathy in the cubital tunnel.

1. Clawing will not occur, as the imbalanced pull of the flexor on the interphalangeal joints will have been eliminated.
2. The examiner will have further confirmation that the lesion lies proximal to the canal of Guyon, indeed certainly lies at or above the elbow.

However, as emphasized above, flexor digitorum profundus is often unaffected, even in the presence of complete paralysis of ulnar innervated intrinsics.

For the purpose of prognosis and evaluation, patients with cubital tunnel syndromes can be classified thus (McGowan[146]):

I Recent, mild, intermittent dysaesthesias
II Persistent dysaesthesia, early motor loss
III Marked atrophy and weakness

Electrophysiological changes

These are often present; indeed, they help to determine the need for surgery and the level at which the exploration is indicated much more in ulnar neuropathy than in affections of the median nerve. Slowing of the nerve conduction velocity across the elbow suggests the need for exploration of the cubital tunnel.

Radiologic examination

The elbow should be examined radiologically, both standard anteroposterior and lateral, and also a cubital tunnel view, taken with the elbow flexed (Fig. 3.30).

The features of ulnar neuropathy at the elbow by which it is distinguished from compression at Guyon's canal and at the thoracic outlet are summarized below.

1. Dysaesthesia in the dorsal sensory branch of the ulnar nerve.
2. A strongly positive Tinel at the cubital tunnel, especially if it is elicited by elbow flexion.
3. Slowing of nerve conduction across the elbow.
4. Absence of wasting or weakness in the thenar muscles.
5. Lack of dysaesthesia in the C8, T1 dermatomes, that is, the inner aspect of the forearm and elbow.

INDICATIONS[147]

The results of surgical release are less predictable than one would wish. For this reason, provided no impingeing pathology is suspected in the tunnel, a trial of splintage should be discussed with the patient. The splint should be long-arm with the elbow set at whatever angle less than 90° suits the patient. The wrist should be supported. The splint serves to protect the nerve from direct contact and from the friction and compression of flexion. It should be worn at all times, apart from bathing and while at work if the splint impedes necessary function or offers a hazard, until one week after all symptoms have resolved.

Where this fails, then the surgeon has the problem of selecting the appropriate surgical procedure[148]. Osborne[149,150] has shown that simple neurolysis with division of the aponeurosis which joins the humeral and ulnar origins of the flexor carpi ulnaris is effective treatment in many cases (Fig. 3.31). Transposition of the nerve with or without medial epicondylectomy has been widely practised but is not without morbidity, especially in heavy manual workers. If the nerve appears to be

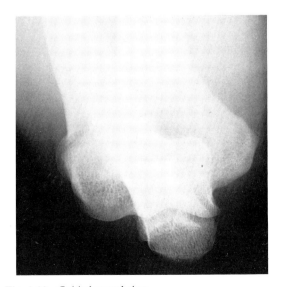

Fig. 3.30 Cubital tunnel view.

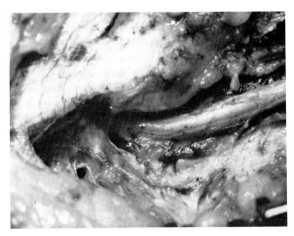

Fig. 3.31 The ulnar nerve is seen here in the cubital tunnel passing beneath the aponeurosis of the flexor carpi ulnaris to enter the forearm.

subject to fibrosis, epineurotomy should also be performed. Internal neurolysis should *not* be done for there are many interfascicular cross-connections here.

Anterior transposition is indicated in the following instances: cubitus valgus, arthritis with osteophyte formation, recurrent dislocation of the nerve, pain and recurrent symptoms after simple neurolysis, provided other causes have been eliminated.

When performed, transposition beneath the entire flexor mass as described by Learmonth[151,152], subcutaneous and intramuscular[153] translocation and medial epicondylectomy[154-159] all have their advocates and their critics. Whatever procedure is selected, the medial intermuscular septum must be split above the elbow at the point where the ulnar nerve passes posteriorly through the septum or the angulation compression may simply be moved proximally[160].

See Green D P 1993 Operative Hand Surgery, 3rd edn. Churchill Livingstone, New York, p. 1357.

OTHER REPORTED CAUSES OF ULNAR NERVE COMPRESSION

Developmental and anatomical
Triceps[161-163]
Flexor carpi ulnaris — mid-forearm[164]
— 5 cm distal to medial epicondyle[165]
Adductor pollicis[166]
Supracondylar process[167]
Trochlear hypoplasia[168,169]
Vascular bands in the forearm[170]

Traumatic
Wrist fractures[171-173]
Carpometacarpal dislocation[174]
Heterotopic bone following burns[175]

Tumours
Giant cell[176,177]
Lipoma[178,179]
Intraneural cyst[180]
Synovial osteochondromatosis[181]

Rheumatoid
At the wrist[182,183]

Thoracic outlet syndrome

The brachial plexus and the subclavian artery emerge from the neck and the thorax into the supraclavicular region through a narrow, triangular space — the thoracic outlet[184] — bounded

below by the first rib
anteriorly by scalenus anterior
behind by scalenus medius.

They then pass beneath the clavicle and coracoid process[185] in turn, with the rib cage, in the form of the first and second ribs, lying immediately below the neuro-

vascular structures. To join the plexus and proceed through this course the cervical root T1 passes upwards through the thoracic outlet, across the first rib to turn

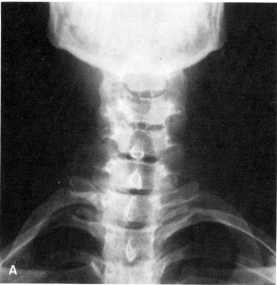
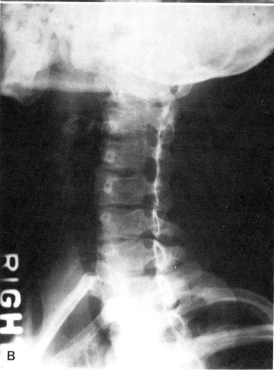

Fig. 3.32 A, B. This patient shows a cervical rib, more evident in the oblique view. In this instance, the rib was responsible for thoracic outlet syndrome which resolved after its removal.

down again towards the arm. Just medial to the rib it is joined by the C8 root to form the lower trunk.

Any structure which encroaches on this narrow space or any process which in some other way reduces its dimension will be likely to compress the roots or the trunks of the brachial plexus and may also narrow the subclavian artery[186]. From whatever sources comes the compression, T1 and the lower trunk bear the brunt of problems. Such compression has been described in association with:

Cervical rib[187], or *rudimentary first rib*[188]. While this may indeed produce compression it is often innocent, but may delude the surgeon into undertaking its removal to no avail (Fig. 3.32).

Fibromuscular, tendinous or ligamentous bands. Roos[189], in the course of over 1000 operations, has identified nine types of band associated with the first rib, scalenus anterior and scalenus medius. He believes them to be the major cause of the syndrome. No direct evidence of their presence is available preoperatively other than a C7 transverse process extending beyond that of T1 in AP or oblique cervical spine views.

Swellings. Seddon described a chondroma causing a thoracic outlet syndrome.

Trauma. Severe fractures of the clavicle may cause costo-clavicular compression of the plexus and artery (Fig. 3.33). In addition, relatively minor trauma to the neck or shoulder may induce the syndrome through muscle spasm which causes the outlet to narrow and bands to impinge on the plexus.

Postural changes. The 'military brace' position, in which the shoulders are held back in an exaggerated posture, has been shown to produce thoracic outlet syndrome. The opposite extreme of posture, namely, slumping of the shoulders, is believed to contribute to the increased incidence of thoracic outlet syndrome in patients in their fourth decade, with or without the presence of a cervical rib. Any sustained activity of the arm may aggravate the patient's symptoms. Examples of such troublesome actions include holding a steering wheel and combing and setting the hair.

SYMPTOMS

Pain is usually present and is described as being of a persistent, 'gnawing' or 'burning' nature. More aching than sharp in quality, it is usually located in the shoulder and inner aspect of the upper arm, radiating down into the hand. Unlike root compression at the intervertebral foramen, the pain rarely radiates upwards into the head. It becomes worse in the course of a day's work, especially if the patient's occupation demands repetitive movements of the hands with the shoulders in an exaggerated position, either reaching forward or upwards. The pain may then be relieved briefly by shrugging the shoulders and exercising the hands, but return to the prevailing posture produces renewed discomfort.

The pain may be worse at night, especially if the patients is accustomed to sleeping on the affected side, and may be relieved by swinging the arm around.

Sensory disturbance

Tingling and *numbness* are common, usually in the C8 and T1 distribution, although they may involve the entire hand. The symptoms in the ulnar two fingers and on the ulnar dorsum of the hand may be confused with ulnar nerve compression. If the numbness can clearly be shown to extend on to the ulnar border of the forearm or upper arm then the likelihood of a thoracic outlet or root aetiology is increased, since these are the territories of the medial cutaneous nerves of forearm and arm respectively, not of the ulnar nerve.

Motor loss

Heralded by a complaint of *swift fatigue* in the arm, wasting and weakness affects mainly those muscles innervated by the first thoracic root, namely, the intrinsic muscles of the hand. The patient may complain of incoordination in all fine movements, especially pinch manoeuvres.

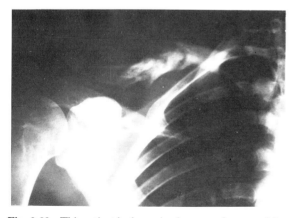

Fig. 3.33 This patient had sustained a severe fracture of the clavicle in falling from a horse, and this came to non-union. Severe compression of the lower cords of the brachial plexus resulted and were relieved by removal of the excess callus from the clavicle during internal fixation.

Vascular changes

A minority of patients may present because of the vascular effects of the thoracic outlet syndrome. These may be due to direct compression of the vessel or due to thrombosis in or embolization from a post-stenotic aneurysm just distal to the point of compression. In vascular compression patients may complain of:

venous congestion[190] in the form of swelling, heaviness and cyanosis

cold intolerance

colour changes in the digits occurring most commonly in the index finger but often involving all. These may take the form of attacks of complete pallor, followed by painful hyperaemia or cyanosis, characteristic of *Raynaud's phenomenon* (p. 263).

If significant thrombosis or embolization ensues *necrosis* of the tips of the digits will result.

EXAMINATION

Sensory disturbance

Localization of areas of dysaesthesia, that is, where sensation 'feels different' from adjacent regions, should be made using light touch or a pinwheel. Commonly the usual distribution of the ulnar nerve will be involved. To differentiate thoracic outlet syndrome from ulnar neuropathy, particular attention should be paid to the forearm and upper arm (Fig. 3.34). Sensitivity here

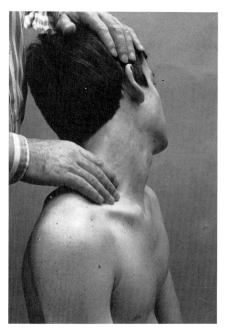

Fig. 3.35 Pressure applied to the brachial plexus in the posterior triangle will produce symptoms in the form of paraesthesia and discomfort in the appropriate dermatome in thoracic outlet syndrome.

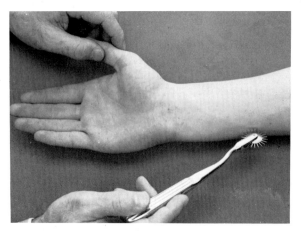

Fig. 3.34 In testing for sensory disturbance in possible thoracic outlet syndrome, particular attention should be paid to the ulnar aspect of the upper arm and forearm since the cutaneous supply, while deriving from a lower cervical root, does not travel in the ulnar nerve but rather in the medial cutaneous nerves of arm and forearm. Dysaesthesia in this location, therefore, serves to eliminate the possibility of ulnar neuropathy.

is much less acute than in the hand and time should be allowed for the patient to be clear which areas are involved. This may require repeated tests and comparison should be made with the other upper limb, while remembering that thoracic outlet syndrome may well be bilateral.

Dysaesthesia of the ulnar nerve
+ medial cutaneous of arm
+ medial cutaneous of forearm

suggests thoracic outlet syndrome.

Tingling and pain may be elicited by direct palpation or *percussion over the brachial plexus* which can be felt in the posterior triangle as it emerges from behind scalenus anterior (Fig. 3.35). These paraesthesiae radiate into the distribution of which the patient complains and should be compared with the contralateral side. They may also be produced by movements of the neck, in which event distinction must be made from cervical root, as opposed to trunk, compression. As classically described lateral flexion can distinguish between thoracic outlet and root compression syndromes:

Symptoms on lateral flexion towards the affected side are due to root compression.

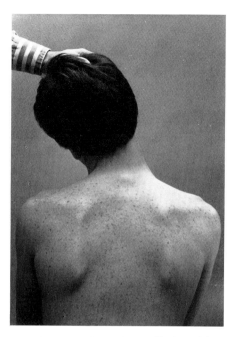

Fig. 3.36 Thoracic outlet syndrome. Flexion of the neck away from the affected side produces discomfort by stretching the compressed nerves.

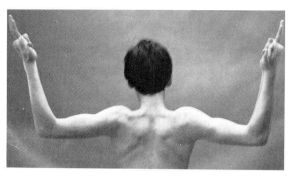

Fig. 3.37 Roos test. The shoulders are braced, the arms elevated, and the hands exercised. In thoracic outlet syndrome, the patient is unable to continue this for 3 minutes.

Symptoms on lateral flexion away from the affected side are due to thoracic outlet syndrome (Fig. 3.36).

Motor loss

Wasting is detected by inspection.

Weakness is detected by active muscle testing.

In both instances particular attention should be paid to the thenar muscles for therein lies an important distinguishing feature from ulnar neuropathy: palsy of the intrinsic muscles of the hand *including* the median-innervated thenar muscles suggest thoracic outlet syndrome.

Commonly the triceps (C7) is weak but the reflexes are normal. This may be a point of distinction from the patient with cervical disc disease in whom strength may be normal but reflexes not.

Three-minute elevated arm exercise test[189] (Fig. 3.37). This simple test has proved the most reliable in diagnosing thoracic outlet syndrome. With the patient sitting with the arms abducted to 90° and the elbow flexed to 90°, he is asked to open and close his hands repeatedly while keeping the shoulders gently braced backwards. The patient with thoracic outlet syndrome will be quite unable to complete this test due to recurrence of all the symptoms of which he complains. If he is able to complete 3 minutes he does not have outlet compression.

Vascular compromise

In those few cases with peripheral evidence of circulatory disturbance of some magnitude, vascular signs will be detected:

colour and temperature difference — when compared with the opposite limb, the affected hand may clearly be pale, blue or cold;

diminished pulses — the radial pulse may be more difficult to palpate, and an *Allen test* (p. 259) may show significantly slower filling than in the opposite limb;

lower blood pressure — the blood pressure should be recorded in both limbs for comparison. When the possibility of bilateral involvement exists, the pressure should be taken in the lower limbs also, using an oscillometer;

thrill and bruit — gentle palpation over the subclavian artery in the posterior triangle may reveal a palpable thrill. More often a bruit may be heard in the same location through the stethoscope.

Vascular compromise through change of position

Several other tests have been described to demonstrate neurological and vascular compromise due to thoracic outlet syndrome. *These have proved unreliable and misleading*[191] and the author never uses them. They are included here because they are still widely practised. It should be emphasized that, if performed, the most significant finding in any of these tests is reproduction of the symptoms of which the patient complains.

Adson's sign[192,193]. The patient is asked to brace the shoulders backwards, rotate his head to the affected side, elevate the chin and hold his breath in full inspiration. The radial pulse may disappear in this position or be palpably reduced in volume. This may be evidence of thoracic outlet syndrome but the examiner must be aware that this test is positive in one out of every four or five normal subjects.

Hyperabduction (Wright) test[194] (Fig. 3.38). With the patient in the same posture as for the Adson test, the arm is abducted to 90° in full external rotation of the shoulder. Diminution or disappearance of the radial pulse should again be sought. In

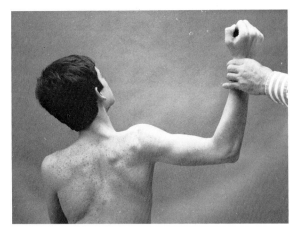

Fig. 3.38 Hyperabduction test. The arm is hyperabducted, the patient's head is turned towards the side of the lesion and the chin tilted upwards. Disappearance of the pulse represents a positive hyperabduction test but may be present in as many as 25% of the normal population.

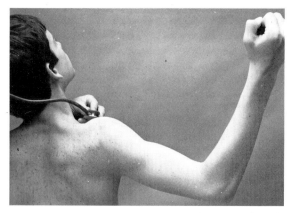

Fig. 3.39 While maintaining the arm in the hyperabducted position auscultation over the subclavian artery may reveal a distinct bruit.

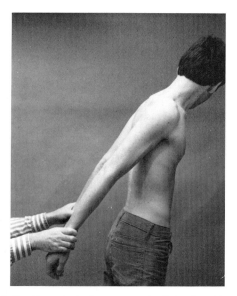

Fig. 3.40 Costoclavicular compression is produced by having the patient relax the shoulders completely while the examiner draws the arms downward and posteriorly while palpating the radial pulses. The pulses may be diminished or disappear and the patient may complain of numbness and tingling.

SPECIAL STUDIES

All patients suspected of having a thoracic outlet syndrome should have the following studies performed.

Radiologic examination of cervical spine: AP and both obliques, lateral views in flexion and extension. The presence of a cervical rib, as emphasized above, does not necessarily mean that it is the cause of the patient's complaints. Vague symptoms and imprecise signs are most unlikely to be cured by resection of a cervical rib simply because it is there. Cervical spondylosis and osteoarthritis, especially with encroachment on the intervertebral foramen by osteophytes, may lead the surgeon to revise his diagnosis from trunk to root compression and he should review his records with this possibility in mind. Spasm of the paravertebral muscles which may result from, or predispose to, outlet compression — hence creating a vicious cycle — may be evidenced by loss of the normal lordotic curve on the otherwise normal lateral radiograph (Fig. 3.41).

Electrophysiological studies may well reveal slowing of nerve conduction velocities across the supraclavicular fossa. Even when this is not the case, such studies are necessary to eliminate more peripheral neuropathies which may remain a possible cause of symptoms. There is some evidence that slowing may be precipitated in outlet compression by adopting the abducted position during testing[195]. This is true of other intermittent com-

this position auscultation over the subclavian artery may reveal a bruit due to partial occlusion (Fig. 3.39).

Claudication. Keeping the patient in the same position, but allowing him to breathe normally, he is asked to exercise the hand vigorously. Forearm pain and tingling will ensue within a few seconds in the presence of compression and the patient will soon lower the arm, complaining of considerable discomfort. An extremity without neurovascular compression, by contrast, can be exercised for over a minute with little or no distress.

Costoclavicular compression (Fig. 3.40). The patient is asked to stand, allow his shoulders to slump and put his extended, supinated arms down alongside and a little behind his thighs. While palpating both radial arteries, the surgeon applies gentle downward traction to the arms. The pulse may be diminished or occluded and the patient may complain of pain and tingling in the affected limb.

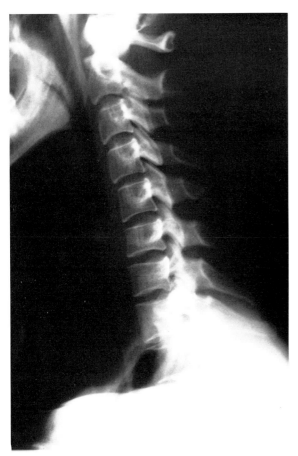

Fig. 3.41 Loss of the normal lordotic curve in an otherwise normal cervical spine is evidence of paravertebral muscle spasm which often occurs in thoracic outlet syndrome.

pression such as pronator syndrome and radial tunnel syndrome. In all patients, relaxed and provocative conduction studies should be performed.

Transfemoral subclavian angiography is indicated only in the small minority of cases showing predominantly vascular signs. It may reveal narrowing of the subclavian artery, poststenotic dilatation, vascular anomalies (Fig. 3.42) or vascular occlusion. Narrowing may not be evident on standard studies and it is important that angiograms be obtained in the posture in which the patient normally experiences symptoms (Fig. 3.43).

[Note: emphasis has been laid in examination on distinguishing ulnar neuropathy from thoracic outlet syndrome producing compression of the *lower* trunk of the plexus, by far the most frequent involvement and certainly the most difficult diagnostic problem. The 'military brace syndrome'[196,197] may produce an Erb's palsy by compressing the *upper* trunk. A cervical rib,

scalenus medius band[198] or swelling may compress the *middle* trunk. The characteristics of such compressions have been detailed in the chapter on Reconstruction (p. 243) and do not present any diagnostic confusion with a more peripheral lesion as does the more common lower trunk compression.]

INDICATIONS[199]

Conservative measures include postural and stretching exercise, weight loss and a period of rest from the provoking occupation[200]. Intensively followed under encouraging supervision, this regime cures more than half of the patients with outlet disease. If it fails, or if vascular compromise is a major element of the disorder, surgical intervention is indicated.

Anterior scalenotomy[201], originally favoured by Adson, has not proved as successful as he first reported. However, the procedure allows visualization of the entire plexus and may reveal unexpected causes of compression, including soft-tissue tumours and, more commonly, fascial bands passing to the first rib. *Resection of a cervical rib* seen to be impingeing on the plexus can be performed through the scalenotomy incision. Release of the anterior scalene is easily undertaken together with removal of all fibromuscular bands which can be found. It is important that these be sought with the arm held in a variety of positions.

All patients to whom this procedure is recommended should be warned of the possibility of failure to relieve the presenting symptoms. In the event of failure or recurrence *first rib resection*[202], best performed by the transaxillary route, may prove effective.

See Green D P 1993 Operative Hand Surgery, 3rd edn. Churchill Livingstone, New York, p. 1372.

Cervical root compression

We have progressed well outwith the domain of the hand surgeon in pursuit of the cause of symptoms in the ulnar nerve distribution in the upper extremity. Although we are about to abandon the chase with a few cautionary words regarding our responsibility to pass on the task to others where appropriate, complaints relative to the hand so commonly come from the neck that cervical root compression must be briefly considered.

Root compression may arise from a tumour of the cervical cord, acute herniation of a disc, chronic herniation with associated spondylosis or intervertebral foraminal osteophyte formation.

In dealing with any neurological disorder radiating from neck to forearm the possibility of a space-occupying lesion should always be remembered and investigated appropriately.

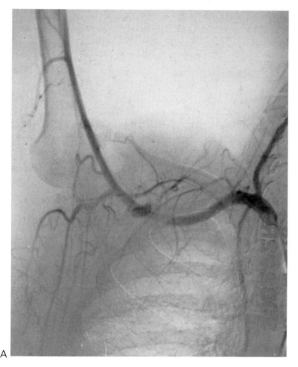

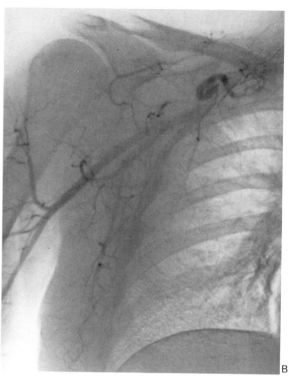

A   B

Fig. 3.42   A, B. The patient presented with severe symptoms and signs of thoracic outlet compression. Hyperabduction angiogram was performed which revealed normal flow but an abnormal vascular structure which filled late (B) and remained filled. Exploration revealed a hamartoma in the region of the plexus causing severe compression.

Acute herniation of a cervical disc is usually associated with a definite injury, which may be a vertebral compression or less frequently a 'whiplash' type of road traffic accident. Pain is the predominant symptom. It is very severe, producing marked limitation in neck motion and radiating into the upper limb. Usually one root alone is involved and paraesthesia, motor

Fig. 3.43   Transfemoral subclavian angiography here reveals total occlusion of the subclavian artery in the hyperabducted position.

weakness and alteration in reflexes help to localize that one involved (p. 238). This patient rarely presents to the hand surgeon.

Chronic cervical root compression by slow disc extrusion or by bony encroachment on the intervertebral foremen may produce symptoms predominantly in the forearm and hand and therefore requires more detailed consideration.

SYMPTOMS

Pain is a major complaint. This usually commences in the neck, involving in turn shoulder, forearm and hand, often becoming sufficiently severe distally as to completely mask more proximal components. The pain is aching in character, made worse by extreme neck movements, by poor sleeping posture and by maintaining one position for prolonged periods as is commonly required in industry. It is typically subject to acute exacerbations, when pain may be excruciating. Such exacerbations may be brought about by uncontrolled movements such as coughing or sneezing, which also act by raising the spinal fluid pressure. The cessation of pain may be

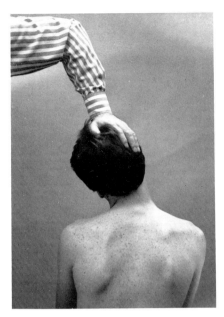

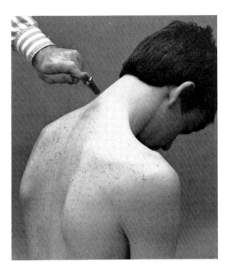

Fig. 3.45 Percussion over the spinous process of the affected vertebrae may produce root pain in cervical root compression.

Fig. 3.44 Spurling test. The head is tilted towards the affected side and direct compression on the vertex is applied. If increase in symptoms results the test is positive.

a sign of significant root damage; if the regression is accompanied by continuing signs in the appropriate myotome and dermatome, myelography is indicated.

Radiation into the occipital region is commonly present and distinguishes radicular pain from more peripheral compression.

Dysaesthesia, wasting and weakness may present and all show a specific root distribution. The points of greatest strain in the cervical spine are discs C5–6 which produces C6 root compression, and C6–7 which produces C7 root compression. Knowledge of this arrangement which differs from the thoracic and lumbar spine is necessary if radiological changes and clinical findings are to be correlated.

EXAMINATION

Sensory disturbance

In more advanced cases typical dermatome dysaesthesia may be found. Clinical evidence of sensory loss may, however, be completely absent despite the patient's complaints of numbness. In these cases the symptoms may be reproduced by *Spurling's test*[203] in which the head is tilted toward the involved side and pressure applied to the top of the head (Fig. 3.44).

Tenderness posteriorly over the vertebra involved may be present. Percussion over the appropriate spinous process may produce radicular pain (Fig. 3.45).

Motor weakness may be present and this shows a specific root distribution as does any reduction in tendon reflexes:

C5–6 disc — weakness of biceps, reduced biceps reflex
C6–7 disc — weakness of triceps, reduced triceps reflex.

Special studies

A *radiograph* of the *cervical spine*, especially the oblique views, may well show significant narrowing of the intervertebral foramina (Fig. 3.46). The lateral view may show loss of intervertebral disc space with loss of the normal lordotic curve even in the hyperextended position and 'beaking' of the vertebral bodies anteriorly.

Electromyography, apart from implicating the muscle of the appropriate myotome, has been reported to provide absolute evidence of root involvement, as opposed to more peripheral lesions, by showing denervation patterns in the paraspinal muscles which can occur only if the neuropathy lies proximal to the posterior primary ramus. However, it is difficult to perform and interpret on account of significant interference.

Myelography is essential in root lesions to eliminate cervical cord tumours. It also commonly confirms the presence of a herniated disc by revealing obliteration of the sleeve which is normally seen passing into the intervertebral foramen.

Discography and *nerve root infiltration*[204] help to localize cervical disc degeneration.

Computerized tomography can be of value in studying the bony elements of the cervical spine and can de-

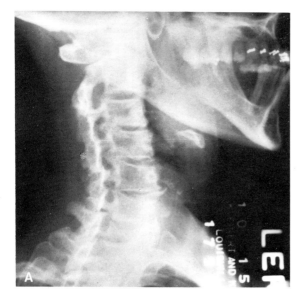

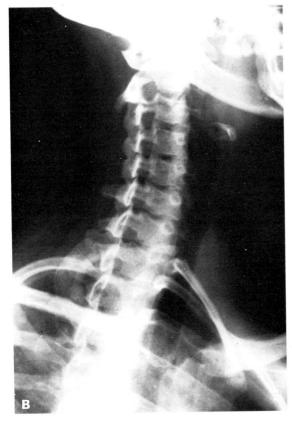

lineate soft-tissue lesions, when used in conjunction with subarachnoid water soluble contrast medium.

Magnetic resonance imaging.

RADIAL NERVE

The radial nerve arises from the posterior cord of the brachial plexus and gains the posterior aspect of the humerus by passing through the triangular space created by the teres major above, the long head of triceps medially and the humerus laterally. It comes to lie in the spiral radial groove beneath the lateral head of triceps and immediately proximal to the origin of the medial head. It then gains the anterior aspect of the arm by piercing the lateral intermuscular septum 10–12 cm proximal to the lateral epicondyle where it can be easily rolled by the finger against the humerus in most limbs. It then lies between the brachialis and biceps tendon medially and the muscles arising from the lateral supracondylar ridge laterally, brachioradialis, extensors carpi radialis longus and brevis. The nerve passes directly over the anterior ligament of the elbow joint or, more specifically, the articulation between the capitulum of the humerus and the head of the radius. At some point between 3 cm above and below that joint the nerve divides into the sensory superficial radial nerve and the motor posterior interosseous nerve. The two diverge gradually at first but to a degree which bodes ill for the motor nerve. While the superficial radial nerve adheres securely to the deep surface of the brachioradialis, the posterior interosseous nerve passes deep and laterally to gain the extensor surface of the

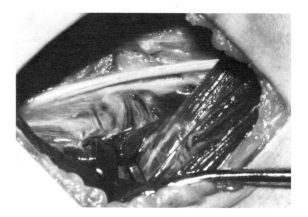

Fig. 3.47 Radial tunnel syndrome. The fan of radial recurrent vessels which crosses the deep posterior interosseous nerve is clearly demonstrated after splitting the brachioradialis muscle. Superficially, the sensory radial nerve is seen overlying the vessels.

Fig. 3.46 Oblique views of the cervical spine in this patient show significant narrowing of the intervertebral foramina together with narrowing of the disc spaces and beaking of the anterior aspect of the vertebral bodies. A normal oblique view is shown for comparison (B).

forearm, encountering as it does so three potentially constricting structures.

Extensor carpi radialis brevis, arising from the common extensor origin, often has a sharp tendinous medial border which overlies the posterior interosseous nerve.

A *'fan' of vessels* from the radial recurrent artery crosses, or passes through, the nerve to supply the structures lateral to it (Fig. 3.47).

The *arcade of Frohse*[205] is the free, aponeurotic proximal margin of the superficial portion of the supinator beneath which the posterior interosseous nerve passes (Fig. 3.48). Spinner[206], whose studies of this area are definitive, states that the size of the space beneath the arcade varies greatly and that the arch is thickened and fibrous in 30% of adults examined. He also notes that it is never fibrous in infants. In the release of over one hundred and fifty radial tunnels, this author has *always* found the arch to be largely fibrous. Whether this is a developmental feature or an occupational adaptation it is impossible to say. Certainly it would appear to be a prerequisite to the onset of nerve compression.

The radial nerve and its posterior interosseous termination run close to bone throughout much of their course, the former on the humerus[207,208], the latter on the radius. They are thus prone to injuries of all degrees in fractures and the management[209] thereof.

While radial palsy has been ascribed to compression of the nerve by a fibrous arch in the lateral head of triceps[210-212] — the author has operated on one in ten years (Fig. 3.49) — and by the lateral intermuscular septum[213] the major compression syndromes of the radial nerve without fracture are related to the posterior interosseous nerve in the region of the supinator.

While two distinct such syndromes have been described, as Roles and Maudsley[214] emphasized in de-

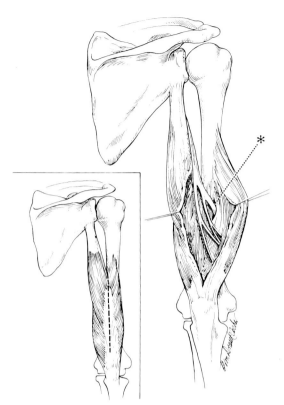

Fig. 3.49 Compression of the radial nerve beneath a fibrous arch in the lateral head of the triceps.

scribing the radial tunnel syndrome, they are simply two points in a spectrum extending from simple 'tennis elbow' (p. 347) to irreversible paralysis of the muscles supplied by the posterior interosseous nerve.

Radial tunnel syndrome (pain)[215,216]

The compressive factors in radial tunnel syndrome are all anatomical:

fibrous bands tethering the nerve to the radiohumeral joint
extensor carpi radialis brevis
the radial recurrent 'fan' of vessels
the arcade of Frohse.

These anatomical structures compress the nerve only when, with the elbow extended, the wrist is passively flexed and pronated, or conversely, when the wrist is extended or supinated against resistance. Occupation therefore plays a major role, since employment requiring frequent repetitive movements of the wrist and forearm in this position may well cause compression. For example, one of the author's patients repeatedly

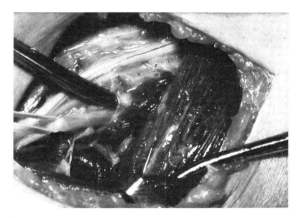

Fig. 3.48 The scissors in this photograph are inserted along the posterior interosseous nerve beneath the arcade of Frohse in the supinator.

reached over into the back of his car to lift out a heavy case of sample materials. When encouraged to keep the case on the passenger seat and lift it with a supinated arm with the wrist in neutral position, his symptoms regressed.

Men and women appear to be affected equally, mainly between the ages of 30 and 50 and in the dominant hand in the great majority of cases.

SYMPTOMS

Pain is usually the *only* presenting symptom. Well localized to the extensor mass just below the elbow, the pain may radiate to the wrist dorsally. Described as aching in character, it can be made more severe by certain movements. Analysis of those movements always reveals elbow extension, wrist flexion and forearm pronation. Typically the pain is absent on awakening but becomes progressively more severe as the arm is used, leaving the patient with a persistent ache in the evening.

The patient has very frequently been diagnosed as having 'tennis elbow' and may have had several injections to or surgical procedures on the lateral epicondylar region with temporary relief. Werner, in a thorough study of the relationship between lateral elbow pain and nerve entrapment, found the latter to be present in 5% of 'tennis elbows'[217].

Weakness may be a complaint, when it will be in extending the wrist and fingers. The wrist extension weakness may result in *reduced grip strength*, a troublesome problem especially for manual workers. This extensor weakness may be due entirely to the pain which these movements elicit or may be early evidence of a posterior interosseous nerve syndrome.

EXAMINATION

In radial tunnel syndrome, there is *no sensory disturbance or motor loss.*

Tenderness is located along the line of the radial nerve over the radial head. The nerve winds around the neck so pressure can be applied over the head anteriorly through the muscles of the 'mobile wad' of Henry[218], or over the neck laterally behind those muscles (Fig. 3.50). This tenderness should always be compared with the opposite side since the region of the radial tunnel is sensitive to pressure even in normal limbs. Tenderness is often also located over the lateral epicondyle but, unlike tennis elbow, is less severe than over the course of the nerve. Three points, which lie in line and equidistant from one another, should be palpated: the lateral epicondyle, the radial head and the radial tunnel.

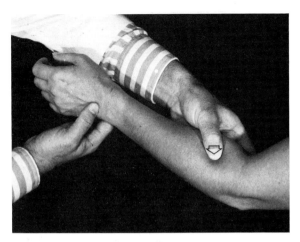

Fig. 3.50 Palpation along the course of the radial nerve in the region of the anterior aspect of the radial head in the 'mobile wad' may show tenderness over the radial tunnel.

Middle finger test (Fig. 3.51). If the patient is asked to extend each finger in turn against resistance with the elbow fully extended pain is experienced over the radial tunnel, sometimes with all fingers but always and most severely on stressing the middle finger. This is accounted for by the fact that extensor carpi radialis brevis inserts into the base of the metacarpal of the middle finger, and the stress drives its tendinous medial edge down on to the posterior interosseous nerve.

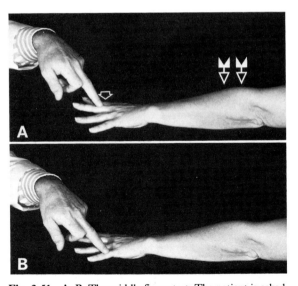

Fig. 3.51 A, B. The middle finger test. The patient is asked to maintain the elbow, wrist, and all fingers in full extension against counter-pressure exerted by the examiner. In the radial tunnel syndrome, the pain experienced on this manoeuvre is significantly greater when pressure is exerted on the middle finger than on any other digit.

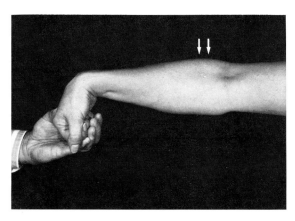

Fig. 3.52 With the elbow extended, the examiner carries the wrist and fingers into full flexion. In radial tunnel syndrome, this may well produce pain but this is less than that experienced with the middle finger test.

Full passive wrist and finger flexion with the elbow extended usually produces pain but, unlike lateral epicondylitis it is less severe in radial tunnel syndrome than that elicited by the 'middle finger' test (Fig. 3.52).

Resisted supination of the extended arm may also produce pain over the radial tunnel (Fig. 3.53). The arm should be extended during this test to eliminate the powerful supinating effect of biceps and place all the load on the supinator proper.

Electrophysiological changes were described in those patients in whom Roles and Maudsley performed nerve conduction studies. They took the form of a significant delay in motor latency in the radial nerve from the spiral groove to the extensor digitorum. The proportion of patients in whom such tests were performed was not stated. Changes may also be provoked by resisted supi-

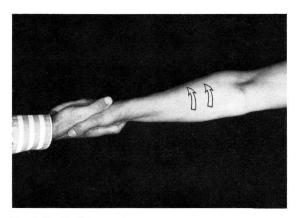

Fig. 3.53 Radial tunnel syndrome. Resisted supination may also produce pain in the patient with compression of the radial nerve in its tunnel.

nator contraction during the study[219]. The author has found that several patients with convincing clinical signs subsequently relieved by surgery showed no electrophysioligical changes whatsoever. This would be compatible with the intermittent nature of the stress.

INDICATIONS

Surgical exploration is indicated on entirely clinical grounds and the examiner comes to depend heavily on accurate localization of the tenderness and the 'middle finger' test.

Even when these are present conservative measures should be adopted initially. These include rest from repetitive movements likely to stress the nerve, the wearing of a wristlet to prevent wrist flexion, and judicious injection of limited quantities of steroid into the common tendinous origin of the extensor muscles to eliminate any element of lateral epicondylitis. If the clinician is convinced of the diagnosis and these measures fail, exploration of the radial tunnel with release of the medial border of extensor carpi radialis brevis and the arcade of Frohse together with ligation and division of the 'fan' of vessels can give dramatic relief. No macroscopic evidence of compression is found in most cases, although there are always microscopic changes[220].

Compression of the posterior interosseous nerve may also occur at the *distal* edge of the supinator[221], which the author now therefore releases in all cases (Fig. 3.54).

See Green D P 1993 Operative Hand Surgery, 3rd edn. Churchill Livingstone, New York, p. 1368.

Posterior interosseous nerve syndrome (palsy)

This entity has become recognized increasingly since four papers on the topic appeared in the November 1966 issue of the *Journal of Bone and Joint Surgery*[222–225]. However, the possibility of paralysis through compression of this nerve had been recorded over one hundred years previously and the various cases reported during that century are well documented in those four papers. Unlike the radial tunnel syndrome, many causes of posterior interosseous nerve syndrome other than the purely anatomical have been inculpated:

Trauma — dislocation of the elbow or, more commonly, fracture or dislocation of the radial head as in the displacement encountered in the Monteggia fracture of the forearm[226–227]. The palsy may be immediate or delayed[228–229].

Inflammation — synovitis associated with rheumatoid disease commonly affects the radiohumeral joint[230–232].

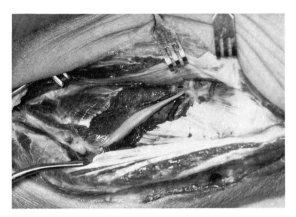

Fig. 3.54 (The hand is to the left of the photograph.) In this patient with persistent evidence of both lateral epicondylitis and radial tunnel syndrome, a long posterior approach was used. All of the compressive forces are displayed. The extensor carpi radialis brevis is lifted by the rake retractor. The superficial head of the supinator has been divided throughout its length to reveal the posterior interosseous nerve. In the depths of the wound at the point where the nerve is first seen proximally, the branches of the radial recurrent vessels are seen in close relationship to the nerve, which shows compression at the proximal edge of the supinator with some distal post-compressive swelling.

Compression of the posterior interosseous nerve and the resultant paralysis of the extensors by the synovium or by subluxation of the radial head (Fig. 3.55) may be mistaken for rupture of the tendons at the wrist (p. 373). Inflammatory swelling of the bicipital bursa which lies between the tendon and the radius was the first cause of this syndrome described, by Agnew at the Pathological Society of Philadelphia in 1863[233].

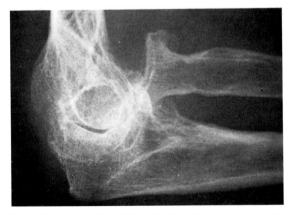

Fig. 3.55 Subluxation of the radial head in this rheumatoid patient produced compression of the posterior interosseous nerve.

Swelling — benign swelling of any kind may compress the nerve in the region of the radial tunnel. Those reported include ganglion[234,235], lipoma[236,237] and fibroma.

Anatomical, postural and *occupational* as described in radial tunnel syndrome.

Iatrogenic — injections in the region of the radial tunnel for tennis elbow have caused temporary, and rarely permanent, posterior interosseous nerve paralysis. Compression may also result from plating of fractures of the radius.

SYMPTOMS

Pain is frequently the first complaint and is similar in nature to that of radial tunnel syndrome. This is later accompanied or replaced by *weakness* and *paralysis* which may develop slowly over a period of two to six weeks or dramatically overnight, usually after a bout of unaccustomed exercise. The sequence in which muscles are affected follows no pattern, the ulnar three fingers, the index finger and the thumb all having been reported as first affected. When fully developed the patient complains of inability to extend the fingers and weakness in extension of the wrist.

In no instance does sensory disturbance occur. This serves to distinguish this syndrome symptomatically from higher lesions of the radial nerve.

EXAMINATION

Sensory disturbance
Dysaesthesia should be carefully excluded, particular attention being paid to the area of absolute radial nerve innervation over the dorsum of the first web and the thumb. Its presence would indicate a more proximal radial nerve lesion.

Motor loss
Wasting of the extensor mass may be evident, contrasting with the normal bulk of the 'mobile wad' of Henry which consists of brachioradialis and the radial extensors of the wrist supplied by the radial nerve before its division.

The posture of the hand is affected little when compared with complete radial palsy, for the wrist can be extended. However, the extension is weak and the attitude diagnostic, the wrist being radially deviated on attempted full extension (Fig. 3.56).

Attempted extension of the fingers produces a characteristic posture in which the interphalangeal joints are fully extended but the metacarpophalangeal joints cannot be extended beyond 45° and often not that far. This posture may mimic intrinsic tightness, and indeed

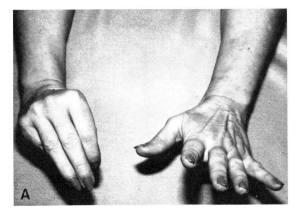

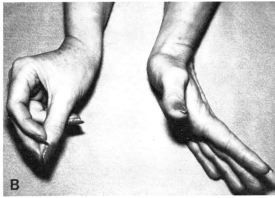

Fig. 3.56 A, B. On the morning after moving some heavy furniture, this patient woke with pain over the extensor aspect of her forearm and associated loss of extension of her fingers and of her thumb. Wrist extension was still present but less strongly with quite evident radial deviation when compared with the normal hand. In each photograph the patient is attempting full extension of both wrist and fingers with the involved and the normal hand.

the posture is produced by intrinsic action unaided by long extensor pull — an 'extrinsic minus' rather than an 'intrinsic plus' hand. True intrinsic tightness can be quickly excluded by testing (p. 251).

Partial paralysis of the muscles supplied by the posterior interosseous nerve may result in lack of extension of the joints of the ring and little fingers alone. This produces the appearance of a 'false ulnar claw hand'. The metacarpophalangeal joints are not hyperextended as in the true ulnar claw and the ulnar innervated intrinsics function normally.

Radial abduction of the thumb is also weakened. Some modest extension of the interphalangeal joint may be retained by virtue of the contributions made via the lateral bands by abductor pollicis brevis and adductor pollicis.

Active testing shows weakness or paralysis in some or all of the muscles innervated by the branches of the posterior interosseous nerve

short	—	extensor digitorum
		extensor carpi ulnaris
		extensor digiti minimi
long—lateral	—	abductor pollicis longus
		extensor pollicis brevis
— *medial* —		extensor pollicis longus
		extensor indicis

Rarely the long branch passes over rather than through the supinator and if the cause of compression lies therein, the relevant muscles are spared.

Electrophysiological changes will show denervation of paralysed muscles and increased distal latency in the radial nerve in patients showing weakness.

Differential diagnosis from *high radial nerve lesions* is made by the lack of sensory disturbance and normal strength of brachioradialis, the radial wrist extensors and the supinator. *Lead poisoning* may produce radial palsy with no sensory loss but it is a high lesion, showing paralysis of brachioradialis and the radial wrist extensors. The diagnosis can be confirmed by seeking the characteristic gingival discoloration and by haematological and urinary studies. *Hysterical drop wrist* shows persistent inability to extend the interphalangeal joints of the fingers even with the metacarpophalangeal joint held in flexion.

(A *distal posterior interosseous nerve syndrome* has been described[238], in which patients present with dorsal wrist pain. They have tenderness over the fourth dorsal compartment and are relieved by selective nerve block and resection of the enlarged fibrotic posterior interosseous nerve at the wrist.)

INDICATIONS

Appropriate splintage should be provided to support the paralysed muscles and permit something approaching normal function. Many will show recovery with time and repeated evaluation should be performed. It will often demonstrate progressive return of individual muscles. Surgical exploration is indicated in all persistent cases of posterior interosseous nerve syndrome.

See Green D P 1993 Operative Hand Surgery, 3rd edn. Churchill Livingstone, New York, p. 1368.

Radial sensory nerve entrapment[239] (Wartenberg's disease)[240,241]

Originally described as cheiralgia paraesthetica, this entrapment occurs at the point at which the sensory branch of the radial nerve emerges from beneath the edge of the brachioradialis tendon 6–8 cm proximal to the radial styloid. The majority of patients give a history of previous trauma which, in almost half, is of a repetitive nature, involving repeated supination and pronation[242].

SYMPTOMS

Complaints of pain over the radial aspect of the dorsum of the hand exacerbated by movement of the wrist causes this condition to mimic de Quervain's disease (p. 343) to a degree that some sufferers have undergone release of the first dorsal compartment with no relief. Pain is often accompanied by dysaesthesia in the radial nerve distribution.

EXAMINATION

Pressure over the sensory branch of the radial nerve reproduces the complaints. The sensory examination shows a reduced two-point discrimination in the radial nerve distribution. Finkelstein's test (p. 344) for de Quervain's disease is misleadingly positive. Nerve conduction studies by the 'inching' technique may accurately localize the site of compression.

INDICATIONS

Splintage may relieve symptoms permanently. When this is not successful, exploration, neurolysis and, where the compression is clearly due to the tendon, step-cut

lengthening of the brachioradialis will provide relief in the majority of cases (Fig. 3.57).

See Green D P 1993 Operative Hand Surgery, 3rd edn. Churchill Livingstone, New York, p. 1371.

OTHER REPORTED CAUSES OF RADIAL NERVE COMPRESSION
Anatomical
Fibrous band in the supinator[243]
Tumour
Hamartoma[244]
Angioleiomyoma[245]
Synovial chondromatosis[246]
Polyarteritis[247]
Localized constrictive neuropathy[248]

Nerves, other than radial, ulnar and median, have rarely been reported as compressed — the suprascapular[249–251], the long thoracic[252], the axillary[253], the musculocutaneous[254] and the supraclavicular[255]. All were the cause of pain, and the compression of the first two was associated with appropriate muscular weakness and paralysis.

MUSCLE COMPRESSION SYNDROMES

Some of the nerve compression syndromes described above may be caused by the presence of an anomalous muscle in the nerve tunnel, such as a reversed palmaris longus, palmaris profundus or an origin in the forearm of the abductor digiti minimi.

Anomalous muscles may in themselves produce discomfort, mainly with use. This difficulty usually arises in the fourth and fifth decades and much more commonly in females, which may be due to occupational stress or hormonal fluid retention.

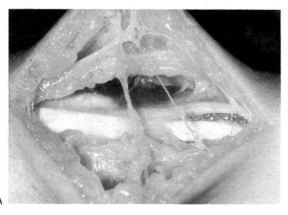
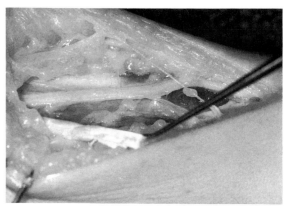

A   B

Fig. 3.57 Radial sensory nerve entrapment (Wartenburg's disease). A. The radial sensory nerve is seen emerging from beneath the brachioradialis tendon to pass distally to the right of the photograph from where it carries sensibility from the dorsal aspect of the thumb and the first web space. There is some tethering and mild fibrosis where the nerve emerges in this symptomatic patient. B. Step-cut lengthening of the brachioradialis tendon and neurolysis of the radial cutaneous nerve have been performed. Symptoms were relieved.

That apart, compression syndromes have been described in which nerves are not involved, but in which a normal or anomalous muscle becomes hypertrophied or inflamed within a tight tunnel, resulting in pain and discomfort.

Chronic exertional compartment syndrome

Such chronic compartment syndromes have been described in the forearm[256,257] and in the first dorsal interosseous muscle[258-260]. Associated in both syndromes with aching on repetitive exercise and in the former with tingling in the median nerve distribution, both are confirmed by pressure studies and relieved by simple fasciotomy. The first dorsal interosseous syndrome may be accompanied by appreciable hypertrophy in the muscle[261].

Extensor indicis syndrome

Originally described by Ritter and Inglis in 1969[262], this syndrome is due to inflammation associated with a normal or anomalous extensor indicis at the point at which it passes through the fourth dorsal compartment beneath the extensor retinaculum.

SYMPTOMS

Pain in the wrist, which shows a normal pain-free range of motion is characteristic of the disorder. Point tenderness over the fourth compartment at the wrist has often been localized by the patient before presentation.

EXAMINATION

Extensor indicis test (Fig. 3.58). Spinner[263] reported in 1973 that if, with the wrist fully flexed, the patient is asked to extend the proximal phalanx of the index finger against resistance, he will complain of sharp pain well localized to the fourth compartment at the wrist. If the tender area is palpated during this resisted extension, crepitation can frequently by felt.

Surgical release of the tunnel is indicated only if splintage, local steroids and anti-inflammatory agents fail to produce relief.

Extensor digiti minimi[264]

A syndrome similar to the extensor indicis syndrome, but related to the extensor digiti minimi in the fifth compartment has recently been reported. The muscle was anomalous in that it had a musculotendinous slip to the ring finger. Pain, elicited on movement of the small finger, was the presenting symptom, and excision of the anomalous slip resulted in improvement.

Extensor digitorum brevis manus[265,266]

This anomalous muscle was first named by Wood in the Proceedings of the Royal Society of London in 1864[267]. Originating on the distal radius, carpus and wrist capsule, it may become troublesome because of pain or swelling. The muscle occurs in 1.1% of patients examined[268] and 3.0% of cadavers dissected[269]. Often mistaken for a ganglion, it is recognized if the surgeon is aware of the entity, for it quite evidently contracts on resisted extension of the fingers. The correct treatment, if troublesome, is surgical excision, although simple division of the retinaculum has also been advocated[270].

NON-COMPRESSIVE CAUSES OF NEUROPATHY

Because their symptoms are confined to the upper limb, many patients with conditions outwith the realm of the hand surgeon will nonetheless understandably present themselves to him for help. A considerable responsibility rests on him to remain aware of the other possibilities, which are legion:

Generalized neuropathy
Spinal cord disease
Spinal tumours
Intracranial disorders
Intrathoracic pathology — 'Pancoast's syndrome'[271].

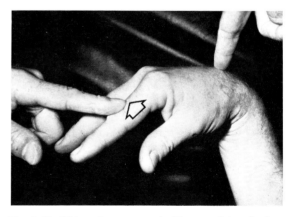

Fig. 3.58 This patient presented with a complaint of pain over the dorsal aspect of the right wrist. Examination revealed a full pain-free range of motion in the wrist, but, when extension of the index finger was attempted against resistance, he experienced pain in the site indicated by the examiner's other finger. This discomfort was associated with crepitus in the region of the fourth dorsal compartment.

The hand surgeon should keep a high index of suspicion in talking to and examining any patient complaining of pain, weakness or paralysis of the upper limb. The history should seek out evidence of familial disorders, of metabolic disturbance, of weakness elsewhere, of visual or cranial nerve disorder or other symptoms apparently unrelated in the patient's estimation. In examination, the signs of upper motor neurone involvement should be sought in the form of increased reflexes and spasticity, the muscles should be observed for fibrillation, the blood pressure should always be recorded and the urine subjected to analysis.

If careful examination suggest that the source lies proximal to the shoulder all patients should undergo radiologic examination of the chest, including apical lordotic views, radiographs of the cervical spine and neurological consultation, pending appropriate study by electroencephalography, brain scan, myelography, CT scan or MRI. Only by remaining constantly mindful of where the nerves which are disturbed in the hand and arm come from and go to can the hand surgeon avoid the tragedy of a missed diagnosis compounded by inappropriate treatment.

REFERENCES

1. Masear V R, Hayes J M; Hyde A G 1986 An industrial cause of carpal tunnel syndrome. J Hand Surg (Am) 11: 222–227
2. Szabo R M, Gelberman R H 1987 The pathophysiology of nerve entrapment syndromes. J Hand Surg (Am) 12: 880–884
3. Feldman R G, Travers P H, Chirico-Post J, Keyserling WM 1987 Risk assessment in electronic assembly workers: carpal tunnel syndrome. J Hand Surg (Am) 12: 849–855
4. Szabo R M, Chidgey L K 1989 Stress carpal tunnel pressures in patients with carpal tunnel syndrome and normal patients. J Hand Surg (Am) 14: 624–627
5. Frymoyer J W, Bland J 1973 Carpal tunnel syndrome in patients with myxedematous arthropathy. J Bone Joint Surg 55A: 78–82
6. Howard F M 1986 Compression neuropathies in the anterior forearm. Hand Clin 2: 737–745
7. Ekerot L 1977 Postanesthetic ulnar neuropathy at the elbow. Scand J Plastic Reconstr Surg Hand Surg 11: 225–229
8. Seyfer A E, Grammer N Y, Bogumill G P, Provost J M, Chandry U 1985 Upper extremity neuropathies after cardiac surgery. J Hand Surg (Am) 10: 16–19
9. Mackinnon S E, Dellon A L 1986 Experimental study of chronic nerve compression. Clinical implications. Hand Clin 2: 639–650
10. Curtis R M, Eversmann W W 1973 Internal neurolysis as an adjunct to the treatment of the carpal tunnel syndrome. J Bone Joint Surg 55A: 733–740
11. Mackinnon S E, Dellon A L 1988 Evaluation of microsurgical internal neurolysis in a primate median nerve model of chronic nerve compression. J Hand Surg (Am) 13: 345–351
12. Upton A R M, McComas A J 1973 The double crush and nerve entrapment syndromes. Lancet ii: 359–362
13. Nemoto K, Matsumoto N, Tazaki K, Horiuchi Y et al 1987 An experimental study on the 'double crush' hypothesis. J Hand Surg (AM) 12: 552–559 (An erratum appears in J Hand Surg (Am) 1987 12: 1011.)
14. Lanz U 1977 Anatomical variations of the median nerve in the carpal tunnel. J Hand Surg 2: 44–53
15. Seradge H, Seradge E 1990 Median innervated hypothenar muscle: anomalous branch of median nerve in the carpal tunnel. J Hand Surg (Am) 15: 356–359
16. Kornberg M, Aulicino P L, DuPuy T E 1983 Bifid median nerve with three thenar branches — case report. J Hand Surg (Am) 8: 583–584
17. Amadio P C 1987 Bifid median nerve with a double compartment within the transverse carpal canal. J Hand Surg (Am) 12: 366–368
18. Mumford J, Morecraft R, Blair W F 1987 Anatomy of the thenar branch of the median nerve. J Hand Surg (Am) 12: 361–365
19. Tountas C P, Bihrle D M, MacDonald C J, Bergman R A 1987 Variations of the median nerve in the carpal canal. J Hand Surg (Am) 12: 708–712
20. Schuind F, Ventura M, Pasteels J L 1990 Idiopathic carpal tunnel syndrome: histologic study of flexor tendon synovium. J Hand Surg (Am) 15: 497–503
21. Lavey E B, Pearl R M 1981 Patent median artery as a cause of carpal tunnel syndrome. Ann Plastic Surg 7: 3236–3238
22. Barfred T, Hjlund A P, Bertheussen K 1985 Median artery in carpal tunnel syndrome. J Hand Surg (Am) 10: 864–867
23. Barton N J 1979 Another cause of median nerve compression by a lumbrical muscle in the carpal tunnel. J Hand Surg 4:189–191
24. Schultz R J, Endler P M, Huddleston H D 1973 Anomalous median nerve and an anomalous muscle belly of the first lumbrical associated with carpal tunnel syndrome. J Bone Joint Surg 55A: 1744–1746
25. Butler B, Bigley E C 1971 Aberrant index (first) lumbrical tendinous origin associated with carpal tunnel syndrome. J Bone Joint Surg 53A: 160–162
26. Robinson D, Aghasi M, Halperin N 1989 The treatment of carpal tunnel syndrome caused by hypertrophied lumbrical muscles. Case reports. Scand J Plastic Reconstr Surg Hand Surg 23: 149–151
27. Asai M, Wong A C, Matsunaga T, Akahoshi Y 1986 Carpal tunnel syndrome caused by aberrant lumbrical muscles associated with cystic degeneration of the tenosynovium: a case report. J Hand Surg (Am) 11: 218–221
28. Smith R J 1971 Anomalous muscle belly of the flexor digitorum superficialis causing carpal tunnel syndrome. J Bone Joint Surg 53A: 1215–1216
29. Ametewee K, Harris A, Samuel M 1985 Acute carpal tunnel syndrome produced by anomalous flexor

digitorum superficialis indicis muscle. J Hand Surg (Br) 10: 83–84

30. Meyer F N, Pflaum B C 1987 Median nerve compression at the wrist caused by a reversed palmaris longus muscle. J Hand Surg (Am) 12: 369–371

31. Schlafly B, Lister G 1987 Median nerve compression secondary to bifid reversed palmaris longus. J Hand Surg (Am) 12: 371–373

32. Backhouse K M, Churchill-Davidson D 1975 Anomalous palmaris longus muscle producing carpal tunnel-like compression. Hand 7: 22–24

33. Brones M, Wilgis E 1978 Anatomical variations of the palmaris longus, causing carpal tunnel syndrome. Plastic Reconstr Surg 62: 798–800

34. Carroll M P, Montero C 1980 Rare anomalous muscle cause of carpal tunnel syndrome. Orthopaedic Rev 9: 83–85

35. Still J M, Kleinert H E 1973 Anomalous muscles and nerve entrapment in the wrist and hand. Plastic Reconstr Surg 52: 394–400

36. Floyd T, Burger RS, Sciaroni CA 1990 Bilateral palmaris profundus causing bilateral carpal tunnel syndrome. J Hand Surg (Am) 15: 364–366

37. Adamson J E, Srouji S J, Horton C E, Mladick R A 1971 The acute carpal tunnel syndrome. Plastic Reconstr Surg 47: 332–336

38. Fissette J, Onkelirx A, Fandi N 1981 Carpal and Guyon tunnel syndrome in burns at the wrist. J Hand Surg 6: 13–15

39. Harvey F J, Bosanquet J S 1981 Carpal tunnel syndrome caused by simple ganglion. Hand 13: 164–166

40. Desai S S, Pearlman H S, Patel M R 1986 Clicking at the wrist due to fibroma in an anomalous lumbrical muscle: a case report and review of literature. J Hand Surg (Am) 11: 512–514

41. Toranto I R 1989 Aneurysm of the median artery causing recurrent carpal tunnel syndrome and anatomic review. Plastic Reconstr Surg 84: 510–512

42. Lee K E 1985 Tuberculosis presenting as carpal tunnel syndrome. J Hand Surg (Am) 10: 242–245

43. Prince H, Ispahani P, Baker M 1988 A *Mycobacterium malmoense* infection of the hand presenting as carpal tunnel syndrome. J Hand Surg (Br) 13: 328–330

44. Suso S, Peidro L, Ramon R 1988 Tuberculous synovitis with 'rice bodies' presenting as carpal tunnel syndrome. J Hand Surg (Am) 13: 574–576

45. DeHertogh D, Ritland D, Green R 1988 Carpal tunnel syndrome due to gonococcal tenosynovitis. Ortho 2: 199–200

46. Barr W G, Blair S J 1988 Carpal tunnel syndrome as the initial manifestation of scleroderma. J Hand Surg (Am) 13: 366–368

47. Short W H, Palmer A K 1981 Amyloidosis and the carpal tunnel syndrome Ortho Rev 10: 89–94

48. Fluhr J E, Farrow A, Nelson S 1989 Vitamin B6 levels in patients with carpal tunnel syndrome. Arch Surg 124: 1329–1330

49. Clayburgh R H, Beckenbaugh R D, Dobyns J H 1987 Carpal tunnel release in patients with diffuse peripheral neuropathy. J Hand Surg (Am)12: 380–383

50. Kummel B M, Zazanis G A 1973 Shoulder pain as the presenting complaint in carpal tunnel syndrome. Clin Orthopaedics Rel Res 92: 227–230

51. Szabo R M, Gelberman R H, Dimick M P 1984 Sensibility testing in patients with carpal tunnel syndrome. J Bone Joint Surg (Am) 66: 60–64

52. Silver M A, Gelberman R H, Gellman H, Rhoades C E 1985 Carpal tunnel syndrome: associated abnormalities in ulnar nerve function and the effect of carpal tunnel release on these abnormalities. J Hand Surg (Am) 10: 710–713

53. Phalen G S 1951 Spontaneous compression of the median nerve at the wrist. J Am Med Assoc 145: 1128–1133

54. Phalen G S 1966 The carpal tunnel syndrome: 17 years experience in diagnosis and treatment of 654 hands. J Bone Joint Surg 48A: 211–228

55. Phalen G S 1981 The birth of a syndrome, or carpal tunnel revisited. J Hand Surg 6: 109–111

56. Gelberman R H, Hergenroeder P T, Hargens A R, Lundburg G N, Akeson W H 1981 The carpal tunnel syndrome — study of carpal pressures. J Bone Joint Surg 63A: 380–383

57. Paley D, McMurtry R Y 1985 Median nerve compression test in carpal tunnel syndrome diagnosis. Ortho Rev 15: 41–45

58. Melvin J L, Schuchmann J A, Lanese R R 1973 Diagnostic specificity of motor and sensory nerve conduction variables in the carpal tunnel syndrome. Arch Phys Med Rehab 54: 69–74

59. Grundberg A B 1983 Carpal tunnel decompression in spite of normal electromyography. J Hand Surg (Am) 8: 348–349

60. Louis D S, Hankin F M 1987 Symptomatic relief following carpal tunnel decompression with normal electroneuromyographic studies. Ortho 10: 434–436

61. Hart V L, Gaynor V 1941 Roentgenographic study of the carpal canal. J Bone Joint Surg 23: 382–383

62. Amadio P C 1985 Pyridoxine as an adjunct in the treatment of carpal tunnel syndrome. J Hand Surg (Am) 10: 237–241

63. Green D P 1984 Diagnostic and therapeutic value of carpal tunnel injection. J Hand Surg 9A: 850–854

64. Wood M R 1980 Hydrocortisone injections for carpal tunnel syndrome. Hand 12: 62–64

65. Gelberman R H, Aronson D, Weisman M H 1980 Carpal tunnel syndrome. J Bone Joint Surg 62A: 1181–1184

66. Heckler F R, Jabaley M E 1986 Evolving concepts of median nerve decompression in the carpal tunnel. Hand Clin 2: 723–736

67. Nalebuff E A, Smith J 1979 Preservation of terminal branches of the median palmar cutaneous nerve in carpal tunnel surgery. Orthopaedics 2: 369–372

68. Lilly C J, Magnell T D 1985 Severance of the thenar branch of the median nerve as a complication of carpal tunnel release. J Hand Surg (Am) 10: 399–402

69. Seiler J G 3rd, Milek M A, Carpenter G K, Swiontkowski M F 1989 Intraoperative assessment of median nerve blood flow during carpal tunnel release with laser Doppler flowmetry. J Hand Surg (Am) 14: 986–991

70. Richman J A, Gelberman R H, Rydevik B L, Hajek P C et al 1989 Carpal tunnel syndrome: morphologic changes after release of the transverse carpal ligament. J Hand Surg (Am) 14: 852–857

71. Gellman H, Kan D, Gee V, Kuschner S H, Botte M J

1989 Analysis of pinch and grip strength after carpal tunnel release. J Hand Surg (Am) 14: 863–864

72. Shurr D G, Blair W F, Bassett G 1986 Electromyographic changes after carpal tunnel release. J Hand Surg (Am) 11: 876–880

73. Gartsman G M, Kovach J C, Crouch C C, Noble P C, Bennett J B 1986 Carpal arch alteration after carpal tunnel release. J Hand Surg (Am) 11: 372–374

74. Garcia-Elias M, An K N, Cooney W P 3rd, Linscheid R L, Chao E Y 1989 Stability of the transverse carpal arch: an experimental study. J Hand Surg (Am) 14: 277–282

75. Seyffarth H 1951 Primary myoses in the m. pronator teres as a cause of lesion of the n. medianus (the pronator syndrome). Acta Psych Scand suppl 74: 251

76. Vichare N A 1968 Spontaneous paralysis of the anterior interosseous nerve. J Bone Joint Surg 50B: 806–808

77. Johnson R K, Spinner M, Shrewsbury M M 1979 Median nerve entrapment syndrome in the proximal forearm. J Hand Surg 4: 48–52

78. Hartz C R, Linscheid R L, Gramse R R, Daube J R 1981 The pronator teres syndrome: compressive neuropathy of the median nerve. J Bone Joint Surg 63A: 885–890

79. Farrell H F 1979 Pain and the pronator teres syndrome. Bull Hosp Joint Dis 37: 59–62

80. Swiggett R, Ruby L K 1986 Median nerve compression neuropathy by the lacertus fibrosus: report of three cases. J Hand Surg (Am) 11: 700–703

81. Buchthal F, Rosenfalck A, Trojaborg W 1974 Electrophysiological findings in entrapment of the median nerve at wrist and elbow. J Neurol Neurosurg Psych 37: 340–360

82. Spinner M 1978 Injuries to the major branches of peripheral nerves of the forearm 2nd edn. W B Saunders Co, Philadelphia

83. Maeda K, Miura T, Komada T, Chiba A 1977 Anterior interosseous nerve paralysis. Report of 13 cases and review of Japanese literature. Hand 9: 165–171

84. Hill N A, Howard F M, Huffer B R 1985 The incomplete anterior interosseous nerve syndrome. J Hand Surg (Am) 10: 4–16

85. Jabaley M E 1978 Personal observations on the role of the lumbrical muscles in carpal tunnel syndrome. J Hand Surg 3: 82–84

86. Nather A, Pho R W H 1981 Carpal tunnel syndrome produced by an organising haematoma within the anomalous second lumbrical muscle. Hand 13: 87–91

87. Wiss D 1979 Aberrant lumbrical muscles causing carpal tunnel syndrome. Orthopedics 2: 357–358

88. Hutton P, Kernohan J, Birch R 1981 An anomalous flexor digitorum superficialis indicis muscle presenting as carpal tunnel syndrome. Hand 13: 85–86

89. Chalmers J 1978 Unusual causes of peripheral nerve compression. Hand 10: 168–175

90. Levy M, Pauker M 1978 Carpal tunnel syndrome due to thrombosed persisting median artery. A case report. Hand 10: 65–68

91. Jones N F, Ming N L 1988 Persistent median artery as a cause of pronator syndrome. J Hand Surg (Am) 13: 728–732

92. Spinner M 1976 Cryptogenic infraclavicular brachial plexus neuritis. Bull Hosp Joint Dis 37: 98–104

93. Laha R K, Dujovny M, DeCastro S C 1977

94. Wolfe J S, Eyring E J 1974 Median nerve entrapment within a greenstick fracture. J Bone Joint Surg 56A: 1270–1272

95. Nunley J A, Ubaniak J R 1980 Partial bony entrapment of the median nerve in a greenstick fracture of the ulna. J Hand Surg 5: 557–559

96. Macnicol M 1978 Roentgenographic evidence of median nerve entrapment in a greenstick humeral fracture. J Bone Joint Surg 60A: 998–1000

97. Lewis M H 1978 Median nerve decompression after Colles' fracture. J Bone Joint Surg 60B: 195–196

98. Manske P 1976 Fracture of the hook of the hamate presenting as carpal tunnel syndrome. Hand 10: 181–183

99. Sturim H S, Edmond J A 1980 Carpal tunnel compression syndrome secondary to a retracted flexor digitorum sublimis tendon. Plastic Reconstr Surg 66: 846–848

100. Weiland A J, Lister G D, Villarreal–Rios A 1976 Volar fracture dislocations of the second and third carpometacarpal joints associated with acute carpal tunnel syndrome. J Trauma 16: 672–675

101. Matev I 1976 A radiological sign of entrapment of the median nerve in the elbow joint after posterior dislocation. J Bone Joint Surg 58B; 353–355

102. Hallett J 1981 Entrapment of the median nerve after dislocation of the elbow: a case report. J Bone Joint Surg 63B: 408–412

103. Floyd W E 3rd, Gebhardt M C, Emans J B 1987 Intra-articular entrapment of the median nerve after elbow dislocation in children. J Hand Surg (Am) 12: 704–707

104. Lazaro L 1972 Carpal tunnel syndrome from an insect sting. J Bone Joint Surg 54A: 1095–1096

105. Short H, Palmer A K 1981 Amyloidosis and the carpal tunnel syndrome. Orthopaedic Rev 10: 89–94

106. MacDougal B, Weeks P M, Wray R C 1977 Median nerve compression and trigger finger in the mucopolysaccharidoses and related disease. Plastic Reconstr Surg 59: 260–263

107. Johnson R J, Bonfiglio M 1969 Lipofibromatous hamartoma of the median nerve. J Bone Joint Surg 51A: 984–990

108. Louis D S, Dick H M 1973 Ossifying lipofibroma of the median nerve. J Bone Joint Surg 55A: 1082–1084

109. Kojima T, Ide Y, Marumo E, Ishikawa E, Yamashita H 1976 Haemangioma of median nerve causing carpal tunnel syndrome. Hand 8: 62–65

110. Engel J, Zinneman H, Tsur H, Farin I 1978 Carpal tunnel syndrome due to carpal osteophyte. Hand 10: 283–284

111. Pritsch M, Engel J, Horowitz A 1980 Cystic change in the wrist, causing carpal tunnel syndrome. Plastic Reconstr Surg 65: 494–495

112. Linscheid R L 1979 Carpal tunnel syndrome secondary to ulnar bursa distention from the intercarpal joint: report of a case. J Hand Surg 4: 191–193

113. Seddon H J 1952 Carpal ganglion as a cause of paralysis of the deep branch of the ulnar nerve. J Bone Joint Surg 34B: 386–390

114. Wood V E 1980 Nerve compression following opponensplasty as a result of wrist anomalies. Report of a case. J Hand Surg 5: 279–280

115. Mancusi-Ungaro A, Corres J J, Di Spaltro F 1976 Case reports: median carpal tunnel syndrome following a vascular shunt procedure in the forearm. Plastic Reconstr Surg 57: 96–97

116. Kenzora J E 1978 Dialysis carpal tunnel syndrome. Orthopaedics 1: 195–203

117. Jain V K, Cestero R V M, Baum J 1979 Carpal tunnel syndrome in patients undergoing maintenance hemodialysis. J Am Med Assoc 242: 2868–2869

118. Semer N B, Goldberg N H, Cuono C B 1989 Upper extremity entrapment neuropathy and tourniquet use in patients undergoing hemodialysis. J Hand Surg (Am) 14: 897–900

119. Gilbert M S, Robinson A, Baez A, Gupta S et al 1988 Carpal tunnel syndrome in patients who are receiving long-term renal hemodialysis. J Bone Joint Surg (Am) 70: 1145–1153

120. Minami A, Ogino T 1987 Carpal tunnel syndrome in patients undergoing hemodialysis. J Hand Surg (Am) 12: 93–97

121. DeLuca F N, Cowen N J 1975 Median nerve compression complicating a tendon graft prosthesis. J Bone Joint Surg 57A: 553

122. Hunt J R 1908 Occupation neuritis of the deep palmar branch of the ulnar nerve. J Neurol Mental Dis 35: 673–689

123. Kleinert H E, Hayes J E 1971 The ulnar tunnel syndrome. Plastic Reconstr Surg 47: 21–24

124. Hayes J R, Mulholland R C, O'Connor B T 1969 Compression of the deep palmar branch of the ulnar nerve. J Bone Joint Surg 51B: 469–472

125. Leslie I J 1980 Compression of the deep branch of the ulnar nerve due to edema of the hand. Hand 12: 271–272

126. Kuschner S H, Gelberman R H, Jennings C 1988 Ulnar nerve compression at the wrist. J Hand Surg (Am) 13: 577–580

127. Seddon H J 1952 Carpal ganglion as a cause of paralysis of the deep branch of the ulnar nerve. J Bone Joint Surg 34B: 386–390

128. Subin G D, Mallon W J, Urbaniak J R 1989 Diagnosis of ganglion in Guyon's canal by magnetic resonance imaging. J Hand Surg (Am) 14: 640–643

129. Salgeback S 1977 Ulnar tunnel syndrome caused by anomalous muscles. Scand J Plastic Reconstr Surg 11: 255–258

130. Turner M S, Caird D M 1977 Anomalous muscles and ulnar nerve compression at the wrist. Hand 9: 140–141

131. Weeks P M, Young V L 1982 Ulnar artery thrombosis and ulnar nerve compression associated with an anomalous hypothenar muscle (case report). 69: 130–131

132. Jeffery A K 1971 Compression of the deep palmar branch of the ulnar nerve by an anomalous muscle. J Bone Joint Surg 53B: 718–723

133. Tonkin M A, Lister G D 1988 The palmaris brevis profundus. An anomalous muscle associated with ulnar nerve compression at the wrist. J Hand Surg (Am) 10: 862–864

134. Dodds G A 3rd, Hale D, Jackson W T 1990 Incidence of anatomic variants in Guyon's canal. J Hand Surg (Am) 15: 352–355

135. O'Hara J J, Stone J H 1988 Ulnar neuropathy at the wrist associated with aberrant flexor carpi ulnaris insertion. J Hand Surg (Am) 13: 370–372

136. Zook E G, Kucan J O, Guy R J 1988 Palmar wrist pain caused by ulnar nerve entrapment in the flexor carpi ulnaris tendon. J Hand Surg (Am) 13: 732–735

137. Fahrer M, Millroy P J 1981 Ulnar compression neuropathy due to an anomalous abductor digiti minimi — clinical and anatomic study. J Hand Surg 6: 266–268

138. Uriburu I J F, Morchio F J, Marin J C 1976 Compression syndrome of the deep motor branch of the ulnar nerve (piso–hamate hiatus syndrome). J Bone Joint Surg 58A: 145–147

139. Stern P J, Vice M 1983 Compression of the deep branch of the ulnar nerve — a case report. J Hand Surg (Am) 8: 72–74

140. Panas J 1878 Sur une case pas connue de paralysie du neuf cubital. Arch Gen Med 2: 5–22

141. Apfelberg D B, Larson S J 1973 Dynamic anatomy of the ulnar nerve at the elbow. Plastic Reconstr Surg 51: 76–81

142. Leffert R D, Dorfman H D 1972 Antecubital cyst in rheumatoid arthritis — surgical findings. J Bone Joint Surg 53A: 1555–1557

143. Hirasawa Y, Sawamura H, Sakakida K 1979 Entrapment neuropathy due to bilateral epitrochleoanconeus muscles: a case report. J Hand Surg 4: 181–185

144. Dahners L E, Wood F M 1984 Anconeus epitrochlearis, a rare cause of cubital tunnel syndrome: a case report. J Hand Surg (Am) 9: 579–580

145. Masear V R, Hill J J Jr, Cohen S M 1989 Ulnar compression neuropathy secondary to the anconeus epitrochlearis muscle. J Hand Surg (Am) 13: 720–724 (Comment in: J Hand Surg (Am) 1989 14: 917–919.)

146. McGowan A J 1950 The results of transposition of the ulnar nerve for traumatic ulnar neuritis. J Bone Joint Surg 32B: 293–301

147. Dellon A L 1989 Review of treatment results for ulnar nerve entrapment at the elbow. J Hand Surg (Am) 14: 688–700

148. Adelaar R S, Foster W C, McDowell C 1984 The treatment of the cubital tunnel syndrome. J Hand Surg (Am) 9A: 90–95

149. Osborne G 1957 The surgical treatment of tardy ulnar neuritis. J Bone Joint Surg 39B: 782

150. Osborne G 1970 Decompression of ulnar nerve at elbow. Hand 2: 10–13

151. Learmonth J R 1942 A technique for transplanting the ulnar nerve. Surg Gynecol Obstet 75: 792–793

152. Dellon A L 1988 Operative technique for submuscular transposition of the ulnar nerve. Cont Ortho 16: 17–24

153. Kleinman W B, Bishop A T 1989 Anterior intramuscular transposition of the ulnar nerve. J Hand Surg (Am) 14: 972–979

154. Craven P R, Green D P 1980 Cubital tunnel syndrome. Treatment by medial epicondylectomy. J Bone Joint Surg 62A: 986–989

155. Froimson A I, Zahrawi F 1980 Treatment of compression neuropathy of the ulnar nerve at the elbow by epicondylectomy and neurolysis. J Hand Surg 5: 391–395

156. Neblett C, Ehni G 1970 Medial epicondylectomy for ulnar palsy. J Neurosurg 32: 55–62

157. Heithoff S F, Millender L H, Nalebuff E A, Petruska A J Jr 1990 Medial epicondylectomy for the treatment

of ulnar nerve compression at the elbow. J Hand Surg (Am) 15: 22–29

158. Goldberg B J, Light T R, Blair S J 1989 Ulnar neuropathy at the elbow: results of medial epicondylectomy. J Hand Surg (Am) 14: 182–188

159. Craven P R, Green D P 1980 Cubital tunnel syndrome. Treatment by medial epicondylectomy. J Bone Joint Surg (Am) 62: 986–989

160. Spinner M, Kaplan E B 1976 The relationship of the ulnar nerve to the medial intermuscular septum in the arm and its clinical significance. Hand 8: 239–242

161. Reis N D 1980 Anomalous triceps tendon as a cause for snapping elbow and ulnar neuritis: a case report. J Hand Surg 5: 361–362

162. Rolfsen L 1970 Snapping triceps tendon with ulnar neuritis. Acta Orthopaedica Scand 41: 74–76

163. Hayashi Y, Kojima T, Kohno T 1984 A case of cubital tunnel syndrome caused by the snapping of the medial head of the triceps brachii muscle. J Hand Surg (Am) 9A: 96–99

164. Harrelson J M, Newmann M 1975 Hypertrophy of the flexor carpi ulnaris as a cause of ulnar nerve compression in the distal part of the forearm. J Bone Joint Surg 57A: 554–555

165. Amadio P C, Beckenbaugh R D 1986 Entrapment of the ulnar nerve by the deep flexor-pronator aponeurosis. J Hand Surg (Am) 11: 83–87

166. Comtet J, Quicot L, Moyen B 1978 Compression of the deep palmar branch of the ulnar nerve by the arch of the adductor pollicis. Hand 10: 176–180

167. Thomsen B 1977 Processus supracondyloidea humeri with concomitant compression of median nerve and ulnar nerve. Acta Orthopaedica Scand 48: 391–393

168. Murakami Y, Komiyama Y 1978 Hypoplasia of the trochlea and the medial epicondyle of the humerus associated with ulnar neuropathy. J Bone Joint Surg 60B: 225–227

169. Hirotani H 1975 An unusual cause of ulnar nerve compression. Hand 7: 266–268

170. Holtzman R N, Mark M H, Patel M R, Wiener L M 1984 Ulnar nerve entrapment neuropathy in the forearm. J Hand Surg (Am) 9: 576–578

171. Vance R, Gelberman R 1978 Acute ulnar neuropathy with fractures at the wrist. J Bone Joint Surg 60A: 962–965

172. Poppi M, Padovani R, Martinelli P, Pozzati E 1978 Fracture of the distal radius with ulnar nerve palsy. J Trauma 18: 276–278

173. Howard F M 1961 Ulnar nerve palsy in wrist fractures. J Bone Joint Surg 43A: 1197-1201

174. Gore D R 1971 Carpometacarpal dislocation producing compression of the deep branch of the ulnar nerve. J Bone Joint Surg 53A: 1387–1390

175. Vorenkamp S E, Nelson T L 1987 Ulnar nerve entrapment due to heterotopic bone formation after a severe burn. J Hand Surg (Am) 12: 378–380

176. Milberg P, Kleinert H E 1980 Giant cell tumor compression of the deep branch of the ulnar nerve. Ann Plastic Surg 4: 426–429

177. Hayes C 1978 Ulnar tunnel syndrome from giant cell tumor of tendon sheath: a case report. J Hand Surg 3: 187–188

178. McFarland G B, Hoffer M M 1971 Paralysis of the intrinsic muscles of the hand secondary to lipoma in Guyon's canal. J Bone Joint Surg 53A: 375–376

179. Zahrawi F 1984 Acute compression ulnar neuropathy at Guyon's canal resulting from lipoma. J Hand Surg (Am) 9: 238–239

180. Bowers W, Doppelt S 1979 Compression of the deep branch of the ulnar nerve by an intraneural cyst. Case report. J Bone Joint Surg 61A: 612–613

181. Fahmy N R M, Noble J 1981 Ulnar nerve palsy as a complication of synovial osteochondromatosis of the elbow. Hand 13: 308–310

182. Taylor A R 1974 Ulnar nerve compression at the wrist in rheumatoid arthritis. J Bone Joint Surg 56B: 142–143

183. Dell P C 1979 Compression of the ulnar nerve at the wrist secondary to a rheumatoid synovial cyst: case report and review of the literature. J Hand Surg 4: 468–473

184. Sanders R J, Roos D B 1989 The surgical anatomy of the scalene triangle. Cont Surg 35: 11–16

185. McIntyre D I 1975 Subcoracoid neurovascular entrapment. Clin Orthopaedics 108: 27–30

186. Poitevin L A 1988 Proximal compressions of the upper limb neurovascular bundle. An anatomic research study. Hand Clin 4: 575–584

187. Brannon E W 1963 Cervical rib syndrome. J Bone Joint Surg 45A: 977–998

188. Baumgartner F, Nelson R J, Robertson J M 1989 The rudimentary first rib — a cause of thoracic outlet syndrome with arterial compromise. Arch Surg 124: 1090–1092

189. Roos D B 1979 New concepts of thoracic outlet syndrome that explain etiology, symptoms, diagnosis, and treatment. Vasc Surg 13: 313–321

190. Siegel R S, Steichten F M 1967 Cervicothoracic outlet syndrome. J Bone Joint Surg 49A: 1187–1192

191. Warrens A N, Heaton J M 1987 Thoracic outlet compression syndrome: the lack of reliability of its clinical assessment. Ann R Coll Surg Eng 69: 203–204

192. Adson A W 1947 Surgical treatment for symptoms produced by cervical ribs and the scalenus anticus muscle. Surg Gynecol Obstet 85: 687–700

193. Adson A W 1951 Cervical ribs: symptoms, differential diagnosis and indications for section of the insertion of the scalenus anticus muscle. J Internat Coll Surg 16: 546–559

194. Wright I S 1945 The neurovascular syndrome produced by hyperabduction of the arms. Am Heart J 29: 1–19

195. Rainer W G, Mayer J, Sadler T R, Dirks D 1973 Effect of graded compression on nerve conduction velocity. Arch Surg 107: 719–721

196. Lain T M 1969 The military brace syndrome. J Bone Joint Surg 51A: 557–560

197. Lain T M 1969 The military brace syndrome: a report of sixteen cases of Erb's palsy occurring in military cadets. J Bone Joint Surg 51A: 557–560

198. Bonney G 1965 Scalenus medius band. J Bone Joint Surg 47B: 268–272

199. Urschel H C, Razzuk M A 1972 Management intelligence. Management of the thoracic outlet syndrome. New Engl J Med 286: 1140–1143

200. Smith K F 1979 The thoracic outlet syndrome: a protocol of treatment. J Orthopaedic Sports Phys Therapy 2: 89–99

201. Adson A W, Colley J R 1927 Cervical rib. A method of anterior approach for relief of symptoms by division of

the scalenus anticus. Ann Surg 85: 839–857

202. Roos D B 1966 Experience with first rib resection for thoracic outlet syndrome. Ann Surg 163: 354–358
203. Spurling R G, Scoville W R 1944 Lateral rupture of the cervical intervertebral discs. Surg Gynecol Obstet 78: 350–357
204. Kikuchi S, Macnab I, Moreau P 1981 Localisation of the level of symptomatic cervical disc degeneration. J Bone Joint Surg 63B: 272–277
205. Frohse F, Frankel M 1908 Die Muskaln des Menschlichen Aunes. Bardelehen's Handbuch der Anatomie des Manschlichen. Fischer, Jena
206. Spinner M 1968 The arcade of Frohse: its relationship to posterior interosseous nerve paralysis. J Bone Joint Surg 50B: 809–812
207. Pollock F H, Drake D, Bovill E G, Day L, Trafton P G 1981 Treatment of radial neuropathy associated with fractures of the humerus. J Bone Joint Surg 63A: 239–243
208. Kaiser T E, Sim F H, Kelly P J 1981 Radial nerve palsy associated with humeral fractures. Orthopedics 4: 1245–1251
209. Strachan J C H, Ellis B W 1971 The vulnerability of the posterior interosseous nerve during radial head resection. J Bone Joint Surg 53B: 320–323
210. Lotem M, Fried A, Levy M, Solzi P, Najenson T, Nathan H 1971 Radial palsy following muscular effort. J Bone Joint Surg 53B: 500–506
211. Manske P R 1977 Compression of the radial nerve by the triceps muscle. Case report. J Bone Joint Surg 59A: 835–836
212. Lubahn J D, Lister G D 1983 Familial radial nerve entrapment syndrome: a case report and literature review. J Hand Surg (Am) 8: 297–299
213. Wilhelm A 1976 Radialis kompressions syndrome. Handchirurgie 8: 113–116
214. Roles N C, Maudsley R 1972 Radial tunnel syndrome: resistant tennis elbow as a nerve entrapment. J Bone Joint Surg 54B: 499–508
215. Lister G D, Belsole R B, Kleinert H E 1979 The radial tunnel syndrome. J Hand Surg 4: 52–60
216. Lister G D 1991 Radial tunnel syndrome. In: Gelberman R H (ed) Operative nerve repair and reconstruction. Lippincott, Philadelphia, pp 1023–1037
217. Werner C 1979 Lateral elbow pain and posterior interosseous nerve entrapment. Acta Orthopaedica Scand 50: suppl 174
218. Henry A K 1973 Extensile exposure, 2nd edn. Churchill Livingstone, Edinburgh
219. Rosen, I, Werner C 1980 Neurophysiological investigation of posterior interosseous nerve entrapment causing lateral elbow pain. Electroencephalog Clin Neurophysiol 50: 125–133
220. Hagert C G, Lundborg G, Hansen T 1977 Entrapment of the posterior interosseous nerve. Scand J Plastic Reconstr Surg 11: 205–212
221. Sponseller P D, Engber W D 1983 Double-entrapment radial tunnel syndrome. J Hand Surg (Am) 8: 420–423
222. Bowen T L, Stone K H 1966 Posterior interosseous nerve paralysis caused by a ganglion at the elbow. J Bone Joint Surg 48B: 774–776
223. Mulholland R C 1966 Nontraumatic progressive paralysis of the posterior interosseous nerve. J Bone Joint Surg 48B: 781–785

224. Capener N 1966 The vulnerability of the posterior interosseous nerve of the forearm. J Bone Joint Surg 48B: 770–783
225. Sharrard W J W 1966 Posterior interosseous neuritis. J Bone Joint Surg 48B: 777–780
226. Spinner M, Freundlich B D, Teicher J 1968 Posterior interosseous nerve palsy as a complication of Monteggia fractures in children. Clin Orthopaedics 58: 141–145
227. Holst-Nielsen F, Jensen V 1984 Tardy posterior interosseous nerve palsy as a result of an unreduced radial head dislocation in Monteggia fractures: a report of two cases. J Hand Surg (Am) 9: 572–575
228. Lichter R L, Jacobson T 1975 Tardy palsy of the posterior interosseous nerve with a Monteggia fracture. J Bone Joint Surg 57A: 124–125
229. Austin R 1976 Tardy palsy of the radial nerve from a Monteggia fracture. Injury 7: 303–304
230. Popelka S, Vainio K 1974 Entrapment of the posterior interosseous branch of the radial nerve in rheumatoid arthritis. Acta Orthopedica Scand 45: 370–372
231. Millender L H, Nalebuff M D, Edward A, Holdsworth D E 1973 Posterior interosseous nerve syndrome secondary to rheumatoid synovitis. J Bone Joint Surg 55A: 753–757
232. White S H, Goodfellow J W, Mowat L A 1988 Posterior interosseous nerve palsy in rheumatoid arthritis. J Bone Joint Surg (Br) 70: 468–471
233. Agnew D H 1863 Bursal tumour producing loss of power of forearm. Am J Med Sci 46: 404–405
234. Mass D P, Tortosa R, Newmeyer W L, Kilgore E S Jr 1982 Compression of posterior interosseous nerve by a ganglion. Case report. J Hand Surg 7: 92–94
235. McCollam S M, Corley F G, Green D P 1988 Posterior interosseous nerve palsy caused by ganglions of the proximal radioulnar joint. J Hand Surg (Am) 13: 725–728
236. Blakemore M E 1979 Posterior interosseous nerve paralysis caused by a lipoma. J Roy Coll Surg Edin 24: 113–117
237. Bieber E J, Moore J R, Weiland A J 1986 Lipomas compressing the radial nerve at the elbow. J Hand Surg (Am) 11: 533–535
238. Carr D, Davis P 1985 Distal posterior interosseous nerve syndrome. J Hand Surg (Am) 10: 873–878
239. Dellon A L, Mackinnon S E 1986 Radial sensory nerve entrapment in the forearm. J Hand Surg (Am) 11: 199–205
240. Wartenberg R 1932 Cheiralgia paresthetica (Isolierte Neuritis des Ramus Superficialis Nerve Radialis). Z Ges Neurol Psychiatr 141: 145–155
241. Ehrlich W, Dellon A L, Mackinnon S E 1986 Classical article: Cheiralgia paresthetica (entrapment of the radial nerve). (A translation in condensed form of Robert Wartenberg's original article published in 1932) J Hand Surg (Am) 11: 196–199
242. Saplys R, Mackinnon S E, Dellon A L 1987 The relationship between nerve entrapment versus neuroma complications and the misdiagnosis of de Quervain's disease. Cont Ortho 15: 51–56
243. Derkash R S, Niebauer J J 1981 Entrapment of the posterior interosseous nerve by a fibrous band in the dorsal edge of the supinator muscle and erosion of a groove in the proximal radius. J Hand Surg 6: 524–526

244. Herrick R T, Godsil R D, Widener J H 1980 Lipofibromatous hamartoma of the radial nerve. A case report. J Hand Surg 5: 211–213

245. Sunram F, Hippe P 1979 Radial nerve paralysis by congenital angioleiomyoma. Hand Chirurgia 11: 27–29

246. Field J H 1981 Posterior interosseous nerve palsy secondary to synovial chondromatosis of the elbow joint. J Hand Surg 6: 336–338

247. Belsole R, Lister G, Kleinert H 1978 Polyarteritis: a cause of nerve palsy in the extremity. J Hand Surg 3: 320–325

248. Burns J, Lister G D 1984 Localized constrictive radial neuropathy in the absence of extrinsic compression: three cases. J Hand Surg (Am) 9A: 99–103

249. Garcia G, McQueen D 1981 Bilateral suprascapular nerve entrapment syndrome. Case report and review of the literature. J Bone Joint Surg 63A: 491–492

250. Rask M R 1977 Suprascapular nerve entrapment: a report of two cases treated with suprascapular notch resection. Clin Orthopaedics 123: 73–75

251. Swafford A R, Lichtman D H 1982 Suprascapular nerve entrapment. Case report. J Hand Surg 7: 57–60

252. Gozna E R, Harris W R 1979 Traumatic winging of the scapula. J Bone Joint Surg 61A: 1230–1233

253. Cahill B R, Palmer R E 1983 Quadrilateral space syndrome. J Hand Surg (Am) 8: 65–69

254. Bassett F H, Nunley J A 1982 Compression of the musculocutaneous nerve at the elbow. J Bone Joint Surg 64A: 1050–1052

255. Gelberman R H, Verdeck W N, Brodhead W T 1975 Supraclavicular nerve-entrapment syndrome. J Bone Joint Surg 57A: 119

256. Kutz J E, Singer R, Lindsay M 1985 Chronic exertional compartment syndrome of the forearm: a case report. J Hand Surg (Am) 10: 302–304

257. Pedowitz R A, Toutounghi F M 1988 Chronic exertional compartment syndrome of the forearm flexor muscles. J Hand Surg (Am) 13: 694–696

258. Phillips J H, Mackinnon S E, Murray J F, McMurtry R Y 1986 Exercise-induced chronic compartment syndrome of the first dorsal interosseous muscle of the hand: a case report. J Hand Surg (Am) 11: 124–127

259. Styf J, Forssblad P, Lundborg G 1987 Chronic compartment syndrome in the first dorsal interosseous muscle. J Hand Surg (Am) 12: 757–762

260. Abdul-Hamid A K 1987 First dorsal interosseous compartment syndrome. J Hand Surg (Br) 12: 269–272

261. Clay N R, Austin S 1988 Idiopathic thenar muscle hypertrophy. J Hand Surg (Br) 13: 100–101

262. Ritter M A, Inglis A E 1969 The extensor indicis proprius syndrome. J Bone Joint Surg 51A: 1645–1648

263. Spinner M, Olshansky K 1973 The extensor indicis proprius syndrome. Plastic Reconstr Surg 51: 134–138

264. Ambrose J, Goldstone R 1975 Anomalous extensor digiti minimi proprius causing tunnel syndrome in the dorsal compartment. J Bone Joint Surg 57A: 706–707

265. Hart J A L 1972 Extensor digitorum brevis manus. Hand 4: 265–267

266. Reef T C, Brestin S G 1975 The extensor digitorum brevis manus and its clinical significance. J Bone Joint Surg 57A: 704–706

267. Wood J 1864 On some varieties in human myology. Proc Roy Soc Lond 13: 299–303

268. Gama C 1983 Extensor digitorum brevis manus: a report on 38 cases and a review of the literature. J Hand Surg (Am) 8: 578–582

269. Ogura R, Inoue H, Tanabe G 1987 Anatomic and clinical studies of the extensor digitorum brevis manus. J Hand Surg (Am) 12: 100–107

270. Patel M R, Desai SS, Bassini-Lipson L, Namba T, Sahoo J 1989 Painful extensor digitorum brevis manus muscle. J Hand Surg (Am) 14: 674–678

271. Pancoast H K 1932 Superior pulmonary sulcus tumor. J Am Med Assoc 99: 1391–1396

4. Inflammation

Inflammation occurs in association with many disorders of the hand, several of which are not considered here. Indeed some have a chapter to themselves — injury, previous trauma, rheumatoid disease and swellings. Inflammation may present as acute or chronic, and these descriptions may be pathologic or temporal, pathologic referring to the nature of the tissue response, temporal to the speed of onset and the duration. Inflammation may be associated with infection or may be sterile, and both may be acute or chronic. For the purposes of organization all *infections* are considered below under the heading of acute inflammatory conditions, although in some instances the arrangement is awkward, even inaccurate.

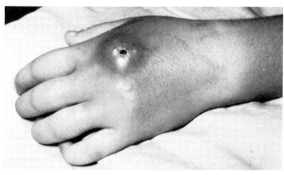

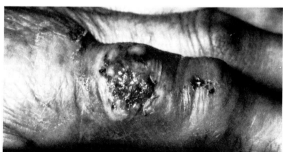

Fig. 4.1 A, B. Infection on the dorsum of the hand forms a *whitlow*. The pus-filled cavities are multilocular, and care must be taken to evacuate all pockets.

ACUTE INFLAMMATORY CONDITIONS

Classification

Hand infections[1-3] may be bacterial, viral, fungal, protozoal or metazoal. Although in one series of bacterial infections 63.5% of patients grew out multiple organisms[4], the most common are *Staphylococcus* (60%), *Streptococcus* and *Enterobacter* (16% each) and *Pseudomonas* (2%). This represents a change in the distribution over the past ten years, a change which continues[5]. Infections could be classified according to the causative organism, but one glance at the selected list of reported pathogens given on page 334 will persuade the reader that such a catalogue would contribute little more than confusion.

Rather are infections classified by their anatomic distribution in the hand, be that generalized or restricted to one area. Localization to one area is a function both of the type of infecting organism and of the fact that the hand has distinct anatomical compartments which tend to contain the spread of sepsis.

LEVEL IN THE TISSUES

Abscesses may develop at differing levels in the tissue:

Subcuticular — lying immediately beneath the epidermis; this is easily recognized, being a thinly covered pocket of pus under very little tension (Fig. 4.11)
Intracutaneous — most common on the dorsum of the fingers in the form of a boil (Fig. 4.1)
Subcutaneous
Subfascial — beneath the palmar aponeurosis.

The deeper abscesses may, in the necrotic process of the overlying tissue known as 'pointing', communicate with more superficial layers. *Collar-stud abscesses* are so formed. The term indicates that two loci of pus communicate with one another through a narrow channel.

323

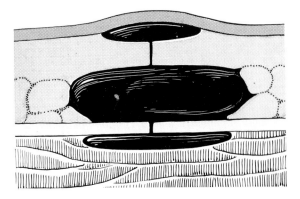

Fig. 4.2   Collar-stud abscess. In this, the accumulation of pus is at two or more sites between natural tissue layers (see text).

In the case of subfascial abscesses, there may develop an abscess with three pockets, one beneath the fascia, one subcutaneous and one subcuticular. The implications surgically are quite clear — the more superficial abscess may be drained and the deeper not recognized, resulting in continued infection (Fig. 4.2).

ANATOMICAL COMPARTMENTS

The palmar surface of the hand and the tissues around the distal phalanx are divided into compartments which serve to limit the spread of infection.

Nail fold
The eponychium, which is the fold of skin overlying the root of the nail, is defined distally by its free margin and proximally by the fascial attachment of the skin to the base of the distal phalanx just distal to the insertion of the extensor tendon. Laterally, the area is defined by the firm attachment of the margin of the nail to the lateral interosseous ligament of the distal phalanx[6].

The nail fold is especially susceptible to injury, often in the course of manicuring or in the form of a 'hangnail'. Infection of such minor wounds is very common, probably because they are initially neglected and the area is subjected to repeated trauma. Infections of the nail fold are called *paronychia*.

Apical spaces
The skin of the very tip of the finger is very firmly attached to the distal phalanx by numerous fibrous

septa which divide the soft tissue immediately beneath the nail into a large number of virtually closed compartments.

Digital pulps
The middle and distal digital creases, which overlie the joints, are attached respectively to the A3 and A5 pulleys of the tendon sheath. This can be confirmed at surgery or more simply by observing the relative immobility of the creases to tangential movement when compared with the adjacent pulps. The pulps therefore become confined compartments. Infection in these pulps remains localized, rarely extending into adjacent compartments. Indeed, soft-tissue necrosis and phalangeal osteitis will develop sooner.

Tendon sheath
The attachment of the skin to the A3 and A5 pulleys and the adjacent cruciate sheath means that there is no intervening fat between skin and sheath to absorb puncture wounds. In addition, the cruciate portion of the sheath is much more flimsy than the annular. Injuries to the digital creases are therefore more likely to result in tendon sheath infections.

In over 80% of hands the tendon sheath of the small finger communicates with the ulnar bursa, which is the major part of the flexor synovial sheath at the wrist. That of the thumb is almost invariably continuous with the radial bursa, which is the synovial sheath of flexor pollicis longus at the wrist. Infection involving the sheaths of these digits may easily communicate with the wrist and lower forearm. They may also connect one with the other, creating the so-called 'horseshoe' abscess which involves the tendon sheaths of both thumb and small finger. The tendon sheaths of the other fingers may communicate with the ulnar bursa — 2.7 to 3.5% in different fingers, other than the small — but more commonly end proximally at the metacarpophalangeal joint, that is, beneath the palmar creases.

Distally, the tendon sheaths end at the insertion of the flexor digitorum profundus.

Web space
Less well-defined anatomically than the other compartments, the web space is nonetheless clearly circumscribed when infected. It is bounded by the margin of the web containing the natatory (or superficial transverse palmar) ligament distally, by the deep attachments of the palmar fascia proximally and by its attachment to the tendon sheaths laterally. The deep transverse metacarpal ligament forms the floor of the space which extends dorsally between the fingers around the distal edge of that ligament.

Deep palmar space

This lies deep to the palmar fascia. The rigid nature of the fascia allied to its resistance to penetration by pus results in considerable tension, and consequent pain, in the relatively rare infection of this space. Kanavel described 'thenar' and 'mid-palmar' spaces. While these can be defined anatomically, deep infection is not always confined to one or other.

History

PREDISPOSING FACTORS

After inoculation with a pathogen, whether or not clinically evident sepsis develops depends on the size and content of the inoculum and on the level of host resistance. A careful history may reveal factors which predispose to sepsis, by reducing that resistance, or which are likely to have exposed the patient to a specific organism or type of infection:

occupation   dentists and nurses[7] — herpes simplex
　　　　　　　barbers　　　　　　 — interdigital
　　　　　　　　　　　　　　　　　　pilonidal sinus[8]
　　　　　　　work in water　　　 — *Mycobacterium*
　　　　　　　　　　　　　　　　　　marinum
　　　　　　　work in slaughterhouse
　　　　　　　　　　　　　　　　 — *Erysipelothrix*
　　　　　　　　　　　　　　　　　　rhusiopathiae, or
systemic disease — diabetes[9-12] and any condition suppressing natural immunity, notably AIDS[13] and organ transplantation
previous injury to the area, notably a bite, human, animal or insect, or a needle stick, incidental or self-inflicted, as in drug abuse
infection elsewhere[14].

TIME LAPSE

The time since injury after which symptoms occur will often differ according to the infection:

cellulitis　　　　　　　within 24 hours
tendon sheath　　　　　within 48 hours
web
deep palmar　　　}　　days
paronychia
pulp　　　　　　　}　　4–5 days
septic arthritis　　　　up to 2 weeks after injury

SYMPTOMS

Pain and *loss of function* are two of the five cardinal signs of inflammation and are always present in the patient

with a hand infection. If pus is present within a confined compartment, the pain will be of a throbbing nature. Accurate localization of pain will already have been made by the patient. This should be determined by questioning. It will invariably correspond with the point of maximum tenderness. While function will be impaired wherever the infection is seated, the disability is greatest in tendon sheath infection, where no movements whatsoever of the involved digit can be tolerated.

Tenderness radiating up the arm, even to the axilla, is evidence of ascending lymphangitis. Usually associated with streptococcal infection, lymphangitis is often present in cases of cellulitis and sometimes in tendon sheath infections and septic arthritis.

General malaise, often with associated *pyrexia*, as a general rule accompanies only those hand infections which show ascending lymphangitis. It is particularly marked in those with cellulitis.

Loss of sleep is an important symptom to seek, for it invariably indicates pus gathering in the tissues.

Examination

The three other cardinal signs of inflammation are found on examination, the affected part being *red*, *swollen* and *hot*.

LOCALIZED

Paronychia[15, 16] (Fig. 4.3)
This presents as a typical lesion usually confined to one

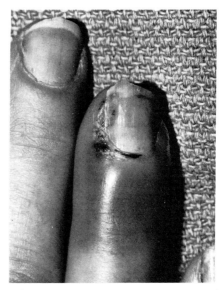

Fig. 4.3   Paronychia, with inflammation around the full extent of the eponychium.

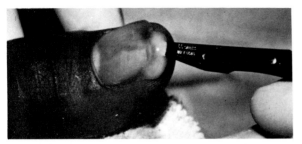

Fig. 4.4 Apical abscess. This is localized to the tip just beneath the nail, and, if advanced, dissects under the nail. Here the track can be seen passing all the way up to the lunula.

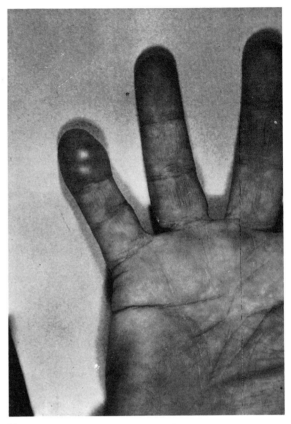

Fig. 4.5 Felon. A terminal pulp infection of the right small finger. It is important to note that while the inflammation is very marked in the terminal pulp, there is little evidence of involvement of the digit over the middle phalanx.

or other corner of the nail fold. Where it runs around to the other corner it is known as just that — a 'run-around'. Later a paronychia may pass beneath the nail around the cul-de-sac of the nail bed, and pus will be evident beneath the nail.

A subungual haematoma may produce inflammation in the eponychium and therefore be mistaken for a paronychia in its early stages.

A *chronic paronychia*[17] is characterized by swollen, red, indurated eponychium with loss of the cuticle which normally adheres to the superficial surface of the nail. From the resultant open cul-de-sac small quantities of pus can be expressed. Such chronic paronychia are often encountered in those whose employment involves repeated and prolonged immersion in water.

Apical pulp infection

These show a very small area of acute tenderness immediately beneath the free margin of the nail. This may be overlooked and a mistaken diagnosis of a full-blown, but as yet unlocalized, terminal pulp infection may be made and observation instituted. Later, apical pulp infection tracks beneath the nail which may be completely detached by a pocket of pus (Fig. 4.4).

Felon

The *terminal pulp* of the normal digit is fluctuant. When infection develops in this closed compartment, fluctuation is lost initially and does not appear until sepsis has destroyed the fibrous septa which bind the skin to the periosteum of the terminal phalanx. If neglected until that stage, terminal pulp infection — a *felon* — (Fig. 4.5) is often associated with osteitis and destruction of the terminal phalanx (Fig. 4.6).

A crush injury of the finger tip with fracture of the distal phalanx may be mistaken for a pulp infection in its early stages.

Web space infecton (Fig. 4.7)

Like those of the deep palm, these are located primarily on the palmar surface but are most easily recognized from the dorsal aspect. Oedema is very evident on the dorsum, and the infection understandably forces the adjacent fingers apart. This fixed separation is absolutely diagnostic of a web space infection.

Deep palmar space infection[18] (Fig. 4.8)

Deep infections are characterized by severe pain, gross dorsal oedema, loss of normal palmar concavity, and fixed posture of the fingers. This results from oedema in the periarticular structures of the metacarpophalangeal joints and from the splinting which this partly voluntary posture provides to the extremely painful hand. Despite their fixed posture, the fingers can be moved at the interphalangeal joints without undue pain, distinguishing deep palmar from tendon sheath infections, except in

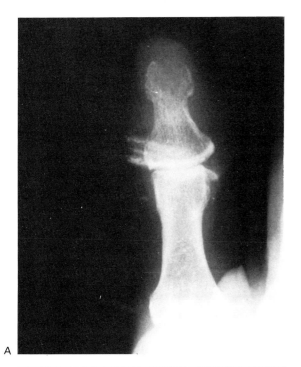

A

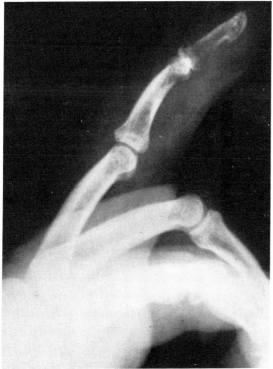

B

Fig. 4.6 A, B. Osteitis of the distal phalanx is seen in these two cases with destruction in (A) of the distal tuft, and in (B) of the juxta articular region. (The opacity across the interphalangeal joint in (A) is ingrained dirt in an old wound).

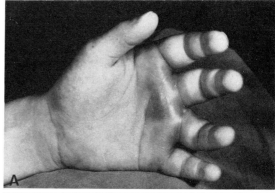

A

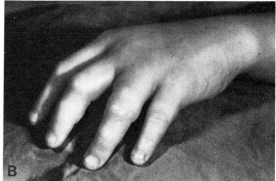

B

Fig. 4.7 A. Web space infection. B. This diagnosis is emphasized by the unnatural separation of middle from ring fingers when viewed from the dorsum.

those cases when the sepsis spreads from the sheath to the palmar space, a common route.

Tendon sheath infection[19, 20] (Fig. 4.9)
Affecting only one digit, these invariably show the four classical signs as stated by Kanavel[21]:

1. The finger is held fixed in slight flexion, the hand being well guarded
2. The finger is uniformly swollen and red
3. There is intense pain on attempted extension
4. Tenderness is present along the line of the sheath.

The tenderness is very accurately localized, little being evident in the distal digital pulp while the metacarpophalangeal joint can be moved with little pain, albeit through a limited range. Rarely, extensor tenosynovitis may be suppurative[22].

Dorsal infections
These are easily recognized by the presence of all the cardinal signs and by their location.

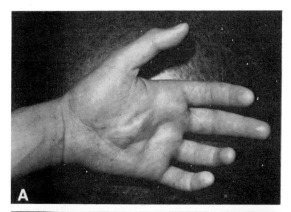

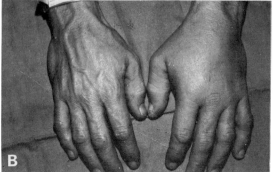

Fig. 4.8 A. A deep palmar space infection producing fullness of the radial aspect of the palm with alteration of posture in the middle finger. B. The major part of the oedema in a deep palmar space infection is to be seen on the dorsum.

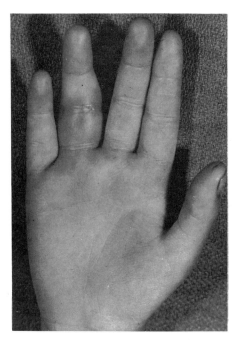

Fig. 4.9 Tendon sheath infection. The ring finger is uniformly swollen and red. Intense pain was present on any attempt to extend the finger.

The dorsum of the hand has no anatomical compartments of significance in containing sepsis. In the matter of infection it behaves like the skin elsewhere in the body. Thus, sepsis is most common in those areas which are hairbearing, one or more follicles becoming involved, a boil or carbuncle developing accordingly. The carbuncle of the dorsum of a finger is also known as a *whitlow* (Fig. 4.1).

Dorsal infections are of significance mainly when they develop over a joint. Unlike boils and carbuncles these infections usually follow recognized injuries, often puncture wounds, often inflicted by animal or human teeth. They carry the danger of *septic arthritis*.

Septic arthritis[23, 24]
An infected joint should be suspected in the presence of a wound overlying the finger joints dorsally. If such a wound continues to discharge small quantities of seropurulent fluid more than a week after the original injury then suspicion should approach certainty.

By far the most common cause of septic arthritis is a human 'bite' (p. 331). Septic arthritis can develop without such a wound or indeed without any recent injury. In such a situation, the surgeon should be mindful of less common causes of septic arthritis, such as gonorrhoea, and of the non-infective causes of acute arthritis, including gout and rheumatoid disease. The clinical features of septic arthritis are:

swelling out of proportion to the inflammation present in the skin around the wound and, at later stages,
restricted motion in the joint; this is often surprisingly slow to develop but eventually both flexion and extension will produce pain;
instability will be evidenced in the later stages by increased laxity in the collateral ligaments; this motion may be accompanied by crepitus;
discharging sinuses will develop if drainage is not instituted;
radiologic changes (Fig. 4.10), only the first of which is apparent in the initial two weeks; they are, in sequence:
— dorsal soft-tissue swelling evident on lateral views
— decalcification of the juxta articular bone
— narrowing of the joint space
— progressive fragmentation of the bone ends.

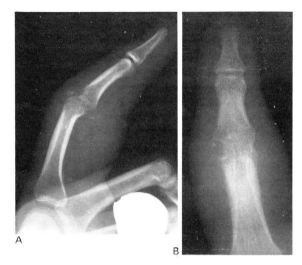

Fig. 4.10 A, B. The radiograph of this patient with septic arthritis of the proximal interphalangeal joint demonstrates extensive soft-tissue swelling, decalcification of the bone adjacent to the joint, and narrowing of the joint space with early fragmentation of the bones.

It should be emphasized that instability, sinuses, radiographic changes and even severe pain on motion may not be present at the stage when the patient with septic arthritis can best be helped[25]. The surgeon must therefore have a high degree of awareness when disproportionate swelling accompanies a wound in the appropriate site and which continues to discharge long after injury. Culture of the effusion from the wound and also of the synovial fluid when the wound is explored is mandatory.

It is not always easy to distinguish septic arthritis from non-infective disorders, particularly if no wound is evident. The differential diagnosis includes osteoarthritis, gout and rheumatoid arthritis. These present a problem mainly when they are monoarticular since inspection of other joints in polyarthritic forms will reveal characteristic signs. Radiographs, while not showing evidence of infective arthritis for more than two weeks after onset, may identify any of the non-infective alternatives.

Wound infection[26]
Wound infection, following trauma or surgery, is more common in those with evident predisposing factors (see above). Setting aside this important, but small, group, it can be said that all infection arises because something in the patient is inadequately perfused with the blood which is the source of most host defenses. Such circumstances can be enumerated:

1. Inanimate objects
   (a) those inserted by the surgeon — these include pins, plates, joint replacements, and rods to permit later tendon grafting
   (b) those deposited by the injury — these include glass, metal and wooden fragments, road dirt, oil and grease, paint, indeed all substances with which the patient may have come in contact before or during the injury
2. Tissues devitalized by the injury or surgery
   (a) well-defined — any part to which the sole blood supply has been arrested and not restored
   (b) ill-defined — skin, muscle, bone and other soft and hard tissues which have been crushed and thereby deprived of circulation by thrombosis, vessel avulsion or local oedema
3. Tissues devitalized by post-traumatic oedema
4. Haematoma
5. Tissues devitalized by post-traumatic ischaemic events
   (a) wound margins
   (b) skin grafts and flaps
   (c) muscle compartments
   (d) parts, be they individual digits or the entire limb.

Rapidly spreading sepsis. Streptococcus spreads rapidly on account of its intrinsic enzymes, producing cellulitis and lymphangitis. *Clostridia*, though rare, swiftly extend along muscle planes producing the gas which can be seen on standard radiographs In all patients with unconfined infection, systemic symptoms and signs will be uppermost. They will show general malaise, often to the point of disorientation. There may be evidence of circulatory disturbance similar to hypovolaemic shock, with cold, sweating extremities and hypotension. The temperature may exceed 103° Fahrenheit, or may be below normal. While it should be emphasized that the diagnosis is clinical and requires emergency surgical care, blood cultures should be taken, optimally at the height of systemic symptoms and signs, which fluctuate.

In extensive injuries, especially if badly contaminated or if the treatment has been long delayed, the surgeon must be alert to the possibility of *gas gangrene*. Largely a clinical and radiologic diagnosis, any evidence of gas in the tissues must be vigorously treated. Bessman and Wagner[62] drew attention to the high incidence of *non-clostridial gas gangrene*, especially in diabetics. It differs from the classical variety in that, while radical debridement is still required as an emergency measure, the extent of amputation necessary is somewhat less and cephalosporins and Kanamycin are more effective than the massive doses of penicillin required for clostridial gas gangrene.

Local sepsis. Though less hazardous to the patient's survival and therefore less dramatic, local wound infection is more common and has serious implications for the function of the injured limb. The patient will complain of an increase of pain, which, in the presence of pus, may be throbbing in nature, reflecting the increased tissue tension. She will complain also of inability to sleep due to the pain, even despite the use of analgesics and hypnotics. This is a cardinal sign of pus in the hand. There may be systemic complaints of fever, chills and rigors but these occur in a minority of localized wound infections. On examination, the dressing may be stained and malodorous. The experienced observer may draw some accurate conclusions regarding the nature of the infection from the colour of the staining and the distinctive odour of the discharge. For example, *Pseudomonas* may cause a greenish-blue stain with the smell of rotting vegetation. The part will be swollen. Wound erythema, which normally will have diminished steadily since surgery, will be more evident and extensive. The area will be tender, most exquisitely so over an accumulation of pus.

Treatment of a *threatening* wound infection will start with elimination of any identifiable cause from those enumerated above. To this will be added rest, elevation and antibiotics, selected on an educated guess as to the infecting organism and its sensitivity.

An *established* infection will be managed by drainage and culture of all pockets of pus, often the insertion of irrigation catheters, and again, rest, elevation and antibiotics.

Osteomyelitis

Osteomyelitis has been distinguished from *osteitis* by some, considering the first to be primarily a blood-borne infection of the metaphysis in children, the latter a chronic infection at any site in any age group due to direct bacterial seeding of bone which has been rendered avascular by trauma. However, the former term, osteomyelitis, is used by most to describe all bone infections.

Blood-borne osteomyelitis of childhood is very rare distal to the elbow; while most cases are staphylococcal, many organisms, including mycobacteria, fungi and viruses have been implicated. It should be considered in any child presenting with pyrexia, malaise, disuse of the limb and localized bone tenderness. Radiologically, acute osteomyelitis may be confused with bone tumour (Ch. 6), showing patchy rarefaction and a periosteal reaction. It can be distinguished by the presence of an elevated white cell count, by isotope bone scan and CT or MRI.

Adult osteomyelitis is similarly uncommon in the upper extremity, which is rarely afflicted by the major vessel disease, venous stasis and/or chronic lymphoedema which so compromises the lower limb. However, in the presence of extensive scarring consequent upon a major wound, scarring which reduces the local vascularity, and especially if there is systemic compromise in the form of diabetes or immune deficiency, osteomyelitis may develop. Its recognition is straightforward, for it should be assumed that all exposed bone is infected, but its extent is impossible to determine with absolute certainty. Such certainty is necessary if debridement is to be total. Total debridement of dead and infected bone is essential for cure. It follows that, despite our best efforts, some treated cases will show later relapse. It is valuable to classify the type of osteomyelitis, for that assists in planning management, which consists in most cases of antibiotic therapy, radical debridement of scarred soft tissue and bone, free flap coverage and bone replacement by cancellous or vascularized graft (see Fig. 2.40).

Type I	medullary
Type II	superficial
Type III	cortex and medulla — localized
Type IV	cortex and medulla — diffuse

Blistering distal dactylitis

Probably the forerunner of full-blown streptococcal cellulitis, this presents as a subcuticular blister over the terminal phalanx. Associated with very little local or generalized reaction, the blister contains whitish, watery pus which grows *Streptococcus* on culture. Easily treated — for the blister can be trimmed away painlessly without anaesthesia (Fig. 4.11) — its significance lies in the need for a full course of penicillin therapy to ensure that no cellulitis, or worse, rheumatic fever or acute glomerulonephritis follows this otherwise minor disorder.

Herpetic whitlow[27-31] (Fig. 4.12)

Despite its name, this occurs mainly on the digital pulp. Commencing with pain, redness and swelling, it may be mistaken for a distal pulp infection in its initial stages. After 24–36 hours, the characteristic vesicles appear, clear at first, quickly becoming opaque and apparently purulent. Culture is sterile but the causative virus can be demonstrated within six hours if there is cause for doubt. The importance is to recognise the nature of the condition, for incision and drainage is contraindicated. With observation the lesion will regress spontaneously.

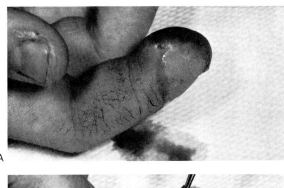

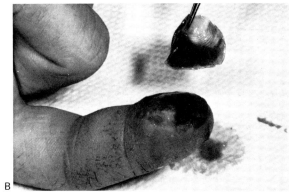

A

B

Fig. 4.11 A, B. Blistering distal dactylitis. This streptococcal infection is subcuticular and can be evacuated without anaesthesia simply by trimming away the skin.

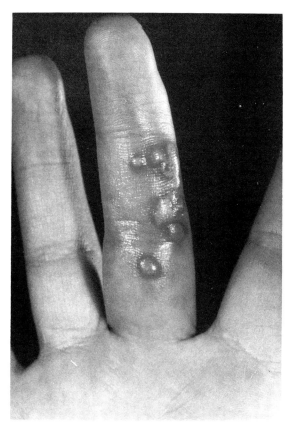

Fig. 4.12 Herpetic whitlow. The characteristic vesicles are pathognomonic of herpes simplex.

Gonorrhoea[27, 34]

Although not its customary territory, *Neisseria gonorrhoeae* (the 'gonococcus') may cause a septic arthritis or acute tendon sheath infection. In a more chronic form it may involve the synovium around the extensors on the wrist, resembling rheumatoid disease. In either event, the importance to the hand surgeon is to remember the possibility and to seek evidence in the form of cultures from either the pus released by incision, which may however fail to reveal the gonococcus, or from skin lesions, prostatic smears, vaginal or rectal swabs. Gonococcal complement fixation tests should provide confirmation, although these may be weakly positive in rheumatoid patients also, and obviously care must be taken to make firm the diagnosis before discussing the matter with the patient.

Cat scratch disease[35, 36]

This should be considered when the patient, usually a child, develops papules or vesicles at the site of a cat scratch or bite. These lesions are in themselves unimpressive but are associated with significant epitrochlear and axillary lymphadenitis and often with high fever.

Human[37–43] *and animal bites*[44, 45]

Because of the organisms encountered in the oral cavity, these are serious injuries which require vigorous treatment. The majority of human 'bites' are not in fact bites but are rather tooth wounds sustained while punching the 'biter' in the mouth! For this reason patients may be late in seeking treatment and may lie about how the injury was sustained. It should always be assumed that a wound over the knuckle communicates with the joint space and it should be explored with that in mind. The wound should be excised at each level, remembering that the posture at exploration is entirely different from that at the time of the blow. For this reason the successive wounds in skin, extensor apparatus, joint capsule and metacarpal head do not correspond, indeed are far removed one from the other (Fig. 4.13). The injury to the metacarpal head will not be seen on the radiograph for it is a *chondral 'divot' fracture*. In the author's experience such a chondral injury is found in the large majority of human fist bites (Fig. 4.14). With early adequate excision and a period

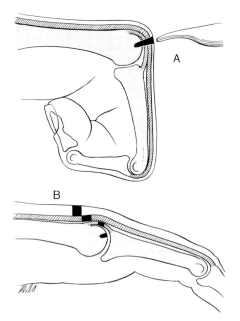

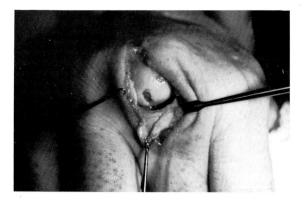

Fig. 4.14 A cartilaginous 'divot' fracture resulting from a human bite.

Fig. 4.13 In this diagrammatic representation it can be seen (A) that the tooth pierces the clenched fist of the attacker penetrating skin, tendon, joint capsule, and the metacarpal head. B. When the finger is extended by swelling and at surgery, the four puncture wounds do not correspond.

of wound irrigation bite injuries do not live up to their evil reputation[46].

While the organisms may vary, and routine cultures should always be supplemented by anaerobic[47] and 10% carbon dioxide[48] preparations, a common growth in human bites is *Eikenella corrodens*[49–52] and in animal bites *Pasteurella multocida*[53–56]. By happy coincidence, both are sensitive to crystalline penicillin, which should therefore be given in appropriate doses[57].

Drug addiction[58]

This has become an increasing source of infection, and for similar reasons of guilt to those above, enhanced by the effects of drug abuse, the patient presents late and gives an inaccurate history[59]. Dorsal abscesses are most common, but septic arthritis may be the presenting disorder, with many cases due to *Serratia* and *Pseudomonas*[60,61]. It is very unlikely that the infection will follow the first use of intravenous or 'main-line' drugs by the patient, and therefore extensive soft-tissue changes will be present in the limb due to previous insults. The typical hand of the established addict shows extensive indurated puffy oedema, chronic tenosynovitis or inflexible ankylosis of the small joints.

GENERALIZED

Cellulitis

When present in the hand cellulitis is dramatic in onset. The patient presents with a history of very acute onset of swelling, redness and pain following often a minor injury. He arrives within 12 to 24 hours of the start of infection.

Examination shows that the patient appears ill, pale and sweating, often with a marked elevation of temperature. The most striking feature in the hand is the extensive puffy redness with streaks of lymphangitis often obvious in the forearm. The axillary nodes are enlarged on occasion, but are more often simply tender in the early stages. There may be a *haemorrhagic blister* present which can be removed without pain. If a wound is present it is usually unremarkable, exuding only a few drops of serous fluid. Culture of the serous fluid from either the blister or the wound usually yields haemolytic streptococci.

Incision and drainage is never indicated in cellulitis and is indeed meddlesome.

Necrotizing fasciitis[62] (= synergistic gangrene, Fournier's gangrene, necrotizing cellulitis, Meleney's haemolytic streptococcal gangrene)

This is a rapidly progressive bacterial infection characterized by extensive necrosis of subcutaneous fat and fascia. Originally thought to be primarily streptococcal it is now known to be a mixed infection in the majority of patients. Commonly associated with alcohol and drug abuse, it initially presents as a low-grade cellulitis, but rapidly becomes fulminant with cyanosis of skin progressing to extensive areas of gangrene. The development of gangrene leads to hyperpyrexia, shock and a high mortality rate. Diagnosis is based on clinical findings and dictates swift, radical debridement. Hyperbaric oxygen may be beneficial in systemically compromised patients[60], but should only supplement surgical treatment.

Purpura fulminans[63, 64]

In its early phases purpura fulminans could be confused with cellulitis or incipient necrotizing fasciitis. It is a rare form of non-thrombocytopenic purpura which occurs mainly in children following a benign infectious process located anywhere in the body. Disseminated intravascular coagulopathy in those who have undergone splenectomy is the underlying pathological event. It is rapid and often fatal. The onset is heralded by fever, tachycardia and an increased respiratory rate. Extensive ecchymoses appear dramatically on both lower limbs and less frequently on the torso and upper extremities, progressing to haemorrhagic necrosis, with loss of areas of skin and of digits. Blood pressure, haemoglobin, platelets and coagulation all become grossly abnormal in a matter of hours. Multidisciplinary treatment is required, of which heparinization is a central feature. Acute debridement is not necessary, unlike necrotizing fasciitis, and the local areas are treated rather like burns.

Pyoderma gangrenosum[65]

This is a neutrophilic dermatosis and therefore non-infective. However, it presents as pustules or bullae and may be diagnosed as multiple staphylococcal whitlows. It occurs in conjunction with inflammatory bowel disease and rarely with myelofibrosis, chronic hepatitis and rheumatoid disease. Any patient with multiple, apparently infected lesions should receive consultations with the internist and dermatologist.

Sarcoidosis

Sarcoidosis is a systemic granulomatous disorder of unknown origin[66]. It may present in the hand as pathological fractures[67], involvement of muscle[68] or tenosynovitis[69]. Diagnosis depends on the presence of bilateral hilar adenopathy on standard lung radiographs, an elevated angiotensin-converting enzyme (ACE) level, a positive Kveim skin test and histological study of biopsied material.

Toxic shock syndrome (TSS)

This has been described following hand infection[70, 71]. It is characterized by fever, rash, hypotension and involvement of at least three of the following systems: gastrointestinal, muscular, renal, hepatic, haemato-logical or CNS. Treatment involves wound drainage, fluid therapy, steroids and broad-spectrum antibiotics.

General indications

With the discovery of antibiotics, infections of the hand, formerly crippling and even life-endangering, have become less significant. The classic work of Kanavel[21] published in 1912 still holds good with regard to diagnosis and conservative management. His formal incisions, designed to decompress extensive areas, have however been supplanted by more simple rules of drainage:

1. Do not wait for a fluctuant swelling in hand infections.
2. Pus is present, even when it cannot be seen, if
   (a) the patient complains of throbbing pain
   (b) he has lost a night's sleep.
3. In the presence of pus, always incise over the point of maximum tenderness. If pus cannot be seen through the skin, the point of maximum tenderness should be sought by the gentlest pressure with a blunt probe.

The establishment of a protocol[72] for infection management involving incision, drainage, irrigation and intravenous antibiotic therapy has been shown to have beneficial results with respect to shortening hospital stay and improving the rate of healing with fewer complications. Early institution of rehabilitation[73] also improves the outcome.

See Green D P 1993 Operative Hand Surgery, 3rd edn. Churchill Livingstone, New York, p. 1021.

PERSISTENT INFECTION

Apart from unusual organisms, there are several factors which cause infection to persist despite treatment.

Inadequate drainage is by far the most common and is most likely to occur:

1. When incision has been performed too early, that is, before throbbing and sleep loss indicated pus accumulation
2. When the incision has not been made over the point of maximum tenderness
3. When all pockets have not been drained — this is especially common when a collar-stud abscess has developed (Fig. 4.2).
4. Where the drainage incision has been allowed to heal too soon, leaving a cavity. This is prevented by copious, repeated irrigation through an indwelling catheter introduced through adjacent healthy skin[74,75] (Fig. 4.15).

Presence of a foreign body, sequestrum of bone or slough. Ischaemia of the limb.

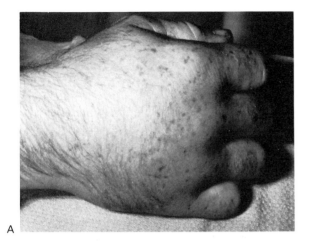

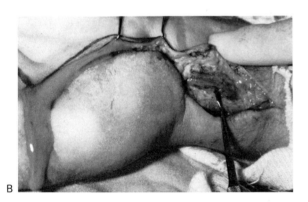

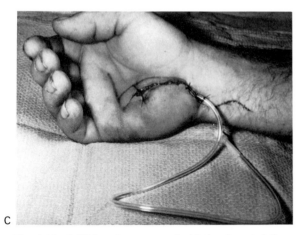

Fig. 4.15 A. This patient presented with the characteristic features of pus in the hand, and the dorsal swelling was marked. B. The point of maximal tenderness was over the Guyon's canal, and for this reason exploration was commenced by proximal exposure of the ulnar nerve and artery. Pus was released from the region of the canal, and (C) an irrigating catheter was inserted to wash out the cavity at regular intervals during the subsequent 3 days.

Continued trauma to the part — this may be iatrogenic, unintentional or factitious.

Generalized systemic disorders sufficiently severe as to prevent wound healing should be immediately apparent. However, a full physical examination with special laboratory studies should be undertaken in all persistent infections where no cause is located.

Uncommon organisms[76] have been recorded as causing hand infections:

Mycobacterium[77–79] (*chelonei*[80], *fortuitum*,[81–83] *kansasii*,[84–88] *marinum*,[89–95] *terrae*[96,97], *tuberculosis*[98–102]) have been reported in recent years involving tendon sheaths, bursae, joints, fascia and bone in that order of frequency. The more chronic forms may be mistaken for gout or rheumatoid disease. Difficult to culture — *marinum* for example, grows at 30–32°C — the diagnosis may be suspected if the tuberculin skin tests are strongly positive.

Histoplasma capsulatum[103]
Coccidioides immitis[104–106] both of the tendon sheath.

These are merely examples of a much wider range of uncommon flora which may complicate the management of a hand infection. In all instances of infection resistant to treatment the active guidance and participation of the bacteriologist should be sought in establishing the diagnosis.

Other uncommon organisms and infectious diseases reported in the hand

Bacteria
  Aeromonas hydrophila[107–111]
  Anthrax[112]
  Bacteroides fragilis (arthritis)[113]
  Clostridium botulinum[114]
  Clostridium septicum[115]
  Clostridium perfringens (arthritis)[116]
  — Gas gangrene[117]
  — Non-clostridial gas gangrene[118, 119]
  Haemophilus influenzae (cellulitis)[120]
  Mycoplasma[121]
  Nocardia[122–124]
  Serratia perfringens (arthritis)[125]
  Vibrio[126–128]
Fungi[129]
  Actinomycosis[130–135]
  Aspergillosis[136, 137]
  Blastomycosis[138]
  Candida albicans[139]
  Chromohyphomycosis[140]
  Maduromycosis[141,142]
  Mucormycosis[143]

Sporotrichosis[144–146]
Alga — Prototheca[147–149]
Larva[150, 151]
Parasite — onchocerciasis[152]

Non-infective causes of acute inflammation

Calcific deposits[153–157] are well known to produce acute inflammation in regions other than the hand but that they may do so in the hand is less well recognized. The patient presents with a complaint of pain and consequently reduced function. Examination reveals a tense, red, shiny, warm area which is acutely tender. The location of the calcium deposits varies but it often presents as an acute calcific tendinitis. Unless aware of the possibility, the surgeon may resort to incision to no avail.

Radiographs so taken as to throw the inflamed area into relief may show calcium deposits as flecks of radio-opaque material in the soft tissues. Rest and support are indicated.

Acute gout may show all the symptoms and signs of septic arthritis. Suspicion should be aroused by the great severity of the pain which is unrelieved by immobilization. A positive history of gout, evidence of chronic disease in other joints or an elevated serum uric acid will confirm the diagnosis in the majority of cases. In the remainder, however, diagnosis is possible only by the detection of birefringent needle-like crystals of monosodium urate monohydrate in the joint fluid or synovium, usually within polymorphonuclear leucocytes.

CHRONIC INFLAMMATORY DISORDERS

The patient with any of the chronic inflammatory disorders presents with a complaint of pain, made worse by use and always relieved by total rest of the afflicted part. The pain may not be present at all times, showing flares of activity, often initiated by unremembered minor trauma. Depending upon the patient's occupation and on the severity or frequency of the attacks of pain, the disorder may be simply a nuisance or may force the patient to forsake his employment increasingly, often resulting in his being labelled a malingerer or in the loss of his job. Chronic inflammation, therefore, constitutes a major cause of loss of work time and may result eventually in social dependency. While specific causes may be identified, such as gout, rheumatoid disease or any of the rheumatoid variants (Ch. 5) the majority of cases come about as the result of trauma. The injury may be clearly remembered and may have been adequately treated (Ch. 2). More commonly, the afflicted part has

been repeatedly subjected to forgotten minor stresses to which it has not proved equal.

The structures affected by these 'chronic inflammatory disorders' are most commonly the joints and the musculotendinous units.

Joints — osteoarthritis[158–160]

It is estimated that 40% of the adult population are afflicted by osteoarthritis in one form or another, but that of these only 10% seek medical advice and only 1% are severely disabled.

It is probable that multiple genetic factors predispose certain patients to the development of osteoarthritis, factors which influence the structure and maintenance of articular cartilage. However, the development of osteoarthritis is due mainly to ageing, major injuries and the microtrauma of daily stress.

Any joint in the hand may be affected by chronic inflammation. Some may proceed to full-blown osteoarthritis, but the majority do not. Those joints which do would appear to be subjected to unavoidable daily stress, while the others are either very well supported or it is possible for the patient to protect them during use.

Joints which are chronically inflamed cause *pain on stress*. Characteristically, the patient states that he has no problems in the morning on rising, in contrast to the rheumatoid patient, but as the day progresses his discomfort increases. In the evening the affected joint is the seat of a dull ache, which may interfere with sleep.

Examination
Examination of such patients should be directed at locating the point of maximal tenderness and detecting any laxity in supporting ligamentous structures. Pain or crepitus on grinding movements of the joint, early evidence of ensuing osteoarthritis, should also be sought.

The primary disorder in osteoarthritis is loss of articular surface, which is seen on radiograph as narrowing of the joint space. Increasingly the bare bones denuded of cartilage make contact with one another. This causes pain, the bone becomes more dense or eburnated and this is shown by sclerosis on radiograph. Cystic erosions occur in the bone ends and bone spurs, osteophytes or exostoses build up around the bony margins of the joint.

Laboratory studies should be performed on all such patients to exclude rheumatoid disease or variants (see Ch. 5). Radiographs will show any early osteoarthritic changes. Stress films should be taken to detect any ligamentous instability.

General indications

Even in patients who have no clear evidence of frank osteoarthritis, surgery is indicated where marked laxity of ligaments is present or where pain is preventing work, is clearly localized to one joint and has not responded to conservative therapy. A common example of such chronic inflammation due to instability which later progresses to established osteoarthritis is found in the basal joint of the thumb. Where the joint surface is still good but a ligament is incompetent it can frequently be replaced by tendon graft or transfer. Where the surface is irretrievably damaged, the choice lies between arthrodesis and arthroplasty. While osteoarthritis may develop in any of the joints in the hand, those most commonly affected and which most come to surgical treatment are the distal interphalangeal joints and certain carpal articulations. Of the latter, the deterioration is clearly related to one injury, such as a scaphoid fracture or scapho-lunate dissociation, in the majority of joints. Those problems are considered in Chapter 2 (pp. 215 and 219), leaving arthritis around the trapezium and in the pisotriquetral joint to be considered here.

See Green D P 1993 Operative Hand Surgery, 3rd edn. Churchill Livingstone, New York, pp. 99 and 143.

TRAPEZIUM

The key structures in the trapeziometacarpal joint are the palmar or ulnar ligament which holds the beak of the thumb metacarpal down to the ridge on the trapezium and the dorsal intermetacarpal ligament which holds the first to the second matacarpal[161]. The alternative names for the first ligament emphasize the differing relationships of the ligament to the planes of the thumb and the hand, respectively. The ligament is on the palmar aspect of the thumb, that is, directly opposite the thumb nail, but because the plane of the relaxed thumb lies at right angles to that of the hand, the ligament is ulnar when the plane of the hand is taken as reference. In normal flexion and extension of the thumb, the joint and the two ligaments are little stressed. In opposition and power pinch however, the joint surfaces twist one on the other[162], threatening to come apart, only the ligaments preventing them[163]. In this position, stresses are unequally distributed over the joint surfaces. With time, wear results. If, in addition, injury damages the joint surface making it incongruous or, worse still, disrupts the ligaments, arthrosis — as the initial stage of the disorder is called — and osteoarthritis become inevitable.

Use of the thumb is unavoidable in the human hand and therefore arthrosis and osteoarthritis of the trapezio-metacarpal joint develop relatively early in life,

usually in the fifth decade. Disease in this joint is much more common in the female than in the male patient. It may follow recognized trauma, develop as a consequence of rheumatoid arthritis, or, in most instances, arise for no apparent reason. To quote Eaton and Littler, 'whatever the underlying cause, once hypermobility is present a painful synovitis is common and the possibility of accelerated articular attrition is increased[164].' This hypermobility is present from birth in patients with Ehlers–Danlos syndrome[165,166] in whom changes occur early.

Symptoms

Pain with use is the patient's one complaint in the early stages. The pain is localized to the base of the thumb, the patient usually pointing to the radial aspect of the thenar eminence just anterior and distal to the anatomical snuff box. Later marked instability with resultant weakness of pinch grip further reduces the patient's capacity to use the affected hand.

Examination

Tenderness is well localized with thumb or fingertip pressure applied exactly over the joint on its anterior aspect. The joint is located at the proximal margin of the thenar eminence 1 to 2 cm radial and slightly distal to the scaphoid tubercle (p. 203). It can best be located by adducting the thumb, when the base of the first metacarpal becomes prominent.

The *torque test* serves further to distinguish basal joint arthrosis from other disorders. Axial rotation is applied to the thumb with the basal joint alternately distracted and compressed and the metacarpophalangeal joint gently flexed. Pain on this manoeuvre is pathognomonic. Later, instability of the joint is evidenced by the prominence of the metacarpal base when compared with a normal thumb. It can be confirmed by applying intermittent pressure to the base while asking the patient to pinch strongly. Considerable motion and often crepitus will be detected. Finally, stress applied to the dorsal intermetacarpal ligament will sometimes reveal marked laxity and will always be painful. This is achieved by fixing the first metacarpal with a thumb on the radial side of its head and then applying radially directed force to the ulnar border of the shaft with the middle finger of the same hand (Fig. 4.16).

Collapse of the thumb may eventually occur with adduction of the first metacarpal and hyperextension of the metacarpophalangeal joint. This produces a 'swan-neck' deformity, similar to a rheumatoid Nalebuff type III thumb (p. 377) (Fig. 4.17).

Pinch strength will progressively decrease and should be recorded with a dynamometer.

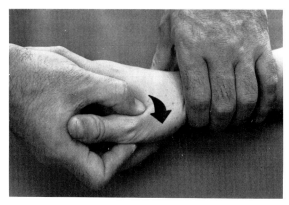

Fig. 4.16 The basal joint of the thumb is stressed by blocking the metacarpal head and applying pressure to the shaft.

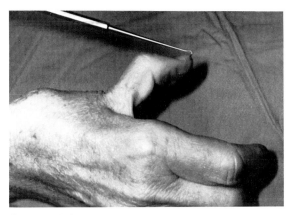

Fig. 4.17 A hyperextension deformity of the metacarpophalangeal joint is demonstrated. The subluxation of the basal joint can be seen to the left of the first metacarpal.

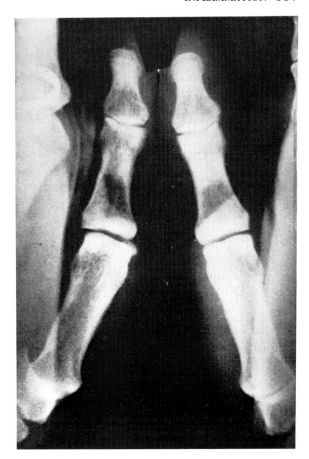

Fig. 4.18 Employing the Eaton stress view in which the two thumbs are driven firmly against one another, subluxation of the basal joint on the left can be seen (stage II).

Radiologic examination

While the basal joint can be seen on standard antero-posterior views, it and the other articulations of the trapezium are best studied on a Robert view (p. 74) and even these views are not entirely representative of the existing disease process[167]. Radiologic changes have been divided into four stages[168]:

Stage I — widening of the joint space (evidence of effusion); less than one-third subluxation in any projection

Stage II— more than one-third subluxation demonstrated especially on stress films; small bone or calcific deposits 2 mm in diameter are to be seen (Fig. 4.18)

Stage III — larger fragments present; joint space narrowing evident (Fig. 4.19)

Stage IV — advanced changes: major subluxation, cystic and sclerotic bone changes, lipping and osteophyte formation (Fig. 4.20).

Involvement of other trapezial joints

While description has thus far been confined to the trapeziometacarpal joint, osteoarthritis is confined to that joint in only a minority of cases. In one series[169], the other articulations of the trapezium were involved as follows:

with the second metacarpal	86.2%
with the scaphoid	48.3%
with the trapezoid	34.6%

Such involvement cannot be diagnosed clinically but can be seen on radiograph. Careful study is therefore

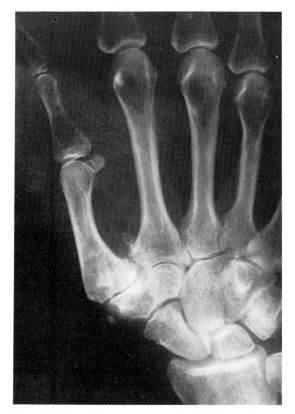

Fig. 4.19 Stage III carpometacarpal arthritis (see text).

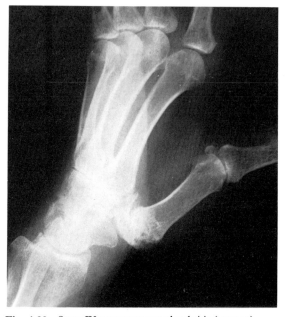

Fig. 4.20 Stage IV carpometacarpal arthritis (see text).

necessary if the correct treatment is to be prescribed to relieve the patient's symptoms (Fig. 4.21).

Infrequently patients will be seen in whom changes are entirely limited to a trapezial articulation other than that with the first metacarpal, most commonly that with the scaphoid[170] (Fig. 4.22).

Indications

At any point in the deterioration of the joint, some temporary relief may be provided by fitting the patient with a hand-based, or better forearm-based, thumb support splint, injecting the joint with steroid and exhibiting non-steroidal anti-inflammatory drugs[171,172]. Most patients eventually come to surgery.

In the early stages, before any evidence of loss of articular cartilage is present, discomfort can be eliminated and further deterioration prevented or at least postponed by stabilizing the joint[173]. The most-used procedure has been that of Eaton and Littler[164] in which half of the flexor carpi radialis, left attached distally, is passed through the base of the metacarpal to replace the attenuated ulnar collateral ligament (Fig. 4.23). Recently, the author has been strengthening the attenuated dorsal intermetacarpal ligament with a strip of extensor carpi radialis longus[174] — a simpler and so far effective procedure.

In late stages with established osteoarthritis the choice lies, as in other joints so afflicted, between arthrodesis[175,176] and arthroplasty. If arthritis clearly involves other trapezial joints, arthrodesis of the trapeziometacarpal joint will give only limited, if any, relief of symptoms, as will any interpositional arthroplasty of that joint alone. Excision of the trapezium becomes necessary and good results have been reported from that alone[177,178]. However, others found that simple excision relieved pain but gave an unstable and therefore weak thumb. Replacement of the excised trapezium by tendon[179,180] or fascia[181] has been advocated. Others report good, long-term results with tendon interposition supplemented by a ligament reconstruction using part of the flexor carpi radialis, which 'suspends' the base of the first metacarpal from the second[182,183]. These techniques, which avoid the use of implants[184-192], are now preferred. Silicone implants, which some still recommend for use in older, low-demand rheumatoid patients[193,194], have proved to be either unstable or subject to fracture and/or wear with resultant silicone synovitis[195-203] (Fig. 4.24). They are no longer recommended for routine use. When they are, specially informed consent should be documented. Whatever excisional procedure is selected, it is important to correct any Z hyperextension deformity of the metacarpophalangeal joint by simultaneous tenodesis,

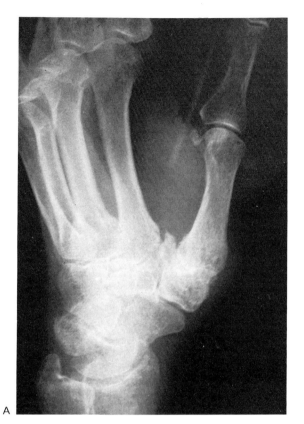

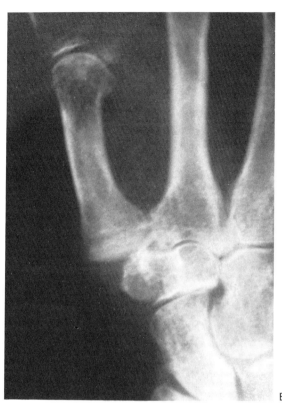

A

B

Fig. 4.21 These patients have been treated (A) by fusion and (B) interpositional arthroplasty of the basal joint. Their pain persists because of evident osteoarthritis between the trapezium and the first metacarpal, the trapezoid, and the scaphoid.

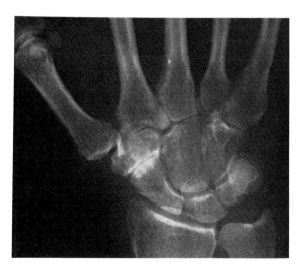

Fig. 4.22 Scaphotrapezial arthritis. This patient presented with symptoms similar to those of trapeziometacarpal disease. Radiographs, however, revealed that the arthritis existed only between the scaphoid and trapezium. Intercarpal fusion cured her symptoms.

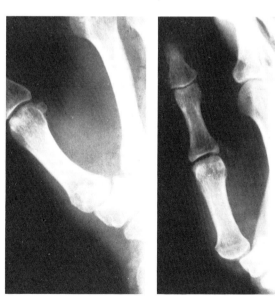

Fig. 4.23 This patient has undergone an Eaton–Littler reconstruction shown on the left for the stage II subluxation shown on the right.

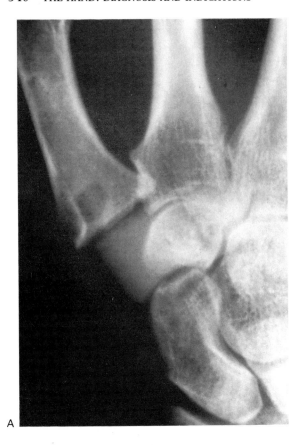

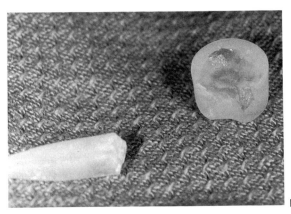

Fig. 4.24 Implant fracture and silicone synovitis. Eighteen months following trapezial resection and implant arthroplasty, this patient presented with increasing pain. A. Radiologic examination showed probable fracture of the implant and silicone synovitis in the scaphoid and capitate. B. The implant was indeed fractured and the wear pattern of the head is evident.

A

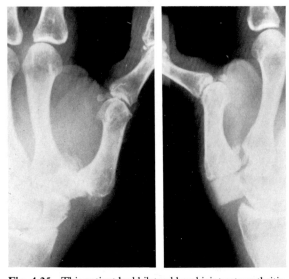

Fig. 4.25 This patient had bilateral basal joint osteoarthritis with severe hyperextension of the metacarpophalangeal joints. The significance of correcting the latter deformity was not appreciated when the trapezial implant was placed in the right. The resulting deformity was worse than the original problem, and pain and weakness persisted.

capsulodesis or arthrodesis. Otherwise, subluxation will occur at the basal joint with recurrence of pain and weakness (Fig. 4.25). Isolated scaphotrapezial disease[170,204] is treated by intercarpal fusion or interpositional arthroplasty[205].

See Green D P 1993 Operative Hand Surgery, 3rd edn. Churchill Livingstone, New York, p. 162.

PISOTRIQUETRAL JOINT

Pisotriquetral arthritis[206] causes wrist pain which may be largely referred to the dorsum of the hand. Ulnar neuropathy was an associated feature in one-third of patients. Instability, due to loss of integrity in the supporting structures of the pisiform, appears to be the cause of pisotriquetral disease[207]. The diagnosis is made by *tenderness* produced by stressing the joint. This can be done in two ways:

(i) direct radial pressure over the ulnar aspect of the pisiform
(ii) resisted combined flexion and ulnar deviation of the wrist.

A radiograph of the joint is taken with the hand supinated 30°–40° from true lateral (Fig. 4.26). Mild problems can be alleviated by injection with local anaesthetic and soluble steroid; those more severe are cured by excision of the pisiform.

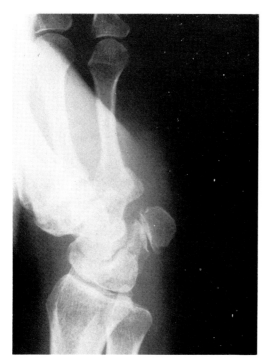

Fig. 4.26 Pisotriquetral osteoarthritis (see text).

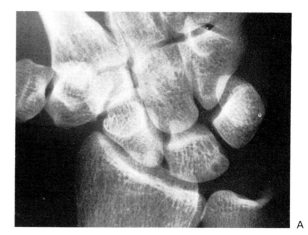

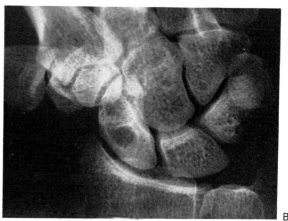

Fig. 4.27 Isolated carpal cysts (A) in the lunate, and (B) in the scaphoid (see text).

ISOLATED CARPAL CYSTS

Occasionally a patient may be seen complaining of poorly localized wrist pain in whom the only positive finding is a cyst in a carpal bone (Fig. 4.27). In a characteristically thorough review[208], Eiken has determined that such bone cysts are the cause of pain only if they have *sclerotic margins* or they *communicate with the joint space*. Such cysts are most common in the scaphoid and lunate and are treated by curettage and bone grafting, providing the joint surfaces are otherwise in good condition.

DISTAL INTERPHALANGEAL JOINT

The patient with distal interphalangeal joint disease may present during the initial phases but more commonly has full-blown osteoarthritis when she consults the surgeon.

The symptoms are those of pain on use, worsening as the day progresses, and instability of the joint.

Examination in the fully developed case is conclusive. The development of *exostoses* is especially florid around the distal interphalangeal joint and these are immediately apparent, giving a knobbly appearance to the

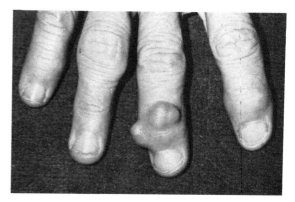

Fig. 4.28 Heberden's nodes. Osteoarthritis of the distal interphalangeal joint with gross osteophyte formation.

joint. Heberden (1710–1801)[209] first described these osteophytes 'Little hard knobs, the size of a small pea, frequently seen upon the fingers, particularly a little below the top, near the joint' and they are named after him — *Heberden's nodes* (Fig. 4.28). (In the much less frequent osteoarthritis of the proximal interphalangeal joint, the osteophytes are known as *Bouchard's nodes*[210].)

Exostoses develop at an early phase in the distal interphalangeal joints and some articular cartilage may still remain despite their presence. Its loss should be confirmed by attempting to elicit crepitus, moving the joint while applying longitudinal compression. The joint often shows additional deformity, with lateral instability or the development of a mallet finger deformity due to erosion of the extensor tendon. The stability of the joint should be checked by stressing the joint laterally using three point leverage.

Radiologic examination confirms the diagnosis (Fig. 4.29).

Ganglion — the 'so-called' mucous cyst[211]. Until recently the pathogenesis of these lesions was disputed. However, it is now evident that the 'mucous cyst' is always a ganglion arising from the distal interphalangeal joint, usually in association with osteoarthritis of that joint (Fig. 4.30). Small ganglions may be mistaken for osteophytes.

Indications

By the time most patients present for help with interphalangeal osteoarthritis, surgery is necessary to give relief[212]. Most surgeons recommend arthrodesis and this is certainly the only treatment in the presence of gross

instability or significant bone destruction (Fig. 4.29) especially now that silicone[213,214] has fallen into disfavour. In cases where the joint is stable and the bone ends are of good contour, however, some have adopted a more conservative approach, performing osteophytectomy and synovectomy, with an acceptable pain-free range of motion resulting[215]. When a ganglion cyst is the reason for surgery, great care must be taken to track the neck of the cyst back to the joint and to perform an adequate synovectomy. Only thus can recurrence be minimized.

The *metacarpophalangeal joint*, especially of the thumb, and the *proximal interphalangeal joint* are the seat of osteoarthritis much less frequently than is the distal interphalangeal joint. The metacarpophalangeal joint of the thumb is best treated by arthrodesis[216] which gives

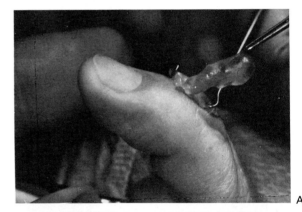

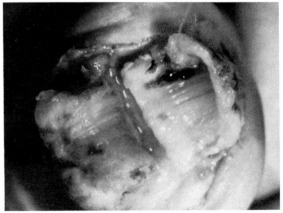

Fig. 4.30   A. A ganglion of the distal interphalangeal joint which had developed in association with osteoarthritis, this presented as a 'mucous cyst' with grooving of the nail. Care is taken at surgery to trace the ganglion down to its origin in the joint. B. This joint shows marked osteoarthritic grooving in association with a ganglion cyst of the distal interphalangeal joint.

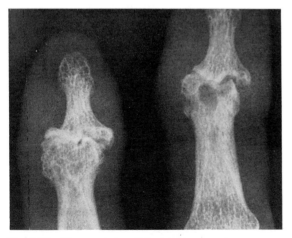

Fig. 4.29   Characteristic radiologic appearance in osteoarthritis of the distal interphalangeal joints, with loss of joint space, formation of exostoses and associated soft-tissue swelling.

excellent results. Management of the proximal interphalangeal joint is much more problematic[217–219]. While attempts are frequently made to preserve motion by silicone arthroplasty, such implants lead in due course to deviation and failure, requiring a later, technically more difficult, arthrodesis. Primary arthrodesis is the only reliable answer, which many patients will understandably reject until the pain becomes intolerable and motion increasingly limited.

Sesamoid arthritis (sesamoiditis)[220,221] at the metacarpophalangeal joint of the thumb is an obscure but very real source of pain in that joint. It is diagnosed by eliciting pain with pressure over the palmar plate of the thumb while holding the main joint immobile. If the joint space of the metacarpophalangeal joint is good and pain is relieved by filling that joint with local anaesthetic, the diagnosis is assured. Excision of the sesamoid — not as easy as it sounds — gives relief to the majority.

See Green D P 1993 Operative Hand Surgery, 3rd edn. Churchill Livingstone, New York, pp. 99 and 143.

Chronic gout

Gout is a disorder primarily of middle-aged and older men and of postmenopausal women. There is often a family history of affliction. It develops as a result of prolonged periods of hyperuricaemia. Uric acid is only sparingly soluble in tissue fluids and is therefore precipitated as monosodium urate monohydrate crystals.

Acute gouty arthritis occurs when these crystals form in the synovial fluid. As the disease progresses, gross deposits of sodium urate, known as *tophi*, appear in the joints, in the periarticular tissues, in the kidneys and in ectopic deposits beneath the skin. One classical site for such ectopic tophi is around the helical margin of the ear.

While early acute monoarticular gout may be difficult to distinguish from septic arthritis (p. 328), the established case has no mimics. The history is one of an onset of monoarticular arthritis usually in the lower extremity, followed by increasingly severe and frequent attacks of joint pain affecting more and more regions. In the upper limb these include the elbow, wrist and fingers. Although at first appearing to return to normal after each attack, the swelling and disability persist for longer periods, eventually becoming permanent. Gouty tenosynovitis affects the wrist extensors and finger flexors[222].

Examination of the upper limbs of the patient with chronic gout reveals tophi, earliest around the olecranon and on the extensor surface of the forearms and later as tumour-like swellings around the joint (Fig. 4.31). These may cause ulceration of the skin and discharge white material with the consistency of wet cement. Tophaceous deposits may also form in the tendon sheaths.

Considerable limitation of motion results and this, or ulceration, may be an indication for surgical intervention, as much of the sodium urate being removed as possible[223]. This is a messy operation, which provokes some anxiety when performed on the interphalangeal joints, for the white material is often all around the finger encasing and camouflaging all structures, including both neurovascular bundles. Arthrodesis is often necessary to stabilize the joint.

Radiologic changes are typical, the bone ends adjacent to the joints showing translucent defects which are deposits of sodium urate, with the later development of an appearance similar to osteoarthritis.

The serum uric acid is consistently elevated in most patients, but not in all.

Musculotendinous units[224]

Considering the significant distances travelled daily around pulleys and through tunnels by the tendons of the upper limb, *chronic tendinitis* is surprisingly uncommon. It is, however, increasingly recognized as one form of *cumulative trauma disorder*[225] (p. 156).

The shoulder will not be considered since it is more the province of the orthopaedic than of the hand surgeon. Musculotendinous units become painful primarily at two sites — when they pass through tight tunnels and are therefore lubricated by synovium and where they attach to bone. There are four sites which frequently give trouble: abductor pollicis longus (de Quervain's disease), digital flexors (trigger finger), flexor carpi radialis (tendinitis) and the extensor origin from the lateral epicondyle (tennis elbow); and four others which rarely do: the tendon sheaths of the wrist extensors[226–229], the extensor pollicis longus[230], the extensor digiti minimi[231] and the anomalously conjoined flexors of thumb and index[232].

STENOSING TENOVAGINITIS AT THE RADIAL STYLOID — DE QUERVAIN'S DISEASE[233]

The abductor pollicis longus and extensor pollicis brevis pass through the first dorsal compartment beneath the extensor retinaculum. The first compartment is more radial than dorsal in position and can be located on the examiner's own hand by tracing the two tendons back on to the radius from their prominent position as the anterior boundary of the anatomical snuff box. Each compartment is lined by synovium and that in the first compartment is particularly prone to become inflamed.

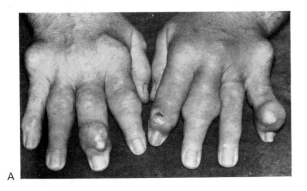

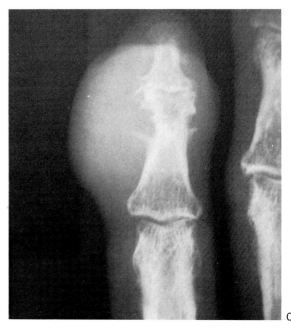

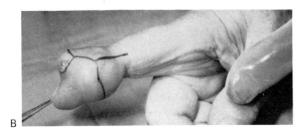

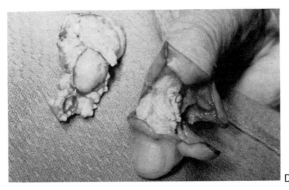

Fig. 4.31   A. Extensive gouty deposits involving many of the joints in the hand. B. In another patient the circumferential nature of the gouty deposit can be seen. C. The deposits are entirely radiolucent. D. Excision involved dissection around the circumference of the joint. Not all material could be removed, and arthrodesis was necessary.

Symptoms

Acute pain on any movement of the thumb is the primary symptom. The pain is located over the tunnel but often radiates into the forearm. Weakness of any hand function involving the wrist or thumb accompanies the pain. Triggering of the thumb may occur[234–235].

Examination

Tenderness over the first dorsal compartment in the acute phase is well localized. In less severe cases it may be difficult to distinguish de Quervain's from arthrosis of the basal joint of the thumb and from flexor carpi radialis tendinitis.

The *Finkelstein test*[236] (Fig. 4.32) is performed by asking the patient to grasp the thumb firmly in the palm of his hand. The examiner then abruptly deviates the hand in an ulnar direction. This places maximum stress on the involved tendons and produces severe pain in de Quervain's disease. The test should be interpreted with some caution. The examiner can confirm on his own hand that the Finkelstein manoeuvre is not comfortable and therefore anxious patients may over-react to normal discomfort. Comparison with the opposite limb should aid in confirming a positive test. The Finkelstein test may also be positive in basal joint arthrosis. This can be differentiated from de Quervain's disease by precise

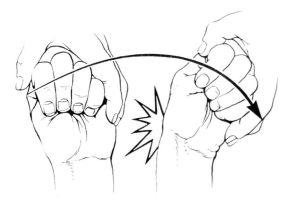

Fig. 4.32 The Finkelstein test. The patient's thumb is enclosed in the palm. The wrist is then abruptly deviated ulnarwards by the examiner. In a positive test pain is produced on the radial border of the wrist.

localization of tenderness and by radiograph (p. 338). Inflammation in the radial aspect of the wrist proper and radial sensory nerve entrapment (p. 313) may also produce a falsely positive test but will produce identical pain if the test is repeated with the thumb *excluded* during ulnar deviation.

Abductor pollicis longus bursitis[229,237] (intersection syndrome) may mimic de Quervain's disease. It presents as a tender swelling localized to the region where the abductor pollicis longus crosses the radial wrist extensors on the radiodorsal aspect of the wrist. Distinct *creptitance* can be felt in the swelling. The Finkelstein test produces pain, referred to the area of the bursitis. Injection and splintage cures most, but some require exploration and may prove to have stenosing tenosynovitis of the radial wrist extensors[229].

Indications

If injection with steroids and splintage[238,239] fail to give permanent relief in de Quervain's then surgical release of the first compartment should be performed. Abductor pollicis longus commonly has multiple tendons. On occasion, one or more of them or the tendon of extensor pollicis brevis may have a separate compartment. Failure to release this may result in a persistence of symptoms. When this is the case, the Finkelstein test will still be positive. If the metacarpal is held immobile and the metacarpophalangeal joint sharply flexed, pain will result if the extensor pollicis brevis is in a separate, unreleased and inflamed compartment[240]. Other problems following release are rare, but do occur[241]. Some may be due to palmar subluxation of the tendon[242].

While technique is outwith the scope of this text, a

cautionary word on the radial nerve in de Quervain's release is always appropriate. Division of radial nerve in the process of this procedure is probably the most common error of commission in hand surgery and is probably the iatrogenic disorder most frequently seen by the hand surgeon. Radial nerve neuroma at the wrist can be a most crippling disorder and one very difficult to treat. The solution, of course, is to carefully identify all branches of the nerve — and three or more may be found — and preserve them during this otherwise simple procedure.

See Green D P 1993 Operative Hand Surgery, 3rd edn. Churchill Livingstone, New York, p. 1990.

FLEXOR TENOSYNOVITIS

Synovitis of the flexor tendons occurs most frequently in rheumatoid patients or those suffering from variants of that disease. It may also occur in other patients for no clear reason, although a higher incidence is recognized in the diabetic patient. The patient does not present with symptoms of chronic synovitis but rather with the consequence — *trigger finger*.

The triggering comes about by the formation of a nodule on the tendon which passes through the proximal pulley of the tendon sheath in a proximal direction with some discomfort (Fig. 4.33). When the extensors, weak relative to the finger flexors, attempt to straighten the digit the nodule jams in the pulley, arresting motion of that finger. It may release suddenly as further extensor force is applied — hence the name.

Trigger thumb also occurs, but a large minority are congenital in origin[243] (p. 479). When so, trigger thumb must be distinguished from congenital shortness of flexor pollicis longus.

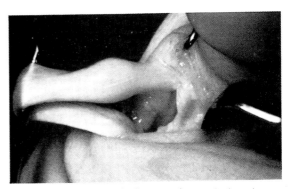

Fig. 4.33 A nodule on the flexor tendon producing trigger finger.

Symptoms

Locking in flexion is the major complaint. Initially present merely as a 'slow finger', in time this comes to the stage where it is necessary to release the locked finger with an adjacent digit or even with the opposite hand. In either event release is painful and may in time prove impossible. The patient then presents with one finger acutely flexed into the palm. Alternatively, the patient becomes understandably more reluctant to bend the digit and may not have done so for some considerable time prior to consultation.

Examination

Tenderness is almost always present over the proximal pulley region. If the patient then flexes the finger over that of the examiner a *nodule* within the tendon may be palpable (Fig. 4.34)

In some patients flexion has become impossible and the examiner must eliminate other possible causes:

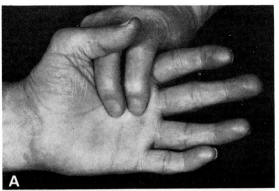
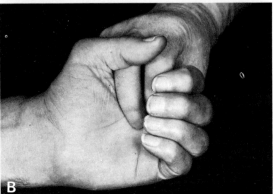

Fig. 4.34 A. Testing a patient for the presence of trigger finger. The examiner's fingers are placed over the region of the proximal pulley at the palmar crease and (B) the patient is invited to flex the fingers over those of the examiner. This may be impossible. If flexion can be achieved the examiner may feel a small nodule passing beneath his fingers and the patient will complain of concomitant pain.

Absent or ruptured tendon. This can usually be excluded by asking the patient to attempt flexion during palpation, when an intact tendon can be felt to become tense.

Fixed joints. A detailed history of onset and the absence of previous injury usually provide the diagnosis. Radiologic examination excludes any articular cause of immobility.

Laboratory studies of a simple nature should be undertaken in all cases of trigger finger on account of the recognized higher incidence in rheumatoid and diabetic patients. Initially, a sedimentation rate and a two-hour postprandial blood sugar estimation are sufficient, any abnormality so detected being investigated further.

Surgery is indicated if steroid injection[244-246] does not provide lasting relief. A simple release of the proximal pulley will be successful in all cases — but should *not* be done in rheumatoid patients (p. 393). A synovectomy where the synovium appears overabundant or inflamed will probably reduce the amount of subsequent tenderness.

FLEXOR CARPI RADIALIS TENDINITIS[247]

Although a distinct clinical entity, this condition is not widely recognized and is difficult to treat with permanent success. The patient complains of discomfort in the wrist, particularly after strenuous exercise. Diagnosis is simple, there being acute localized tenderness over the flexor carpi radialis just proximal to the scaphoid tubercle (Fig. 4.35). Once again, comparison should be made with the normal wrist to confirm that

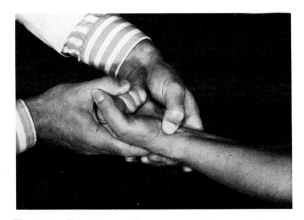

Fig. 4.35 Palpation over flexor carpi radialis just proximal to the scaphoid tubercle may well reveal acute tenderness when compared with the normal side. This is diagnostic of flexor carpi radialis tendinitis.

the tenderness on pressure is greater than normal. A *modified Finkelstein test* has proved useful in making this diagnosis. The relaxed wrist is abruptly deviated as in the Finkelstein, but in a true dorsal direction. Acute pain results in the presence of tendinitis. The scapho-trapezial joint should be studied on appropriate radiographs for it is immediately deep to the tendon and disease there may mimic or cause flexor carpi radialis tendinitis[248] or even rupture[249] of that tendon. Surgery is rarely performed for this condition unless scapho-trapezial arthritis requires fusion. Otherwise it is treated conservatively with steroid injection and splintage.

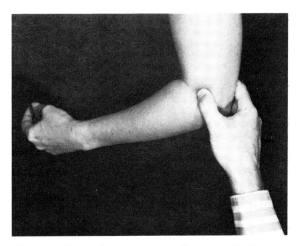

Fig. 4.36 The tenderness in tennis elbow is localized over the anterior aspect of the lateral condyle of the humerus.

LATERAL EPICONDYLITIS — TENNIS ELBOW

The pathogenesis of this common condition is multiple and often a matter of conjecture. Postulated causes include chronic periostitis of the lateral condyle with spur formation[250], partial tears of the common extensor origin[251,252] or granulation tissue therein[253], traumatic capsulitis of the radiohumeral joint, chondromalacia of the radial head[254,255], radio-ulnar bursitis, cervical spine disease[256] and radial tunnel syndrome, which is dealt with elsewhere (p. 309).

The condition is characteristic of a chronic inflammatory disorder as it usually occurs on the first occasion as an acute attack of differing intensity, often following on a period of vigorous extensor activity. Treatment or simply rest causes the acute attack to abate, but less severe trouble persists with increasingly frequent attacks of an acute nature, often initiated by the original causative activity. The patient either ceases engaging in that activity, which may alone eliminate the problem, or he consults his physician.

Symptoms
Despite the name which it is commonly given, the majority of cases occur in the fourth decade in patients who never play tennis. In one series, less than 5% of those afflicted played any sport.

The patient complains of pain centred at the elbow but radiating both proximally and distally, mainly the latter, along the extensor muscles. In the acute phase, extension of the arm and flexion of the wrist are avoided as they exacerbate the pain.

Examination
Tenderness is sought at three anatomical points which are in line proximal to distal over the lateral aspect of the elbow (Fig. 4.36):

lateral epicondyle — periostitis, partial tears

radial head (while rotating the forearm) — synovitis, capsulitis
neck of the radius — posterior interosseous nerve

The patient is asked which of the three elicits the most discomfort, remembering that multiple pathology is possible, indeed likely, in this condition. In this examination it is particularly important to compare the affected with the normal side, for pressure at these points normally produces fairly marked discomfort.

Postural discomfort is produced by flexing the wrist and fingers passively, while the patient holds the arm in extension (Fig. 4.37). Pain referred to the epicondyle will frequently cause the patient to ask the examiner to desist before the fingers and wrist have been fully flexed.

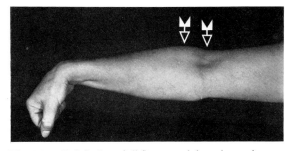

Fig. 4.37 Full flexion of all fingers and the wrist produces discomfort in the patient with tennis elbow more severe than that produced by the middle finger test (p. 310). This contrasts with the findings in a patient with radial tunnel syndrome.

The *middle finger test* should be performed (p. 310). If epicondylitis is the primary problem, pressure on the extended middle finger should cause little more pain than pressure on any of the others. It certainly should not produce as much discomfort as the postural test described above. If this is not so, then radial nerve compression must be considered, especially if the patient has not responded to conservative therapy.

Radiologic examination of the elbow should always be undertaken, which may reveal disorders of the humerus or radial head.

Indications

Surgery is indicated when severe symptoms persist despite rest and repeated injections with steroid. Some authors recount that they almost always find a tear, resection and suture providing a cure. Others have designed a number of procedures including removal of calcifications, release of the extensor origin and excision of a portion of the annular ligament. The very multiplicity of procedures indicates that universal success has been achieved with none.

See Green D P 1993 Operative Hand Surgery, 3rd edn. Churchill Livingstone, New York, p. 2001.

REFERENCES

1. Mann R J 1989 Hand infections. Hand Clin 5: 515–667
2. Kilgore E S Jr 1983 Hand infections. J Hand Surg (Am) 8: 723–762
3. Leddy J P 1986 Infections of the upper extremity. J Hand Surg (Am) 11: 294–297
4. Stern P J, Staneck J L, McDonough J J, Neale H W, Tyler G 1983 Established hand infections: a controlled, prospective study. J Hand Surg (Am) 8: 553–559
5. Stromberg B V 1985 Changing bacteriologic flora of hand infections. J Trauma 25: 530–533
6. Shrewsbury M, Johnson R K 1975 The fascia of the distal phalanx. J Bone Joint Surg 57A: 784–788
7. Bleicher J N, Blinn DL, Massop D 1987 Hand Infections in dental personnel. Plastic Reconstr Surg 80: 420–422
8. Hueston J T 1952 Pathology of the inter-digital pilonidal sinus. Aust NZ J Surg 21: 226–229
9. Mandel M 1978 Immune competence and diabetes mellitus: pyogenic human hand infections. J Hand Surg 3: 458–461
10. Mann R J, Peacock J M 1977 Hand infections in patients with diabetes mellitus. J Trauma 17: 376–380
11. Sneddon J 1970 The care of hand infections. Williams & Wilkins, Baltimore
12. Sneddon J 1969–70 Sepsis in hand injuries. Hand 1–2: 58–62
13. Glickel S Z 1988 Hand infections in patients with acquired immunodeficiency syndrome. J Hand Surg (Am) 13: 770–775
14. Pruzansky M E, Remer S 1986 Abscesses of the hand associated with otopharyngeal infections in children. J Hand Surg (Am) 11: 844–846
15. Keyser J J, Littler J W, Eaton R G 1990 Surgical treatment of infections and lesions of the perionychium. Hand Clin 6: 137–153, discussion 155–157
16. Canales F L, Newmeyer W L 3rd, Kilgore E S Jr 1989 The treatment of felons and paronychias. Hand Clin 5: 515–523
17. Barlow A, Chattaway F, Holgate M, Aldersley T 1970 Chronic paronychia. Br J Dermatol 82: 448–453
18. Burkhalter WE 1989 Deep space infections. Hand Clin 5: 553–559
19. Neviaser R J 1989 Tenosynovitis. Hand Clin 5: 525–531
20. Schecter W P, Markison R E, Jeffrey R B, Barton R M, Laing F 1989 Use of sonography in the early detection of suppurative flexor tenosynovitis. J Hand Surg (Am) 14: 307–310
21. Kanavel A B 1925 Infections of the hand. Lea & Febiger, Philadelphia
22. Newman E D, Harrington T M, Torretti D, Bush D C 1989 Suppurative extensor tenosynovitis caused by Staphylococcus aureus. J Hand Surg (Am) 14: 849–851
23. Freeland A E, Senter B S 1989 Septic arthritis and osteomyelitis. Hand Clin 5: 533–552
24. Wittels N P, Donley J M, Burkhalter W E 1984 A functional treatment method for interphalangeal pyogenic arthritis. J Hand Surg (Am) 9: 894–898
25. Howard J B, Highgenboten C L, Nelson J D 1976 Residual effects of septic arthritis in infancy and childhood. J Am Med Assoc 236: 932–935
26. Thompson L 1991 Postoperative care. In: Kasdan M L (ed) Occupational hand and upper extremity injuries and diseases. Hanley & Belfus, Philadelphia, pp 433–442
27. Berkowitz R L, Hentz V R 1977 Herpetic whitlow — a non-surgical infection of the hand. Plastic Reconstr Surg 60: 125–127
28. Larossa D, Hamilton R 1971 Herpes simplex infections of the digits. Arch Surg 102: 600–603
29. Louis D S, Silva J Jr 1979 Herpetic whitlow: herpetic infections of the digits. J Hand Surg 4: 90–94
30. Walker L G, Simmons B P, Lovallo J L 1990 Pediatric herpetic hand infections. J Hand Surg (Am) 15: 176–180
31. Widenfalk B, Wallin J 1988 Recurrent herpes simplex virus infections in the adult hand. Scand J Plastic Reconstr Surg Hand Surg 22: 177–180
32. Ogiela D M, Peimer C A 1981 Acute gonococcal flexor tenosynovitis. Case report and literature review. J Hand Surg 6: 470–472
33. Rosenfeld N, Kurzer A 1978 Acute flexor tenosynovitis caused by gonococcal infection. A case report. Hand 10: 213–214

34. Thompson S E, Jacobs N F, Zacarias F, Rein M F, Shulman J A 1980 Gonococcal tenosynovitis — dermatitis and septic arthritis. Intravenous penicillin vs oral erythromycin. J Am Med Assoc 244: 1101–1102

35. Carithers H A, Carithers C M, Edwards R O 1969 Cat scratch disease: its natural history. J American Med Assoc 207: 312–316

36. Margileth A M 1968 Cat scratch disease. Pediatrics 42: 803–818

37. Chuinard R G, D'Ambrosia R D 1977 Human bite infections of the hand. J Bone Joint Surg 59A: 416–418

38. Farmer C, Mann R 1966 Human bite infections of the hand. Southern Med J 59: 515–518

39. Hooper G 1978 Tooth fragment in a metacarpophalangeal joint. Hand 10: 215–216

40. Malinowski R, Strate R G, Perry J F, Fischer R 1979 The management of human bite injuries of the hand. J Trauma 19: 655–659

41. Peeples E, Boswick J A, Scott F A 1980 Wounds of the hand contaminated by human or animal saliva. J Trauma 20: 383–389

42. Faciszewski T, Coleman D A 1989 Human bite wounds. Hand Clin 5: 561–569

43. Dreyfuss U Y, Singer M 1985 Human bites of the hand: a study of one hundred six patients. J Hand Surg (Am) 10: 884–889

44. Snyder C C 1989 Animal bite wounds. Hand Clin 5: 571–590

45. Rayan G M, Flournoy D J, Cahill S L 1984 Aerobic mouth flora of the rhesus monkey. J Hand Surg (Am) 12: 299–301

46. Zook E G, Miller M, VanBeek A L, Wavek P 1980 Successful treatment protocol for canine fang injuries. J Trauma 20: 243–247

47. Mann R J, Hoffeld T A, Farmer C B 1977 Human bites of the hand: twenty years of experience. J Hand Surg 2: 97–104

48. Goldstein E, Miller T, Citron D, Finegold S 1978 Infections following clenched-fist injury: a new perspective. J Hand Surg 3: 455–457

49. McDonald I 1979 Eikenella corrodens infection of the hand. J Hand Surg 11: 224–227

50. Rayan G M, Putnam J L, Cahill S L, Flournoy D J 1988 Eikenella corrodens in human mouth flora. J Hand Surg (Am) 13: 953–956

51. Schmidt D R, Heckman J D 1983 Eikenella corrodens in human bite infections of the hand. J Trauma 23: 478–482

52. Goldstein E J, Barones M F, Miller T A 1983 Eikenella corrodens in hand infections. J Hand Surg (Am) 8: 563–567

53. Arons M S, Fernando L, Polayes I M 1982 Pasteurella multocida — the major cause of hand infections following domestic animal bites. Journal Hand Surg 7: 47–52

54. Lucas G L, Bartlett D H 1981 Pasteurella multocida infection in the hand. Plastic Reconstr Surg 67: 49–53

55. Lee B 1960 Dog bites and local infection with Pasteurella septica. Br Med J i: 1969–1976

56. Veitch J M, Omer G E 1979 Case report: treatment of catbite injuries of the hand. J Trauma 19: 201–203

57. Goldstein E, Miller T, Citron D, Wield B, Finegold S 1979 Clenched-fist injuries: infection and empiric antibiotic selection. Contemp Orthopaedics 1: 30–33

58. Reyes F A 1989 Infections secondary to intravenous drug abuse. Hand Clin 5: 629–633

59. Whitaker L A 1973 Management of hand infections in the narcotic addict. Plastic Reconstr Surg 52: 384–389

60. Ross G N, Baraff L J, Quismorio F P 1975 Serratia arthritis in heroin users. J Bone Joint Surg 57A: 1158–1160

61. Gifford D B, Patzakis M, Ivler D, Swezey L 1975 Septic arthritis due to Pseudomonas in heroin addicts. J Bone Joint Surg 57A: 631–635

62. Schechter W, Meyer A, Schechter G, Giuliano A, Newmeyer W, Kilgore E 1982 Necrotizing fasciitis of the upper extremity. J Hand Surg 7: 15–20

63. Singer R M, Gorosh J E 1990 Purpura fulminans. J Hand Surg (Am) 15: 172–175

64. Canale S T, Ikard S T 1984 The orthopaedic implications of purpura fulminans. J Bone Joint Surg (Am) 66: 764–769

65. Ferlic D C 1983 Pyoderma gangrenosum presenting as an acute suppurative hand infection — a case report. J Hand Surg (Am) 8: 573–575

66. Adelaar R S 1983 Sarcoidosis of the upper extremity: case presentation and literature review. J Hand Surg (Am) 8: 492–496

67. Terranova W A, Williams G S, Kuhlman T A, Morgan R F 1985 Acute phalangeal fractures due to undiagnosed sarcoidosis. J Hand Surg (Am) 10: 902–903

68. Landi A, Brooks D, De Santis G 1983 Sarcoidosis of the hand — report of two cases. J Hand Surg (Am) 8: 197–200

69. Stambough J L, Bora F W Jr, DuShuttle R P 1986 Sarcoid flexor tenosynovitis of the finger: a case report. J Hand Surg (Am) 11: 436–438

70. Long W T, Filler B C, Cox E 2nd, Stark H H 1988 Toxic shock syndrome after a human bite to the hand. J Hand Surg (Am) 13: 957–959. (Comment in J Hand Surg (Am) 1989 14: 1036–1037.)

71. Grayson M J, Saldana M J 1987 Toxic shock syndrome complicating surgery of the hand. J Hand Surg (Am) 12: 1082–1084

72. Spiegel J D, Szabo R M 1988 A protocol for the treatment of severe infection of the hand. J Hand Surg (Am) 13: 254–259

73. Mancini L H, Fort L K 1989 Rehabilitation of the infected hand. Hand Clin 5: 635–641

74. Carter S, Mersheimer W 1970 Infections of the hand. Orthopaedic Clin North Am 1: 455–466

75. Neviaser R 1978 Closed tendon sheath irrigation for pyogenic flexor tenosynovitis. J Hand Surg 3: 462–466

76. Linscheid R, Dobyns J 1975 Common and uncommon infections of the hand. Orthopaedic Clin North Am 6: 1063–1103

77. Gunther S F, Elliott R C, Brand R L, Adams J P 1977 Experience with atypical mycobacterial infection in the deep structures of the hand. J Hand Surg 2: 90–96

78. Gunther S F, Levy C S 1989 Mycobacterial infections. Hand Clin 5: 591–598

79. Dixon J H 1981 Non-tuberculous mycobacterial infection of the tendon sheaths in the hand. A report of six cases. J Bone Joint Surg (Br) 63B: 542–544

80. Stern P J, Gula D C 1986 Mycobacterium chelonei tenosynovitis of the hand: a case report. J Hand Surg (Am) 11: 596–599

81. Herndon J H, Lanoue A M 1972 *Mycobacterium fortuitum* infections involving the extremities. J Bone Joint Surg 54A: 1279–1282

82. Ariel I, Haas H, Weinberg H, Rousso M, Rosenmann E 1983 *Mycobacterium fortuitum* granulomatous synovitis caused by a dog bite. J Hand Surg (Am) 8: 342–343

83. Crick J C, Vandevelde A G 1986 *Mycobacterium fortuitum* midpalmar space abscess: a case report. J Hand Surg (Am) 11: 438–440

84. Gunther S F, Elliott R C 1976 *Mycobacterium kansasii* infection in the deep structures of the hand. Report of two cases. J Bone Joint Surg 58A: 140–142

85. Zvetina J R, Foster J, Reves C V 1979 *Mycobacterium kansasii* infection of the elbow joint. J Bone Joint Surg 61A:1090–1102

86. Parker M D, Irwin R S 1975 Mycobacterium kansasii tendinitis and fasciitis. J Bone Joint Surg 57A: 557–559

87. Minkin B I, Mills C L, Bullock D W, Burke F D 1987 *Mycobacterium kansasii* osteomyelitis of the scaphoid. J Hand Surg (Am) 12: 1092–1094

88. Sanger J R, Stampfl D A, Franson T R 1987 Recurrent granulomatous synovitis due to *Mycobacterium kansasii* in a renal transplant recipient. J Hand Surg (Am) 12: 436–441

89. Williams C S, Riordan D C 1973 *Mycobacterium marinum* (atypical acid-fast bacillus) infections of the hand. J Bone Joint Surg 55A: 1042–1050

90. Chow S P, Stroebel A B, Lau J H, Collins R J 1983 *Mycobacterium marinum* infection of the hand involving deep structures. J Hand Surg (Am) 8: 568–573

91. Wendt J R, Lamm R C, Altman D I, Cruz H G, Achauer B M 1986 An unusually aggressive *Mycobacterium marinum* hand infection. J Hand Surg (Am) 11: 753–755

92. Jones M W, Wahid I A 1988 *Mycobacterium marinum* infections of the hand and wrist. J Bone Joint Surg (Am) 70: 631–632

93. Chow S P, Ip F K, Lau J H, Collins R J et al 1987 *Mycobacterium marinum* infection of the hand and wrist. Results of conservative treatment in twenty-four cases. J Bone Joint Surg (Am) 69: 1161–1168

94. Jones M W, Wahid I A, Matthews J P 1988 Septic arthritis of the hand due to *Mycobacterium marinum*. J Hand Surg (Br) 13: 333–334

95. Hurst L C, Amadio P C, Badalamente M A, Ellstein J L, Dattwyler R J 1987 *Mycobacterium marinum* infections of the hand. J Hand Surg (Am) 12: 428–435

96. Love G L, Melchior E 1985 *Mycobacterium terrae* tenosynovitis. J Hand Surg (Am) 10: 730–732

97. Deenstra W 1988 Synovial hand infection from *Mycobacterium terrae*. J Hand Surg (Br) 13: 335–336

98. Bush D C, Schneider L H 1984 Tuberculosis of the hand and wrist. J Hand Surg (Am) 9: 391–398

99. Borgsmiller W K, Whiteside L A 1980 Tuberculous tenosynovitis of the hand ('compound palmar ganglion'): literature review and case report. Orthopedics 3: 1093–1096

100. Ekerot L, Eiken O 1981 Tuberculosis of the hand. Scand J Plastic Reconstr Surg 15: 77–79

101. Leung P 1978 Tuberculosis of the hand. Hand 10: 285–291

102. Pinstein M L, Scott R L, Sebes J I 1981 Tuberculous arthritis of the wrist: differential diagnosis and case report. Orthopaedics 4: 1016–1018

103. Perlman R, Jubelirer A, Schwarz J 1972 Histoplasmosis of the common palmar tendon sheath. J Bone Joint Surg 54A: 676–678

104. Winter W G, Larson R K, Honeggar M H, Jacobesen D, Pappagianis D M, Huntington R W 1975 Coccidioidal arthritis and its treatment. J Bone Joint Surg 57A: 1152–1157

105. Iverson R E, Vistnes L M 1973 Coccidioidomycosis tenosynovitis in the hand. J Bone Joint Surg 55A: 413–417

106. Gropper P T, Pisesky W A, Bowen V, Clement P B 1983 Flexor tenosynovitis caused by *Coccidioides immitis*. J Hand Surg (Am) 8: 344–347

107. Liseki E J, Curl W W, Markey K L 1980 Hand and forearm infections caused by *Aeromonas hydrophila*. J Hand Surg 5: 605

108. Hanson P G, Standridge J, Jarrett F, Mali D 1977 Freshwater wound infections due to *Aeromonas hydrophila*. J Am Med Assoc 238: 1053–1054

109. Geller H S, Tofte R W, Cunningham B L 1983 *Aeromonas hydrophila* wound infection of the hand initially presenting as clostridial myonecrosis. J Hand Surg (Am) 8: 333–335

110. Sanger J R, Yousif N J, Matloub H S 1989 *Aeromonas hydrophila* upper extremity infection. J Hand Surg (Am) 14: 719–721

111. Lowen R M, Rodgers C M, Ketch L L, Phelps D B 1989 *Aeromonas hydrophila* infection complicating digital replantation and revascularization. J Hand Surg (Am) 14: 714–718

112. Wylock P, Jaeken R, Deraemaecker R 1983 Anthrax of the hand: case report. J Hand Surg (Am) 8: 576–578

113. Childers J C 1980 Pyogenic arthritis due to *Bacteroides fragilis* infection. Orthopedics 3: 319–320

114. Thorne F L, Kroop R J 1983 Wound botulism: a life-threatening complication of hand injuries. Plastic Reconstr Surg 71: 548–551

115. Neimkin R J, Jupiter J B 1985 Metastatic nontraumatic *Clostridium septicum* osteomyelitis. J Hand Surg (Am) 10: 281–284

116. Korn J A, Gilbert M S, Siffert R S, Jacobson J H 1975 *Clostridium welchii* arthritis. J Bone Joint Surg 57A: 555–557

117. Fee N F, Dobranski A, Bisla R S 1977 Gas gangrene complicating open forearm fractures. Report of five cases. J Bone Joint Surg 59A: 135–138

118. VanBeek A, Zook E, Yaw P, Gardner R, Smith R, Glover J 1974 Nonclostridial gas-forming infections. Arch Surg 108: 552–557

119. Bessman A N, Wagner W 1975 Nonclostridial gas gangrene. J Am Med Assoc 233: 958–963

120. Scott F A, German C, Boswick J A 1981 *Haemophilus influenzae* cellulitis of the hand. J Hand Surg 6: 506–509

121. McCabe S J, Murray J F, Ruhnke H L, Rachlis A 1987 *Mycoplasma* infection of the hand acquired from a cat. J Hand Surg (Am) 12: 1085–1088

122. Smith J, Ruby L K 1977 *Nocardia asteroides* thenar space infection: a case report. J Hand Surg 2: 109–110

123. Petersen D P, Wong L B 1981 *Nocardia* infection of the hand. Case report. J Hand Surg 6: 502–505

124. Nahas L F, Bennett J E 1981 Case reports: nocardiosis of the upper limb. Plastic Reconstr Surg 68: 593–595

125. Donovan T L, Chapman M W, Harrington K D, Nagel D A 1976 *Serratia* arthritis. Report of seven cases.

J Bone Joint Surg 58A: 1009–1011

126. Zielinski C J, Bora F W Jr 1984 *Vibrio* hand infections: a case report and review of the literature. J Hand Surg (Am) 9: 754–757

127. Kaye J J 1990 *Vibrio vulnificus* infections in the hand. Report of three patients. J Bone Joint Surg (Am) 72: 283–285

128. Hung L K, Kinninmonth AW, Woo ML 1988 *Vibrio vulnificus* necrotizing fasciitis presenting with compartment syndrome of the hand. J Hand Surg (Br) 13: 337–339

129. Hitchcock T F, Amadio P C 1989 Fungal infections. Hand Clin 5: 599–611

130. Southwick G, Lister G D 1979 Actinomycosis of the hand: a case report. J Hand Surg 4: 360–362

131. Robinson R A 1945 Actinomycosis of the subcutaneous tissue of the forearm secondary to a human bite. J Am Med Assoc 142: 1049–1051

132. Eastridge C E 1972 Actinomycosis: a 24 year experience. Southern Med J 65: 839–843

133. Fayman M, Schein M, Braun S 1985 A foreign body related actinomycosis of a finger. J Hand Surg (Am) 10: 411–412

134. Bromley G S, Solender M 1986 Hand infection caused by *Actinobacillus actinomycetemcomitans*. J Hand Surg (Am) 11: 434–436

135. Burgess R C 1987 Chronic tenosynovitis caused by *Actinobacillus actinomycetemcomitans*. J Hand Surg (Am) 12: 294–295

136. Goldberg B, Eversmann W W, Eitzen E M 1982 Invasive aspergillosis of the hand. J Hand Surg 7: 38–42

137. Jones N F, Conklin W T, Albo V C 1986 Primary invasive aspergillosis of the hand. J Hand Surg (Am) 11: 425–428

138. Monsanto E H, Johnston A D, Dick H M 1986 Isolated blastomycotic osteomyelitis: a case simulating a malignant tumor of the distal radius. J Hand Surg (Am) 11: 896–898

139. Yuan R T, Cohen M J 1985 *Candida albicans* tenosynovitis of the hand. J Hand Surg (Am) 10: 719–722

140. Monroe P W, Floyd W E 1981 Chromohyphomycosis of the hand due to *Exophiala jeanselmei*, (*Phialophora jeanselmei, Phialophora gougerotii*) Case report and review. J Hand Surg 6: 370–373

141. Lichtman D, Johnson D, Mack G, Lack E 1978 Maduromycosis (*Allescheria boydii*) infection of the hand: a case report. J Bone Joint Surg 60A: 546–548

142. Martinez R E, Couchel S, Swartz W M, Smith M B 1989 Mycetoma of the hand. J Hand Surg (Am) 14: 909–912

143. Hennessy M J, Mosher T F 1981 Mucormycosis infection of an upper extremity. J Hand Surg 6: 249–252

144. DeHaven K E, Wilde A H, O'Duffy J D 1972 Sporotrichosis arthritis and tenosynovitis. Report of a case cured by synovectomy and amphotericin B. J Bone Joint Surg 54A: 874–877

145. Hay E L, Collawn S S, Middleton F G 1986 *Sporothrix schenckii* tenosynovitis: a case report. J Hand Surg (Am) 11: 431–434

146. Janes P C, Mann R J 1987 Extracutaneous sporotrichosis. J Hand Surg (Am) 12: 441–445

147. Holcomb H S III, Behrens F, Winn W C Jr, Hughes

I M, McCue F C III 1981 *Prototheca wickerhamii* — an alga infecting the hand. J Hand Surg 6: 595–599

148. Ahbel D E, Alexander A H, Lichtman D M 1980 Prototothecal olecranon bursitis. J Bone Joint Surg 62A: 835–836

149. Sirikulchayanonta V, Visuthikosol V, Tanphaichitra D, Prajaktham R 1989 Protothecosis following hand injury. A case report. J Hand Surg (Br) 14: 88–90

150. Belsole R, Fenske N 1980 Cutaneous larva migrans in the upper extremity. J Hand Surg 5: 178–180

151. Raturi U, Burkhalter W 1986 Gnathostomiasis externa: a case report. J Hand Surg (Am) 11: 751–753

152. Simmons E H, Peteghem K V, Tramell T R 1980 Onchocerciasis of the flexor compartment of the forearm: a case report. J Hand Surg 5: 502–504

153. Carroll R E, Sinton W, Carcis A 1955 Acute calcium deposits in the hand. J Am Med Assoc 157: 422–426

154. Resnik C S, Miller B W, Gelberman R H, Resnick D 1983 Hand and wrist involvement in calcium pyrophosphate dihydrate crystal deposition disease. J Hand Surg (Am) 8: 856–863

155. Ames E L, Posch J L 1984 Calcinosis of the flexor and extensor tendons in dermatomyositis — case report. J Hand Surg (Am) 9: 876–879

156. Mercer, Newman J H, Watt I 1984 Acute calcific periarthritis in a child. J Hand Surg (Br) 9: 351–352

157. Jones F E 1986 Calcification simulating infection in congenital brachydactyly. J Hand Surg (Am) 11: 35–37

158. Swanson A B, Swanson G D 1983 Osteoarthritis in the hand. J Hand Surg (Am) 8: 669–675

159. Dray G J, Jablon M 1987 Clinical and radiologic features of primary osteoarthritis of the hand. Hand Clin 3: 351–369

160. Bora F W Jr, Miller G 1987 Joint physiology, cartilage metabolism, and the etiology of osteoarthritis. Hand Clin 3: 325–336

161. Pagalidis T, Kuczynski K, Laatnb D W 1981 Ligamentous stability of the base of the thumb. Hand 13: 29–35

162. Cooney W P 3rd, Lucca M J, Chao E Y, Linscheid R L 1981 The kinesiology of the thumb trapeziometacarpal joint. J Bone Joint Surg (Am) 63: 1371–1381

163. Kuczynski K 1975 The thumb and the saddle. Hand 7: 120–122

164. Eaton R G, Littler J W 1973 Ligament reconstruction for the painful thumb carpometacarpal joint. J Bone Joint Surg 55A: 1655–1666

165. Gamble J G, Mochizuki C, Rinsky L A 1989 Trapeziometacarpal abnormalities in Ehlers–Danlos syndrome. J Hand Surg (Am) 14: 89–94

166. Moore J R, Tolo V T, Weiland A J 1985 Painful subluxation of the carpometacarpal joint of the thumb in Ehlers–Danlos syndrome. J Hand Surg (Am) 10: 661–663

167. North E R, Eaton R G 1983 Degenerative joint disease of the trapezium: a comparative radiographic and anatomic study. J Hand Surg 8: 160–166

168. Eaton R G, Glickel S Z 1987 Trapeziometacarpal osteoarthritis. Staging as a rationale for treatment. Hand Clin 3: 455–471

169. Swanson A B 1972 Disabling arthritis at the base of the thumb. J Bone Joint Surg 54A: 456–471

170. Rogers W D, Watson H K 1990 Degenerative arthritis at the triscaphe joint. J Hand Surg (Am) 15: 232–235

171. Palmieri T J, Grand F M, Hay E L, Burke C 1987 Treatment of osteoarthritis in the hand and wrist. Nonoperative treatment. Hand Clin 3: 371–383

172. Docken W P 1987 Clinical features and medical management of osteoarthritis at the hand and wrist. Hand Clin 3: 337–349

173. Eaton R G, Lane L B, Littler J W, Keyser J J 1984 Ligament reconstruction for the painful thumb carpometacarpal joint: a long-term assessment. J Hand Surg (Am) 9: 692–699

174. Biddulph S L 1985 The extensor sling procedure for an unstable carpometacarpal joint. J Hand Surg (Am) 10: 641–645

175. Carroll R E, Hill N A 1973 Arthrodesis of the carpometacarpal joint of the thumb. J Bone Joint Surg 55B: 292–294

176. Stark H H, Moore J F, Ashworth C R, Boyes J H 1977 Fusion of the first metacarpotrapezial joint for degenerative arthritis. J Bone Joint Surg 59A: 22–26

177. Dell P C, Brushart T M, Smith R J 1978 Treatment of trapeziometacarpal arthritis: results of resection arthroplasty. J Hand Surg 3: 243–249

178. Gervis W H 1973 A review of excision of the trapezium for osteoarthritis of the trapezio-metacarpal joint after 25 years. J Bone Joint Surg 55B: 56

179. Menon J, Schoene H, Hohl J 1981 Trapeziometacarpal arthritis — results of tendon interpositional arthroplasty. J Hand Surg 6: 442–446

180. Froimson A I 1987 Tendon interposition arthroplasty of carpometacarpal joint of the thumb. Hand Clin 3: 489–505

181. Wilson J H 1972 Arthroplasty of the trapezio-metacarpal joint. Plastic Reconstr Surg 49: 143–148

182. Eaton R G, Glickel S Z, Littler J W 1985 Tendon interposition arthroplasty for degenerative arthritis of the trapeziometacarpal joint of the thumb. J Hand Surg (Am) 10: 645–654

183. Burton R I, Pellegrini V D Jr 1986 Surgical management of basal joint arthritis of the thumb. Part II. Ligament reconstruction with tendon interposition arthroplasty. J Hand Surg (Am) 11: 324–332

184. Ferlic D C, Busbee G A, Clayton M L 1977 Degenerative arthritis of the carpometacarpal joint of the thumb: a clinical follow-up of eleven Neibauer prostheses. J Hand Surg 2: 212–215

185. Lister G D, Kleinert H E, Kutz J E, Atasoy E 1977 Arthritis of the trapezial articulations treated by prosthetic replacement. Hand 9: 117–129

186. Poppen N, Niebauer J 1978 'Tie-in' trapezium prosthesis: long-term results. J Hand Surg 3: 445–450

187. Swanson A B, Swanson G, Watermeier J I 1981 Trapezium implant arthroplasty — long-term evaluation of 150 cases. J Hand Surg 6: 125–141

188. Kessler F B, Epstein M J, Culver J E Jr, Prewitt J, Homsy C A 1984 Proplast stabilized stemless trapezium implant. J Hand Surg 9: 227–231

189. Adams B D, Unsell R S, McLaughlin P 1990 Niebauer trapeziometacarpal arthroplasty. J Hand Surg (Am) 15: 487–492

190. Ho P K, Jacobs J L, Clark G L 1985 Trapezium implant arthroplasty: evaluation of a semiconstrained implant. J Hand Surg (Am) 10: 654–660

191. Boeckstyns M E, Sinding A, Elholm K T, Rechnagel K 1989 Replacement of the trapeziometacarpal joint with a cemented (Caffiniere) prosthesis. J Hand Surg (Am) 14: 83–89

192. Ferrari B, Steffee A D 1986 Trapeziometacarpal total joint replacement using the Steffee prosthesis. J Bone Joint Surg (Am) 68: 1177–1184

193. Hofammann D Y, Ferlic D C, Clayton M L 1987 Arthroplasty of the basal joint of the thumb using a silicone prosthesis. Long-term follow-up. J Bone Joint Surg (Am) 69: 993–997

194. Burton R I 1987 Basal joint implant arthroplasty in osteoarthritis. Indications, techniques, pitfalls, and problems. Hand Clin 3: 473–487

195. Pellegrini V D Jr, Burton R I 1986 Surgical management of basal joint arthritis of the thumb. Part I. Long-term results of silicone implant arthroplasty. J Hand Surg (Am) 11: 309–324

196. Burton R I 1986 Complications following surgery on the basal joint of the thumb. Hand Clin 2: 265–269

197. Carter P R, Benton L J, Dysert P A 1986 Silicone rubber carpal implants: a study of the incidence of late osseous complications. J Hand Surg (Am) 11: 639–644

198. Peimer C A, Medige J, Eckert B S, Wright J R, Howard C S 1986 Reactive synovitis after silicone arthroplasty. J Hand Surg (Am) 11: 624–638

199. Smith R J, Atkinson R E, Jupiter J B 1985 Silicone synovitis of the wrist. J Hand Surg (Am) 10: 47–60

200. Atkinson R E, Smith R J 1986 Silicone synovitis following silicone implant arthroplasty. Hand Clin 2: 291–299

201. Kleinert J M, Lister G D 1986 Silicone implants. Hand Clin 2: 271–290

202. Swanson A B, Swanson G G, Maupin B K, Hynes D E, Jindal P 1989 Failed carpal bone arthroplasty: causes and treatment. J Hand Surg 14: 417–424

203. Paplanus S H, Payne C M 1988 Axillary lymphadenopathy 17 years after digital silicone implants: study with X-ray microanalysis. J Hand Surg (Am) 13: 399–400

204. Crosby E B, Linscheid R L, Dobyns J H 1978 Scaphotrapezial trapezoidal arthrosis. J Hand Surg 3: 223–234

205. Eiken O 1979 Implant arthroplasty of the scapho-trapezial joint. Scand J Plastic Reconstr Surg 13: 461–468

206. Carroll R E, Coyle M P Jr 1985 Dysfunction of the pisotriquetral joint: treatment by excision of the pisiform. J Hand Surg (Am) 10: 703–707

207. Paley D, McMurtry R Y, Cruickshank B 1987 Pathologic conditions of the pisiform and pisotriquetral joint. J Hand Surg (Am) 12: 110–119

208. Eiken O, Jonsson K 1980 Carpal bone cysts. A clinical and radiographic study. Scand J Plastic Reconstr Surg 14: 285–290

209. Heberden W 1802 Commentaries on history and cure of disease. T Payne, London

210. Bouchard C 1891 Semaine Med (Paris) 11: 387

211. Kleinert H E, Kutz J E, Fishman I H, McCraw L H 1972 Etiology and treatment of the so-called mucous cyst of the finger. J Bone Joint Surg 54A: 1455–1458

212. Culver J E, Fleegler E J 1987 Osteoarthritis of the distal interphalangeal joint. Hand Clin 3: 385–403

213. Brown LG 1989 Distal interphalangeal joint flexible implant arthroplasty. J Hand Surg (Am) 14: 653–656

214. Zimmerman N B, Suhey P V, Clark G L, Wilgis E F

1989 Silicone interpositional arthroplasty of the distal interphalangeal joint. J Hand Surg (Am) 14: 882–887

215. Eaton R G, Dobranski A I, Littler J W 1973 Marginal osteophyte excision in treatment of mucous cysts. J Bone Joint Surg 55A: 570–574

216. Hagan H J, Hastings H 2nd 1988 Fusion of the thumb metacarpophalangeal joint to treat posttraumatic arthritis. J Hand Surg (Am) 13: 750–753

217. Peimer C A, Putnam M D 1987 Proximal interphalangeal joint following traumatic arthritis. Hand Clin 3: 415–427

218. Stern P J, Ho S 1987 Osteoarthritis of the proximal interphalangeal joint. Hand Clin 3: 405–413

219. Pellegrini V D, Jr, Burton R I 1990 Osteoarthritis of the proximal interphalangeal joint of the joint: arthroplasty or fusion? J Hand Surg (Am) 15: 194– 209

220. Trumble T E, Watson H K 1985 Posttraumatic sesamoid arthritis of the metacarpophalangeal joint of the thumb. J Hand Surg (Am) 10: 94–100

221. Parks B J, Hamlin C 1986 Chronic sesamoiditis of the thumb: pathomechanics and treatment. J Hand Surg (Am) 11: 237–240

222. Moore J R, Weiland A J 1985 Gouty tenosynovitis in the hand. J Hand Surg (Am) 10: 291–295

223. Straub L R, Smith I W, Carpenter G K, Dietz G H 1961 The surgery of gout in the upper extremity. J Bone Joint Surg 43A: 731

224. Rosenthal E A 1987 Tenosynovitis: tendon and nerve entrapment. Hand Clin 3: 585–609.

225. Armstrong T J, Fine L J, Goldstein S A, Lifshitz Y R, Silverstein BA 1987 Ergonomic considerations in hand and wrist tendinitis. J Hand Surg (Am) 12: 830–837

226. Williams J G P 1977 Surgical management of traumatic non-effective tenosynovitis of the wrist extensors. J Bone Joint Surg 59B: 408–410

227. Lemon R A, Engber W D 1985 Trigger wrist: a case report. J Hand Surg (Am) 10: 61–63

228. Hajj A A, Wood M B 1986 Stenosing tenosynovitis of the extensor carpi ulnaris. J Hand Surg (Am) 11: 519–520

229. Grundberg A B, Reagan D S 1985 Pathologic anatomy of the forearm: intersection syndrome. J Hand Surg (Am) 10: 299–302

230. Mogensen B A, Mattsson H S 1980 Stenosing tendovaginitis of the third compartment of the hand. Scand J Plastic Reconstr Surg 14: 127–128

231. Hooper G, McMaster M J 1979 Stenosing tenovaginitis affecting the tendon of extensor digiti minimi at the wrist. Hand 11: 299–301

232. Lombardi R M, Wood M B, Linscheid R L 1988 Symptomatic restrictive thumb-index flexor tenosynovitis: incidence of musculotendinous anomalies and results of treatment. J Hand Surg (Am) 13: 325–328

233. De Quervain F 1895 Ueber eine form von chronischer tendovaginitis. Correspondenz-Blatt F Schweizer Aerzte 25: 389–394

234. Viegas S F 1986 Trigger thumb of de Quervain's disease. J Hand Surg (Am) 11: 235–237

235. Witczak J W, Masear V R, Meyer R D 1990 Triggering of the thumb with de Quervain's stenosing tendovaginitis. J Hand Surg (Am) 15: 265–268

236. Finkelstein H 1930 Stenosing tendovaginitis at the radial styloid process. J Bone Joint Surg 12: 509–540

237. Wood M B, Linscheid R L 1973 Abductor pollicis longus bursitis. Clin Orthopedics Rel Res 93: 293–296

238. Harvey F J, Harvey P M, Horsley M W 1990 De Quervain's disease: surgical or nonsurgical treatment. J Hand Surg (Am) 15: 83–87

239. McGrath M H 1984 Local steroid therapy in the hand. J Hand Surg (Am) 9: 915–921

240. Louis D S 1987 Incomplete release of the first dorsal compartment — a diagnostic test. J Hand Surg (Am) 12: 87–88

241. Arons M S 1987 de Quervain's release in working women: a report of failures, complications, and associated diagnoses. J Hand Surg (Am) 12: 540–544

242. White G M, Weiland A J 1984 Symptomatic palmar tendon subluxation after surgical release for de Quervain's disease: a case report. J Hand Surg (Am) 9: 704–706

243. Dinham I M, Meggitt B F 1974 Trigger thumbs in children. J Bone Joint Surg 56B: 153–155

244. Carlson C S Jr, Curtis R M 1984 Steroid injection for flexor tenosynovitis. J Hand Surg (Am) 9: 286–287

245. Marks M R, Gunther S F 1989 Efficacy of cortisone injection in treatment of trigger fingers and thumbs. J Hand Surg (Am) 14: 722–727

246. Freiberg A, Mulholland R S, Levine R 1989 Nonoperative treatment of trigger fingers and thumbs. J Hand Surg (Am) 14: 553–558

247. Weeks P 1978 A cause of wrist pain: non-specific tenosynovitis involving the flexor carpi radialis. Plastic Reconstr Surg 62: 263–266

248. Fisson J M, Shea F W, Goldin W 1968 Lesions of the flexor carpi radialis tendon and sheath causing pain at the wrist. J Bone Joint Surg 50B: 359

249. Bowe A, Doyle L, Millender L H 1984 Bilateral partial ruptures of the flexor carpi radialis tendon secondary to trapezial arthritis. J Hand Surg (Am) 9: 738–739

250. Begg R E 1980 Epicondylitis or tennis elbow. Orthopaedic Rev 9: 33–42

251. Coonrad R W, Hooper W R 1973 Tennis elbow: its source, natural history, conservative and surgical management. J Bone Joint Surg 55A: 1177–1182

252. Garden R S 1961 Tennis elbow. J Bone Joint Surg 43B: 100–106

253. Nirschl R P, Pettrone F A 1979 Tennis elbow. J Bone Joint Surg 61A: 823–839

254. Bosworth D M 1965 Surgical treatment of tennis elbow. J Bone Joint Surg 47A: 1533–1536

255. Newman J H, Goodfellow J W 1975 Fibrillation of head of radius as one cause of tennis elbow. Br Med J 1: 328–330

256. Gunn C, Milbrandt W E 1976 Tennis elbow and the cervical spine. Can Med Assoc J 114: 803–809

5. Rheumatoid

Although the fundamental cause is not known, rheumatoid disease is ultimately an auto-immune process. Over 70% of patients with rheumatoid disease demonstrate rheumatoid factor, a macroglobulin, in their serum[1]. This seropositivity leads to arteritis, which, in the digital vessels, may be obliterative, producing Raynaud's phenomenon, with ulceration or even necrosis, and resulting more proximally in the hand in ischaemic neuropathy and muscle wasting[2]. Despite this fact, seropositivity is associated with a more predictable outcome of the surgical procedures performed on rheumatoid patients. Absence of rheumatoid factor from the

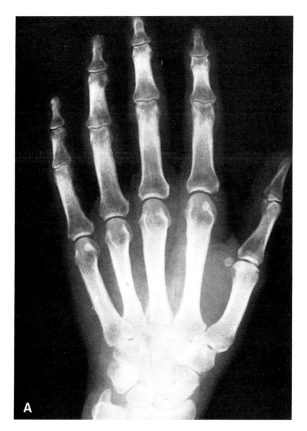
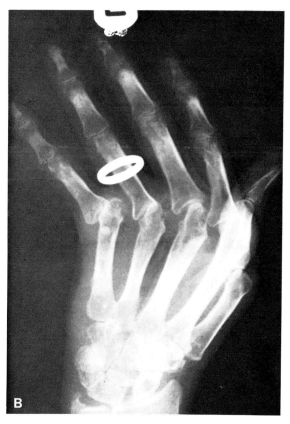

Fig. 5.1 A, B. The progression of rheumatoid disease is illustrated by these two radiographs of a young woman in her twenties taken at an interval of four years. At the time of her first radiograph, she had been diagnosed as having seropositive rheumatoid disease but little evidence of deformity was present. Four years later, rheumatoid disease is all too evident in the radial shift at the wrist and the ulnar deviation of the fingers with metacarpophalangeal joint destruction.

serum (seronegativity) and hence a more guarded surgical prognosis, is associated with a number of conditions which may show joint changes similar to those of pure rheumatoid disease. These are known as rheumatoid variants (p. 395).

In the hands, rheumatoid disease affects primarily the synovium which is found in all the joints and around portions of the flexor and extensor tendons. Tendons are covered with synovium wherever they pass beneath pulleys. They pass beneath pulleys wherever they run across the concavity of a joint or series of joints. Thus, synovium is present around both flexor and extensor tendons at the wrist beneath their respective retinacula, and also around the flexor tendons in the fibrous sheaths along the fingers. These digital sheaths commence over the metacarpophalangeal joints, that is, beneath the proximal palmar crease on the radial side of the palm of the hand and beneath the distal palmar crease on the ulnar side. The small finger is an exception, for the synovial sheath extends proximally to join the wrist synovial bursa, as does that of the thumb. Distally, the digital sheaths end at the tendon insertion.

There are three stages in rheumatoid disease:

1. *Proliferative*, characterized by synovial swelling which produces pain on motion, limitation of movements and nerve compression.
2. *Destructive*, in which synovial erosion causes irreversible changes — tendon rupture, capsular weakness and disruption, bone erosion and joint subluxation and deformity.
3. *Reparative*. Synovial activity has now 'burnt out', and fibrosis replaces chronic inflammation, causing tendon adhesions, fibrous ankylosis and finally fixed deformity.

These three stages produce differing and characteristic problems for the patient. Examination is directed at identifying these and determining the appropriate management.

HISTORY

Time of onset and pattern of disease
The duration of the disease process should be ascertained. The patient should be questioned regarding exacerbations and remissions of his symptoms, from which the pattern of his disease will be appreciated. Three general patterns are recognised:

Monocyclic — only one attack followed by permanent remission; 10% of rheumatoid patients
Polycyclic — attacks of varying duration and of differing severity occurring at unpredictable intervals; 45%

Progressive — an unremitting, inexorable course; 45% (Fig. 5.1).

Major problems
The patient should be asked to identify those aspects of his disease which give him most trouble. These may well not be those most apparent on inspection of the upper limb. Nonetheless *these* problems should receive particular attention in the treatment plan, even at the expense of temporarily disregarding more obvious and challenging deformities. Although terribly disabled, the patient is often functionally very competent (Fig. 5.2).

Other problem areas
A brief summary should be made of the regions other than the hand and arm which are troublesome. The name of the physician or surgeon treating those problems should be noted so that early cooperative management can be established. If the patient is receiving no medical help with other disabilities then referral should be offered. Surgery previously performed should be recorded. Future plans for other regions should be discussed and, at a later stage, priorities determined.

Functional grading
The patient should be asked to explain his or her difficulties in both occupation and domestic life. This can often best be achieved by asking a series of questions regarding everyday acts which cover all functions of the hand. Alternatively these acts can be used as tests performed by the patient at the examination or during a preliminary assessment by a physical or occupational therapist.

A simple grading of ability to fulfil everyday needs of locomotion and manipulation can now be made according to the following scale:

1. No incapacity
2. Manages all but the heaviest tasks
3. Manages none but the lightest duties
4. Chair- or bed-bound.

Pain
The pain of rheumatoid disease is characteristically most severe during the proliferative and early destructive stages of the disease. A recent increase in pain should make the surgeon suspect that a 'flare-up' in the disease is commencing. Except during such exacerbations, the pain is usually not present at rest but is provoked by movement. The patient should be asked to demonstrate the movements which cause pain to aid in localization of the most active synovitis.

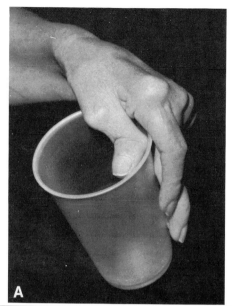

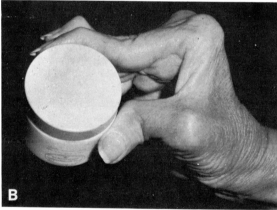

Fig. 5.2 Despite severe disability, rheumatoid patients contrive to perform everyday functions (A). Not only is compensation due to trick movements but also to the development of additional deformities as seen in (B). Palmar subluxation of the metacarpophalangeal joints and a boutonniere deformity in the thumb has been compensated to some extent by the development of a swan-neck deformity in the fingers and of radial instability at the interphalangeal joint of the thumb, giving an otherwise unobtainable grasp on a small jar.

Stiffness

It is necessary to distinguish between stiffness and limitation of active joint movements. The latter is a relatively constant feature throughout the day and can be measured. The former is difficulty in movement which cannot be measured and which varies during the course of the day. Attempts have been made to place a value on stiffness by asking the patient how long it takes him to loosen up after getting out of bed in the morning — the time at which stiffness is characteristically present. This has been named the 'limber-up time' (LUT).

Numbness and paraesthesia

Compression, especially of the median nerve, is more common in rheumatoid patients than in the general population due to the increase in the volume of synovium in, or adjacent to, the rigid confines of the nerve tunnels. The symptoms and signs are the same as those described in the chapter on compression. Very often the rheumatoid patient will not volunteer the symptoms of compression, their presence only being revealed by direct questioning.

Generalized neuropathy, common in the lower limbs of rheumatoid patients, is unusual in the upper.

Weakness

Weakness is often generalized and is believed to be part of the systemic disturbance of rheumatoid disease. Localized weakness may be due to pain, to the loss of mechanical advantage resulting from joint collapse, to the blocking of tendon gliding due to synovitis, or to the disuse resulting from any or all of these afflictions. Weakness of grasp may be due to nerve compression. Rarely, polymyositis masquerading as muscular dystrophy may complicate longstanding rheumatoid disease[3].

Appearance

On occasion the patient's main complaint is of the ugliness of the deformity. To some the deformed hands are an understandable social embarrassment, to others a disability which prevents them following their occupation.

MEDICATION AND ITS EFFECT

It is necessary to know what treatment the patient has previously received and what he is currently taking. The duration of adequate treatment is of significance to the surgeon in timing any planned intervention. For example, synovectomy during the proliferative stage should probably be withheld until a three to six months trial of medication has been shown to be ineffective in giving relief. This general rule applies unless damage threatens function which it would be difficult to restore, as in gross peritendinous synovitis or marked dorsal subluxation of the ulnar head which may at any stage cause tendon rupture.

Steroid intake should be recorded, especially its duration, since therapy for more than 3 years has been shown to delay wound healing[4].

NON-ARTICULAR EFFECTS OF RHEUMATOID DISEASE[5]

Iritis or *uveitis* occurs in 3–5% of the patients.

Scleromalacia perforans is rupture of the globe due to necrosis in a rheumatoid nodule.

Anaemia and apparent lack of nutrition are frequently present; 25% show a normocytic normochromic anaemia typical of chronic infection.

Polyneuropathy. As stated above, this is confined mainly to the lower limbs.

Lung changes may[6] be any one of the following:

'Rheumatoid lung' has a characteristic honeycombed appearance on radiographs due to multiple rheumatoid nodules.

Caplan's syndrome[7] is found in patients with concomitant pneumoconiosis and produces massive pulmonary fibrosis.

Idiopathic pulmonary fibrosis.

Cardiac manifestations include pericarditis, myocarditis and valvular disease.

Arteritis is uncommon but may rarely be of a fulminating variety.

RHEUMATOID SYNDROMES

Felty's syndrome[8]
Classical rheumatoid polyarthritis
Lymphadenopathy
Splenomegaly   → granulocytopenia
               → anaemia

Rheumatoid seropositive, these patient's haematological problems can be relieved by steroids and cured by splenectomy, which has no effect, however, on the arthritis.

Sjogren's syndrome[9]
Classical rheumatoid polyarthritis
Keratoconjunctivitis sicca   } any 2 out of 3
Xerostomia

Seropositive for rheumatoid factor, these patients also show several other tissue antibodies. Confirmation of the diagnosis is made by estimating the tear production using the *Schirmer test* or by labial salivary gland biopsy.

SOCIAL HISTORY

At the juncture at which the examiner feels he is beginning to establish rapport with the patient, a picture should be obtained of the patient's social background. Rheumatoid arthritis is economically as well as physi-

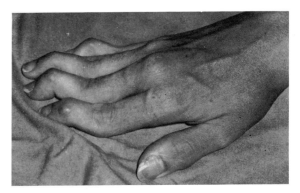

Fig. 5.3 Swan-neck deformity of the fingers with hyperextension of the proximal interphalangeal joints and flexion of the distal interphalangeal joints of all fingers.

cally crippling and the number of dependants whom the victim supports may have a great influence upon the time he can devote to surgery. The attitude of employers varies greatly and this must be known to the surgeon for he may be able to influence that attitude to the patient's benefit simply by an explanatory letter or telephone call. In later stages of disease, the availability, health and attitude of relatives is of great importance in helping the patient to conduct a normal daily life.

Allied to the functional assessment already made, knowledge of the home circumstances will clarify the way in which the patient can best be helped by social and welfare services, often by the provision of simple mechanical aids or the management of more elaborate structural alterations to assist the patient in dressing, toilet, cooking and moving about his home.

EXAMINATION

While due attention is paid to sensory loss and motor weakness, skin cover and joint ranges, examination of the rheumatoid hand is conducted more by region than by system. Further, the rheumatoid hand is characterized by certain deformities which would be complex to record by range of motion and degrees of deviation and then difficult to comprehend even for the well-trained reader. These characteristic deformities have consequently been standardized by the use of generally accepted terms, such as 'ulnar drift' (Fig. 5.1B), 'swan neck' (Fig. 5.3) and 'boutonniere' (Fig. 5.4).

The author personally organizes this complexity, and often multiplicity, by summarizing all information on one sheet of paper. Down the left hand side are written all the areas of potential involvement — neck, shoulders, elbows, radial head, ulnar head, wrist, extensors, thumb, MP joints, PIP joints, DIP joints, flexors, and

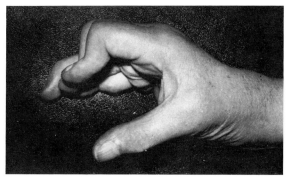

Fig. 5.4 Boutonniere deformity with flexion deformity of the proximal interphalangeal joints and compensatory hyperextension of the distal interphalangeal joints.

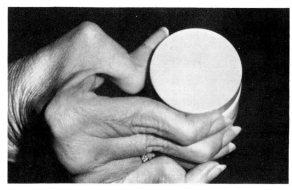

Fig. 5.5 Boutonniere deformity of the thumb with palmar subluxation of the metacarpophalangeal joint and hyperextension of the interphalangeal joint. This is the same patient as seen in Fig. 5.1.

nerve compression — in the order in which they are examined. The remainder of the sheet is divided into two columns, the left-hand one headed RIGHT, the right-hand one LEFT, because the surgeon is facing the patient. On this sheet all the problems can be marked in shorthand, giving an overall view from which a quick recollection of the patient can be gained and on which a rational surgical agenda can be planned[10].

One feature of rheumatoid disease is its *symmetrical distribution*. As a result, the examiner frequently finds the same joints involved in both hands and the same apparently spared. Progression often differs, the dominant hand usually being more advanced in disease than the other.

General inspection

An early indication of the patient's main problems may be obtained by inspection of the upper extremity.

DEFORMITY

Several deformities may be evident:

Posterior subluxation of the elbow
Palmar subluxation of the wrist
Ulnar translocation of the carpus
Radial deviation of the wrist
Ulnar drift of the fingers
Palmar subluxation of the metacarpophalangeal joints
'Swan neck' }
'Boutonniere' } deformities of the fingers
Z-deformity of the thumb, either into 'swan neck' or 'boutonniere' (Fig. 5.5)
Lateral dislocation of any of the interphalangeal joints
Misalignment of digits suggestive of tendon rupture.

The Z mechanism

This phenomenon underlies the development of many of the characteristic deformities of the rheumatoid hand. It can be defined: when a joint, for whatever reason, persistently adopts an angulation in one direction, the joints on either side of it will tend to go in the opposite direction, provided other local conditions in those joints permit it. The mechanism is due to the changes in relative mechanical advantage of the tendons acting on

Table 5.1

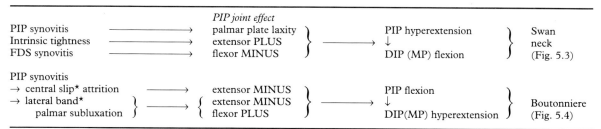

*Read 'extensor pollicis brevis' for 'central slip' and 'extensor hood' for 'lateral band' and the mechanism of boutonniere in the *thumb* is explained (Fig. 5.5.).

a series of joints. It is seen in the hand in several instances (Table 5.1). The pathogenesis of the swan-neck and boutonniere deformities of the thumb can best be understood if the metacarpophalangeal joint of the thumb is considered rather as being the proximal interphalangeal joint (which indeed it is in some respects, for example, the location of the epiphyses).

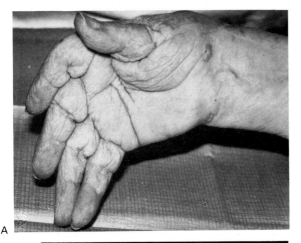

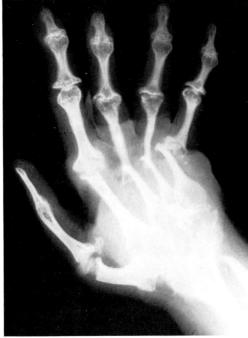

Fig. 5.6 A. Gross destruction of the metacarphophalangeal and interphalangeal joints, particularly on the right hand, in this patient has resulted in the collapse of the skeleton with consequent excess of skin. Traction on the digits produces marked telescoping, hence the term 'opera-glass hands'. B. Arthritis mutilans (see text).

Gross instability; arthritis mutilans[11]; 'opera-glass hands'[12] (Fig. 5.6)

This degree of instability results when the bone ends are excessively eroded. In later stages the diaphyses become tapered. This results in totally flail joints with marked digital shortening. Grasp of almost any object becomes impossible. The excess of skin falls into folds which telescope out as the digit is restored to its original length by traction — hence the term 'opera-glass hands' or *'la main en lorgnette'*. Occasionally ankylosis of a joint arrests the shortening, so that one digit may be disproportionately long. This effect is the aim of surgery, which should be performed relatively early and consists of arthrodesis of all effected interphalangeal joints, adding bone grafts for length wherever appropriate. Only the carpometacarpal joint of the thumb and the metacarpophalangeal joints of the fingers can be kept mobile in the most advanced cases.

Swellings

Rheumatoid nodules. These subcutaneous swellings may be found at any site over the hands and arms, but are by far most commonly located over the subcutaneous ulnar border (Fig. 5.7) just distal to the elbow. They may be present in conjunction with a swollen olecranon bursa from which they should be distinguished. Rheumatoid nodules are firm and rubbery, not fluctuant as is a swollen olecranon bursa. The presence of rheumatoid nodules has been shown to be a poor prognostic factor in rheumatoid disease. Nodules are uncomfortable and may ulcerate. They should be excised and this is usually undertaken in conjunction with other procedures on the hand.

Benign pseudorheumatoid nodules, identical histologically, but without other stigmata of rheumatoid disease, have been reported[13,14].

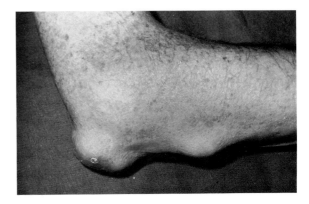

Fig. 5.7 Rheumatoid nodules are most commonly found over the subcutaneous border of the ulna.

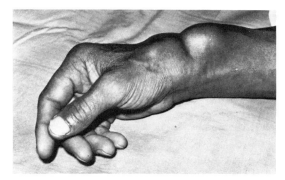

Fig. 5.8 Synovial swelling associated with extensor compartment disease is often prominent and extends over the wrist proximally and the dorsum of the hand distally.

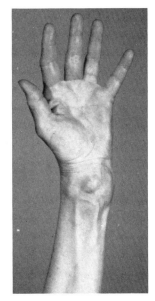

Fig. 5.10 An accumulation of flexor tenosynovitis can be seen in the wrist proximal to the carpal tunnel.

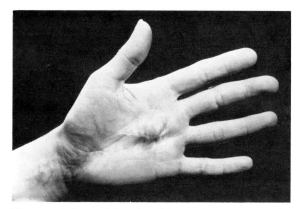

Fig. 5.9 Fullness of the palm of the hand along the line of the middle finger is most evident just proximal to the fibrous tendon sheath. This is indicative of flexor tendon synovitis.

Rheumatoid nodulosis[15] differs from benign pseudo-rheumatoid nodules in that it appears in seropositive adults. The nodules are histologically rheumatoid in character. While the patient may experience mild arthralgia and there may be multiple small radiolucent bone cysts on radiologic examination, typical rheumatoid destruction and deformity rarely occurs.

Prominent ulna head — see p. 369.

Synovial swelling. Markedly swollen joints can be detected on inspection, as can any associated inflammation. Redness is seen only in the presence of very severe, active synovitis. On the dorsum of the wrist the extent of the synovial swelling indicates whether the extensor tendon synovial sheaths are involved or the wrist joint alone. In the former case, the swelling extends well on to the dorsum of the hand distally and on to the forearm proximally (Fig. 5.8). It is also a much more clearly delineated swelling than that in the wrist joint proper where swelling is difficult to see and may be detected only on palpating and moving the joint. Undue fullness

on the palmar aspect over the proximal phalanx, in the palm (Fig. 5.9), and above the wrist (Fig. 5.10) suggests flexor synovitis.

SKIN

The skin of the rheumatoid patient is typically thin and papery, especially susceptible to trauma. This is particularly so in the patient who has been treated for some time with steroids. As a result, the skin frequently shows *bruising*, *petechiae* and *finger-tip haemorrhages* and *infarcts*, especially at the nail folds. Other causes should be sought; for example, petechiae may be evidence of the thrombocytopenia of Felty's splenomegaly.

Psoriasis. The characteristic skin lesion should be sought and is most commonly found around the elbow. Deformity of the nails may also help in establishing the diagnosis (Fig. 5.11). If the patient proves to be seronegative then one is dealing with psoriatic rather than rheumatoid arthritis and surgery should be approached more guardedly as the outcome is often less satisfactory (p. 356).

Palmar erythema. Not associated with hepatic dysfunction, this is seen in many rheumatoid patients, mainly over the thenar and hypothenar eminences.

Intertrigo. This is often encountered in the grossly deformed hand and is due to the accumulation of moisture, most often between the fingers and in the palm in the presence of severe metacarpophalangeal joint disease. Every effort, including splinting, regular cleansing

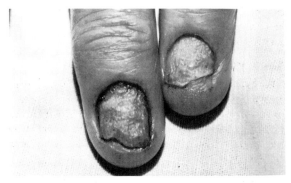

Fig. 5.11 The characteristic nail deformity of psoriasis.

and drying, and the application of appropriate local medication, should be made to heal the skin before surgery.

MUSCLE WASTING

A common general feature in rheumatoid disease, excessive wasting of the thenar eminence should suggest possible median nerve compression. The first dorsal interosseous commonly shows marked atrophy evidenced by the deep concavity on the dorsal aspect of the first web space (Fig. 5.12), masked only by the equally common adduction deformity of the thumb. This wasting results in unusual prominence of the second metacarpal head and allows ulnar drift (p. 382).

SYSTEMATIC REGIONAL ASSESSMENT

The surgeon should now proceed to assess the upper extremity joint by joint, tendon by tendon, nerve by

nerve. In assessing joints, certain facts are determined in almost all of them. These are:

Pain
Synovial swelling
Tenderness
Range of motion — active
                 — passive
                 — associated pain
Stability
Crepitus
Deformity — fixed
          — mobile

Although the patient was asked generally about pain while his history was being taken, this question should be asked specifically at the start of examination of each joint and during passive range of motion. If pain is experienced equally throughout the range and worsened by applying some longitudinal compression during motion, the cause is probably articular erosion. If the pain is mainly at the extremes of the range then compression and tension on inflamed synovium is much more probable (Fig. 5.13). The passive movement in all joints must be produced slowly and gently. Pain is much more severe if produced by rapid movement, and the recorded range therefore less.

Neck

Rheumatoid involvement of the joints in the cervical spine is common. Three deformities occur as a result:

atlanto-axial subluxation
superior migration of the odontoid process into the foramen magnum
subaxial subluxation of the vertebral bodies.

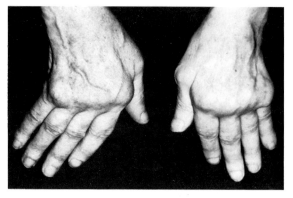

Fig. 5.12 The wasting of the first dorsal interosseous especially evident in the right hand was due to rheumatoid atrophy, ulnar nerve function being intact.

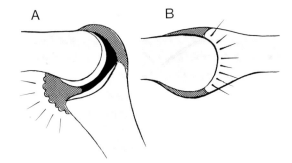

Fig. 5.13 This diagram shows how (A) in the presence of inflamed synovium, compression of and tension on the synovium on opposite aspects of the joint produce pain, where as (B) where the cartilaginous surface has been completely worn down, the pain is due to rubbing of one bone end on another.

These may result in *pain* of varying degree characteristically radiating into the occiput, *instability* of the cervical spine and *neurological disturbance* which at worst can result in fatal cord transection. This may well occur during general anaesthesia and full assessment of the neck before anaesthesia of any rheumatoid patient is therefore mandatory.

Examination should include:

Passive range of movement. In most patients with cervical spine disease this will be limited, and in about three-quarters of them will produce pain characteristically in the distribution of the greater occipital nerve[16]. Audible and palpable crepitation may be present. Stressing the neck at extremes may produce pain but must be hazardous and *should not be attempted.*

Trigeminal nerve testing. Due to involvement of the descending tract of the fifth cranial nerve, about 20% of the patients with narrowing of the canal will show suppressed sensation in the area of the ophthalmic division of the trigeminal nerve, readily assessed on the forehead.

Lower limb reflexes. Patients may show reduced reflexes due to peripheral neuropathy but in narrowing of the spinal canal *hyperreflexia* occurs in about one-third of the patients due to involvement of the pyramidal tracts.

If any of these tests suggests the presence of atlantoaxial subluxation full neurological assessment should be undertaken and the patient fitted immediately with a hard cervical collar pending more detailed evaluation.

At the Hospital for Special Surgery in New York[17] they classify neural deficit as follows:

    I   — nil
    II — subjective weakness, hyperreflexia, dysaesthesia
    IIIa — objective long tract signs
    IIIb — quadriparesis

All patients with rheumatoid disease should have anteroposterior and lateral radiographs in extension and flexion performed (Fig. 5.14).

The following relationships should be studied:

(i) The gap between the dens and the arch — this should not exceed 3 mm in any position[18] — it is most likely to be detected on the flexed lateral view

(ii) McGregor's line — from the upper surface of the hard palate to a point most caudal on the curve of the occiput — the distance by which the dens is above that line should not exceed 4.5 mm[19]

(iii) The C2–C3 relationship.

Changes progress with time[20]. Only 1% of patients come to posterior fusion, which is indicated for in-

tractable pain, significant instability and grade II or certainly IIIa neural deficit.

Shoulder

The shoulder is the hub around which the hand moves, and disease will indirectly but seriously limit hand function. The range of motion in the shoulder can quickly be tested by inviting the patient to touch the interscapular region in three ways with the hand being examined:

over the ipsilateral shoulder — abduction, external rotation
over the contralateral shoulder — flexion, adduction
beneath the ipsilateral axilla — extension, internal rotation (see Fig. 2.15).

Difficulty in performing any of these movements should be followed by more detailed clinical and radiological assessment, which falls within the province of the orthopaedic rather than the hand surgeon.

Elbow[21]

Subcutaneous rheumatoid nodules[14] are most commonly found about the elbow joint, usually situated over the subcutaneous border of the ulna about 5 cm from the olecranon. They may, however, be in the wall of an olecranon bursa and if this is the seat of effusion a double swelling of differing pathology may present.

Synovium
In extension of the normal elbow, there is a depression just above the radial head. This depression overlies the joint space between the radial head and the capitulum of the humerus and is largely obliterated by swelling in the presence of active synovitis of the joint. With the elbow flexed to 90 degrees, it is also possible to feel synovial swelling to the medial side of the olecranon. Fluid, if present, can be felt to fluctuate from the lateral to the medial aspect.

Range of motion: pain
The elbow should now be moved through a full range of active and passive movements, recording the results obtained. The normal range is 0°–145° extension to flexion.

Active synovitis is suggested by pain towards the extremes of the range, increasing as they are reached and indeed often being itself the limiting factor. These patients tend to have less range of active than passive movement. Synovectomy has been shown to be effective in relieving pain but unpredictable in improving the

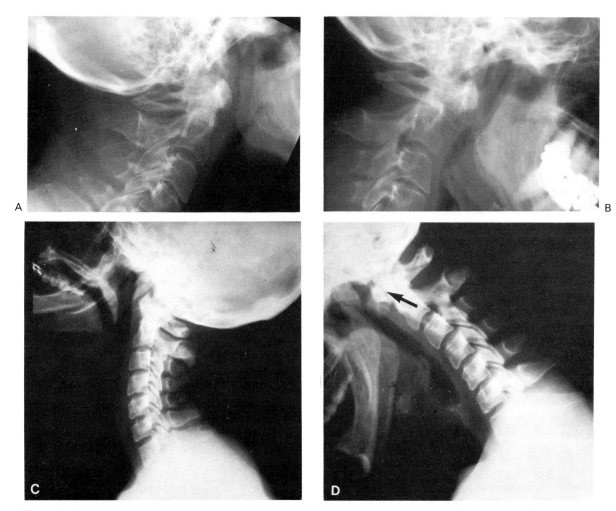

Fig. 5.14   The contrast in the distance between the dens and the arch of the atlas in extension (A) and flexion (B) is very marked in this patient, being some 11 mm when measured on a true lateral view. The dens was not the seat of erosion on a transoral film and this very hazardous subluxation was therefore due to laxity of the transverse ligament of the atlas. (C) and (D) show that the space in a non-rheumatoid patient does not alter with flexion.

range of motion[22,23]. The approach appears to make little difference — bilateral incisions[24], transolecranon[25] or by excising the radial head[26] — provided all synovium is removed from both humero-radial and humero-ulnar compartments[27]. It can now, with benefit, be performed arthroscopically.

Pain experienced throughout the range, especially if associated with crepitus and worsened by longitudinal compression, indicates probable erosion of articular cartilage (Fig. 5.15). Provided the joint is relatively stable, such patients may be considerably relieved by synovectomy and fascial interposition arthroplasty[28]. Reduction in range of motion due to joint destruction

may be very pronounced, even to the point of spontaneous ankylosis. Where neither hand can be used to eat or to perform toilet activities, total elbow joint replacement can restore function in a large proportion of patients[29–31], although the procedure is attended by a high rate of complications[32,33] and reoperation[34].

Crepitus
If the elbow joint is cupped in the palm of one hand and the joint is then slowly moved passively through a short arc, creaking or grinding may be felt by the supporting hand. This may be due to marked synovitis or more frequently to advanced erosion of the articular surfaces.

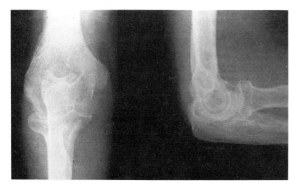

Fig. 5.15 This AP and lateral radiograph of the elbow reveals loss of joint space and was associated with pain experienced throughout the range of flexion and extension of the elbow joint.

Stability

Dislocation of the elbow is relatively rare in rheumatoid disease since it requires not only disruption of the ligaments of the joint and weakening of the muscles but also considerable erosion of the humerus and ulna. If it does occur the clinical picture is similar to that of trauma in that posterior dislocation of the olecranon is the common displacement and can be detected by increase in the distance from olecranon to either epicondyle when compared with the interepicondylar distance. It differs from traumatic dislocation in that any of these bony landmarks may be destroyed by erosion and in the fact that the dislocation in the rheumatoid is usually remarkably painless.

The much less severe instability of the subluxed joint can be detected by grasping both upper and forearms with the elbow joint at 90 degrees and attempting to displace the ulnar first backwards and then forwards in relation to the trochlea of the humerus. Being a perfect hinge joint, the normal elbow cannot be subluxed at all by this manoeuvre (Fig. 5.16).

Gross instability of one or other collateral ligament should be assessed by holding the arm in full extension and supination, placing the palm of one hand over the opposite side of the joint as a fulcrum and then stressing the collateral ligament with force applied laterally with the other hand just above the wrist, using the forearm as a lever. Instability is a contraindication to interpositional arthroplasty. The one compensation for instability is that it is usually accompanied by a functional range of motion.

RADIAL HEAD

With the patient's arm abducted somewhat and the forearm flexed to 90 degrees, the arm should be sup-

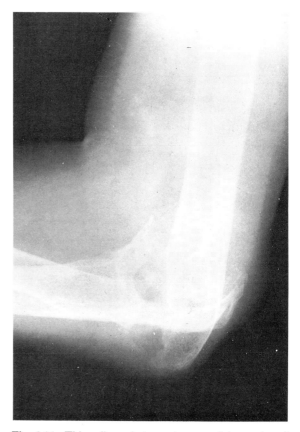

Fig. 5.16 This radiograph shows almost total destruction of the elbow joint associated with gross instability on clinical examination.

ported beneath the elbow with the palm of the hand while the radial head is sought with the thumb of that hand (Fig. 5.17). Its identification can be greatly facilitated by passively pronating and supinating the forearm with the other hand, causing the radial head to rotate.

Crepitus

During this movement crepitus may be detected and this may be accompanied by discomfort. This is due to loss of articular cartilage in the superior radioulnar joint. Excision of the radial head is indicated (Fig. 5.18). This procedure relieves pain and increases the range of motion in the majority of patients[35]. Replacement of the head with a silicone prosthesis appears to give inferior results and is associated with a significant incidence of prosthesis fracture[36-38].

Range of motion

Supporting the elbow with the palm of the hand, the

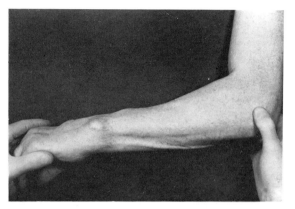

Fig. 5.17 With the elbow flexed some 90 degrees, the radial head is sought with the examiner's thumb while the arm is carried into pronation and supination with the other hand.

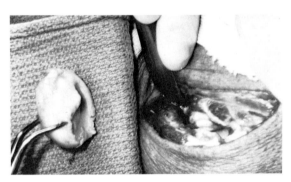

Fig. 5.18 At excision, the radial head is seen to be the site of erosive arthritis.

patient's hand should be held and the forearm carried into full pronation and supination, and the passive and then active ranges recorded. These ranges are measured taking 0° to be with the plane of the hand vertical. The average normal range is pronation 70°, supination 85°. Care should be taken to immobilize the elbow during this test for the apparent ranges can be greatly increased by movement of the shoulder and trunk.

Pain

With the elbow stabilized, passive pronation and supination of the forearm are very commonly accompanied by pain, especially on extreme supination (Fig. 5.19). This should be accurately localized by the patient. The pain may be experienced at the elbow, which suggests superior radio-ulnar joint disease, but much more commonly it is very accurately referred to the ulnar head (see below).

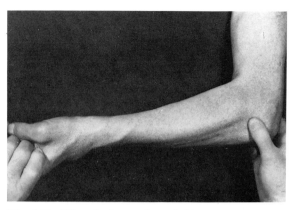

Fig. 5.19 When the forearm is carried into extreme supination, the patient very commonly complains of pain, usually at the ulnar head.

Wrist[39]

Synovitis occurs in two regions of the wrist:

The *extensor compartment*, more so on its ulnar aspect. Synovitis here is easily observed during examination, extending as it does on to the forearm and dorsum of the hand. It is characterized by an hour-glass constriction caused by the overlying extensor retinaculum. Synovitis around the extensor tendons contributes to their dysfunction and rupture (see below).

The *joints of the wrist*, where the synovitis wreaks its effects particularly around the attachments of the major ligaments, resulting in deformities unique to the rheumatoid hand, deformities which have great impact on the fingers, both in form and function.

All ligaments may be effected, and their resultant incompetence produces specific changes in the wrist architecture.

The *ulnar carpal complex* (UCC) (p. 79) is commonly the first afflicted.

Synovitis damages the structures around the ulnar head:

Laterally where, by eroding the sigmoid notch of the radius with which the ulnar head articulates, it produces typical 'scalloping' (Fig. 5.20), evident on plain films.

Distally in the prestyloid recess, where it causes attrition and eventual rupture of the triangular fibrocartilaginous complex (TFCC).

This allows the ulnar carpus to drop forward, or supinate relative to the forearm, leaving the ulnar head behind as a marked prominence — if erosion of the head has produced sharp edges, the threat to the extensors of the fourth and fifth fingers is evident.

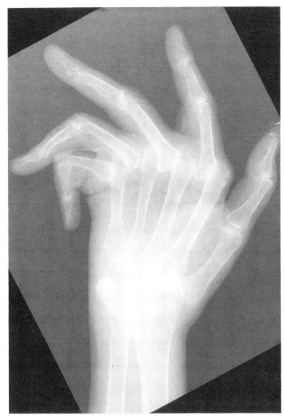

Fig. 5.20 'Scolloping' of the radius at the sigmoid notch produced by synovitis in the distal radio-ulnar joint.

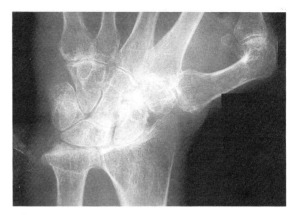

Fig. 5.21 Ulnar translocation (type I) with loss of radial height. The Shapiro angle is 145 degrees (normal 112 degrees) (the Shapiro angle equals that between the radial cortex of the index metacarpal and the line drawn from the radial styloid to the distal ulnar margin of the radius).

Medially around the *extensor carpi ulnaris*, causing the tendon initially to become a less efficient motor for both dorsiflexion and ulnar deviation (A, below), and later, as it subluxes anteriorly, to function as a wrist flexor.

The *radioscaphocapitate* (RSC) or 'sling' ligament (p. 79), which crosses the waist of the carpus, is next most frequently involved. The synovitis may produce 'scaphoid grooving', which can be seen on radiograph. Once it fails it is quickly joined by incompetence of the *radioscapholunate* (RSL) ligament of Testut. As in trauma, the loss of this ligamentous support causes *rotatory subluxation of the scaphoid* and consequently *loss of radial carpal height* (B, below).

If, as often occurs, loss of RSC and RSL support is joined by failure of the *radiolunatotriquetral* (RLT) ligament, then all the major supports of the palmar aspect of the radiocarpal joint have gone and the wrist subluxes in an anterior direction (Fig. 5.22).

The RLT ligament is one of two major ligaments preventing the carpus from sliding down the natural incline of the radius. The other is the *dorsal radiocarpal* (DRC) (p. 79) ligament. When that also fails, *ulnar translocation* of the carpus results (C, below). If the whole carpus moves this is termed type I translocation (Fig. 5.21). If the scaphoid remains behind, possibly due to its rotatory subluxation, the translocation is type II (Fig. 5.23).

Considering the damage in the radiocarpal joint detailed above, it is remarkable that the midcarpal joint is largely spared, but that is a feature of the rheumatoid wrist. It is not always so, however. Attrition of the *triquetrohamatocapitate* (THC) ligament does occur on occasion, resulting in a marked VISI pattern. If this precedes the more common anterior subluxation at the radiocarpal joint described above (Fig. 5.22), the laxity may result in anterior dislocation at the midcarpal joint — but this is uncommon.

To summarize this havoc, one can tabulate the clinically apparent effects of incompetence in each of the ligamentous structures:

UCC ⟶ *prominent ulnar head*
⟶ supinated carpus
⟶ ineffective ECU (A)
RSC
+ RSL ⟶ loss rad. hght. (B) } *radial carpal rotation*
+ RLT ⟶ *ant wrist subluxation*
+ DRC → uln trnslctn (C)

The combination of A, B and C produces the last of the three clinically apparent deformities, *radial carpal rotation*. Radial carpal rotation is recorded by measuring the angle between a line drawn along the radial cortex of the index metacarpal and the line of radial inclination

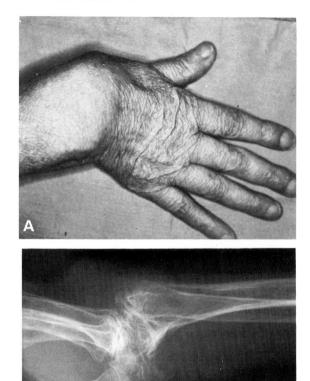

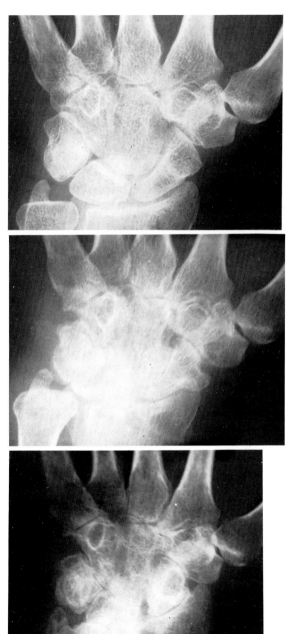

Fig. 5.22 A. Total anterior dislocation of the wrist joint is evident even on clinical examination, the radius and ulna being abnormally prominent on the dorsum of the wrist. B. Anterior subluxation. The subluxation is here at the radiocarpal joint and has produced a considerable increase in the radial tilt which here measures 40 degrees (normal 10 to 15 degrees).

(that is, the line from the tip of the radial styloid to the ulnar corner of the distal radius)[40]. This 'Shapiro angle' measures 112° in the normal hand, significantly more in radial carpal rotation. Each of the three clinical manifestations of wrist collapse has an impact on digital function: the prominent ulnar head by rupturing extensor tendons; radial carpal rotation by changing the alignment of the metacarpus and, by the Z phenomenon, encouraging ulnar drift; anterior wrist subluxation by reducing the efficiency of the extrinsic tendons, which not only weakens grasp, but makes the hand, relatively, 'intrinsic plus', which encourages the development of 'swan neck' deformity[41].

Fig. 5.23 A, B. The progressive deterioration in the wrist of a patient in her 30s is seen in these radiographs taken four years apart. The later shows scapholunate dissociation, ulnar translocation (Type II) and radial carpal rotation (Shapiro angle over 120°). Erosive cysts are noted in two significant locations: the radius at the attachment of the RSL ligament of Testut, and the ulnar styloid at the attachment of the TFCC.

Synovium

The synovium on the dorsum of the wrist and ulnar aspect should be palpated using the three-finger test for fluctuation to confirm its relatively fluid nature (Fig. 5.24). By placing the wrist in flexion, the boundaries of the synovial swelling are made more apparent. In the case of dorsal swelling, the exact location of the diseased synovium can often be deduced by the wider and obviously superficial extent of that around the extensor tendons compared with that in the radiocarpal joint.

Range of motion

The wrist joint should be carried into maximum flexion, extension, radial deviation and ulnar deviation, both actively and passively. The average normal range is flexion 75°, extension 70°, ulnar deviation 35°, radial deviation 20°.

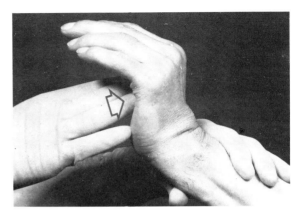

Fig.5.25 By carrying the hand into extremes of wrist joint motion the presence of pain most marked at either end of the arc is suggestive of synovitis.

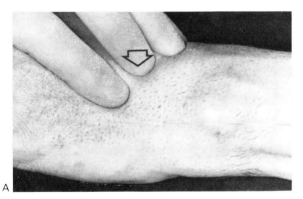

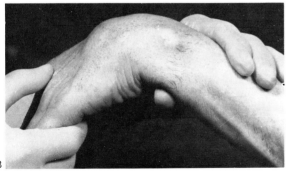

Fig. 5.24 A. The presence of synovium in the wrist joint and the extensor compartment can be palpated by fixing the swelling with two fingers of one hand and palpating it with a finger of the examiner's other hand, thereby eliciting fluctuation. B. By carrying the wrist into palmar flexion the precise boundaries of the synovial swelling can be made more apparent.

Pain

If pain is experienced in the more extreme arcs of the range and is accompanied by joint swelling, synovitis of the composite radiocarpal and midcarpal joint is the most likely cause (Fig. 5.25). To distinguish between the two components of the joint is difficult.

If on the other hand, pain is experienced throughout a limited arc with little or no swelling present, then loss of articular cartilage is the more likely cause. This is supported by the detection of crepitus.

Crepitus

As with the elbow crepitus can best be detected by cradling the joint in the palm of one hand while gently flexing and extending the joint.

Instability

Minor degrees of subluxation may not be detectable on inspection, being masked by dorsal synovitis. The lower forearm should be grasped firmly in one hand and the hand and carpus in the other. Alternate dorsal and palmar movement of one hand relative to the other in a shearing manner will reveal instability (Fig. 5.26). In the normal wrist little or no movement can be achieved by this manoeuvre.

ULNAR HEAD[42]

Extreme supination of the forearm, usually performed while examining the radial head, commonly produces pain at the wrist. It is evidence of ulnar head subluxation. With either the thumb of the supporting hand or the index finger of the other, the surgeon should firmly depress the prominent ulnar head. It may be stable, in

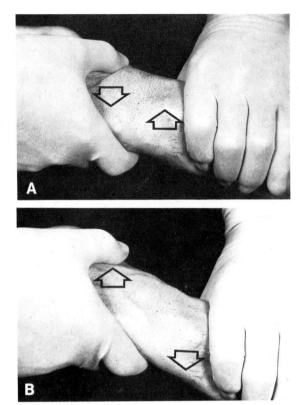

Fig. 5.26 A, B. By grasping the forearm and hand and attempting to produce a shearing action at the wrist joint which in normal patients is stable, the early stages of subluxation can be demonstrated.

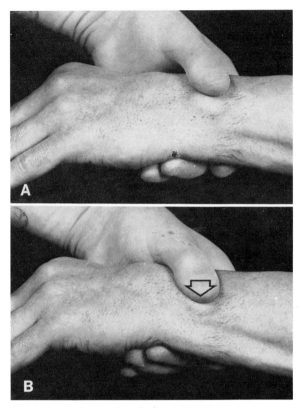

Fig. 5.27 A, B. The piano-key sign. Pressure exerted over the ulnar head will cause distinct motion in the presence of dislocation and surrounding synovitis. On release the ulnar head jumps back into its original position.

which event the patient simply has a naturally large ulnar head. In rheumatoid patients, however, the prominence can often be depressed by 5 mm or more, usually with accompanying pain (Fig. 5.27). This movement has been described as the *'piano key' sign* for, like a piano key, when the bone is released it springs back into its original position.

Depression of the ulnar head often has two effects apart from producing pain:

1. Recurrence of radial deviation of the wrist. As the ulnar head is depressed the carpus can often be felt to rotate radially with a grinding sensation.
2. Increased prominence of synovial swelling on the ulnar border of the wrist.

INDICATIONS (Fig. 5.28)

Synovectomy is appropriate when synovitis has persisted for six months despite adequate medication and where no more advanced changes require more complex procedures. It has been shown to be beneficial in reducing

wrist pain[43] and thereby improving motion, but it appears to have no merit in reducing the progress of wrist deformity.

Ulnar head resection (Darrach procedure) is indicated for subluxation of the ulnar head causing extensor tendon rupture or painful pronation and supination. It is customary to attempt reduction of the supinated carpus at the same procedure by re-aligning the extensor carpi ulnaris using a radially based sling of extensor retinaculum. This may be further strengthened, and the propensity to radial carpal rotation reduced, by transfer of the extensor carpi radialis longus to the extensor carpi ulnaris. Significant problems may be encountered after the Darrach procedure, including painful clicking between the radius and ulna and ulnar instability, the latter often proving intractable[44,45]. To prevent this occurring a silicone cap was designed, but this has proved to have problems of its own, including implant fracture (Fig. 5.29), bone erosion and silicone synovitis[46,47]. Alternative operations which achieve similar results to the Darrach have therefore been described,

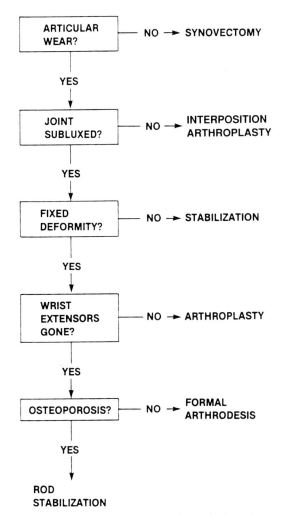

Fig. 5.28 This flow chart illustrates the method of selecting the appropriate procedure in rheumatoid disease of the wrist (see text).

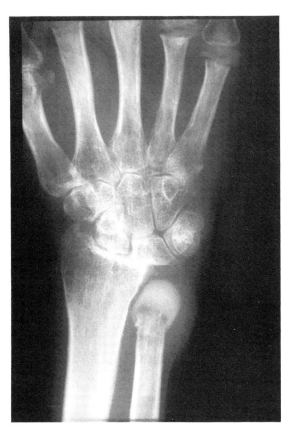

Fig. 5.29 Fracture of an ulnar head implant. Also evident is type I ulnar translocation, rotatory subluxation of the scaphoid, loss of radial carpal height and erosions at the attachment of the radioscapholunate ligament to the radius and of the radioscaphocapitate ligament to the radius.

including *hemiresection–interposition* arthroplasty[48] and *'matched' distal ulnar resection*[49]. The author uses the latter in patients with negative or neutral ulnar variance, a Darrach in those who are ulnar-positive. These procedures carry a high satisfaction rating, removing pain and increasing the range of motion[50,51].

When the wrist is stable but painful due to cartilage loss, *interposition arthroplasty* using a 3 mm sheet of silicone[52] has proved effective with no reported cases of silicone synovitis. Those concerned about it should employ soft tissue as an interposition[56–58].

Once instability in the form of ulnar translocation commences, this can be corrected and stabilized effectively by *radiolunate arthrodesis*[53], originally described by Chamay. If the radioscaphoid joint also shows wear, it may also be fused, leaving motion at the midcarpal joint, which is often relatively normal[54].

If the joint is anteriorly subluxed or otherwise in a state of advanced derangement, surgery is indicated only if the joint is symptomatic or threatens tendon integrity. A joint which looks disastrous on a radiograph may function well and with minimal discomfort. If surgery is required, the choice lies between arthrodesis and arthroplasty[55]. In general terms, arthroplasty is indicated in older patients who do no heavy manual work and have intact wrist motors, and particularly where tendon transfers are required to replace ruptured *digital* flexor or extensor tendons, for wrist motion will aid the transfers. The choice of arthroplasty lies between *soft-tissue arthroplasty*[56–58], establishing a *fibrous ankylosis*[59], *total wrist replacement*[60–62] and *silicone interposition arthroplasty*[63]. The latter two both have problems. Total wrist replacement has been followed by dislocation[64], fracture

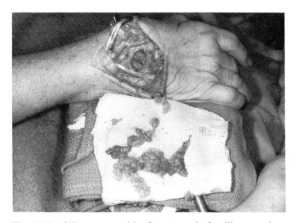

Fig. 5.30 Silicone synovitis. On removal of a silicone wrist implant, which had been in place for three years, florid synovitis was evident, showing silicone fragments on histological examination. Stabilization of the wrist was performed.

of the radius[65] and damage to tendons and nerve[66]. It also requires very accurate alignment if instability is to be avoided. The silicone wrist may develop silicone synovitis (Fig. 5.30) and is followed in a high proportion of patients by fracture or settling of the implant (Fig. 5.31), both of which result in pain and limitation of movement[67-69]. If the bone stock is good, *arthrodesis* can be done by standard techniques[70], but if it is osteoporotic, stabilization with a Rush[71,72] or Steinmann[73] pin can give excellent results with few complications. The author, who has considerable experience with the silicone spacer and none with total wrist replacement, strongly favours Steinmann pin stabilization in the large majority of patients, for even bilateral arthrodeses do well[74]. The rheumatoid patient faces many trials. There is no need to add problems with implants if they offer no clear benefits.

See Green D P 1993 Operative Hand Surgery, 3rd edn. Churchill Livingstone, New York, p. 1624.

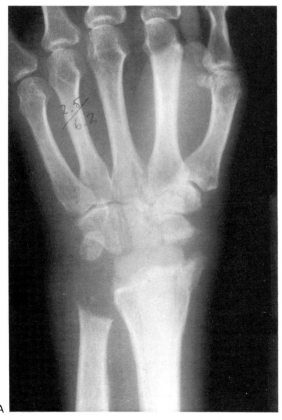

A

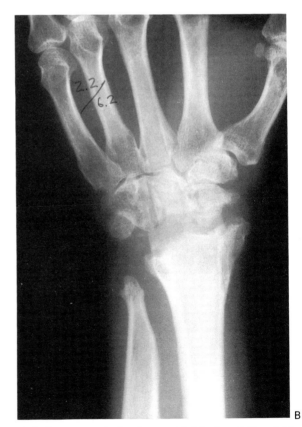

B

Fig. 5.31 A, B. Silicone wrist implant settling developed over a period of one year reducing the carpal height from 0.40 to 0.35 (normal 0.54 ± 0.03) with coincident loss of motion and increase in wrist pain.

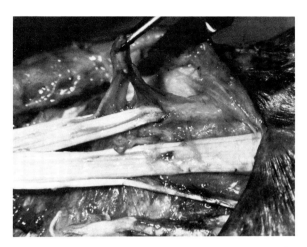

Fig. 5.32 Diseased synovium is here shown being dissected off the extensor tendons during exploration of a tendon rupture.

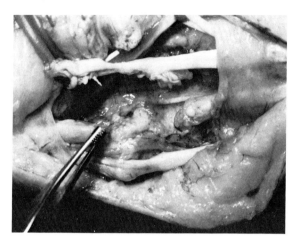

Fig. 5.34 The erosion produced in this tendon by the ulnar head which has here been removed can clearly be seen to conform to the hemispherical shape of that head.

Extensor tendons

Synovium

The distinguishing features of synovitis around the extensor tendons at the wrist have already been stated: discrete, well-demarcated, often prominent swelling, extension of the swelling on to the dorsum of the hand, thumb and forearm, absence of pain, even on passive movement of the wrist, bogginess to palpation, crepitus on palpation during finger motion.

Significant synovitis requires synovectomy as it is a major factor in producing tendon rupture (Fig. 5.32).

TENDON RUPTURE[75-77]

The most apparent cause of rupture of tendons, namely attrition against rough or prominent bone (Fig. 5.33)

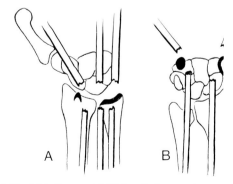

Fig. 5.33 This diagram highlights the bony points at which tendinous rupture is likely to occur: on the left, dorsally, the radial tubercle and the dislocated ulnar head, and on the right, anteriorly, the ridge on the trapezium and the hook of the hamate.

has been refuted by some who emphasize the importance of synovitis within the tendon and interference with its blood supply. Certainly tendon disruptions in rheumatoid disease occur only where the tendon lies within a synovial sheath. Nonetheless, the most common sites for rupture are related to bony prominences:

extensor pollicis longus at the tubercle on the radius
extensor digiti minimi and extensor digitorum of small and ring fingers over the dorsally subluxed ulna head (Fig. 5.34).

These ruptures are usually evident on inspection but may require active testing when pain elicited by resistance offered by the examiner suggests that the tendon is partially worn.

Extensor pollicis longus

Posture: flexion of both metacarpophalangeal and interphalangeal joints of the thumb (Fig. 5.35).

Active test: resisted extension of the interphalangeal joint of the thumb (Fig. 5.36). Partial rupture may be present with little effect on the normal posture. However, active testing reveals weakness and often pain over the site of partial rupture.

Extensor digiti minimi
Extensor digitorum

Posture: drooping of the affected fingers at the metacarpophalangeal joint (Fig. 5.37). This becomes increasingly apparent as the patient actively attempts to straighten the fingers, for this results in unbalanced action of the intrinsic muscles which extend the interphalangeal joints but flex the metacarpophalangeal joint.

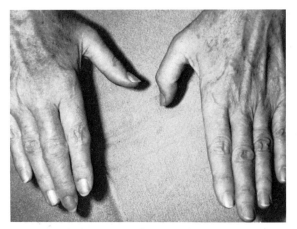

Fig. 5.35   Extensor pollicis longus rupture is revealed by the posture of the metacarpophalangeal and interphalangeal joints on the right.

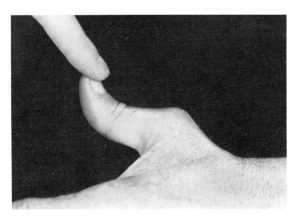

Fig. 5.36   This patient with rheumatoid disease is able to perform extension against resistance indicating a normal extensor pollicis longus, which is palpable over the metacarpal of the thumb.

Active test: resisted extension of the metacarpophalangeal joint (Fig. 5.38).

A mistaken diagnosis of extensor tendon rupture may be made for any one of three reasons:

1. *Subluxation of the metacarpophalangeal joint* with intrinsic contracture and palmar plate shortening may make the joint incapable of extension. This possibility can be eliminated by testing passive extension of the metacarpophalangeal joints (Fig. 5.39).
2. *Ulnar displacement of the extensor tendons* (Fig. 5.40) at the metacarpophalangeal joints may be so

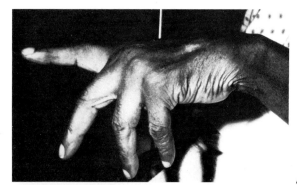

A

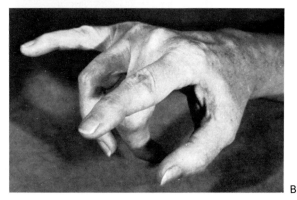

B

Fig. 5.37   A. The most common order of rupture of the extensor tendons has occurred in this patient with progressive loss of extension in the small, ring and middle fingers.
B. This patient shows rupture of extensor digitorum and pollicis longus. Extensors indicis and digiti minimi are intact.

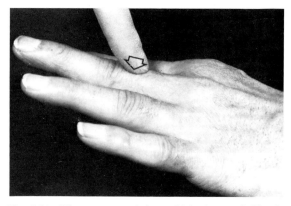

Fig. 5.38   The metacarpophalangeal joint is extended by the long extrinsic extensor and this should be tested in each finger.

marked that they fall below the axis of that joint losing all power to extend it. In extreme cases they become weak flexors. This is more difficult to detect but should be suspected if the tendons can be felt to tighten on attempted extension and if

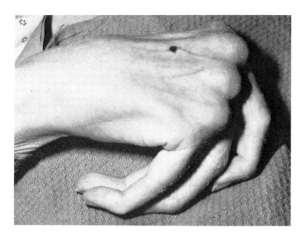

Fig. 5.39 The fixed flexion contracture of these metacarpophalangeal joints is due to severe palmar subluxation of the proximal phalanges.

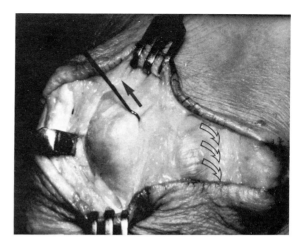

Fig. 5.40 In this patient about to undergo metacarpophalangeal replacement, the ulnar displacement of the extensor tendon to the middle finger is clearly shown. The tendon has fallen into the space between the metacarpophalangeal joints and here is being pulled up into its normal position using a skin hook.

their line passes towards the ulnar aspect of the relevant metacarpophalangeal joint. In early stages of this extensor tendon dislocation, the patient cannot initiate finger extension but can maintain it if the fingers are first placed in that position.

3. *Posterior interosseous nerve palsy*[78,79] resulting from compression of that nerve by synovitis of the radiohumeral joint may mimic extensor tendon rupture (see Ch. 3, p. 311).

INDICATIONS

Ruptured extensor tendons require early surgical reconstruction lest joint flexion contractures ensue. In those cases in which too much tendon length has been destroyed to allow direct repair, early intervention *may* allow reconstruction using a tendon graft[80] while power remains in the motor unit. Tendon transfers[81,82] are usually required and the integrity of appropriate tendons should be determined during examination — extensor indicis, extensor carpi ulnaris, flexor digitorum superficialis and others. The transfers commonly employed are:

```
for EPL — EI[83] or EDM or EPB
    EDM — EI
    1 ED — link to an adjacent intact tendon
    2 ED — EI + adjacent
    3 or 4 ED — FDS[84] or ECU or FCU
```

See Green D P 1993 Operative Hand Surgery, 3rd edn. Churchill Livingstone, New York, pp. 1595 and 1612.

Thumb

At each joint — trapeziometacarpal, metacarpophalan-

geal and interphalangeal — the presence of pain and of the signs of rheumatoid disease should be noted.

Synovium
In all the small joints of the hand active synovitis can be felt as a 'boggy' swelling between the finger and thumb of the examining hand or, perhaps more precisely, between the two index fingers of the examiner (Fig. 5.41). The synovium may be made more evident and obviously fluctuant by gently flexing the joint under examination. Because of the relative resistance of the palmar plate all joint synovitis in the hand is more evident dorsally.

Tenderness
Tenderness should be recorded during palpation.

Range of motion
The range of motion should be recorded both actively and passively. The normal range of motion in the joints of the thumb varies very widely from a combined range in normal metacarpophalangeal and interphalangeal joints of 120 degrees to over 300 degrees. The average accepted by the American Academy of Orthopedic Surgeons is:

	CM	MP	IP
extension	20°	10°	−15°
flexion	15°	55°	80°
abduction	60°	–	–

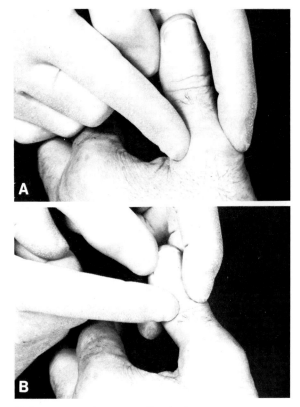

Fig. 5.41   A,B. Synovial swelling in the metacarpophalangeal and interphalangeal joints of the thumb can best
be palpated by using two fingers. Its presence is evidenced by
a 'boggy' fluctuance between two digits.

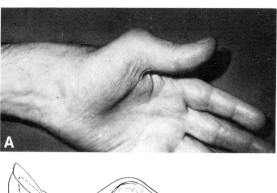

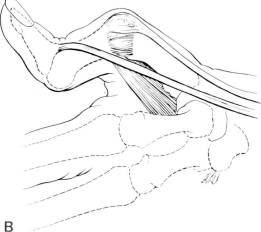

Fig. 5.42   A. An early boutonniere deformity of the thumb is
demonstrated with palmar subluxation of the
metacarpophalangeal joint and the commencement of
hyperextension of the interphalangeal joint. B. The
mechanism is here diagrammatically illustrated. The synovial
swelling in the metacarpophalangeal joint results in
attenuation of the extensor pollicis brevis with resultant loss
of extension of that joint. It also causes distal shift of the
intrinsic tendons going to the extensor expansion.
Contrasting with their normal neutral function, the intrinsics
become flexors of the metacarpophalangeal joint.

Of greater significance than recording the active and
passive ranges is careful observation of specific points:

pain: throughout range, emphasized by compression —
   articular loss; at extremes of range — synovitis;
passive range: the examiner must be able to correct
   passively any deformity of the thumb joints, if soft-
   tissue reconstruction is to prove effective;
instability.

Stability
Collapse of the skeleton of the thumb in rheumatoid
disease is very common. The resultant deformity tends
to conform to one of four patterns, which have been
classified and described by Nalebuff[85].

TYPE I (= 'BOUTONNIERE') (Fig. 5.42)

Disease commences at the metacarpophalangeal joint.
Synovial expansion of the dorsal capsule produces attrition of extensor pollicis brevis and ulnar displacement

of extensor pollicis longus. Thus the thumb becomes
'extrinsic-minus' and progressive metacarpophalangeal
flexion results. The consequent palmar subluxation of
the base of the proximal phalanx in addition to the dorsal synovial expansion causes distal and palmar displacement of the intrinsics — abductor pollicis brevis
and adductor pollicis — which further increases the
metacarpophalangeal flexion and hyperextends the
interphalangeal joint (Fig. 5.43).

Indications in type I [86]
If (i)   joints can be reduced passively
   (ii) joints are stable laterally in the reduced position
   (iii) articular surfaces are adequate on radiologic
        examination

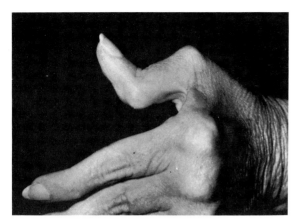

Fig. 5.43 An advanced boutonniere deformity of the thumb known also as an intrinsic plus or '90–90' thumb.

> → *synovectomy + insertion of extensor pollicis longus* into the base of the proximal phalanx

If any of (i), (ii) or (iii) not present:
> → *stabilization* of the metacarpophalangeal joint by arthrodesis or peg[87]

Millender[88] has recorded a 64% recurrence after reconstruction and recommends fusion for most, with replacement arthroplasty[89,90] reserved for the low-demand patient with advanced disease who requires IP joint fusion.

See Green D P 1993 Operative Hand Surgery, 3rd edn. Churchill Livingstone, New York, pp. 1671 and 1676.

TYPE II — uncommon

Type II is identical to type I but is consequent upon disease in the trapeziometacarpal joint with adduction of the first metacarpal.

TYPE III (= 'SWAN-NECK') (Fig. 5.44)

Disease commences at the trapeziometacarpal joint resulting in adduction and flexion of the first metacarpal. In the presence of concomitant disease in the metacarpophalangeal joint, the Z-mechanism (p. 359) produces hyperextension of that joint and hyperflexion of the interphalangeal joint.

Indications in type III
1. Correct adduction of first metacarpal[91] by release of adductor pollicis, or first dorsal interosseous, or the overlying fascia, or all three;
2. Maintain correction by attending to the trapeziometacarpal disease (see Ch. 4, p. 336). It is highly desirable to maintain motion at this joint in

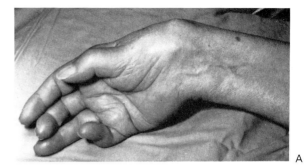

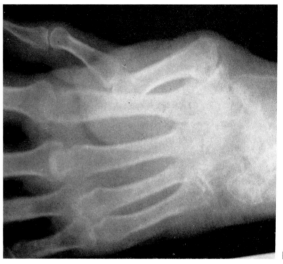

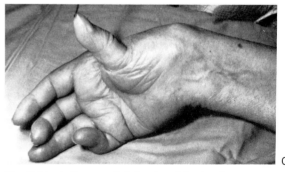

Fig. 5.44 A. Swan-neck deformity of the thumb seen on radiograph (B) to be due to basal joint disease followed by adduction contracture and hyperextension deformity. The deformity is fixed as is shown in (C), resulting in severe loss of first web space span.

rheumatoid disease, therefore fusion is rarely performed.

If (i) articular surfaces adequate on radiological examination and peroperative inspection
   (ii) no evident disease in other trapezial joints
> → *synovectomy*
>   + *ligament reconstruction* with FCR or ECRL

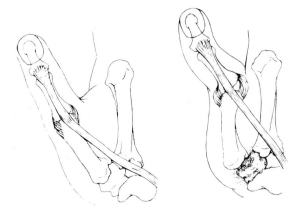

Fig. 5.45 The mechanism of a type IV deformity of the thumb is here illustrated diagrammatically. Disease at the trapeziometacarpal joint results in adduction deformity of the first metacarpal towards the second. This is compensated for by stretching of the collateral ligaments of either the metacarpophalangeal joint as illustrated here or of the interphalangeal joint. The normal relationships are demonstrated in the diagram on the left.

If articular surfaces not adequate
    → *basal joint arthroplasty* (see p. 338, Ch. 4)

3. Once the adduction contracture has been overcome the metacarpophalangeal and interphalangeal joint deformities can be corrected:

If (i) joints reducible passively
  (ii) joints stable laterally in the reduced position
 (iii) articular surfaces adequate on radiological examination
    → *synovectomy* and soft tissue stabilization by palmar *capsulodesis* or *tenodesis*[92–94]
If any of (i), (ii) (iii) not present
    → *stabilization*

See Green D P 1993 Operative Hand Surgery, 3rd edn. Churchill Livingstone, New York, pp. 1673 and 1676.

TYPE IV (Fig. 5.45)

Disease again commences at the trapeziometacarpal joint, resulting in adduction of the first metacarpal. However, in this instance collateral ligament laxity at the metacarpophalangeal and/or interphalangeal joint produces radial deviation at either or both of these articulations (Fig. 5.46).

Indications in type IV
1. Correct adduction and basal joint disease as in type III
2. Manage the metacarpophalangeal and/or interphalangeal joints as follows:

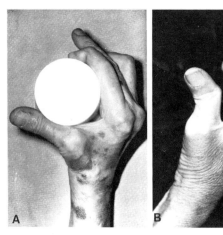

Fig. 5.46 A. Radial deviation has occurred at the metacarpophalangeal joint following adduction deformity in a type IV rheumatoid thumb. B. The radial deviation has here occurred at the interphalangeal joint.

If articular surfaces adequate on radiograph (uncommon)
    → *synovectomy + collateral ligament reconstruction*

If articular surfaces poor (common)
    → *stabilization* of the metacarpophalangeal joint ± *stabilization* of the interphalangeal joint.

As has been emphasized previously, the pathogenesis of type I and type III can be understood in the terms of the pathological anatomy of the rheumatoid finger if the metacarpophalangeal joint of the thumb is equated to the proximal interphalangeal joint of the finger. Substitutions would then be made as in Table 5.2. In those cases in which a full-blown deformity of types I–IV has not occurred, stability should be assessed at each joint in turn.

Trapeziometacarpal. As subluxation develops, the base of the first metacarpal moves radially and anterior relative to the trapezium (these directions are referred to the plane of the palm of the hand). Such subluxation can be detected by the examiner placing his thumb over the metacarpal base and his index finger on the flexor

Table 5.2

Thumb	Finger
Metacarpophalangeal joint	Proximal interphalangeal joint
Abductor pollicis brevis and adductor pollicis	Intrinsic lateral bands
Extensor pollicis brevis	Central slip of extensor digitorum
Interphalangeal joint	Distal interphalangeal joint

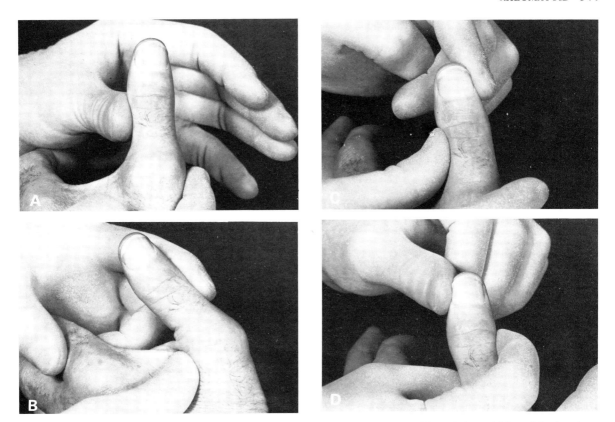

Fig. 5.47 A–D. The integrity of the collateral ligaments of the metacarpophalangeal and interphalangeal joints of the thumb should be tested by laterally stressing these when held in maximum extension. (B) shows that there is some laxity of the radial collateral ligament of the metacarpophalangeal joint.

aspect of the patient's thumb. Pressing with both digits will reduce any subluxation usually with accompanying pain. No movement is present in the normal joint with this manoeuvre.

Metacarpophalangeal and interphalangeal joints. Each collateral ligament should be stressed in turn with the joint held in maximum extension (Fig. 5.47). In the normal hand this produces only a few degrees of pain-free movement. The palmar plate should be stressed by firm extension. The normal hyperextension in these joints of the thumb is very variable.

Crepitus. If the whole thumb is grasped in one hand and the wrist in the other with the examiner's thumb over the trapeziometacarpal joint and the joint rotated while applying some force along the axis of the thumb, crepitus can be detected. This is evidence of loss of articular cartilage, especially if the movement is accompanied by pain. It should be treated as indicated above (type III; 2).

See Green D P 1993 Operative Hand Surgery, 3rd edn. Churchill Livingstone, New York, p. 1676.

Metacarpophalangeal joints[95]

SYNOVIUM

As in all other digital joints, the capsule of the metacarpophalangeal joint is most substantial on its palmar and lateral aspects, where it is thickened into the palmar plate, accessory collateral and collateral ligaments. These structures allow motion while providing strong stability. Synovitis is therefore best detected on the dorsal aspect where swelling can be felt as fluctuation between two of the examiner's digits with the joints held in gentle flexion of some 40 to 50 degrees (Fig. 5.48).

In time the synovium erodes through the capsule and comes to bear on the extensor expansion. The expansion is significantly thinner on the radial aspect than on the ulnar, especially in the index finger. Stretching of the expansion results in ulnar dislocation of the tendons. This displacement should be noted for it is one of the factors responsible for the production of ulnar drift. In the normal hand, the extensor tendons are held over the metacarpophalangeal joints by the dorsal hood.

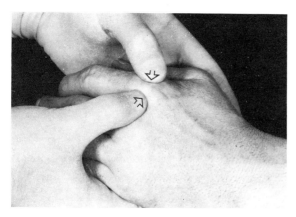

Fig. 5.48 Synovitis in the metacarpophalangeal and interphalangeal joints of the digits can be detected by the two thumbs of the examiner with the joint held in gentle flexion. Its presence is revealed by a 'boggy' fluctuance between the two examining digits.

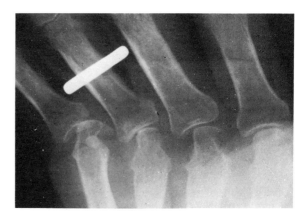

Fig. 5.50 A Brewerton view of the metacarpophalangeal joints demonstrates very clearly the erosions of the metacarpal heads, particularly beneath the radial collateral ligaments of these joints. This occurs at an area of bare bone within the capsule of the joint.

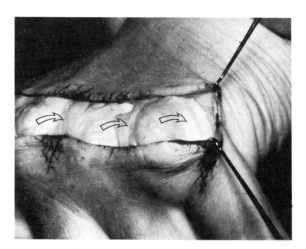

Fig. 5.49 The extreme ulnar subluxation of the extensor tendons is seen here prior to metacarpophalangeal joint replacement. The extensor digiti minimi can be seen on the ulnar aspect of the neck of the metacarpal.

Indeed, in power grasp they can be seen to shift radially as full force is applied. As the dorsal hood is weakened and stretches this radial movement is replaced by ulnar dislocation of the extensor tendons. In late stages, the extensor tendons fall between the metacarpal heads (Fig. 5.49). In this position they are unable to extend the fingers and a mistaken diagnosis of tendon rupture may be made.

In periods of active synovitis, palpation of the synovium will produce marked *tenderness*.

Indications

Synovectomy of the metacarpophalangeal joints is indicated in the following situations:

1. Persistent painful swelling despite adequate medical therapy;
2. Early erosions evident on radiologic examination; these are most likely to be seen on Brewerton views (p. 394) (Fig. 5.50).
3. Displacement of the extensor tendons in the presence of synovitis. The radial extensor hood can be reefed following synovectomy, but care must be taken not to limit flexion. Release of the ulnar hood and intrinsic tendon is often necessary to achieve recentralization[96].

In one review, synovectomy was effective in relieving pain in about half of the patients while almost all lost motion[97], with an average reduction of 20°.

All patients being prepared for synovectomy should be warned of the possible need for joint replacement, since the condition of the bone ends cannot be fully assessed clinically or by radiograph (Fig. 5.51). Only 18% of patients in one series[98] were seen to have erosions on radiologic examination, whereas they were found to be present on exploration in 81%.

See Green D P 1993 Operative Hand Surgery, 3rd edn. Churchill Livingstone, New York, p. 1647.

RANGE OF MOTION

The range of both active and passive motion in each metacarpophalangeal joint should be recorded with the

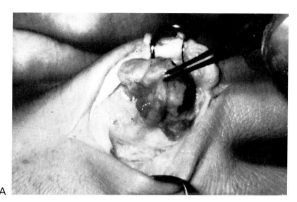

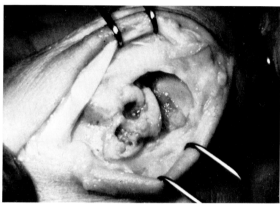

Fig. 5.51 A, B. Synovium frequently obscures large erosions in the underlying metacarpal head.

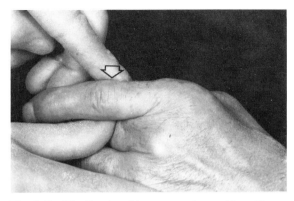

Fig. 5.52 The first dorsal interosseous is tested by asking the patient to abduct the index finger against pressure exerted by the examiner.

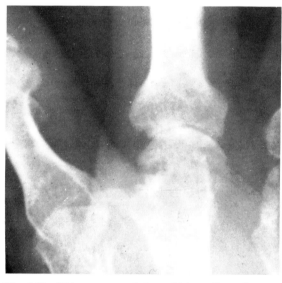

Fig. 5.53 This metacarpophalangeal joint radiograph illustrates the erosion on the radial aspect of the metacarpal head of the index finger. It results in disruption of the collateral ligament attachment on that side which permits the development of ulnar drift.

goniometer, taking note of whether or not motion is limited by pain.

STABILITY[99]

While the normal metacarpophalangeal joint shows a wide range of motion both in flexion and extension and, when the fingers are extended, in a lateral direction, their stability is essential for normal hand function. In the extended position, where stability is required for strong lateral pinch, it is provided mainly by the interosseous muscles and that primarily by the powerful first dorsal interosseous. When the joints are flexed, and stability is necessary for power grasp, the normal metacarpophalangeal joint is locked in lateral immobility by its collateral ligaments. This laxity in extension and immobility in flexion is provided by virtue of the eccentric attachment of the ligament to the cam-shaped metacarpal head. The metacarpal head is also wider on its palmar aspect than dorsally and this also serves to tighten the collateral ligaments.

Instability in rheumatoid disease results from:

Weakness of the first dorsal interosseous, which should therefore be tested in all cases to detect early loss of stability (Fig. 5.52)

Disruption of the collateral ligaments[100]. This results from synovial erosion of the only area of bare bone within the joint capsule, namely that beneath the proximal attachment of the collateral ligament. A deep erosion is commonly detected in this situation, both radiologically (Fig. 5.53) and during synovectomy (Fig. 5.54). This eventually causes detachment of the collateral ligament from its insertion with significant loss of stability. This

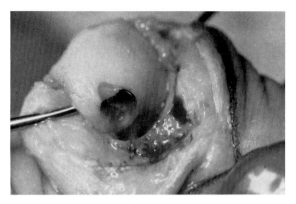

Fig. 5.54 Significant erosions may be detected only at the time of synovectomy.

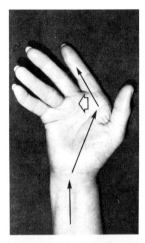

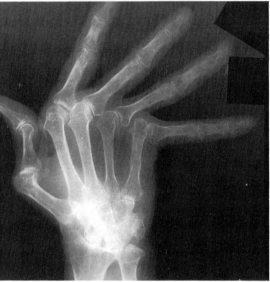

can be detected by flexing the index finger at the meta-carpophalangeal joint and exerting lateral pressure. In the normal hand no motion results. In the advanced rheumatoid there is considerable movement, while in the incipient case the patient complains of pain on this manoeuvre.

When these two stabilizing factors have been eliminated or significantly weakened, other forces, mechanical and pathological, produce the characteristic deformities of the rheumatoid metacarpophalangeal joints, *ulnar drift* and *palmar subluxation*.

Ulnar drift[101]
Flatt describes ulnar drift as having two components[102]:

Ulnar deviation, an ulnar rotation of the phalanx around the metacarpal head, is present in the normal hand and only pathological when uncorrectable.
Ulnar shift, an ulnar translocation of the base of the phalanx on the metacarpal head, is always abnormal.

The normal usage and structure of the hand impose pressures on the metacarpophalangeal joints which displace them into ulnar deviation:

Thumb pressure in all pinch grips.
The ulnar inclination of the head of the metacarpal bone.
The action of abductor digiti minimi which is a strong ulnar deviator of the small finger proximal phalanx. Its action is increased by a slip of tendon from extensor digiti minimi which becomes increasingly powerful as the extensor becomes dislocated in an ulnar direction.

These forces produce the *ulnar deviation* seen in the normal hand in extension and which increases in power grasp.

Fig. 5.55 A. As was emphasized in the section on surface anatomy, the flexor tendons cross the wrist joint to the ulnar side of the midline. With progressive radial deviation of the wrist the angle of incidence of these tendons to the index finger in particular is increasingly from an ulnar direction. As laxity in the flexor tendon sheath develops so the force of the flexor tendons on the metacarpophalangeal joint is applied further out on the proximal phalanx and becomes progressively more and more powerful in its ulnar moment. B. Ulnar drift of the metacarpophalangeal joints, to the point of complete dislocation in the case of the small finger. Note also the ulnar translocation of the wrist with loss of radial carpal height and the boutonniere deformity of the thumb.

The pathological forces which produce *ulnar drift* once stability has been lost should be sought at the appropriate stage in the examination:
r*adial deviation of the wrist*, which, by the Z-mechanism, induces ulnar drift of the metacarpophalangeal joints[103];

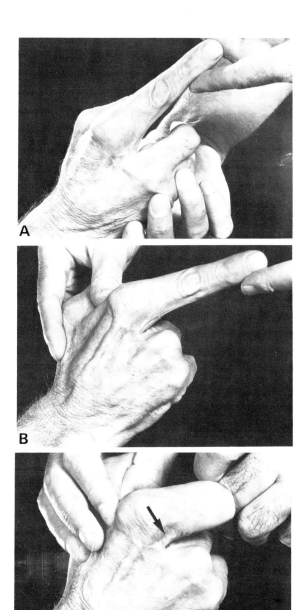

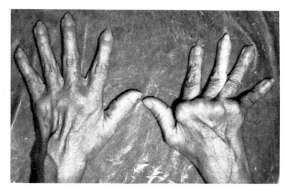

Fig. 5.57 Palmar subluxation of the metacarpophalangeal joints is clearly evident in the right hand of this patient, the metacarpal heads being evident as a ridge across the dorsum of the hand.

ulnar shift of the extensor tendons;
ulnar applied force of the flexor tendons (Fig. 5.55)[104];
intrinsic tightness (p. 385).

All of these abnormal ulnar deviating forces are self-perpetuating. That is, in each instance, once ulnar drift has arisen as a result of removal of the radial stabilizing factors and application of the ulnar deviating forces, the mechanical advantage of those forces to produce further ulnar drift is enhanced (Fig. 5.56).

Palmar subluxation
This displacement can occur only when the collateral ligaments have been stretched or their attachments disrupted. It is further encouraged by the stretching of the dorsal expansion of the extensor mechanism with dislocation of the extrinsic extensor tendons to lie between the metacarpal heads. These changes remove the dorsal structures which normally resist palmar subluxation and often create a flexion deformity of the metacarpophalangeal joints. The forces which then produce the subluxation are *intrinsic tightness* and the powerful palmar moment of the *extrinsic flexor tendons*.

Palmar subluxation is commonly evident on inspection, the metacarpal heads being prominent dorsally (Fig. 5.57). In less apparent cases, usually where florid synovitis still persists, the presence of subluxation can be demonstrated by stabilizing the metacarpal with one hand, gripping the proximal phalanx with the other and testing the motion of one on the other in a palmar–dorsal direction (Fig. 5.58). In the normal hand, little or no motion is possible. In the extreme case of palmar subluxation, the joint cannot be reduced (Fig. 5.59). Proximal–distal motion of the proximal phalanx may then be present and, when extreme, is referred to as *telescoping*.

Fig. 5.56 This patient who does not suffer from rheumatoid disease but has been subjected to a ray resection of the middle finger with subsequent scarring illustrates well two of the factors which play a part in producing ulnar drift of the fingers. In (A) the finger is held extended without any active effort by the patient. In (B) active extension shows that the extensor tendon is lying to the ulnar aspect of the metacarpophalangeal joint and that active extension results in ulnar deviation of the finger. C. Here the intrinsic test is being applied and it can be seen how the patient's finger swings into ulnar drift on account of tightness of the intrinsic on the ulnar aspect of his index finger.

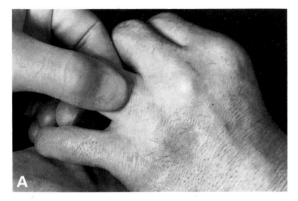

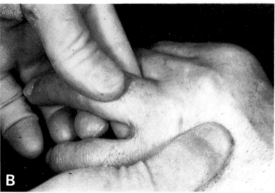

Fig. 5.58 A, B. By gripping the hand and proximal phalanx of the digit under examination, subluxation of the phalanx on the metacarpal head can be detected by moving the proximal phalanx alternately dorsally and palmarwards on the metacarpal head.

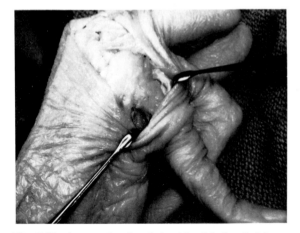

Fig. 5.59 At operation the relationship of the head of the metacarpal to the base of the proximal phalanx can be seen. Stress being applied to the tip of the small finger (bottom left) is placing this metacarpophalangeal joint in maximum *extension*.

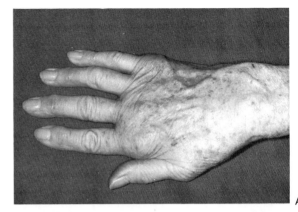

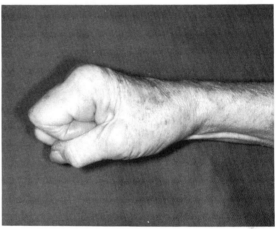

Fig. 5.60 One year prior to these photographs, this patient had marked ulnar drift and palmar subluxation of the metacarpophalangeal joints. She underwent a Wood reconstructive arthroplasty with the early result shown here.

INDICATIONS

The various agents producing ulnar drift should be dealt with as detailed in their respective sections.

Crossed intrinsic transfer has been shown to be beneficial and longlasting[105] despite prior reservations expressed by the same author[106]. Dissatisfaction with the results of resection interposition arthroplasty and concerns over the use of silicone has led to renewed efforts to reconstruct the metacarpophalangeal joint. The procedure described by *Wood*[107] has been used by the author in a small number of patients and given surprisingly good results (Fig. 5.60), although the longevity of the satisfaction is not yet determined. Where the metacarpal head is destroyed, renewed efforts are being made to employ the techniques of interpositional arthroplasty described by *Vainio*[108], *Fowler*[109] and *Tupper*[110]. *Implant resection arthroplasty* still has a role,

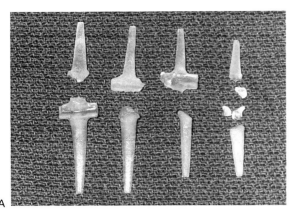

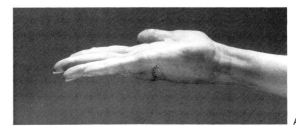

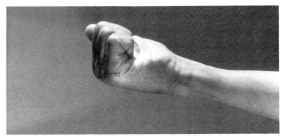

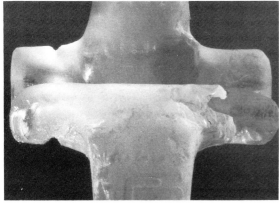

Fig. 5.61 A. Fracture of silicone implants. B. Wear pattern on a silicone metacarpophalangeal joint implant which was removed for associated silicone synovitis.

Fig. 5.62 Three weeks previously this patient underwent silicone implant arthroplasty for palmar subluxation and ulnar drift of the metacarpophalangeal joints. Studies show that this will be the best motion she will have, with progressive loss over subsequent years.

whichever implant is used[111–113]. Problems do arise[114–116] including recurrence of ulnar drift, settling with loss of initial motion, implant fracture and surface wear (Fig. 5.61), the latter leading to silicone synovitis. However, such synovitis is much less common at this joint than in the carpus and patient satisfaction is high[115,116] (Fig. 5.62). The author schedules most patients for a possible Wood arthroplasty, possible implant resection arthroplasty and makes the decision during surgery.

See Green D P 1993 Operative Hand Surgery, 3rd edn. Churchill Livingstone, New York, pp. 151 and 1651.

Intrinsic muscles

Tightness of the intrinsic muscles of the hand contributes to several of the major problems of the rheumatoid patient:

weakness of power grasp (Fig. 5.63)
ulnar drift

palmar subluxation of the metacarpophalangeal joints
swan-neck deformity of the fingers.

The muscles primarily involved are the interossei and the lumbricals. The pathogenesis of intrinsic tightness has not been clearly established, but spasm provoked by the inflamed metacarpophalangeal joints is the probable cause. Secondary fibrosis results in the fixed intrinsic contracture. In testing for intrinsic tightness, the examiner should first assess the range of passive joint motion and the extent to which that is impaired by joint disease or tendon adhesions.

The intrinsics flex the metacarpophalangeal joints and extend the interphalangeal joints. Therefore the test for tightness should be performed as follows:

1. Hold the metacarpophalangeal joint in full passive extension (Fig. 5.64).
2. Gently flex the proximal interphalangeal joint with the other hand. In the normal hand, full proximal interphalangeal joint flexion will be possible.

By contrast, in the presence of intrinsic tightness, firm, rather resilient, resistance will be encountered (see Fig. 2.59, p. 194). The angle of the proximal interphalangeal joint at which this is met should be recorded (p. 195).

3. The metacarpophalangeal joint should now be allowed to fall progressively into flexion while keeping pressure applied to the middle phalanx.

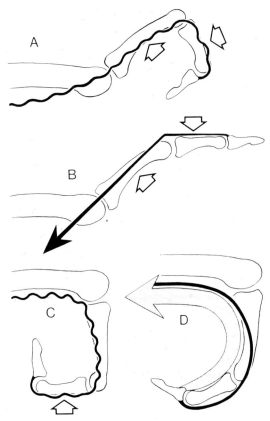

Fig. 5.63   This diagram illustrates the mechanism of intrinsic tightness. A. In the normal finger the intrinsics are sufficiently loose to permit flexion of the proximal interphalangeal joint when the metacarpophalangeal joint is fully extended. B. In intrinsic tightness the proximal interphalangeal joint cannot be flexed with the metacarpophalangeal in that position. C. In relaxed flexion the intrinsics are loose in both the normal circumstance and also in the presence of intrinsic tightness. D. In intrinsic tightness powerful flexion draws the flexor digitorum profundus proximally and therefore translocates the origin of the lumbrical. The intrinsic tightness then serves to para-doxically extend the interphalangeal joints, thereby resisting the power of flexion and resulting in weakness of grip.

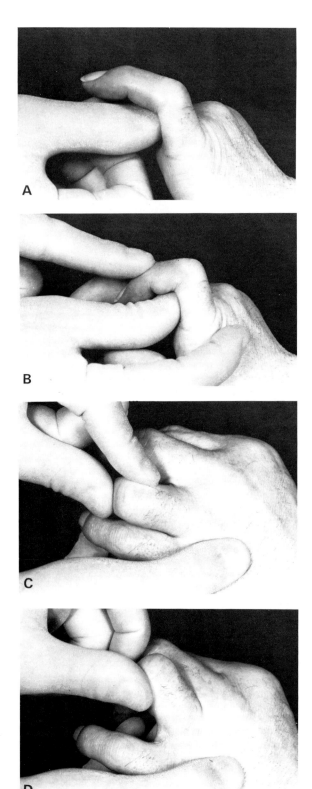

Fig. 5.64   Testing for intrinsic tightness. A. The metacarpophalangeal joint is held in full extension. B. The proximal interphalangeal joint is then fully flexed and resistance to this movement suggests tightness of the intrinsics. Differentiation between tightness in the radial and ulnar intrinsics can be achieved by deviating the digit in both radial and ulnar directions while in this intrinsic minus position (C, D).

The proximal interphalangeal joint will flex further as the metacarpophalangeal joint is lowered from extension.

In pure intrinsic tightness, the proximal interphalangeal joint will flex fully once the metacarpophalangeal joint has been allowed to pass into flexion. The extent by which it fails to achieve full flexion is a measure of proximal interphalangeal joint disease or extrinsic tendon adhesion.

The test should then be repeated while deviating the finger both radially and ulnarwards. This will reveal whether the tightness in the initial test is primarily of the ulnar or radial intrinsics:

ulnar — when more tightness is encountered with the finger deviated radially

radial — when there is greater tightness in ulnar deviation.

Commonly, the ulnar intrinsics are significantly tighter than the radial.

INDICATIONS

Intrinsic release is possibly one of the swiftest and most effective procedures in surgical practice. Complete excision of the wing tendon (Fig. 5.65) as advocated by Littler should be employed, as its removal eliminates not only the lateral band tightness which causes the weakness of grasp and contributes to the swan-neck deformity, but also that of the dorsal digital expansion which passes over the extrinsic extensor to form an extensor hood. Tightness of this expansion, together with the palmar moment of the flexor tendons, are the subluxing forces which dislocate the unstable metacarpophalangeal joint.

See Green D P 1993 Operative Hand Surgery, 3rd edn. Churchill Livingstone, New York, p. 1649.

Proximal interphalangeal joints

SYNOVIUM

The proximal interphalangeal joint of the rheumatoid patient is one of the earliest and most commonly afflicted. The synovium is driven dorsally by intra-articular pressures during flexion, where, as in other joints, it encounters less resistance. The central slip and the more medial and deep fibres of the lateral bands of the extensor tendon insert into the base of the middle phalanx. This firm tendinous insertion drives the bulging synovium proximally along the dorsum of the proximal phalanx. This has been called descriptively 'the synovial snail' (Fig. 5.66). The presence of

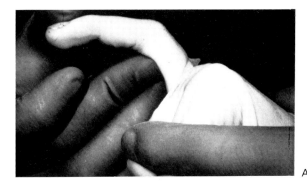

A

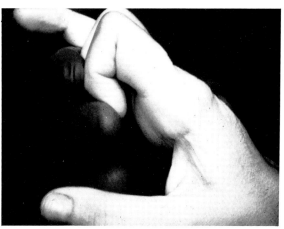

B

Fig. 5.65 The effect of intrinsic release. In (A) an unreleased finger is being stressed into flexion at the proximal interphalangeal joint with the metacarpophalangeal extended. In (B) two digits previously equally tight are being placed in the same position. The improvement in range is apparent.

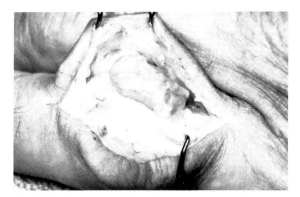

Fig. 5.66 The mass of diseased synovium is seen here being dissected from beneath the extensor apparatus at the proximal interphalangeal joint. The tip of the finger is to the left of the picture and the lateral bands and central slip are being supported by a retractor. The synovial mass has been dissected out entirely and is being gripped by the forceps in the lower part of the illustration.

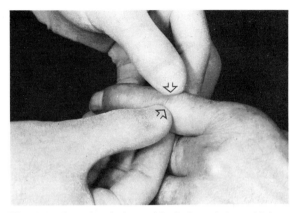

Fig. 5.67   Synovium is detected in the interphalangeal joint as a fluctuant swelling between the examiner's thumbs.

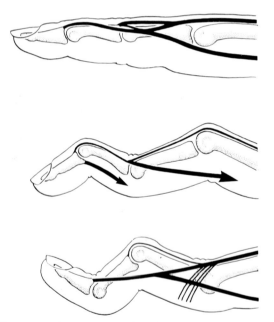

Fig. 5.68   The mechanism of development of swan-neck and boutonniere deformities is shown here in diagrammatic form. In the upper figure the extrinsic and intrinsic tendons, the central slip and lateral bands bear their normal relationship to the finger joints. In the centre illustration, tightness of the intrinsic associated with disease in the proximal interphalangeal joint has resulted in hyperextension of the proximal interphalangeal joint with compensatory flexion at the distal interphalangeal joint. In the lowermost diagram, disease in the proximal interphalangeal joint has caused weakness in the central slip and disruption of the aponeurosis between the central slip and lateral bands which have consequently fallen below the axis of the joint and become flexors rather than extensors. As a result the proximal interphalangeal joint has gone into flexion and the distal interphalangeal joint assumed compensatory hyperextension.

synovium can be detected as in other joints, by fluctuation beneath the examiner's thumbs with the joint held in gentle flexion to some 45 degrees (Fig. 5.67).

The destructive effect of synovitis on the soft tissues around the proximal interphalangeal joint depends on other forces acting on the joint and may take one of several forms:

boutonniere deformity
swan-neck deformity   } (Fig. 5.68)
joint destruction
lateral instability.

BOUTONNIERE DEFORMITY[117,118] (Fig. 5.69)

The extensor apparatus of the proximal interphalangeal joint is braced against the joint by the transverse retinacular ligament. This thin but distinct structure overlies the collateral and accessory collateral ligaments laterally. Dorsally it blends with the surface of the extensor components and ventrally with the cruciate part of the fibrous flexor tendon sheath. In resisted finger flexion, this cruciate portion moves away from the skeleton, as can be palpated quite distinctly in the normal hand, and this serves to stabilize the extensor apparatus and, by its embracing nature, the entire joint structure. In rheumatoid disease the 'synovial snail' stretches and often herniates through the weakest portion of the expansion which is that on either side of the central slip, between it and the lateral bands (Fig. 5.70). As this weakness increases, the lateral bands are pulled further anteriorly with each finger flexion by the transverse retinacular ligament. Flexor tenosynovitis, by stretching the flexor sheath, allows the flexor tendon to move further away from the skeleton, increasing the subluxing force applied to the lateral bands. The synovial erosion continues dorsally and, as in the metacarpophalangeal joint of the thumb, causes weakening and eventually complete disruption of the central slip. This results in loss of extensor power.

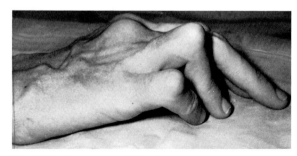

Fig. 5.69   Boutonniere deformity.

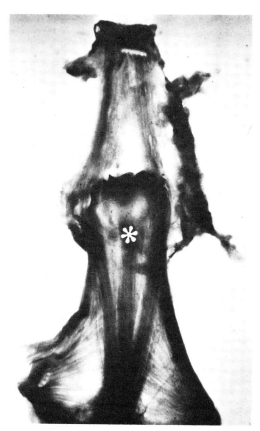

Fig. 5.70 This transilluminated specimen of the entire extensor apparatus shows the central slip marked with an asterisk. Distal to the asterisk, towards the upper part of the photograph, there is a weak point evident in the central slip. On either side of that point the connection between the central slip and lateral bands can also be seen to be somewhat thinner than the other parts of the extensor apparatus. These thin areas are those which are eroded by synovium in the proximal interphalangeal joint allowing the lateral bands to slip palmarwards. Attached to the lateral bands are the transverse retinacular ligaments which connect the bands to the cruciate part of the fibrous flexor tendon sheath (dissection by Dr D. C. Riordan).

Imbalance in favour of flexion at the proximal interphalangeal joint results in a flexion deformity and the Z-mechanism produces compensatory hyperextension at the metacarpophalangeal and distal interphalangeal joints. This deformity is initially *mobile*, that is, the joint shows a normal passive range of motion but later becomes *fixed*[119]. Only the former is amenable to soft-tissue reconstruction.

SWAN-NECK DEFORMITY (Fig. 5.71)[120,121]

This deformity also has its basis in weakening of the periarticular structures of the proximal interphalangeal

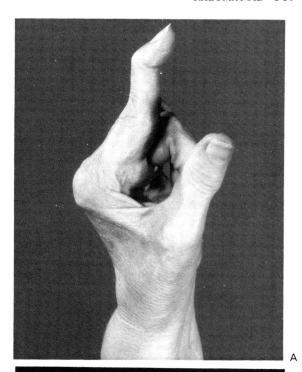

A

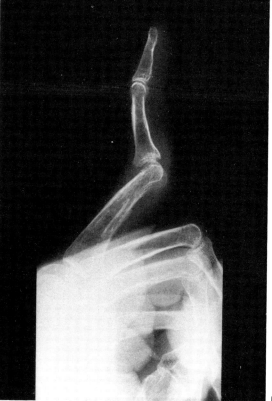

B

Fig. 5.71 Swan-neck deformity.

joint by active synovitis. The abnormal force applied to the joint is tightness of the intrinsic muscles. Some believe that swan neck will develop only with decreased flexor power, this resulting from synovitis around the flexor digitorum superficialis. The resultant hyperextension of the joint is initially added to a normal range of motion. However, joint disease allied to the inability of the weakened flexors to pull the middle phalanx around the head of the proximal phalanx from the increasingly hyperextended position results in a decreased range of motion. The Z-mechanism causes flexion in both distal interphalangeal and metacarpophalangeal joints.

RANGE OF MOTION

The range of motion should be recorded with a goniometer in each joint in turn. Hyperextension is recorded as a negative value. This may be misleading if the negative sign is misunderstood or overlooked. This problem can be overcome by illustrating the measurement with a small stick diagram.

INSTABILITY

The proximal interphalangeal joint is often unstable in swan-neck deformity as described above. Lateral stability should be tested by applying three-point stress with the finger in extension (Fig. 5.72). If the joint cannot be fully extended, too much importance should not be laid on minor degrees of apparent lateral instability (p. 63).

INDICATIONS

Early *swan-neck* deformity, that is before irreversible changes occur in the articular surface, can be corrected by:

1. Intrinsic release to eliminate the deforming force
2. Flexor synovectomy when synovitis is present
3. Correction of the hyperextension, which may be achieved by capsulodesis or by tenodesis.

Early, mobile *boutonniere* deformity may be improved by synovectomy and reconstruction of the extensor apparatus. This is an operation in which it is difficult to achieve improvement as is attested to by the large number of described procedures[122-131].

Advanced proximal interphalangeal deformities are amongst the most difficult to correct. Thus, the indications for synovectomy and intrinsic release are applied at an early juncture. Those for synovectomy are:

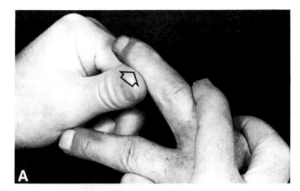

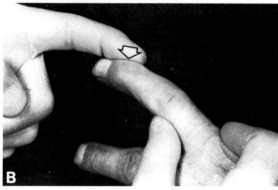

Fig. 5.72 A, B. Lateral stress should be applied in a three-point fashion to test the collateral ligaments on both the ulnar and radial aspects of all interphalangeal joints in maximum extension.

1. Persistent intractable painful synovitis
2. Early erosions seen on radiologic examination. These are best seen on true anteroposterior and lateral views using a dental film (Fig. 5.73).
3. Incipient boutonniere deformity as evidenced by synovitis associated with some lag to proximal interphalangeal joint extension.

Synovectomy of the proximal interphalangeal joint has been shown to result in significant relief of pain and improvement of grip strength in 60% of patients five years after surgery[132] and even to result in the healing of small erosions[133]. Flexor tendon disease has great significance in limiting motion of the proximal interphalangeal joint (p. 192).

Advanced swan-neck or boutonniere with articular changes, lateral instability or joint destruction precludes soft-tissue reconstruction. The choice lies between:

stabilization — by formal arthrodesis or by peg stabilization[134], and

replacement arthroplasty[135].

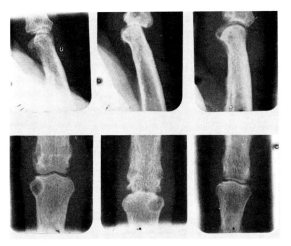

Fig. 5.73 Radiologic examination of the interphalangeal joints in the rheumatoid patient is best performed using dental films which allow true anteroposterior and lateral films to be obtained.

The choice is made according to the extent of disease in other parts of the hand, especially in the metacarpophalangeal joints and in the tendons acting on the proximal interphalangeal joint, the age and occupation of the patient and the digit which requires treatment. The index finger most requires stability for pinch manoeuvres, and stabilization there is more often indicated than in the ulnar digits where a range of motion is required for power grasp. In those digits therefore, the poorer the range of motion in the metacarpophalangeal joint, the more replacement arthroplasty is indicated.

See Green D P 1993 Operative Hand Surgery, 3rd edn. Churchill Livingstone, New York, p. 1654.

Distal interphalangeal joint

Rheumatoid synovitis is uncommon in the distal interphalangeal joint when compared with its incidence in other joints of the hand. Indeed, the presence of synovitis in the distal joint should arouse the examiner's suspicion that the patient is suffering not from rheumatoid disease but from *psoriasis* which is especially likely to cause distal joint disease.

The distal joint is certainly affected by classical rheumatoid but mainly in a secondary manner consequent upon proximal interphalangeal joint deformities. Deformity of the distal joint in both swan-neck and boutonniere deformities of the proximal interphalangeal joint is initially mobile, but later fixed. In the boutonniere especially, correction of a fixed contracture of the proximal interphalangeal joint must often be ac-

companied by atttention to the distal interphalangeal joint. In almost all instances arthrodesis or peg stabilization is the procedure most likely to aid function. The angle at which fusion is performed increases from radial to ulnar across the four digits.

Flexor tendons

SYNOVIUM

A smoothly contoured swelling proximal to the wrist creases is evidence of increase in the volume of synovium beneath the flexor retinaculum. This swelling can be seen to move a little proximally as the fingers are flexed. The presence of synovium in the digital sheaths is suggested if the skin over the proximal phalanges especially is unnaturally tense and shiny.

By supporting the supinated hand with his thumbs and placing the index and middle fingers of both hands across the palm so that the middle fingers are in contact with one another at the level of the palmar creases, the examiner is able to palpate the region of the flexor tendons as they emerge from the digital sheaths (Fig. 5.74). If the patient is then asked to close slowly all the fingers over those of the examiner, the crepitus created by increased, diseased synovium can be detected. By adjusting the finger tips to lie over each sheath in turn, the examiner can localize which tendons are involved. Not uncommonly, one or two fingers are involved and the others not. Further evidence of this selective involvement is gained by then asking the patient to open and close the hand repetitively as rapidly as possible. This may reveal that there is a 'slow finger' which flexes out of phase with the others, indicating active flexor synovitis even to the extent of causing a 'trigger finger'.

Trigger finger in rheumatoid disease may be due to locking at the proximal pulley as in non-rheumatoid patients. However, it may equally be caused by a nodule of synovium in the tendon, catching in the bifurcation of the flexor digitorum superficialis (Fig. 5.75).

A 'slow finger' can also be caused by a swan-neck deformity, flexion of the proximal interphalangeal joint being delayed until sufficient force has been generated by the flexor tendon to pull the middle phalanx around the head of the proximal phalanx (Fig. 5.76).

Palpation of the wrist in similar manner to that described above during finger flexion will detect crepitations due to diseased synovium.

NERVE COMPRESSION

Significant increase in the volume of synovium around the flexor tendons in the carpal tunnel may cause

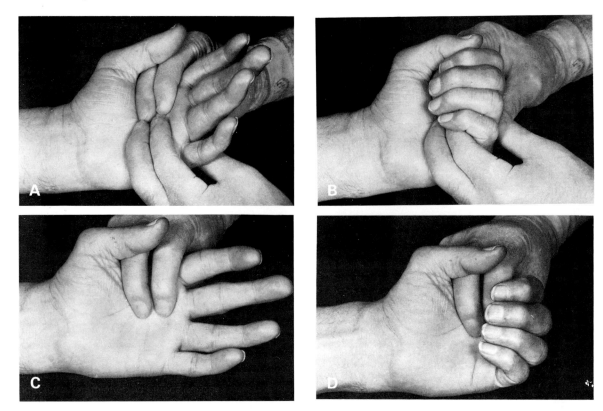

Fig. 5.74 A. The index and middle fingers of both hands of the examiner are placed across the palm of the patient and the patient is then asked to flex the fingers strongly, B. Crepitation can be detected in those synovial sheaths in which synovitis is present. This can be further localized by palpating the sheaths individually as in (C) and (D), while the patient repeats the manoeuvre.

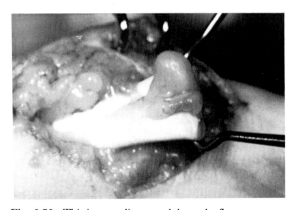

Fig. 5.75 This intratendinous nodule on the flexor digitorum profundus produced locking of the finger by blocking on the bifurcation of the flexor digitorum superficialis.

compression of the median nerve with typical symptoms of carpal tunnel syndrome (p. 285) — numbness and paraesthesia in the median nerve distribution and weakness and atrophy of the thenar muscles. More rarely, the sensory and motor loss will be in the distribution of the ulnar nerve indicating compression in Guyon's canal (p. 295).

It is important to seek these pathognomonic symptoms and signs in the rheumatoid patient who will frequently fail to volunteer them, either because they have been masked by his many other problems or because he or she believes that they are of little consequence by comparison.

TENDON RUPTURE[136,137]

Rupture of tendons occurs as a result of interference

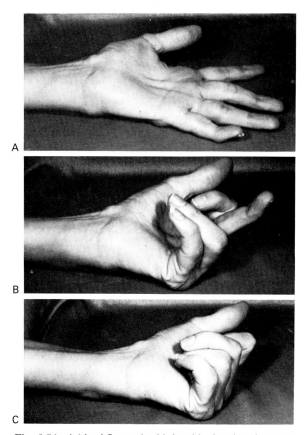

A

B

C

Fig. 5.76 A 'slow' finger. As this hand is closed so the swan-neck deformity of the middle finger causes it to delay (B) until increasing force of the flexor tendons pulls it suddenly and painfully around the head of the proximal phalanx into flexion (C).

with their blood supply and also of intratendinous infiltration of synovium. At surgery, smooth, relatively firm nodules of visceral synovium are found penetrating deeply between the tendon fibres. Individual testing of each flexor tendon should therefore be performed as described elsewhere. Weakness and pain on resisted flexion have less significance than in the injured tendon, since it is not possible to determine to what extent they are due to the synovitis itself or to impending rupture. Frequently tendon adhesions coexist with ruptures and incomplete tendon erosions. Thus the surgeon undertaking flexor synovectomy must prepare the patient for possible tendon graft and distal interphalangeal joint fusion and prepare himself for an often perplexing encounter.

INDICATIONS

Release of the carpal tunnel with complete *flexor syno-*

vectomy is indicated in the presence of median nerve compression. Trigger fingers should be treated by synovectomy where indicated, particular attention being paid to the presence of intratendinous nodules of synovium which may be the primary cause of the triggering. The A1 pulley should always be preserved for its excision will increase the force of the ulnar moment of the flexor on the metacarpophalangeal joint. Where meticulous synovectomy does not eliminate triggering, one slip of the superficialis should be excised rather than incur that risk[138]. When triggering alone is being treated, surgery should be done under wrist block to ensure full active function after treatment

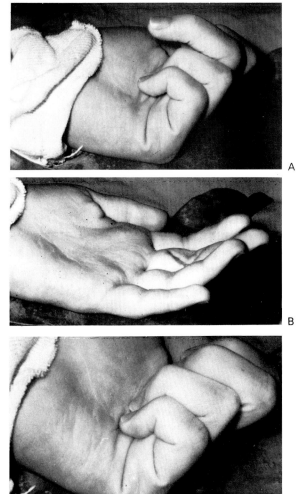

A

B

C

Fig. 5.77 Exploration of a trigger finger under local anaesthesia. A. The patient is unable to form a full fist. B. A nodule could be palpated over the proximal interphalangeal joint (Fig. 5.75). Excision resulted in full flexion (C).

(Fig. 5.77). The efficacy of flexor tenosynovectomy[139] is considerable in improving motion in the proximal interphalangeal joint — in one series[140] the range increased from 40 to 84°.

Synovectomy is indicated whenever a significant bulk of synovium is detected around the flexor tendons (Fig. 5.78). Delay in this situation is not justified, largely because it is not possible to determine clinically to what extent tendon erosion has progressed and also because the results of tendon graft in the rheumatoid patient are too poor to justify the risk of delay. When rupture is encountered, it should be managed as follows:

flexor pollicis longus — graft

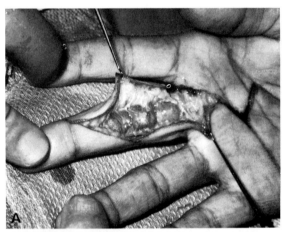

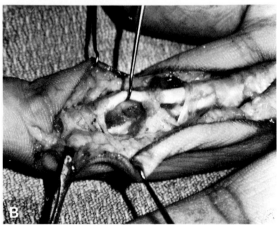

Fig. 5.78 Through a Bruner incision the flexor tendon sheath has been displayed in this patient with rheumatoid flexor synovitis. A. The bulging, particularly of the cruciate part of the tendon sheath, is clearly to be seen. B. When the tendon sheath is opened the extensive nature of the diseased synovium can be appreciated.

flexor digitorum profundus — fuse distal interphalangeal joint
both FDS and FDP — transfer intact FDS from adjacent finger to FDP.

See Green D P 1993 Operative Hand Surgery, 3rd edn. Churchill Livingstone, New York, pp. 1603 and 1618.

Radiologic assessment

All patients complaining of rheumatoid disease in the upper limb should undergo radiological examination of:

neck — especially requesting lateral views taken in extension and flexion
elbow
wrist and *hands*, including Brewerton views of the metacarpophalangeal joints.

As emphasized above, all rheumatoid patients are in danger of cervical cord compression and transection (p. 362).

The *Brewerton view*[141] of the metacarpophalangeal joints is taken with the fingers flat on the plate, the metacarpals at 65 degrees inclination to them and the tube at 15 degrees from the ulnar side of the hand (Fig. 5.79). In early rheumatoid disease, when the standard anteroposterior view of the hand shows little change, the Brewerton view may show a surprising amount of bony erosion beneath the collateral ligaments of the metacarpophalangeal joints.

Apart from these standard views, radiographs should be taken of any other joints of which the patient specifically complains. In the severely diseased hand, the standard views do not always demonstrate the proximal interphalangeal joints clearly, in which case true individual anteroposterior and lateral views should be taken of each proximal interphalangeal joint.

In all joints involved by rheumatoid disease, the changes are similar on radiologic examination, in order of appearance:

Loss of joint space. Due to loss of articular surface, this may be seen relatively early in the patient's clinical course, but is evidence of fairly advanced disease.
Bony erosions. Bony erosion is always evidence of advanced rheumatoid disease.
Subluxation.
Ankylosis.

'*Egg-cup' deformity* is encountered on occasion in the metacarpophalangeal joint (Fig. 5.80). This nomenclature is used when the erosion in that joint is into the base of the proximal phalanx, the head of the metacarpal being bluntly conical. No subluxation or ulnar

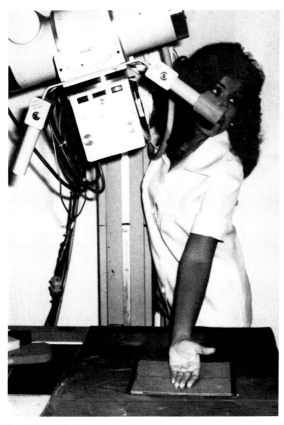

Fig. 5.79 The Brewerton view (see text).

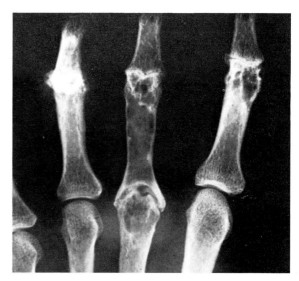

Fig. 5.80 This radiograph demonstrates an 'egg cup deformity' of the metacarpophalangeal joint of the middle finger. In this, no subluxation or deviation has occurred, and the erosion in the metacarpophalangeal joint is at the base of the proximal phalanx. This commonly results in a pain-free joint having an excellent range of motion. No surgical intervention is indicated.

drift of significance accompanies this deformity, and the patient usually has a good range of motion with little pain. No surgical intervention is indicated.

Giant bone cysts may occur in conjunction with rheumatoid disease, most commonly in the ulnar head[142].

As several authors have emphasized, the assessment of rheumatoid disease is made clinically, not radiologically.

RHEUMATOID VARIANTS

Certain patients, while having polyarthritis apparently indistinguishable from rheumatoid arthritis, show certain features which set them in a different category.

Juvenile rheumatoid arthritis (JRA)[143,144]

This presents in three different clinical forms:

1. *Systemic onset type JRA* (Still's disease[145]) — 20% — is characterized by polyarthritis associated with systemic manifestations such as *uveitis, pericarditis, splenomegaly, hepatomegaly* and *fever*.

2. *Polyarticular JRA* — 40% — is very similar to the adult form of the disease by distribution, although having different effects as outlined below. This is the most likely form to continue unabated into adult rheumatoid disease.

3. *Mono-articular or pauci-articular JRA* — 40% — affects four or less joints. In one series[146], 32% progressed to involve other joints at a later stage. Eye problems were common.

Some 80% of children with JRA are seronegative. The deformities in the upper extremity are often quite different from the adult form:

shortening of the ulna
flexion and *ulnar* deviation of the wrist, often progressing to ankylosis
radial deviation and loss of flexion of the metacarpophalangeal joints (Fig. 5.81)
boutonniere common (swan-neck rare)
altered growth due to premature epiphyseal fusion

Unlike adult disease, tendon rupture and nerve compression rarely occur.

The key to management is splintage of the wrist in good position at virtually all times. Regular therapy to maintain finger motion during the day, allied to night resting splints, will help to prevent deformity.

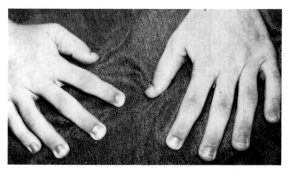

Fig. 5.81 Juvenile rheumatoid arthritis. The ulnar deviation at the wrist with radial drift of the fingers is commonly encountered in juvenile rheumatoid disease.

Synovectomy can give pain relief and has been shown to cause no harm[147]. Once deformity is established, corrective surgery may improve function although, as with the arthrogrypotic child (p. 483), caution should be exercised for these intelligent people have adjusted to their limitations with great skill. Osteotomy of the radius will align the wrist, as may proximal row carpectomy. Capsular release at the metacarpophalangeal joints may improve flexion. Once skeletal maturity has been reached, arthrodesis of the digital joints may improve position. Implant arthroplasty has little part to play — in the young it would transgress epiphyses, in the skeletally mature the implants rarely fit into the very narrow bones.

Ankylosing spondylitis

This condition usually commences at the sacroiliac joints and involves the spine. Clinically, the diagnosis can be made on the basis of five specific historical features[148]:

back pain of insidious onset
patient under 40 (M/F = 10/1)
present for more than 3 months
morning stiffness
stiffness improves with exercise.

Some 20% show peripheral arthritis indistinguishable from rheumatoid disease, although there is a much greater tendency to ankylosis of joints than to their destruction. Less than 10% show positive tests for rheumatoid factor. The HLA type B27[149] is present in the serum of well over 90% of patients with ankylosing spondylitis as compared with 4% of the general population.

Systemic lupus erythematosus[150,151] (SLE)

Almost all patients have a positive fluorescent antinuclear antibody test (ANA). SLE causes painful, swollen, but rarely destroyed, joints. If deformity does occur it is due to ligamentous laxity and takes the form of subluxation, with *little evidence of radiologic changes*. Swan-neck deformities and hyperextension of the interphalangeal joint of the thumb are common, but the first is not accompanied by intrinsic tightness or the latter by a flexion contracture of the metacarpophalangeal joint. In the rare cases in whom destruction and radiologic changes do occur then some 'overlap' of rheumatoid and systemic lupus erythematosus is probable.

Raynaud's phenomenon is found in some 50% of these patients (p. 263) and may be responsible for the major part of the symptoms in the hand.

Where ligamentous laxity becomes extreme to the point of impairing hand function, resection of a subluxed ulnar head and stabilization of the basal joint of the thumb are of value. Other, soft-tissue, procedures are generally not successful, and in severe deformities arthroplasty of the wrist or metacarpophalangeal joints may be necessary[152].

Systemic sclerosis[153]

Scleroderma shows polyarthritis but the joint deformities result from fibrous contractures of skin and muscle

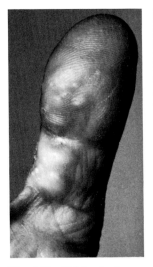
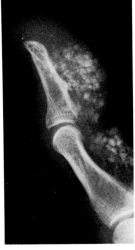

Fig. 5.82 Calcinosis circumscripta in a patient with systemic sclerosis. Excision of the calcific nodular deposits may relieve the discomfort they cause, but caution is required since healing in scleroderma is not normal.

rather than from erosive synovitis. However, when it presents as a polyarthritis without any of its other features, it may not be possible to distinguish it from rheumatoid, especially since 20–40% will be seropositive. Other manifestations should therefore be sought in patients presenting with joint deformity, muscle wasting but little bony change. *Calcinosis circumscripta* can occur independently, but in the majority of cases is associated with scleroderma[154] (Fig. 5.82).

In scleroderma the hand surgeon can be of assistance by:

1. Prescribing careful splintage and active and passive exercise to prevent contracture
2. Urgently treating early infections which will otherwise progress to extensive ulceration
3. Performing digital sympathectomy and vascular reconstruction in attempts to save digits
4. Fuse digital joints when contractures become too extreme. (Ulcers exposing bone may heal remarkably if placed completely at rest.)

Mixed connective tissue disease (MCTD)[155]

This disorder has features in common with both lupus and scleroderma; the majority of patients show Raynaud's phenomenon and also decreased oesophageal motility. Serology can distinguish between the three disorders, of which MCTD appears most responsive to steroid therapy.

The striking feature in the hands of patients with MCTD is *tightness of the long flexors*, resulting in a significant decrease in finger extension, which progressively worsens with wrist extension. Less common manifestations are intrinsic tightness and boutonniere deformity of the thumb.

Psoriatic arthritis

Psoriatic arthritis[156,157] may resemble rheumatoid very closely. However, it is distinguished by several features:

negative rheumatoid factor
absence of rheumatoid nodules
presence of a typical skin rash
involvement of the distal interphalangeal joints

and radiologically:

osteolysis of the distal phalanges
cortical erosions of the phalangeal shafts
periosteal new bone formation near the joints.

Usually the deformity shows much less destruction of articular cartilage, and deformities are due more to

contracture than collapse, although a small minority may show *arthritis mutilans* (p. 360). Surgery is undertaken later than in rheumatoid disease and is designed to overcome deformity, for example of the metacarpophalangeal joints by metacarpal osteotomy[158].

Ulcerative colitis; regional enteritis (Crohn's)

Patients with colitis or enteritis often show transient arthritis of the peripheral joints. Only 10% of these progress to classic rheumatoid-like changes. Seronegative, if these patients are cured of their visceral disorder, their arthritis invariably shows marked improvement.

Behçet's syndrome (= mucocutaneous ocular syndrome)

This condition, probably a cell-mediated immunologic response, has many varied manifestations, major amongst which are recurrent oral and genital ulceration and relapsing iritis.

Arthritis is common, usually occurring long after the onset, and resembling the arthropathy of ulcerative colitis. It usually affects the elbow and wrist and is not associated with permanent changes. The sedimentation rate is increased and the patients are seronegative for rheumatoid factor.

Reiter's syndrome

Polyarthritis
Non-gonococcal urethritis
Conjunctivitis

Mucocutaneous papules, vesicles or pustules are often encountered on the glans penis, the soles and palms and in the mouth. Seronegative, their joint changes are usually transitory but may show recurrent exacerbations. Diagnosis then rests on the other manifestations. As with ankylosing spondylitis, the incidence of B27-positive cases is very high.

Other forms of so-called *reactive arthritis* have been described in association with infections by *Salmonella*, *Yersinia*, *Brucella* and *Neisseria gonorrhoeae*.

SURGICAL PLANNING

The aim of surgical treatment is to restore better function: improve mobility, provide adequate stability, correct deformity, increase power, relieve pain and facilitate the patient's return to normal activity[159].

Choosing the time at which to operate on the rheumatoid patient depends upon the stage of their disease, the degree of their disability, priority with respect to other parts of the body and convenience in their normal work and social schedule. This latter consideration is of more importance in the rheumatoid than in others, for several surgical assaults can be anticipated over the years. Urgency exists with respect to nerve compression and tendon rupture or the threat of it, most commonly by extensor synovitis and a dislocated ulnar head. Synovectomy is prophylactic in protecting tendons at the dorsal wrist and in the proximal interphalangeal joint. It appears to improve function and may have some protective value in the elbow joint and in the flexor tendons. Its merits in other areas are unproven. Soft tissue reconstruction is of benefit in the presence of good articular cartilage in deformities of the thumb and in mobile boutonniere or swan-neck deformities.

Once joints are irrevocably deformed or destroyed, the surgeon must be aware of the functional needs in each joint. *Stability* is required in the wrist, the metacarpophalangeal and interphalangeal joints of the thumb and the distal interphalangeal joints of the fingers. *Mobility* is required in *one* elbow, the basal joint of the thumb and the metacarpophalangeal joints of the fingers. Hence, ankylosis in the first group and instability in the second is not nearly as disabling as if the situation were reversed. It follows further that arthrodesis of the first group and arthroplasty of the second are the required procedures, modified only by considerations such as the need for one wrist to reach the perineum. Only the proximal interphalangeal joints remain in limbo: they do well with arthrodesis in the index finger and in the others if the metacarpophalangeal joints show a good range; they require arthroplasty if those metacarpophalangeal joints do not show motion and cannot be made to do so. The minimal aims in treating the rheumatoid finger is to achieve coordinate motion of all fingers at one of the joints at least, with the non-mobile joints in a functional position and the whole finger complex showing good lateral stability.

Consulting the summary sheet (p. 358) and remembering the need for compatibility of simultaneous operations during postoperative care and therapy, the surgeon should construct a surgical programme with the patient. If to do so would not ignore priorities imposed by specific patient problems, the programme should work from proximal to distal. It should combine procedures which are complementary and serve to remove at the same operation mutually deforming disorders. For example, the correction of radial deviation of the wrist with metacarpophalangeal joint replacement is logical[160]. Finally, the necessary work under tourniquet control should be limited to one inflation time, that is, a maximum of two hours. Second inflation greatly increases oedema, with resultant difficulty in skin closure and in early postoperative mobilization. It is also likely that the rheumatoid patient, resourceful and uncomplaining though he undoubtedly is, suffers untold discomfort in other parts from prolonged periods on the operating table. Further, recovery, rehabilitation and therefore return for other necessary surgery are all speeded by so limiting our endeavours.

As to the outcome of our work, Souter[161] has placed a realistic 'score' on the surgical armamentarium available to the surgeon treating rheumatoid disease. This is expressed below as a 'percentage of satisfaction'.

Fusion of the MP joint of the thumb	85
Extensor synovectomy and excision ulnar head	83
Wrist stabilization	73
Flexor synovectomy	68
PIP fusion	68
IP fusion in the thumb	68
MP arthroplasty	65
Correction of swan-neck	65
MP and proximal interphalangeal synovectomy	53
PIP arthroplasty	43
Correction of boutonniere	35

REFERENCES

1. Nicolle F V, Dickson R A 1979 Surgery of the rheumatoid hand. Heinemann Medical Books, London
2. Bywaters E G L, Scott J T 1963 The natural history of vascular lesions in rheumatoid arthritis. J Chronic Dis 16: 905
3. Labbate V A, Ehrlich E E 1976 Rheumatoid arthritis with unusual myositis resembling muscular dystrophy. J Bone Joint Surg 58A: 571–572
4. Garner R W, Mowat A G, Hazleman B L 1973 Wound healing after operations on patients with rheumatoid arthritis. J Bone Joint Surg 55B: 134–144
5. Schneller S 1989 Medical considerations and perioperative care for rheumatoid surgery. Hand Clin 5: 115–126
6. Cervantes-Perez Col P, Toro-Perez Col A H, Rodriguez Jurado P 1980 Pulmonary involvement in rheumatoid arthritis. J Am Med Assoc 243: 1715–1719
7. Caplan A 1953 Certain unusual appearances in the chest of coal miners suffering from rheumatoid arthritis. Thorax 8: 29–37
8. Felty A R 1924 Chronic arthritis in the adult associated with splenomegaly and leukopenia. Bull Johns Hopkins Hosp 35: 16–20
9. Sjogren H 1933 A new conception of kerato

conjunctivitis sicca. Acta Ophthal Kbh suppl 2: 1

10. Miller-Breslow A, Millender L H, Feldon PG 1989 Treatment considerations in the complicated rheumatoid hand. Hand Clin 5: 279–289

11. Froimson A I 1971 Hand reconstruction in arthritis mutilans. J Bone Joint Surg 53A: 1377–1382

12. Nalebuff E A, Garrett J 1976 Opera glass hand in rheumatoid arthritis. J Hand Surg 1: 210–220

13. Williams H J, Biddulph E C, Coleman S S, Ward I R 1977 Isolated subcutaneous nodules (pseudorheumatoid). J Bone Joint Surg 59A: 73–76

14. McGrath M H, Fleischer A 1989 The subcutaneous rheumatoid nodule. Hand Clin 5: 127–135

15. Fleischer E, McGrath M H 1984 Rheumatoid nodulosis of the hand. J Hand Surg (Am) 9: 404–411

16. Sadegbpour E, Noer H R, Mahinpour S 1981 Skull-C2 fusion in rheumatoid patients with atlantoaxial subluxation. Orthopedics 4: 1369–1374

17. Ranawat C S, O'Leary P, Pellicci P, Tsairis P, Marchisello P, Dorr L 1979 Cervical spine fusion in rheumatoid arthritis. J Bone Joint Surg 61A: 1003–1010

18. Rana N A, Hancock D O, Taylor A R, Hill A G S 1973 Atlanto-axial subluxation in rheumatoid arthritis. J Bone Joint Surg 55B: 458–470

19. Rana N A, Hancock D O, Taylor A R, Hill A G S 1973 Upward translocation of the dens in rheumatoid arthritis. J Bone Joint Surg 55B: 471–477

20. Pellicci P M, Ranawat C S, Tsairis P, Bryan W I 1981 A prospective study of the progression of rheumatoid arthritis of the cervical spine. J Bone Joint Surg 63A: 342–350

21. Boyd A D Jr, Thornhill T S 1989 Surgical treatment of the elbow in rheumatoid arthritis. Hand Clin 4: 645–655

22. Brumfield R H, Resnick C T 1985 Synovectomy of the elbow in rheumatoid arthritis. J Bone Joint Surg 67A: 16

23. Eichenblat M, Wass A, Kessler I 1982 Synovectomy of the elbow in rheumatoid arthritis. J Bone Joint Surg 64A: 1074

24. Copeland S A, Taylor I G 1979 Synovectomy of the elbow in rheumatoid arthritis. J Bone Joint Surg 61B: 69–74

25. Inglis A E, Ranawat C S, Straub L R 1971 Synovectomy and debridement of the elbow in rheumatoid arthritis. J Bone Joint Surg 53A: 652–662

26. Marmor L 1972 Surgery of the rheumatoid elbow. Follow-up study on synovectomy combined with radial head excision. J Bone Joint Surg 54A: 573–578

27. Wilson D W 1973 Synovectomy of the elbow in rheumatoid arthritis. J Bone Joint Surg 55B: 106–111

28. Wright P E, Stewart M J 1985 Fascial arthroplasty of the elbow. In: Morrey B F (ed) The elbow and its disorders. WB Saunders Co, Philadelphia, p 530

29. Pritchard R 1979 Semiconstrained elbow prosthesis. A clinical review of five years of experience. Orthopaedic Rev 8: 33–43

30. Kudo H, Iwano K, Watanabe S 1980 Total replacement of the rheumatoid elbow with a hingeless prosthesis. J Bone Joint Surg 62A: 277–285

31. Pritchard R 1981 Long-term follow-up study: semi-constrained elbow prosthesis. Orthopedics 4: 151–155

32. Ewald F C, Scheinberg R D, Poss R, Thomas W H, Scott R D, Sledge C B 1980 Capitellocondylar total

elbow arthroplasty. J Bone Joint Surg 62A: 1259–1263

33. Morrey B F, Bryan R S, Dobyns I H, Linscheid R L 1981 Total elbow arthroplasty. A five year experience at the Mayo Clinic. J Bone Joint Surg 63A: 1050–1063

34. Inglis A E, Pellicci P A M 1980 Total elbow replacement. J Bone Joint Surg 62A: 1252–1258

35. Taylor A R, Mukerjea S K, Rana N A 1976 Excision of the head of the radius in rheumatoid arthritis. J Bone Joint Surg 58B: 485–487

36. Mayhall W S T, Tiley F T, Paluska D I 1981 Fracture of silastic radial-head prosthesis. Case report. J Bone Joint Surg 63A: 459–460

37. Morrey B F, Askew L, Chao E T 1981 Silastic prosthetic replacement for the radial head. J Bone Joint Surg 63A: 454–458

38. Bohl W R, Brightman E 1981 Fracture of a silastic radial-head prosthesis: diagnosis and localization of fragments by xerography. J Bone Joint Surg 63A: 1482–1483

39. Taleisnik J 1989 Rheumatoid arthritis of the wrist. Hand Clin 5: 257–278

40. Shapiro J S 1970 A new factor in the etiology of ulnar drift. Clin Orthop 68: 32

41. Shapiro J S 1982 Wrist involvement in rheumatoid swan-neck deformity. J Hand Surg 7: 484

42. O'Donovan T M, Ruby L K 1989 The distal radioulnar joint in rheumatoid arthritis. Hand Clin 5: 249–256

43. Thirupathi R G, Ferlic D C, Clayton M L 1983 Dorsal wrist synovectomy in rheumatoid arthritis — a long-term study. J Hand Surg (Am) 8: 848–856

44. Bieber E J, Linscheid R L, Dobyns J H, Beckenbaugh R D 1988 Failed distal ulna resections. J Hand Surg (Am) 13: 193–200

45. Breen T F, Jupiter J B 1989 Extensor carpi ulnaris and flexor carpi ulnaris tenodesis of the unstable distal ulna. J Hand Surg (Am) 14: 612–617

46. White R E Jr 1986 Resection of the distal ulna with and without implant arthroplasty in rheumatoid arthritis. J Hand Surg (Am) 11: 514–518

47. McMurtry R Y, Paley D, Marks P, Axelrod T 1990 A critical analysis of Swanson ulnar head replacement arthroplasty: rheumatoid versus nonrheumatoid. J Hand Surg (Am) 15: 224–231

48. Bowers W H 1985 Distal radioulnar joint arthroplasty: the hemiresection–interposition technique. J Hand Surg (Am) 10: 169–178

49. Watson H K, Ryu J Y, Burgess R C 1986 Matched distal ulnar resection. J Hand Surg (Am) 11: 812–817

50. Rana N A, Taylor A R 1973: Excision of the distal end of the ulna in rheumatoid arthritis. J Bone Joint Surg 55B: 96–105

51. Ansell B M, Harrison S H 1974 The results of ulna styloidectomy in rheumatoid arthritis. Scand Rheumatol 3: 67

52. Jackson I T, Simpson R G 1979 Interpositional arthroplasty of the wrist in rheumatoid arthritis. Hand 11: 169–175

53. Linscheid R L, Dobyns J H 1985 Radiolunate arthrodesis. J Hand Surg (Am) 10: 821–829

54. Taleisnik J 1987 Combined radiocarpal arthrodesis and midcarpal (lunocapitate) arthroplasty for treatment of rheumatoid arthritis of the wrist. J Hand Surg (Am) 12: 1–8

55. Vicar A J, Burton R I 1986 Surgical management of the

rheumatoid wrist — fusion or arthroplasty. J Hand (Am) 11: 790–797

56. Straub L R, Ranawat C S 1969 The wrist in rheumatoid arthritis. J Bone Joint Surg 51A: 1–20
57. Clayton M L 1965 Surgical treatment at the wrist in rheumatoid arthritis. J Bone Joint Surg 47A: 741–750
58. Kulick R G, DeFiore I C, Straub L R, Ranawat C S 1981 Long-term results of dorsal stabilization in the rheumatoid wrist. J Hand Surg 6: 272–280
59. Ryu J, Watson H K, Burgess R C 1985 Rheumatoid wrist reconstruction utilizing a fibrous nonunion and radiocarpal arthrodesis. J Hand Surg (Am) 10: 830–836
60. Lamberta F I, Ferlic D C, Clayton M L 1980 Volz total wrist arthroplasty in rheumatoid arthritis: a preliminary report. J Hand Surg 5: 245–252
61. Figgie M P, Ranawat C S, Inglis A E, Sobel M, Figgie H E 3rd 1990 Trispherical total wrist arthroplasty in rheumatoid arthritis. J Hand Surg (Am) 15: 217–223
62. Dennis D A, Ferlic D C, Clayton M L 1986 Volz total wrist arthroplasty in rheumatoid arthritis: a long-term review. J Hand Surg (Am) 11: 483–490
63. Goodman M I, Millender L H, Nalebuff E A, Philips C A 1980 Arthroplasty of the rheumatoid wrist with silicone rubber: an early evaluation. J Bone Joint Surg 5: 114–121
64. Dennis D A, Clayton M L, Ferlic D C, Patchett C E 1985 Bilateral traumatic dislocations of Volz total wrist arthroplasties: a case report. J Hand Surg (Am) 10: 503–504
65. Dawson W J 1989 Radius fracture after total wrist arthroplasty. J Hand Surg (Am) 14: 630–634
66. Siemionow M, Lister G D 1987 Tendon ruptures and median nerve damage after Hamas total wrist arthroplasty. J Hand Surg (Am) 12: 374–377
67. Comstock C P, Louis D S, Eckenrode J F 1988 Silicone wrist implant: long-term follow-up study. J Hand Surg (Am) 13: 201–205
68. Fatti J F, Palmer A K, Mosher J F 1986 The long-term results of Swanson silicone rubber interpositional wrist arthroplasty. J Hand Surg (Am) 11: 166–175
69. Brase D W, Millender L H 1986 Failure of silicone rubber wrist arthroplasty in rheumatoid arthritis. J Hand Surg (Am) 11: 175–183
70. Haddad R I, Riordan D C 1967 Arthrodesis of the wrist. J Bone Joint Surg 49A: 950–954
71. Mikkelsen O T 1980 Arthrodesis of the wrist joint in rheumatoid arthritis. Hand 12: 149–153
72. Vahvanen V, Tallroth K 1984 Arthrodesis of the wrist by internal fixation in rheumatoid arthritis: a follow-up study of forty-five consecutive cases. J Hand Surg (Am) 9: 531–536
73. Millender L H, Nalebuff E A 1973 Arthrodesis of the rheumatoid wrist. J Bone Joint Surg 55A: 1026–1234
74. Rayan G M, Brentlinger A, Purnell D, Garcia-Moral C A 1987 Functional assessment of bilateral wrist arthrodeses. J Hand Surg (Am) 12: 1020–1024
75. Rana N A, Taylor A R 1973 Excision of the distal end of the ulna in rheumatoid arthritis. J Bone Joint Surg 55B: 96–105
76. Straub L R, Wilson E H 1956 Spontaneous rupture of extensor tendons in the hand associated with rheumatoid arthritis. J Bone Joint Surg 38A: 1208–1217
77. Leslie B M 1989 Rheumatoid extensor tendon ruptures. Hand Clin 5: 191–202

78. Millender L H, Nalebuff E A, Holdsworth D E 1973 Posterior interosseous nerve syndrome secondary to rheumatoid synovitis. J Bone Joint Surg 55A: 753–757
79. White S H, Goodfellow J W, Mowat A 1988 Posterior interosseous nerve palsy in rheumatoid arthritis. J Bone Joint Surg (Br) 70: 468–471
80. Bora F W Jr, Osterman A L, Thomas V J, Maitin E C, Polineni S 1987 The treatment of ruptures of multiple extensor tendons at wrist level by a free tendon graft in the rheumatoid patient. J Hand Surg (Am) 12: 1038–1040
81. Mannerfelt L G 1988 Tendon transfers in surgery of the rheumatoid hand. Hand Clin 4: 309–316
82. Moore J R, Weiland A J, Valdata L 1987 Tendon ruptures in the rheumatoid hand: analysis of treatment and functional results in 60 patients. J Hand Surg (Am) 12: 9–14
83. Moore J R, Weiland A J, Valdata L 1987 Independent index extension after extensor indicis proprius transfer. J Hand Surg (Am) 12: 232–236
84. Nalebuff E A, Patel M R 1973 Flexor digitorum superficialis transfer for multiple extensor tendon ruptures in rheumatoid arthritis. Plastic Reconstr Surg 52: 530–533
85. Nalebuff E A 1968 Diagnosis classification and management of rheumatoid thumb deformities. Bull Hosp Joint Dis 29: 119–137
86. Inglis A E, Hamlin C, Sengelmann R P 1972 Reconstruction of the metacarpophalangeal joint of the thumb in rheumatoid arthritis. J Bone Joint Surg 54A: 704–712
87. Harrison S, Smith P, Maxwell D 1977 Stabilization of the first metacarpophalangeal and terminal joints of the thumb. Hand 9: 242–249
88. Terrono A, Millender L 1989 Surgical treatment of the boutonniere rheumatoid thumb deformity. Hand Clin 5: 239–248
89. Swanson A B, Herndon J H 1977 Flexible (silicone) implant arthroplasty of the metacarpophalangeal joint of the thumb. J Bone Joint Surg 59A: 362–368
90. Figgie M P, Inglis A E, Sobel M, Bohn W W, Fisher D A 1990 Metacarpal-phalangeal joint arthroplasty of the rheumatoid thumb. J Hand Surg (Am) 15: 210–216
91. Kessler R 1973 Aetiology and management of adduction contracture of the thumb in rheumatoid arthritis. Hand 5: 170–174
92. Kessler I 1979 A simplified technique to correct hyperextension deformity of the metacarpophalangeal joint of the thumb. J Bone Joint Surg 61A: 903–905
93. Eaton R G, Floyd W E 3rd 1988 Thumb metacarpophalangeal capsulodesis: an adjunct procedure to basal joint arthroplasty for collapse deformity of the first ray. J Hand Surg (Am) 13: 449–453
94. Posner M A, Langa V, Ambrose L 1988 Intrinsic muscle advancement to treat chronic palmar instability of the metacarpophalangeal joint of the thumb. J Hand Surg (Am) 13: 110–115
95. Wilson R L, Carlblom E R 1989 The rheumatoid metacarpophalangeal joint. Hand Clin 5: 223–237
96. Zancolli E 1970 Arthritic ulnar drift. An operation for metacarpophalangeal dislocation before cartilage destruction. J Bone Joint Surg 52A: 1067
97. Ellison M R, Kelly K I, Flatt A E 1971 The results of

surgical synovectomy of the digital joints in rheumatoid disease. J Bone Joint Surg 53A: 1041–1060

98. McMaster M 1972 The natural history of the rheumatoid metacarpophalangeal joint. J Bone Joint Surg 54B: 687–697

99. Smith R I, Kaplan E B 1967 Rheumatoid deformities at the metacarpophalangeal joints of the fingers. J Bone Joint Surg 49A: 31–47

100. Hakstian R W, Tubiana R 1968 Ulnar deviation of the fingers. J Bone Joint Surg 49A: 299–316

101. Backhouse K M 1968 Mechanics of normal digital control in the hand and an analysis of ulnar drift of the rheumatoid hand. Ann Roy Coll Surg Engl 43: 154–173

102. Flatt A E 1983 Care of the arthritic hand, 4th edn. C V Mosby, St Louis

103. Pahle J A, Raunio P 1969 Influence of wrist position on finger deviation in rheumatoid arthritis. J Bone Joint Surg 51B: 664–676

104. Wise K S 1975 The anatomy of the metacarpophalangeal joints, with observations of the aetiology of ulnar drift. J Bone Joint Surg 578: 485–490

105. Oster L H, Blair W F, Steyers C M, Flatt A E 1989 Crossed intrinsic transfer. J Hand Surg (Am) 14: 963–971

106. Ellison M R, Flatt A E, Kelly K I 1974 Ulnar drift of the finger in rheumatoid disease. J Bone Joint Surg 53A: 1061–1082

107. Wood V E, Ichtertz D R, Yahiku H 1989 Soft tissue metacarpophalangeal reconstruction for treatment of rheumatoid hand deformity. J Hand Surg (Am) 14: 163–174

108. Vainio K 1989 Vainio arthroplasty of the metacarpophalangeal joints in rheumatoid arthritis. J Hand Surg (Am) 14: 367–368

109. Riordan D C, Fowler S B 1989 Arthroplasty of the metacarpophalangeal joints: review of resection-type arthroplasty. J Hand Surg (Am) 14: 368–371

110. Tupper J W 1989 The metacarpophalangeal volar plate arthroplasty. J Hand Surg (Am) 14: 371–375

111. Swanson A B 1973 Flexible implant arthroplasty in the hand and extremities. C V Mosby, St Louis

112. Swanson A F, Leonard J B, deGroot Swanson G 1986 Implant resection arthroplasty of the finger joints. Hand Clin 2: 107–117

113. Derkash R S, Niebauer J J Jr, Lane C S 1986 Long-term follow-up of metacarpal phalangeal arthroplasty with silicone Dacron prostheses. J Hand Surg (Am) 11: 553–558

114. Beckenbaugh R D, Dobyns J H, Linscheid R L, Bryan R S 1976 Review and analysis of silicone-rubber metacarpophalangeal implants. J Bone Joint Surg 58A: 483–487

115. Blair W F, Shurr D G, Buckwalter J A 1984 Metacarpophalangeal joint implant arthroplasty with a silastic spacer. J Bone Joint Surg 66A: 365–370

116. Vahvanen V, Viljakka T 1986 Silicone rubber implant arthroplasty of the metacarpophalangeal joint in rheumatoid arthritis: a follow-up study of 32 patients. J Hand Surg (Am) 11: 333–339

117. Nalebuff E A, Millender L H 1975 Surgical treatment of the boutonniere deformity in rheumatoid arthritis. Orthopedic Clin North Am 6: 753–763

118. Ferlic D C 1989 Boutonniere deformities in rheumatoid arthritis. Hand Clin 5: 215–222

119. Heywood A E B 1969 Correction of the rheumatoid boutonniere deformity. J Bone Joint Surg 51A: 1309–1314

120. Nalebuff E A, Millender L H 1975 Surgical treatment of the swan-neck deformity in rheumatoid arthritis. Orthopedic Clin North Am 6: 733–752

121. Nalebuff E A 1989 The rheumatoid swan-neck deformity. Hand Clin 5: 203–214

122. Dolphin J A 1965 Extensor tenotomy for chronic boutonniere deformity of the finger. J Bone Joint Surg 47A: 161–164

123. Harris C, Rutledge G L 1972 The functional anatomy of the extensor mechanism of the finger. J Bone Joint Surg 54A: 713–726

124. Kilgore E S, Graham W P 1968 Operative treatment of boutonniere deformity. Surgery 64: 999–1000

125. Littler J W, Eaton R G 1967 Redistribution of forces in the correction of the boutonniere deformity. J Bone Joint Surg 49A: 1267–1274

126. Matev I 1964 Transposition of the lateral slips of the aponeurosis of long-standing boutonniere deformity of the fingers. Br J Plastic Surg 17: 281–286

127. Salvi V 1969 Technique for the buttonhole deformity. Hand 1: 96–97

128. Snow J W 1976 A method for reconstruction of the central slip of the extensor tendon of a finger. Plastic Reconstr Surg 57: 455–459

129. Souter W A 1974 The problem of boutonniere deformity. Clin Orthopaedics 104: 116–133

130. Urbaniak J R, Hayes M G 1981 Chronic boutonniere deformity: an anatomic reconstruction. J Hand Surg 6: 379–383

131. Weeks P M 1967 The chronic boutonniere deformity: a method of repair. Plastic Reconstr Surg 40: 248–251

132. Ansell B, Harrison S 1975 A five year follow-up of synovectomy of the proximal interphalangeal joint in rheumatoid arthritis. Hand 7: 34–36

133. Ansell B M, Harrison S H, Little H, Thouas B 1970 Synovectomy of proximal interphalangeal joints. Br J Plastic Surg 23: 380–385

134. Harrison S H 1974 The Harrison Nicolle intramedullary peg. Follow-up study of 100 cases. Hand 6: 304–307

135. Swanson A B, Maupin B K, Gajjar N V, Swanson G D 1985 Flexible implant arthroplasty in the proximal interphalangeal joint of the hand. J Hand Surg (Am) 10: 796–805

136. Ertel A N 1989 Flexor tendon ruptures in rheumatoid arthritis. Hand Clin 5: 177–190

137. Ertel A N, Millender L H, Nalebuff E, McKay D, Leslie B 1988 Flexor tendon ruptures in patients with rheumatoid arthritis. J Hand Surg (Am) 13: 860–866

138. Ferlic D, Clayton M 1978 Flexor tenosynovectomy in the rheumatoid finger. J Hand Surg 3: 364–367

139. Stirrat C R 1989 Treatment of tenosynovitis in rheumatoid arthritis. Hand Clin 5: 169–175

140. Mills M B, Millender L H, Nalebuff E A 1976 Stiffness of the proximal interphalangeal joints in rheumatoid arthritis. The role of flexor tenosynovitis. J Bone Joint Surg 58A: 801–805

141. Brewerton D A 1967 A tangential radiographic projection for demonstrating involvement of metacarpal heads in rheumatoid arthritis. Br J Radiol 40: 233–234

142. Magyar E, Talerman A, Feher M, Wouters H W 1974

Giant bone cyst in rheumatoid arthritis. J Bone Joint Surg 56B: 121–129

143. Granberry W M, Mangum G L 1980 The hand in the child with juvenile rheumatoid arthritis. J Hand Surg 5: 105–113

144. Simmons B P, Nutting J T 1989 Juvenile rheumatoid arthritis. Hand Clin 5: 157–168

145. Still G F 1897 On a form of chronic joint disease in children. Med Chir Trans 80: 47–59

146. Blockey N J, Gibson A A M, Goel K M 1980 Monarticular juvenile rheumatoid arthritis. J Bone Joint Surg 62B: 368–371

147. Eyring E J, Longert A, Bass J C 1971 Synovectomy in juvenile rheumatoid arthritis. J Bone Joint Surg 53A: 638–651

148. Calin A, Ports J, Fries J F, Schurman D J 1977 Clinical history as a screening test for ankylosing spondylitis. J Am Med Assoc 237: 2613–2614

149. Constantz R, Bluestone R 1980 Diagnosis of the seronegative spondyloarthropathies: HL-A B27 testing as an aid to diagnosis. Contemp Orthopaedics 2: 141–147

150. Bleifeld C J, Inglis A E 1974 The hand in systemic lupus erythematosis. J Bone Joint Surg 56A: 1207–1215

151. Dray G J 1989 The hand in systemic lupus erythematosus. Hand Clin 5: 145–155

152. Dray G J, Millender L H, Nalebuff E A, Philips C 1981 The surgical treatment of hand deformities in systemic lupus erythematosis. J Hand Surg 6: 339–345

153. Jones N F, Imbriglia J E, Steen V D, Medsger T A 1987 Surgery for scleroderma of the hand. J Hand Surg (Am) 12: 391–400

154. Schlenker J D, Clark D D, Weckesser E C 1973 Calcinosis circumscripta of the hand in scleroderma. J Bone Joint Surg 55A: 1051–1056

155. Lewis R A, Adams J P, Gerber N L, Decker I L, Parsons D B 1978 The hand in mixed connective tissue disease. J Hand Surg 3: 217–222

156. Loebl D, Kirby S, Stephenson R, Cook E, Mealing H, Bailey J 1979 Psoriatic arthritis. J Am Med Assoc 242: 2447–2451

157. Rose J H, Belsky M R 1989 Psoriatic arthritis in the hand. Hand Clin 5: 137–144

158. Stern H S, Lloyd G J 1978 Metacarpal shortening. Hand 10: 202–204

159. Nicolle F V 1973 Recent advances in the management of joint disease in the rheumatoid hand. Hand 5: 91

160. Millender L H, Philips C 1978 Combined wrist arthrodesis and metacarpophalangeal joint arthroplasty in rheumatoid arthritis. Orthopedics 1: 43–48

161. Souter W A 1989 Planning treatment of the rheumatoid hand. Hand 11: 3

6. Swelling

Swellings may arise from any tissue in the hand[1,2,4-11]:

bone and cartilage
muscle
nerve
skin and its adnexa
subcutaneous tissue
synovium and tendon
vessel

(this alphabetic order is being used in the text and the references in this chapter).

A few are common — ganglion, giant cell tumour of tendon sheath, epidermoid inclusion cysts, haemangiomas and lipomas — and together constitute 95% of the masses encountered in the hand. They are readily recognized. The remaining 5% derive from a wide variety of uncommon lesions arising from any of the tissues listed above. Their multiplicity and rarity means that each one is not often familiar to the individual surgeon to whom it is presented. This unfamiliarity, allied to the fact that the swelling may be of any degree of malignancy, dictates that the examiner must pursue a disciplined approach to diagnosis if errors of both omission and commission are to be avoided. This discipline is called *staging*. The staging system most commonly employed for musculoskeletal tumours is that of Enneking[3], in which the stage is derived from the *surgical grade (G)* — of which there are three (0, 1 and 2) — the *anatomical location (T)* or surgical site (1 or 2), and the presence or absence of *metastases (M)* (0 or 1). The evaluation is summarized here, detailed later. The surgical grade depends on three determinants:

Clinical presentation — pain and rapid growth suggest G2

Imaging — radiograph — marked destruction — G2
isotope bone scan — extensive uptake — G2.
CT scan — cortical disruption — G2
MRI — satellite lesions — G2

angiogram — considerable neovascular response — G2
Biopsy — frequent mitoses, cellular atypia, poor differentiation and necrosis indicate G2 .

The biopsy is conducted according to strict rules:

longitudinal incision
no violation, if possible, of fascial planes or of bone
haemostasis, no drains
frozen section mainly to ensure a representative tissue specimen
histology plus electron microscopy, special stains and studies
culture for infection.

The anatomical location is either *intracompartmental (T1)* or *extracompartmental (T2)*. A compartment is bounded by natural anatomical barriers to local tumour spread. In the extremities the compartments are intraosseous, paraosseous, intra-articular and intramuscular. Extension through the barriers converts a T1 lesion to T2. This is best assessed by *CT scan* or *MRI*. Some locations are not within compartments, and tumours therein are T2 from their inception — those locations are the vascular planes, the mid-hand, the antecubital fossa and the axilla.

Metastases are sought by physical examination of the *regional nodes* supplemented by *CT of the chest*.

The sequence of these steps in individual cases is determined by consultation between surgeon, oncologist and radiologist, who should seek maximum information for minimum cost.

Once the grade, location and the presence or absence of metastases have been decided, the lesion can be staged:

Musculoskeletal tumour staging
All benign lesions are G0, Stage 0
All with metastases are M1, Stage III

Anatomical location

	Intracompartmental (T1)	Extracompartmental (T2)
GRADE		
Low (G1)	IA	IB
High (G2)	IIA	IIB

This staging system pays no heed to tumour size, but otherwise leads to a logical choice of surgical indication (see page. 411).

Sarcomatous change in pre-existing benign lesions occurs in the four instances listed below, each in 10% of cases and in each only when they are multiple[3].

fibrous dysplasia	$\longrightarrow$	fibrosarcoma
osteochondroma	$\longrightarrow$	chondrosarcoma
Paget's disease	$\longrightarrow$	osteosarcoma
neurofibromatosis	$\longrightarrow$	neurosarcoma

HISTORY

Age
The age of the patient may be significant. Malignant change in neurofibromatosis occurs most commonly between 30 and 40. Primary osteogenic sarcoma is most prevalent in the second decade; some other bony tumours are more common under the age of thirty — aneurysmal bone cyst, chondroblastoma, Ewing's sarcoma, osteoblastoma, osteoid osteoma — as are some bony swellings which are hard to distinguish from tumours — eosinophilic granuloma, fibrous dysplasia, giant-cell reparative granuloma and simple bone cyst. By contrast, only a few bony tumours are more prevalent in older age groups — chondrosarcoma, malignant fibrous histiocytoma and secondary osteosarcoma. Unlike the tumours of skin and viscera, which are the blights of our advancing years and which tend to be impressed upon us in our early medical training, musculoskeletal tumours are more common in the young. Tragically, they are all too often malignant.

Duration
Presence since birth, increasing in size with the patient, suggests a *hamartoma*.

Swift growth indicates inflammation or high-grade malignancy.

Bursts of growth at puberty and during pregnancy are characteristic of *cavernous haemangioma*. Growth in previously quiescent lesions should be viewed with suspicion. For example, a plexiform neurofibroma may develop a neurosarcoma, evidenced by sudden enlargement in one area, and often accompanied by distal motor and sensory changes. These changes are identical to those of nerve compression and may tragically be mistaken for them.

Pain
The sudden onset of pain, throbbing in nature, coincident with the appearance of swelling indicates infection (Ch. 4).

Pain without swelling, severe and episodic, suggests *glomus tumour* or *osteoid osteoma*. If cold temperatures precipitate paroxysmal pain, a glomus tumour is the likely cause. If the pain is initially nocturnal, is accompanied by vasomotor symptoms and is relieved by aspirin, osteoid osteoma is probable.

Aching, unremitting pain with a bony swelling has sinister implications.

Neurological effects
Sensory and motor change, such as dysaesthesia, numbness and weakness, suggest nerve compression (Ch. 3). A tumour located in a snug tunnel, such as Guyon's canal, may well precipitate the compression and should be part of the differential diagnosis until excluded by examination, imaging and/or surgery.

Nature of onset
If sudden and related to injury, but persisting after much of the associated oedema has gone, vascular involvement is probable, in the form of a traumatic aneurysm. *Epidermoid* cysts follow minor trauma to the skin (Fig. 6.1).

Foreign body granulomas likewise follow minor injury.

Patients presenting with *bone tumours*, especially those which are malignant, not infrequently give a history of trauma, usually minor, which first drew their attention to the swelling.

Pathological fracture may be the first event to draw

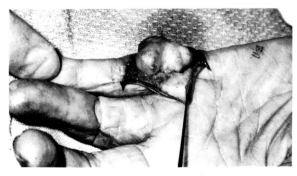

Fig. 6.1 The lesion which had developed over the course of two to three years at the proximal digital crease was attached to the skin and was an *epidermoid* or *implantation cyst*.

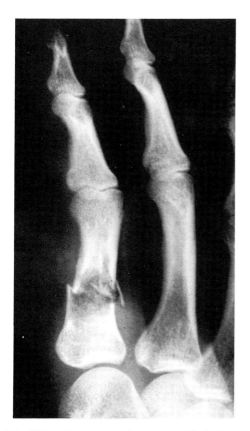

Fig. 6.2 This patient sustained a fracture while bed-making. As she had previously been asymptomatic, and because of the radiologic appearances, the fracture was allowed to heal. Curettage and bone graft of this enchondroma were then performed.

attention to the osteolytic lesion which precipitated it (Fig. 6.2). Minor trauma resulting in an unstable fracture should make the examiner suspicious even before radiologic examination.

Variation in size
This is characteristically a feature of *ganglion cysts* which develop to a significant size, then disperse, often as a result of a forgotten blow, only to recur at a later date.

Although one thinks of malignancy as relentlessly growing in size, some may apparently regress only to enlarge again. This is true particularly of the epithelioid sarcoma.

Previous similar swellings
Recurrence following apparently adequate previous excision should always arouse concern with the one exception of the ganglion cyst. The original histological sections should be reviewed before further surgery.

Similar swellings elsewhere
Neurofibromatosis, lymphangioma and osteochondroma produce multiple swelling.

Lesions associated with *systemic disorders* may be multiple, such as *xanthoma* in patients with hyperlipidaemia.

Symptoms related to other systems
Metastatic tumours in the hand are rare[362-380] but they do occur and the examiner should seek evidence of the primary focus (Fig. 6.3).

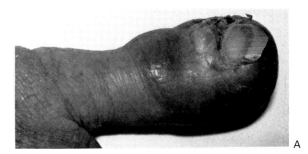

A

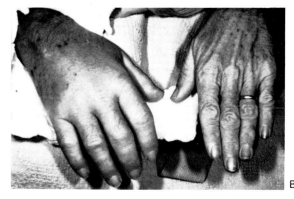

B

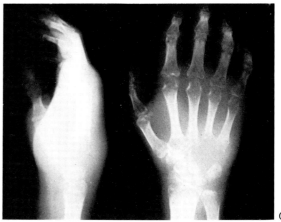

C

Fig. 6.3 Metastatic tumours. A. Consequent upon renal carcinoma. B, C. Consequent upon bronchogenic carcinoma.

EXAMINATION

Swellings

A system for examination of swellings should be adopted from which the examiner never strays. The mnemonic ascribed to Learmonth is useful:

$S^3 C^2 M$ site   colour   mobility
             size   consistency
             shape

To this could well be added NI, for *nodes* and *imaging*.

SITE

The location of a swelling may be virtually diagnostic. For example, a swelling located over the distal phalanx in the region of the nail-bed, especially if grooving of the nail is apparent, can only be a ganglion of the distal interphalangeal joint, the so-called 'mucous cyst' (pp. 342, 435). A firm swelling on the palmar aspect of the proximal phalanx of the thumb of the dominant hand which is mobile transversely but not longitudinally, is a neuroma on the digital nerve — a 'bowler's thumb' (p. 234). A firm, small, immobile swelling beneath the proximal digital crease of the finger is almost always a ganglion of the tendon sheath (p. 436).

A skin lesion on the dorsum of the hand or forearm, especially of those who have worked a lifetime in the sun, is likely to be actinic keratosis, basal or squamous-cell carcinoma. These may exist together and are usually multiple.

Determining the site also requires the examiner to attempt to localize the swelling to a particular tissue. This is considered further under mobility.

SIZE

The size of a lesion should be recorded and the swelling photographed. In the unusual case where the decision is made not to excise the lesion — as for example in haemangioma or Bowen's disease — then the record will be of value in monitoring growth or regression between visits (see Figs 6.74 and 6.75).

SHAPE

To determine the shape of a swelling, the surgeon must be able to define its margins. Spherical lesions are commonly ganglia or epidermoid inclusion cysts. Some swelling may appear to be multilocular and some indeed are. However, the many rigid structures in the hand, especially tendons and fascia, may mould a benign lesion growing beneath them into an irregular form (Fig. 6.4).

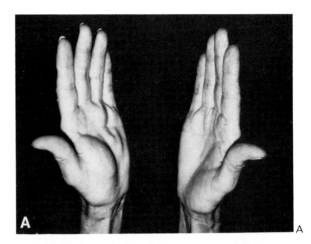

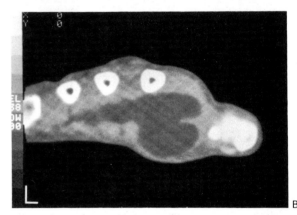

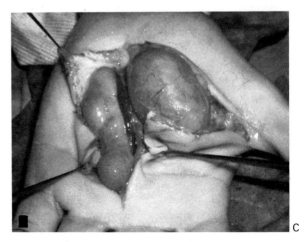

Fig. 6.4 A. This patient presented with a history of a gradually developing mutilocular lesion in the palm of the left hand. While it appeared clinically that this was composed of several lesions it was appreciated on CT scan (B) and at surgery (C) that because this *lipoma* arose beneath the tendons and nerves of the palm of the hand, it had been distorted by them from its basic unilocular form.

COLOUR

Any pigmented lesion, especially beneath the nail or on the palms of the hand should be considered as dangerous. Mitotic activity in a malignant melanoma is classically indicated by any of the following: alteration in colour, increase in size, elevation of a previously flat lesion, bleeding and itching. In short, any change in a pigmented lesion should be treated as prima facie evidence of malignancy. The subungual *melanoma* may be a relatively slow-growing tumour, the patient often giving a lengthy history only of an increasing dark spot beneath the nail.

All *naevi* of the palm of the hand are *junctional* in location and therefore excision should be recommended in all cases.

The typical appearance of a '*strawberry naevus*' in the newborn is well-known — raised and pinkish-red.

CONSISTENCY

To determine whether the swelling is *fluctuant*, the consistency should be assessed with two fingers fixing the lesion and a third exerting intermittent pressure (Fig. 6.5). At body temperature in the relatively unyielding surroundings of the hand, a *lipoma*[237-245] is a fluctuant swelling.

The ganglion is fluctuant but the resistance offered varies with the site. The anterior wrist ganglion clearly contains fluid, while the ganglion of flexor tendon sheath is so firm as to be non-fluctuant. When first encountered it is often thought to be bony, but the location is pathognomonic.

When the consistency is yielding and apparently fluid, steady pressure should be applied to it. If this

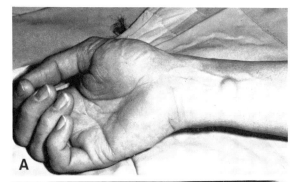

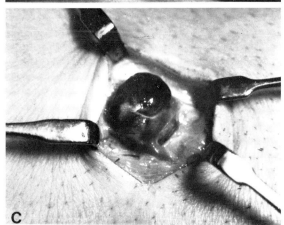

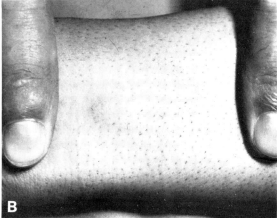

Fig. 6.6 This swelling on the forearm (A) could be completely evacuated by pressure (B). The diagnosis of a *varicocele* was confirmed at operation (C).

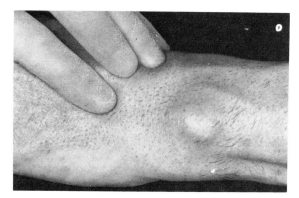

Fig. 6.5 Fluctuance in a swelling is elicited by fixing it with two fingers of one hand and exerting pressure with a third digit. Although usually evidence of free fluid, fluctuance is encountered in lipomata at body temperature.

serves to empty the swelling which then *refills*, it is clearly a *vascular lesion* (Fig. 6.6). If hard and unyielding, a swelling is probably arising from bone, although *gouty tophi* and the calcium deposits of *calcinosis* are of similar consistency. However they are both craggy, irregular and usually show some mobility.

MOBILITY

The tissues to which the swelling is attached can often be determined by checking its mobility with respect to skin, bone and tendon. The skin overlying the lesion should be lifted and the fingers rolled to detect whether or not the swelling moves with the skin inseparably. Certain lesions which do not involve the skin surface are nonetheless always attached to it — *epidermoid cyst*, *Dupuytren's disease* (p 193) and *juvenile dermatofibroma* are the most common.

If fully developed to contracture, Dupuytren's offers no diagnostic difficulties. However, a patient may complain of a tender palmar nodule with no evidence of contracture. Examination will reveal a smooth rounded mass firmly attached to the skin in most instances in the line of the ring finger between the proximal and distal palmar creases. Provided the possibility occurs to the examiner no doubt will exist regarding the diagnosis.

Garrod's knuckle pads, fibrous thickening over the dorsum of the proximal interphalangeal joints, appear to be related to Dupuytren's disease and to have the same familial tendency.

If the swelling is not attached to the skin, it may appear to be attached to bone, being firmly immobile in all directions. If such a lesion is well-defined it is unlikely to arise from the bone itself but rather from the tendon sheath, a *ganglion* or *giant-cell tumour* being most likely.

Some swellings may be mobile in one direction and not in another implying that they arise from, or are attached to, a longitudinally running structure. This is the case, for example, with a *neurilemmoma* of a digital nerve, a fusiform swelling which moves freely from side to side but very little along the axis of the finger. Other lesions may move as the patient moves the hand, a feature which is pathognomonic of a *ganglion on the extensor tendon*, most commonly seen in children (Fig. 6.7).

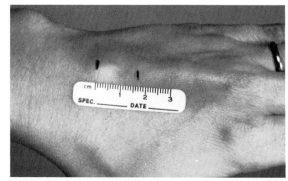

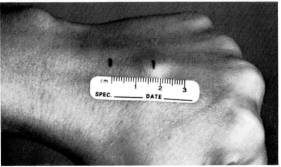

Fig. 6.7   A, B. The movement of this small, hard mass through a distance of 1.5 cm is characteristic of a ganglion of the extensor tendon.

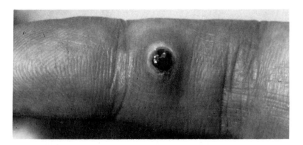

Fig. 6.8   This pyogenic granuloma shows the flat uninvolved surrounding skin and exuberant granulation which is characteristic.

Ulcers

If the swelling has ulcerated, certain features of the ulcer should be examined.

EDGE

The characteristically heaped-up margins of a *squamous carcinoma* (Figs 6.35B, 6.36, 6.41) contrast with the flat, normal skin which surrounds a *pyogenic granuloma* (Fig. 6.8). *Basal cell carcinoma* is rarely encountered in the hand and the 'pearly edge' with which it is credited is not always apparent. If the surgeon places the skin on stretch, however, and inspects the edge of the ulcer, preferably with magnification, the typical pearly appearance becomes more evident, the whiteness being interrupted by fine telangiectatic vessels coursing across the margin.

A 'punched-out' edge is characteristic of a *factitious ulcer* (Fig. 6.9) (see p. 165). If active bleeding or congealed blood is present, that confirms the diagnosis, as does healing when treated with prolonged occlusion.

When doubt is present, the edge is the site from which lesions should be biopsied.

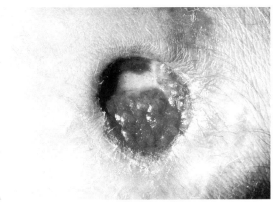

A

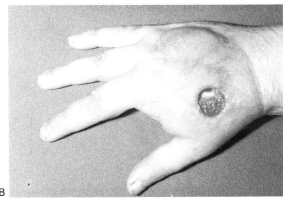

B

Fig. 6.9 Factitious ulcer. A.This wound has the characteristic 'punched-out' margin of a factitious ulcer. There is no reaction other than erythema in the surrounding skin. The bed shows normal granulation tissue and exposed bone. B. The ulcer had already been treated by ray resection and application of a free tissue transfer. When treated with a totally occlusive cast, the lesion healed uneventfully. The patient then disappeared from care.

FLOOR

The floor of an ulcer is that portion which the examiner can inspect. A red, overgrown granulating floor which overflows the edge of the ulcer is found most frequently in a *pyogenic granuloma*. The surgeon must be aware, however, that the relatively rare totally *amelanotic melanoma* (Fig. 6.44) may have a very similar appearance. He should explain the remote possibility to patients, thereafter undertaking early surgery.

The floor of an ulcer is often crusted over. If it can be done without pain, this crust should be removed. Should this produce brisk bleeding and there be no evidence of attempts at marginal re-epithelialization, *squamous carcinoma* is likely.

Keratocanthoma with a characteristic circular plug of keratin should be excised for it may rarely be a swiftly growing carcinoma (p. 429 and Fig. 6.41).

BASE

The base of an ulcer is that part underlying it which the examiner can palpate. If the base is thickened and indurated, and especially if it is fixed to underlying tissues, the possibility of malignancy is considerable.

An ulcer arising in the nail-bed will declare itself only by the presence of discharge from beneath the nail. Should such a discharge persist for more than three weeks biopsy must be performed and may reveal an unsuspected *squamous-cell carcinoma* (see p. 428 and Fig. 6.38).

Regional nodes

These should always be examined, taking care not to omit the supratrochlear node.

The axillary nodes can best be palpated with the examiner standing behind the sitting patient. The patient's arm should be raised, and the examining hand placed with the fingertips high in the axillary vault. The patient's arm is then lowered. The examiner's contralateral hand passed across the front of the patient's chest is best used to palpate the medial wall of the axilla. The ipsilateral hand passed around the involved arm feels the lateral wall. From this position, the examiner should proceed to examine the contents of the posterior triangle of the neck and the nodes of the head and neck. These are located in a circle from the suboccipital to the pre-auricular to the submandibular to the submental, and down the line of the internal jugular vein. When doubt exists about the nature of a swelling, the mandatory full physical examination will include the nodes of the lower extremity and the groin.

Imaging

Radiologic examination may reveal:

1. The presence of lesions arising primarily from bone
2. Any effects produced on the bone by soft-tissue swellings
3. The presence of calcification in the soft tissue.

Calcification in the soft tissue is seen in acute calcific tendinitis (p. 335), calcinosis circumscripta, and quite frequently in atherosclerotic vessels, subcutaneous haemangioma, juvenile aponeurotic fibroma, synovial chondromatosis, synovial sarcoma, lipoma and liposarcoma.

Calcinosis circumscripta[24,25] presents as tender calcific deposits which quite commonly afflict the finger pads (Fig. 6.10), in which position they are troublesome to the patient. They give no diagnostic difficulties, but are

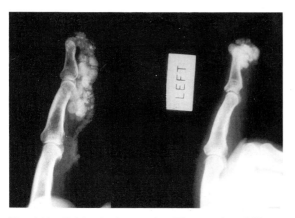

Fig. 6.10   Calcinosis circumscripta.These tender calcific deposits in the pulp were displayed on a patient with scleroderma.

mentioned here because of the high incidence of *scleroderma* in patients with this condition (p. 396).

Despite the development of sophisticated imaging techniques, the analysis of the plain radiographs of bone tumours remains of paramount importance in diagnosis, staging and planning management[14]. The key features to be observed are:

anatomical location
changes in bony architecture produced by the lesion
response of the host bone as in the periosteal reaction
the internal contents of the lesion.

These are detailed below with some examples illustrating the importance of each observation. (While no illustrations are provided here, by glancing onward to the section on specific lesions of bone (p. 413) the reader can study several of the features listed.)

ANATOMICAL LOCATION

Tubular bones or carpus?
While other tumours may involve the carpus, *enchondroma* is invariably confined to tubular bones.

Epiphysis, metaphysis or diaphysis?
Chondroblastoma is epiphyseal, *chondrosarcoma* and *giant-cell tumour* are in the equivalent of the epiphysis in the adult; *osteochondroma, simple bone cyst* and most *osteosarcomas* arise from the metaphysis; *giant-cell reparative granuloma* is a diaphyseal lesion.

Central or eccentric? (with respect to the transverse plane of the bone)
Enchondroma is a central lesion, while *aneurysmal bone cyst* (ABC), *giant-cell tumour* (GCT) and *osteosarcoma*

are eccentric in origin. In practice this is often difficult to determine in the small bones of the hand.

CHANGES IN ARCHITECTURE

Osteolytic or bone-producing?
Osteoblastoma, osteoid osteoma and *osteosarcoma* are the tumours which produce bone. This may not be apparent in the latter two, for they may produce bone which is not mineralized and therefore is not seen on routine radiographs. Osteosarcoma, while producing new bone, simultaneously destroys pre-existing bony architecture, hence having an appearance which lies anywhere within a wide spectrum. All primary lesions other than the three named above are osteolytic.

Expansile or not?
Enchondroma, ABC and *GCT* are expansile in that they appear to 'inflate' the bone. *Metastatic* lesions do not. *Osteosarcoma*, while producing new bone, does not. The presence of expansile change indicates the passage of time and therefore implies a more benign lesion than does its absence.

Margins well-defined or not?
Of similar import as 'expansile or not?'. *Chondroma* has a well-defined margin, *malignant fibrous histiocytoma* does not.

Cortex intact or broken?
Pathological fractures may occur through benign, expansile osteolytic lesions, but where the cortex is disrupted without fracture it implies spread into the soft tissues.

HOST REACTION

Some tumours, notably giant-cell tumours, are characterized by minimal periosteal reaction. In others, the uninterrupted deposition of new bone implies a benign lesion, or one of low-grade malignancy, while disruptive bone deposition suggests a more aggressive neoplasm — this takes one or more of three forms:

Spiculation. Often at right angles to the bone, this produces the 'sunburst' appearance of *osteosarcoma*.

Linear, multilayered deposits giving the appearance of an onion skin are characteristic of *Ewing's sarcoma*.

Codman's triangle: triangular deposits of non-lesional reactive bone which blend with the cortex at either end of the lesion, this is seen in *osteosarcoma*, but also in some examples of *aneurysmal bone cyst* and other benign lesions.

INTERNAL CONTENTS

Lucency
Typically *ABC* shows no trabeculation or calcification.

Calcific deposits
Taking various forms, these are characteristic of *enchondroma*, but are absent from *ABC* and *GCT*.

Trabeculation
This is seen in *giant-cell reparative granuloma*.

Central nidus
A central nidus of bone is typical of *osteoid osteoma*.

More sophisticated studies of swellings may be required, either because the lesion is poorly seen on standard views or to assist in staging or to delineate a tumour more exactly.

Xeroradiography is valuable in demonstrating details of internal topography and in delineating the extent of the tumour by 'edge enhancement'.

Bone scan is of value in revealing skip lesions in the involved bone, and foci in other parts of the skeleton in multicentric tumours or where metastasis has occurred. As CT scan and MRI can give more information regarding the local site, bone scan may be confined to those patients in whom involvement elsewhere seems likely due to the nature of the tumour, once that has been established.

Tomography and, better, *CT scan*, will distinguish between osteomyelitis and tumour, determine the extent of the tumour in both bone and soft tissue, and demonstrate satellite nodules and skip lesions.

Magnetic resonance imaging is indicated when a tumour is not clearly visualized on routine radiographs, when there is a soft-tissue component or when improved delineation of location and content is required. It provides even greater accuracy that CT scan in determining the extent of the tumour, clearly important in ensuring total resection, but also essential if limb-saving procedures are planned for malignant lesions.

Angiography[3] is used to study potentially malignant lesions which arise from or have spread to the soft tissues. The *early arterial phase* will demonstrate the relationship to major neurovascular bundles of the reactive peripheral zone around a tumour. Various views and several injections of dye may be required to achieve maximum accuracy (ideally the surgeon should be present to advise). The *late venous phase* produces the 'tumour blush' which persists after other dye has disappeared, giving an outline of the tumour which can be 'fitted inside' the reactive zone demonstrated by the early arterial phase. The late venous phase also shows intravenous tumour thrombi and skip lesions larger than 1 cm in diameter. The value of angiography, still advocated by some, has been challenged by sophisticated interpretation of modern CT and MRI studies, which can provide the same information in non-invasive fashion.

Radiologic examination of the chest, or, better, CT scan, is required if the lesion is believed to be malignant.

If the lesion is shown by biopsy to be a malignant primary, a lymphoma or a round-cell tumour of bone, *lymphangiography*, *staging abdominal CT* and a *liver–spleen scan* should be performed.

If a hand swelling is believed to be a metastatic deposit, appropriate consultation should be sought. Studies directed especially at lung, breast, kidney, thyroid and prostate will be required.

LABORATORY STUDIES

CBS and urine analysis are routine tests and they should be supplemented as deemed necessary with some or all of the following: sedimentation rate, BUN, fasting blood sugar, Ca, P, alkaline phosphatase, IEP, T3, T4 and SGOT.

Indications[11]

Complete excision of any benign swelling presenting in the hand usually proves curative although some lesions have a propensity to occur locally, as detailed below.

SKIN MALIGNANCY

Squamous-cell carcinoma in the hand is considered by most as relatively benign, by some not so[176]. Excision of the lesion with a 1 cm margin is indicated: the deep margin is at the plane in which dissection is free — this can best be determined by preliminary injection of fluid beneath the tumour. When no such plane can be demonstrated, indicating involvement of bone or tendon, appropriate amputation is required. This is most likely to occur in the 'danger area' of the interdigital clefts[163].

Carcinomata of the hand are frequently infected and this may result in reactive lymphadenopathy (Fig. 6.35C). For this reason the presence of enlarged nodes should not lead to gloom or even immediate node dissection. Rather should the nodes be left for six weeks after excision of the primary, at which stage dissection should be undertaken in the cases in which they are still enlarged.

Squamous-cell carcinoma of the *nailbed* requires ablation of the distal phalanx.

Many factors have been cited as influencing the

prognosis, and therefore the appropriate surgical treatment, of *malignant melanoma* — age, sex, size, ulceration, presence of satellites, absence of melanin and nodularity. Certainly, if a suspected lesion is ulcerated or nodular, the prognosis is poorer and the excision should be wider. However, more accurate guidance can be obtained by histological examination: Breslow[193,194] has shown that the incidence of metastases is directly related to the maximal thickness of the tumour; for example, those less than 0.76 mm thick rarely, if ever, metastasize. Where deemed desirable incisional biopsy for staging followed by later wide resection has been shown to carry no added danger, contrary to previous teaching. Where nodes are involved, dissection is indicated and may be effective, in inverse proportion to the number of nodes found to be involved.

MUSCULOSKELETAL TUMOURS

Four types of surgical excision are recognized and can be assigned to the stages of musculoskeletal tumours determined by the discipline detailed above:

Intralesional, in which tumour is exposed (stage 0);

Marginal, in which the lesion is 'shelled out' (Stage 0 or IA) — in lesions more malignant than IA, marginal excision will leave microscopic extensions of tumour immediately adjacent, called *'satellites'* (*daughter nodules*), and lesions further removed but within the same compartment, known as *'skip lesions'*;

Wide resection takes with it a cuff of normal tissue likely to include 'satellites' but not 'skips' (stage IB);
Radical excision takes the whole compartment (stage IIA).

Stage IIB lesions, which by definition are aggressive and have infiltrated outside the compartment, require still wider excision. One of the more exquisitely important decisions the surgeon must make is whether this can be done with safety by a limb-sparing procedure or whether amputation must be recommended.

These indications are adjusted to accommodate the value or otherwise of chemotherapy and radiation, considerations of the age and condition of the patient and his or her wishes once all has been explained. In this surgery, concern must primarily be for the survival of that patient, which is achieved by good ablative cancer surgery. Only once that is ensured can attention be paid to function and appearance.

Much of the above has been distilled from the writings of Mankin[8], who also offers the following axioms regarding swellings of the hand:

Primary bone tumours are usually benign.

The most common bone tumours are enchondroma and osteocartilaginous exostoses, except in the terminal phalanx where the most prevalent is the epidermoid inclusion cyst.

The distal radius is the third most common site in the body for giant cell tumour of bone, which is rare in the hand itself, but when found there is often aggressive, both locally and in causing metastases.

Chondrosarcoma is very rare in the metacarpals or phalanges.

Deep soft-tissue tumours — if not ganglia, lipomata or giant-cell tumours of the tendon sheath — are often malignant.

Epithelioid sarcoma, synovial sarcoma and clear-cell sarcoma are common in the hand and forearm and are highly malignant even when the histology suggests otherwise. All three may metastasize to lymph nodes.

Synovial chondromatosis, synovial sarcoma, liposarcoma (juvenile aponeurotic fibroma and subcutaneous haemangioma) may show calcification on radiograph.

Metastatic carcinoma (except that from the lung), lymphoma and myeloma are rarely seen in the hand.

Unlike other chapters, here surgical indications are included with each specific lesion below.

See Green D P 1993 Operative Hand Surgery, 3rd edn. Churchill Livingstone, New York, pp. 2158, 2173, 2203 and 2225.

SPECIFIC LESIONS

By selectively applying the diagnostic techniques outlined above it should be possible to identify virtually all lesions and select the safe surgical treatment.

It is appropriate to offer more details on the common swellings which make up 95% of those encountered.

Brief summaries, in shorthand style, of relevant data on less common tumours may be helpful.

Both are offered in this section, which is organized alphabetically, with first-generation headings for tissue and, below them, second generation headings for tumours. The references are arranged in similar fashion. (Where alphabetical sequence is transgressed for the purpose of juxtaposing lesions often confused, this is also done in the references.) For the purposes of comparison and contrast, the data in the brief summaries on bone tumours can, with benefit, be arranged in spread sheet format, which is how this section was prepared. By its very nature, the spread sheet does not lend itself to publication, but the reader may find it entertaining and instructive to prepare such a layout.

Bone and cartilage[12–16]

In presenting the following somewhat cryptic abstracts of information, brevity necessarily dictates simplification. It should be understood that bone tumours may not present all, or indeed any, of their 'characteristic' features. They may then require the retrospective confirmation which only histological examination of the full specimen can provide. In some differential diagnoses that is required more frequently than in others, for example, with the 'giant-cell-bearing' lesions of bone — giant-cell tumour, giant-cell reparative granuloma and aneurysmal bone cyst[12].

ANEURYSMAL BONE CYST[17–23] (Fig. 6.11)

Peak incidence – the second decade; pain and rapid growth, especially in pregnancy; metaphyseal; eccentric; lytic, 'soap-bubble' appearance with no calcification; uniformly expansile; a sharp interface but often no marginal sclerosis; cortex intact (often haemorrhage will

cause a 'blow-out' (Fig. 6.11) which can be alarming); MRI may show fluid levels. Intralesional curettage may lead to recurrence; when feasible, marginal excision and bone grafting are recommended[20].

BROWN TUMOUR OF HYPERPARATHYROIDISM (Fig. 6.12)

Osteolytic, often multiple lesions in generally osteopenic bone, these may be confused with fibrous dysplasia, giant-cell reparative granuloma or giant-cell tumours. They are readily diagnosed by changes in blood calcium, phosphate, alkaline phosphatase and parathormone.

CHONDROBLASTOMA[28] (Fig. 6.13)

The humerus is the third most common location, but this lesion is very rare in the hand; peak incidence the second decade; pain with little local swelling but

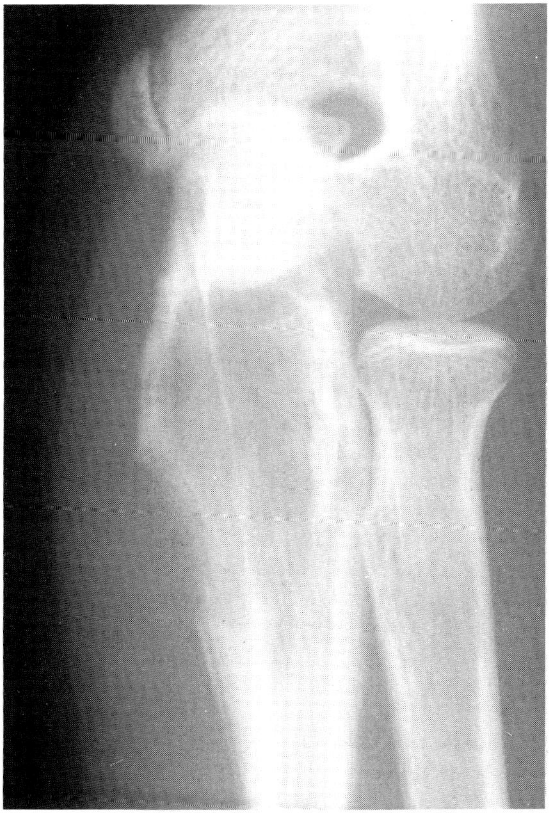

Fig. 6.11 Aneurysmal bone cyst (see text for features). (Case of Dr Sherman Coleman.)

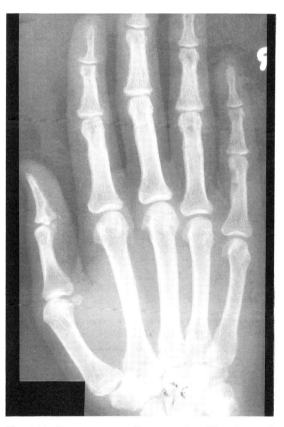

Fig. 6.12 Brown tumour of hyperparathyroidism (see text). Lesions in proximal phalanx of small, distal phalanx of thumb and the third metacarpal head. (Case of Dr Sherman Coleman.)

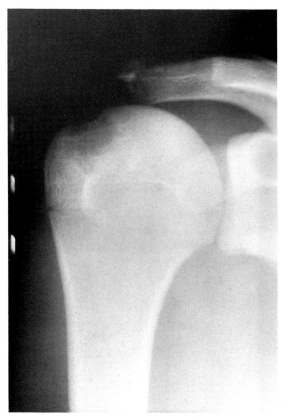

Fig. 6.13 Chondroblastoma of humeral epiphysis (see text).(Case of Dr Sherman Coleman.)

complaints related to the adjacent joint; epiphyseal, but may cross the growth plate; eccentric; lytic, with fuzzy calcification; expansile; marginal sclerosis; cortex intact; CT defines the extent of this benign but locally aggressive tumour. Intralesional curettage and bone graft usually initiates resolution.

CHONDROMA[29,30]

Enchondroma[31–33](Fig. 6.14)
Benign hyaline cartilage growth within the medullary cavity of a bone; most common bony tumour in the hand; peak presentation the third and fourth decades; painless swelling, often discovered fortuitously on radiologic examination, less often by pathological fracture; central location, usually in tubular bones; lytic, with calcification; expansile; margins well-defined; cortex intact but often very thin and difficult to see on standard radiographs. Rarely an enchondroma undergoes malignant degeneration, heralded by unremitting pain, rapid growth and cortical disruption. The benign

majority are treated by intralesional curettage and bone graft.

Juxtacortical chondroma
A benign cartilaginous growth beneath the periosteum and outside the cortex; rare; peak incidence third decade; painful, hard, well-localized swelling; outside the cortex, sitting in a sclerotic depression; lytic; expansile, no margin seen in soft tissue; no cortex. Marginal excision cures.

Soft-tissue chondroma (syn. synovial chondromatosis)[34–41]
Benign hyaline cartilaginous masses found in the soft tissues, usually associated with the flexor sheaths; hard, of limited mobility; some calcification on radiograph. Marginal excision carries 10% recurrence which can again be marginally excised[39].

CHONDROSARCOMA[42–53]

Although 10% occur in the humerus (Fig. 6.15), this tumour is rare in the hand (Fig. 6.16), but is still the most common primary malignant bone tumour found there[15]; one-quarter arise secondarily to *multiple* enchondroma. Peak incidence in the hand seventh and eighth decades[47]; pain; lies in the epiphyseal equivalent in the adult, that is, the subchondral bone; central; scattered lysis with punctate calcification; non-expansile; no marginal sclerosis; cortical destruction but late; associated soft-tissue shadow with radiating spicules which are flattened at the end unlike osteosarcoma; Codman's triangle. Radical excision is required.

EOSINOPHILIC GRANULOMA[57]

Benign tumour-like disorder very rarely seen in the hands, but does occur in the humerus; peak incidence the first two decades; pain; rapid growth, and regression; diaphyseal; multiple, 'punched-out' lytic lesions; non-expansile; no sclerosis, but 'bevelling' of the margin, giving the optical illusion of depth; cortical thinning; 'onion-skin' periosteal new bone formation. Solitary lesions are treated by curettage, multiple with vigilant observation, for they are believed to be self-limiting.

EWING'S SARCOMA[58,59]

Rarely affects the upper limb, and then almost exclusively in the humerus; pain and swelling; fever, anaemia, leucocytosis, elevated sedimetation rate; peak incidence second decade; diaphyseal or metaphyseal; 'motheaten' appearance, likened to 'cracked ice'; sym-

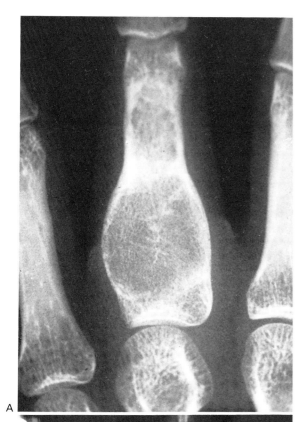

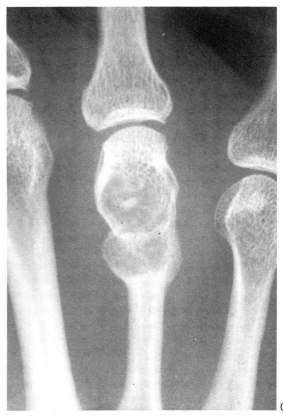

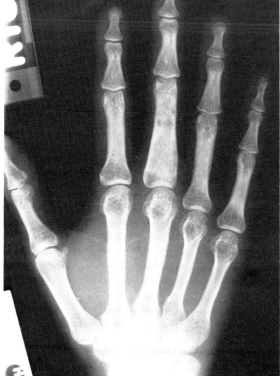

Fig. 6.14 A. Enchondroma. The margins of the smooth, hard swelling of the proximal phalanx were difficult to define, seeming to merge into adjacent bone. The features are characteristic: metaphyseal, central, lytic with calcification, expansile marginal sclerosis, intact cortex. After curettage and packing with cancellous bone remodelling occurred as seen two years later (B). C. A second lesion showing similar characteristics.

metrical, fusiform modest expansion; poorly defined margins; cortical breakthrough; soft-tissue spread; 'onion-skin' periosteal reaction; metastases to lymph nodes and lung; angiography and CT scan assist in determining extent. Treatment is by high-dose chemotherapy, radiation and surgical excision.

FIBROUS DYSPLASIA[60]

Monostotic (70%) or polyostotic arrest of bone maturation, with resulting deformity, such as bowing of the shaft; pathological fracture often the presentation; peak incidence below 20; diaphyseal; eccentric; 'frosted glass' lytic lesions; modestly expansile; well-defined, sclerotic margins; cortical thinning.

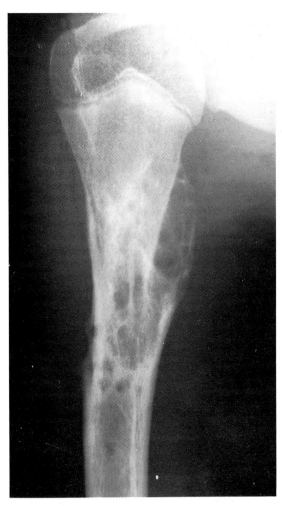

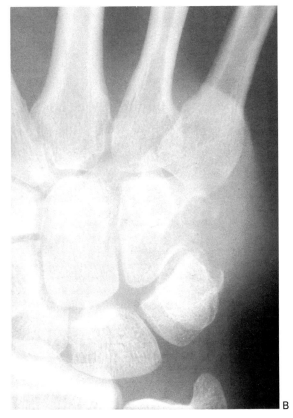

Fig. 6.16 (*continued*)

Fig. 6.15   Low-grade chondrosarcoma (see text). Note satellite lesions. (Case of Dr Sherman Coleman.)

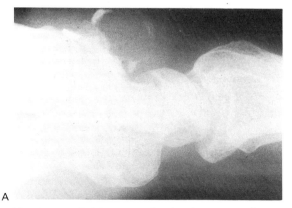

Fig. 6.16   A, B. More aggressive chondrosarcoma of hamate. (Case of Dr Sherman Coleman.)

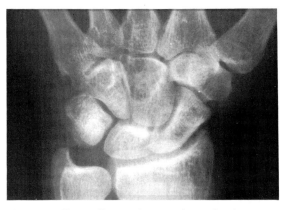

Fig. 6.17   Giant-cell reparative granuloma of capitate. (Case of Dr Sherman Coleman.)

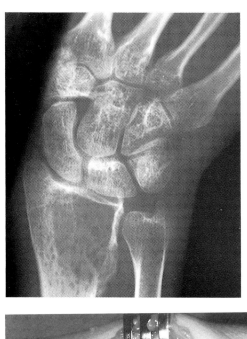

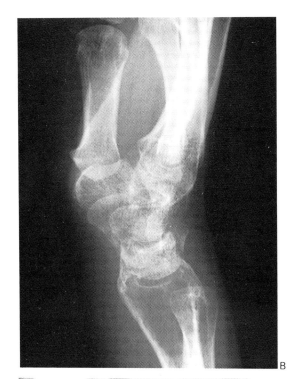

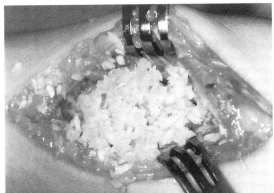

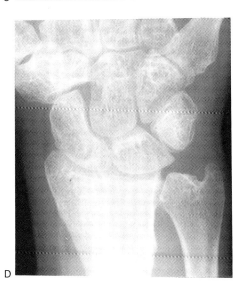

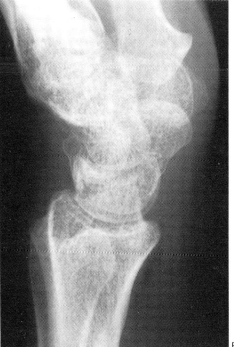

Fig. 6.18 Stage II giant-cell tumour; A, B. This patient presented with a fracture through a giant-cell tumour of the distal radius. A biopsy was taken through a longitudinal incision; inspection while the tourniquet was still inflated showed this to be a low-grade lesion histologically.
C. The lesion was curretted and packed with allograft.
D, E. Satisfactory resolution was achieved, although with some loss of radial inclination.

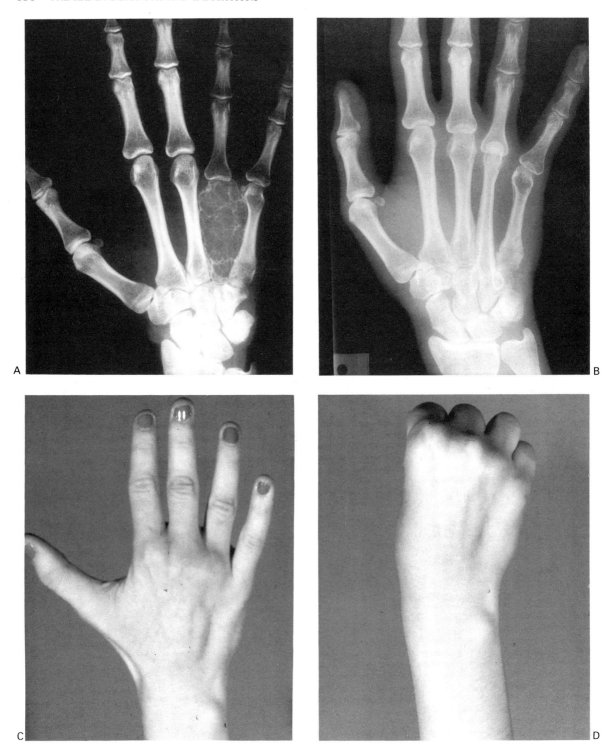

Fig. 6.19 Stage II giant-cell tumour. A. Although this tumour had entirely replaced the fourth metacarpal, the cortex was intact. Excision with the contents of the interosseus spaces showed this to be a low-grade lesion. B. The metacarpal was replaced with the non-vascularized fourth metatarsal which was fused to the hamate. C, D. Function three years later was satisfactorily maintained with only some limitation of extension and flexion.

GIANT-CELL REPARATIVE GRANULOMA[61-63] (Fig. 6.17)

Rare, benign lesion more common in the jaw; diaphyseal; lytic; trabeculated; expansile; cortical thinning. Treatment requires curettage or marginal resection.

GIANT-CELL TUMOUR (GCT)[64-78]

Occurring in the skeletally mature, peak incidence is in the third and fourth decades; intermittent pain and local swelling; epiphyseal equivalent; eccentric; central radiolucency with fine trabeculation; expansile; no marginal sclerosis; cortical erosion and soft-tissue extension in late or aggressive lesions; has been classified:

Stage I   normal bony contour
Stage II   expanded contour, intact cortex (Figs 6.18, 6.19)
Stage III   cortical disruption; Codman's triangle; neovascularity; metastatic potential (Figs 6.20, 6.21)

CT scan best displays cortical integrity, MRI soft-tissue extension and arthrotomography penetration of articular cartilage. Multiple GCT are especially common in the hand[73], and bone scan is required to locate all lesions. Secondary aneurysmal bone cysts may develop in GCT. Treatment is problematic, for success, and conversely recurrence and metastasis, has been reported after both curettage and wide resection[71]. Only one-third of GCT throughout the body are cured after one therapy, one-third after two, while one-third require three to five attempts[16]. The recurrence rate is even higher in small bones, having an incidence at the Mayo Clinic of two-thirds[12]. Recurrence usually occurs early, but may take up to five years, and is more common in women. As a result of these statistics some have advocated routine cryotherapy if curettage is employed[70]. Others[72] advocate fairly radical management from the outset for phalangeal GCT, ranging from wide resection for stage I to ray amputation for stage III.

MALIGNANT FIBROUS HISTIOCYTOMA (MFH)[79]

An aggressive, metastasizing lesion identical to that encountered in soft tissues, where it is the most common sarcoma of adults; 30% arise in bone compromised by infarcts or radiation. Any age group, though MFH secondary to infarcts is more common in older patients; insidious onset by tender swelling or pathological fracture; metaphyseal; marked osteolysis, with no internal structure; no expansion; margins very ill-defined with significant intramedullary spread; no periosteal reaction; early soft-tissue involvement (see Fig. 6.16). CT

scan and MRI delineate extent. The minority are relatively, and only relatively, low grade and can be treated by radical excision alone, while the majority require adjuvant chemotherapy.

OSTEOBLASTOMA[82,83]

Akin to osteoid osteoma, but larger; metaphyseal or diaphyseal; central or eccentric; well-defined osteolytic; granular opacities; variable marginal sclerosis. Curettage may be followed by recurrence; some therefore recommend wide excision if feasible[82].

OSTEOCHONDROMA[84-93]

A bony protrusion on the outer surface of the bone capped by cartilage; solitary or multiple; asymptomatic, usually detected as a hard lump in adolescence, or may cause progressive deformity due to impingement on the joint [87,89,92,93]; juxtaepiphyseal, rotates away from the epiphysis with growth; bony protuberance merging with the adjacent normal cortex (Fig. 6.22). Excision is unnecessary unless causing problems, unless sudden rapid growth suggests the development of chondrosarcoma, which occurs very rarely.

OSTEOID OSTEOMA[94-112] (Fig. 6.23)

Benign osteoblastic lesion; pain, especially at night and preferentially relieved by aspirin, is the key feature in diagnosis, but does not always occur[112]; local vasomotor changes with increased temperature and sweating; most cases under 25 years of age; occasionally multiple; cortical or medullary; central, highly vascular nidus is initially lytic but with maturation ossifies; surrounding sclerosis or cortical thickening marked (Fig. 6.24), and may obscure nidus. Angiography shows highly vascular lesion, distinguishing it from an abscess; bone scan highlights location of presenting and any other lesions; tomography displays nidus, confirming diagnosis. Treatment dictates curettage, but in larger bones the difficult task may be in finding the lesion[111]! Intraoperative radiologic control is essential. Even if the nidus is not found, removing overlying sclerosed cortex may give relief from pain.

OSTEOSARCOMA[113-119]

A heterogeneous group of malignant neoplasms; primary osteosarcoma has its peak incidence between 10 and 25 years of age, while osteosarcoma secondary to Paget's, radiation or benign bony lesions occurs in the fifth and sixth decades; aching, constant pain, worse at

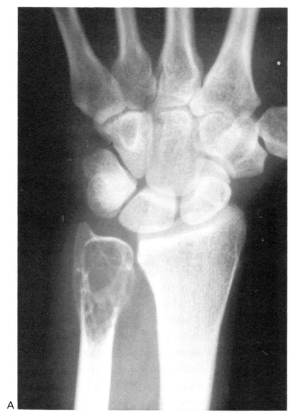

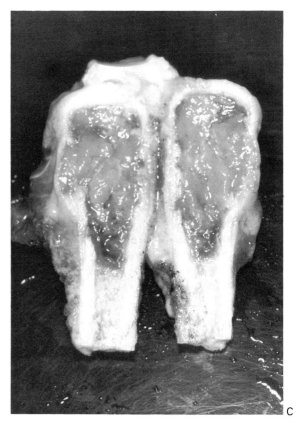

A

C

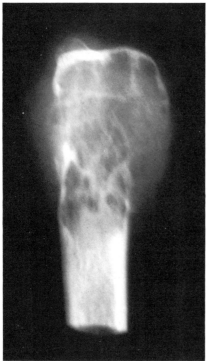

B

Fig. 6.20 Stage III giant-cell tumour. A. This lesion appeared to disrupt the cortex. B. This was confirmed on wide resection. C. The surgical specimen showed the cortical disruption.

night; metaphyseal; destructive lytic lesion associated with a widely variable amount of new bone formation; cortical destruction; spiculation; Codman's triangle; skip lesions; metastases. Bone scan and CT or MRI are necessary to delineate the tumour and define skip lesions; chest CT determines whether metastasis has occurred. Staging biopsy is advisable. Chemotherapy and radical resection are mandatory. Prognosis, which is poor, depends on the duration of symptoms, the location of the tumour (lesions distal on the extremity fare better than those proximal), the size of the lesion, its histological grade and, of course, the presence of metastases.

SIMPLE (UNICAMERAL) BONE CYST[120]

Asymptomatic, this presents by chance or by pathological fracture; peak incidence in childhood; metaphyseal;

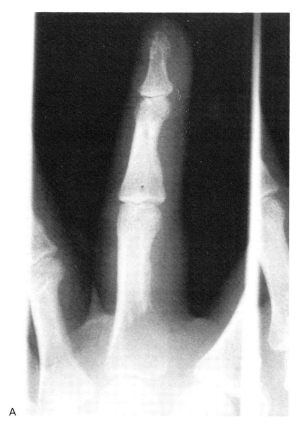

A

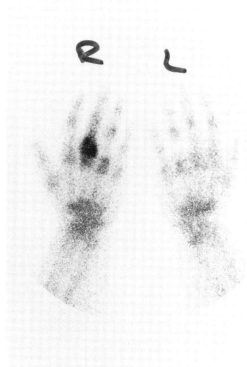

B

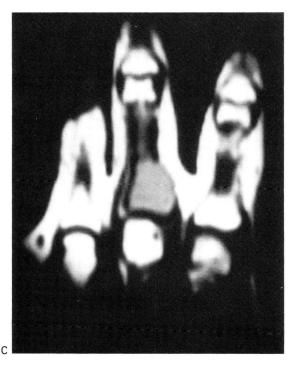

C

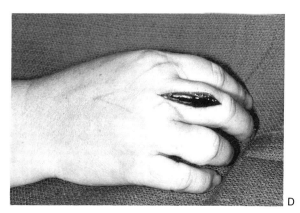

D

Fig. 6.21 Stage III giant-cell tumour. A. This lesion presented disturbing radiologic findings in that there was little evidence of cortex and no marginal sclerosis. This appearance was suggestive of a malignant fibrous histiocytoma. B. Bone scan showed that it was an isolated lesion. C. MRI suggested that it was confined to the immediate phalangeal area. D. Frozen section under tourniquet was considered by the pathologist too difficult to classify histologically.

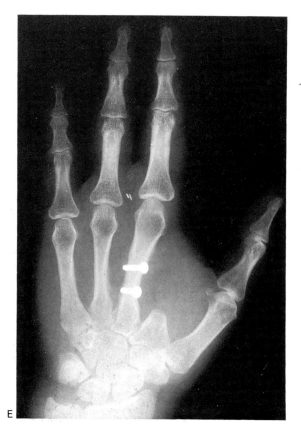

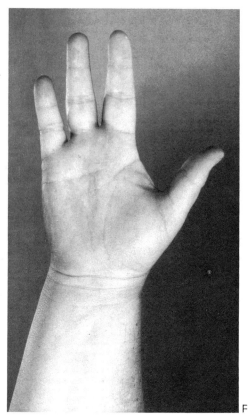

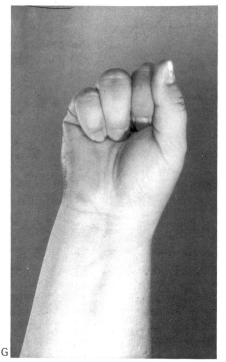

Fig. 6.21   E, F, G. Ray amputation with immediate transposition resulted in good function. On permanent sections the lesion was deemed to be a giant-cell tumour.

central; lytic, trabeculated, contains fluid; expansile as it progresses down the shaft, but only to the width of the epiphyseal plate; sharp interface with marginal sclerosis; cortex thin but always intact. Treatment is problematic, ranging from injection of methylprednisolone acetate to segmental resection and bone grafting.

Muscle

When one considers how much of the upper extremity is muscle, tumours in that tissue are surprisingly rare. Ones which arise in the smooth muscle of vessel walls — *leiomyoma* and *leiomyosarcoma*[355-359] — are rare indeed and are considered no further. While others may occur with reportable rarity, only three swellings arising from muscle need be recalled in diagnosing soft-tissue and bony swellings.

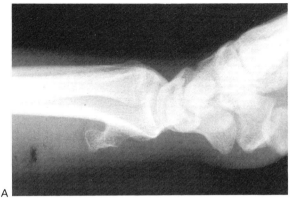

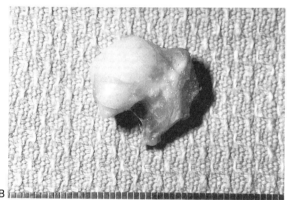

Fig. 6.22   Osteochondroma. A. A bony protuberance merging with adjacent normal cortex, a protuberance which rotates away from the epiphysis in this eighteen-year-old. B. The excised specimen shows the cartilaginous cap.

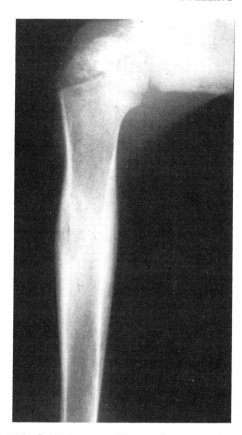

Fig. 6.24   Osteoid osteoma. The significant cortical thickening is smooth and of benign appearance. (Case of Dr Sherman Coleman.)

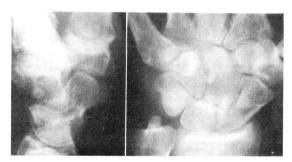

Fig. 6.23   Osteoid osteoma. On standard radiographs this was seen as a radio-opaque area to the ulnar, cortical aspect of the capitate.

GRANULAR CELL MYOBLASTOMA[121,122]

Histological origin in dispute; 15% multifocal; peak incidence fourth to sixth decade; firm, slow-growing lesion in subcutaneous tissue; rarely recurrent; very rarely malignant. Marginal excision curative.

PSEUDOMALIGNANT MYOSITIS OSSIFICANS[123-125] (heterotopic ossification)

Extraosseous bone formation that can easily by mistaken for osteosarcoma; commonly follows mechanical trauma, but may not; association with extensive third degree burns (Fig. 6.25); peak incidence second and third decades; rapid enlargement and severe pain; radiographically no trace for the first two weeks, then ossification, commencing at the periphery of the lesion, being alarmingly undifferentiated in its centre — 'zonal architecture'. Distinction from osteogenic sarcoma: myositis ossificans progresses much more quickly and its zonal architecture is centripetal as opposed to centrifugal.

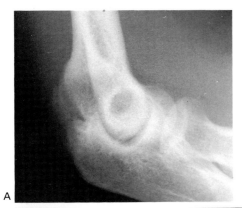

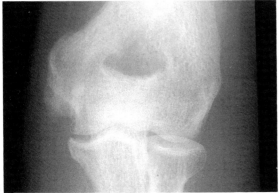

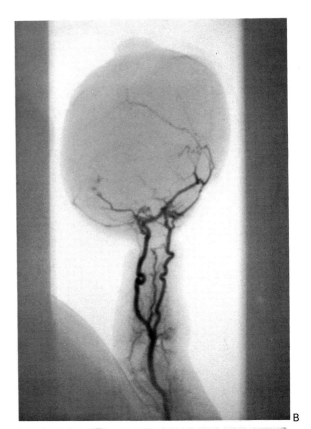

Fig. 6.25   A, B. Pseudomalignant myositis ossificans following third-degree burns in the olecranon fossa and cubital tunnel limited the elbow to 30 degrees of motion. Excision when mature permitted an almost full range.

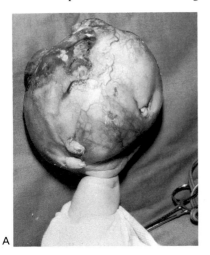

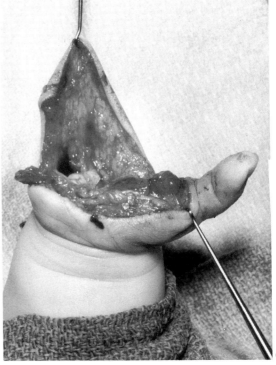

Fig. 6.26   Embryonal rhabdomyosarcoma. A. Present at birth, this lesion was initially felt to be a haemangioma or vascular malformation. B. Angiography demonstrated a relatively avascular lesion. C. After staging and consultation, limb-sparing wide resection was undertaken in conjunction with radiotherapy and chemotherapy.

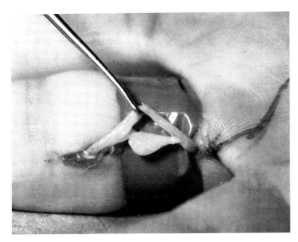

Fig 6.27 This patient came with a somewhat tender, small nodular swelling over the proximal phalanx of her middle finger. This was freely mobile in the transverse direction but not at all in the longitudinal and could therefore be adjudged to be attached to either nerve or artery. At operation it appeared to be intimately involved in the structure of the digital nerve but careful dissection under the microscope showed that it could be completely separated from the fascicles of the nerve. It was a *neurilemmoma*.

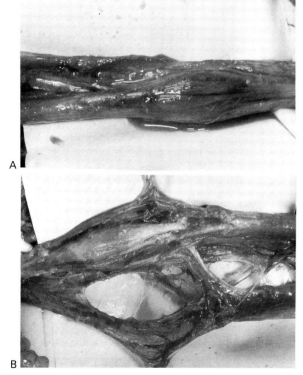

A

B

Fig. 6.28 A, B. Solitary neurofibroma. This patient presented with a painless growth he had noticed in the line of his radial nerve. Exploration, including intraneural dissection, showed a lesion which was in continuity with the fascicles. Biopsy showed this to be a benign neurofibroma.

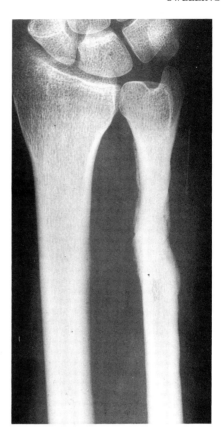

Fig. 6.29 Solitary neurofibroma. Radiographic changes observed in the ulna adjacent to a solitary neurofibroma.

RHABDOMYOSARCOMA[126–128]

'Embryonal' and adult forms, with different peak incidences, the first in infancy and childhood (Fig. 6.26), the second in young adults; actively growing, tender soft-tissue masses; routine radiographs show spread to bone, which can be more precisely determined by bone scan; angiograms show tumour blush; MRI determines extent and defines daughter nodules and skip lesions which are common in rhabdomyosarcoma. Both require radical extracompartmental excision, although the mandatory chemotherapy may permit more limb-sparing in the embryonal lesion. Radiotherapy is a necessary adjunct in the treatment of both forms. No tissue is spared in metastatic spread. The formerly dismal prognosis has been improved by modern team management. Over 50% five-year survival in embryonal, and over 30% in adult rhabdomyosarcoma, can be achieved but to do so requires that none in the medical team may set a foot wrong in walking the tightrope of diagnosis, staging and treatment.

Nerve[136,140,150,158]

Tumours found in peripheral nerves fall into two distinct groups: those of non-neural origin, and those which arise from the Schwann cell. There are three in each group, lipoma, lipofibromatous hamartoma and haemangioma in the former, neurilemmoma, neurofibroma and neurosarcoma in the latter.

Solitary tumours in peripheral nerves usually present as swellings which have the characteristic that they can be freely moved at right angles to the axis of the nerve, but not along that axis. Unless they lie in canals commonly associated with nerve compression (Ch. 3), pain and distal sensory changes and motor weakness have sinister import.

All such lesions require exploration for the purposes of identification, doubly so if they are symptomatic. The first in each of the above groups, *lipoma*[143,145,154,159] and *neurilemmoma*[131,132,135,139,151,152] are readily recognized for they can be easily removed in toto by epineurotomy and interfascicular dissection aided by magnification, without interfering with the functional fascicles of the nerve (Fig. 6.27). Staging studies are of no assistance. Marginal excision by enucleation cures.

The second in each of the groups, *lipofibromatous hamartoma*[129,130,137,138,141,146,148,153] and *solitary neurofibroma* cannot, for they are intimately involved within most or all of the fascicles (Fig. 6.28). Staging studies are of no assistance, although if a neurofibroma is close to periosteum it may produce cortical sclerosis (Fig. 6.29). Once tissue has been taken to ensure the diagnosis they can be left alone, provided they were asymptomatic, for malignant change in either is exceedingly rare. If symptomatic, and they lie in a compressive site, decompression of the canal will suffice. If symptomatic and no cause for compression can be demonstrated, resection is justified, for only histological inspection of the whole lesion will exclude early malignancy (Fig. 6.30).

INTRANEURAL HAEMANGIOMA[147,149]

Like the last pair, haemangioma may well present with peripheral neurological changes. Unlike them, simple decompression of a canal does not give lasting relief. As with all vascular lesions (see below), partial excision, in this case to save the involved nerve, does not work and recurrence is inevitable. Total excision of the haemangioma with grafting of the nerve is more likely to be curative and, partly because these lesions arise in children, partly because grafting is done immediately after surgical division of the nerve, partly because motor-sensory identification of fascicles can be done, recovery of function is remarkably good (Fig 6.31).

NEUROFIBROMATOSIS (NF)[133,134,142,144,151,157]

Autosomal dominant, this condition takes two forms — bilateral acoustic NF and von Recklinghausen's disease (VRD). The latter is a neurocutaneous syndrome affecting the skin, the eye and the peripheral nerves to a degree that is highly variable. The National Neurofibromatosis Foundation Inc, 141 Fifth Avenue, New York 10010 (1.800.323.7938) has established criteria for the diagnosis and, more importantly, set up support groups for patients with this condition, which can be crippling both physically and psychologically. 'Cafe-au-lait' spots, brown macules on the skin, are a distinctive but not essential criterion.

The hand surgeon comes in contact with NF patients either because of macrodactyly (p. 494) or because of peripheral nerve involvement in the upper extremity. Because of the multiplicity of the lesions, prophylactic excision of neurofibromata is not practical. Unlike solitary neurofibroma, NF has an incidence of malignant change[155,160] of 10%, dictating the need for prompt intervention with the onset of pain, tumour enlargement or peripheral nerve symptoms.

NEUROSARCOMA (= fibrosarcoma of nerve sheath = Schwannoma = neurogenic sarcoma)

Some 40% arise de novo, the remainder in pre-existing neurofibromatosis; secondary neurosarcoma arises most commonly in the fourth decade; pain, enlargement, dysaesthesia, weakness in the presence of a pre-existing lesion; angiography shows the extent in the early arterial phase by defining the reactive zone, but 'tumour blush' is not marked; MRI can define the primary neurosarcoma but cannot distinguish benign from malignant in neurofibromatosis. Preoperative and, indeed, peroperative definition of the neurosarcomatous lesion amongst the several neurofibromata which may be present is difficult. Prognosis after radical extracompartmental excision is worse in secondary, compared with primary, partly perhaps because the patient who has had a swelling for many years may present less early than the one who has found a new lump, partly because of the differing histology, the primary being cellular, the secondary fibrous.

Skin and adnexae

Factors which increase the incidence of skin tumours on the hand are radiation, chronic open wounds, scars, chronic exposure to sunlight or arsenical compounds and a deficient immune system, such as occurs in AIDS and following organ transplant. By far the most common of these factors is sunlight, or actinic exposure.

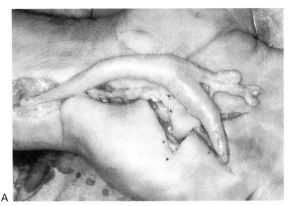

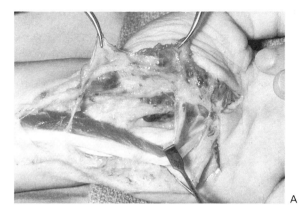

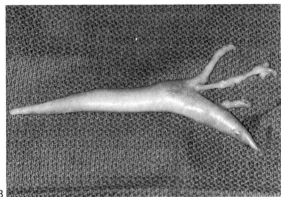

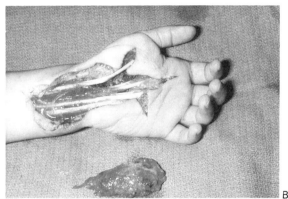

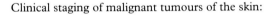

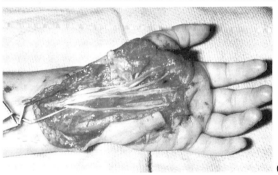

Fig. 6.30 Solitary neurofibroma. This patient presented with pain, fairly rapid growth of the swelling in the hand and diminution in two-point discrimination in the ulnar nerve distribution. Excision was deemed appropriate but the lesion proved benign. Immediate grafting was performed.

Clinical staging of malignant tumours of the skin:

Stage I	no nodes or metastases
Stage II	involvement of regional nodes, no metastases elsewhere
Stage III	metastases other than locally or to regional nodes

ACTINIC LESIONS[161-163]

When sun exposure of those with light skin pigment is occupational, and prolonged, it leads to hyperkeratosis and thence to basal cell carcinoma or, more frequently, squamous-cell carcinoma. Since most people working in the sun wear clothes, these changes occur most frequently on the head and neck, hands and forearms. *Xeroderma pigmentosum* accelerates the response

Fig. 6.31 Intraneural haemangioma. A. The median nerve was infiltrated throughout its course in the carpal tunnel by haemangioma. Attempts at interfascicular dissection failed. B. The haemangioma was excised in toto and replaced (C) with immediate interfascicular nerve grafts. Median nerve recovery was excellent.

so that the tumours develop in childhood (Fig. 6.32). When there is field change, with lesions at various stages present, excision of the whole area and resurfacing with skin graft is advisable (Fig. 6.33). There is evidence that when the sun exposure is recreational,

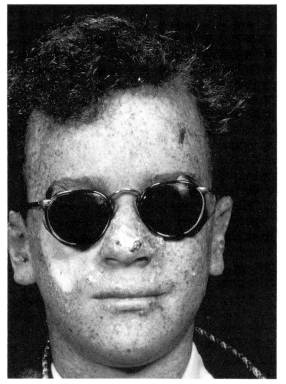

Fig. 6.32   Xeroderma pigmentosum. This teenage boy presented with multiple basal and squamous-cell carcinomata.

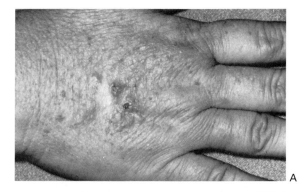

A

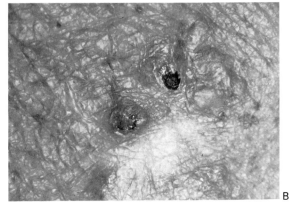

B

Fig. 6.34   A, B. Basal cell carcinoma of the 'self-healing, cicatrizing, or field fire' variety.

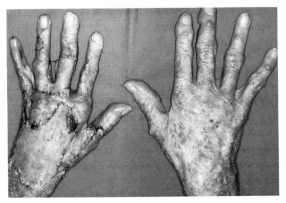

Fig. 6.33   Actinic field change affecting both hands, of which the one of the left of the photograph was excised and grafted three weeks previously.

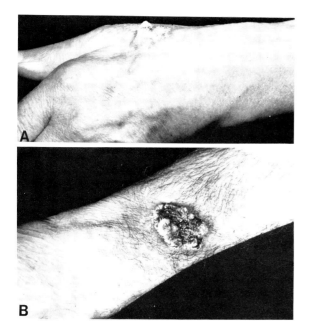

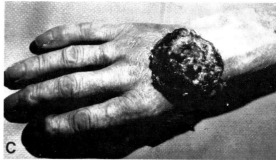

Fig. 6.35 Squamous-cell carcinoma on the hand may be encountered at a very early hyperkeratotic stage (A), in a more florid but excrescent form with little involvement of the underlying tissues (B), or quite commonly in an advanced stage with some involvement of the underlying tissue, usually with superadded infection (C). In this last case, quite marked lymphadenopathy was present. This was observed for a period of six weeks after excision of the primary tumour and disappeared completely. This phenomenon is often encountered with squamous-cell carcinoma and is due to secondary infection.

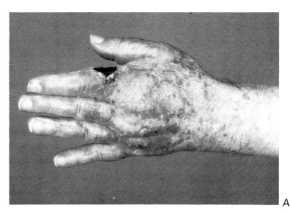

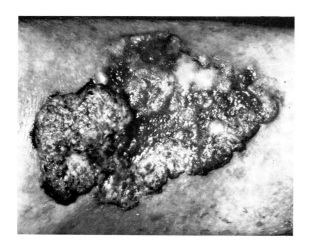

Fig 6.36 Marjolin's ulcer. This ulcer had been present for some sixteen years and showed change in that the edges began to become heaped up in appearance. A crust formed over the ulcer which, on removal, produced brisk bleeding. Subsequent histological examination showed this to be *squamous-cell carcinoma*.

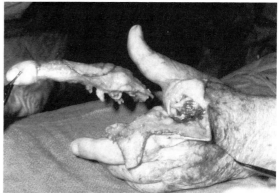

Fig. 6.37 Infiltrating squamous-cell carcinoma. A. The lesion was firmly fixed to deep structures. B. Ray amputation was performed.

and therefore intermittent but intense, the incidence of malignant melanoma is increased.

Hyperkeratosis

Superficial, dry crusty lesions on the dorsum of the hand; while of the skin, that skin is freely mobile over the underlying tissue; frequently present with the next two lesions. Excision not necessary, but observation for change required.

Basal cell carcinoma (BCC)[164]

This may have the characteristic appearance, a heaped up lesion with pearly borders, but may be less evident with a 'field fire' or 'self-healing' morphology (Fig. 6.34): it is almost always mobile over underlying tissues and very rarely metastasizes. Excision with 5 mm clearance confirmed by frozen section is adequate.

Squamous-cell carcinoma (SCC)[165–177]

By far the most common malignant tumour encountered on the hand, this may be:

dry and crusty, barely distinguishable from hyperkeratosis (Fig. 6.35A),
a florid granulomatous lesion which is infected with surrounding erythema (Fig. 6.35C), or
an open ulcer, with heaped edges, a red floor which easily bleeds and an indurated base which is rarely attached to deep structures.

Lymph node metastases are more common in the hand than in SCC of the skin elsewhere, especially when the tumour follows arsenical dermatosis, burns or chronic wounds (Marjolin's ulcer is a tumour arising in a pre-existing chronic wound [Fig. 6.36], occurring in 5–15%). Excision with a 1 cm. margin is curative. If the lesion is fixed to deep structures, such clearance may require amputation (Fig. 6.37). Lymphadenectomy in the presence of lymphadenopathy is indicated, except when the primary is clearly infected, when the enlarged nodes may regress within six weeks. Recurrence should probably be accompanied by prophylactic lymphadenectomy[176].

SCC of the *nail* presents most commonly as an intractable infection. If subungual suppuration persists for more than two weeks, the nail should be removed and the nail-bed biopsied (Fig. 6.38). As the nail-bed is fixed to the distal phalanx, disarticulation at the interphalangeal joint is the correct resection.

BOWEN'S DISEASE[178–181] (Fig. 6.39)

This dry, sessile, often scaly, lesion is carcinoma in situ. Previously reported as being associated with an increased incidence of visceral carcinoma, this is not so. Excision or observation is appropriate.

EPIDERMOID INCLUSION CYST[182–186]

Due to a minor wound which drives skin cells below the skin surface, this forms a smooth, spherical tumour which is attached to skin, but mobile over the underlying tissues. Found almost exclusively on the palmar surface, it is most common around the fingertips, especially after digital amputation. In the latter situation it commonly erodes into the terminal phalanx, producing a smoothly lytic lesion; no mineral deposition; very mildly expansile; marginal sclerosis; cortex intact; no periosteal reaction (Fig. 6.40). Enucleation cures.

KERATOACANTHOMA[187–189]

A volcano-like lesion, its crater filled with a keratin plug, this lesion is found on the dorsum of the hand, where it grows with alarming speed, only to regress and disappear if left alone. This rarely happens, however, before the patient seeks medical advice and the pathologist may have difficulty in distinguishing its edge from that of a squamous-cell carcinoma, which indeed it may be (Fig. 6.41). If it is, then it is unusually aggressive. For this reason most keratoacanthomata are excised with a 5 mm margin.

MALIGNANT MELANOMA[190–199]

Change in a previously existing pigmented lesion should always be viewed with great suspicion. The change may take the form of increase in size, change in colour, development of nodules, bleeding or the onset of itching. Melanoma has been classified morphologically:

Superficial spreading melanoma
Lentigo maligna melanoma develops within a Hutchison's freckle, a patch of pigmentation on exposed skin in older patients (Fig. 6.42) (Both of the above have a similar prognosis.)
Nodular melanoma, unlike the first two, grows vertically from the outset and therefore has a worse prognosis

Acral lentiginous melanoma occurs in the palms and beneath the nails[191,197–199] (Fig. 6.43) and is the most common type seen in black patients; it carries the worst prognosis.

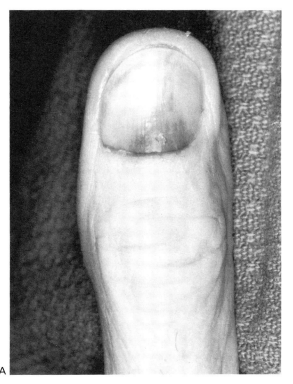
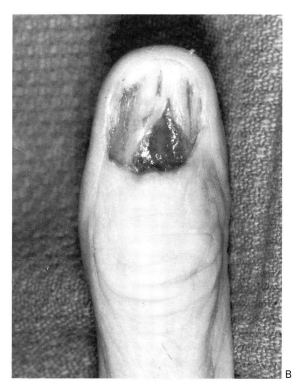

A B

Fig. 6.38 Carcinoma of the nail bed. A. Subungual discoloration and surrounding inflammation that persisted despite antibiotic treatment for some weeks. B. Removal of the nail and biopsy revealed a squamous-cell carcinoma which was treated by disarticulation through the interphalangeal joint.

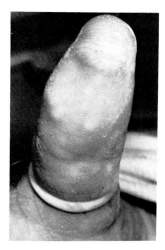

Fig. 6.39 This patient presented with the nodular lesion beneath the thumb pulp with multiple seed nodules further proximal. Biopsy showed this to be *Bowen's disease* which was thereafter observed, and showed no progression.

Amelanotic melanoma is an entirely unpigmented, rather granulomatous lesion which may be confused with a pyogenic granuloma (Fig. 6.44).

Stage I melanoma may be accompanied by 'satellite' lesions in the skin surrounding the primary tumour, very akin to the 'skip lesions' of musculoskeletal tumours; such lesions are ominous[196].

The *Breslow system*[193,194]. The thickness of a melanoma at its deepest part when viewed histologically has been found to be most reliable both in establishing a prognosis and guiding treatment:

< 0.76 mm   uniformly curable; marginal excision by 1 cm
< 2.00 mm   margin 2 cm of skin; interphalangeal amputation
> 2.00 mm   margin 3–5 cm skin; ray amputation.

Whether prophylactic lymphadenectomy is beneficial in thicker lesions is still controversial[195]. Lymph node resection is mandatory in the presence of palpable nodes and should be radical, not simply the removal of enlarged nodes. The prognosis in clinical stage II has been found to be worse the more nodes are found to

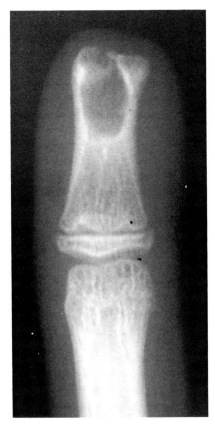

Fig. 6.40 Epidermoid inclusion cyst of the bone. Some years after traumatic amputation this patient has a lesion which shows characteristic features: smoothly lytic; no mineral deposition; mildly expansile; marginal sclerosis; cortex intact; no periosteal reaction.

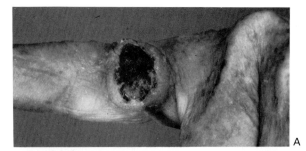

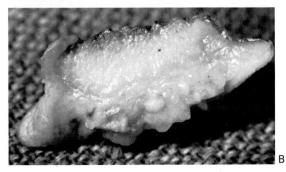

Fig. 6.41 A, B. Kerato-acanthoma or squamous-cell carcinoma? This lesion proved on excisional biopsy to be a squamous-cell carcinoma of the index finger.

be involved at lymphadenectomy. Stage III lesions are usually fatal, but resection of isolated metastases has yielded prolonged survival in some cases. Isolated limb perfusion may prove beneficial in eliminating in-transit metastases[191]. Absence of antigen-specific immune complexes in the serum of the patient after excision is predictive of a disease-free status[200].

An occasional patient will present with secondary melanoma for which no primary can be found despite an exhaustive search (Fig. 6.45).

Patients who have been treated for malignant melanoma must be followed at intervals throughout their lives, for recurrence after fifteen or more disease-free years has been reported.

The increased potential for the development of malignant melanoma in *giant hairy nevus* is still debated. It appears to be valid, and is more likely in lesions which are thick, darkly pigmented and have a wart-like surface (Fig. 6.46). Since malignant change appears to be maximal during the first five years of life, early excision, including a generous margin to avoid further pigmentation, with skin graft is appropriate.

PYOGENIC GRANULOMA

Pyogenic granuloma is a florid, haemorrhagic overgrowth of granulation tissue presumably at the site of a forgotten minor laceration, usually on the finger (Fig. 6.8). Its only significance is its similarity to amelanotic melanoma. It should be excised promptly, both to stop the bleeding and to reassure all that it is indeed benign. Rarely a counterpart may occur intravenously[201].

SWEAT GLAND TUMOURS[202–205] (acrospiroma, cylindroma, eccrine tumour, hidradenoma, spiradenoma, syringoma, any of the former preceded by the word 'malignant', sweat gland carcinoma)

Since the apocrine glands in the upper extremity are confined to the axilla, all sweat gland tumours encountered by the hand surgeon arise from eccrine glands. Some 90% are benign and present as firm,

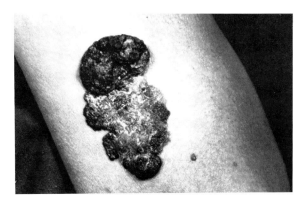

Fig. 6.42 This patient presented with a history of having a previously flat pigmented lesion on the inner aspect of the upper arm. This subsequently underwent an increase in size, the development of an excrescent area in the upper part of the lesion, changes in colour, persistent irritation, and recent bleeding on contact with clothing. As anticipated, it proved to be a *lentigo maligna melanoma*.

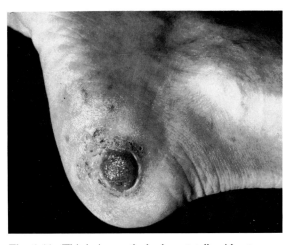

Fig. 6.44 This lesion on the heel was totally without pigment even after careful examination under magnification. Suspicions were entertained regarding its nature and wide excision performed. It was indeed an *amelanotic melanoma*.

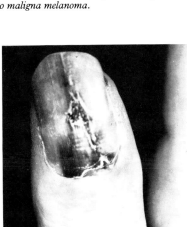

Fig. 6.43 Acral lentiginous melanoma. This patient presented with a history of a dark lesion deep to the nail of the thumb present for some twelve months.

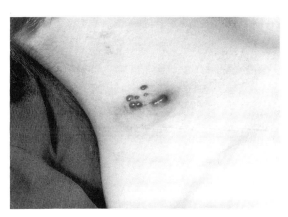

Fig. 6.45 Secondary malignant melanoma. This patient presented with a pigmented lesion in the right posterior triangle. Histology showed this to be a secondary malignant melanoma deposit in a lymph node. No primary was ever found.

nodular masses attached to the skin but mobile over the underlying tissue. Malignant change is seen so rarely in these rare lesions that no 'red flags' have been identified. All swellings which the surgeon cannot identify with confidence must be subjected to excisional biopsy obeying the rules enunciated at the beginning of this chapter. If malignancy is detected in a sweat gland tumour, it requires grading. If grade 1, wide re-excision is required; if grade 2, radical excision is indicated, dictating ray amputation if a digit is involved.

Subcutaneous tissue

EPITHELIOID SARCOMA[206–213]

A soft-tissue mass which slowly enlarges, most often found in the extremities and usually in the second and third decades, epithelioid sarcoma is distinguished by inflammatory reaction. This causes pain and tenderness, but no systemic manifestations, and often results in its being treated as an infection, with antibiotics and incision, often repeated (Fig. 6.47). It becomes in-

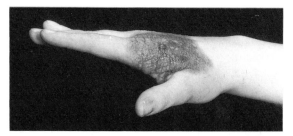

Fig. 6.46 Giant hairy nevus. This lesion, although not visibly hairy, was thick, showed variable dark pigmentation and had a wart-like surface. Excision with a 5 mm margin and full-thickness skin graft was performed.

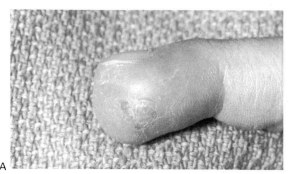

A

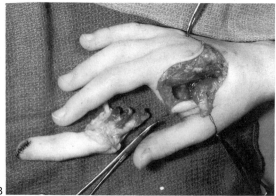

B

Fig. 6.47 Epithelioid sarcoma. A. This teenage girl had undergone numerous incisions of the lesion in the tip of her finger. B. Incisional biopsy performed under tourniquet (the wound of biopsy is shown in the tip of the finger) showed this to be an epithelioid sarcoma. Ray amputation has resulted in prolonged survival.

creasingly aggressive but is late to metastasize. When it does, it is more prone to go to regional lymph nodes than other sarcomata. Staging studies are unrewarding, bone scan showing remarkably little increase in uptake, angiograms showing a tumour blush, but CT and MRI failing to show a clear margin with normal tissue, partly due to the common previous incisions. Wide

excision of untouched lesions is curative; this may require ray amputation. Radiotherapy and chemotherapy have no role.

FIBROMA[214-234]

There is a wide and confusing spectrum of fibromatoses which includes keloid, torticollis and Dupuytren's amongst over thirty variants[7].

Dermatofibroma
Dermatofibroma is a small, spherical, firm nodule found on the dorsum, the palm or the wrist in children attached either to the skin or the underlying tissue (Fig. 6.48). Simple excision is effective.

Juvenile aponeurotic fibroma[214-216,224,231,232,234]
This, again is found in children but more commonly on the palmar surface. Of similar consistency to the dermatofibroma, it is multinodular and more likely to be fixed to the deeper tissues. Radiologic examination may show some calcification, and it often contains cartilage[231]. Marginal excision is very likely to result in recurrence, so wide excision with preservation of normal structures is recommended.

This gradually increasing aggression is a feature of fibromatous lesions of children, until one reaches tumours so locally aggressive and so unrelenting in their local recurrence that repeated, more radical amputation becomes the unhappy course (Fig. 6.49). Rarely, metastatic fibrosarcoma may be the outcome[224].

FIBROSARCOMA[235,236]

Believed by some to be precipitated by injury or scar, fibrosarcoma develops as a deep soft-tissue mass, most

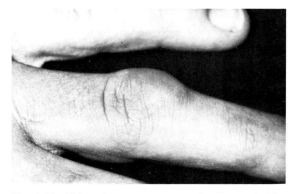

Fig. 6.48 This patient was a teenager who presented with a history of a swelling which had developed over the proximal interphalangeal joint of his left ring finger. This was firmly attached to skin and proved to be a *dermatofibroma*.

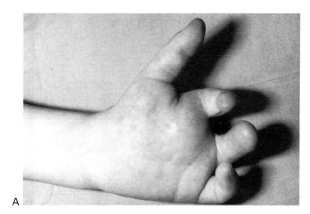

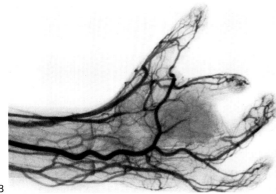

Fig. 6.49 Aggressive juvenile fibromatosis.
A. A fibromatous lesion developed in this child's hand
following syndactyly release. This was followed by ray
amputation, but the recurrence shown here ensued some 12
months later. B. The late arterial, early venous phase already
shows a tumour blush present in the metacarpophalangeal
region. Less noticeable is the blush at the level of the carpus.
Wrist disarticulation, though depressingly radical, failed to
eliminate this lesion. Recurrence in the forearm occurred
some two years later.

prevalent in the fifth and sixth decades. Metastasis is
mainly to the lung, with little propensity to spread to
regional lymph nodes. Staging is aided by angiogram,
CT and MRI, for the lesion shows distinct boundaries.
It has been suggested that histological grade varies with
the degree of uptake on isotope scan and that prognosis
depends on histological grade. Excision is determined
by staging.

MALIGNANT FIBROUS HISTIOCYTOMA (MFH)[248-258]

Dermatofibrosarcoma protuberans represents the superficial form of MFH, stage IA; presents as a multinodular, firm, reddish lesion immediately beneath the skin
to which it is attached and which readily ulcerates,

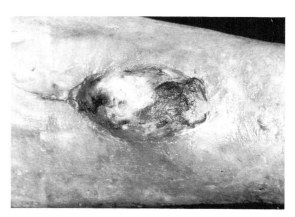

Fig. 6.50 Dermatofibrosarcoma protuberans. This
represents stage I malignant fibrous histiocytoma. Repeated
marginal excision failed to cure this patient. The lesion
resolved after radical removal of the tumour and underlying
tissue.

displaying greyish-white, relatively avascular tumour
(Fig. 6.50). Often fixed to underlying tissue, it is characterized by bursts of rapid growth and high recurrence
following excision. Metastasizes but rarely and never
involves the regional nodes. Wide excision is necessary
to prevent recurrence.

The deep form of MFH represents stage IIB and
presents as a large mass with a rapid growth rate often
with involvement of the regional lymph nodes. MFH
invades adjacent bone, and pathological fracture may
occur. Isotope scans show increased uptake, *especially in
radiologically uninvolved adjacent bone*; angiograms show
a marked reactive zone and tumour blush at the lesion
and will also show node involvement. So aggressive is
the deep MFH that it has been recommended that it be
treated in the manner appropriate for one stage worse
than that revealed by staging studies. Radical resection, preceded by radiotherapy and supplemented with
chemotherapy may be required.

Synovium and tendon

GANGLION[259-284]

Ganglion is the most common swelling encountered in
the hand. It may arise virtually anywhere in the limb
and be significant more for its effects than its mere
presence, as in Guyon's canal where it produces nerve
compression (see Ch. 3). It is most commonly found in
one of four sites:

Distal phalanx (Fig. 6.51). Overlying the nail-bed,
this ganglion from the distal interphalangeal joint,
formerly considered to be a mucous cyst, invariably

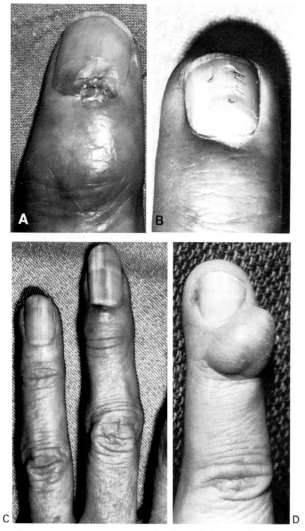

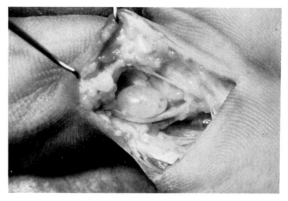

Fig. 6.52   Ganglion of the flexor tendon sheath.

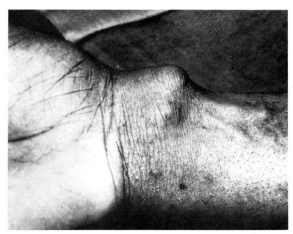

Fig. 6.53   A common site for a *ganglion* of the wrist is on the radial side of the anterior aspect. Most of these ganglia arise from the intercarpal joints and pass along the tendon of flexor carpi radialis in its tunnel under the ridge of the trapezium before emerging on the wrist. This should be carefully pursued at the time of surgery if recurrence is to be avoided.

Fig. 6.51   A. A ganglion over the distal phalanx arising from the distal interphalangeal joint in the presence of osteoarthritis commonly produces distortions of the nail which grow out after excision (B). This is the so-called 'mucous cyst'. C, D. Two other presentations of a *ganglion* of the distal interphalangeal joint.

produces a groove or even a split in the nail. Not infrequently this ganglion erodes the overlying skin or is incised. It is then often the seat of chronic or recurrent infection[280]. A local flap may be required to cover the defect created by excision.

Proximal digital crease. The ganglion here emerges from the tendon sheath just distal to the proximal pulley. It presents as a small, very firm, immobile and often tender mass palpable to one or other side of the mid-

line (Fig. 6.52). It is most commonly encountered in the middle finger and in one series more than 25% of the patients were full-time typists.

Anterior aspect of the wrist (Fig. 6.53). Ganglia in this site are almost always found just lateral to the flexor carpi radialis tendon, in close proximity to the radial artery which they may occlude[269,271] (Fig. 6.54). Although in some instances they arise from the radiocarpal or inferior radioulnar joint, they usually have their origin in the scapholunate and pass along the tunnel of flexor carpi radialis. The surgeon must be aware of this fact so that he may pursue it and thereby reduce the chances of recurrence.

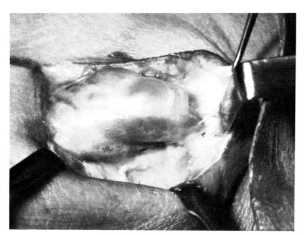

Fig. 6.54 The anterior wrist ganglion is very commonly closely adherent to the radial artery. In these instances, the integrity of the ganglion should be sacrificed if any danger exists of entering the wall of the radial artery.

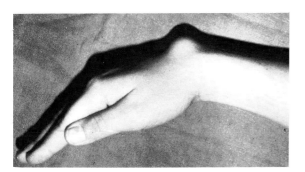

Fig. 6.55 A dorsal swelling not attached to the skin characteristic of a cystic *ganglion*.

Dorsal aspect of the wrist (Fig. 6.55). All the ganglia so far considered are cystic, well-defined masses. The dorsal ganglion may also be so, but not uncommonly is a more sessile, ill-defined swelling. Commonly arising from the scapholunate joint, this ganglion is intimately involved in the dorsal capsule and is often associated with complaints of pain and weakness of the wrist [264] (Fig. 6.56).

Because of similar aching, its position and its sessile character, an anomalous *extensor digitorum brevis manus* is often misdiagnosed as a dorsal ganglion. A *carpometacarpal boss*[26,27] also presents in a similar site, being an excess of bone at the second or, less commonly, third metacarpal. However, its consistency and radiographic appearance (Fig. 6.57) distinguish it from a ganglion.

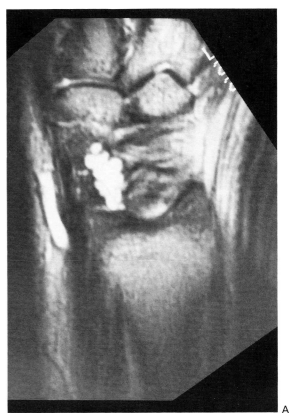

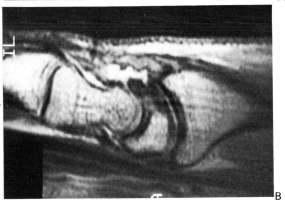

Fig. 6.56 A, B. Occult ganglion. Persistent pain and weakness of grip strength led to bone scan which was hot. MRI revealed the lesion.

Films of the appropriate area should always be taken. The distal interphalangeal joint is often the seat of osteoarthristis. Any pathology of the carpus must be excluded before surgery, since excision involves dissection amongst the ligaments of the wrist and postoperative problems will be thought to be due to the surgery if not detected before surgery. Ganglia may

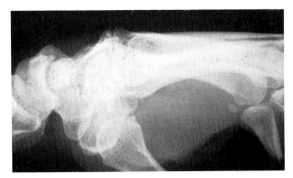

Fig. 6.57   Carpometacarpal boss.

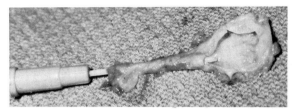

Fig. 6.59   The neck to a ganglion is frequently longer than the width of the ganglion itself.

be *intraosseus*[261,262,266,268,270,276, 278], especially in the carpus (Fig. 6.58). Like osteoid osteoma, locating the lesion at surgery may prove difficult.

Recurrence of a ganglion after excision is not uncommon. The best safeguard is to pursue the neck of the ganglion to its very source, often a lengthy chase (Fig. 6.59). It is possible, of course, that the recurrence may be a second, new lesion.

GIANT-CELL TUMOUR (= pigmented villonodular synovitis)[285–294]

This is the second most common swelling encountered in the hand following ganglion cyst. The aetiology is not clear, but it is always found in the presence of synovial tissue, most commonly arising from the flexor tendon sheath or interphalangeal joints. It presents therefore on the finger, somewhat more often on the palmar than on the dorsal surface. Because it is usually symptomless, the patient may present late, by which time there may be a visible, irregular swelling. On palpation, it has the consistency of soft rubber and it may be difficult to define its boundaries.

On occasion it produces radiologic changes by pressure (Fig. 6.60), by eroding the osteochondral junction like rheumatoid pannus, or by migrating along the foramina of bony vessels. Exploration reveals the very characteristic yellow and brown mottled tumour which surrounds normal structures rather than displacing them (Fig. 6.61).

Excision cures the condition only if the lesion is pursued throughout its often tortuous path, which may

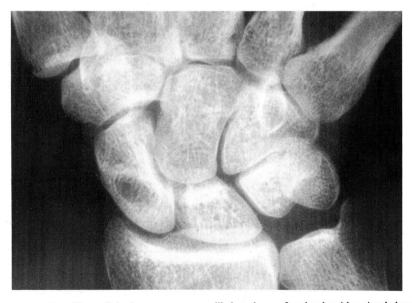

Fig. 6.58   Intraosseous ganglion. The radiologic appearances are likely to be confused only with a simple bone cyst. However, the location of this lytic lesion in the carpus makes an intraosseous ganglion more likely.

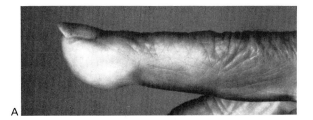

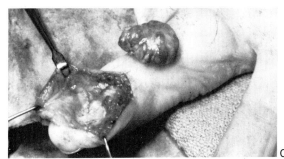

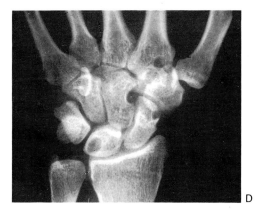

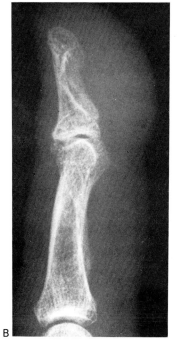

Fig. 6.60 A. A rubbery, ill-defined swelling in the terminal pulp produced (B) scalloping of the distal phalanx. The lesion proved to be a well-localized *giant-cell tumour* (C). D. In its more widespread form as pigmented villonodular synovitis, it produces multiple bony erosions in the carpus. (Case of Dr Sherman Coleman.)

be circumferential and also involve the entire flexor tendon sheath. Otherwise recurrence is common[285] (Fig. 6.62).

SYNOVIAL SARCOMA[295-298]

Most common in the extremities, this tumour need not arise from synovial membrane. A minority present as relatively indolent lumps beneath the skin of the hand, in stark contrast to the majority which arise in muscle bulk, are larger, have a more rapid growth rate and are painful. About one-third of synovial sarcomata have fine granular calcification which is pathognomonic when taken in conjunction with the factors previously mentioned. Early spread to regional nodes is a feature shared with MFH. In the larger lesions, isotope scans demonstrate an unusually vigorous reactive zone; angiograms and CT scan further delineate the lesion and node involvement. By contrast the smaller lesions

appear relatively benign and are often diagnosed only by excisional biopsy. Wide excision will cure the small peripheral lesions, but recurrence after inadequate excision will often require amputation (Fig. 6.63). Preoperative radiotherapy plays an important role, followed by radical excision supplemented by chemotherapy.

XANTHOMA[299-302]

This lesion represents a collection of lipid material, usually on extensor tendons, found in patients with hypercholesterolaemia[299]. It is not a tumour, and is mentioned here first to distinguish it from giant-cell tumour of tendon sheath, which has on occasion been called xanthoma, and secondly because the finding of these lesions may presage the more serious consequences of atherosclerosis which may be offset by appropriate management.

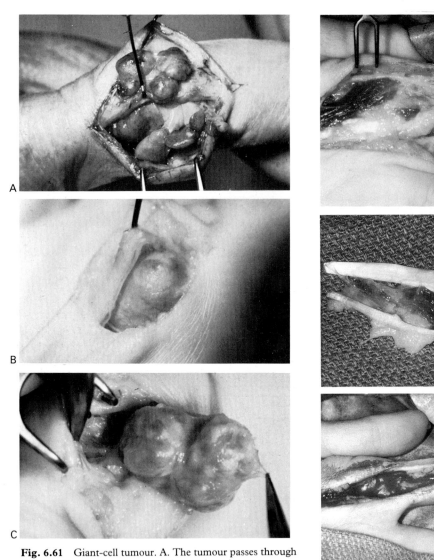

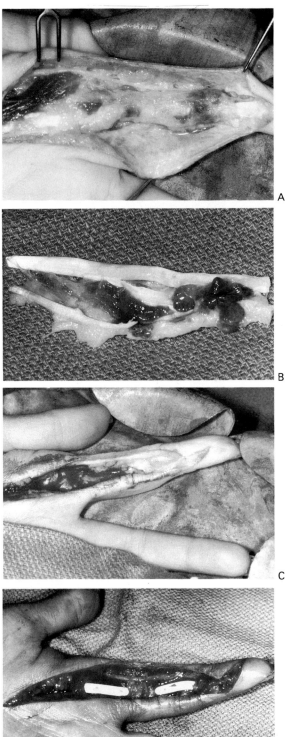

Fig. 6.61 Giant-cell tumour. A. The tumour passes through the interstices in the extensor tendon, and can be seen emerging from various aspects of the proximal interphalangeal joint. B, C.The giant-cell tumour characteristically envelops normal structures, here the digital nerve, which has grooved the tumour.

Fig. 6.62 Recurrent giant-cell tumour of tendon sheath. A. This patient had undergone 13 previous attempts to remove the giant-cell tumour of the tendon sheath. Amputation was discussed and declined. B. All structures on the anterior surface of the finger were excised. C. Release of the tourniquet revealed absent circulation. D. Arterial graft, pulley reconstruction and two-stage tendon graft restored function with no evidence of recurrence after two years.

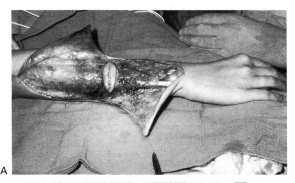
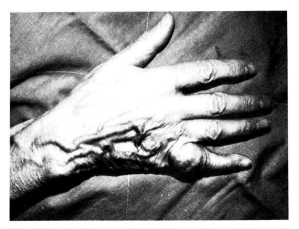

Fig. 6.63 Synovial sarcoma. A. This patient had undergone an enucleation of a painful swelling in the muscle of the extensor compartment. The histology showed synovial sarcoma. B. On referral, and after refusal of amputation by the patient, radical compartment excision was performed in conjunction with radiotherapy and chemotherapy. The patient died of miliary sarcomatosis of the lung nine months later.

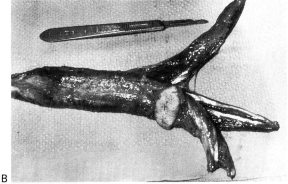

Fig. 6.64 Arteriovenous fistula. The swelling at the base of the small finger was pulsatile and the temperature of the overlying skin was significantly higher than that of the adjacent normal fingers. The grossly varicose veins on the ulnar aspect of the dorsum of the hand made the diagnosis virtually certain.

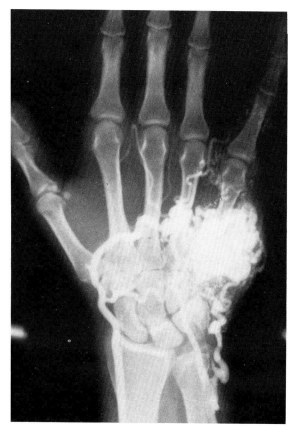

Fig. 6.65 All of the angiographic features of arteriovenous fistulae are shown in this examination, with dilatation of the arteries, absence of normal filling distal to the fistula, 'snowflake' pooling of the medium in the fistula and the presence of contrast in the veins in this early film in the angiographic series.

Vessel

ACQUIRED ARTERIOVENOUS FISTULA (Fig. 6.64)

Such arteriovenous fistulae may arise as a result of trauma — commonly a penetrating wound — or iatrogenically. Iatrogenic fistulae may of course be intentional for the purposes of dialysis or they may arise as a complication of cardiac catheterization (p. 48). Blood flow through such fistulae has been recorded as being as much as forty times normal. The patient may consult the physician because of the pulsatile swelling or because of a recent wound to another part of the hand which has failed to heal. This arose because of a 'steal' phenomenon whereby the flow through the fistula is so high that less blood than normal reaches the more distal circulation to the digits. Examination reveals obvious

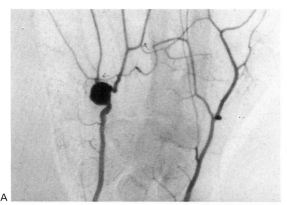

A

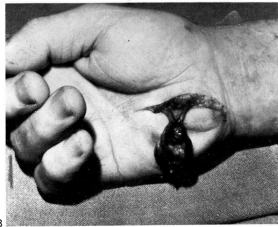

B

Fig. 6.66 A. Traumatic aneurysm. B. This patient gave a history of having struck his hand very forcibly over the ulnar aspect some two weeks previously and presented with a painful, pulsatile swelling. Angiography showed an evident aneurysm, which was excised and grafted.

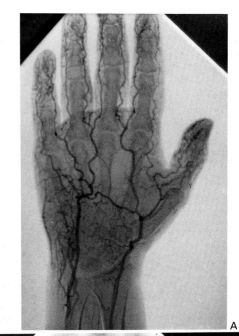

A

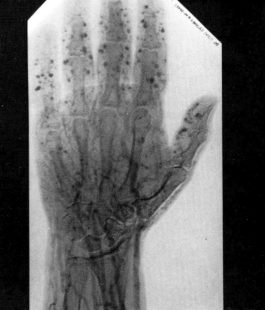

B

Fig. 6.67 Venous aneurysms. During the arterial phase (A) these lesions are not evident, but once the angiogram enters the venous phase, the multiple small venous aneurysms can be seen.

varicosities in a limb which may or may not be hypertrophied. The skin temperature over the lesion is elevated, in the digits subject to 'steal', lowered. The varicosities can be emptied by firm pressure but quickly refill. A thrill should be sought with the palpating hand and auscultation performed to detect a bruit. When the arteriovenous shunt is severe, the pulse pressure is greatly increased and the patient is in danger of developing high-output cardiac failure. Occlusion of the main artery to the limb in such circumstances will result in appreciable slowing of the pulse (the *Branham reaction*). Studies of the oxygen saturation of the venous blood should be performed. In the presence of an arteriovenous fistula the saturation will exceed that of central venous samples.

Angiographic signs (Fig. 6.65) in arteriovenous fistula are:

1. Dilatation of arteries leading to the fistula
2. Absence of normal filling distal to the fistula
3. Pooling of the medium in the fistula, referred to as 'snowflakes'

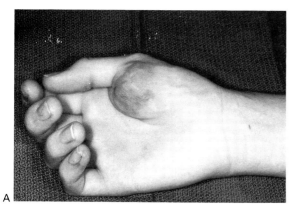

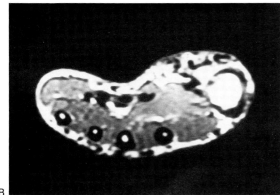

Fig. 6.68 'Low-flow' venous malformation. A. This patient presented with sudden increase in symptoms at puberty. B. MRI showed that the lesion was relatively superficial and therefore resectable.

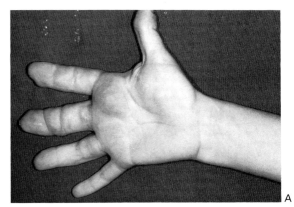

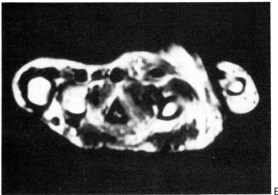

Fig. 6.69 'Low-flow' venous malformation. A. This patient presented with increased symptoms at puberty. B. MRI showed that the lesion was around the third metacarpal and involved both dorsal and palmar spaces. It was not *resectable*. A compression garment was recommended and worn.

4. The presence of contrast medium in the veins on the first film in the angiographic series.

The dialysis patient with 'shunt steal' problems has a swollen, blue, cold hand with ulceration on one or more fingertips. Surprisingly on examination, bounding pulses can be felt throughout the hand, especially marked in the dilated, tortuous veins.

Indications
Revision of the shunt in the dialysis patient resolves the situation. In the traumatic AV fistula, as opposed to most congenital AVM, it is usually possible to locate the abnormal communication and ligate or reconstruct it.

See Green D P 1993 Operative Hand Surgery, 3rd edn. Churchill Livingstone, New York, p. 2294.

ANEURYSM[304-313]

Three types of aneurysm are encountered:

mycotic — which is rare[305]
atherosclerotic — uncommon, usually dorsal[313]
traumatic — most common, invariably palmar.

The *traumatic aneurysm* (Fig. 6.66), which is *not* the result of a penetrating injury (p. 46) comes about as a result of repeated blows to the hand and has a similar aetiology to the ulnar artery thrombosis encountered in the 'hypothenar hammer syndrome' (p. 262). In the latter the injury is to the intima, while aneurysm formation follows disruption of the media. Penetrating injuries tend to result in *false* aneurysms, in which the 'wall' of the swelling is blood clot, whereas blunt trauma causes *true* aneurysms in which the wall is weakened vessel. The most common sites for such aneurysmal formation are:

The ulnar artery where it is exposed between Guyon's canal and the palmar fascia and overlies the hook of the hamate.

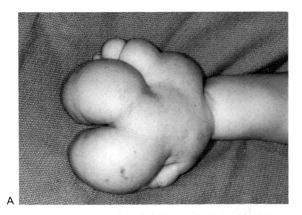

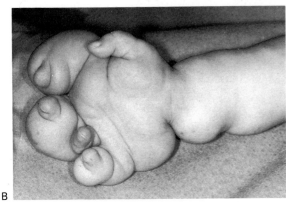

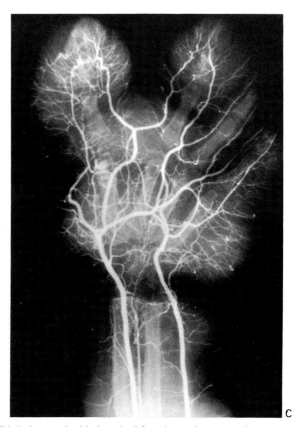

Fig. 6.70 'Low-flow' lymphatico-venous malformation. A, B. This lesion resulted in impaired function and concern about appearance with overgrowth of the underlying skeleton of the index and middle fingers.C. Angiography showed a significant relatively early blush suggesting a lymphatico-venous lesion.

The superficial branch of the radial artery as it enters the thenar eminence over the tubercle of the scaphoid.

The diagnosis is suggested when the patient complains of the development of a painful swelling after sustaining a blow to the hand. He may also complain of coolness in his fingers, most commonly the ring, and cold intolerance may progress as far as ulceration of the digital pulp. Rarely he may give symptoms indicative of ulnar nerve compression (p. 295).

The presence of a pulsatile mass is pathognomonic. When no pulsation is detectable, a positive Allen test (p. 259) will confirm the diagnosis. Angiography will provide further evidence but is not required in the presence of the stated symptoms and signs.

Excision is indicated and if circumstances allow, a reversed vein graft should be inserted.

Rarely, multiple small venous aneurysms may present, usually in middle-aged women (Fig. 6.67). There is no treatment possible or necessary.

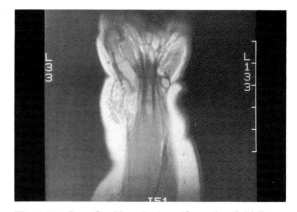

Fig. 6.71 'Low-flow' lymphatic malformation. Initially thought to be a well localized lesion and so demonstrated on MRI following excision, this lesion showed recurrence further proximally in the limb. A compression garment was recommended.

CONGENITAL VASCULAR SWELLINGS

Such lesions present with swelling, or changes in the skin colour, or evident disturbances in blood flow through the involved limb or any combination of the three. The often difficult decisions to be made in the management of these lesions are further complicated by confused nomenclature. Organization has been brought to the confusion by the concept of *cellular dynamics*[321]. Those vascular swellings which grow by cellular proliferation are recognized by the suffix '-oma', and are considered below under haemangioma. As discussed there, such swellings show growth greater than that experienced by the child, followed later by regression. Other vascular lesions which show no such propensities are termed malformations. Both haemangiomas and malformations may be rheologically dynamic, making it difficult or impossible to distinguish clinically between the two. Whether or not there is flow disturbance is the basis for classification of congenital vascular malformations.

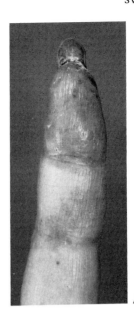

A

Congenital vascular malformation[315-322]

'Low-flow' (*capillary*). These are characterized by pink to purple discoloration of the skin and include portwine stains and naevus flammeus; small or very extensive; frequently present in association with other malformations, low- or high-flow, which are responsible for any symptoms. No treatment is required, but excision may be requested for reasons of appearance.

'Low-flow' (*venous*). These may be of any size; if large they may be associated with skeletal overgrowth; complaints may be of pain due to distension with dependency or due to localized subcutaneous thrombi, or may be related to the bulk of a large lesion; angiography is more useful than more sophisticated studies in defining the lesion. Excision of small lesions carries few problems (Fig. 6.68); staged 'debulking' carries no haemodynamic complications, but may cause problems with vital structures and with wound healing. Ligation is worthless. Compressive garments are effective in relieving pain due to dependency (Fig. 6.69).

'Low-flow' (*lymphatic* and *lymphatico-venous*). Wrongly called lymphangioma, these may, like venous malformations, be small or large, involving one digit, the hand or the entire arm and chest wall. Skeletal overgrowth may be present. Problems are primarily ones of impaired function and appearance (Fig. 6.70), but troublesome, recurrent cellulitis requiring hospitalization may present. Definition of large lesions is impossible (Fig. 6.71); lymphangiography is unwise for it may yield little and precipitate cellulitis. Excision of

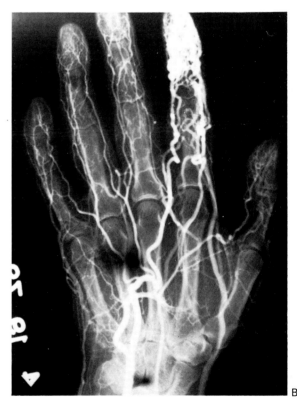

B

Fig. 6.72 This patient presented with cold intolerance and incipient necrosis of the tip of the finger shortly after puberty. A. Examination revealed that the finger was pulsatile, and arteriography (B) showed a traumatic arteriovenous fistula. Ray amputation was curative.

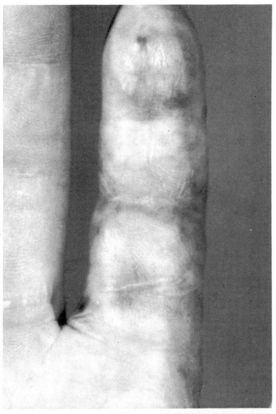

A

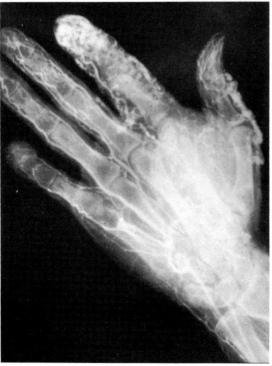

B

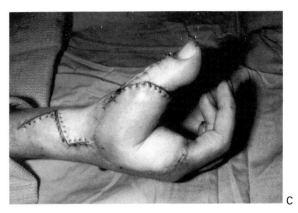

C

Fig. 6.73 'High-flow' arteriovenous malformation. A. This patient presented in middle age with sudden increase in a pre-existing malformation following a minor injury, with intractable continuous pain in his dominant hand such as to prevent work and sleep. B. Angiograms revealed involvement of the thumb and index finger. C. Pain was relieved by amputation of the index and thumb and function restored by reconstruction using a pedicle groin flap and great toe transfer.

small lesions is simple. Compression does not give the relief afforded those with purely venous lesions. Staged debulking or even amputation may be required.

'High-flow' (arterial) (= arteriovenous malformation, AVM). Similar in most respects to acquired arteriovenous fistula (see above), these malformations may present at birth, puberty (Fig. 6.72), pregnancy or following trauma (Fig. 6.73). The latter three may also precipitate symptomatic change in previously asymptomatic malformations. The lesions are warm, pulsatile and have a 'thrill' to the touch and a 'bruit' on auscultation. Uninvolved digits are cold as a result of poor perfusion due to the *'steal'* phenomenon, and may show *ulceration* or non-healing wounds. *Pain,* due both to swelling and ischaemia, is unremitting. *Consumption coagulopathy* may occur, and this contributes to the uncontrolled bleeding which may result from an injury to the malformation. *Congestive heart failure* may result from the high cardiac output induced by the shunt (Fig. 6.74). In such cases the Branham reaction will be positive — a slowing of the pulse with tourniquet occlusion of flow to the affected limb. Any of the four — steal, coagulopathy, bleeding or failure — may necessitate treatment. Compressive garments are used initially. Ligation is of no value. Selective angiography should be used in an attempt to define the lesion; tomography or CT will define any bony involvement. Selective embolization has, as yet, little part to play in the extremity for fear of digital ischaemia. Partial excision results in 100% recurrence, often with proximal extension of the

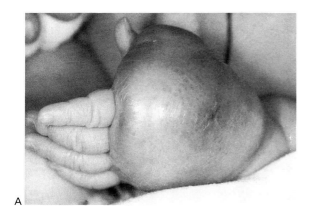

A

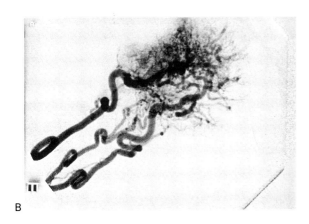

B

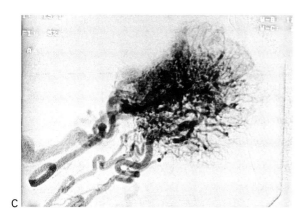

C

Fig. 6.74 'High-flow' arterial malformation, or haemangioma? A. This child presented at birth with a pulsatile swelling over the dorsum of the left hand. She had mild congestive cardiac failure which was controlled with medication. B, C. Angiography shows considerable tortuosity in the radial, ulnar and intraosseous arteries with rapid filling of, and rapid venous outflow from, this lesion. It later resolved following conservative treatment, proving it to be a haemangioma.

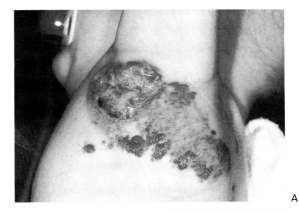

A

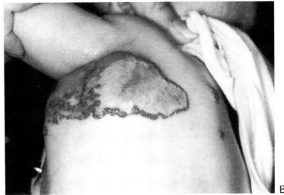

B

Fig. 6.75 Haemangioma. A. Ulceration and bleeding caused concern over this large lesion in the axilla of a child three months old. Conservative management was pursued. B. Six months later, the lesion had grown somewhat smaller, showed some grey areas and a marginal red line. No surgery was necessary and the child now is two years old with no problems.

lesion and worsening of the symptoms. Excision believed to be total also has a distressingly high recurrence rate[318], may require complex reconstruction and is complicated by wound breakdown and reduced limb function. Amputation may be the only alternative — and it may fail.

Haemangioma[323–327]

Haemangioma are characterized by a proliferative phase, usually during the first year of life, and a regressive or involutional phase lasting for some years. In the proliferative phase, the lesion clearly grows more rapidly than the child, shows increased ³H-thymidine uptake and mast cell activity. If the lesion is in the superficial dermis, a 'strawberry haemangioma' results. If they involve deeper, larger vessels they are termed 'cavernous haemangiomas' and may have all the

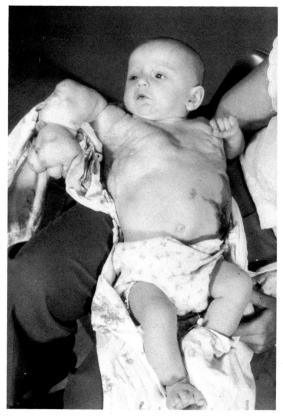

Fig. 6.76 A huge cavernous haemangioma involved the upper extremity and entire thorax. The child died before any surgery could be designed. The design of a *successful* procedure would have been impossible.

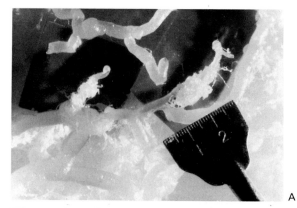

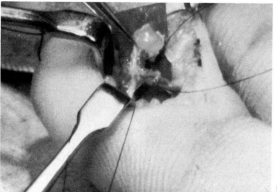

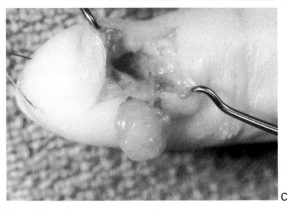

Fig. 6.77 Glomus tumour. A. A glomus body in an injection specimen of the human pulp. The scale shown alongside is in tenths of a millimetre. B, C. Glomus tumours at the time of excision.

complications of a high-flow arterial malformation — steal, coagulopathy, bleeding, congestive failure — and may indeed be indistinguishable from one clinically (Fig. 6.74). Although involution may lie in the future, these complications of the proliferating, larger lesion may prove fatal. Ulceration and secondary infection is common in more superficial haemangiomas (Fig. 6.75A). At about 12 months of age, grey areas appear, called 'herald spots', the colour lightens with often a marginal red line (Fig. 6.75B), and involution ensues. Management is conservative, with repeated reassurance of the parents who watch the growth of the haemangioma with understandable alarm and distrust. Compression may help. If cavernous lesions cause failure or thrombocytopenia, systemic steroids may accelerate involution. In rare, extensive, complicated tumours radical excision, including amputation, may be forced on the reluctant surgeon in an attempt to save life — and that may fail (Fig. 6.76).

GLOMUS TUMOUR[328-344] (Fig. 6.77)

Glomus tumour is usually solitary, but may be multiple. It may present as a swelling, and Riddell and Martin[340] reported one of unusual size. However, more commonly the patient presents with no swelling but

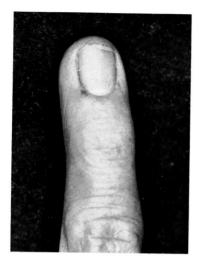

Fig. 6.78 Glomus tumour. This patient complained of excruciating pain in the right small finger. Examination revealed a small and insignificant purple patch on the eponychial fold which was however extremely tender.

only *pain* of spasmodic and excruciating nature. Sometimes triggered by trauma or mere contact, it is more often entirely spontaneous, radiating from the site of the tumour in a lancinating manner. It is characteristically precipitated by exposure to cold and relieved by warmth, although it may be sensitive to any temperature change.

Examination, if the tumour can be located — for its most common situation is beneath the nail — reveals an unimpressive, small, purplish patch in the skin (Fig. 6.78). The characteristic pain can be elicited by the use of ethyl chloride spray.

Tenderness is extreme and very well localized. This is best demonstrated by *Love's pin test*[335], in which the head of a pin is pressed around the area, finally coming on the tumour. Only then is pain elicited.

HAEMANGIOPERICYTOMA[351,352]

A distinct entity sometimes confused with glomus tumour, this rare tumour has a propensity to pursue a malignant course with some 50% showing metastases; peak incidence fourth and fifth decades; may occur in bone — lytic, expansile, non-reactive. Wide excision is curative.

KAPOSI'S SARCOMA[353,354]

Associated with deficient immune responses, this lesion is now more common as a result of increased transplant surgery and more widespread AIDS; raised, violaceous, non-tender cutaneous nodules. Excision of isolated lesions is curative. Multiple nodules are treated by irradiation.

REFERENCES

These references are presented differently from those in other chapters. After the initial survey, sections on tissues are headed in **bold type**, with subsections on specific tumours in each tissue in SMALL CAPITALS, with subsets in *italics*.

Survey
1. Butler E D, Hamill J P, Seipel R S, DeLorimier A A 1960 Tumors of the hand. A ten-year survey and report of 437 cases. Am J Surg 100: 293–302
2. Clifford R H, Kelly A P 1959 Diagnosis and treatment of tumors of the hand. Clin Orthopaedics 13: 204–212
3. Enneking W F 1983 Musculoskeletal surgery. Churchill Livingstone, Edinburgh
4. Froimson A I 1987 Benign solid tumors. Hand Clin 3: 213–217
5. Gaisford J C 1960 Tumors of the hand. Surg Clin North Am 40: 549
6. Haber M H, Alter A H, Whellock M C 1965 Tumors of the hand. Surg Gynecol Obstet 121: 1073–1080
7. Hajdu S J 1979 Pathology of soft tissue tumors. Lea & Febiger, Philadelphia
8. Mankin H J 1987 Principles of diagnosis and management of tumors of the hand. Hand Clin 3: 185–195

9. Mason M L 1937 Tumors of the hand. Surg Gynecol Obstet 64: 129
10. Posch J L 1956 Tumors of the hand. J Bone Joint Surg 38A: 517–540
11. Smith R J 1977 Tumors of the hand. Who is best qualified to treat tumors of the hand? J Hand Surg 2: 251–255

Bone and Cartilage
12. Dahlin D C 1987 Giant-cell-bearing lesions of bone of the hands. Hand Clin 3: 291–297
13. Dick H M, Angelides A C 1989 Malignant bone tumors of the hand. Hand Clin 5: 373–381
14. Feldman F 1987 Primary bone tumors of the hand and carpus. Hand Clin 3: 269–289
15. Frassica F J, Amadio P C, Wold L E, Dobyns J H, Linscheid R L 1989 Primary malignant bone tumors of the hand. J Hand Surg (Am) 14: 1022–1028
16. Huvos A G 1991 Bone Tumors, 2nd end. Saunders, Philadelphia

ANEURYSMAL BONE CYST
17. Barbieri C H 1984 Aneurysmal bone cyst of the hand. An unusual situation. J Hand Surg (Br) 9: 89–92

18. Burkhalter W, Schroeder F, Eversmann W 1978 Aneurysmal bone cysts occurring in the metacarpals. J Hand Surg 3: 579
19. Chalmers J 1981 Aneurysmal bone cysts of the phalanges. Hand 13: 296–300
20. Frassica F J, Amadio P C, Wold L E, Beabout J W 1988 Aneurysmal bone cyst: clinicopathologic features and treatment of ten cases involving the hand. J Hand Surg (Am) 13: 676–683
21. Fuhs S E, Herndon J H 1979 Aneurysmal bone cysts involving the hand: a review and report of two cases. J Hand Surg 4: 160–164
22. Johnston A D 1987 Aneurysmal bone cyst of the hand. Hand Clin 3: 299–310
23. Lin E, Engel J, Bubis J J, Herman O 1984 Aneurysmal bone cyst of the hamate bone. J Hand Surg (Am) 9: 847–850

CALCINOSIS
24. Haher T R, Devlin V J, Haher J N, Freeman B, Smith A G 1984 A case report of calcinosis universalis. J Hand Surg 9A: 243–245
25. Viegas S F, Evans E B, Calhoun J, Goodwillier S E 1985 Tumoral calcinosis: a case report and review of the literature. J Hand Surg 10A: 744–748

CARPOMETACARPAL BOSS
26. Artz D, Posch J L 1973 The carpometacarpal boss. J Bone Joint Surg 55A: 747–752
27. Cuono C B, Watson H K 1979 The carpal boss: surgical treatment and etiological considerations. Plastic Reconstr Surg 63: 88–94

CHONDROBLASTOMA
28. Neviaser R J, Wilson J N 1972 Benign chondroblastoma in the finger. J Bone Joint Surg 54A1: 389–392

CHONDROMA
29. Takigawa K 1971 Chondroma of the bones of the hand. J Bone Joint Surg 53A: 1591–1600
30. Takigawa K 1971 Carpal chondroma. J Bone Joint Surg 53A: 1601–1604

Enchondroma
31. Jewusiak E M, Spence K, Sell K 1971 Solitary benign enchondroma of the long bones of the hand. J Bone Joint Surg 53A: 1587–1590
32. Mosher J F 1976 Multiple enchondromatosis of the hand. A case report. J Bone Joint Surg 58A: 717–719
33. Zimmy M L, Redler I 1984 Ultrastructure of solitary enchondromas. J Hand Surg (Br) 9: 95–97

Soft-tissue chondroma
34. Armin A, Blair S J, Demons T C 1985 Benign soft tissue chondromatous lesion of the hand. J Hand Surg (Am) 10: 895–899
35. Ballet F L, Watson H K, Ryu J 1984 Synovial chondromatosis of the distal radioulnar joint. J Hand Surg (Am) 9: 590–592
36. Dellon A L, Weiss S W, Mitch W E 1978 Bilateral extraosseous chondromas of the hand in a patient with chronic renal failure. J Hand Surg 3: 139–141
37. Harvey F J, Negrine J 1990 Synovial chondromatosis in the distal interphalangeal joint. J Hand Surg (Am) 15: 102–105
38. Lucas G L, Sponsellar P D 1984 Synovial chondrometaplasia of the hand: case report and review of the literature. J Hand Surg (Am) 9: 269–272
39. Mahoney J L 1987 Soft tissue chondromas in the hand. J Hand Surg (Am) 12: 317–320
40. Sim F H, Dahlin D C, Ivins J C 1977 Extra-articular synovial chondromatosis. J Bone Joint Surg 59A: 492–495
41. Strong M L 1975 Chondromas of the tendon sheath of the hand. Report of a case and review of the literature. J Bone Joint Surg 57A: 1164–1165

CHONDROSARCOMA
42. Block R S, Burton R I 1977 Multiple chondrosarcomas in a hand. A case report. J Hand Surg 2: 310–313
43. Gottschalk R G, Smith R T 1963 Chondrosarcoma of the hand. J Bone Joint Surg 45A: 141–150
44. Granberry W M, Bryan W 1978 Chondrosarcoma of the trapezium: a case report. J Hand Surg 3: 277–279
45. Jokl P, Albright J A, Goodman A H 1971 Juxtacortical chondrosarcoma of the hand. J Bone Joint Surg 53A: 1370–1376
46. Justis E J Jr, Dart R C 1983 Chondrosarcoma of the hand with metastasis: a review of the literature and case report. J Hand Surg (Am) 8: 320–324
47. Palmieri T J 1984 Chondrosarcoma of the hand. J Hand Surg (Am) 9: 332–338
48. Patel M R, Pearlman H S, Engler J, Wollowick B S 1977 Chondrosarcoma of the proximal phalanx of the finger. Review of the literature and report of a case. J Bone Joint Surg 59A: 401–403
49. Roberts P H, Price C H G 1977 Chondrosarcoma of the bones of the hand. J Bone Joint Surg 59B: 213–221
50. Stackhouse T G, Weiland A J 1984 Extraosseous chondrosarcoma of the wrist: a case report. J Hand Surg (Am) 9: 338–342
51. Wu K K, Collon D J, Guise E R 1980 Extraosseous chondrosarcoma. Report of five cases and review of the literature. J Bone Joint Surg 62A: 189–194
52. Wu K K, Frost H M, Guise E E 1983 A chondrosarcoma of the hand arising from an asymptomatic benign solitary enchondroma of 40 years' duration. J Hand Surg (Am) 8: 317–319
53. Wu K K, Kelly A P 1977 Periosteal (juxta-cortical) chondrosarcoma. Report of a case occurring in the hand. J Hand Surg 2: 314–315

ECTOPIC OSSIFICATION
54. Altner P C, Singh S K 1981 An unusual case of ectopic ossification in a finger. J Hand Surg 6: 142–145
55. Johnson M K, Lawrence J F 1975 Metaplastic bone formation (myositis ossificans) in the soft tissue of the hand. Case report. J Bone Joint Surg 57A: 999–1000
56. Wissiner H A, McClain E J, Boyes J H 1966 Turret exostosis. Ossifying hematoma of the phalanges. J Bone Joint Surg 48A: 105

EOSINOPHILIC GRANULOMA
57. Palmer R E 1984 Eosinophilic granuloma of the hand: case report. J Hand Surg (Am) 9: 283–285

EWING'S SARCOMA
58. Dreyfuss U Y, Auslander L, Bialik V, Fishman J 1980 Ewing's sarcoma of the hand following recurrent trauma. A case report. Hand 12: 300–303
59. Dryer R, Buckwalter J, Flatt A, Bonfiglio M 1979 Ewing's sarcoma of the hand. J Hand Surg 4: 372–374

FIBROUS DYSPLASIA
60. Hayter R G, Becton J L 1984 Fibrous dysplasia of a metacarpal; a case report. J Hand Surg (Am) 9: 587–589

GIANT CELL REPARATIVE GRANULOMA
61. Bertheussen K J, Holck S, Schidt T 1983 Giant cell lesion of bone of the hand with particular emphasis on giant cell reparative granuloma. J Hand Surg (Am) 8: 46–49
62. Merkow R L, Bansal M, Inglis A E 1985 Giant cell reparative granuloma in the hand: report of three cases and review of the literature. J Hand Surg 10A 733–739
63. Wenner S M, Johnson K 1987 Giant cell reparative granuloma of the hand. J Hand Surg (Am) 12: 1097–1101

GIANT CELL TUMOUR
64. Averill R M, Smith R J, Campbell C J 1980 Giant cell tumors of the bones of the hand. J Hand Surg 5: 39–50
65. Fitzpatrick D J, Bullough P G 1977 Giant cell tumor of the lunate bone: a case report. J Hand Surg 2: 269–270
66. Gupta S, Kumar A, Gupta I 1980 Giant cell tumor of the first metacarpal bone. Hand 12: 288–292
67. Henard D C 1984 Giant cell tumor of the thumb metacarpal in an elderly patient: a case report. J Hand Surg (Am) 9: 343–345
68. Howard F M, Lassen K 1984 Giant cell tumor of the capitate. J Hand Surg (Am) 9: 272–274
69. Larsson S E, Lorentzon R, Boquist L 1975 Giant cell tumor of bone. J Bone Joint Surg 57A: 167–173
70. Meals R A, Mirra J M, Bernstein A J 1989 Giant cell tumor of metacarpal treated by cryosurgery. J Hand Surg (Am) 14: 130–134
71. Murray J A, Schlafly B 1986 Giant-cell tumors in the distal end of the radius. Treatment by resection and fibular autograft interpositional arthrodesis. J Bone Joint Surg (Am) 68: 687–694
72. Patel M R, Desai S S, Gordon S L, Nimberg G A et al 1987 Management of skeletal giant cell tumors of the phalanges of the hand. J Hand Surg 12: 70–77
73. Peimer C A, Schiller A L, Mankin H J, Smith R J 1980 Multicentric giant-cell tumors of bone. J Bone Joint Surg (Am) 62: 652–656
74. Peimer C A, Schiller A L, Mankin H J, Smith R J 1980 Multicentric giant-cell tumor of bone. J Bone Joint Surg 62A: 652–656
75. Serra J M, Muirragui A, Tadjalli H 1985 Extensive distal subcutaneous metastases of a 'benign' giant cell tumor of the radius. Plastic Reconstr Surg 75: 263–267
76. Shaw J A, Mosher J F 1983 A giant-cell tumor in the hand presenting as an expansile diaphyseal lesion. Case report. J Bone Joint Surg (Am) 65: 692–695
77. Smith J A, Millender L H 1979 Treatment of recurrent giant cell tumor of the digit by phalangeal excision and

toe phalanx transplant. A case report. J Hand Surg 4: 164–168
78. Smith R J, Mankin H J 1977 Allograft replacement of distal radius for giant cell tumor. J Hand Surg 2: 299–309

MALIGNANT FIBROUS HISTIOCYTOMA
79. Kerr R 1986 Malignant fibrous histiocytoma of bone. Ortho 9: 910–913

MELORHEOSTOSIS
80. Caudle R J, Stern P J 1987 Melorheostosis of the hand. A case report with long-term follow-up. J Bone Joint Surg (Am) 69: 1229–1231
81. Kawabata H, Tsuyuguchi Y, Kawai H, Yasui N 1984 Melorheostosis of the upper limb: a report of two cases. J Hand Surg (Am) 9: 871–876

OSTEOBLASTOMA
82. Menon J, Rankin D, Jacobson C 1988 Recurrent osteoblastoma of the carpal hamate. Ortho 11: 609–611
83. Mosher J, Peckham A 1978 Osteoblastoma of the metacarpal: a case report. J Hand Surg 3: 358–360

OSTEOCHONDROMA
84. Callan J E, Wood V E 1975 Spontaneous resolution of an osteochondroma. J Bone Joint Surg 57A: 723
85. Ganzhorn R W, Baliri G, Horowitz M 1981 Osteochondroma of the distal phalanx. J Hand Surg 6: 625–626
86. Ishizuki M, Isobe Y, Arai T, Nagatsuka Y, Tanabe K, Okumura S 1977 Osteochondromatosis of the finger joints. Hand 9: 198–200
87. Karr M A, Aulicino P L, DuPuy T E, Gwathmey F W 1984 Osteochondromas of the hand in hereditary multiple exostosis: report of a case presenting as a blocked proximal interphalangeal joint. J Hand Surg (Am) 9: 264–268
88. Medlar R C, Sprague H H 1979 Osteochondroma of the carpal scaphoid. J Hand Surg 4: 150–152
89. Moore J R, Curtis R M, Wilgis E F 1983 Osteocartilaginous lesions of the digits in children: an experience with 10 cases. J Hand Surg (Am) 8: 309–315
90. Murphy A F, Wilson J N 1958 Tenosynovial osteochondroma in the hand. J Bone Joint Surg 40A: 1236
91. Sowa D T, Moore J R, Weiland A J 1987 Extraskeletal osteochondromas of the wrist. J Hand Surg (Am) 12: 212–217
92. Stern P J, Phillips D 1986 Phalangeal osteochondroma: an unusual cause of swan-neck deformity. J Hand Surg (Am) 11: 70–73
93. Wood V E, Sauser D, Mudge D 1985 The treatment of hereditary multiple exostosis of the upper extremity. J Hand Surg (Am) 10: 505–513

OSTEOID OSTEOMA
94. Allieu Y, Lussiez B, Benichou M, Cenac P 1979 A double nidus osteoid osteoma in a finger. J Hand Surg (Am) 14: 538–541
95. Ambrosia J M, Wold L E, Amadio P C 1987 Osteoid osteoma of the hand and wrist. J Hand Surg (Am) 12: 794–800

96. Aulicino P L, Dupuy T E, Moriarity R P 1981 Osteoid osteoma of the terminal phalanx of finger. Orthopaedic Rev 10: 59–63
97. Carroll R E 1953 Osteoid osteoma in the hand. J Bone Joint Surg 35A: 888–893
98. Crosby L A, Murphy R P 1988 Subperiosteal osteoid osteoma of the distal phalanx of the thumb. J Hand Surg (Am) 13: 923–925
99. Doyle L K, Ruby L K, Nalebuff E G, Belsky M R 1985 Osteoid osteoma of the hand. J Hand Surg (Am) 10: 408–410
100. Gartsman G M, Ranawat C S 1984 Treatment of osteoid osteoma of the proximal phalanx by use of cryosurgery. J Hand Surg (Am) 9: 275–277
101. Ghiam G F, Bora F W 1978 Osteoid osteoma of the carpal bones. J Hand Surg 3: 280–283
102. Giannakis A, Papachristou G, Tiniakos G, Chrysafidis G, Hartofilakidis-Garofalidis G 1977 Osteoid osteoma of the terminal phalanges. Hand 9: 295–300
103. Grundberg A B 1977 Osteoid osteoma of the thumb. Report of a case. J Hand Surg 2: 266
104. Jensen E G 1979 Osteoid osteoma of the capitate bone. Hand 11: 102–105
105. Lamb D W, Castillo F D 1981 Phalangeal osteoid osteoma in the hand. Hand 13: 291–295
106. Murray J A, Thaggard A, Wallace S, Benmenachem G 1979 Arteriography of osteoid osteoma: an aid in differentation and management. Orthopedics 2: 359–365
107. O'Hara J P, Tegtmeyer C, Sweet D E, McCue F C 1975 Angiography in the diagnosis of osteoid osteoma of the hand. J Bone Joint Surg 57A: 163–166
108. Riester J, Mosher J F 1984 Osteoid osteoma of the capitate: a case report. J Hand Surg (Am) 9: 278–280
109. Rosenfeld K, Bora F W, Lane J M 1973 Osteoid osteoma of the hamate. J Bone Joint Surg 55A: 1085–1087
110. Shaw J A 1987 Osteoid osteoma of the lunate. J Hand Surg (Am) 12: 128–130
111. Sim F H, Dahlin D C, Beabout J W 1975 Osteoid osteoma: diagnostic problems. J Bone Joint Surg 57A: 154–159
112. Wiss D A, Reid B S 1983 Painless osteoid osteoma of the fingers — report of three cases. J Hand Surg (Am) 8: 914–917

OSTEOSARCOMA
113. Bickerstaff D R, Harris S C, Kay N R 1988 Osteosarcoma of the carpus. J Hand Surg (Br) 13: 303–305
114. Brostrom L, Harris M, Simon M, Cooperman D, Nilsonne U 1979 The effect of biopsy on survival of patients with osteosarcoma. J Bone Joint Surg 61B: 209–212
115. Campanacci M, Bacci G, Pagani P, Giunti A 1980 Multiple drug chemotherapy for the primary treatment of osteosarcoma of the extremities. J Bone Joint Surg 62B: 93–101
116. Fleegler E J, Marks K E, Sebek B A, Groppe C W, Belhobek G 1980 Osteosarcoma of the hand. Hand 12: 316–322
117. Gebhardt M C, Mankin H J 1988 Osteosarcomas: a review and update — Part I. Surg Rounds Ortho 21–30

118. Gebhardt M C, Mankin H J 1988 Osteosarcomas: the treatment controversy — Part II. Surg Rounds Ortho 25–42
119. Stark H H, Jones F E, Jernstrom P 1971 Parosteal osteogenic sarcoma of a metacarpal bone. J Bone Joint Surg 53A: 147–153

SIMPLE BONE CYST
120. Baruch A, Haas A, Lifschitz-Mercer B, Zeligowsky A 1987 Simple bone cyst of the metacarpal. J Hand Surg (Am) 12: 1103–1106

Muscle
GRANULAR CELL MYOBLASTOMA
121. Bielejeski T R 1973 Granular cell tumor (myoblastoma) of the hand. J Bone Joint Surg 55A: 841–843
122. Maher D P 1987 Granular cell tumor in the hand. J Hand Surg (Am) 12: 800–803

PESUDOMALIGNANT MYOSITIS OSSIFICANS
123. Kay Y, Masuda S, Ushijima M, Kojima T, Sugioka Y 1987 Pseudomalignant myositis ossificans occurring in the hand. J Hand Surg (Am) 12: 634–638
124. Ogilvie-Harris D J, Fornasier V L 1980 Pseudomalignant myositis ossificans: heterotopic new bone formation without a history of trauma. J Bone Joint Surg 62A: 1274–1283
125. Schecter W P, Wong D, Kilgore E S, Newmeyer W L, Howes E L, Clark G 1982 Peripartum pseudomalignant myositis ossificans of the finger. J Hand Surg 7: 44–46

RHABDOMYOSARCOMA
126. Cohen M, Ghosh L, Schafer M E 1987 Congenital embryonal rhabdomyosarcoma of the hand and Apert's syndrome. J Hand Surg (Am) 12: 614–617
127. Mutz S B, Curl W 1977 Alveolar cell rhabdomyosarcoma of the hand. Case report with four year survival and no evidence of recurrence. J Hand Surg 2: 283–284
128. Potenza A D, Winslow D J 1961 Rhabdomyosarcoma of the hand. J Bone Joint Surg 43A: 700–708

Nerve
(To conform with the structure employed in the text, all nerve tumours are grouped together.)
129. Abu Jamra F N, Rebeiz J J 1979 Lipofibroma of the median nerve. J Hand Surg 4: 160–164
130. Amadio P C, Reiman H M, Dobyns J H 1988 Lipofibromatous hamartoma of nerve. J Hand Surg (Am) 13: 67–75
131. Barre P S, Shaffer J W, Carter J R, Lacey S H 1987 Multiplicity of neurilemmomas in the upper extremity. J Hand Surg (Am) 12: 307–311
132. Blair W F 1980 Granular cell schwannoma of the hand. J Hand Surg. 5: 51–52
133. Bloem J J A M, Van Der Meulen J C 1978 Neurofibromatosis in plastic surgery. Br J Plastic Surg 31: 50–53
134. Claman H N 1877 New hope for neurofibromastosis — the mast cell connecion. JAMA 258–283
135. Davidson S F, Das S K, Smith E E 1989 Cellular schwannoma of the hand. J Hand Surg (Am) 14: 907–909

136. Holdsworth B J 1985 Nerve tumours in the upper limb. A clinical review. J Hand Surg (Br) 10: 236–238
137. Houpt P, Storm van Leeuwen J B, van den Bergen H A 1989 Intraneural lipofibroma of the median nerve. J Hand Surg (Am) 14: 706–709
138. Langa V, Posner M A, Steiner G E 1987 Lipofibroma of the median nerve: a report of two cases. J Hand Surg (Br) 12: 221–223
139. Lewis R C, Nannini L H, Cocke W M 1981 Multifocal neurilemmomas of median and ulnar nerves of the same extremity — case report. J Hand Surg 6: 406–408
140. Louis D S 1987 Peripheral nerve tumours in the upper extremity. Hand Clin 3: 311–318
141. Louis D S, Hankin F M, Greene T L, Dick H M 1985 Lipofibromas of the median nerve: long-term follow-up of four cases. J Hand Surg (Am) 10: 403–408
142. Match R M, Leffert R D 1987 Massive neurofibromatosis of the upper extremity with paralysis. J Hand Surg (Am) 12: 718–722
143. Mikhail I K 1964 Median nerve lipoma in the hand. J Bone Joint Surg 46B: 726
144. Monballiu G 1981 Plexiform neurofibroma of the median nerve. Chirurgia Plastica 6: 141–145
145. Morely G H 1964 Intraneural lipoma of the median nerve in the carpal tunnel. Report of a case. J Bone Joint Surg 46B: 734–735
146. Paletta F X, Senay L C 1981 Lipofibromatous hamartoma of median nerve and ulnar nerve: surgical treatment. Plastic Reconstr Surg 68: 915–926
147. Patel C B, Tsai T M, Kleinert H E 1986 Hemangioma of the median nerve: a report of two cases. J Hand Surg (Am) 11: 76–79
148. Patel M, Silver J, Lipton D, Pearlman H 1979 Lipofibroma of the median nerve in the palm and digits of the hand. J Bone Joint Surg 61A: 393–397
149. Peled I, Iosipovich Z, Rousso M, Wexler M R 1980 Hemangioma of the median nerve. J Hand Surg 5: 363–365
150. Pulvertaft R G 1964 Unusual tumours of the median nerve. Report of two cases. J Bone Joint Surg 46B: 731–733
151. Rinaldi E 1983 Neurilemmomas and neurofibromas of the upper limb. J Hand Surg (Am) 8: 590–593
152. Rowland S A 1978 Trigger finger due to neurilemmoma in the carpal tunnel. Hand 10: 229–301
153. Rowland S A 1977 Case report: ten-year follow-up of lipofibroma of the median nerve in the palm. J Hand Surg 2: 316–317
154. Rusko R A, Larsen R D 1981 Intraneural lipoma of the median nerve — case report and literature review. J Hand Surg 6: 388–391
155. Sands M J, McDonough M T, Cohen A M, Rutenberg H L, Elsner J W 1975 Fatal malignant degeneration in multiple neurofibromatosis. J Am Med Assoc 233: 1381–1382
156. Schiffman K L, Harris D C, Hooper G 1988 Hemangiopericytoma of the median nerve. J Hand Surg (Am) 13: 75–78.
157. Shereff M J, Posner M A, Gordo M H 1980 Upper extremity hypertrophy secondary to neurofibromatosis: a case report. J Hand Surg 5: 355–357
158. Strickland J W, Steichen J B 1977 Nerve tumors of the hand and forearm. J Hand Surg 2: 285–291
159. Terzis J K, Daniel R K, Williams H B, Spencer P S 1978 Benign fatty tumors of the peripheral nerves. Ann Plastic Surg 1: 193–216
160. Williams G D, Hoffman S, Schwartz I S 1984 Malignant transformation in a plexiform neurofibroma of the median nerve. J Hand Surg (Am) 9: 583–587

Skin

ACTINIC LESIONS

161. Fleegler E J 1987 Tumors involving the skin of the upper extremity. Hand Clin 3: 197–212
162. Glass A G, Hoover R N 1989 The emerging epidemic of melanoma and squamous cell cancer. JAMA 262: 2097–2100
163. Rayner C R W 1981 The results of treatment of two hundred and seventy-three carcinomas of the hand. Hand 13: 183–186

Basal-cell carcinoma
164. Enna C 1978 Adenoid basal cell epithelioma involving a finger. Hand 10: 309–311

Squamous-cell carcinoma
165. Attiyeh F F, Shah J, Booher R J, Knapper W H 1979 Subungual squamous cell carcinoma. J Am Med Assoc 241: 262–263
166. Belinkie S A, Swats W M, Zitelli J A 1986 Invasive squamous cell carcinoma of the carpus: malignant transformation of epidermis dysplasia verruciformis. J Hand Surg (Am) 11: 273–275
167. Bunkis J, Mehrohof A I, Stayman J W 1981 Radiation induced carcinoma of the hand. J Hand Surg. 6: 384–387
168. Canipe T L, Howell J A, Howell C M 1964 Subungual carcinoma. Plastic Reconstr Surg 33: 263–265
169. Carroll R E 1976 Squamous cell carcinoma of the nail bed. J Hand Surg 1: 92–97
170. Eichenholtz S N, Deangelis C 1965 Squamous cell carcinoma of nail bed. J Am Med Assoc 191: 102–104
171. Fitzgerald R H, Brewer N S, Dahlin D C 1976 Squamous cell carcinoma complicating chronic osteomyelitis. J Bone Joint Surg 58A: 1146–1148
172. Forsythe R L, Bajaj P, Engeron O, Shadid E A 1978 The treatment of squamous cell carcinoma of the hand. Hand 10: 104–108
173. Long P I, Espiniella J L 1978 Squamous cell carcinoma of the nail bed. J Am Med Assoc 239: 2154–2155
174. Neilson D, Dundas S, Page RE 1988 Carcinoma cuniculatum of the hand. J Hand Surg (Br) 13: 218–220
175. Onukak E E 1980 Squamous cell carcinoma of the nail bed: a diagnostic and therapeutic problem. Br J Surg 67: 893–894
176. Schiavon M, Mazzoleni F, Chiarelli A, Matano P 1988 Squamous cell carcinoma of the hand: fifty-five case reports. J Hand Surg (Am) 13: 401–404
177. Silverman I 1935 Epithelioma following chronic paronychia. Am J Surg 19: 141–142, 151

Bowen's disease
178. Bowen J T 1912 Precancerous dermatoses: study of two cases of chronic atypical epithelial proliferation. J Cancer Dis 30: 241–255

179. Defiebre B K 1978 Bowen's disease of the nail bed: a case representation and review of the literature. J Hand Surg 3: 184–186
180. Stilwell J H, Maisels D O 1981 Subungual Bowen's disease. Hand 13: 287–290
181. Strong M L 1983 Bowen's disease in multiple nail beds — case report. J Hand Surg (Am) 8: 329–330

EPIDERMOID INCLUSION CYST
182. Carroll R E 1955 Epidermoid (epithelial) cyst of the hand. Am J Surg 85: 327–334
183. O'Hara J J, Stone J H 1990 An intratendinous epidermoid cyst after trauma. J Hand Surg (Am) 15: 477–479
184. St Onge R A, Jackson I T 1977 An uncommon sequel to thumb trauma: epidermoid cyst. Hand 9: 52–56
185. Sieracki J C, Kelly A P 1959 Traumatic epidermoid cysts involving digital bones: epidermoid cysts of the distal phalanx. Arch Surg 78: 597–703
186. Zadek I, Cohen H G 1953 Epidermoid cyst of the terminal phalanx of a finger with a review of literature. American Journal of Surgery 85: 771

KERATOACANTHOMA
187. Lamp J C, Graham J H, Urbach F, Burgoon C F 1964 Keratoacanthoma of the subungual region. A clinicopathological and therapeutic study. J Bone Joint Surg 46A: 1721–1731, 1752
188. Patel MR, Desai S 1989 Subungual keratoacanthoma in the hand. J Hand Surg (Am) 14: 139–142
189. Pellegrini V D Jr, Tompkins A 1986 Management of subungual keratoacanthoma. J Hand Surg (Am) 11: 718–724

MALIGNANT MELANOMA
190. Annamaria C, Singletary S E, Balch C M 1989 Patterns of relapse in 1001 consecutive patients with melanoma nodal metastases. Arch Surg 124: 1051–1055
191. Baas P C, Hoekstra H J, Koops H S 1989 Isolated regional perfusion in the treatment of subungual melanoma. Arch Surg 124: 373–376
192. Banzet P, Glicenstein J, Dufourmentel C 1975 Melanotic tumors of the hand. Hand 7: 183–184
193. Breslow A 1975 Tumor thickness, level of invasion and node dissection in state I cutaneous melanoma. Ann Surg 182: 572–575
194. Breslow A, Macht S D 1978 Evaluation of prognosis in Stage I cutaneous melanoma. Plastic Reconstr Surg 61: 342–346
195. Heller R, Becker J, Wasselle J et al 1991 Detection of submicroscopic lymph node metastases in patients with melanoma. Arch Surg 126: 1455–1460
196. Leon P, Daly J M, Synnestvedt M et al 1991 The prognostic implications of microscopic satellites in patients with clinical stage I melanoma. Arch Surg 126: 1461–1468
197. Patterson R H, Helwing E L 1980 Subungual melanoma: a clinical pathological study. Cancer 46: 2074–2087
198. Rushfort G F 1971 Two cases of subungual malignant melanoma. Br J Surg 58: 451
199. Ware J W 1977 Subungual malignant melanoma presenting as sub-acute paronychia following trauma. Hand 9: 49–51

200. Wong J H, Xu S H, Skinner K A et al 1991 Prospective evaluation of the use of antigen-specific immune complexes in predicting the development of recurrent melanoma. Arch Surg 126: 1450–1454

PYOGENIC GRANULOMA
201. DiFazio F, Mogan J 1989 Intravenous pyogenic granuloma of the hand. J Hand Surg 14A: 310–312

SWEAT GLAND TUMOURS
202. Lopez-Burbano L F, Cimorra G A, Gonzalez-Peirona E, Alfora J 1987 Malignant clear-cell hidradenoma. Plastic Reconstr Surg 80: 300–303
203. Terrill R Q, Groves R J, Cohen M B 1987 Two cases of chondroid syringoma of the hand. J Hand Surg (Am) 12: 1094–1097
204. Wilson K M, Jubert A V, Joseph J I 1989 Sweat gland carcinoma of the hand (malignant acrospiroma). J Hand Surg (Am) 14: 531–535
205. Yaremchuk M J, Elias L S, Graham R R, Wilgis E F 1984 Sweat gland carcinoma of the hand: two cases of malignant eccrine spiradenoma. J Hand Surg (Am) 9: 910–914

Subcutaneous tissue
EPITHELOID SARCOMA
206. Archer I A, Brown R B, Fitton J M 1984 Epithelioid sarcoma in the hand. J Hand Surg (Br) 9: 207–209
207. Boyes J, Marroum M 1978 Epithelioid sarcoma of hand and forearm. Hand 10: 302–305
208. Bryan R S, Soule E H, Dobyns J H, Pritchard D J, Linscheid R L 1974 Primary epithelioid sarcoma of the hand. J Bone Joint Surg 56: 458
209. Button M 1979 Epithelioid sarcoma: a case report. J Hand Surg 4: 368–371
210. Enzinger F M 1970 Epithelioid sarcoma. Cancer 26: 1029–1040
211. Hoopes J E, Graham W P 3rd, Shack R B 1985 Epithelioid sarcoma of the upper extremity. Plastic Reconstr Surg 75: 810–813
212. Patel M R, Desai S S, Gordon S L 1986 Functional limb salvage with multimodality treatment in epithelioid sarcoma of the hand: a report of two cases. J Hand Surg (Am) 11: 265–269
213. Peimer C A, Smith R J, Sirota R L, Cohen B E 1977 Epithelioid sarcoma of the hand and wrist: patterns of extension. J Hand Surg 2: 275–282

FIBROMA
214. Adeyemi-Doro H O, Olude O 1985 Juvenile aponeurotic fibroma. J Hand Surg (Br) 10: 127–128
215. Carroll R E 1987 Juvenile aponeurotic fibroma. Hand Clin 3: 219–224
216. Eisenbaum S L, Eversmann W W Jr 1985 Juvenile aponeurotic fibroma of the hand. J Hand Surg (Am) 10: 622–625
217. Goldstein S A, Imbriglia J E 1986 Fibrous hamartoma of the wrist in infancy. J Hand Surg (Am) 11: 847–849
218. Greene T L, Strickland J W 1984 Fibroma of tendon sheath. J Hand Surg (Am) 9: 758–760
219. Grenga T E 1990 Intratendinous fibroma of flexor tendon. J Hand Surg (Am) 15: 92–93
220. Kapff P D, Hocken D B, Simpson R H 1987

Elastofibroma of the hand. J Bone Joint Surg (Br) 69: 468–469

221. Kawabata H, Masada K, Aoki Y, Ono K 1986 Infantile digital fibromatosis after web construction in syndactyly. J Hand Surg (Am) 11: 741–743
222. Kernohan J, Dakin P K, Quain J S, Helal B 1984 An anomalous flexor digitorum superficialis indicis muscle in association with a fibroma presenting as a stiff painful finger. J Hand Surg (Br) 9: 335–336
223. Kojima T, Nagano T, Uchida M 1987 Periungual fibroma. J Hand Surg (Am) 12: 465–470
224. Lafferty K A, Nelson E L, Demuth R J, Miller S H, Harrison M W 1986 Juvenile aponeurotic fibroma with disseminated fibrosarcoma. J Hand Surg (Am) 11: 737–740
225. Lauri G, Santucci M, Ceruso M, Innocenti M 1990 Recurrent digital fibromatosis of childhood. J Hand Surg (Am) 15: 106–109
226. Lee B S 1983 Desmoid tumor of the hand — case report and literature review. J Hand Surg (Am) 8: 95–97
227. Moloney S R, Cabbabe E B, Shively R E, deMello D E 1986 Recurring digital fibroma of childhood. J Hand Surg (Am) 11: 584–587
228. Moskovich R, Posner M A 1988 Intratendinous aponeurotic fibroma. J Hand Surg (Am) 13: 563–566
229. Poppen N K, Niebauer J J 1977 Recurring digital fibrous tumor of childhood. J Hand Surg 2: 256–257
230. Schenkar D L, Kleinert H E 1977 Desmoplastic fibroma of the hand. Plastic Reconstr Surg 59: 128–133
231. Specht E E, Konkin L A 1976 Juvenile aponeurotic fibroma. The cartilage analogue of fibromatosis. J Am Med Assoc 236: 626–628
232. Specht E E, Staheli L T 1877 Juvenile aponeurotic fibroma. J Hand Surg 2: 258–260
233. Sugiura I 1976 Desmoplastic fibroma. Case report and review of the literature. J Bone Joint Surg 58A: 126–130
234. Zeide M S, Wiessel S, Terry R 1978 Juvenile aponeurotic fibroma. Plastic Reconstr Surg 61: 922–923

FIBROSARCOMA
235. Akbarnia B A, Wirth C R, Colman N 1976 Fibrosarcoma arising from chronic osteomyelitis. Case report and review of the literature. J Bone Joint Surg 58A: 123–125
236. Rasi H B, Mascardo T, Jinkdrak K 1980 Congenital fibrosarcoma of hand. Orthopaedic Rev 9: 49–54

LIPOMA
237. Booher R J 1965 Lipoblastic tumors of the hands and feet. Review of the literature and report of thirty–three cases. J Bone Joint Surg 47A: 727–740
238. Brand M G, Gelberman R H 1988 Lipoma of the flexor digitorum superficialis causing triggering at the carpal canal and median nerve compression. J Hand Surg (Am) 13: 342–344
239. Hart J A L 1973 Intraosseus lipoma. J Bone Joint Surg 55B: 624–632
240. Kernohan J, Dakin R P, Quain J S, Helal B 1984 An unusual 'giant' lipofibroma in the palm. J Hand Surg (Br) 9: 347–348
241. Leffert R D 1972 Lipomas of the upper extremity. J Bone Joint Surg 54A: 1262–1266
242. Oster L H, Blair W F, Steyers C M 1989 Large

lipomas in the deep palmar space. J Hand Surg (Am) 14: 700–704
243. Schmitz R L, Keeley J L 1957 Lipomas of the hand. Surgery 42: 696–700
244. Strauss A 1922 Lipoma of the tendon sheaths: with report of case and review of the literature. Surg Gynecol Obstet 35: 161
245. Sullivan C R, Dahlin D C, Bryan R S 1956 Lipoma of the tendon sheath. J Bone Joint Surg 38A: 1275–1280

LYMPHOMA
246. Ellstein J, Xeller C, Fromowitz F, Elias J M et al 1984 Soft tissue T cell lymphoma of the forearm: a case report. J Hand Surg (Am) 9: 346–350
247. Hung L K, Cheng J C, McGuire L J, Tsao S Y 1988 Primary malignant lymphoma of the deep tissues of the hand. J Hand Surg (Am) 13: 683–686

MALIGNANT FIBROUS HISTIOCYTOMA
248. Bullon A, Nistal M, Razquin S, Novo A et al 1986 Malignant fibrous histiocytoma in a child's hand. J Hand Surg (Am) 11: 744–748
249. Coles M, Smith M, Rankin E A 1989 An unusual case of dermatofibrosarcoma protuberans. J Hand Surg (Am) 14: 135–138
250. Dick H M 1987 Malignant fibrous histiocytoma of the hand. Hand Clin 3: 263–268
251. Hankin F M, Hankin R C, Louis D S 1987 Malignant fibrous histiocytoma involving a digit. J Hand Surg (Am) 12: 83–86
252. Hubbard L F, Burton R I 1977 Malignant fibrous histiocytoma of the forearm. Report of a case and review of the literature. J Hand Surg 2: 292–296
253. Karev A 1979 Malignant histiocytoma of the arm in a four year old boy. Hand 11: 106–108
254. Karev A, Stahl S 1990 Spontaneous rupture of the biceps muscle due to a concealed malignant fibrous histiocytoma. J Hand Surg (Am) 15: 94–97
255. McDowell C L, Hencreoth D 1977 Malignant fibrous histiocytoma of the hand. A case report. Journal of Hand Surgery (Am) 2: 297–298, 345
256. Schvarcz L W 1977 Congenital dermatofibrosarcoma protuberans of the hand. Hand 9: 182–185
257. Spector D, Miller J, Viloria J 1979 Malignant fibrous histiocytoma. J Bone Joint Surg 61B: 190–193
258. Wirman J A, Sherman S, Sullivan M R 1981 Dermatofibrosarcoma protuberans arising on the hand. Hand 13: 187–190

Synovium and tendon
GANGLION
259. Andren L, Eiken O 1971 Arthrographic studies of wrist ganglions. J Bone Joint Surg 53A: 299–302
260. Angelides A C, Wallace P F 1976 The dorsal ganglion of the wrist: its pathogenesis, gross and microscopic anatomy, and surgical treatment. J Hand Surg 1: 228–235
261. Bowers H, Hurst L 1979 An intra-articular intraosseous carpal ganglion. J Hand Surg 4: 375–377
262. Brown I, Huffstadt A J C 1981 Intraosseous ganglia. Hand 13: 51–54
263. Dodge L D, Brown R L, Niebauer J J, McCarroll H R Jr 1984 The treatment of mucous cysts: longterm follow-up in sixty-two cases. J Hand Surg 9A: 901–904

264. Gunther S F 1985 Dorsal wrist pain and the occult scapholunate ganglion. J Hand Surg (Am) 10: 697–703
265. Grange W J 1978 Subperiosteal ganglion: a case report. J Bone Joint Surg 60B: 124–125
266. Helal B, Vernon-Roberts B 1976 Intraosseous ganglion of the pisiform bone. Hand 8: 150–154
267. Janzon L, Niechajev I A 1981 Wrist ganglia. Scand J Plastic Reconstr Surg 15: 53–56
268. Kambolis C, Bullough P G, Jaffe H I 1973 Ganglionic cystic defects of bone. J Bone Joint Surg 55A: 496–505
269. Kelly G L 1973 Radial artery occlusion by a carpal ganglion. Plastic Reconstr Surg 52: 191–193
270. Kenan S, Graham S, Lewis M, Yabut S M Jr 1987 Intraosseous ganglion in the first metacarpal bone. J Hand Surg (Am) 12: 471–473
271. Lister G D, Smith R R 1976 Ideas and innovations. Protection of the radial artery in the resection of adherent ganglions of the wrist. Plastic Reconstr Surg 61: 127–129
272. Loder R T, Robinson J H, Jackson W T, Allen D J 1988 A surface ultrastructure study of ganglia and digital mucous cysts. J Hand Surg (Am) 13: 758–762
273. MacCollum M S 1977 Dorsal wrist ganglions in children. J Hand Surgery 2: 325
274. McEvedy B V 1962 Simple ganglion. Br J Surg 49: 585–594
275. Matthews P 1973 Ganglia of the flexor tendon sheaths in the hand. J Bone Joint Surg 55B: 612–617
276. Mogan J V, Newberg A H, Davis P H 1981 Intraosseous ganglion of the lunate. J Hand Surg 6: 61–63
277. Nelson C L, Sawmiller S, Phalen G S 1984 Ganglions of the wrist and hamartoma of the hand. J Hand Surg (Br) 9: 349–350
278. Posner M A, Green S M 1984 Intraosseous ganglion of a phalanx. J Hand Surg (Am) 9: 280–282
279. Richman J A, Gelberman R H, Engber W D, Salamon P B, Bean D J 1987 Ganglions of the wrist and digits: results of treatment by aspiration and cyst wall puncture. J Hand Surg (Am) 12: 1041–1043
280. Rangarathnam C S, Linscheid R L 1984 Infected mucous cyst of the finger. J Hand Surg 9A: 245–247
281. Rosson J W, Walker G 1989 The natural history of ganglia in children. J Bone Joint Surg (Br) 71: 707–708
282. Watson H K, Rogers W D, Ashmead D 4th 1989 Reevaluation of the cause of the wrist ganglion. J Hand Surg (Am) 14: 812–817
283. Young S C, Freiberg A 1985 A case of an intratendinous ganglion. J Hand Surg (Am) 10: 723–724
284. Zubowicz V N, Ishii C H 1987 Management of ganglion cysts of the hand by simple aspiration. J Hand Surg (Am) 12: 618–620

GIANT CELL TUMOUR OF TENDON SHEATH
(pigmented villonodular synovitis; benign synovioma)
285. Adamson B E, Lucas G L 1985 Multiple recurrence of digital pigmented villonodular tenosynovitis: a case report. J Hand Surg (Am) 10: 278–280
286. Crawford G P, Offerman R J 1980 Pigmented villonodular synovitis in the hand. Hand 12: 282–287
287. Fletcher A G, Horn R C 1951 Giant cell tumors of tendon sheath origin. A consideration of bone

involvement and report of two cases with extensive bone destruction. Ann Surg 133: 374–385
288. Fyfe I S, MacFarlane A 1980 Pigmented villonodular synovitis of the hand. Hand 12: 179–188.
289. Hansen P, Nielsen P T, Wahlin A B 1988 Pigmented villonodular synovitis of the extensor tendon sheaths in a child. J Hand Surg (Br) 13: 313–314
290. Matthews R E, Gould J S, Kashlan M B 1981 Diffuse pigmented villonodular tenosynovitis of the ulnar bursa — a case report. J Bone Joint Surg 6: 64–69
291. Moore J R, Weiland A J, Curtis R M 1984 Localized nodular tenosynovitis: experience with 115 cases. J Hand Surg (Am) 9: 412–417
292. Patel M R, Zinberg E M 1984 Pigmented villonodular synovitis of the wrist invading bone — report of a case. J Hand Surg (Am) 9: 854–858
293. Phalen G S, McCormack L J, Gazale W J 1959 Giant cell tumor of tendon sheath (benign synovioma) in the hand. Evaluation of 56 cases. Clin Orthopedics 15: 140–151
294. Zook E G 1977 Extensive giant cell tumor of the finger. A case history. Orthopedics 2: 267–268

SYNOVIAL SARCOMA
295. Dick H M 1987 Synovial sarcoma of the hand. Hand Clin 3: 241–245
296. Dreyfuss U Y, Boome R S, Kranold D H 1986 Synovial sarcoma of the hand — literature study. J Hand Surg (Br) 11: 471–474
297. Kazayeri M, Gallo G 1979 Synovial sarcoma: a case report. Orthopedics 2: 496–498
298. Louis D S, Hankin F M, Hankin R C, Brennan M, Greene T L 1986 Synovial cell sarcoma: a case report with a comment on 27 years of treatment. J Hand Surg (Am) 11: 578–581

XANTHOMA
299. Doyle J R 1988 Tendon xanthoma: a physical manifestation of hyperlipidemia. J Hand Surg (Am) 13: 238–241
300. Gunther S F, Gunther A G, Hoeg J M, Kruth H S 1986 Multiple flexor tendon xanthomas and contractures in the hands of a child with familial hypercholesterolemia. J Hand Surg (Am) 11: 588–593
301. Hamilton W C, Ramsey P L, Hanson S M, Schiff D C 1975 Osseous xanthoma and multiple hand tumors as a complication of hyperlipidemia. J Bone Joint Surg 57A: 551–553
302. Hoehn J 1978 Multiple fibrous xanthomas of tendon sheath. Hand 10: 306–308

Vessel
303. Booher R J 1961 Tumors arising from blood vessels in the hands and feet. Clin Orthopedics 19: 71–98

ANEURYSM
304. Baxt S, Mori K, Hoffman S 1975 Aneurysm of the hand secondary to Kaposi's sarcoma. Case report. J Bone Joint Surg 57A: 995–997
305. Berrettoni B A, Seitz W H Jr 1990 Mycotic aneurysm in a digital artery: case report and literature review. J Hand Surg 15A: 305–308

306. Carneiro R D S 1974 Aneurysm of the wrist. Plastic Reconstr Surg 54: 483–489
307. Dangles C J 1984 True aneurysm of a thumb digital artery. J Hand Surg (Am) 9: 444–445
308. Dormandy J A, Barkley H 1979 Bilateral axillary artery aneurysms in a child. Br J Surg 66: 650
309. Ho P K, Weiland A J, McClinton M A, Wilgis E F 1987 Aneurysms of the upper extremity. J Hand Surg (Am) 12: 39–46
310. Jenkins A McL, Macpherson A I S, Nolan B, Housely E 1976 Peripheral aneurysms in Behcet's disease. Br J Surg 63: 199–202
311. Kleinert H E, Burget G C, Morgan J A, Kutz J E, Atasoy E 1973 Aneurysms of the hand. Arch Surg 106: 554–557
312. Swanson E, Freiberg A, Salter D R 1990 Radial artery infections and aneurysms after catheterization. J Hand Surg (Am) 15: 166–171
313. Thorrens S, Tripple O H, Bergan J J 1966 Arteriosclerotic aneurysms of the hand. Arch Surg 92: 937–939

ANGIOMYOMA
314. Neviaser R J, Newman W 1977 Dermal angiomyoma of the upper extremity. J Hand Surg 2: 271–274

CONGENITAL VASCULAR MALFORMATION
315. Bogumill G P 1977 Clinico-pathological correlation in a case of congenital arterio-venous fistula. Hand 9: 60–64
316. Cabbabe E B 1985 Xeroradiography as an aid in planning resection of arteriovenous malformation of the upper extremities. J Hand Surg (Am) 10: 670–674
317. Curtis R M 1953 Congenital arteriovenous fistulae of the hand. J Bone Joint Surg 35A: 917–928
318. Gelberman R, Goldner J L 1978 Congenital arteriovenous fistulas of the hand. J Hand Surg 3: 451–454
319. Griffin J M, Vasconcz L O, Schatten W E 1978 Congenital arteriovenous malformations of the upper extremity. Plastic Reconstr Surg 62: 49–58
320. Moore J R, Weiland A J 1985 Embolotherapy in the treatment of congenital arteriovenous malformations of the hand: a case report. J Hand Surg (Am) 10: 135–139
321. Upton J, Mulliken J B, Murray J E 1985 Classification and rationale for management of vascular anomalies in the upper extremity. J Hand Surg (Am) 10: 970–975
322. Veal J R, McCord W M 1936 Congenital abnormal arteriovenous anastomoses of the extremities with special reference to diagnosis by arteriography and by the oxygen saturation test. Arch Surg 33: 848–866

HAEMANGIOMA
323. Geister J H, Eversmann W W 1978 Closed system venography in the evaluation of upper extremity hemangiomas. J Hand Surg 3: 173–178
324. Palmieri T J 1983 Subcutaneous hemangiomas of the hand. J Hand Surg (Am) 8: 201–204
325. Milner R H, Sykes P J 1987 Diffuse cavernous haemangiomas of the upper limb. J Hand Surg (Br) 12: 199–200
326. Pezehski C, Daneshbod K, Faghihi E 1980 Multiple hemangiomas of bone of upper extremity. Orthopaedic Rev 9: 67–69

327. Tunon J B, Gonzalez F P 1977 Angiomatosis of the metacarpal skeleton. Hand 9: 88–91

GLOMUS TUMOUR
328. Carroll R E, Berman A T 1972 Glomus tumors of the hand. Review of the literature and report of 28 cases. J Bone Joint Surg 54A: 691–703
329. Chan C W 1981 Intraosseous glomus tumor — case report. J Hand Surg 6: 368–369
330. Cornell S J 1981 Multiple glomus tumors in one digit. Hand 13: 301–302
331. Davis T S, Graham W P, Blomain E W 1981 A ten-year experience with glomus tumors. Ann Plastic Surg 6: 297–299
332. Jablon M, Horowitz A, Bernstein D A 1990 Magnetic resonance imaging of a glomus tumor of the fingertip. J Hand Surg (Am) 15: 507–509
333. Joseph F R, Posner M A 1983 Glomus tumors of the wrist. J Hand Surg (Am) 8: 918–920
334. Kline S C, Moore J R, deMente S H 1990 Glomus tumor originating within a digital nerve. J Hand Surg (Am) 15: 98–101
335. Love J G 1944 Glomus tumors: diagnosis and treatment. Mayo Clin Proc 19: 113–116
336. Maley E D, McDonald C J 1975 Bilateral subungual glomus tumors. Plastic Reconstr Surg 55: 488–489
337. Maxwell G P, Curtis R, Wilgis F 1979 Multiple digital glomus tumors. J Hand Surg 4: 363–367
338. Mullis W F, Rosato E F, Butler C J, Mayer L J 1972 The glomus tumor. Surg Gynecol Obstet 135: 705–707
339. Rettig A C, Strickland J W 1977 Glomus tumor of the digits. J Hand Surg 2: 261–265
340. Riddell D H, Martin R S 1951 Glomus tumor to unusual size. Ann Surg 133: 401–403
341. Riveros M, Pack T 1951 The glomus tumor. Report of 20 cases. Ann Surg 133: 394–400
342. Serra J M, Muirragui A, Tadjalli H 1985 Glomus tumor of the metacarpophalangeal joint: a case report. J Hand Surg (Am) 10: 142–143
343. Sugiura I 1976 Intra-osseous glomus tumor. J Bone Joint Surg 58B: 245–247
344. Varian J P, Cleak D K 1980 Glomus tumors in the hand. Hand 12: 293–299

HAEMANGIOENDOTHELIOMA
345. Acharya G, Merritt W H, Theogaraj S D 1980 Hemangioendotheliomas of the hand. Case reports. J Hand Surg 5: 181–182
346. Ekerot L, Eiken O, Jonsson K, Lindstrom C 1981 Malignant hemangioendothelioma of metacarpal bones. Scand J Plastic Reconstr Surg 15: 73–76
347. Finsterbush A, Husseini N, Rousso M 1981 Multifocal hemangioendothelioma of bones in the hand — a case report. J Hand Surg 6: 353–356
348. Larsson S E, Lorentzon R, Boquist L 1975 Malignant haemangioendothelioma of bone. J Bone Joint Surg 57A: 84–89
349. Moss L D, Stueber K, Hafiz M A 1982 Congenital hemangioendothelioma of the hand — case report. J Hand Surg 7: 53–56
350. Patel M, Srinivasion K, Pearlman H 1978 Malignant hemangioendothelioma in the hand. J Hand Surg 3: 585

HAEMANGIOPERICYTOMA

351. Ratna S 1976 Case reports: hemangiopericytoma of the hand. Plastic Reconstr Surg 57: 746–748
352. Vathana P 1984 Primary hemangiopericytoma of bone in the hand: a case report. J Hand Surg (Am) 9: 761–764

KAPOSI'S SARCOMA

353. Baxt S, Mori K, Hoffman S 1975 Aneurysm of the hand secondary to Kaposi's sarcoma. Case report. J Bone Joint Surg 57A: 995–997
354. Keith J E Jr, Wilgis E F 1986 Kaposi's sarcoma in the hand of an AIDS patient. J Hand Surg (Am) 11: 410–413

LEIOMYOMA

355. Brenton G E, Johnson D E, Eady J L 1986 Leiomyosarcoma of the hand and wrist. Report of two cases. J Bone Joint Surg (Am) 68: 139–142
356. Duinslaeger L, Vierendeels T, Wylock P 1987 Vascular leiomyoma in the hand. J Hand Surg (Am) 12: 624–627
357. Freeman A M, Meland N B 1989 Angioleiomyomas of the extremities: report of a case and review of the Mayo clinic experience. Plastic Reconstr Surg 83: 328–331
358. Hauswald K R, Kasdan M L, Weis D L 1975 Vascular leiomyoma of the hand. Plastic Reconstr Surg 55: 89–91
359. Sanders J O, Weiland A J, Moore J R 1986 Leiomyosarcoma of the forearm: treatment with wide local excision and a lateral arm flap. J Hand Surg (Am) 11: 906–910

LYMPHANGIOMA

360. Blair W F, Buckwalter J A, Mickelson M R, Omer G E 1983 Lymphangioma of the forearm and hand. J Hand Surg (Am) 8: 399–405
361. Moss A L, Ibrahim N B 1985 Lymphangiosarcoma of the hand arising in a pre-existing non-irradiated lymphangioma. J Hand Surg (Br) 10: 239–242

Metastatic

362. Aggarwal N D, Mittal R L, Bhalla B 1972 Delayed solitary metastasis to the radius of renal-cell carcinoma. J Bone Joint Surg 54A: 1314–1316
363. Amadio P C, Lombardi R M 1987 Metastatic tumors of the hand. J Hand Surg (Am) 12: 311–316
364. Bevan D A, Ehrlich G E, Gupta V P 1977 Metastatic carcinoma simulating gout. J Am Med Assoc 237: 2746–2747
365. Craigen M A, Chesney R B 1988 Metastatic adenocarcinoma of the carpus: a case report. J Hand Surg (Br) 13: 306–307
366. Creighton J J Jr, Peimer C A, Mindell E R, Boone D C et al 1985 Primary malignant tumors of the upper extremity: retrospective analysis of one hundred twenty-six cases. J Hand Surg (Am) 10: 805–814
367. Healey J H, Turnbull A D, Miedema B, Lane J M 1986 Acrometastases. A study of twenty-nine patients with osseous involvement of the hand and feet. J Bone Joint Surg (Am) 68: 743–746
368. Heymans M, Jardon-Jeghers C, Vanwijck R 1990 Hand metastases from urothelial tumor. J Hand Surg (Am) 15: 509–511
369. Hindley C J, Metcalfe J W 1987 A colonic metastatic tumor in the hand. J Hand Surg (Am) 12: 803–805
370. Huber D F, Weis L D 1985 Metastatic carcinoma of the distal ulna from an occult pancreatic carcinoma. J Hand Surg (Am) 10: 725–727
371. Kent K W, Guise E R 1978 Metastatic tumors of the hand: a report of six cases. J Hand Surg 3: 271–276
372. Kerin R 1958 Metastatic tumors of the hand. J Bone Joint Surg 40A: 263
373. Kerin R 1983 Metastatic tumors of the hand. A review of the literature. J Bone Joint Surg (Am) 65: 1331–1335
374. Kerin R 1987 The hand in metastatic disease. J Hand Surg (Am) 12: 77–83
375. McGraw J M, Stern P J 1989 Flexion contracture of the thumb: a malignant etiology. J Hand Surg (Am) 14: 736–738
376. Marmor L, Horner R L 1959 Metastasis to a phalanx simulating infection in a finger. Am J Surg 97: 236
377. Prystowsky S D, Herndon J H, Freeman R G 1975 Bronchogenic carcinoma metastatic to the hand. Cutis 16: 678–681
378. Rose B A, Wood F M 1983 Metastatic bronchogenic carcinoma masquerading as a felon. J Hand Surg (Am) 8: 325–328
379. Uriburu I J F, Morchio F J, Mario J C 1976 Metastases of carcinoma of the larynx and thyroid gland to the phalanges of the hand. Report of two cases. J Bone Joint Surg 58A: 134–136
380. Wu K K, Winkelman N Z, Guise E R 1980 Metastatic bronchogenic carcinoma to the finger simulating acute osteomyelitis. Orthopedics 3: 25–28

7. Congenital

The classification indicated above by Roman numerals is that adopted by the International Federation of Hand Societies and by the International Society for Prosthetics and Orthotics[1]. Those conditions presented in italics are considered in this chapter. This is not a complete list of congenital differences. It does, however, represent 98.1% of one large series of affected hands[2]. Greek and Latin 'unpronounceables' are avoided where possible for it seems unfair to copy them from another book into this. Should the reader encounter them or be invited by a learned geneticist to see a patient with a multi-eponymous syndrome, then he is referred to the Glossary and the Index of Syndromes in Adrian Flatt's excellent book, *The Care of Congenital Hand Anomalies*[2].

And so to the task in hand. It is different, challenging and rewarding. Firstly, before becoming preoccupied with the deformity of the hand, the examiner should inquire about other associated anomalies[3,4] and ensure that they are being properly handled. If a full examination has not been undertaken it should be performed or arranged. Consultation and planning may be necessary with other treating physicians.

Secondly, diagnosis is made more difficult by the total lack of active participation of the patient. The history must be taken from the parents who may seem surprisingly uncertain about the manual capabilities and limitations of their child. This is because they are of course untrained in clinical observation. Where the information is required, they must be trained to look for particular features, such as use of a part or its active motion. No facts can be obtained where patient co-operation is required, for example, two-point discrimination, active motion and the Allen test. Thus, much more weight comes to rest on *inspection*; on *palpation* and *passive motion*, both normal and abnormal (Fig. 7.1); on *radiologic evaluation*. Clinical examination should be appropriately prolonged to permit observation, supplemented and stimulated by the provision of two-handed toys if the child is old enough. An occupational therapist can greatly expedite this assessment. Some tricks may help — *active motion* is indicated by the presence of normal skin creases; its absence by their absence (Fig. 7.2). Active motion can be revealed sometimes by holding the digit or limb at the extremes of the range for some moments and then releasing it. Thus, holding the fingers in full flexion may cause the child to keep them there momentarily after release, or, holding them in full extension may induce reflex flexion when freed. Clearly only positive observations are valid. In the few situations where sensation is in doubt — for example, in constriction ring syndrome — tactile adhesion and the wrinkling test (pp. 230, 233) can be used. Radiologic evaluation is made more difficult, sometimes worthless, by the fact that much of the infant hand is present only in cartilage. Ossification centres appear at different ages (Table 7.1)[5]. These ages vary

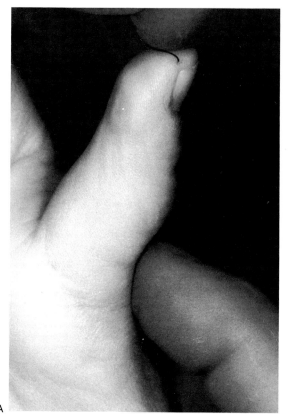

A

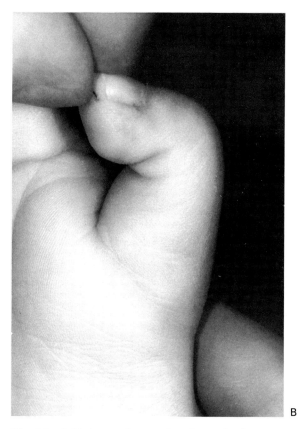

B

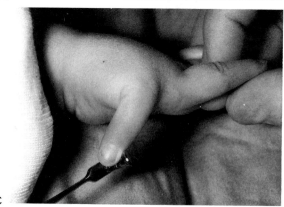

C

Fig. 7.1 A, B. A normal range of passive motion is demonstrated in this thumb which has no active function. This demonstrates clearly that the tendons are anomalous; pollex abductus (p. 499). C. Abnormal motion is demonstrated passively here, demonstrating laxity of the ulnar collateral ligament in this Blauth type II thumb. (From Lister G 1991 Pollex abductus in hypoplasia and duplication of the thumb: J Hand Surg 16A: 626–633.)

Table 7.1 Age of appearance of ossification centres. (Figures are for the 50th percentile in girls; centres appear later in boys by a multiplication factor of 1.55 ± 0.14 SD.)

Carpus	
Capitate and hamate	2 months
Triquetral	1.7 years
Lunate	2.6 years
Scaphoid, trapezium, trapezoid	4.1 years
Metacarpus and phalanges (epiphyseal centres)	
Metacarpophalangeal joints	
of the fingers (both centres) all by	1.5 years
Metacarpal of thumb	1.6 years
Proximal phalanx of thumb	1.7 years
Middle phalanges	all by 2.0 years
Distal phalanges	all by 2.5 years

considerably in the normal individual, but knowledge of them — as of other radiologic variables[6] — is of value, both in routine reading of films and also because there are specific causes of *advanced, retarded* and *dysharmonic maturation* which are outwith the scope of this text. For the above and other reasons — changes with growth, establishment of rapport — it is often desirable to see the child on two or more occasions before making surgical plans.

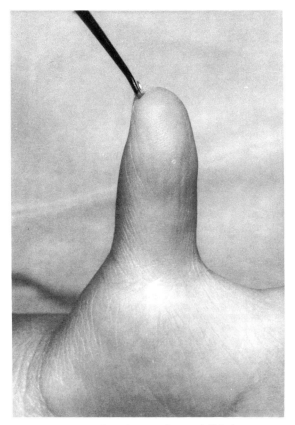

Fig. 7.2 The complete absence of normal digital creases on the palmar surface of this thumb which was allied to good passive motion, as demonstrated in Fig. 7.1 (A and B), indicates tendon anomalies. (From Lister G 1991 Pollex abductus in hypoplasia and duplication of the thumb. J Hand Surg 16A: 626–633.)

Finally, the surgeon should remember that while he examines and operates upon the baby, he is treating the parents. For the infant is sublimely unaware that he has any problem and he certainly does not present with a complaint. The parents by contrast are distraught to a degree that may seem out of all proportion. But it is not, for their concern is heightened by the potential of personal guilt, by the disappointment of having other than the expected perfect child, by the fear of anaesthesia and surgery at an age they believe to be so delicate, by the possibility of further abnormal children. They must therefore be informed with clarity and precision, reassured with honesty and compassion. From an early stage in the relationship, they must be told, with tact and sympathy, of the limitations of surgical endeavour. They must be brought as far as possible to view function as beauty, regardless of uncorrectable deviations from the norm. They should not be given false hopes, either by too glowing or inadequate a prognosis. Restoration, manufacture rather, of a normal hand is possible in only the most simple of defects. In rare and complex cases there is much to be said for a second opinion arranged by the surgeon. It gives support and often information to the doctor, and reassurance to the parents with invariably a perceptible increase in their confidence about their first choice of physician.

The surgeon may do much less surgery to the child with more informed consent than he could to the parents themselves. This is only right and proper for such protectiveness is an expression of their biologic function. Having performed that surgery he must maintain the information link: speaking to the parents immediately on completion of their child's operation; telling them at what time rounds are made so that they may be there; inviting them if concerned to the office or clinic at any time in the post-operative period; sharing plans for future management. Only in these ways will the surgeon gain that which he needs in addition to knowledge and technical skill in dealing with congenital deformity — the trust of the family.

Congenital differences in adults

The adult who presents with a congenital difference uncorrected requires evaluation of an entirely different kind. Evidently, they have functioned efficiently to that stage. Why then do they now come forward seeking surgical correction? The possibility of underlying psychiatric disturbance must never be overlooked. The evident symbolism of the unseparated complete syndactyly of the left middle and ring fingers in an unmarried 28-year-old woman is very clear (Fig. 7.3). The subconscious reliance that another patient may be placing on surgical correction may be less evident, but nonetheless devastating when it fails to yield the desired social result. Psychiatric consultation should always be suggested — the patient who readily assents in order to have surgery is well balanced and does not need the consultation! (see Fig. 7.42).

FAILURE OF FORMATION OF PARTS

Failure of formation has been divided into transverse and longitudinal. Transverse deficiencies have been restricted to include all congenital amputations, from absence of the fingers — aphalangia — to absence of the entire upper extremity — amelia. All other failures of formation are considered to be longitudinal deficiencies. Hence intercalated defects — phocomelia — are classified as longitudinal, since the peripheral limb which is present invariably shows anomalies.

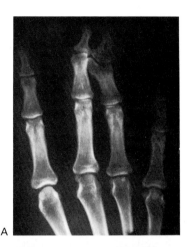

A

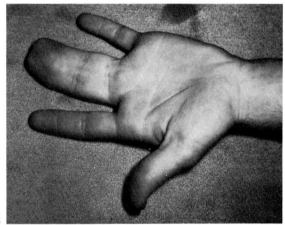

B

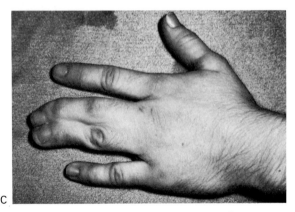

C

Fig. 7.3 A–C. Adult presentation congenital difference. This patient with a complete simple syndactyly and concealed distal central polydactyly of the left middle and ring fingers presented at the age of 28. Some months following correction the patient became sufficiently disturbed psychiatrically as to require prolonged hospital admission. Psychiatric opinion at the time indicated that the patient subconsciously associated her unwed status with the syndactyly (see also Fig. 7.42)

Transverse absence — upper third of forearm

This is the most common transverse absence in the upper limb and is almost entirely a problem for the prosthetist. The length of forearm below the normal elbow joint is usually 5 to 7 cm at birth, but growth is relatively decreased and the adult length rarely exceeds 10 cm[7].

Indications
The child should be fitted with a simple prosthesis at six months which aids considerably in crawling and climbing[8]. More sophisticated devices are provided at 12–18 months, and even myoelectric prostheses are now being fitted in some centres at the age of three. The infant and child does well with prostheses[9], even bilateral, but renewed counselling is required at adolescence when social pressures may cause him to reject it. Surgery may rarely be indicated to lengthen an unduly short forearm[10]. In countries where prostheses are not available, and especially in those both blind and bilaterally involved, the Krukenberg procedure is beneficial[11,12,13].

See Green D P 1993 Operative Hand Surgery, 3rd edn. Churchill Livingstone, New York, p. 256.

Transverse absence — carpus, metacarpus, phalanges

The absence of digits may present as a result of several congenital anomalies, the most common being:

(i)   true transverse absence
(ii) cleft hand (p. 468)
(iii) amputations from constriction ring syndrome
      (p. 506)
(iv) symbrachydactyly.

While the carpus is rarely complete, most of these children have a normal wrist joint and may also have vestigial digits (Fig. 7.4). If left alone, they will become remarkably adroit at crude grasp and release by the age of two to three, using the flexed wrist against the torso. The back of the carpus is also used and when they present at an older age, both the palmar and dorsal two point discrimination are more acute than normal.

Shortness of isolated or multiple metacarpals (brachymetacarpia) and phalanges[14–16] may result in shortening of one or more digits (Fig. 7.5).

Examination
Skeletal parts should be palpated, paying particular attention to *wrist motion* and *vestigial metacarpus*. The former is important for prosthesis design and for possi-

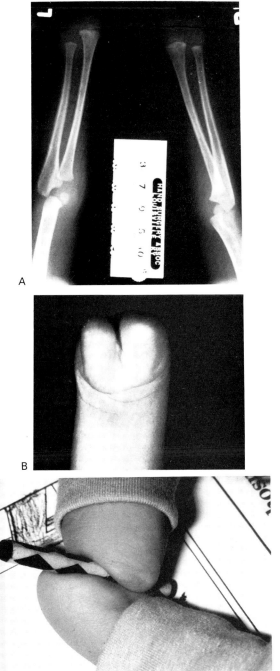

A

B

C

Fig. 7.4 A. This child presented with bilateral transverse absence, on radiograph apparently at the level of the wrist. B. It was evident on clinical examination, however, that there were mobile vestigial metacarpals at the thumb and ring or small finger positions. For this reason, he should be observed for development of bone in those positions and then scheduled for toe-to-hand transfer. C. If he receives no treatment, all grasp will be bimanual or against the torso.

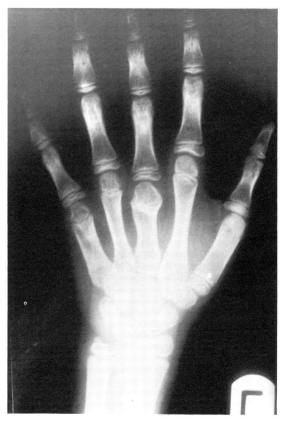

Fig. 7.5 Brachymetacarpia. The short metacarpal results in no functional deficit but the absence of a knuckle may cause the patient or parents to request bony lengthening of the metacarpal.

ble tendon transfers, both because they will probably be of wrist motors and because a full active range of wrist motion will add excursion to such transfers through the tenodesis effect. Good vestigial metacarpals at the thumb position and at the fifth or fourth ray are especially valuable. If any of the thumb metacarpal is present, the thenar area should be examined for passive range of the basal joint and observed for intrinsic muscle function, revealed both by contour and by voluntary active motion.

When vestigial digits are present in symbrachydactyly, they are simply nubbins of tissue often bearing a minute nail (Fig. 7.6). These vestigial digits are retracted into the pad of the transverse absence by the action of rudimentary long extrinsic tendons. These nubbins should be grasped gently and distracted, both to assess the presence and to some degree the strength of these extrinsics and also to evaluate the size of the skin enve-

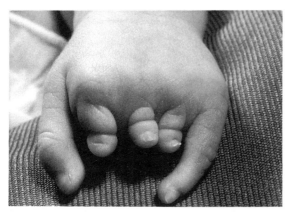

Fig. 7.6 Symbrachydactyly or transverse absence with vestigial digits. This child showed a stable skeleton in the rudimentary thumb, but only rudimentary cartilaginous fragments in the vestigial digits. There were extrinsic tendons evidenced by the retraction of the nubbins when they were drawn distally.

lope of the distal remnant. Radiographs are of limited value at the probable age of first presentation.

Indications
Initially, the infant should be fitted with a palmar plate prosthesis which, by motion of the wrist, permits grasp of smaller objects than otherwise[7]. Management can continue with prostheses, by conversion to a split hook with simple hinge control by the wrist joint.

However, there are some limited possibilities employing surgery, particularly where some metacarpal remnants are present. These include any or all of the following:

distraction manoplasty
free phalangeal transfer
ulnar post construction
microvascular toe to hand transfer.

Armed with the information regarding skeleton, skin, passive and active motion gleaned from examination, the surgical possibilities can be discussed with the parents.

[Transverse absence of the *thumb* at metacarpal level is considered with *constriction ring syndrome* (p. 506).]

Distraction manoplasty has been said to lengthen the skin envelope of the vestigial digits[17]. Done by transfixing the pulps with wire and applying steady traction over some weeks, it is more effective if there are cartilaginous elements in the pulp for they reduce the chance of the wire cutting out and the speed with which it does so. After distraction has been applied for four to six weeks, or if adequate skin envelopes already exist

as is most common in symbrachydactyly, *phalangeal transfer* should be undertaken, with Z-plasty lengthening if necessary of the annular ring constriction which is often present at the base of the vestigial digit. The reports of success with phalangeal transfer vary very widely from highly reputable and experienced authors: Carroll reports no growth in 159 transferred phalanges in 79 cases[18], Watson 90% of expected growth in 20 of 27 cases[19]. Other experience suggests that free bone grafts survive more certainly and are integrated well when they are employed as an interposition rather than a cantilever graft and when they are fixed, cancellous bone to cancellous[20,21]. It is now agreed that phalangeal transfers offer an excellent prospect of survival and future growth provided that three rules are observed (Fig. 7.7):

(i)   transfer must be done before the age of 15 months
(ii) periosteum must be taken
(iii) collateral ligaments must be repaired

If fourth (or fifth) metacarpal remnants are present on examination, these can be put to good use. The ulnar remnant can be lengthened by bony distraction[22-25] with or without subsequent interposition cancellous bone grafting[26], the skin envelope being enlarged by peroperative distraction or — rarely necessary[21] — by advancing the skin cone and applying a full-thickness graft to the base — somewhat akin to a Gillies 'cocked-hat' procedure[27]. An alternative to bone-grafting is the microsurgical transfer of one or more toes[28-30]. While it is technically possible to achieve survival, the acquisition of function is even more difficult in congenital absence than following traumatic loss of fingers[31], because of the vestigial nature of all structures in the hand:

— tendons are rudimentary, often represented by a sheet of fascia; transfer of wrist motors is often required
— the median and ulnar nerves, having nowhere to go, are underdeveloped; digital nerves have to be joined to cutaneous branches such as the terminal radial, the dorsal sensory branch of the ulnar nerve and the palmar cutaneous branch of the median nerve.

All of these surgical alternatives may be tried and are not incompatible. Distraction manoplasty at six months with phalangeal transfer thereafter, using the proximal phalanges of the third and fourth toes, can be followed by a two-year observation period during which phalangeal survival, epiphyseal development and overall growth can be assessed. If no grasp is so restored, ulnar post construction and toe-to-hand transfer can be performed knowing that all less complex avenues have been explored.

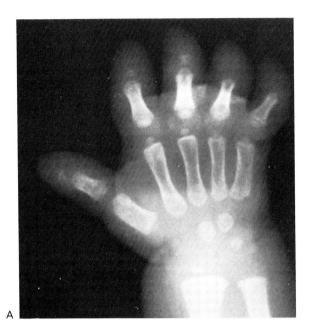

A

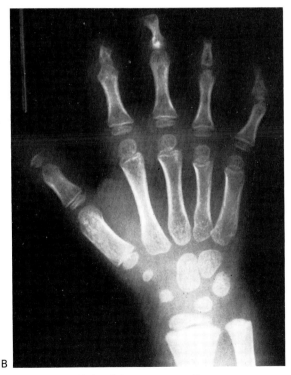

B

Fig. 7.7   A. This hand demonstrates uniform transverse absence of the fingers. After a period of distraction, phalangeal transfers were undertaken to all four fingers from the second and third toes of both feet. It can be seen four years later (B) that the phalanges in the middle, ring, and small have survived but with no clear evidence of a growth centre while that placed in the index finger has not.

This plan potentially exposes the child to several surgical procedures at an early age, which must be made clear to the parents when discussing the choice between prosthesis and surgery.

See Green D P 1993 Operative Hand Surgery, 3rd edn. Churchill Livingstone, New York, pp. 308 and 314.

Longitudinal absence – phocomelia

An intercalary deficiency of varying severity often results in an extremely short limb, characterized by the presence of digital skeletal elements, usually in reduced number and function. Phocomelia has been classified into three types[32]. In *complete* phocomelia the hand attaches to the trunk, in *proximal* phocomelia the forearm to the trunk, and in *distal* phocomelia the hand to the humerus.

Indications
Prosthetic fitting[33] is required for most phocomelic children, who may well activate the device with their terminal digits. Surgery is rarely required and then only to stabilize the limb, to render it of appropriate length for fitting or to improve function in the terminal digits.

Longitudinal absence — distal radial — radial club hand[34]

As a diagnosis, the term 'radial club hand' emphasizes the main feature of the disorder, namely, the hypoplasia or absence of the radius with resultant radial deviation of the hand on the forearm (Fig. 7.8). The condition is commonly associated with other anomalies, and these should not be overlooked during examination (see below). There is no clearly understood aetiology, either genetic or environmental[35]. Both extremities are affected in 50–72% of cases, depending on the series. In unilateral cases the opposite thumb is often hypoplastic[36].

Examination
The *wrist* is radially deviated to a variable degree. Passive motion reveals a significant reduction in the range of motion available, when compared with normal, both in palmar and dorsiflexion of the wrist and in ulnar deviation. The degree to which the radial deviation can be corrected is important, as it may indicate the power of deviating forces which will work against any surgical correction and certainly determines the need for manipulation with or without splintage before surgery. When fully deviated ulnarward, skin webbing on the radial aspect and redundancy on the ulnar will be noted. The former may contain a tight band which may

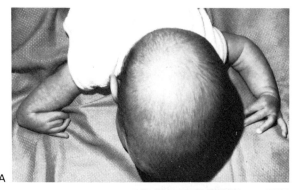

A

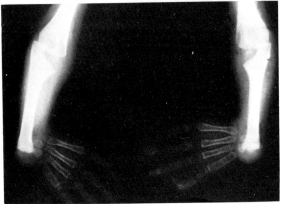

B

Fig. 7.8 Bilateral radial club hand A. Note that the right hand is more severely affected, and the absence of wrinkles on the extensor surface of the fingers indicates the lack of digital motion. The elbow as seen here is in full extension, and passive flexion was markedly limited at birth. With manipulation this improved to a point where centralization could be performed. B. The radius totally absent. The ulna is short and wide, though in this case not curved.

be the fibrous anlage of the radius, which may need to be excised, or, more importantly, the median nerve — this is frequently the most radial structure and in one fourth of cases is duplicated, one branch serving radial and the other median territory.

The *thumb* may be normal, hypoplastic, rudimentary or absent, the incidence varying widely in different series. The *rudimentary* thumb is present, but has no function, being distally located and having neither normal articulations nor motors — a 'pouce flottant'. The *hypoplastic* has function which is impaired to a varying degree (p. 499).

The *elbow* of the child with radial club hand is held in the extended posture, and attempts at passive motion will reveal that this is a fixed extension in many of the cases seen early. The passive motion improves with age and this should be encouraged by manipulation and splintage of both elbow and wrist. Certainly, the hand

should *not* be centralized where lack of elbow flexion would prevent the corrected hand from reaching the head.

Motion in the *finger joints* is most impaired in the radial digits. Thus the passive range of motion is more significantly reduced in the index than in the small finger. The metacarpophalangeal joint, while lacking flexion, usually shows normal or increased hyperextension (Fig. 7.9). The proximal interphalangeal joints in one series[34] showed average active ranges of motion as follows:

index 24°
middle 35°
ring 57°
small 78°

Despite this reduced motion, true symphalangism (p. 475) rarely occurs. It is not known to what extent the reduced motion is due to primary changes in the joint and what to anomalies of the motors, but muscle inadequacies certainly occur. On the extensor aspect, the extensor digitorum may be fused to the wrist extensors. The long flexors, especially the superficial, may be incomplete, atrophic or fused. Here again the degree of involvement is greatest in the index finger.

The *absence of muscles* or their anomalies may be detected in some small part by loss of *contour*, of *flexion creases*, or of *passive range* and evident *lack of voluntary motion* when the child is observed for some time. However, the deficiency may be confirmed only at surgery or at a much later age when the child can co-operate in active testing. While almost all upper extremity muscles may be affected (Table 7.2)[37] those most commonly so are:

pectoralis major
biceps[38]

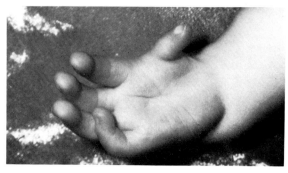

Fig. 7.9 Radial club hand. Following centralization and prior to pollicization, the relative lack of flexion in the index finger when compared with the small can be detected by the relative absence of flexion skin creases.

Table 7.2 Muscle anomalies in radial club hand (after Skerik and Flatt[37])

*MM	ABSENT > 50%	ABERRANT ORIGIN	ABERRANT INSERTION	FUSION with
PM	sterno-costal head		//////////	
D				
BB	long head	//////////		coraco-brachialis, PT
T				
BR	//////////		//////////	ECRL
PT				BB, PL, FCR
PQ	//////////			
S	//////////		//////////	
FCR	//////////			PT
FCU			//////////	ECU
PL	//////////		//////////	FDS, PT
FDS	index	radial head		FDP, PL
FDP	index		//////////	FDS
FPL	//////////		//////////	
FPB	//////////		//////////	
APB	//////////		//////////	
AP	//////////		//////////	
ADM				FDM
FDM				ADM
IO	1st DORSAL			
EPL	//////////		//////////	
EPB	//////////		//////////	
APL	//////////		//////////	
EI	//////////		//////////	
EDM				ED or ECU
ED				ECRL or EDM or ECU
ECU			//////////	ED or FCU or EDM
ECRL	//////////			ECRB, ED, BR
ECRB	//////////			ECRL

*Abbreviations for muscles are those given in the Appendix (pp. 513–526)

brachioradialis
supinator
extensor carpi radialis
flexor carpi radialis
the muscles of the thumb

The nerves and arteries of the radial club hand are also usually abnormal but this cannot be determined on examination of the infant nor need it affect the surgical correction provided the surgeon exercises appropriate caution.

Radiologic examination, depending upon the age of the child, will reveal to a varying degree the following anomalies:

radius — I   deficient distal radial epiphysis
   — II   complete but short = hypoplasia
   — III   present proximally = partial aplasia
   — IV   completely absent = total aplasia
ulna curved, thickened and, on average, only 60% of normal length (Fig. 7.10)
humerus also shorter than normal

carpal bone fusions and absence, the latter especially of the trapezium and scaphoid — other carpal bones may be absent, but are more likely to show fusion or delayed ossification
thumb absence or hypoplasia.(p. 499)

Associated anomalies must be sought either by the surgeon himself or by referral to a paediatrician. These may affect the decision to undertake surgery and its timing. *Cardiac defects* occur in 10–13% of patients with radial club hand[2], most commonly Holt–Oram syndrome[39]. *Blood dyscrosias* are also common. Fanconi's anaemia[40] is the most serious, being associated with progressive pancytopenia and an increased predisposition to malignancy. It is often not apparent in infancy, and less pronounced cases may never be diagnosed. Identification in the pre-anaemic stage can be achieved by tests on the peripheral blood[41] and, indeed, by amniocentesis[42]. All radially dysplastic infants should be so assessed, for early diagnosis will lead not only to appropriate genetic counselling since there is a 1-in-4

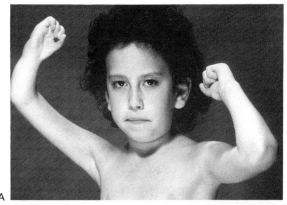

A

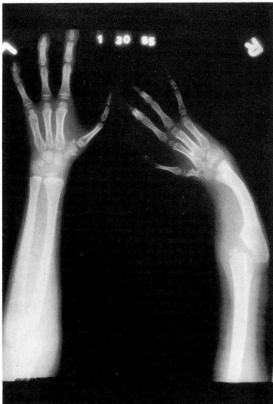

B

Fig. 7.10   Radial club hand. A. Some years after centralization, the ulna is seen to be significantly shorter than that on the contralateral side in which there had only been a Blauth type IV thumb hypoplasia. B. Radiologic examination further emphasizes the difference and also the persistence of curvature in the ulna. Both thumbs were created from index fingers.

chance of later children developing Fanconi syndrome, but also to intrauterine testing during later pregnancies. Such testing both warns of further affected children and

offers the possibility of umbilical cord transfusion, from those not affected, to their older Fanconi sibling.

Indications

Manipulation should be taught to the parents to be undertaken twice daily, emphasizing both ulnar deviation of the wrist and flexion of the elbow. Splintage is difficult to apply and of doubtful value provided manipulation is being faithfully administered.

If elbow flexion has been achieved, centralization, or radialization[43], of the carpus on the ulna should be undertaken at six to twelve months of age[44]. This is achieved by appropriate carpal excision and accompanied by transfer of radial wrist motors to ulnar motors and, where necessary, by angulation closing wedge osteotomy of the curved ulna[21]. Centralization should aim to preserve the distal ulnar epiphysis, although premature fusion is a recognized complication[2]. The limb is however always shorter than normal (Fig. 7.10) and the loss of length is more than balanced by the improvement in appearance and, to a lesser degree, function[45-47].

Where required, pollicization is performed three months after centralization. It is always required in absent or rudimentary thumbs while the indications in hypoplasia are discussed below (p. 499).

While some will centralize and pollicize only in bilateral cases, and then on only one side, current practice increasingly favours surgical treatment of all cases with good elbow motion and no other complicating anomalies.

See Green D P 1993 Operative Hand Surgery, 3rd edn. Churchill Livingstone, New York, p. 266.

Longitudinal absence — distal central — cleft hand[48]

Typical[49]:	bilateral; familial; absent metacarpus; usually middle ray absence; sometimes index, rarely ring; V-shaped defect; foot often involved.
Symbrachydactyly (formerly atypical):	unilateral; non-genetic; metacarpus present; several rays absent; U-shaped defect; no foot involvement (Fig. 7.11)

Atypical cleft hand and symbrachydactyly is identical, such that the first term has been discarded[14,51] (by decision of the Vth Congress of the International Federation of Societies for Surgery of the Hand, Paris, 1992). The embryological aetiology of symbrachydactyly differs from that of the typical cleft hand[52], as do the genetics[53]. Symbrachydactyly is characterized by the presence of

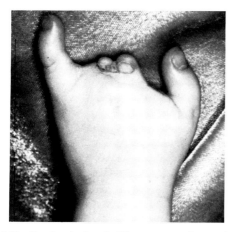

Fig. 7.11 Symbrachydactyly. The presence of normal metacarpals in the cleft is characteristic.

rudimentary nails on very hypoplastic digits with shortened metacarpals, whereas in the typical cleft hand, bones may be absent or malpositioned, but never rudimentary. In more severe cases of typical cleft hand the radial side is more affected, while in symbracydactyly it is the ulnar. Thus, a monodactylous thumb is an advanced form of the latter, a monodactylous fifth finger of the former (Fig. 7.12).

The typical cleft hand can vary in severity:

simple cleft between middle and ring fingers (rarely ring
 and small [54,55]), no absence
    → absent middle (Fig. 7.13)
        → progressive hypoplasia of radial
             digits (Fig. 7.14A)
             → syndactyly of remaining
                  digits (Fig. 7.14A)

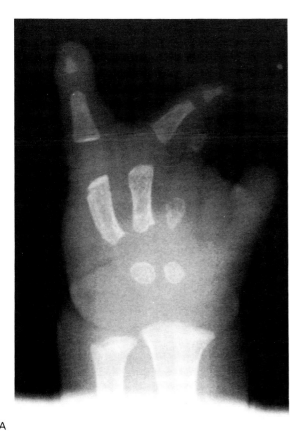

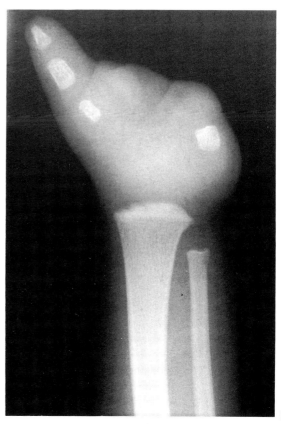

A

B

Fig. 7.12 Oligodactyly. A. As the digits which are present are on the ulnar side, this is a variant of *cleft hand*. B. Since the only relatively normal digit is on the radial aspect of the hand, this would be classified as *symbrachydactyly*.

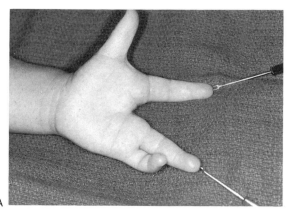

A

Fig. 7.13 Cleft hand. A, B. This relatively mild example shows absence of the middle finger and narrowing of the first web space. By simple transposition, a satisfactory hand can be created, closing the cleft and widening the first web space.

Early forms of radial hypoplasia show a degree of adduction contracture of the thumb with varying hypoplasia of the intrinsic muscles of the thumb. A reduced range of motion, with or without flexion contracture, may limit the function of any of the proximal interphalangeal joints. Transverse bones may be present, usually in the metacarpus (Fig. 7.15), which shows other abnormalities, such as one metacarpal splitting to support two digits, and vice versa.

In the extreme forms of either typical cleft hand or symbrachydactyly there may be only two border digits, either of which may have arisen from fusion — the 'lobster claw' hand[56].

Examination

Observation should be directed at assessing the function in the border digits and in the wrist.

Border digits:

grasp — this may be achieved by the cleft or by the usual mechanism of the thumb-index web space

pinch may be easily performed by two residual border digits, for example, in the U-shaped symbrachydactylous hand or the 'lobster claw' cleft hand, or may be prevented by a number of different factors, namely,

inadequate rotation, the ulnar digit being too pronated or the radial digit too supinated or both

blocking by the remaining metacarpus of the missing digits in symbrachydactyly

impaired digital motion which may be due to poor joint range, to the point of symphalangism, or to anomalous or absent motors — the digit may be flail.

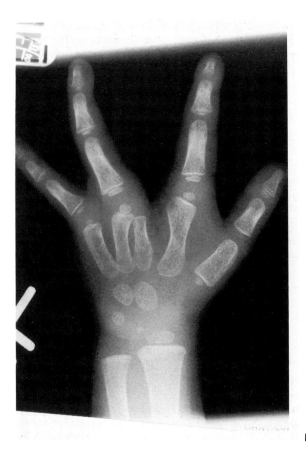

B

The wrist motion is usually normal and its motors may be required for tendon transfers.

Palpation will assess the *passive range of motion*, both normal and abnormal, in the joints, *contracture*, especially of the first web space, and the presence of normal and abnormal *skeleton*. The latter is confirmed by *radiologic evaluation*.

Indications

Since the syndactyly, when it exists, is between digits of unequal length in the first and the fourth web space early correction is required to prevent further deformity of the longer digit. This should be performed at as young an age as the child is deemed fit, when both ulnar and radial components can be separated simultaneously. The tendons and joints in such finger are frequently abnormal, and parents should be warned that separation may lead to intractable deviation, rotation and camptodactyly.

Reconstruction of the thumb may require simple deepening of the first web space, tendon transfers, rotational osteotomy, full pollicization or even toe

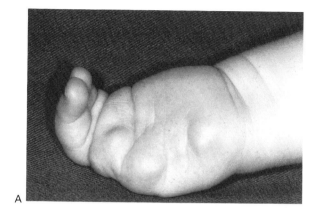

A

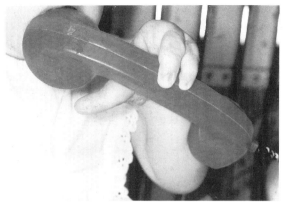

C

Fig. 7.14 Cleft hand. This child and her brother both presented with advanced bilateral cleft hands and feet. A. The hand demonstrates aplasia of the radial digits with syndactyly of the ring and small. B. The foot has a tibial element which is flail and non-functional. C. Microsurgical transfer of the flail element to the hand with separation of the syndactyly establishes grasp which is used and which has recently been improved by two-stage tendon graft.

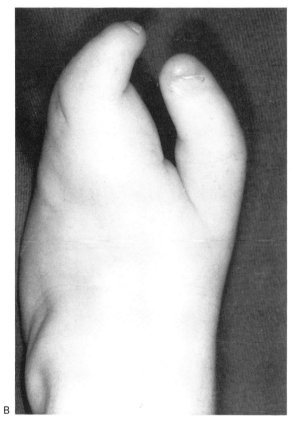

B

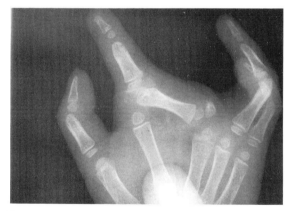

Fig. 7.15 Cleft hand. The transverse bone, by growth, progressively drives the second ray away from the third, fourth and fifth. Removal is complicated by the complex articulation at the metacarpophalangeal level of the second ray which is best left untouched during ostectomy, cleft closure and widening of the first web space.

transfer . The skin from the cleft can be transferred as a palmar based flap into the first web such as described by Snow and Littler[57,58], thus combining the two procedures of *cleft closure* and *first space widening. Rotational osteotomy* of border digits, the radial into pronation and the ulnar into supination, is performed at the metacarpal level and is designed to bring the tips into pinch contact. It is important that the osteotomies be so positioned that active flexion of the digits carries them beyond, and not just into contact with, one another, otherwise no power can be exerted in pinch activities. *Transverse bones* should be removed early as they drive the border digits further apart. As such bones frequently engage in complex joints, careful analysis of the effect of total removal should be made before electing to perform total or subtotal excision. Full *pollicization* is required where the radialmost digit is triphalangeal and supinated into the plane of the fingers. This invariably oc-

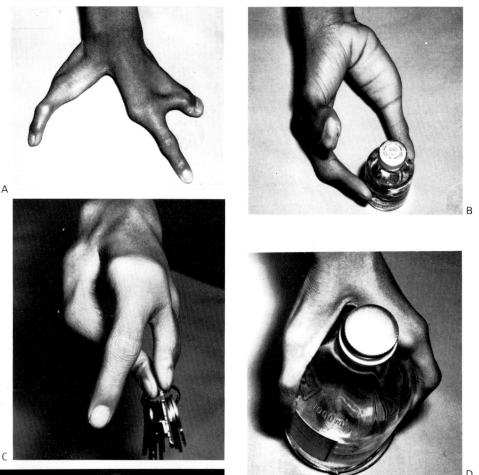

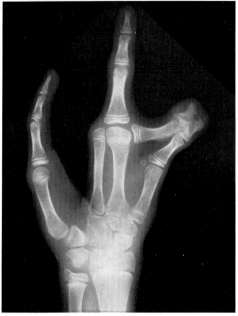

Fig. 7.16 Cleft hand. A. This boy presented for evaluation at the age of 18. B–D. It can be seen he has full prehensile function using the different digits in unique fashion. Such function would only be impaired at this late age by surgical intervention. E. The radiograph reveals a typical cleft with symphalangism and complex syndactyly of the index and thumb and resultant deviation.

curs in association with syndactyly. Caution must be exercised in this circumstance for frequently the blood supply comes from as few as two common digital arteries, one to the radial and one to the ulnar component of the cleft. Prudence dictates that correction be achieved in two stages, first syndactyly separation, second cleft closure and pollicization. The parents must be warned of the potential for vascular compromise.

When the cleft hand is oligodactylous, *toe transfer* may be the only means of creating a thumb. This requires both careful evaluation of the oft-times cleft foot and subsequent reconstruction of the inadequacies of the new thumb (Fig. 7.14).

Where a digit is flail, *tendon transfers* employing wrist motors extended by a tendon graft may restore active function. However, this will not restore more than the pre-existing passive motion and that passive motion can rarely be increased by joint release procedures. Further, where normal tendons are absent, so also are both the pulley mechanism on the flexor surface and the complex extensor apparatus.

By comparison with the anomalies which may occur in the border digits, *closure* of the typical cleft itself is relatively simple. It is important to employ zig-zag incisions, to design a distally based flap to restore the web and to reconstitute the deep transverse metacarpal ligament.

Rather than the closure required in the typical cleft, the symbrachydactylous hand may require *deepening* to facilitate grasp by the border digits. This is achieved by excision of the intervening metacarpus.

The function of cleft hands is often remarkably good (Fig. 7.16) the patient being capable of all manipulative activities, provided of course that all five digits are not required. However, the appearance of the hand is socially unacceptable and may cause great distress to the parents and later to the child. The surgeon must nonetheless be aware of the severe limitations, indeed the sometimes meddlesome nature, of surgical correction. Here as much as in any other congenital anomaly, emphasis must be laid on support and counselling, stressing that the unscarred, functioning, supple hand, however deformed, is much more acceptable aesthetically than a scarred, clumsy and stiff extremity — still deformed.

See Green D P 1993 Operative Hand Surgery, 3rd edn. Churchill Livingstone, New York, p. 278.

Longitudinal absence — distal ulnar — ulnar club hand

Ulnar club hand occurs less frequently than does radial club hand, by a factor varying from 1/3.6 to 1/10, depending upon the source[2,59]. It is characterized by deficiencies on the ulnar side of the hand and forearm and by a varying degree of dysfunction in the elbow. It differs from radial club hand in that in ulnar club hand the wrist is stable, the elbow not. The anomalies associated with ulnar club hand tend to be of the musculoskeletal system as opposed to the visceral and haematopoietic problems which may accompany the radial deficiency. Several classifications of ulnar club hand have been proposed[59-62] and Bayne has rationalized these:

I   Hypoplasia of the ulna (both ulnar epiphyses present)
II   Partial aplasia of the ulna (absence of the distal or middle third) (Fig. 7.17)
III   Total aplasia of the ulna
IV   Radiohumeral synostosis (Fig. 7.18).

Digits are absent from the ulnar side of the hand and in more advanced cases, those present are syndactylized. If digits are absent carpal bones are also, in the order of frequency, pisiform, hamate, triquetrum, capitate. The forearm and wrist are ulnar deviated. This is due both to curvature in the radius and to the tethering force of the ulnar anlage, a fibrocartilaginous band which attaches to the carpus distally and to the ulna, or, if the ulna is absent, the humerus, proximally.

The anlage is present in types II and IV, not in I and III. Because the anlage does not grow and the radius does, the anlage is believed to produce problems that increase as the child grows, although some disagree[63-65]:

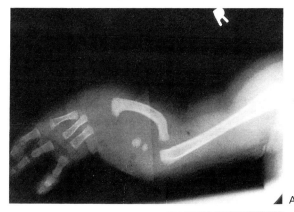

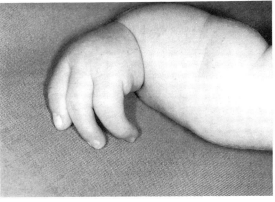

Fig. 7.17 Ulnar club hand. A, B. The partial aplasia of the ulna leaves the proximal portion represented by two small opacities. The radial head is dislocated. The curvature of the radius and the oligodactyly are evident.

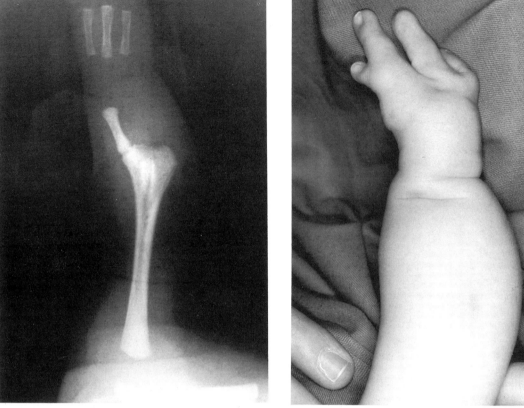

Fig. 7.18 Ulnar club hand; radiohumeral synostosis. A. The ulna is completely absent and despite the vestigial joint, the radius is one with the humerus. B. The complex digital anatomy presents significant problems in the surgical planning.

Deviation of the hand
Ulnar bowing of the radius
Ulnar inclination of the distal radius
Subluxation of the radial head (except in type IV).

Examination
Apart from determining the number and condition of the fingers present, examination is directed towards classifying the type of ulnar dysmelia, for that will determine whether the anlage is present and whether the elbow is stable. This in turn will dictate the operative management. Inspection will give the first clue except in the very young, for ulnar deviation will show the presence of an anlage. Palpation will reveal whether or not the elbow is stable, and if the ulna is present in cartilage and to what extent. Motion will confirm the stability of the wrist and aid in assessment of the elbow. Radiologic examination will show little that is not determined

on examination, indeed may show less, for much that is significant is in cartilage.

Indications
In types II and IV, roughly half of the authorities on this condition maintain that the ulnar anlage should be excised before six months of age[65], the others disagree! In later cases of type IV, an osteotomy of the radius will straighten the arm, and an osteotomy may be required to correct the internal rotation of the humerus which may accompany the radiohumeral synostosis. Syndactyly release and rotation osteotomy of the fingers should be performed during the first year of life[66]. In later cases of type II the subluxation of the radial head may require radial head resection, with creation of a one-bone forearm if there is insufficient proximal ulna to stabilize the forearm.

See Green D P 1993 Operative Hand Surgery, 3rd edn. Churchill Livingstone, New York, p. 298.

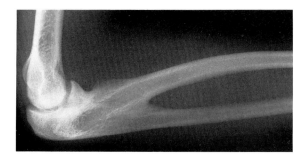

Fig. 7.19 Primary radio-ulnar synostosis. The radial head is absent. The synostosis is extensive. The radius is heavy and bowed, and the ulna is straight and narrow.

FAILURE OF DIFFERENTIATION OF PARTS

Radio-ulnar synostosis

This condition occurs at the proximal forearm in the large majority and is bilateral in 60% of cases. There are two types described — *primary*, in which the radial head is absent and the synostosis is more extensive than in the *secondary* form, in which the radial head is normal, although often dislocated.

Examination
This reveals a fixed pronation deformity which exceeds 50° in about 50%. Some compensation for this limitation is provided by hypermobility of the wrist which permits up to 50° of rotation.

Radiologic evaluation confirms the diagnosis and shows the radius to be heavy and bowed, the ulna to be straight and narrow (Fig. 7.19).

Indications
Attempts to restore active rotation by a variety of methods have proved unsuccessful. Therefore, where a case is unilateral or minor, no treatment is indicated[67,68]. In severe cases, a rotational osteotomy through the synostosis[69,70] should be performed at age 5. In unilateral cases the limb is placed at 10–20° of pronation, in bilateral the dominant is fixed at 30–45° pronation, the non-dominant at 20–35° supination[71].

Synostosis may occur elsewhere in the limb, notably at the metacarpal (Fig. 7.20).

See Green D P 1993 Operative Hand Surgery, 3rd edn. Churchill Livingstone, New York, pp. 324 and 330.

Symphalangism[72]

While strictly defined by Cushing[73] as hereditary stiffness of the proximal interphalangeal joints, sympha-

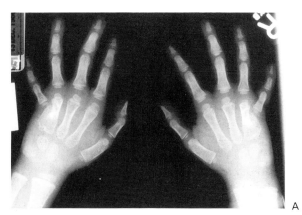

A

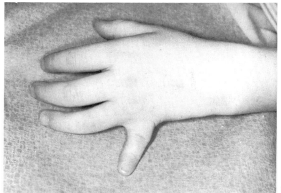

B

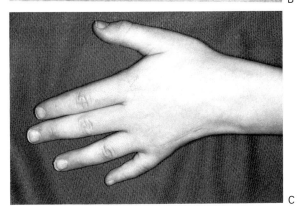

C

Fig. 7.20 Metacarpal synostosis. A. Metacarpal synostosis creates a problem, both in appearance and function. B. Distraction, double-angle osteotomy and bone graft to the vestigial fifth metacarpal can produce an improvement in both (C).

langism has come to mean congenital stiffness of a finger at any joint, genetically transmitted or not. Nonetheless, the condition does affect mainly the proximal interphalangeal joint and is commonly associated with varying degrees of shortness of the middle phalanx.

Hereditary symphalangism is transmitted as a dominant trait: it may affect one digit but usually more: it is more common in ulnar than in radial digits. Where the digit is of normal length, the distal interphalangeal joint commonly shows an increased, compensatory range of motion. More frequently the middle phalanx is short — *symbrachydactyly* — and then the distal joint may also show some stiffness. In either case the patient cannot make a fist. Hereditary symphalangism may be associated with hearing loss[74], which is treatable.

Non-hereditary symphalangism occurs in association with syndactyly, Apert's syndrome (see Fig. 7.35), Poland's syndrome and anomalies of the feet — in that order of incidence.

Examination

The fingers are commonly short and always atrophic, the skin being shiny and unmarked by creases on either dorsal or palmar surface. Attempts at *passive motion* will confirm the absence of motion, usually at the proximal interphalangeal joint and also the relatively slender nature of the bones. *Radiologic evaluation* may be confusing for the middle phalangeal epiphysis may appear to be a joint space.

Indications

Surgery in infancy should not be attempted. Efforts to restore motion by release or arthroplasty will fail, in part due to the lack of normal motors, both flexor and extensor. Surgery also carries the risk of damaging the epiphysis, further shortening an already short finger. Both function and appearance can be improved only by an angulation osteotomy in late adolescence, once the epiphysis has fused. The angles chosen should be those recommended for proximal interphalangeal joint arthrodesis — index 20°, middle 30°, ring 40°, small 50°.

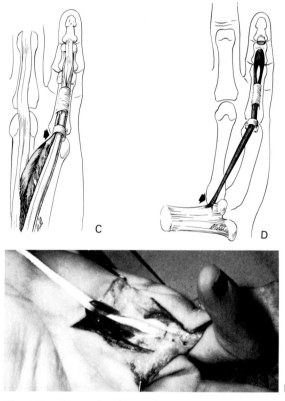

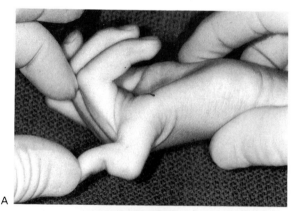

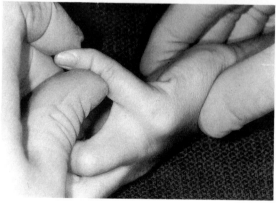

Fig. 7.21 Camptodactyly. A. The contracture of the proximal interphalangeal joint is 90 degrees with the metacarpophalangeal joint extended. B. With metacarpophalangeal joint flexion, the proximal interphalangeal joint can be brought into full extension. Clearly, the contracting structure crosses both joints and proved to be an anomalous lumbrical as shown in E. C, D. Two more common causes of camptodactyly. C. The fourth lumbrical inserting with the superficialis. D. Superficialis arising from the retinaculum or palmar fascia. E. Exploration of this camptodactyly revealed that the lumbrical tendon inserted into the superficialis producing flexion of the proximal interphalangeal joint as demonstrated here, rather than its usual function of extending the proximal interphalangeal joint.

See Green D P 1993 Operative Hand Surgery, 3rd edn. Churchill Livingstone, New York, p. 345.

Camptodactyly[75,76]

This is a congenital flexion deformity of the digit, usually at the proximal interphalangeal joint and encountered most commonly in the small finger (Fig. 7.21). It can occur, with rapidly decreasing frequency, in the ring, middle and very rarely the index fingers, usually in association with camptodactyly of the small. It is commonly bilateral and may be transmitted by an autosomal dominant trait or may occur sporadically.

Debate exists over this simple condition, both with respect to the anatomical cause and also as to whether or not there are two distinct types of camptodactyly. The balance would appear to favour there being two types, one which appears in infancy and affects the sexes equally and one which usually first presents in girls in their early adolescence. Both types of deformity may become much more marked during the teenage growth spurt. Function is rarely if ever affected and therefore it is usually appearance which prompts the patient to present. This, allied with the growth spurt deterioration, probably accounts for the fact that the majority of cases are seen during the second decade of life.

As to the anatomical cause, most structures around the proximal phalanx have been implicated at one time or another[75]. Cases seen by the author, in whom it was possible to establish a cause, have been due to one of two anomalies:

abnormal insertion of the lumbrical[77,78] (Fig. 7.21)
abnormal origin and/or insertion of the superficialis.

Where these cases have been established for some years, secondary changes occur in the proximal interphalangeal joint.

Examination
This should first be directed at determining the number of fingers involved and then measuring the *extension deficit*, both active and passive:

with the metacarpophalangeal joint extended
with the metacarpophalangeal joint held in flexion[75] (Fig. 7.21).

The distal interphalangeal joint is never involved. If it shows fixed hyperextension, a traumatic boutonniere is the likely cause of the flexion contracture of the proximal interphalangeal joint.

Radiologic evaluation should be undertaken on a *true lateral* of the involved proximal interphalangeal joint. Particularly in those cases in which full passive exten

sion could not be attained, characteristic changes are seen (Fig. 7.22):

(i) The neck of the proximal phalanx may show an indentation corresponding to the anterior lip of the base of the middle phalanx when in full flexion.
(ii) The base of the middle phalanx, which is wider than normal in an antero-posterior direction, may also show an indentation of its articular surface, impairing the normal smooth arc of that feature.
(iii) The head of the proximal phalanx, rather than being a full, smooth arc of a circle matching other heads and congruous with the base of the middle phalanx, has a blunt-pointed configuration such as would be produced by grinding off the palmar surface of the head.

Indications
Splintage[79] should be attempted, for some have reported better results than those achieved by surgical correction[80].

Indications for surgical correction depend very largely on the presence or absence of the above radiologic findings[75]. When they are well-established, soft-tissue procedures are unlikely to restore full extension. Where the deformity is pronounced and troublesome, a dorsal angulation osteotomy of the neck of the proximal phalanx can be proposed. It must be made clear to the patient, however, that the procedure only changes the arc of motion of the joint and that for every degree of extension gained, one of flexion and therefore of grasp must be sacrificed.

When the radiograph reveals a normal joint, the palmar aspect of the digit should be explored, seeking in particular anomalies of the lumbrical and/or superficialis. Where flexion of the metacarpophalangeal joint produced full active proximal interphalangeal joint extension only *release* of the abnormal tendon is necessary. Where only passive extension was achieved a tendon transfer to the radial lateral band is needed in addition. This can be of:

(i) An anomalous lumbrical if superficialis is normal
(ii) An anomalous superficialis provided it is normal proximally as demonstrated by normal excursion on traction
(iii) The normal superficialis of the adjacent finger if the superficialis of the affected digit is abnormal proximally as well as distally
(iv) An alternative tendon[81].

Camptodactyly of several digits (Fig. 7.23) is more complex and intractable, often part of arthrogryposis (p. 483).

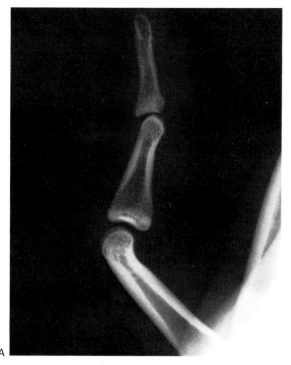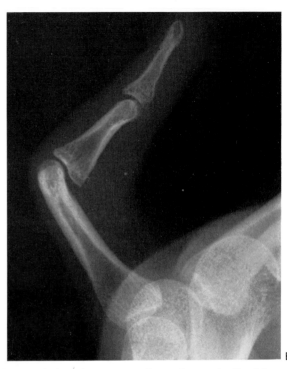

A   B

Fig. 7.22 Camptodactyly. A. The neck of the proximal phalanx shows an indentation corresponding to the anterior lip of the base of the middle phalanx. B. The base of the middle phalanx is wider than normal and also shows an indentation. The head of the proximal phalanx lacks the anterior portions of both condyles. These radiologic changes indicate that a soft-tissue release alone will be unsuccessful.

See Green D P 1993 Operative Hand Surgery, 3rd edn. Churchill Livingstone, New York, p. 413.

Clinodactyly[82]

This is curvature of a digit in a radio-ulnar plane. The condition occurs in conjunction with many syndromes, which must be identified. It is most commonly seen in the small finger and next most frequently in the triphalangeal thumb (p. 491). In most instances the resultant curvature turns the tip of the digit towards the mid-line of the hand and is due to a deformity of the middle phalanx. As emphasized in the assessment of malunited fractures, the two articular surfaces of the phalanx should be parallel. In clinodactyly, they are not. There are three different forms of clinodactyly encountered in the small finger:

(i)   minor angulation: normal length, very common
(ii) minor angulation: short phalanx, present in 25% of mongoloid children, only 3% of normal
(iii) marked angulation: delta phalanx

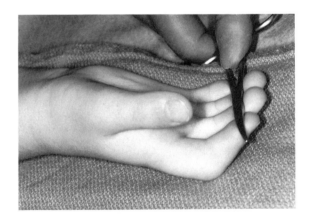

Fig. 7.23 Camptodactyly. All four fingers on both hands were affected in this child who probably represented a form of arthrogryposis. Exploration showed anomalous flexor tendons and significant shortage of skin.

The *delta phalanx*[83,84] comes about as a result of an abnormal epiphysis, which extends from one end of the normal proximal epiphysis around and along the short side — a 'J-shaped epiphysis', sometimes continuing to form an abnormal distal epiphysis to the bone, thus creating a 'C-shaped epiphysis' or *'longitudinally bracketed diaphysis*[85]' (Fig. 7.24).

Examination

Measure the degree of angulation and confirm that all other functions of the digit are normal.

Radiologic evaluation should determine whether the phalanx is short as well as angled and whether or not it is a delta phalanx. During the first 18 months to 2 years of life a delta phalanx is suggested by the location of the diaphyseal portion of the phalanx towards the convex side of the curve. The abnormal epiphysis ossifies thereafter.

Indications

Minor clinodactyly is only of aesthetic importance and surgery should be discouraged. Where the patient, usually an adolescent, is clearly distressed by the deformity, *closing wedge osteotomy* should be performed where the

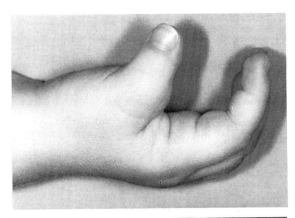

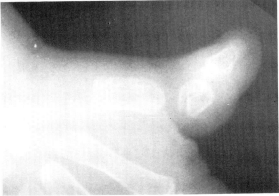

Fig. 7.24 Delta phalanx. A. The marked deviation in this thumb is due to (B) a delta phalanx, demonstrating a 'C-shaped epiphysis', or longitudinally bracketed diaphysis.

phalanx is of normal length, *opening wedge* where the phalanx is short, the necessary cortico-cancellous bone graft being taken from the distal radius (Fig. 7.25). The delta phalanx usually creates much more severe clinodactyly and therefore presents in infancy. When the digit is too long, especially where the phalanx is an additional one, as in triphalangeal thumb, then early excision should be performed (Fig. 7.26). The ligaments should be preserved and repaired and, where possible, the extensor tendon should be shortened appropriately. When the delta phalanx replaces a normal constituent of a consequently short finger, opening wedge osteotomy should be performed. This not only straightens and lengthens the digit — it also breaks the continuity of the abnormal epiphysis. In all instances the possibilities of residual deformity, non-union and tendon adhesions must be made clear to both patient and parents.

Kirner's deformity[86] is palmar and radial curvature of the distal phalanx of the fifth finger, which may be mistaken for clinodactyly[87]. Not truly congenital in that it is first noticed between 7 and 14 years of age, the disease is much more common in girls. It commences with a painless swelling and, once established, shows characteristic radiologic features of curvature, delay in epiphyseal closure, sclerosis of the diaphysis and a radiolucent nidus on the tuft. Treatment can be by splintage, selective epiphyseodesis or wedge osteotomy.

See Green D P 1993 Operative Hand Surgery, 3rd edn. Churchill Livingstone, New York, pp. 426 and 434.

Flexed thumb

The infant's thumb is normally flexed, and for this reason abnormal fixed flexion may not be noticed until some months after birth. The two main causes are *trigger thumb* and *clasped thumb*, distinguished by the fact that the fixed flexion in the first is of the interphalangeal joint alone while in the latter the metacarpophalangeal joint is affected also.

TRIGGER THUMB

Trigger digits may rarely involve the fingers as well as the thumb, may not be due solely to problems at the A1 pulley and may prove relatively intractable. However, by far the majority of congenital cases involve the thumb alone and, if they do not resolve spontaneously, will respond immediately to release of the A1 pulley.

Examination in most cases shows that, contrary to the clicking associated with adult triggering, the thumb is fixed, most commonly in flexion but sometimes in

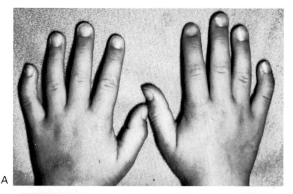

A

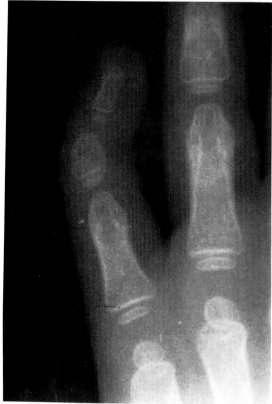

B

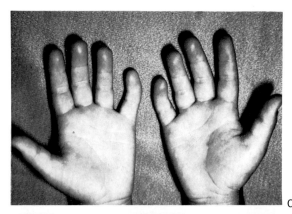

C

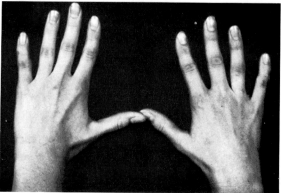

D

Fig. 7.25 Clinodactyly. A–C. The clinodactyly of each small finger is due to an angulated short middle phalanx. D. An opening wedge osteotomy of the middle phalanx with interposition of a small bone graft taken from the distal radius has resulted in normal growth and reasonable correction of the clinodactyly.

extension. On palpation a nodule (Notta's node[88]) can be felt over the metacarpophalangeal joint, a joint which shows free passive motion into hyperextension, in contrast to that of the clasped thumb (see below).

Indications
Trigger thumbs present at birth can be left for one year, for 30% will resolve spontaneously in that time, and joint contracture has not been reported in any child operated on before the age of three[89]. Surgical release of

the pulley at the metacarpophalangeal joint will cure all residual cases (Fig. 7.27).

See Green D P 1993 Operative Hand Surgery, 3rd edn. Churchill Livingstone, New York, p. 376.

Weckesser[90] and others have classified *clasped thumb* as follows:

Group I — deficient extension alone	70%
Group II — + flexion contracture	24%
Group III — + thumb hypoplasia	⎫
Group IV — miscellaneous	⎬ 5%

McCarroll[91] has criticized this system as being of little value, both in explaining the cause and in planning treatment. He suggests a simpler grouping, which in effect separates Weckesser group I from the remainder:

supple   weak or absent extensors pollicis
complex   hypoplastic extensor tendons
            flexion contracture of the metacarpophalan-
            geal joint

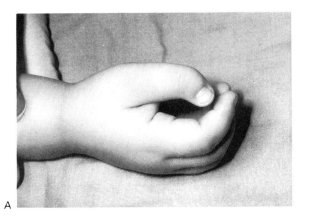

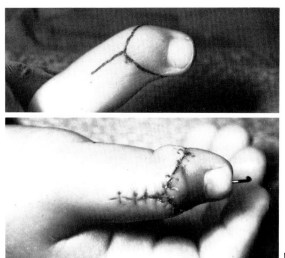

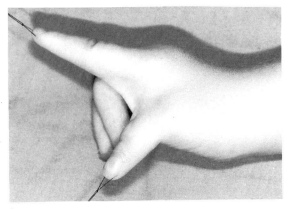

Fig. 7.26   Delta phalanx in a triphalangeal thumb. A. The marked angulation present in this triphalangeal thumb of a nine-month-old was corrected by total excision and reconstruction of the collateral ligaments (B).

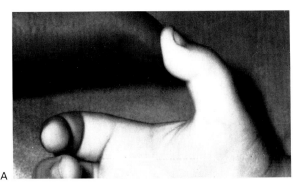

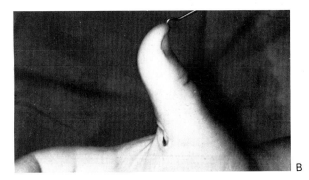

Fig. 7.27   Congenital trigger thumb. This persistent trigger thumb (A) was corrected by release of the A1 pulley at an age of eighteen months (B).

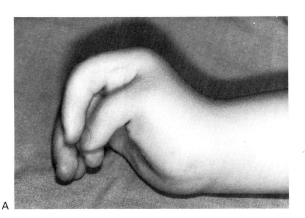

Fig. 7.28   Complex clasped thumb. A, B. All the features are seen: hypoplastic extensor tendons; flexion contracture of the metacarpophalangeal joint; ulnar collateral ligament laxity; thenar muscle hypoplasia; adduction contracture of the carpometacarpal joint; inadequate skin in the first web space; ulnar deviation and flexion contracture at the metacarpophalangeal joints of the fingers; wrist dorsiflexion; lack of the normal skin creases.

ulnar collateral ligament laxity

thenar muscle absence or hypoplasia

adduction contracture of the carpometacarpal joint

inadequate skin in the first web space
(Fig. 7.28).

COMPLEX CLASPED THUMB

The complex clasped thumb is often associated with the
ulnar deviation and flexion contracture at the metacarpophalangeal joints and wrist dorsiflexion characteristic
of a 'wind-blown hand'[92], or congenital ulnar drift of
the fingers[93]. If, in turn, this complex exists in conjunction with typical facial deformities, the condition is
known as 'whistling face syndrome'[94] or Freeman–
Sheldon syndrome[95]. Complex clasped thumb has
been reported to have a high association with
arthrogryposis[96].

Examination

The thumb is in the clasped position and lacks the
normal skin creases on both the palmar and dorsal
aspects. The creases may also be less pronounced on
the fingers if they show significant ulnar drift and
metacarpophalangeal joint contracture. The facies may
be anomalous, having a masklike appearance and
narrowed oral commissure. Attempts at passive motion
of the thumb will give easy hyperextension in supple
cases and in the complex will show a flexion and first
web contracture.

Indications

Supple clasped thumb diagnosed in infancy should be
splinted for three months in extension and then reassessed. If extension is now present, but weak,
splinting should continue. If it is not, then a tendon
transfer will be required. The common choice for
transfer, the extensor indicis, may be absent and an
alternative must be sought during examination.

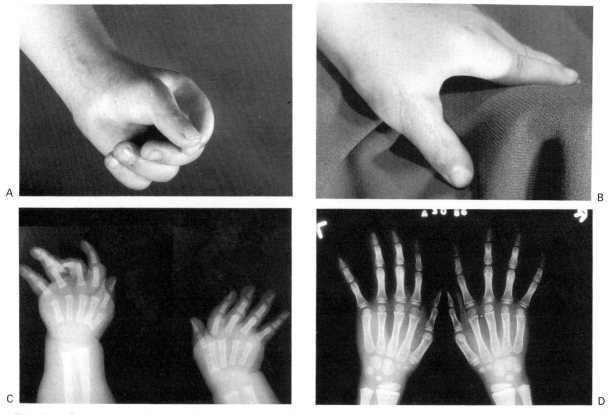

Fig. 7.29   Complex clasped thumb. A, B. Following thumb release, there is improvement of the whole hand. C, D.
Comparative radiographs taken six years apart confirm that correction of the thumb has led to spontaneous improvement in the
posture of the fingers.

Complex clasped thumb requires extensive release on the palmar aspect. Full and free extension may be achieved only when the first dorsal interosseous, the adductor pollicis and both heads of the flexor pollicis brevis have been released. The flexor pollicis longus may be short and require step-cut lengthening. A transposition flap is often required to maintain the release achieved with a full-thickness graft on the secondary defect. The ulnar collateral ligament of the metacarpophalangeal joint of the thumb may need added strength. Finally, transfers may be required both for extension and, in cases with thenar atrophy, opposition.

Once the thumb has been released, any ulnar deviation in and flexion contracture of the fingers may improve spontaneously to a surprising degree (Fig. 7.29). If it does not, then release of the palmar skin and any retaining structures[93], with lengthening of the flexor and centralization of the extensor tendons, may be required[97].

See Green D P 1993 Operative Hand Surgery, 3rd edn. Churchill Livingstone, New York, p. 404.

Arthrogryposis

Arthrogryposis, *curved joints*, is due to a defect in the motor unit as a whole, at some point between the anterior horn cells and the muscle itself. It has thus been divided into *neurogenic* and *myopathic*, the former constituting over 90% of cases[98]. The resultant severe muscle weakness occurs early in fetal life, producing immobility of joints which proceeds to contractures. The contractures are present at birth and do not progress thereafter. Involvement may be minimal, moderate or severe; it is symmetrical; upper and lower extremities are equally impaired.

Weeks[99] has developed a classification useful in planning treatment:

I Single localized deformities
    forearm pronation contracture
    complex clasped thumb
    loss of wrist and/or finger extensors (Fig. 7.30)
    intrinsic contracture

II Full expression of arthrogryposis
    absence of shoulder musculature
    thin tubular limbs
    elbows fixed, usually in extension, sometimes flexion
    wrist fixed in flexion and ulnar deviation
    fingers fixed usually in intrinsic plus posture
    thumb adducted
    skin thick and shiny with no creases

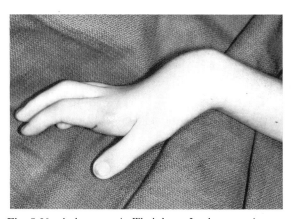

Fig. 7.30 Arthrogryposis. Weeks' type I arthrogryposis demonstrating fixed wrist flexion and metacarpophalangeal joint hyperextension.

III Same as II with added anomalies, including polydactyly and involvement of systems other than the neuromusculoskeletal.

Examination
This quickly yields the diagnosis in groups I and II. Palpation and attempts at passive motion reveal the location and extent of the joint contractures. More subtle is the assessment of active motors, for this may be difficult to detect if the joint on which the muscle acts is fixed in maximum excursion due to the lack of function in the antagonists. It also requires some voluntary or incidental participation of the patient and may have to wait until the child is older. In this respect the arthrogrypotic differs from the cerebral palsy patient in a major way, that is, in the level of intelligence and cooperation. However, this superior intelligence makes the arthrogrypotic child amazingly adaptable. The surgeon must exercise humility in the face of such physical initiative and not offer surgery until he is convinced of its benefits by repeated evaluation of the child's skills and limitations.

Indications
In group I cases, correction of the isolated deformity is usually achieved surgically. In the more complex groups II and III, efforts are directed at overcoming contractures and replacing essential motors which are not functioning. The minimal goal is one of achieving function in elbow extension on at least one side to assist in pushing off and using crutches, and in elbow flexion on at least one side for eating and toilet. Initially, contractures are addressed by progressive casting, splints and stretching exercises. If these are unsuccessful, then

surgical correction may be achieved by capsulectomy or, in more severe cases, skeletal adjustment. For internal rotation of the shoulder this would require a rotational osteotomy, for flexion contracture of the wrist, proximal row carpectomy[100,101]. The most significant active transfer is that to retrieve elbow flexion. This may be achieved with a Steindler flexorplasty, or transfer of pectoralis major[102], latissimus dorsi or triceps[103]. In those cases where these transfers are not available and in the minority which are myopathic in origin, free muscle transfer is a theoretical possibility, if a satisfactory muscle can be found. Wrist extension, once achieved, is maintained by transfer if one is available. Finger posture will be improved by successful management of the wrist and further splinting, but occasionally arthrodesis of the proximal interphalangeal joints will be of value.

Because of the early onset of contracture, the scarring which inevitably follows joint release and the relative weakness of transfers, even the few successful cases will be required to wear night splints for many years.

See Green D P 1993 Operative Hand Surgery, 3rd edn. Churchill Livingstone, New York, p. 365.

Syndactyly[104]

Complete:	the involved digits are united as far as the distal phalanx
Incomplete:	united further than the mid-point of the proximal phalanx but short of the distal phalanx
Complex:	bony union exists between the involved digits
Simple:	no such bony union exists
Acrosyndactyly[105]:	fusion between the more distal portions of the digits; always some proximal fenestration from dorsal to palmar surfaces (Fig. 7.31).

While in the simple, incomplete syndactyly, the union of the involved digits is a web, which may provide sufficient local skin for correction, it is preferable to view the digits as ones which have failed to separate rather than ones which are webbed, for a true web is rarely present. By this approach, the need for additional skin in the form of full-thickness grafts in the surgical separation of the great majority of cases is readily appreciated by all.

Syndactyly is the most common congenital deformity, both in its pure form and more so still when one includes its presentation as one feature of syndromes such as Poland's and Apert's (see below). When syndactyly presents alone — endogenous — it is trans-

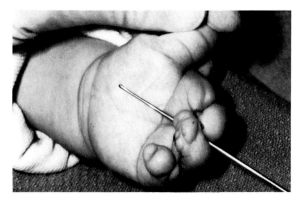

Fig. 7.31 Acrosyndactyly. The index, middle, and ring fingers are here fused at the tips producing the so-called 'rosebud' hand. The proximal fenestration which is always present from dorsal to palmar surfaces is here demonstrated with a probe.

mitted by a dominant gene, but with reduced penetrance and variable expression, so that a family history is present in from 10 to 40% of patients, depending on the series. Fifty per cent of such cases are bilaterally symmetrical.

The incidence of ray involvement also varies according to the source and can best be recalled by the mnemonic 5.15.50.30:

Thumb — index	5%
Index — middle	15%
Middle — ring	50%
Ring — small	30%

Accessory phalanges may be present between the skeletons of syndactylized digits either in an organized form — concealed central polydactyly — or in an apparent jumble of bones, lying transversely and obliquely as well as longitudinally (Fig. 7.32 see also Fig. 7.3).

Anomalies of tendons, nerves and vessels occur with increasing frequency the more complete a syndactyly. Even in the most simple complete syndactyly the bifurcations of both nerve and artery lie distal to the normal location. As the condition becomes more complex, the bifurcation of the common vessel becomes progressively more distal and, as shown in studies of infantile angiograms[106,107], the arteries on the outer aspect become progressively more rudimentary. The implications of vascular compromise at the time of division are self-evident.

Acrosyndactyly is commonly associated with constriction ring syndrome (p. 506) and has been classified by Walsh[108]:

moderate — two phalanges and one interphalangeal joint in each digit

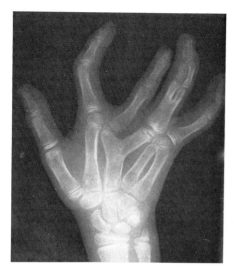

Fig. 7.32 Syndactylized concealed central polydactyly. This hand shows a bifid third metacarpal, an anomalous fourth metacarpal, and an additional digit forming part of a syndactylized duplication of the ring finger.

severe — one phalanx (Fig. 7.33)

The deviation, distortion and 'jumbling' of the involved digits increases with the severity.

Poland's syndrome[109] is a rare, non-genetic disorder characterized by four features[110]:

(i) Unilateral shortening of the digits, mainly the index, long and ring, due largely to shortness or absence of the middle phalanx

(ii) Syndactyly of the shortened digits, usually of a simple, complete type

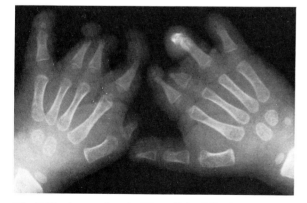

Fig. 7.33 Acrosyndactyly. These digits, following some releases, demonstrate both moderate and severe acrosyndactyly as defined by Walsh, there being digits with two phalanges and other digits with only one.

(iii) Hypoplasia of the hand, and, to a lesser degree, of the forearm (Fig. 7.34)

(iv) Absence of the sternocostal head of the pectoralis major muscle on the same side, associated to a decreasing degree[111] with:

(a) absence of the pectoralis minor

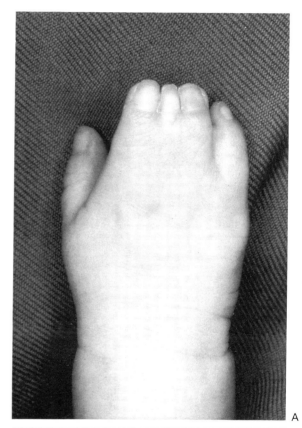

A

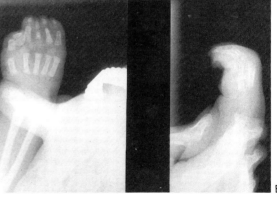

B

Fig. 7.34 Poland's syndrome. A, B. The typical features are seen: Shortening of the digits due to absence of the middle phalanx; complete simple syndactyly; hypoplasia of the hand.

(b) hypoplasia of the breast and nipple (33% of affected females[112])

(c) contraction of the anterior axillary fold

(d) absence of serratus anterior, latissimus dorsi and deltoid

(e) rib deficiencies, thoracic scoliosis and dextrocardia.

The soft tissues of the hand are abnormal such as to suggest an arrest of development at embryological stages XX to XXII[113]. Other anomalies may be associated with Poland's syndrome[114], including the Pierre Robin syndrome[115].

Apert's syndrome[116,117] occurs initially by mutation, but is thereafter a strongly dominant gene, a fact of

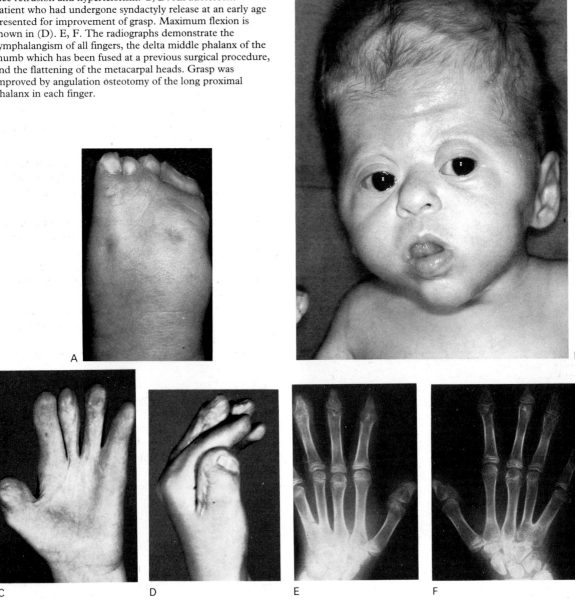

Fig. 7.35 Apert's syndrome. This child shows the total complex syndactyly with a common nail for the thumb and index, so typical of Aperts's syndrome. B. Acrocephaly, mid-face retrusion and hypertelorism. C, D. An adolescent patient who had undergone syndactyly release at an early age presented for improvement of grasp. Maximum flexion is shown in (D). E, F. The radiographs demonstrate the symphalangism of all fingers, the delta middle phalanx of the thumb which has been fused at a previous surgical procedure, and the flattening of the metacarpal heads. Grasp was improved by angulation osteotomy of the long proximal phalanx in each finger.

increasing significance as craniofacial surgery improves the mental and aesthetic status of these patients. The features are:

(i) acrocephaly with hypertelorism
(ii) bilateral complex syndactyly with symphalangism (Fig. 7.35)

The index, middle and ring fingers frequently share a common nail. The thumb is involved in the syndactyly in one-third of cases; it often demonstrates a delta proximal phalanx with resultant radial deviation. Vascular and tendinous anomalies are the rule.

Examination
Examination in syndactyly should determine the rays involved and how complete the involvement. The *nails* should be examined for they are commonly united especially in complex, complete cases. Any deformity in the involved digits should be noted. The *length* of the digits compared with normal may reveal *brachysyndactyly*. *Passive motion* should be undertaken on all joints for *symphalangism* may co-exist. The presence of these latter two conditions — brachydactyly or symphalangism — in conjunction with syndactyly suggests that more than the hand may be involved and a full physical examination is required.

Radiologic evaluation should reveal the number of digits, the number of metacarpals, the number of phalanges, the presence and situation of complex cross-union, delta phalanges and, in later cases the configuration of joint surfaces.

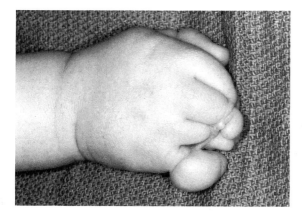

Fig. 7.36 Acrosyndactyly. The initial release performed in acrosyndactyly is simply of the tethering between the fingers which is shown here. The earlier this is done the better, as it permits unrestricted bone growth. Later, formal syndactyly release is performed at the usual age.

Indications
Early separation, whenever the infant is deemed fit, is indicated in certain situations.

1. *Acrosyndactyly* (Fig. 7.36). It is especially important to release distal, tethering bands very early. It permits improved growth. More formal proximal separation can wait.
2. *Syndactyly between rays of unequal length.* If this is not done the longer ray will develop rotation and flexion deformities which may not be corrected even with additional later surgery. The urgency is increased the greater the discrepancy between the digits, thus the rare thumb–index syndactyly should be separated when first seen (Fig. 7.37). It follows that involved border digits in Poland's and Apert's syndrome require early release[116,118].

Other cases should be released as convenient, and certainly by 18 months[2].

While technique is outwith the range of this text, certain points are worthy of emphasis since they involve planning based on examination:

— Where two digits have a common nail, syndactyly separation should be preceded by nail division with introduction of additional skin using a thenar flap[119] (Fig. 7.38).
— The sinus fenestration present in acrosyndactyly is always too far distal to form the new web space, and must always be excised during division.
— Syndactyly release should not be performed simultaneously on adjacent webs, that is, on both sides of one digit.
— The shorter the digit, the more proximal should be the new web, the limit being the level of the metacarpophalangeal joint.
— The new web must always be constructed of local skin (Fig. 7.39).
— Skin grafts will always be required, except in the least of incomplete cases.
— When the thumb is involved, as in Apert's syndrome, simultaneous rotation and angulation osteotomy is required where all metacarpals are in the same plane and there is absence of the thenar musculature[21].
— Bilateral syndactyly can be operated upon by two teams at the same operation in order to reduce the number of procedures.

Patients, and their parents, must be made aware that the limbs in Poland's and Apert's syndrome will always be smaller than normal and the fingers stiff. Where symphalangism exists, angulation osteotomy in adolescence is indicated. Delta phalanges should be dealt with

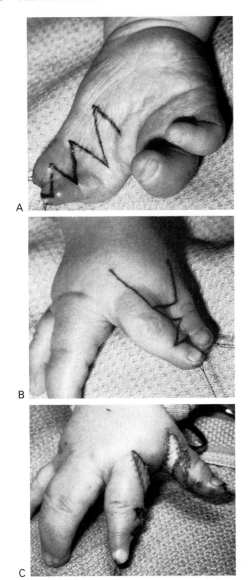

Fig. 7.37 Simple complete syndactyly. A, B. The simple complete syndactyly between the thumb and index finger in this child is here being separated at the age of seven months. Despite this the rotation and angulation of the index finger can be detected in (C) (see same patient in Fig. 7.38).

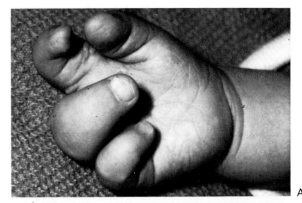

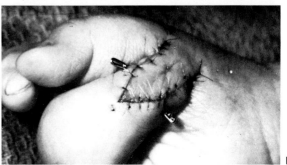

Fig. 7.38 Complex complete syndactyly — nail union. A. The union of the nails of the syndactylized middle and ring fingers is separated in a preliminary procedure with application of a thenar flap (B), providing extra tissue to resurface the contiguous surfaces of the distal phalanges at later division. The Kirschner wires maintain the distal phalangeal separation in order to avoid circulatory embarrassment of the thenar flap. The pronation of the index finger referred to in Fig. 7.37 is seen here more clearly.

by excision or wedge osteotomy as discussed under triphalangeal thumb (below) and clinodactyly (above).

See Green D P 1993 Operative Hand Surgery, 3rd edn. Churchill Livingstone, New York, p. 349.

DUPLICATION

Polydactyly[120,121] is a common congenital disorder, vying with syndactyly for first place[122]. Duplication of the small finger, in strong contrast to that of the thumb, is usually the result of an autosomal recessive trait[123] and is often part of a syndrome. Its presence therefore dictates the need for a full physical examination. The radial aspect of the hand is involved a little more than the ulnar, and both are much more common than central polydactyly. The latter is almost always associated with syndactyly and often shows disorganization of the skeleton. 'Mirror hand' or ulnar dimelia[124–126] presents with multiple digits, duplication of the ulna and absence of the radial ray (see Fig. 7.45F). The varying manifestations of duplication have been classified by Stelling[127]:

Type I: Soft tissue mass containing no skeletal structure[128]; rare in the thumb

Type II: A digit or part thereof, containing all normal

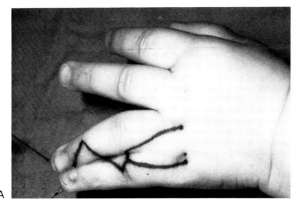

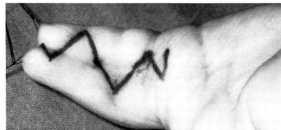

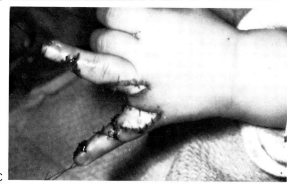

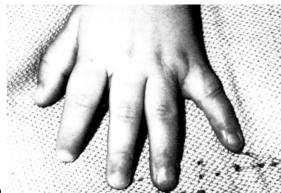

components and articulating with a normal or bifid metacarpal or phalanx (Fig. 7.40)

Type III: A digit, complete with metacarpal; rare (see Wassel VI, below)

Radial duplication

Duplication of the thumb can occur at any level, and clarity has been given by the introduction of the following classification by Wassel[129]:

Type I —	*Bifid* distal phalanx	2%
II —	distal phalanx *duplicated*	15%
III —	*Bifid* proximal phalanx	6%
IV —	proximal phalanx *duplicated*	43%
V —	*Bifid* metacarpal	10%
VI —	metacarpal *duplicated*	4%
VII —	Triphalangia, in either or both of the thumbs and at any level II–VI	20%

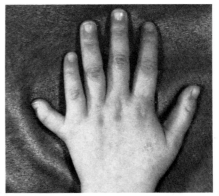

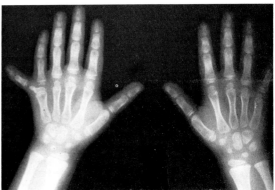

Fig. 7.39 Complete simple syndactyly. A–C. The general principles of release are here illustrated. The new web is constructed entirely of local skin. A number of full-thickness grafts taken from the groin are required. The resultant separation shown in (D) is pleasing — and permanent.

Fig. 7.40 A, B. Ulnar duplication — Stelling type II. The additional digit shown here articulates with a relatively normal metacarpal although the epiphysis and metaphysis are somewhat widened. Reconstruction of the ulnar collateral ligament was necessary at the time of excision.

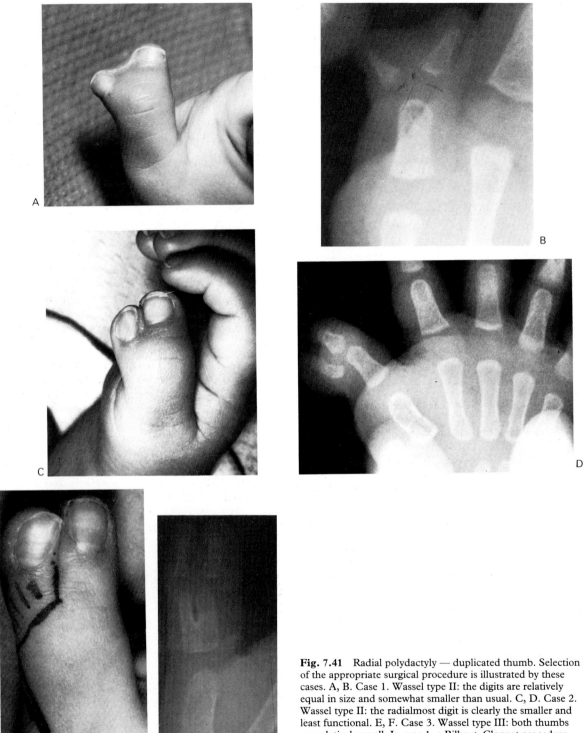

Fig. 7.41 Radial polydactyly — duplicated thumb. Selection of the appropriate surgical procedure is illustrated by these cases. A, B. Case 1. Wassel type II: the digits are relatively equal in size and somewhat smaller than usual. C, D. Case 2. Wassel type II: the radialmost digit is clearly the smaller and least functional. E, F. Case 3. Wassel type III: both thumbs are relatively small. In case 1, a Bilhaut–Cloquet procedure was performed. In case 2, the radial of the two digits was excised. In case 3, the radial of the two digits was excised producing an unsatisfactorily small distal thumb.

It can be seen that confusion may arise between the Stelling and Wassel classifications. In practice, this does not occur since the Wassel classification is used exclusively when describing thumb duplications. By contrast with ulnar polydactyly, thumb duplication is usually unilateral and sporadic, except for type VII triphalangia which results from a dominant gene. The great majority of duplicate thumbs have only one vessel to each component[130].

Examination

Examination should initially place the duplication in the appropriate Wassel category and then, with the exception of the majority of types I and II (see below), should be directed at determining which of the two thumbs should be retained on the basis of the following criteria.

Size (Fig. 7.41). While most duplications are of similar size, and that size somewhat smaller than the normal, unaffected thumb, one of the two may be rudimentary; this is most common in type VI, the radial being small and functionless.

Deviation may be present both at the point of duplication and at joints distal to that point[131]. Where a digit is markedly deviated at its base frequently it deviates in the opposite direction at more distal joints under the influence of anomalous tendon insertions and of the Z-ing phenomenon similar to that seen in rheumatoids (Fig. 7.42).

Function may differ markedly in two thumbs of similar size and this may be revealed only by repeated, quite prolonged observation. Frequently, functions may be shared, extension being good in one, flexion in the other. Even in the youngest infant, complete loss of motion will be revealed by absence of the matching skin creases. The tendon insertions are often anomalous, both flexor and extensor attaching more on the facing aspects of the phalanges in a manner which encourages deviation of the distal phalanges of the two thumbs towards one another. On occasion the flexor may insert into the extensor as in *pollex abductus* (see below) serving then solely as a deviating force.

Passive mobility, both normal and abnormal, should be assessed in all joints. The *first web space* is contracted in certain cases of thumb duplication and this should not be overlooked.

Radiologic evaluation will confirm the classification of the duplication and in triphalangeal thumb should determine the nature of the extra phalanx (see below).

Indications

In types I and II where the thumbs are usually of equal size, the Bilhaut[132]-Cloquet sharing procedure should be performed[133]. Since the thumbs are usually small, a little more than half should be taken from each. The difficulties associated with this procedure are residual nail deformity and unintentional epiphyseodesis. If the thumbs are of almost normal size, the first problem can be avoided by taking the entire nail from only one of them, discarding that from the other. The second problem is avoided by accurate matching of the epiphyseal plate, disregarding any incongruity in the joint surface which can be shaved down later in the procedure — the two epiphyses are rarely of equal thickness.

In the more proximal types, *size, deviation, function* or *passive mobility* may make the choice easy. However, where the thumbs are equal in all respects, the choice may await exploration before a final decision is made on the basis of tendon and nerve anatomy. In the bifid types III and V the surgeon can be entirely unbiased. In the duplicated types IV and VI — especially the former which is also the most common — he should favour retention of the ulnar thumb, thereby avoiding reconstruction of the ulnar collateral ligament so important for thumb stability. In any event certain steps are indicated in type IV to ensure the best result[134,135] (Fig. 7.43):

— Exploration and appropriate realignment of the insertions of both flexor and extensor tendons
— Division of anomalous connections between flexor and extensor tendons
— Shaving of the metacarpal head on the side of excision of the duplicate, in order to eliminate an unsightly prominence, whilst ensuring
— Preservation of both ligaments — that between the two duplicated proximal phalanges and that between the metacarpal and the discarded phalanx — for reconstruction of the one collateral[136]
— Re-attachment of the intrinsic muscles.

Where the first web space is contracted, the skin from the duplicated thumb to be discarded should be preserved as a dorsally based flap to be transposed into the defect created by release (Fig. 7.44).

See Green D P 1993 Operative Hand Surgery, 3rd edn. Churchill Livingstone, New York, p. 444.

TRIPHALANGEAL THUMB

Triphalangeal thumb[137] may present as part of a type VII duplication (Fig. 7.45) or as an isolated entity. It may be inherited as a dominant trait[138]. The additional phalanx lies between the proximal and distal phalanges and may be any one of three types:

— delta phalanx, producing increasing deviation (see also p. 478)

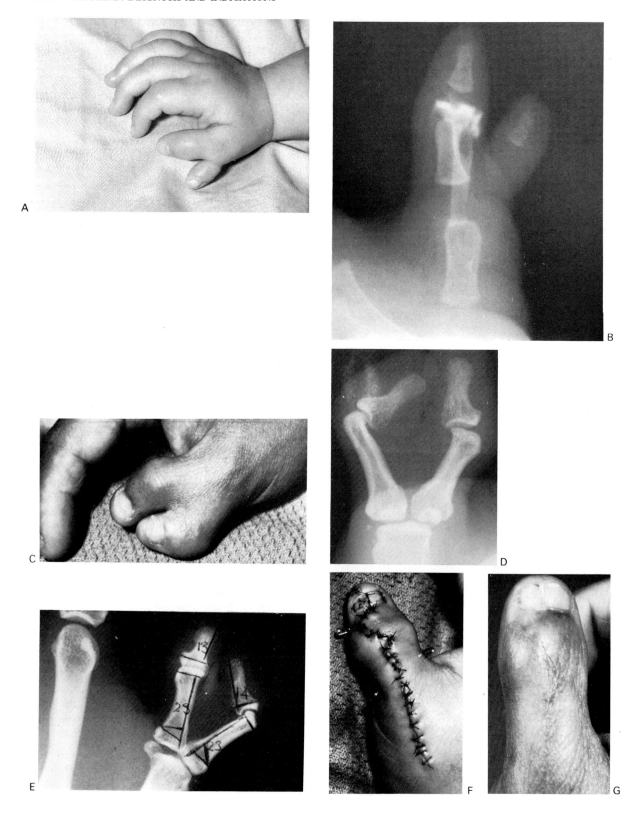

A

B

C

D

E

F

G

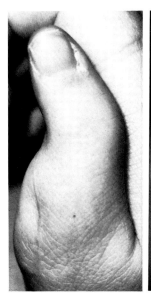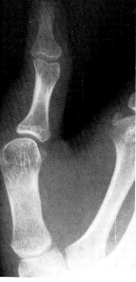

Fig. 7.43 A, B. This patient previously had a radialmost digit excised from a Wassel type IV. This was clearly performed without shaving of the metacarpal head or reconstruction of the radial collateral ligament. This has resulted in the Z-ing deformity shown here affecting both the metacarpophalangeal and the interphalangeal joint. It was found on exploration that there was a communication between flexor and extensor tendons on the radial aspect of the proximal phalanx (see Fig. 7.55).

— rectangular phalanx which is short
— rectangular phalanx of normal length.

In the latter two types the metacarpal is longer than normal, adding even more length to the already lengthened thumb. If in addition, the digit is supinated, the first web space is contracted and the thenar muscles small, then there is little distinction from a five-fingered hand[139], a diagnosis which would be confirmed by finding a deep transverse metacarpal ligament.

Indications[140]

A *delta phalanx* should be totally excised as early as possible and the soft tissues reconstructed. If seen late, arthrodesis of one joint with wedge osteotomy[141] is required. A *rectangular phalanx* is treated by resection and arthrodesis of the distal joint, where necessary ac-

companied by an opponensplasty, widening of the first web space and shortening of the metacarpal. The closer the triphalangeal thumb comes to being a five-fingered hand, the more should formal pollicisation be considered (see below).

See Green D P 1993 Operative Hand Surgery, 3rd edn. Churchill Livingstone, New York, pp. 452 and 465.

Central duplication

This, the least common of the duplications, affects the ring finger in more than half of the cases and the middle and index fingers in about an equal number of cases. Stelling types I and III present little problem requiring simple excision of the supernumerary digit. Type II, which is most common, and is almost invariably associated with syndactyly, thereby producing a '*hidden central polydactyly*', is most difficult to treat. This is both because it is intimately involved anatomically with both of the digits between which it lies and because they also are impaired to a differing degree (Fig. 7.46).

Examination

Inspection may show what appears to be a simple complete syndactyly. The presence of an additional digit may be detected clinically only with *palpation*. Both active and *passive motion* may be impaired and should be carefully assessed.

Radiologic evaluation should determine the Stelling type of polydactyly, the point of duplication with special attention to shared epiphyses, and the condition of the 'normal' digits with particular reference to complex syndactyly, symphalangism, deviation and abnormal phalanges.

Indications[142]

Early surgery is indicated since deviation of the digits to be retained only worsens with time and correction becomes more difficult. It is important to emphasize to the parents a number of points:

(i) Impairment of motion may be due to the interposed extra digit or to an indeterminable degree of limitation in the apparently normal digits alongside, even

Fig. 7.42 Duplicated thumb Wassel type IV. A. This apparently straightforward Wassel type IV had well disguised deviation in the dominant thumb. B. This deviation was, in part, due to the anomalous and eccentric insertion of the flexor tendon as demonstrated by the tenogram during surgery. C, D. This thumb shows deviation both at the metacarpophalangeal joint and also at the interphalangeal joints distally. This is somewhat similar to the Z-ing phenomenon seen in rheumatoids. E. A Bilhaut–Cloquet procedure with multiple osteotomies was undertaken with an acceptable result. F, G. This patient presented at the age of 28. When psychiatric evaluation was suggested, she readily assented. It was therefore not performed. She has had no psychiatric consequences to surgical correction (see also Fig. 7.3).

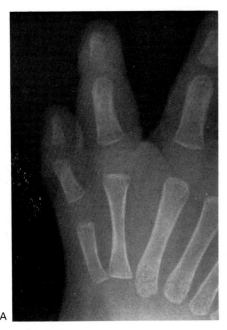

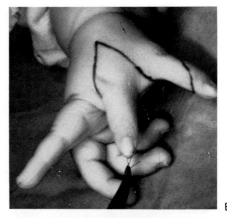

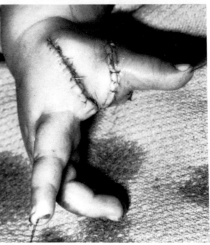

Fig. 7.44   A. Duplicated thumb — Wassel type VI. The radialmost digit here was excised. The first web space was contracted and also showed shortage of skin. This was corrected (B, C) by transposing the skin from the digit to be discarded into the first web space and by translocating the metacarpal which was retained on to the articular surface of the trapezium previously occupied by the excised metacarpal.

to the point of *symphalangism*, the implications of which must be explained.

(ii) *Tendons* and *nerves* may be shared between two, or even three, digits in central polydactyly. The flexor, and more so the extensor, tendons may be a conjoined sheet of tissue difficult to separate and even more difficult to impart with function.

(iii) *Deviation* of the 'normal' digits which may be evident or concealed may require ligament reconstruction with simultaneous or subsequent angulation osteotomy.

(iv) Flatt[2] has pointed out that the anomalies existing within an apparently simple complete syndactyly may be so great that only one functional finger can be obtained from the three digital skeletons available, producing a four-digit hand from the six available; this requires very sympathetic discussion with the parents.

Ulnar duplication is often inherited and is associated with a number of syndromes, demanding full physical examination. The principles outlined above for diagnosis and indications apply.

Hyperphalangism[143] means that a digit has an extra phalanx. A rare occurrence, it usually produces deformity which requires surgical correction[144]

See Green D P 1993 Operative Hand Surgery, 3rd edn. Churchill Livingstone, New York, pp. 485 and 488.

OVERGROWTH

Macrodactyly

Macrodactyly[145] is a non-hereditary congenital enlargement of a digit. It is unilateral in 90% of cases. In 70% of those afflicted the condition affects more than one digit, those always being adjacent and corresponding to the territory of one or more peripheral nerves[146], most commonly the median (Fig. 7.47). The enlargement is more pronounced distally than proximally; thus, phalanges are affected more frequently than meta-

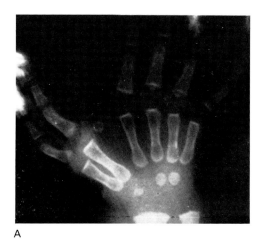

A

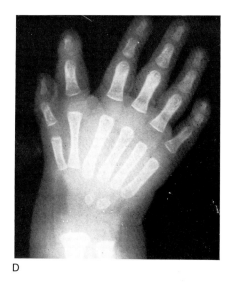

D

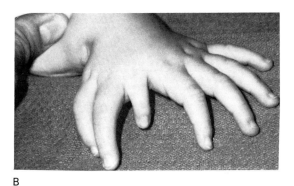

B

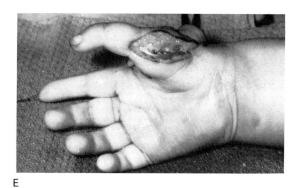

E

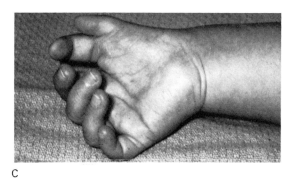

C

Fig. 7.45 Radial polydactyly with triphalangeal thumb.
A, B. The radial polydactyly shown here consists of two
triphalangeal thumbs and a Stelling type II additional radial
duplication. (This is not a mirror hand since the two forearm
bones are of relatively normal nature.) In another Wassel type
VII duplication (C, D) following excision of the radialmost of
these duplicated digits, (E) the excessive length and
additional joint of the triphalangeal remaining thumb is
clearly evident. F. In a true mirror hand, the forearm is
composed of two 'mirror image' ulna bones and no radius.

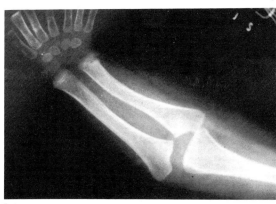

F

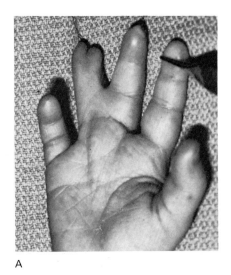

A

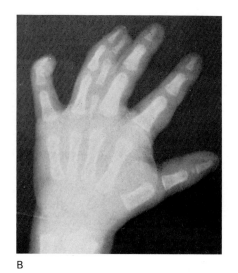

B

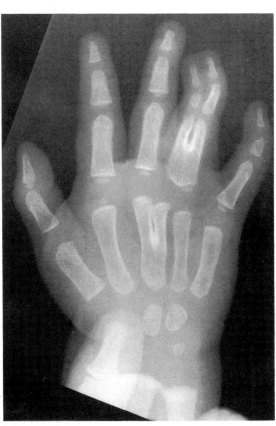

C

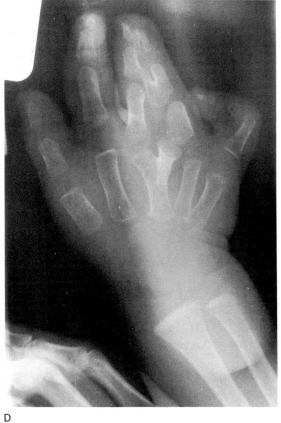

D

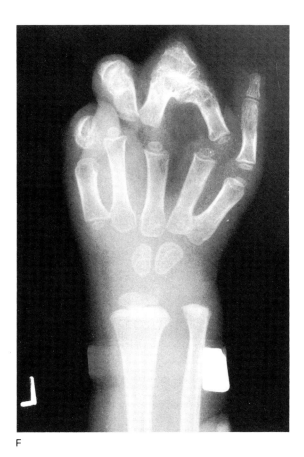

F

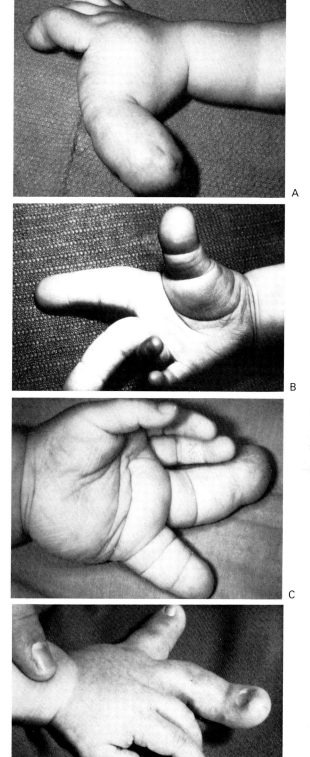

A

B

C

D

Fig. 7.46 A, B. Concealed central polydactyly. Here the Stelling type II additional ring finger is not entirely hidden. There is however, syndactyly between the middle and ring fingers. The radiograph (B) reveals that the main ring finger is somewhat hypoplastic in structure. Indeed, the collateral ligaments had to be reconstructed in this finger which despite that reconstruction, went on to show some rotation and slight deviation. C, D, E. Examples of increasingly complex concealed central polydactyly.

Fig. 7.47 Macrodactyly. It can be seen here that the median (A, B) and ulnar nerve (C, D) distributions are primarily affected in these three cases. Case B is that of Mr Gwyn Morgan FRCS.

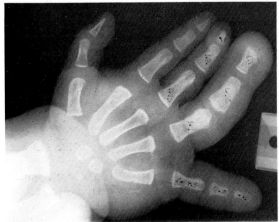

A

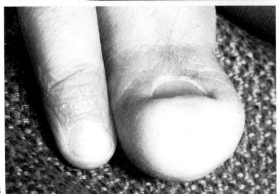

B

Fig. 7.48 It can be seen from the radiograph (A) that the phalanges are markedly enlarged while the metacarpals are of normal size. B. This illustrates the difference between the ring finger of the normal hand and that of the macrodactylous hand of the same patient.

carpals (Fig. 7.48). All tissues that respond late in development to neurogenic influence are enlarged — nerves, fat, skin appendages and bone. Two facts follow from this:

1. The cause of macrodactyly is neurogenic[147] — probably a form of neurofibromatosis[148], the enlarged nerves being similarly infiltrated with fat and fibrous tissue (Fig. 7.49).
2. Tendons and blood vessels are of normal size; the latter fact results in relatively poor blood supply to all tissues, with a consequently higher incidence of avascular necrosis of skin flaps.

Two types of macrodactyly have been described[149]:

static — present at birth, often involving only one digit, the enlargement keeps pace with growth of the normal digits

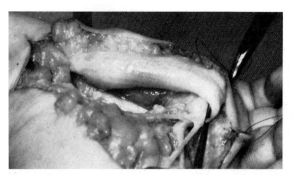

Fig. 7.49 The marked enlargement of the median nerve of the patient shown in Fig. 7.47A.

progressive — much more common, this form is sometimes not apparent until as late as 2 years of age; this form is more aggressive, growing more quickly than adjacent digits and involving the adjacent palm.

Hyperostotic macrodactyly[150] differs from other forms in its late onset and lack of nerve involvement. It is characterized by florid osteochondral enlargement which arrests joint motion.

Examination

Inspection yields a swift diagnosis. The involved digit should be watched during manipulation for it may be excluded either because it is clumsy or because of *joint stiffness* which becomes progressively more severe with age and excessive growth. *Deviation* is a common accompaniment, due to uneven overgrowth of the two borders of the digit. *Palpation* will detect any temperature difference suggestive of locally poor circulation and may also reveal significant increase in tension which in part explains both the stiffness and the diminished blood supply. *Passive motion* should be recorded. While sensation is usually normal in the young, in adult patients, compression of the enlarged median nerve may lead to carpal tunnel syndrome[151]. *Ulceration* of the fingertips may be evidence of impaired neurovascular status. The most likely differential diagnosis — cavernous hemangioma — is excluded by the entirely different consistency of the digit and appropriate vascular observations (p. 447).

Radiologic evaluation plays a significant role. Comparison should be made between the involved fingers and films taken by identical technique of:

(i) the same digits on successive visits
(ii) the corresponding digit on the opposite uninvolved hand
(iii) the corresponding digit on the parent of the same sex (Fig. 7.50)

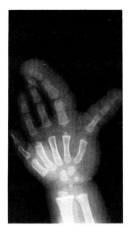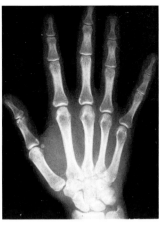

Fig. 7.50 Here on the same radiographs are shown the hands of the patient shown in.Fig. 7.47C and Fig. 7.48 and the mother of that patient. The grossly macrodactylous ring finger of the child is still 1.3 cm shorter than that of the mother. This demonstrates the impracticality in some progressive macrodactyly cases of the recommendation that one should undertake epiphyseal arrest when the digit is equal to that of the same finger in the parent.

Careful measurements should be made and recorded. While of course particular attention should be paid to the involved fingers, adjacent digits should be assessed equally closely for any evidence of incipient macrodactyly.

Indications
Macrodactyly reduces even the giants of hand surgery. The severely affected single digit which has little motion, gross curvature and poor circulation presents only the problem of informing the parents of what they feared — that amputation is the correct treatment. But what of the thumb[152]? And of multiple digits? Reduction is the only answer, and that both time-consuming and inadequate — epiphyseal ablation; osteotomies both shortening to reduce length and angulatory to correct deviation. Even this is insufficient — further shortening with nail preservation as described by Barsky[149,153] or Tsuge[154] and longitudinal narrowing osteotomies are required. Nerve stripping (Tsuge)[154] and extensive defatting to the extent of creating 'flap grafts' (Edgerton) achieve some meagre soft-tissue reduction. Many operations are required and each reduces blood and nerve supply and contributes to scarring and stiffness. The whole is an experience frustrating for the surgeon, painful for the child, harrowing for the parents. A test of rapport.

See Green D P 1993 Operative Hand Surgery, 3rd edn. Churchill Livingstone, New York, p. 501.

UNDERGROWTH

Hypoplasia and aplasia of the thumb

Hypoplasia of the thumb has been classified by Blauth[155]:

Grade I — minor hypoplasia, in which all elements are present, the thumb being overall somewhat smaller than normal

Grade II (Fig. 7.51) — adduction contracture of the first web space
— laxity of the ulnar collateral ligament of the metacarpophalangeal joint
— hypoplasia of the thenar muscles[156,157]
— normal skeleton, with respect to articulations

Grade III (Fig. 7.52) — significant hypoplasia, with aplasia of intrinsics, rudimentary extrinsic tendons, if any
— skeletal hypoplasia, especially of the carpometacarpal joint which is vestigial

Grade IV (Fig. 7.53) — floating thumb (= pouce flottant) a vestigial, totally uncontrolled digit attached just proximal to the metacarpophalangeal joint of the index finger

Grade V (Fig. 7.54) — total absence.

Hypoplasia, especially of grade II, may be associated with[158,159]:

(i) duplication of the thumb
(ii) triphalangia, with or without delta phalanx
(iii) anomalies of tendons and muscles
   (a) flexor pollicis longus, which may be absent[160-163], rudimentary or attached to the extensor tendon — the *pollex abductus*[164-167] (Fig 7.55)
   (b) eccentric insertion of extrinsic motors on the distal phalanx with resultant deviation of the distal phalanx, early or late
   (c) anomalous extensors[157,168]
   (d) aplasia of the thenar muscles[169,170]
   (e) m. lumbricalis pollicis[171]
(iv) a single, midline neurovascular bundle[172]

Examination
Once the grade has been determined, examination is largely directed at the tendon anomalies which may be associated with grade II hypoplasia. *Skin creases* should be sought, indicative of active joint motion, which

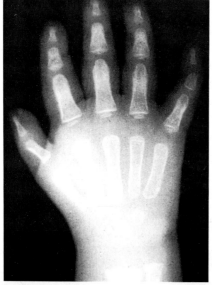

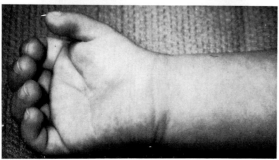

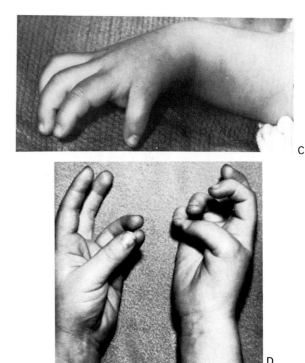

Fig. 7.51 Hypoplasia of the thumb — Blauth grade II. A. The radiograph reveals hypoplasia of the thumb skeleton but an acceptable length to the metacarpal. The same patient is shown in (B) and (C) and illustrates contracture of the web space, hypoplasia of the thenar muscles, and laxity of the ulnar collateral ligament. D. An older patient demonstrates hypoplasia of the thenar muscles and resultant impairment of opposition of the hypoplastic thumb.

should also be observed. Where flexion creases are absent or rudimentary, abduction at the metacarpophalangeal joint may be seen and the tendon of the anomalous flexor pollicis longus of a pollex abductus palpated where it crosses the hypoplastic thenar area. *Passive motion* of all joints should be recorded. Laxity of the collateral ligaments of the interphalangeal and, more probably, the metacarpophalangeal joints should be assessed. *Radiologic evaluation* should confirm the grade, seek abnormal phalanges in the thumb and exclude other anomalies.

Indications
Grade I — no treatment required
Grade II — see below
Grades III–V — pollicization of the index finger[173–176].

Parents, and indeed some surgeons, may express reluctance to sacrifice a hypoplastic thumb, especially of grade III. However, the deficiencies of basal joint, motors and size can never be restored. If the parents are adamant, the child can be left until grasp movements commence, when he will clearly demonstrate that the manipulative potential lies in the index and middle fingers by their use of the so-called 'cigarette grip' for all pick-up manoeuvres (Fig. 7.56). However, where all are agreed, pollicization of the index should be undertaken within the first year of life[174] (Fig. 7.57).

Grade II hypoplasia requires:

1. Exploration of flexor and extensor tendons and correction of any anomalies[177]
2. Release of the first web space[178]
3. Opponensplasty[179]
4. Stabilization of the metacarpophalangeal joint.

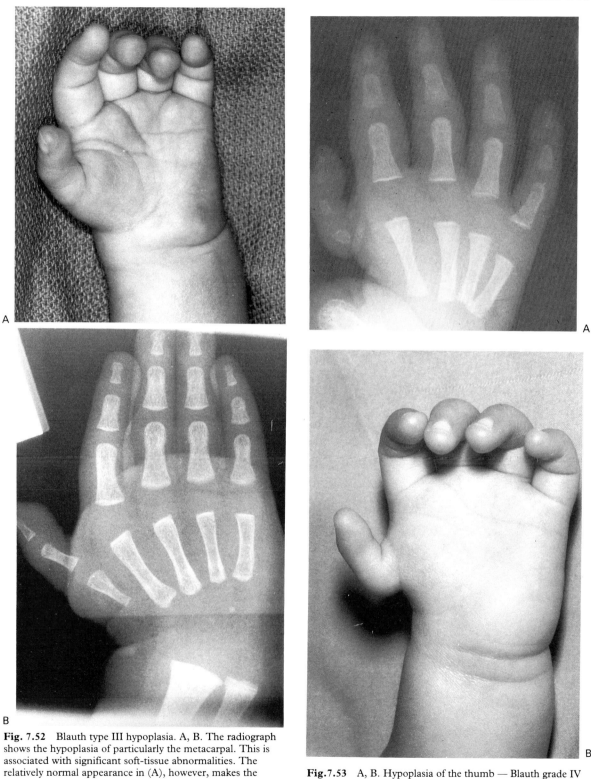

Fig. 7.52 Blauth type III hypoplasia. A, B. The radiograph shows the hypoplasia of particularly the metacarpal. This is associated with significant soft-tissue abnormalities. The relatively normal appearance in (A), however, makes the parents' reluctance to sacrifice this thumb understandable.

Fig.7.53 A, B. Hypoplasia of the thumb — Blauth grade IV 'pouce flottant'.

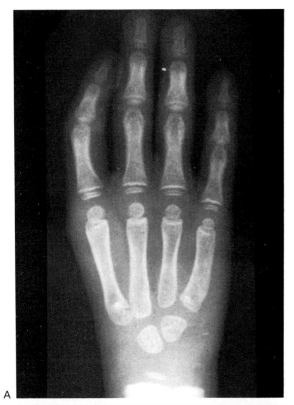

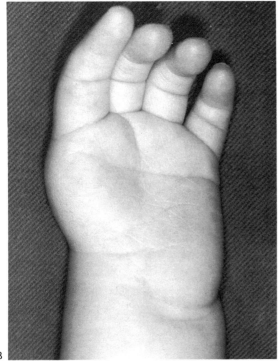

Fig. 7.54 A, B. Aplasia of the thumb — Blauth grade V.

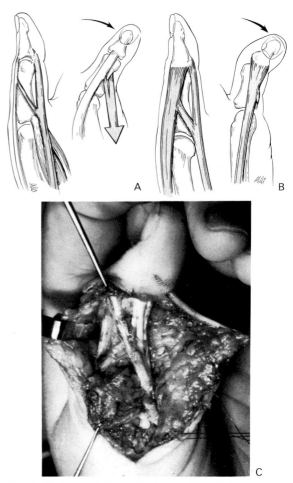

Fig. 7.55 Pollex abductus. In this condition the extensor and flexor tendons are conjoined by a band running from the flexor tendon proximally to the extensor tendon distally. Thus, action of the flexor pollicis results in radial deviation of the thumb. This may occur at the level of the metacarpal (A) or the level of the proximal phalanx (B, C). (The patient shown in (C) is that in Fig. 7.43.)

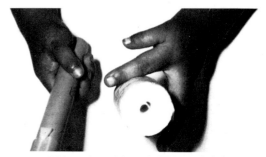

Fig. 7.56 This patient with grade III hypoplasia has undergone pollicization on the right (by Professor Dieter Buck-Gramcko) while on the left illustrates the use of the 'cigarette grip' between the index and middle fingers.

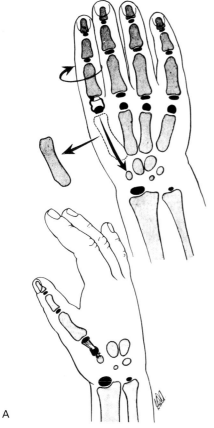

A

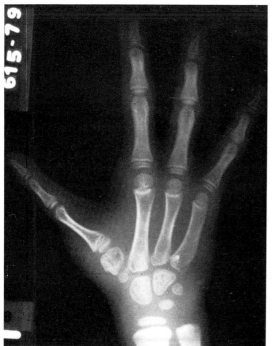

B

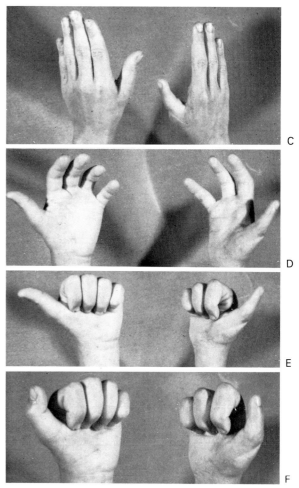

C

D

E

F

Fig. 7.57 A. The elements of skeletal adjustment involved in pollicization are shown diagrammatically. B. The skeletal appearance three years after pollicization of the index finger. C, D, E, F. The appearance and function of the hand shown in (B).

Tendon anomalies are most significant on the flexor surface. Infrequently, an anomalous attachment from flexor to extensor must be divided. Flexor pollicis longus, if absent or grossly anomalous, may require to be replaced using immediate or two stage tendon graft[180], employing either the proximal tendon or a superficialis as motor. In such circumstances, and even in some cases where the flexor is adequate, pulley reconstruction will be required at the level of the proximal phalanx, employing extensor retinaculum or fascia. The m. lumbricalis pollicis[171], if present, runs from an anomalous flexor pollicis longus to join the extensor apparatus of the index fingers (Fig. 7.58A, B). As it

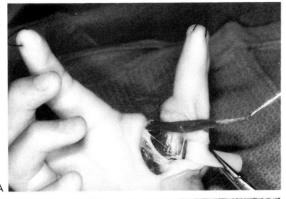

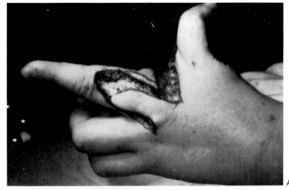

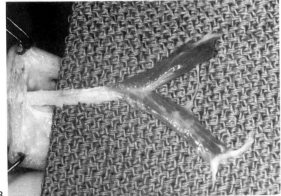

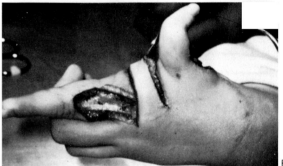

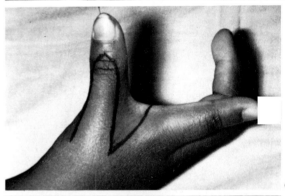

Fig. 7.58   M. lumbricalis pollicis. A. In pollex abductus associated with type II hypoplasia, the anomalous lumbrical passing from the flexor pollicis longus to the extensor of the index is shown. B. In a Blauth type III, in the course of pollicization, the entire lumbrical was excised, the normal from the index profundus and the abnormal from the flexor pollicis longus (From Lister G 1991 Musculus lumbricalis pollicis. J Hand Surg 16A: 622–625.)

narrows the first web space, the anomalous belly should be excised.

Release of the web space may be achieved with a two- or four-flap Z-plasty but frequently additional skin is required[181]. In hypoplasia associated with duplication this is available from the discarded digit. In other cases skin is obtained by sliding or transposition flaps from the index finger or the dorsum of the thumb[182] or by rotation flaps from the dorsum of the hand[183] (Fig. 7.59). Distant flaps are *never* necessary[21].

Opponensplasty can be achieved by use of the flexor digitorum superficialis[179] or the abductor digiti mini-mi[184-187]. The author prefers the former both because it is more powerful and also because, by passing it through the metacarpal, the tendon end can serve a second purpose of reconstructing the ulnar collateral ligament.

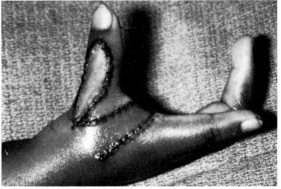

Fig. 7.59   Transposition flaps to the first web space. A B. From the dorsum of the index finger (after Brand). C, D. From the dorsum of the thumb (after Strauch).

Stabilization of the metacarpophalangeal joint is undertaken by one of three techniques (Fig. 7.60):

(i) Fusion[188], taking care to leave the epiphyseal plate undisturbed
(ii) Reconstruction using the end of a superficialis opponensplasty, as indicated above
(iii) Tendon graft attached to the vestigial ligament or through bone.

While preservation of joint motion is clearly desirable, stability of this particular joint is even more important. Where this cannot be achieved by either (ii) or (iii), it is appropriate to resort to (i).

Partial aplasia of the thumb, in which the basal structures are normal but the distal portion absent, arises not from undergrowth but from transverse absence or constriction ring amputation. It is considered with the latter.

See Green D P 1993 Operative Hand Surgery, 3rd edn. Churchill Livingstone, New York, pp. 390, 400, 2046.

Madelung's deformity[189]

This congenital disorder, inherited as an autosomal dominant trait, is due to inadequate development of the distal radial physis in its anterior, ulnar segment. It is therefore not evident at birth, usually presenting between the ages of eight and twelve. The failure of growth results in changes in the radius, ulna and carpus[190]:

radius   decreased length
          increased inclination of the articular surface, often far above the upper limit of normal 20°
ulna   dorsal subluxation
          deformity and enlargement of the ulnar head
carpus   wedge-shaped deformity to conform to the deformed radius.

The result is that the ulnar head is more prominent and the following movements are reduced: dorsiflexion and radial deviation of the wrist, and supination of the forearm. In addition to deformity and limitation of motion the patient may complain of discomfort.

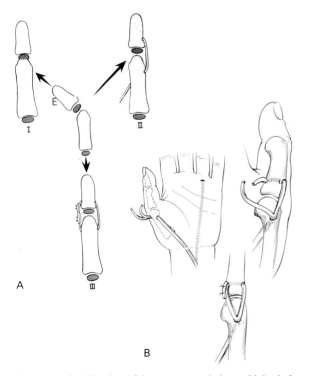

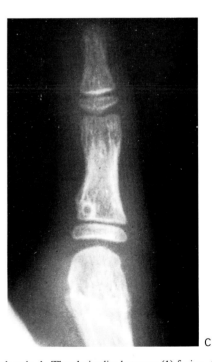

Fig. 7.60 Stabilization of the metacarpophalangeal joint in hypoplastic thumb. A. The choice lies between (1) fusion, (2) reconstruction employing the end of a superficialis opponensplasty or, (3) tendon graft. B. The superficialis opponensplasty is passed through the metacarpal to the ulnar aspect where it is used to reconstruct the collateral ligament in a relatively anatomic V-shape. C. The necessary hole through the metacarpal head and the metaphysis of the proximal phalanx can be seen in this radiograph.

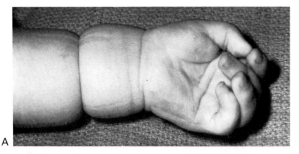

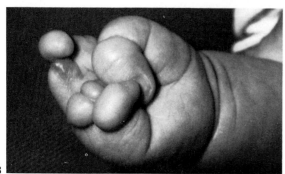

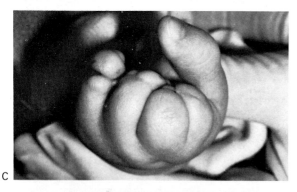

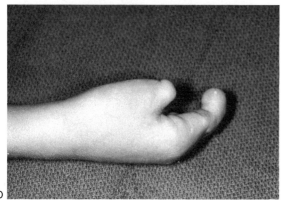

Fig. 7.61 Constriction ring syndrome. A. Simple constriction ring. B. Rings in the index, ring, and small fingers with distal deformity and lymphodema. C. Acrosyndactyly. D. Amputations.

INDICATIONS[191]

As surgery does not appear to improve the range of motion, and discomfort settles in most patients, the sole, doubtful indication for surgery is the deformity. This may be improved by ulna shortening, ulnar head excision, radial epiphyseodesis or wedge osteotomies of the radius[192].

See Green D P 1993 Operative Hand Surgery, 3rd edn. Churchill Livingstone, New York, p. 517.

CONSTRICTION RING SYNDROME

This condition occurs sporadically, there being no evidence of heredity. The debate as to cause, which commenced with Hippocrates, continues[193,194] — but not here! Patterson has classified the cases as follows[195] (Fig. 7.61):

1. Simple constriction rings
2. Rings accompanied by distal deformity, with or without lymphoedema
3. Rings accompanied by distal fusion — acrosyndactyly
4. Amputations.

Examination
This should first assess the urgency of the situation. This is usually indicated by severe distal lymphoedema. In the more severe cases even where no emergency exists, both circulation and neurological function will be impaired[196] and these should be assessed as far as possible by measuring temperature gradients, observing spontaneous movement and assessing sensation by the adherence test (p. 230). The level of amputations should be accurately determined, together with the passive and active motion present in the remaining joints. The presence or absence of intrinsic muscles, especially in the thumb, should be noted from contour, palpation and observation. *Radiologic evaluation* will assist in this determination, particular attention being paid in the thumb to the length of metacarpal remaining and the normal function of the basal joint.

Indications
Early release of constriction rings is required, in the immediate neonatal period where oedema is gross. Contrary to traditional teaching there is no hazard in multiple, circumferential Z-plasties[21] (Fig. 7.62). Amputation fortunately usually occurs in only one or two fingers and good function can be achieved with the remaining digits, which may be enhanced by ray resection

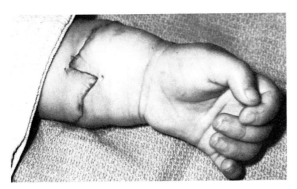

Fig. 7.62 The ring constriction shown in Fig. 7.61A was safely released by multiple Z-plasties circumferentially.

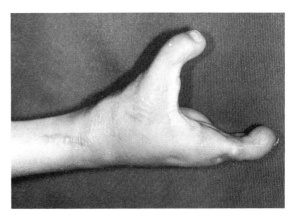

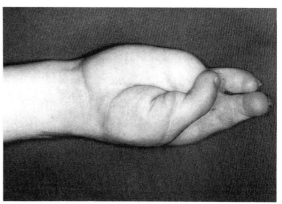

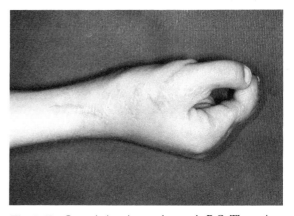

of the residual stumps. Amputation of the thumb is another matter entirely and is the major cause of *partial thumb aplasia*, the other being transverse absence.

Partial aplasia of the thumb is treated by one of the following procedures:

1. Phalangization
2. Metacarpal lengthening[197]
3. Toe-to-hand transfer[32,198] (Fig. 7.63)
4. Digital transfer.

The considerations involved in choosing the correct procedure are *existing length, intrinsic function, presence of a basal joint* and the *condition of the other digits*, some of which have been discussed under post-traumatic thumb reconstruction (p. 176). In partial aplasia, as opposed to congenital hypoplasias, the basal joint and proximal metacarpal are sound. Digital transfer in the affected hand is therefore indicated only in those patients in whom the thumb can be lengthened by transfer of another congenitally amputated digit — 'on-top plasty'. Metacarpal lengthening may be stabilized after distraction either without a bone graft[193], or with an immediate or a secondary bone graft[199]. Second toe-to-hand transfer is often beneficial and relatively straightforward when compared to transfer for other congenital differences, for in constriction ring syndrome the anatomy proximal to the amputation is entirely normal.

See Green D P 1993 Operative Hand Surgery, 3rd edn. Churchill Livingstone, New York, p. 511.

Fig. 7.63 Constriction ring syndrome. A, B C. The patient seen in Fig. 7.61D has been reconstructed by second-toe-to-thumb transfer, improving the span of grasp and providing satisfactory, rudimentary tip-to-tip contact.

TIMING OF SURGERY[21]

Some congenital differences require urgent attention, such as the constriction ring which is causing severe lymphoedema. Some should be treated early although not urgently:

1. Complex syndactyly
2. Syndactyly between digits of differing length
3. Acrosyndactyly
4. Delta phalanges
5. Radial club hand.

Others, like trigger thumb and minor clinodactyly, should be left for they may never require surgical correction. But what of the other, major, proportion of congenital differences of the hand? The immunologists advise us to do urgent surgery in the first five weeks while the child retains decreasing amounts of passive immunity derived from the mother, and to delay other procedures until after five months so that active immune mechanisms are sufficiently mature. The child psychologists tell us not to separate mother and child between the second and fifth birthdays, since the infant is fully aware of the trauma of separation but cannot understand its reason or its finite duration.

What are the disadvantages of early surgery? Firstly, the child of that age cannot co-operate in any rehabilitative programme. However, to wait for that co-operation would mean no surgery until age ten or twelve and, in any event, the lack of co-operation is far outweighed by the enviable healing properties of infancy. Secondly, the anatomy of the hand is very small and delicate at that early age, and the risk of damage must be greater than at a more mature juncture. Here lies a challenge to the surgeon — not the obvious challenge of delicate technique, but the hidden, unrecognized and therefore more potent challenge of self-evaluation. Injuries must be dealt with to the best of our ability for they are emergencies; reconstruction after injury is so influenced by tissue damage as to defy assessment; rheumatoid disease imposes its own influences on our results; release of compression syndromes demands diagnostic and anatomical knowledge more than surgical skill; only in the correction of congenital differences do we hand surgeons see so clearly the distinction between the craftsman and the novice. And so each must examine his training, his experience and his inclinations. There is honour, not shame, in delaying surgery or in referring infants after such honest scrutiny. Where, however, the surgeon is competent, the advantages of early surgery aided by magnification heavily outweigh any disadvantages. The results in the child's function and in the parents' contentment attest to this fact.

REFERENCES

1. Swanson A B 1976 A classification for congenital limb malformation. J Hand Surg 1: 8–22
2. Flatt A E 1977 The care of congenital hand anomalies. C V Mosby, St Louis
3. Goldberg M J, Bartoshesky L E 1985 Congenital hand anomaly: etiology and associated malformations. Hand Clin 1: 405–415
4. Miura T 1981 Congenital hand anomalies, and their association with other congenital abnormalities. Hand 13: 267–270
5. Garn S M, Rohmann C G, Silverman F N 1967 Radiographic standards for postnatal ossification and tooth calcification. Med Radiogr Photogr 43: 45–66
6. Poznanski A K 1974 The hand in radiologic diagnosis. W B Saunders, Philadelphia
7. Lamb D W, Kuczynski K 1981 The practice of hand surgery. Blackwell, Edinburgh
8. MacDonell J A 1968 Age of fitting upper extremity prostheses in children. J Bone Joint Surg 40A: 655–662
9. Swanson A B 1968 Restoration of hand function by the use of partial or total prosthetic replacement. J Bone Joint Surg 45A: 276–283
10. Seitz W H Jr 1989 Distraction osteogenesis of a congenital amputation at the elbow. J Hand Surg (Am) 14: 945–948
11. Nathan P A, Trung N B 1977 The Krukenberg operation: A modified technique avoiding skin grafts. J Hand Surg 2: 127
12. Swanson A B, Swanson G D, Tada K 1983 A classification for congenital limb malformation. J Hand Surg (Am) 8: 693-702
13. Chan K M, Ma G F, Cheng J C, Leung P C 1984 The Krukenberg procedure: a method of treatment for unilateral anomalies of the upper limb in Chinese children. J Hand Surg (Am) 9: 548–551
14. Miura T, Torii S, Nakamura R 1986 Brachymetacarpia and brachyphalangia. J Hand Surg (Am) 11: 829–836
15. Miura T 1988 Congenital absence of the fourth metacarpal bone (congenital dysplasia of the ring finger). J Hand Surg (Am) 13: 93–96
16. Cohn B T, Shall L 1986 Idiopathic bilaterally symmetrical brachymetacarpia of the fourth and fifth metacarpals. J Hand Surg (Am) 11: 735–737
17. Cowen N J, Loftus J M 1978 Distraction augmentation manoplasty technique for lengthening digits of hands. Orthopaedic Rev 7: 45–53
18. Carroll R E, Green D P 1975 Reconstruction of the hypoplastic digits. J Bone Joint Surg 57A: 727
19. Goldberg N H, Watson H K 1982 Composite toe (phalanx and epiphysis) transfers in the reconstruction of the aphalangic hand. J Hand Surg 7: 454–459
20. Rank B K 1978 Long-term results in epiphyseal transplants in congenital deformities of the hand. Plastic Reconstr Surg 61: 321–329
21. Buck-Gramcko D 1988 Congenital malformations. In: Nigst H, Buck-Gramcko D, Millesi H, Lister G (eds) Hand surgery. Georg Thieme, Stuttgart
22. Manktelow R T, Wainwright D J 1984 A technique of distraction osteosynthesis in the hand. J Hand Surg (Am) 9: 858–862
23. Baruch A D, Hecht O A 1983 Treatment of monodactyly by the distraction–lengthening principle: a case report. J Hand Surg (Am) 8: 604–606
24. Dobyns J H 1985 Segmental digital transposition in congenital hand deformities. Hand Clin 1: 475–482
25. Smith R J, Gumley G J 1985 Metacarpal distraction lengthening. Hand Clin 1: 417–429
26. Fultz C W, Lester D K, Hunter J M 1986 Single stage lengthening by intercalary bone graft in patients with congenital hand deformities. J Hand (Br) 11:40–46

27. Reid D A C 1980 The Gillies thumb lengthening operation. Hand 12: 123–129
28. Gilbert A 1985 Reconstruction of congenital hand defects with microvascular toe transfers. Hand Clin 1: 351–360
29. Lister G 1988 Microsurgical transfer of the second toe for congenital deficiency of the thumb. Plastic Reconstr Surg 82: 658–665
30. Gilbert A 1989 Congenital absence of the thumb and digits. J Hand Surg (Br) 14: 6–17
31. Gilbert A 1982 Toe transfers for congenital hand defects. J Hand Surg 7: 118–124
32. Frantz C H, O'Rahilly R 1961 Congenital skeletal limb deficiencies. J Bone Joint Surg 43: 1202
33. Lamb D W 1983 Upper limb dysplasia, form and function. J Roy Coll Surg Edinb 28: 203–213
34. Lamb D W 1977 Radial club hand. A continuing study of sixty-eight patients with one hundred and seventeen club hands. J Bone Joint Surg 59A: 1–13
35. Kelikian H, Doumanian A 1957 Congenital anomalies of the hand. Part I. J Bone Joint Surg 39A: 1002–1019
36. Bayne L G, Lovell W W, Marks T W 1970 The radial club hand (abstract). J Bone Joint Surg 52A: 1065
37. Skerik S K, Flatt A E 1969 The anatomy of congenital radial dysplasia. Clin Orthopaedics 66: 125–143
38. Menelaus M B 1976 Radial club hand with absence of the biceps muscle treated by centralisation of the ulna and triceps transfer. J Bone Joint Surg 58B: 488–491
39. Silverman M E, Copeland A J Jr, Hurst J W 1970 The Holt–Oram syndrome: the long and the short of it. Am J Cardiol 25: 11–17
40. Fanconi G 1967 Familial constitutional panmyelocytopathy, Fanconi's anemia (FA). I. Clin Asp Semin Hematol 4: 233
41. Auerbach A D, Rogatko A, Schroeder-Kurth T M 1989 International Fanconi Anemia Registry: relation of clinical symptoms to diepoxybutane sensitivity. Blood 73: 391–396
42. Auerbach A D, Liu Q, Ghosh M S, Pollack G W, Douglas G W, Broxmeyer H E 1990 Prenatal identification of potential donors for umbilical cord blood transplantation for Fanconi anemia. Transfusion 30: 682–687
43. Buck-Gramcko D 1985 Radialization as a new treatment for radial club hand. Surg (Am) 10: 964–968
44. Riordan D C 1955, 1963 Congenital absence of the radius. J Bone Joint Surg 37A: 1129–1140, 45A: 1783
45. Bora F W, Nicholson J T, Cheema H M 1970 Radial meromelia. J Bone Joint Surg 52A: 966–979
46. Bora F W, Osterman A L, Kaneda R R, Esterhal J 1981 Radial club-hand deformity. J Bone Joint Surg 63A: 741–745
47. Bayne L G, Klug M S 1987 Long-term review of the surgical treatment of radial deficiencies. J Hand Surg (Am) 12: 169–179
48. Nuts J N, Flatt A E 1981 Congenital central hand deficit. J Hand Surg 6: 48–60
49. Barsky A J 1964 Cleft hand: classification, incidence and treatment. J Bone Joint Surg 46A: 1701–1720
50. Sandzen S C Jr 1985 Classification and functional management of congenital central defect of the hand Hand Clin 1: 483–498
51. Buck-Gramcko D 1985 Cleft hands: classification and treatment. Hand Clin 1: 467–473
52. Muller W 1937 Die angeborenen Fehlbildungen der menschlichen Hand. Thieme, Leipzig
53. Jaworska M, Popiolek 1968 Genetic counselling in lobster-claw anomaly: discussion of variability of genetic influence in different families. Clin Pediatr 7: 396-399
54. Kato S, Ishii S, Ogino T, Shiono H 1983 Anomalous hands with cleft formation between the fourth and fifth digits. J Hand Surg (Am) 8: 909–913
55. Miura T 1988 Cleft hand involving only the ring and small fingers. J Hand Surg (Am) 13: 530–535
56. Maisels D O 1970 Lobster-claw deformities of the hands and feet. Br J Plastic Surg 23: 269–282
57. Snow J W, Littler J W 1969 Surgical treatment of cleft hand. Transactions of the Fourth International Congress of Plastic and Reconstructive Surgery 888–893. Excerpta Medica Foundation, Amsterdam
58. Miura T, Komada T 1979 Simple method for reconstruction of the cleft hand with an adducted thumb. Plastic Reconstr Surg 64: 65–67
59. Ogden J A, Watson H K, Bohne W 1976 Ulnar dysmelia. J Bone Joint Surg 58A: 467–475
60. Kummel W 1895 Die Missbildungen der Extremitaten durch defeckt. Verwachsung and Uberzahl. Hefte 3. Bibliotheca Medica, Kassel
61. Riordan D C 1978 Congenital absence of the ulna. In: Lovell W W, Winter R B (eds) Pediatric orthopedics. J B Lippincott, Philadelphia, pp 714–719
62. Swanson A B, Tada K, Yonenobu K 1984 Ulnar ray deficiency: its various manifestations. J Hand Surg (Am) 9: 658–664
63. Johnson J, Omer G E Jr 1985 Congenital ulnar deficiency. Natural history and therapeutic implications. Hand Clin 1: 499–510
64. Miller J K, Wenner S M, Kruger L M 1986 Ulnar deficiency. J Hand Surg (Am) 11: 822–829
65. Khuri S M, Ger E 1979 The ulnar clubhand — congenital ulnar deficiency. Ortho Rev 8: 149–153
66. Broudy A S, Smith R J 1979 Deformities of the hand and wrist with ulnar deficiency. J Hand Surg 4: 304–315
67. Bauer M, Jonsson K 1988 Congenital radioulnar synostosis. Radiological characteristics and hand function: case reports. Scand J Plastic Reconstr Hand Surg 22: 251–255
68. Cleary J E, Omer G E Jr 1985 Congenital proximal radio-ulnar synostosis. Natural history and functional assessment. J Bone Joint Surg (Am) 67: 539–545
69. Simmons B P, Southmayd W W, Riseborough E J 1983 Congenital radioulnar synostosis. J Hand Surg (Am) 8: 829–838
70. Miura T, Nakamura R, Suzuki M, Kanie J 1984 Congenital radio-ulnar synostosis. J Hand Surg (Br) 9: 153–155
71. Green W T, Mital M 1979 Congenital radio-ulnar synostosis: surgical treatment. J Bone Joint Surg 61A: 738–748
72. Flatt A E, Wood V E 1975 Rigid digits or symphalangism. Hand 7: 197–214
73. Cushing H 1916 Hereditary anchylosis of proximal phalangeal joints (symphalangism). Genetics 1: 90–106
74. Gaal A S, Doyle J R, Larsen I J 1988 Symphalangism in Hawaii: a study of three distinct ethnic pedigrees. J Hand Surg (Am) 13: 783–787

75. Smith R J, Kaplan E B 1968 Camptodactyly and similar atraumatic flexion deformities of the PIP joints of the fingers. A study of 31 cases. J Bone Joint Surg 50A: 1187–1203
76. Engber W D, Flatt A E 1977 Camptodactyly: an analysis of sixty-six patients and twenty-four operations. J Hand Surg 2: 216–224
77. McFarlane R M, Curry G I, Evans H B 1983 Anomalies of the intrinsic muscles in camptodactyly. J Hand Surg (Am) 8: 531–544
78. Maeda M, Matsue T 1985 Camptodactyly caused by an abnormal lumbrical muscle. J Hand Surg 10B: 95–96
79. Hori M, Nakamura R, Inoue G, Imamura T et al 1987 Nonoperative treatment of camptodactyly. J Hand Surg (Am) 12: 1061–1065
80. Siegert J J, Cooney W P, Dobyns J H 1990 Management of simple camptodactyly. J Hand Surg (Br) 15: 181–189
81. Gupta A, Burke F D 1990 Correction of camptodactyly. Preliminary results of extensor indicis transfer. J Hand Surg (Br) 15: 168–170
82. Burke F, Flatt A 1979 Clinodactyly — a review of a series of cases. Hand 11: 269–280
83. Watson H K, Boyes J H 1967 Congenital angular deformity of the digits — delta phalanx. J Bone Joint Surg 49A: 333–338
84. Wood V E, Flatt A E 1977 Congenital triangular bones in the hand. J Hand Surg 2: 179–193
85. Theander G, Carstam N 1974 Longitudinally bracketed diaphysis. Ann Radiologie 17: 355–360
86. Kirner J 1927 Doppelseitige Verkrummung des Kleinfingergrundgliedes als selbstandiges Krankheitsbild. Fortschr Rontgenstr 36: 804–806
87. Poznanski A K, Pratt G B, Manson G, Weiss L 1969 Clinodactyly, camptodactyly, Kirner's deformity, and other crooked fingers. Radiology 93: 573–582
88. Notta A 1850 Recherches sur une affection particulière des gaines tendineuses de la main, caracterisee par le developpement d'une nodosité sur le trajet des tendons flechisseurs des doigts et par l'empêchement de leurs movements. Arch Gen Med 24: 142–161
89. Dinham J M, Meggitt D F 1974 Trigger thumbs in children. J Bone Joint Surg 56B: 153
90. Weckesser E C, Reed J R, Heiple K G 1968 Congenital clasped thumb (congenital flexion-adduction deformity of the thumb). J Bone Joint Surg 37A: 1417–1428
91. McCarroll H R Jr 1985 Congenital flexion deformities of the thumb. Hand Clin 1: 567–575
92. Boix E 1984 Deviation des doigts en coup de vent et insuffisance de l'opone' vrose paliciaire d'origine congenitale. Nouv Inconogr Salpet 10: 180–194
93. Zancolli E, Zancolli E Jr 1985 Congenital ulnar drift of the fingers. Pathogenesis, classification, and surgical management. Hand Clin 1:443–456
94. Burian F 1963 The whistling face characteristic in a compound cranio-facio-corporal syndrome. Br J Plast Surg 16: 140
95. Freeman E A, Sheldon J H 1938 Craniocarpotarsal dystrophy. Undescribed congenital malformations. Arch Dis Child 13: 277.
96. Tsuyuguchi Y, Masada K, Kawabata H, Kawai H, Ono K 1985 Congenital clasped thumb: a review of forty-three cases. J Hand Surg (Am) 10: 613–618
97. Wood V E, Boindi J 1990 Treatment of the windblown hand. J Hand Surg (Am) 15: 431–438
98. Banker B Q 1985 Neuropathologic aspects of arthrogryposis multiplex congenita. Clin Orthop Rel Res 194: 30–43
99. Weeks P M 1965 Surgical correction of upper extremity deformities in arthrogrypotics. Plastic Reconstr Surg 36: 459–465
100. Smith R J, Lipke R W 1979 Treatment of congenital deformities of the hand and forearm. N Engl J Med 300: 402–407
101. Wenner S M, Saperia B S 1987 Proximal row carpectomy in arthrogrypotic wrist deformity. J Hand Surg (Am) 12: 523–525
102. Lloyd-Roberts G C, Lettin A W F 1970 Arthrogryposis multiplex congenita. J Bone Joint Surg 52B: 494–508
103. Carroll R E, Hill N A 1970 Triceps transfer to restore elbow flexion. The study of fifteen patients with paralytic lesions and arthrogryposis. J Bone Joint Surg 52A: 239–244
104. Entin M A 1976 Syndactyly of upper limb. Clin Plastic Surg 3: 129–140
105. Maisels D O 1962 Acrosyndactyly. Br J Plastic Surg 15: 166–172
106. Mantero R, Rossello M I, Grandis C 1989 Digital subtraction angiography in preoperative examination of congenital hand malformation. J Hand Surg (Am) 2: 351–352
107. Hadidi A T, Kaddah N T, Zaki M S, Sami A, Aal N A 1990 Congenital malformations of the hand. A study of the vascular pattern. J Hand Surg (Br)15: 171–180
108. Walsh R J 1970 Acrosyndactyly: a study of 27 patients. Clin Orthopaedics 71: 99–111
109. Ravitch M M 1977 Poland's syndrome — a study of an eponym. Plastic Reconstr Surg 59: 508–512
110. Sugiura Y 1976 'Poland's syndrome'. Clinicoroentgenographic study on 45 cases. Cong Anom 16: 17–28
111. Ireland D C R, Takayama N, Flatt A E 1976 Poland's syndrome. A review of forty-three cases. J Bone Joint Surg 58A: 52–58
112. Epstein L I, Bennett J E 1970 Syndactyly with ipsilateral chest deformity. Plastic Reconstr Surg 46: 236–240
113. Senrui H, Egawa T, Horiki A 1982 Anatomical findings in the hands of patients with Poland's syndrome. J Bone Joint Surg (Am) 64: 1079–1082
114. Wilson M R, Louis D S, Stevenson T R 1988 Poland's syndrome: variable expression and associated anomalies. J Hand Surg (Am) 13: 880–882
115. Wood V E, Sandlin C 1983 The hand in the Pierre Robin syndrome. J Hand Surg (Am) 8: 273–276
116. Hoover G H, Flatt A E, Weiss M W 1970 The hand in Apert's syndrome. J Bone Joint Surg 52A: 878–895
117. Upton J, Zuker R M 1991 Apert syndrome. Clin Plastic Surg 18: 217–235
118. Barot L R, Caplan H S 1986 Early surgical intervention in Apert's syndactyly. Plastic Reconstr Surg 77: 282–287
119. Johannson S H 1982 Nagelwallhildung durch Thenarlappen bei Kompletter Syndaktylie. Handchirurgie 14: 199–203
120. Simmons B P 1985 Polydactyly. Hand Clin 1: 545–565
121. Nicolai J P, Schoch S L 1986 Polydactyly in the bible. J Hand Surg 11: 293

122. Cheng J C, Chan K M, Ma G F, Leung P C 1984 Polydactyly of the thumb: a surgical plan based on ninety-five cases. J Hand Surg (Am) 9: 155–164

123. Miura T, Nakamura R, Imamura T 1987 Polydactyly of the hands and feet. J Hand Surg (Am) 12: 474–476

124. Gropper P T 1983 Ulnar dimelia. J Hand Surg (Am) 8: 487–491

125. Barton N J, Buck-Gramcko D, Evans D M, Kleinert H et al 1986 Mirror hand treated by true pollicization. J Hand Surg (Br) 11: 320–336

126. Barton N J, Buck-Gramcko D, Evans D M 1986 Soft-tissue anatomy of mirror hand. J Hand Surg (Br) 11: 307–319

127. Stelling F 1963 The upper extremity. In: Ferguson A B (ed) Orthopaedic surgery in infancy and childhood, vol 2. Williams & Wilkins, Baltimore, pp 304–308

128. Kitayama Y, Tsukada S, Ishikura N, Ide Y, Kojima M 1985 Rudimentary polydactyly: report of five cases. J Hand Surg (Am) 10: 382–385

129. Wassel H D 1969 The results of surgery for polydactyly of the thumb. Clin Orthopaedics 64: 175–193

130. Kitayama Y, Tsukada S 1983 Patterns of arterial distribution in the duplicated thumb. Plastic Reconstr Surg 72: 535–542

131. Marks T W, Bayne L G 1978 Polydactyly of the thumb: abnormal anatomy and treatment. J Hand Surg 3: 107–116

132. Bilhaut M 1890 Guerison d'un pouce bifide par un nouveau procede operatoire. Congr Fr Chir 4: 576

133. Hartrampf C R, Vasconez L O, Mathes S 1975 Construction of one good thumb from both parts of a congenitally bifid thumb. Plastic Reconstr Surg 54: 148–152

134. Miura T 1977 An appropriate treatment for post-operative Z-formed deformity of the duplicated thumb. J Hand Surg 2: 380–386

135. Tada K, Yonenobu K , Tsuyuguchi Y, Kawai H, Egawa T 1983 Duplication of the thumb. A retrospective review of two hundred and thirty-seven cases. J Bone Joint Surg (Am) 65: 584–598

136. Manske P R 1989 Treatment of duplicated thumb using a ligamentous/periosteal flap. J Hand Surg (Am) 14: 728–733

137. Miura T 1976 Triphalangeal thumb. Plastic Reconstr Surg 58: 587–594

138. Wood V 1978 Polydactyly and the triphalangeal thumb. J Hand Surg 3: 436–444

139. Lamb D W, Wynne-Davies R, Whitmore J M 1983 Five-fingered hand associated with partial or complete tibial absence and pre-axial polydactyly. A kindred of 15 affected individuals in five generations. J Bone Joint Surg (Br) 65: 60–63

140. Wood V E 1976 Treatment of the triphalangeal thumb. Clin Orthop 120: 188–200

141. Peimer C A 1985 Combined reduction osteotomy for triphalangeal thumb. J Hand Surg (Am) 10: 376–381

142. Wood V E 1971 Treatment of central polydactyly. Clin Orthopaedics 74: 196–205

143. Wood V E 1988 Different manifestations of hyperphalangism. J Hand Surg (Am) 13: 883–887

144. Klug M S, Ketchum L D, Lipsey J H 1983 Symmetric hyperphalangism of the index finger in the palatodigital syndrome: a case report. J Hand Surg (Am) 8: 599–603

145. Dell P C 1985 Macrodactyly. Hand Clin 1: 511–524

146. Frykman G, Wood V 1978 Peripheral nerve hamartoma with macrodactyly in the hand: report of three cases and review of the literature. J Hand Surg 3: 307–312

147. Pho R W, Patterson M, Lee Y S 1988 Reconstruction and pathology in macrodactyly. J Hand Surg (Am) 13: 78–83

148. Edgerton M T, Tuerk D B I 1974 Macrodactyly (digital gigantism): its nature and treatment. In: Littler J W, Cramer L M, Smith J W (eds) Symposium on reconstructive hand surgery. C V Mosby Co, St Louis, pp 157–172

149. Barsky A 1967 Macrodactyly. J Bone Joint Surg 49A: 1255–1266

150. Schuind F, Merle M, Dap F, Bour C, Michon J 1988 Hyperostotic macrodactyly. J Hand Surg (Am) 13: 544–548

151. Allende B T 1967 Macrodactyly with enlarged median nerve associated with carpal tunnel syndrome. Plastic Reconstr Surg 39: 578–582

152. Rousso M, Katz S, Khodadadi D 1976 Treatment of a case of macrodactyly of the thumb. Hand 8: 131–133

153. Tsuge K 1967 Treatment of macrodactyly. Plastic Reconstr Surg 39: 590–599

154. Tsuge K 1985 Treatment of macrodactyly. J Hand Surg (Am) 10: 968–969

155. Blauth W 1967 Der hypoplastische Daumen. Arch Orthop Unfall Chir 62: 225–246

156. Fromont M J 1895 Anomalies musculaires multiples de la main. Absence du flechisseur propre du pouce. Absence des muscles de l'eminence thenar; lombricaux supplementaires. Bull Soc Anat Paris 70: 395–401

157. Neviaser R 1979 Congenital hypoplasia of the thumb with absence of the extrinsic extensors, abductor pollicis longus and thenar muscles. J Hand Surg 4: 301–304

158. Edgerton M T, Snyder C B, Webb W L 1965 Surgical treatment of congenital thumb deformities. J Bone Joint Surg 47A: 1453–1474

159. Tajima T 1985 Classification of thumb hypoplasia. Hand Clin 1: 577–594

160. Miura T 1977 Congenital absence of the flexor pollicis longus. Hand 9: 272–274

161. Tsuchida Y, Kasai S, Kojima T 1976 Congenital absence of flexor pollicis longus and flexor pollicis brevis: a case report. Hand 8: 294–297

162. Usami F 1987 Bilateral congenital absence of the flexor pollicis longus with craniofacial abnormalities. J Hand Surg (Am) 12: 603–604

163. DeHaan M R, Wong L B, Petersen D P 1987 Congenital anomaly of the thumb: aplasia of the flexor pollicis longus. J Hand Surg (Am) 12: 108–109

164. Tupper J W 1969 Pollex abductus due to congenital malposition of the flexor pollicis longus. J Bone Joint Surg 51A: 1285–1290

165. Blair W F, Buckwalter J A 1983 Congenital malposition of flexor pollicis longus — an anatomy note. J Hand Surg (Am) 8: 93–94

166. Fitch R D, Urbaniak J R, Ruderman R 1984 Conjoined flexor and extensor pollicis longus tendons in the hypoplastic thumb. J Hand Surg (Am) 9: 417–419

167. Lister G 1991 Pollex abductus in the hypoplastic and duplicated thumb. J Hand Surg 16A: 626–633

168. Kobayashi A, Ohmiya K, Iwakuma T, Mitsuyasu M 1976 Unusual congenital anomalies of the thumb extensors. Hand 8: 17–21

169. Dellon A L, Rayan G 1981 Congenital absence of the thenar muscles. Report of two cases. J Bone Joint Surg (Am) 63: 1014–1015

170. McCarrol H R Jr, Manske P R 1982 Congenital absence of the thenar muscles (letter). J Bone Joint Surg (Am) 64: 153

171. Lister G 1991 Musculus lumbricalis pollicis. J Hand Surg 16A: 622–625

172. Rayan G M 1984 Congenital hypoplastic thumb with absent thenar muscles: anomalous digital neurovascular bundle. J Hand Surg (Am) 9: 665–668

173. Buck-Gramcko D 1971 Pollicisation of the index finger. J Bone Joint Surg 53A: 1605–1617

174. Buck-Gramcko D 1977 Thumb reconstruction by digital transposition. Orthopaedic Clin North Am 8: 329–342

175. Egleff D V, Verdan C 1983 Pollicization of the index finger for reconstruction of the congenitally hypoplastic or absent thumb. J Hand Surg (Am) 8: 839–848

176. Manske P R, McCaroll H R Jr 1985 Index finger pollicization for a congenitally absent or nonfunctioning thumb. J Hand Surg (Am) 10: 606–613

177. Blair W F, Omer G E 1981 Anomalous insertion of the flexor pollicis longus. J Hand Surg 6: 241–244

178. Strauch B, Spinner M 1976 Congenital anomaly of the thumb: absent intrinsics and flexor pollicis longus. J Bone Joint Surg 58A: 115–118

179. Su C T, Hoopes J E, Daniel R 1972 Congenital absence of the thenar muscles innervated by the median nerve. J Bone Joint Surg 54A: 1087–1090

180. Arminio J A 1979 Congenital anomaly of the thumb: absent flexor pollicis longus tendon. J Hand Surg 4: 487–488

181. Lister G D, Milward T M 1976 Skin contracture of the first web space. Transactions Sixth International Congress of Plastic and Reconstructive Surgery, Masson, Paris, pp 594–604

182. Strauch B 1975 Dorsal thumb flap for release of adduction contracture of the first web space. Bull Hos Joint Dis 36: 34–39

183. Flatt A E, Wood V 1970 Multiple dorsal rotation flaps from the hand for thumb web contractures. Plastic Reconstr Surg 45: 258–262

184. Huber E 1921 Hilssoperation bei medianuslahmung. Deutsche Zeitschrift fur Chirurgie 162: 271–275

185. Littler J W, Cooley S G E 1963 Opposition of the thumb and its restoration by abductor digiti quinti transfer. J Bone Joint Surg 45A: 1389–1396

186. Manske P, McCarroll H 1978 Abductor digiti minimi opponensplasty in congenital radial dysplasia. J Hand Surg 3: 552–559

187. Dunlap J, Manske P R, McCarthy J A 1989 Perfusion of the abductor digiti quinti after transfer on a neurovascular pedicle. J Hand Surg (Am) 14: 992–995

188. Kowalski M F, Manske P R 1988 Arthrodesis of digital joints in children. J Hand Surg (Am) 13: 874–879

189. Madelung V 1975 Die spontane subluxation der hand nach norne Verh Dtsch Ges Chir 7: 259, 1878. Arch Klin Chir 23: 395

190. Ranawat C S, DeFiore J, Straub L R 1975 Madelung's deformity: an end-result study of surgical treatment. J Bone Joint Surg 57A: 772

191. Nielsen J B 1977 Madelung's deformity: a follow-up study of 26 cases and a review of the literature. Acta Orthopaedica Scand 48: 379–384

192. White G M, Weiland A J 1987 Madelung's deformity: treatment by osteotomy of the radius and Lauenstein procedure. J Hand Surg (Am) 12: 202–204

193. Field J H, Krag D O 1973 Congenital constricting bands and congenital amputation of the fingers: placental studies. J Bone Joint Surg 55A: 1035–1041

194. Yoshitake K 1975 Clinical and experimental studies of the congenital constriction band syndrome, with an emphasis on its etiology. J Bone Joint Surg 57A: 636–642

195. Patterson T J S 1961 Congenital ring-constrictions. Br J Plastic Surg 14: 1–31

196. Moses J M, Flatt A E, Cooper R R 1979 Annular constricting bands. J Bone Joint Surg 61A: 562–565

197. Matev J 1979 Thumb reconstruction in children through metacarpal lengthening. Plastic Reconstr Surg 64: 665–669

198. Yoshimura M 1980 Toe-to-hand transfer. Plastic Reconstr Surg 66: 74–83

199. Kessler I, Baruch A, Hecht O 1977 Experience with distraction lengthening of digital rays in congenital anomalies. J Hand Surg 2: 394–401

Appendix: Muscle testing

Figure No.	Muscle	Abbreviation	Action	Nerve	Cord	Root
A.1(a)	Supraspinatus	SS	External rotation of arm fixes shoulder in carrying	Suprascapular (from upper trunk)	—	C5 (6)
A.1(b)	Infraspinatus	IS	External rotation of arm	Suprascapular	—	C5 (6)
A.1(c)	Teres major	TMa	Internal rotation of arm adduction, extension	Lower subscapular	Posterior	C6 (7)

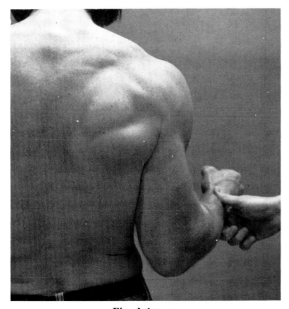
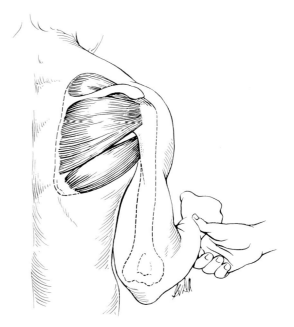

Fig. A.1 a–c

Figure No.	Muscle	Abbreviation	Action	Nerve	Cord	Root
A.2	Pectoralis major	PM	Internal rotation of arm	Lateral pectoral Medial pectoral	Lateral Medial	C5 6 C7 8
A.3	Latissimus dorsi	LD	Adduction of arm	Thoracodorsal	Posterior	C6 7 8
A.4	Deltoid	D	Abduction of arm	Axillary	Posterior	C5 (6)
A.5	Serratus anterior (seen under LD)	SA	Forward rotation of scapula (absence produces 'winging')	Arises directly from roots	—	C5 6 7

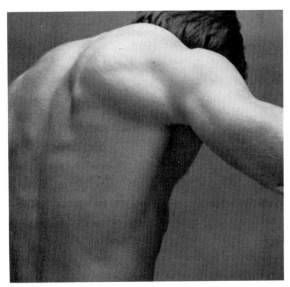
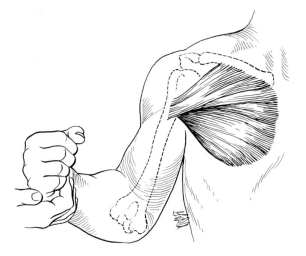

Fig. A.2

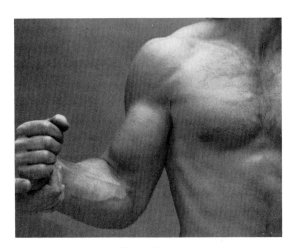
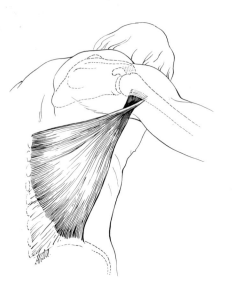

Fig. A.3

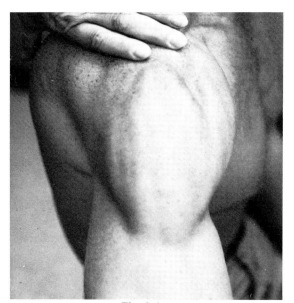
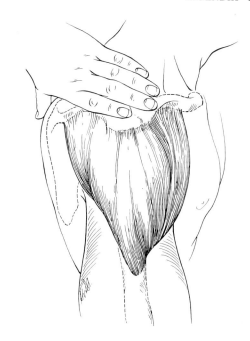

Fig. A.4

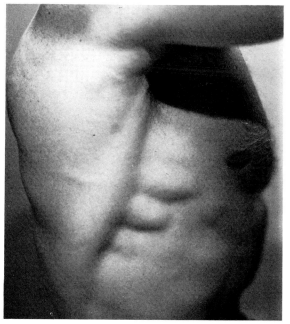
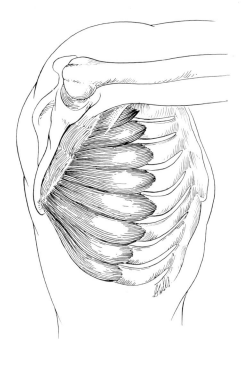

Fig. A.5

Figure No.	Muscle	Abbreviation	Action	Nerve	Cord	Root
A.6	Biceps	BB	Flexion of elbow supination of forearm (flexed)	Musculocutaneous	Lateral	C5 (6)
A.7	Triceps	T	Extension of elbow	Radial	Posterior	C(6) 7
A.8	Brachioradialis	BR	Flexion of elbow	Radial	Posterior	C6
A.9	Pronator teres	PT	Pronation of forearm (extended)	Median	Lateral	C6 7
A.10	Pronator quadratus	PQ	Pronation of forearm (flexed)	Ant. interosseous (median)	Lateral	C7
A.11	Supinator	S	Supination of forearm (extended)	Post. interosseous (radial)	Posterior	C6
A.12	Flexor carpi radialis	FCR	Flexion of wrist	Median	Lateral	C6 7

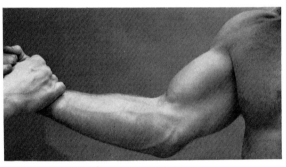
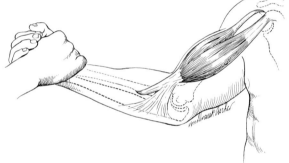

Fig. A.6

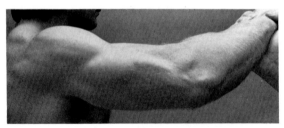
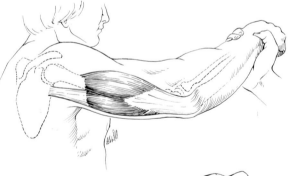

Fig. A.7

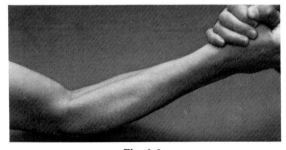
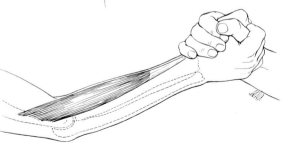

Fig. A.8

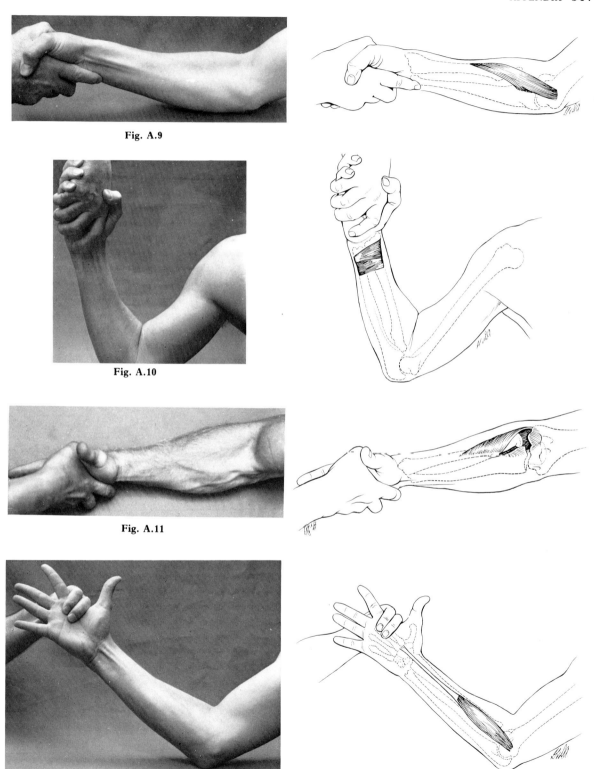

Fig. A.9

Fig. A.10

Fig. A.11

Fig. A.12

Figure No.	Muscle	Abbreviation	Action	Nerve	Cord	Root
A.13	Flexor carpi ulnaris	FCU	Flexion of wrist Ulnar deviation of wrist	Ulnar	Medial	C8
A.14	Palmaris longus	PL	—	Median	Medial	C8
A.15(a)	Flexor digitorum superficialis	FDS	Flexion of PIP joints	Median	Medial	C7 8
A.15(b)	Flexor digitorum superficialis (index)					
A.16	Flexor digitorum profundus	FDP	Flexion of DIP joints	Anterior interosseous (index and middle)	Medial	C8
				Ulnar (ring and small)	Medial	C8
A.17	Flexor pollicis longus	FPL	Flexion of thumb IP joint	Ant. interosseous	Medial	C8

(see page 35 for explanation of A.15, a and b)

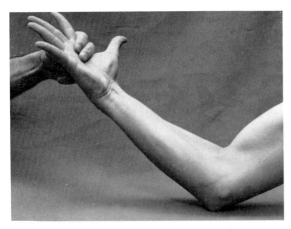
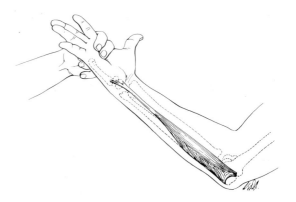

Fig. A.13

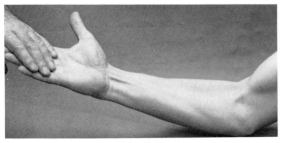
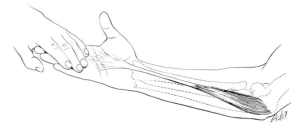

Fig. A.14

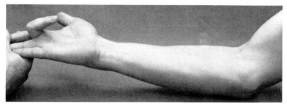

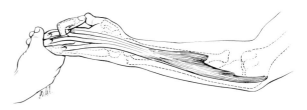

Fig. A.15a

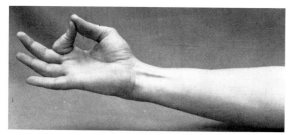

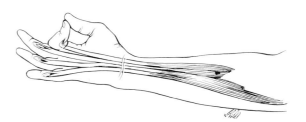

Fig. A.15b

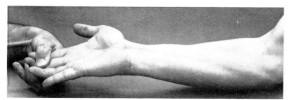

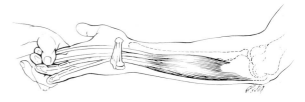

Fig. A.16

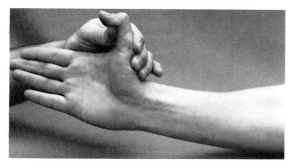

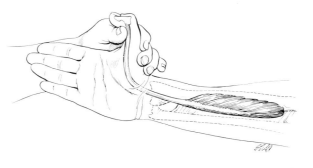

Fig. A.17

Figure No.	Muscle	Abbreviation	Action	Nerve	Cord	Root
A.18	Flexor pollicis brevis	FPB	Flexion of MP joint of thumb	Median (superficial head) Ulnar (deep head)	Medial	T1
A.19	Abductor pollicis brevis	APB	Abduction of thumb (extension of IP joint)	Median	Medial	T1
A.20	Adductor pollicis	AP	Adduction of thumb (extension of IP joint)	Ulnar	Medial	T1
A.21	Abductor digiti minimi	ADM	Abduction of small finger	Ulnar	Medial	T1
A.22	Flexor digiti minimi	FDM	Flexion of MP joint of small finger	Ulnar	Medial	T1

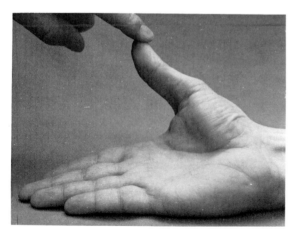
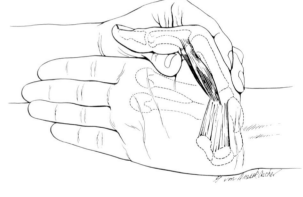

Fig. A.18

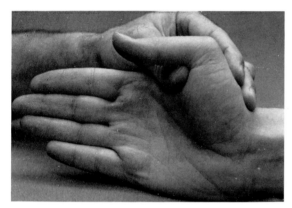
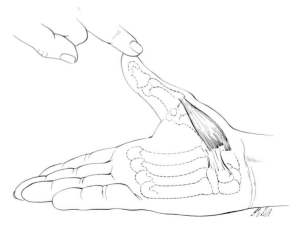

Fig. A.19

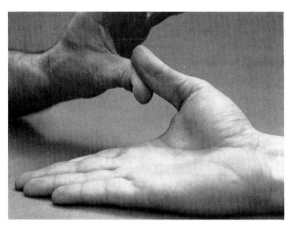
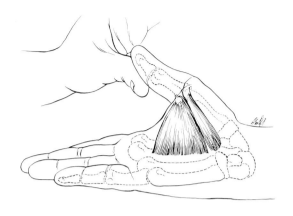

Fig. A.20

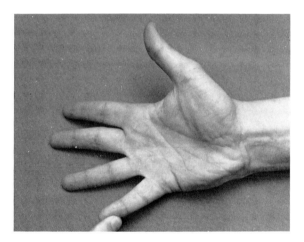
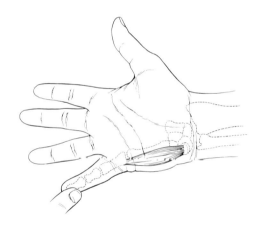

Fig. A.21

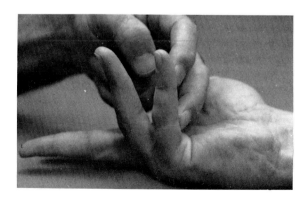
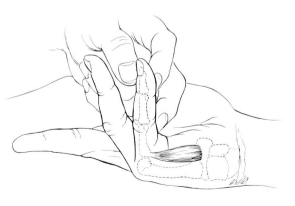

Fig. A.22

Figure No.	Muscle	Abbreviation	Action	Nerve	Cord	Root
	Interosseous		*Line of reference is axis of middle finger*			
	Dorsal		*Dorsal ABduct 'DAB'*			
A.23	1st	1st DIO	Abducts index finger	Ulnar	Medial	T1
A.24	2nd	2nd DIO	Abducts middle finger radially	Ulnar	Medial	T1
A.25	3rd	3rd DIO	Abducts middle finger ulnar-wards	Ulnar	Medial	T1
A.26	4th	4th DIO	Abducts ring finger	Ulnar	Medial	T1
	Palmar		*Palmar ADduct 'PAD'*			
A.27	1st	1st PIO	Adducts index finger	Ulnar	Medial	T1
A.28	2nd	2nd PIO	Adducts ring finger	Ulnar	Medial	T1
A.29	3rd	3rd PIO	Adducts small finger	Ulnar	Medial	T1

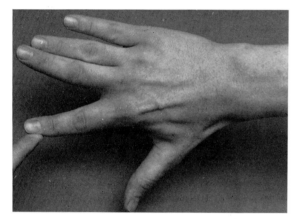

Fig. A.23

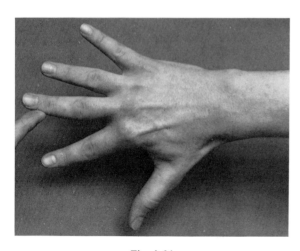

Fig. A.24

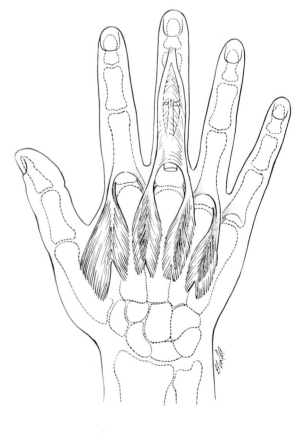

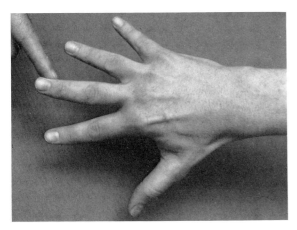

Fig. A.25

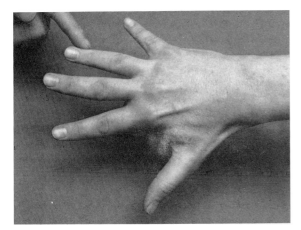

Fig. A.26

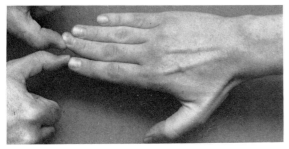

Fig. A.27

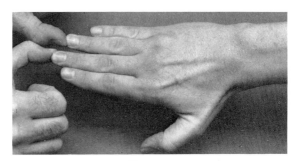

Fig. A.28

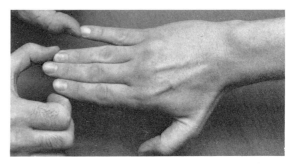

Fig. A.29

Figure No.	Muscle	Abbreviation	Action	Nerve	Cord	Root
A.30	Extensor pollicis longus	EPL	Extension of IP joint of thumb (with AP and APB)	Posterior interosseous (radial)	Posterior	C7 8
A.31	Extensor pollicis brevis	EPB	Extension of MP joint of thumb	Posterior interosseous	Posterior	C7 8
A.32	Abductor pollicis longus	APL	Extension of CM joint of thumb Radial deviation of wrist	Posterior interosseous	Posterior	C7 8
A.33	Extensor digitorum	ED	Extension of MP joints	Posterior interosseous	Posterior	C7 (8)
A.34	Extensor indicis	EI	Extension of index	Posterior interosseous	Posterior	C7 8
A.35	Extensor digiti minimi	EDM	Extension of small	Posterior interosseous	Posterior	C7 8

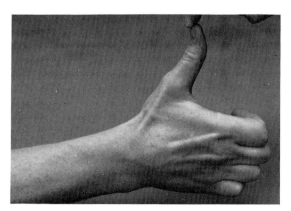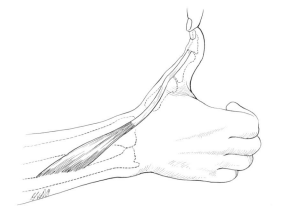

Fig. A.30

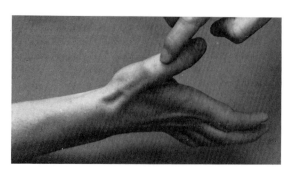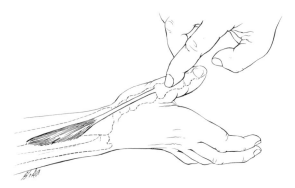

Fig. A.31

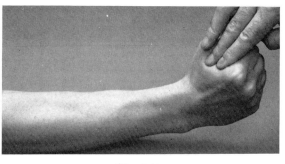
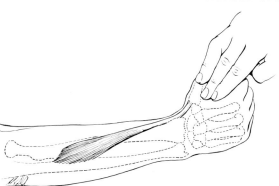

Fig. A.32

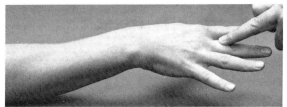
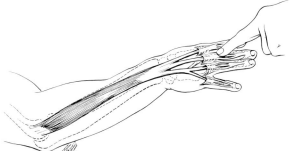

Fig. A.33

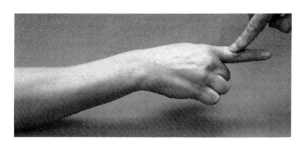
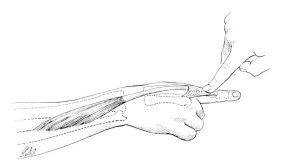

Fig. A.34

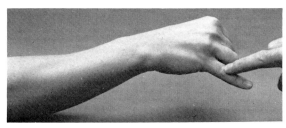
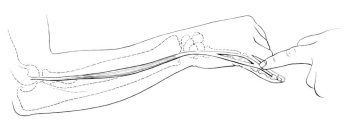

Fig. A.35

Figure No.	Muscle	Abbreviation	Action	Nerve	Cord	Root
A.36	Extensor carpi ulnaris	ECU	Extension of wrist Ulnar deviation of wrist	Posterior interosseous	Posterior	C7 (8)
A.37	Extensor carpi radialis longus and brevis	ECRL ECRB	Extension of wrist Radial deviation of wrist	Radial	Posterior	C6 7

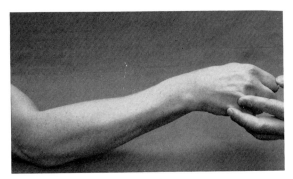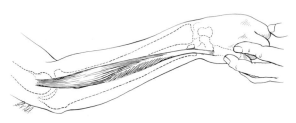

Fig. A.36

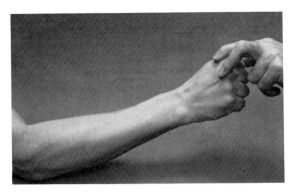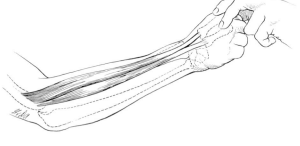

Fig. A.37

Cumulative bibliography

Abdul-Hamid A K 1987 First dorsal interosseous compartment syndrome. J Hand Surg (Br) 12: 269–272

Abrahamsson S O, Sollerman C, Lundborg G, Larsson J, Egund N 1990 Diagnosis of displaced ulnar collateral ligament of the metacarpophalangeal joint of the thumb. J Hand Surg (Am) 15: 457–460

Abu Jamra F N L, Akel S R, Shamma A R 1981 Repair of major defect of the upper extremity with a latissimus dorsi myocutaneous flap: a case report. Br J Plastic Surg 34: 121–123

Abu Jamra F N, Rebeiz J J 1979 Lipofibroma of the median nerve. J Hand Surg 4: 160–164

Acharya G, Merritt W H, Theogaraj S D 1980 Hemangioendotheliomas of the hand. Case reports. J Hand Surg 5: 181–182

Achauer B M, Brody G S, Wilson-Mackby L 1979 A classification of burned hand deformities. Orthopaedic Rev 8: 71–77

Adams B D, Blair W F, Reagan D S, Grundberg A B 1988 Technical factors related to Herbert screw fixation. J Hand Surg (Am) 13: 893–899

Adams B D, Unsell R S, McLaughlin P 1990 Niebauer trapeziometacarpal arthroplasty. J Hand Surg (Am) 15: 487–492

Adams J T, McEvoy R K, DeWeese J A 1965 Primary deep venous thrombosis of upper extremity. Arch Surgery 91: 29–42

Adamson B E, Lucas G L 1985 Multiple recurrence of digital pigmented villonodular tenosynovitis: a case report. J Hand Surg (Am) 10: 278–280

Adamson J E, Horton C E, Crawford H H 1967 Sensory rehabilitation of the injured thumb. Plastic Reconstr Surg 40: 53–57

Adamson J E, Srouji S J, Horton C E, Mladick R A 1971 The acute carpal tunnel syndrome. Plastic Reconstr Surg 47: 332–336

Adar R, Schramek A, Khodadadi J, Zweig A, Golcman L, Romanoff H 1980 Arterial combat injuries of the upper extremity. J Trauma 20: 297–302

Adelaar R S 1983 Sarcoidosis of the upper extremity: case presentation and literature review. J Hand Surg (Am) 8: 492–496

Adelaar R S, Foster W C, McDowell C 1984 The treatment of the cubital tunnel syndrome. J Hand Surg (Am) 9A: 90–95

Adeyemi-Doro H O, Olude O 1985 Juvenile aponeurotic fibroma. J Hand Surg (Br) 10: 127–128

Adson A W 1947 Surgical treatment for symptoms produced by cervical ribs and the scalenus anticus muscle. Surg Gynecol Obstet 85: 687–700

Adson A W 1951 Cervical ribs: symptoms, differential diagnosis and indications for section of the insertion of the scalenus anticus muscle. J Internat Coll Surg 16: 546–559

Adson A W, Colley J R 1927 Cervical rib. A method of anterior approach for relief of symptoms by division of the scalenus anticus. Ann Surg 85: 839–857

Aggarwal N D, Mittal R L, Bhalla B 1972 Delayed solitary metastasis to the radius of renal-cell carcinoma. J Bone Joint Surg 54A: 1314–1316

Agnew D H 1863 Bursal tumour producing loss of power of forearm. Am J Med Sci 46: 404–405

Agris J, Simmons C 1978 Factitious (self-inflicted) skin wounds. Plastic Reconstr Surg 62: 686–692

Ahbel D E, Alexander A H, Lichtman D M 1980 Protothecal olecranon bursitis. J Bone Joint Surg 62A: 835–836

Akbarnia B A, Wirth C R, Colman N 1976 Fibrosarcoma arising from chronic osteomyelitis. Case report and review of the literature. J Bone Joint Surg 58A: 123–125

Al-Arabi K M, Sabet N A 1984 Severe mincer injuries of the hand in children in Saudi Arabia. J Hand Surg (Br) 9: 249–250

Albright J A, Linburg R M 1978 Common variations of the radial wrist extensors. J Hand Surg 3: 134–138

Alexander A H, Turner M A, Alexander C E, Lichtman D M 1990 Lunate silicone replacement arthroplasty in Kienbock's disease: a long-term follow-up. J Hand Surg (Am) 15: 401–407

Alldred A 1954 A locked index finger. J Bone Joint Surg 36B: 102–103

Allen B N, Frykman G K, Unsell R S, Wood V E 1987 Ruptured flexor tendon tenorrhaphies in zone II: repair and rehabilitation. J Hand Surg (Am) 12: 18–21

Allen E V 1929 Thromboangitis obliterans: methods of diagnosis of chronic occlusive arterial lesions distal to the wrist with illustrative cases. Am J Med Sci 178: 237–244

Allen M J 1980 Conservative management of fingertip injuries in adults. Hand 12: 257–265

Allende B T 1967 Macrodactyly with enlarged median nerve associated with carpal tunnel syndrome. Plastic Reconstr Surg 39: 578–582

Allieu Y, Cenac P 1988 Is surgical intervention justifiable for total paralysis secondary to multiple avulsion injuries of the brachial plexus? Hand Clin 4: 609–618

Allieu Y, Lussiez B, Benichou M, Cenac P 1979 A double nidus osteoid osteoma in a finger. J Hand Surg (Am) 14: 538–541

Almdahl S M, Saebe-Larsen J, Due J Jr 1989 Injuries to the hand inflicted by rotary snowcutters. J Trauma 29: 227–228

Almquist E E 1987 Kienbock's disease. Hand Clin 3: 141–148

Alnot J Y 1989 Elbow flexion palsy after traumatic lesions of the brachial plexus in adults. Hand Clin 5: 15–22

Altner P C, Singh S K 1981 An unusual case of ectopic ossification in a finger. J Hand Surg 6: 142–145

Amadio P C 1985 Pyridoxine as an adjunct in the treatment of carpal tunnel syndrome. J Hand Surg (Am) 10: 237–241

Amadio P C 1987 Bifid median nerve with a double compartment within the transverse carpal canal. J Hand Surg (Am) 12: 366–368

Amadio P C, Beckenbaugh R D 1986 Entrapment of the ulnar nerve by the deep flexor-pronator aponeurosis. J Hand Surg (Am) 11: 83–87

Amadio P C, Berquist T H, Smith D K, Ilstrup D M et al 1989 Scaphoid malunion. J Hand Surg (Am) 14: 679–687

Amadio P C, Lombardi R M 1987 Metastatic tumors of the hand. J Hand Surg (Am) 12: 311–316

Amadio P C, Reiman H M, Dobyns J H 1988 Lipofibromatous hamartoma of nerve. J Hand Surg (Am) 13: 67–75

Ambrose J, Goldstone R 1975 Anomalous extensor digiti minimi proprius causing tunnel syndrome in the dorsal compartment. J Bone Joint Surg 57A: 706–707

Ambrosia J M, Wold L E, Amadio P C 1987 Osteoid osteoma of the hand and wrist. J Hand Surg (Am) 12: 794–800

Ames E L, Posch J L 1984 Calcinosis of the flexor and extensor tendons in dermatomyositis — case report. J Hand Surg (Am) 9: 876–879

Ametewee K, Harris A, Samuel M 1985 Acute carpal tunnel syndrome produced by anomalous flexor digitorum superficialis indicis muscle. J Hand Surg (Br) 10: 83–84

An H S, Hawthorne K B, Jackson W T 1988 Reflex sympathetic dystrophy and cigarette smoking. J Hand Surg (Am) 13: 458–460

An H S, Southworth S R, Jackson W T, Russ B 1988 Cigarette smoking and Dupuytren's contracture of the hand. J Hand Surg (Am) 13: 872–874

Anderson P A, Chanoski C E, Devan D L, McMahon B L, Whelan E P 1990 Normative study of grip and wrist flexion strength employing a BTE Work Simulator. J Hand Surg (Am) 15: 420–425

Anderson W J, Bowers W H 1985 Congenital absence of the triquetrum: a case report. J Hand Surg (Am) 10: 620–622

Andren L, Eiken O 1971 Arthrographic studies of wrist ganglions. J Bone Joint Surg 53A: 299–302

Andress M R, Peckar V G 1970 Fracture of the hook of the hamate. Br J Radiol 93: 141–143

Angelides A C, Wallace P F 1976 The dorsal ganglion of the wrist: its pathogenesis, gross and microscopic anatomy, and surgical treatment. J Hand Surg 1: 228–235

Annamaria C, Singletary S E, Balch C M 1989 Patterns of relapse in 1001 consecutive patients with melanoma nodal metastases. Arch Surg 124: 1051–1055

Ansell B M, Harrison S H 1974 The results of ulna styloidectomy in rheumatoid arthritis. Scand Rheumatol 3: 67

Ansell B M, Harrison S H, Little H, Thouas B 1970 Synovectomy of proximal interphalangeal joints. Br J Plastic Surg 23: 380–385

Ansell B, Harrison S 1975 A five year follow-up of synovectomy of the proximal interphalangeal joint in rheumatoid arthritis. Hand 7: 34–36

Antrum R M, Solomkin J S 1987 A review of antibiotic prophylaxis for open fractures. Orthopaedic Rev 16: 81–89

Apfelberg D B, Larson S J 1973 Dynamic anatomy of the ulnar nerve at the elbow. Plastic Reconstr Surg 51: 76–81

Apley A G 1956 Test of the power of flexor digitorum sublimis. Br Med J 1: 25–26

Araki S, Ohtani T, Tanaka T 1987 Open dorsal metacarpophalangeal dislocations of the index, long, and ring fingers. J Hand Surg (Am) 12A: 458–460

Archer I A, Brown R B, Fitton J M 1984 Epithelioid sarcoma in the hand. J Hand Surg (Br) 9: 207–209

Argenta L C, Duus E C, Lane G A 1983 Carotid injury and cerebral infarction in a revascularization hand injury case. J Hand Surg (Am) 8: 935–937

Ariel I, Haas H, Weinberg H, Rousso M, Rosenmann E 1983 *Mycobacterium fortuitum* granulomatous synovitis caused by a dog bite. J Hand Surg (Am) 8: 342–343

Armin A, Blair S J, Demons T C 1985 Benign soft tissue chondromatous lesion of the hand. J Hand Surg (Am) 10: 895–899

Arminio J A 1979 Congenital anomaly of the thumb: absent flexor pollicis longus tendon. J Hand Surg 4: 487–488

Armstrong T J 1986 Ergonomics and cumulative trauma disorders. Hand Clin 2: 553–565

Armstrong T J, Fine L J, Goldstein S A, Lifshitz Y R, Silverstein B A 1987 Ergonomic considerations in hand and wrist tendinitis. J Hand Surg (Am) 12: 830–837

Arndt R 1987 Work pace, stress, and cumulative trauma disorders. J Hand Surg (Am) 12: 866–869

Arnulf G 1976 Physiological basis of sympathetic surgery for the upper limb in Raynaud's diseases. J Cardiovasc Surg 17: 354–357

Arons M S 1985 Fingertip reconstruction with a palmar advancement flap and free dermal graft: a report of six cases. J Hand Surg (Am) 10: 230–232

Arons M S 1987 de Quervain's release in working women: a report of failures, complications, and associated diagnoses. J Hand Surg (Am) 12: 540–544

Arons M S, Fernando L, Polayes I M 1982 *Pasteurella multocida* — the major cause of hand infections following domestic animal bites. Journal Hand Surg 7: 47–52

Artz D, Posch J L 1973 The carpometacarpal boss. J Bone Joint Surg 55A: 747–752

Asai M, Wong A C, Matsunaga T, Akahoshi Y 1986 Carpal tunnel syndrome caused by aberrant lumbrical muscles associated with cystic degeneration of the tenosynovium: a case report. J Hand Surg (Am) 11: 218–221

Aschan W, Moberg E 1962 The Ninhydrin finger printing test used to map out partial lesions to hand nerves. Acta Chir Scand 123: 365–370

Ashbell T S, Kleinert H E, Kutz J E 1967 Vascular injuries about the elbow. Clin Orthopaedics 50: 107–127

Aston J N 1960 Locked middle finger. J Bone Joint Surg 42B: 75–79

Atasoy E 1982 Reversed cross-finger subcutaneous flap. J Hand Surg 7: 481–483

Atasoy E, Godfrey A, Kalisman M 1983 The antenna: procedure for the 'hook-nail' deformity. J Hand Surg (Am) 8: 55–58

Atasoy E, Ioakimidis E, Kasdan M, Kutz J E, Kleinert H E 1970 Reconstruction of the amputated fingertip with a triangular volar flap. J Bone Joint Surg 52A: 921–926

Atkins R M, Duckworth T, Kanis J A 1990 Features of

algodystrophy after Colles' fracture. J Bone Joint Surg (Br) 72: 105–110

Atkinson R E, Smith R J 1986 Silicone synovitis following silicone implant arthroplasty. Hand Clin 2: 291–299

Attiyeh F F, Shah J, Booher R J, Knapper W H 1979 Subungual squamous cell carcinoma. J Am Med Assoc 241: 262–263

Auerbach A D, Liu Q, Ghosh M S, Pollack G W, Douglas G W, Broxmeyer H E 1990 Prenatal identification of potential donors for umbilical cord blood transplantation for Fanconi anemia. Transfusion 30: 682–687

Auerbach A D, Rogatko A, Schroeder-Kurth T M 1989 International Fanconi Anemia Registry: relation of clinical symptoms to diepoxybutane sensitivity. Blood 73: 391–396

Aulicino P L, Dupuy T E, Moriarity R P 1981 Osteoid osteoma of the terminal phalanx of finger. Orthopaedic Rev 10: 59–63

Aulicino P L, Klavans S M, DuPuy T E 1984 Digital ischemia secondary to thrombosis of a persistent median artery. J Hand Surg (Am) 9: 820–823

Austin G J, Leslie B M, Ruby L K 1989 Variations of the flexor digitorum superficialis of the small finger. J Hand Surg (Am) 14: 262–267

Austin R 1976 Tardy palsy of the radial nerve from a Monteggia fracture. Injury 7: 303–304

Averill R M, Smith R J, Campbell C J 1980 Giant cell tumors of the bones of the hand. J Hand Surg 5: 39–50

Ayres J R, Goldstrohm G L, Miller G J, Dell P C 1988 Proximal interphalangeal joint arthrodesis with the Herbert screw. J Hand Surg (Am) 13: 600–603

Baas P C, Hoekstra H J, Koops H S 1989 Isolated regional perfusion in the treatment of subungual melanoma. Arch Surg 124: 373–376

Backhouse K M 1968 Mechanics of normal digital control in the hand and an analysis of ulnar drift of the rheumatoid hand. Ann Roy Coll Surg Engl 43: 154–173

Backhouse K M, Churchill-Davidson D 1975 Anomalous palmaris longus muscle producing carpal tunnel-like compression. Hand 7: 22–24

Badalamente M A, Stern L, Hurst L C 1983 The pathogenesis of Dupuytren's contracture: contractile mechanisms of the myofibroblasts. J Hand Surg (Am) 8: 235–243

Baker D S, Gaul S, Williams V K, Graves M 1981 The little finger superficialis — clinical investigation of its anatomic and functional shortcomings. J Hand Surg 6: 374–378

Balas P, Tripolitis A J, Kaklamanis P, Mandalaki T, Paracharalampous N 1979 Raynaud's Phenomenon. Primary and secondary causes. Arch Surg 114: 1174–1177

Ballantyne J P, Campbell M J 1973 Electrophysiological study after surgical repair of sectioned human peripheral nerves. J Neurol Neurosurg Psych 36: 797–805

Ballet F L, Watson H K, Ryu J 1984 Synovial chondromatosis of the distal radioulnar joint. J Hand Surg (Am) 9: 590–592

Banker B Q 1985 Neuropathologic aspects of arthrogryposis multiplex congenita. Clin Orthop Rel Res 194: 30–43

Banzet P, Glicenstein J, Dufourmentel C 1975 Melanotic tumors of the hand. Hand 7: 183–184

Barbieri C H 1984 Aneurysmal bone cyst of the hand. An unusual situation. J Hand Surg (Br) 9: 89–92

Bardsley A F, Soutar D S, Elliot D, Batchelor A G 1990 Reducing morbidity in the radial forearm flap donor site. Plastic Reconstr Surg 86: 287–292

Barfred T, Adamsen S 1986 Duplication of the extensor carpi ulnaris tendon. J Hand Surg (Am) 11: 423–425

Barfred T, Hjlund A P, Bertheussen K 1985 Median artery in carpal tunnel syndrome. J Hand Surg (Am) 10: 864–867

Barlow A, Chattaway F, Holgate M, Aldersley T 1970 Chronic paronychia. Br J Dermatol 82: 448–453

Barot L R, Caplan H S 1986 Early surgical intervention in Apert's syndactyly. Plastic Reconstr Surg 77: 282–287

Barr W G, Blair S J 1988 Carpal tunnel syndrome as the initial manifestation of scleroderma. J Hand Surg (Am) 13: 366–368

Barre P S, Shaffer J W, Carter J R, Lacey S H 1987 Multiplicity of neurilemmomas in the upper extremity. J Hand Surg (Am) 12: 307–311

Barry T P, Linton P 1977 Biophysics of rotary mower and snowblower injuries of the hand: high vs. low velocity 'missile' injury. J Trauma 17: 214–221

Barsky A 1967 Macrodactyly. J Bone Joint Surg 49A: 1255–1266

Barsky A J 1964 Cleft hand: classification, incidence and treatment. J Bone Joint Surg 46A: 1701–1720

Barton N 1989 Conservative treatment of articular fractures in the hand. J Hand Surg (Am) 14: 386–390

Barton N 1989 Internal fixation of hand fractures [editorial]. J Hand Surg (Br) 14: 139–142

Barton N J 1979 Another cause of median nerve compression by a lumbrical muscle in the carpal tunnel. J Hand Surg 4:189–191

Barton N J 1979 Fractures of the phalanges of the hand in children. Hand 11: 134–143

Barton N J 1984 Dupuytren's's disease arising from the abductor digiti minimi. J Hand Surg (Br) 9: 265–270

Barton N J 1984 Fractures of the hand. J Bone Joint Surg (Br) 66: 159–167

Barton N J, Buck-Gramcko D, Evans D M 1986 Soft-tissue anatomy of mirror hand. J Hand Surg (Br) 11: 307–319

Barton N J, Buck-Gramcko D, Evans D M, Kleinert H et al 1986 Mirror hand treated by true pollicization. J Hand Surg (Br) 11: 320–336

Baruch A D, Hecht O A 1983 Treatment of monodactyly by the distraction–lengthening principle: a case report. J Hand Surg (Am) 8: 604–606

Baruch A, Haas A, Lifschitz-Mercer B, Zeligowsky A 1987 Simple bone cyst of the metacarpal. J Hand Surg (Am) 12: 1103–1106

Bassett F H, Nunley J A 1982 Compression of the musculocutaneous nerve at the elbow. J Bone Joint Surg 64A: 1050–1052

Batillas J, Vasilas A, Pizzi W, Gokcebay T 1981 Bone scanning in the detection of occult fractures. J Trauma 21: 564–569

Bauer M, Jonsson K 1988 Congenital radioulnar synostosis. Radiological characteristics and hand function: case reports. Scand J Plastic Reconstr Hand Surg 22: 251–255

Baumgartner F, Nelson R J, Robertson J M 1989 The rudimentary first rib — a cause of thoracic outlet syndrome with arterial compromise. Arch Surg 124: 1090–1092

Baur G, Porter J, Bardana E, Wesche D, Rosch J 1977 Rapid onset of hand ischemia of unknown etiology. Ann Surg 186: 184–189

Baxt S, Mori K, Hoffman S 1975 Aneurysm of the hand secondary to Kaposi's sarcoma. Case report. J Bone Joint Surg 57A: 995–997

Baxt S, Mori K, Hoffman S 1975 Aneurysm of the hand

secondary to Kaposi's sarcoma. Case report. J Bone Joint Surg 57A: 995–997

Bayne L G, Klug M S 1987 Long-term review of the surgical treatment of radial deficiencies. J Hand Surg (Am) 12: 169–179

Bayne L G, Lovell W W, Marks T W 1970 The radial club hand (abstract). J Bone Joint Surg 52A: 1065

Bayon P, Pho R W 1988 Anatomical basis of dorsal forearm flap based on posterior interosseous vessels. J Hand Surg (Br) 13: 435–439

Beasley R W 1983 Principles of soft tissue replacement for the hand. J Hand Surg (Am) 8: 781–784

Beasley R W 1987 Hand and finger prostheses. J Hand Surg (Am) 12: 144–147

Beasley R W, de Beze G M 1990 Prosthetic substitution for fingernails. Hand Clin 6: 105–110

Beatty M E, Zook E G, Russell R C, Kinkead L R 1982 Grain auger injuries: The replacement of the corn picker injury? Plastic Reconstr Surg 69: 96–102

Bechtol C O 1954 Grip test: use of dynamometer with adjustable handle spacings. J Bone Joint Surg 36A: 820–824

Beckenbaugh R D, Dobyns J H, Linscheid R L, Bryan R S 1976 Review and analysis of silicone-rubber metacarpophalangeal implants. J Bone Joint Surg 58A: 483–487

Bedbrook G M 1979 Spinal injuries with tetraplegia and paraplegia. J Bone Joint Surg 61B: 267–284

Bedeschi P, Celli L, Balli A 1984 Transfer of sensory nerves in hand surgery. J Hand Surg (Br) 9: 46–49

Begg R E 1980 Epicondylitis or tennis elbow. Orthopaedic Rev 9: 33–42

Belinkie S A, Swats W M, Zitelli J A 1986 Invasive squamous cell carcinoma of the carpus: malignant transformation of epidermis dysplasia verruciformis. J Hand Surg (Am) 11: 273–275

Bell-Krotoski J, Tomancik E 1987 The repeatability of testing with Semmes–Weinstein monofilaments. J Hand Surg (Am) 12: 155–161

Belsky M R, Eaton R G, Lane L B 1984 Closed reduction and internal fixation of proximal phalangeal fractures. J Hand Surg (Am) 9: 725–729

Belsky M R, Millender L H 1980 Bowler's thumb in a baseball player: a case report. Orthopedics 3: 122–123

Belsole R J, Eikman A, Muroff L R 1981 Bone scintigraphy in trauma of the hand and wrist. J Trauma 21: 163–166

Belsole R J, Quinn S F, Greene T L, Beatty M E, Rayhack J M 1990 Digital subtraction arthrography of the wrist. J Bone Joint Surg (Am) 72: 846–851

Belsole R, Fenske N 1980 Cutaneous larva migrans in the upper extremity. J Hand Surg 5: 178–180

Belsole R, Lister G, Kleinert H 1978 Polyarteritis: a cause of nerve palsy in the extremity. J Hand Surg 3: 320–325

Bendick P J, Mayer J R, Glover J L, Park H M 1979 A photoplethysmographic technique for detecting vascular compromise. J Trauma 19: 398–402

Bendre D V, Baxi V K 1981 Dislocation of trapezoid. J Trauma 21: 899–900

Benkeddache Y, Gottesman H, Fourrier P 1984 Multiple stapling for wrist arthrodesis in the nonrheumatoid patient. J Hand Surg (Am) 9: 256–260

Benner C L, Schilling A D, Klein L 1987 Coordinated teamwork in California industrial rehabilitation. J Hand Surg (Am) 12: 936–939

Bennett E H 1886 On fracture of the metacarpal bone of the thumb. Br Med J 2: 12–13

Bergfield T G, DuPuy T E, Aulicino P L 1985 Fracture-dislocations of all five carpometacarpal joints: a case report. J Hand Surg (Am) 10: 76–78

Berkowitz R L, Hentz V R 1977 Herpetic whitlow — a non-surgical infection of the hand. Plastic Reconstr Surg 60: 125–127

Berrettoni B A, Seitz W H Jr 1990 Mycotic aneurysm in a digital artery: case report and literature review. J Hand Surg 15A: 305–308

Bertheussen K J, Holck S, Schidt T 1983 Giant cell lesion of bone of the hand with particular emphasis on giant cell reparative granuloma. J Hand Surg (Am) 8: 46–49

Bessman A N, Wagner W 1975 Nonclostridial gas gangrene. J Am Med Assoc 233: 958–963

Bevan D A, Ehrlich G E, Gupta V P 1977 Metastatic carcinoma simulating gout. J Am Med Assoc 237: 2746–2747

Bickerstaff D R, Harris S C, Kay N R 1988 Osteosarcoma of the carpus. J Hand Surg (Br) 13: 303–305

Biddulph S L 1985 The extensor sling procedure for an unstable carpometacarpal joint. J Hand Surg (Am) 10: 641–645

Bieber E J, Linscheid R L, Dobyns J H, Beckenbaugh R D 1988 Failed distal ulna resections. J Hand Surg (Am) 13: 193–200

Bieber E J, Moore J R, Weiland A J 1986 Lipomas compressing the radial nerve at the elbow. J Hand Surg (Am) 11: 533–535

Bieber E J, Weiland A J 1984 Traumatic dorsal dislocation of the triquetrum: a case report. J Hand Surg (Am) 9: 840–842

Bieber E J, Wood M B, Cooney W P, Amadio P C 1987 Thumb avulsion: results of replantation/revascularization. J Hand Surg (Am) 12: 786–790

Bielejeski T R 1973 Granular cell tumor (myoblastoma) of the hand. J Bone Joint Surg 55A: 841–843

Bilhaut M 1890 Guerison d'un pouce bifide par un nouveau procede operatoire. Congr Fr Chir 4: 576

Bilos J, Eskestrand T 1979 External fixator use in comminuted gunshot fractures of the proximal phalanx. J Hand Surg 4: 357–359

Bingold A C 1979 On splitting plasters. J Bone Joint Surg 61B: 294–295

Bishop A T, Beckenbaugh R D 1988 Fracture of the hamate hook. J Hand Surg (Am) 13: 135–139

Black D M, Mann R J, Constine R M, Daniels A U 1986 The stability of internal fixation in the proximal phalanx. J Hand Surg (Am) 11: 672–677

Black D M, Watson H K, Vender M I 1987 Arthroplasty of the ulnar carpometacarpal joints. J Hand Surg (Am) 12: 1071–1074

Blacker G J, Lister G D, Kleinert H E 1976 The abducted little finger in low ulnar nerve palsy. J Hand Surg 1: 190–196

Blair S J 1991 Prevention of occupational hand injuries. In: Kasdan M L (ed) Occupational hand and upper extremity injuries and diseases. Hanley & Belfus, Philadelphia

Blair S J, Bear-Lehman J 1987 Prevention of upper extremity occupational disorders. J Hand Surg (Am) 12: 821–822

Blair S J, McCormick E 1985 Prevention of trauma: cooperation toward a better working environment. J Hand Surg (Am) 10: 953–958

Blair W F 1980 Granular cell schwannoma of the hand.
J Hand Surg. 5: 51–52

Blair W F, Berger R A, el-Khoury G Y 1985
Arthrotomography of the wrist: an experimental and
preliminary clinical study. J Hand Surg (Am) 10: 350–359

Blair W F, Buckwalter J A 1983 Congenital malposition of
flexor pollicis longus — an anatomy note. J Hand Surg
(Am) 8: 93–94

Blair W F, Buckwalter J A, Mickelson M R, Omer G E 1983
Lymphangioma of the forearm and hand. J Hand Surg
(Am) 8: 399–405

Blair W F, Omer G E 1981 Anomalous insertion of the flexor
pollicis longus. J Hand Surg 6: 241–244

Blair W F, Shurr D G, Buckwalter J A 1984
Metacarpophalangeal joint implant arthroplasty with a
silastic spacer. J Bone Joint Surg 66A: 365–370

Blakemore M E 1979 Posterior interosseous nerve paralysis
caused by a lipoma. J Roy Coll Surg Edin 24: 113–117

Blanco R H 1985 Excision of the lunate in Kienbock's
disease: long-term results. J Hand Surg (Am)
10: 1008–1013

Blatt G 1987 Capsulodesis in reconstructive hand surgery.
Dorsal capsulodesis for the unstable scaphoid and volar
capsulodesis following excision of the distal ulna. Hand
Clin 3: 81–102

Blauth W 1967 Der hypoplastische Daumen. Arch Orthop
Unfall Chir 62: 225–246

Bleicher J N, Blinn D L, Massop D 1987 Hand infections in
dental personnel. Plastic Reconstr Surg 80: 420–422

Bleifeld C J, Inglis A E 1974 The hand in systemic lupus
erythematosis. J Bone Joint Surg 56A: 1207–1215

Blevens A D, Light T R, Jablonsky W S, Smith D G et al
1989 Radiocarpal articular contact characteristics with
scaphoid instability. J Hand Surg (Am) 14: 781–790

Block R S, Burton R I 1977 Multiple chondrosarcomas in a
hand. A case report. J Hand Surg 2: 310–313

Blockey N J, Gibson A A M, Goel K M 1980 Monarticular
juvenile rheumatoid arthritis. J Bone Joint Surg
62B: 368–371

Bloem J J A M, Van Der Meulen J C 1978 Neurofibromatosis
in plastic surgery. Br J Plastic Surg 31: 50–53

Blomgren I, Blomqvist G, Ejeskar A, Fogdestam I et al 1988
Hand function after replantation or revascularization of
upper extremity injuries. Scand J Plastic Reconstr Surg
Hand Surg 22: 93–101

Blumenthal S M 1987 Vocational rehabilitation with the
industrially injured worker. J Hand Surg (Am) 12: 926–930

Blunt R J, Porter J M 1981 Raynaud syndrome. Semin
Arthrit Rheum 10: 282–308

Bodyns J H, O'Brien E T, Linscheid R L, Farrow G M 1972
Bowler's thumb: diagnosis and treatment. J Bone Joint
Surg 54A: 751–755

Boeckstyns M E, Busch P 1984 Surgical treatment of
scaphoid pseudarthrosis: evaluation of the results after soft
tissue arthroplasty and inlay bone grafting. J Hand Surg
(Am) 9: 378–382

Boeckstyns M E, Kjaer L, Busch P, Holst-Nielsen F 1985
Soft tissue interposition arthroplasty for scaphoid
nonunion. J Hand Surg (Am) 10: 109–114

Boeckstyns M E, Sinding A, Elholm K T, Rechnagel K 1989
Replacement of the trapeziometacarpal joint with a
cemented (Caffiniere) prosthesis. J Hand Surg (Am)
14: 83 89

Bogumill G P 1977 Clinico-pathological correlation in a case
of congenital arterio-venous fistula. Hand 9: 60–64

Bogumill G P 1983 A morphologic study of the relationship
of collateral ligaments to growth plates in the digits. J Hand
Surg (Am) 8: 74–79

Bohl W R, Brightman E 1981 Fracture of a silastic radial-
head prosthesis: diagnosis and localization of fragments by
xerography. J Bone Joint Surg 63A: 1482–1483

Boix E 1984 Deviation des doigts en coup de vent et
insuffisance de l'opone' vrose paliciaire d'origine
congenitale. Nouv Inconogr Salpet 10: 180–194

Bolesta M J, Garrett W E Jr, Ribbeck B M, Glisson R R et al
1988 Immediate and delayed neurorrhaphy in a rabbit
model: a functional, histologic, and biochemical
comparison. J Hand Surg (Am) 13: 352–357

Bonnel F 1985 Histologic structure of the ulnar nerve in the
hand. J Hand Surg (Am) 10: 264–269

Bonney G 1954 The value of axon responses in determining
the site of lesion in traction injuries of the brachial plexus.
Brain 77: 588–609

Bonney G 1965 Scalenus medius band. J Bone Joint Surg
47B: 268–272

Booher R J 1961 Tumors arising from blood vessels in the
hands and feet. Clin Orthopedics 19: 71–98

Booher R J 1965 Lipoblastic tumors of the hands and feet.
Review of the literature and report of thirty–three cases.
J Bone Joint Surg 47A: 727–740

Boome R S, Kaye J C 1988 Obstetric traction injuries of the
brachial plexus. J Bone Joint Surg (Br) 70: 571–576

Bora F W Jr 1985 Wrist arthroscope. J Hand Surg (Am)
10: 308

Bora F W Jr, Bednar J M, Osterman A L, Brown M J,
Sumner AJ 1987 Prosthetic nerve grafts: a resorbable tube
as an alternative to autogenous nerve grafting. J Hand Surg
(Am) 12: 685–692

Bora F W Jr, Miller G 1987 Joint physiology, cartilage
metabolism, and the etiology of osteoarthritis. Hand Clin
3: 325–336

Bora F W Jr, Osterman A L, Thomas V J, Maitin E C,
Polineni S 1987 The treatment of ruptures of multiple
extensor tendons at wrist level by a free tendon graft in
the rheumatoid patient. J Hand Surg (Am)
12: 1038–1040

Bora F W, Nicholson J T, Cheema H M 1970 Radial
meromelia. J Bone Joint Surg 52A: 966–979

Bora F W, Osterman A L, Kaneda R R, Esterhal J 1981
Radial club-hand deformity. J Bone Joint Surg
63A: 741–745

Borgsmiller W K, Whiteside L A 1980 Tuberculous
tenosynovitis of the hand ('compound palmar
ganglion'): literature review and case report. Orthopedics
3: 1093–1096

Boswick J A, Burkhalter W E, Gonzalez R, Kilgore E S,
Watson H K 1988 Symposium: Dupuytren's contracture.
Cont Ortho 16: 71–110

Bosworth D M 1965 Surgical treatment of tennis elbow.
J Bone Joint Surg 47A: 1533–1536

Botte M J, Cooney W P, Linscheid R L 1989 Arthroscopy of
the wrist: anatomy and technique. J Hand Surg (Am)
14: 313–316

Botte M J, Gelberman R H 1987 Modified technique for
Herbert screw insertion in fractures of the scaphoid. J Hand
Surg (Am) 12: 149–150

Botte M J, Gelberman R H, Smith D G, Silver M A, Gellman
H 1987 Repair of severe muscle belly lacerations using a
tendon graft. J Hand Surg (Am) 12: 406–412

Botte M J, Keenan M A 1988 Percutaneous phenol blocks of

the pectoralis major muscle to treat spastic deformities. J Hand Surg (Am) 13: 147–149

Botte M J, Keenan M A, Gellman H, Garland D E, Waters R L 1989 Surgical management of spastic thumb-in-palm deformity in adults with brain injury. J Hand Surg (Am) 14: 174–182

Botte M J, Keenan M A, Korchek J I, Waters R L 1987 Modified technique for the superficialis-to-profundus transfer in the treatment of adults with spastic clenched fist deformity. J Hand Surg (Am) 12: 639–640

Botte M J, Mortensen W W, Gelberman R H, Rhoades C E, Gellman H 1988 Internal vascularity of the scaphoid in cadavers after insertion of the Herbert screw. J Hand Surg (Am) 13: 216–220

Bouchard C 1891 Semaine Med (Paris) 11: 387

Boulas H J, Milek M A 1990 Ulnar shortening for tears of the triangular fibrocartilaginous complex. J Hand Surg (Am) 15: 415–420

Bourne M H, Wood M B, Carmichael S W 1987 Locating the lateral antebrachial cutaneous nerve. J Hand Surg (Am) 12: 697–699

Bourne M H, Wood M B, Cooney W P 1988 Reconstruction by free-tissue transfer of electively amputated parts. Surg Rounds Ortho 56–61

Bouvier M 1851-2 Note sur une paralysie partielle des muscles de la main. Bull Acad Nat Med 18: 125–139 (cited in Zancolli 1979)

Bowe A, Doyle L, Millender L H 1984 Bilateral partial ruptures of the flexor carpi radialis tendon secondary to trapezial arthritis. J Hand Surg (Am) 9: 738–739

Bowen J T 1912 Precancerous dermatoses: study of two cases of chronic atypical epithelial proliferation. J Cancer Dis 30: 241–255

Bowen T L, Stone K H 1966 Posterior interosseous nerve paralysis caused by a ganglion at the elbow. J Bone Joint Surg 48B: 774–776

Bowers H, Hurst L 1979 An intra-articular intraosseous carpal ganglion. J Hand Surg 4: 375–377

Bowers W H 1981 The proximal interphalangeal joint volar plate. A clinical study of hyperextension injury. J Hand Surg 6: 77–81

Bowers W H 1985 Distal radioulnar joint arthroplasty: the hemiresection–interposition technique. J Hand Surg (Am) 10: 169–178

Bowers W H, Carlson E C, Wenner S M, Doyle J R 1989 Nerve suture and grafting. Hand Clin 5: 445–453

Bowers W H, Hurst L C 1977 Gamekeeper's thumb. Evaluation by arthrography and stress roentgenography. J Bone Joint Surg 59A: 519–524

Bowers W H, Wolf J W, Nehil J L, Bittinger S 1980 The proximal interphalangeal joint volar plate. I. An anatomical and biomechanical study. J Hand Surg 5: 79–88

Bowers W, Doppelt S 1979 Compression of the deep branch of the ulnar nerve by an intraneural cyst. Case report. J Bone Joint Surg 61A: 612–613

Boxers D G, Lynch J B 1977 Xeroradiography for nonmetallic foreign bodies. Plastic Reconstr Surg 60: 470–471

Boyd A D Jr, Thornhill T S 1989 Surgical treatment of the elbow in rheumatoid arthritis. Hand Clin 4: 645–655

Boyes J H 1980 The measuring of motions. J Hand Surg 5: 89–90

Boyes J, Marroum M 1978 Epithelioid sarcoma of hand and forearm. Hand 10: 302–305

Brammer A J, Piercy J E, Auger P L, Nohara S 1987 Tactile perception in hands occupationally exposed to vibration. J Hand Surg (Am) 12: 870–875

Brand M G, Gelberman R H 1988 Lipoma of the flexor digitorum superficialis causing triggering at the carpal canal and median nerve compression. J Hand Surg (Am) 13: 342–344

Brand P W 1958 Paralytic claw hand. J Bone Joint Surg 40B: 618–632

Brand P W 1988 Biomechanics of tendon transfers. Hand Clin 4: 137–154

Brand P W, Cranor K C, Ellis J C 1975 Tendon and pulleys at the metacarpophalangeal joint of a finger. J Bone Joint Surg 57A: 779–783

Brand P W, Thompson D E 1982 Relative tension and potential excursion of muscles in the forearm and hand. J Hand Surg 6: 209–219

Brandner M D, Buncke H J, Campagna-Pinto D 1989 Experimental treatment of neuromas in the rat by retrograde axoplasmic transport of ricin with selective destruction of ganglion cells. J Hand Surg (Am) 14: 710–714

Brandsma J W, Birke J A, Sims D S Jr 1986 The Martin-Gruber innervated hand. J Hand Surg (Am) 11: 536–539

Brannon E W 1963 Cervical rib syndrome. J Bone Joint Surg 45A: 977–998

Brase D W, Millender L H 1986 Failure of silicone rubber wrist arthroplasty in rheumatoid arthritis. J Hand Surg (Am) 11: 175–183

Braun R M, Hoffer M M, Mooney V, McKeever J, Roper B 1973 Phenol nerve block in the treatment of acquired spastic hemiplegia in the upper limb. J Bone Joint Surg 55A: 580–585

Braun R M, Rhoades C E 1985 Dynamic compression for small bone arthrodesis. J Hand Surg (Am) 10: 340–343

Breen T F, Gelberman R H, Jupiter J B 1988 Intra-articular fractures of the basilar joint of the thumb. Hand Clin 4: 491–501

Breen T F, Jupiter J B 1989 Extensor carpi ulnaris and flexor carpi ulnaris tenodesis of the unstable distal ulna. J Hand Surg (Am) 14: 612–617

Breidenbach W C 3rd 1989 Emergency free tissue transfer for reconstruction of acute upper extremity wounds. Clin Plastic Surg 16: 505–514

Brent B, Upton J, Acland R D, Shaw W W et al 1985 Experience with the temporoparietal fascial free flap. Plastic Reconstr Surg 76: 177–188

Brenton G E, Johnson D E, Eady J L 1986 Leiomyosarcoma of the hand and wrist. Report of two cases. J Bone Joint Surg (Am) 68: 139–142

Breslow A 1975 Tumor thickness, level of invasion and node dissection in state I cutaneous melanona. Ann Surg 182: 572–575

Breslow A, Macht S D 1978 Evaluation of prognosis in Stage I cutaneous melanoma. Plastic Reconstr Surg 61: 342–346

Brewerton D A 1967 A tangential radiographic projection for demonstrating involvement of metacarpal heads in rheumatoid arthritis. Br J Radiol 40: 233–234

Brody G A, Buncke H J, Alpert B S, Hing D N 1990 Serratus anterior muscle transplantation for treatment of soft tissue defects in the hand. J Hand Surg 15: 322–327

Bromley G S, Solender M 1986 Hand infection caused by *Actinobacillus actinomycetemcomitans*. J Hand Surg (Am) 11: 434–436

Brones M F, Wheeler E S, Lesavoy M A 1982 Restoration of

elbow flexion and arm contour with the latissimus dorsi myocutaneous flap. Plastic Reconstr Surg 69: 329–332

Brones M, Wilgis E 1978 Anatomical variations of the palmaris longus, causing carpal tunnel syndrome. Plastic Reconstr Surg 62: 798–800

Brostrom L, Harris M, Simon M, Cooperman D, Nilsonne U 1979 The effect of biopsy on survival of patients with osteosarcoma. J Bone Joint Surg 61B: 209–212

Broudy A S, Jupiter J, May J W 1979 Management of supracondylar fracture with brachial artery thrombosis in a child. J Trauma 19: 540–544

Broudy A S, Smith R J 1979 Deformities of the hand and wrist with ulnar deficiency. J Hand Surg 4: 304–315

Browett J P, Fiddian N J 1985 Delayed median nerve injury due to retained glass fragments. A report of two cases. J Bone Joint Surg (Br) 67: 382–384

Brown D E, Lichtman D M 1987 Midcarpal instability. Hand Clinics 3: 135–140

Brown F E, Jobe J B, Hamlet M, Rubright A 1986 Induced vasodilation in the treatment of posttraumatic digital cold intolerance. J Hand Surg (Am) 11: 382–387

Brown I, Huffstadt A J C 1981 Intraosseous ganglia. Hand 13: 51–54

Brown LG 1989 Distal interphalangeal joint flexible implant arthroplasty. J Hand Surg (Am) 14: 653–656

Brown R H L, Muddu B N 1981 Scaphoid and lunate dislocation. Hand 13: 303–307

Brown T D 1974 The treatment of hydrofluoric acid burns. J Soc Occup Med 24: 80–89

Browne E Z Jr, Dunn H K, Snyder C C 1976 Ski pole thumb injury. Plastic Reconstr Surg 58: 19–23

Bruch H P, Lanz U, Horl M, Wolter J 1985 Rigor of small human vessels. J Hand Surg (Am) 10: 985–988

Brumfield R H, Resnick C T 1985 Synovectomy of the elbow in rheumatoid arthritis. J Bone Joint Surg 67A: 16

Brunel W, Schecter W P, Schecter G 1988 Hand deformity and sensory loss due to Hansen's disease in American Samoa. J Hand Surg (Am) 13: 279–283

Brunelli G, Monini L 1985 Direct muscular neurotization. J Hand Surg (Am) 10: 993–997

Bryan A S, Ghorbal M S 1988 The long-term results of closed palmar fasciotomy in the management of Dupuytren's contracture. J Hand Surg (Br) 13: 254–256

Bryan R S, Soule E H, Dobyns J H, Pritchard D J, Linscheid R L 1974 Primary epithelioid sarcoma of the hand. J Bone Joint Surg 56: 458

Brys D, Waters R L 1987 Effect of triceps function on the brachioradialis transfer in quadriplegia. J Hand Surg (Am) 12: 237–239

Buchler U, Aiken M A 1988 Arthrodesis of the proximal interphalangeal joint by solid bone grafting and plate fixation in extensive injuries to the dorsal aspect of the finger. J Hand Surg (Am) 13: 589–594

Buchthal F, Rosenfalck A, Trojaborg W 1974 Electrophysiological findings in entrapment of the median nerve at wrist and elbow. J Neurol Neurosurg Psych 37: 340–360

Buck-Gramcko D 1971 Pollicisation of the index finger. J Bone Joint Surg 53A: 1605–1617

Buck-Gramcko D 1977 Denervation of the wrist joint. J Bone Joint Surg 59A: 54–61

Buck-Gramcko D 1977 Thumb reconstruction by digital transposition. Orthopaedic Clin North Am 8: 329–342

Buck-Gramcko D 1985 Cleft hands: classification and treatment. Hand Clin 1: 467–473

Buck-Gramcko D 1985 Radialization as a new treatment for radial club hand. Surg (Am) 10: 964–968

Buck-Gramcko D 1988 Congenital malformations. In: Nigst H, Buck-Gramcko D, Millesi H, Lister G (eds) Hand surgery. Georg Thieme, Stuttgart

Buckle P 1987 Musculoskeletal disorders of the upper extremities: the use of epidemiologic approaches in industrial setting. J Hand Surg (Am) 12: 885–889

Bufalini C, Pescatori G 1969 Posterior cervical electromyography in the diagnosis and prognosis of brachial plexus injuries. J Bone Joint Surg 51B: 627–631

Bullon A, Nistal M, Razquin S, Novo A et al 1986 Malignant fibrous histiocytoma in a child's hand. J Hand Surg (Am) 11: 744–748

Bunkis J, Mehrohof A I, Stayman J W 1981 Radiation induced carcinoma of the hand. J Hand Surg. 6: 384–387

Bunnell S 1931 Physiologic reconstruction of the thumb after total loss. Surg Obstet Gynecol 52: 245–248

Burgess R C 1987 Chronic tenosynovitis caused by *Actinobacillus actinomycetemcomitans*. J Hand Surg (Am) 12: 294–295

Burgess R C 1987 The effect of a simulated scaphoid malunion on wrist motion. J Hand Surg (Am) 12: 774–776

Burgess R C 1987 The effect of rotatory subluxation of the scaphoid on radio-scaphoid contact. J Hand Surg (Am) 12: 771–774

Burgess R C 1990 Anatomic variations of the midcarpal joint. J Hand Surg (Am) 15: 129–131

Burian F 1963 The whistling face characteristic in a compound cranio-facio-corporal syndrome. Br J Plast Surg 16: 140

Burke F, Flatt A 1979 Clinodactyly — a review of a series of cases. Hand 11: 269–280

Burkhalter W E 1989 Closed treatment of hand fractures. J Hand Surg (Am) 14: 390–393

Burkhalter W, Schroeder F, Eversmann W 1978 Aneurysmal bone cysts occurring in the metacarpals. J Hand Surg 3: 579

Burkhalter WE 1989 Deep space infections. Hand Clin 5: 553–559

Burkhart S S, Wood M B, Linscheid R L 1982 Posttraumatic recurrent subluxation of the extensor carpi ulnaris tendon. J Hand Surg 7: 1–3

Burns J, Lister G D 1984 Localized constrictive radial neuropathy in the absence of extrinsic compression: three cases. J Hand Surg (Am) 9A: 99–103

Burton R I 1986 Complications following surgery on the basal joint of the thumb. Hand Clin 2: 265–269

Burton R I 1987 Basal joint implant arthroplasty in osteoarthritis. Indications, techniques, pitfalls, and problems. Hand Clin 3: 473–487

Burton R I, Pellegrini V D Jr 1986 Surgical management of basal joint arthritis of the thumb. Part II. Ligament reconstruction with tendon interposition arthroplasty. J Hand Surg (Am) 11: 324–332

Bush D C, Schneider L H 1984 Tuberculosis of the hand and wrist. J Hand Surg (Am) 9: 391–398

Buterbaugh G A, Palmer A K 1988 Fractures and dislocations of the distal radioulnar joint. Hand Clin 4: 361–375

Butler B, Bigley E C 1971 Aberrant index (first) lumbrical tendinous origin associated with carpal tunnel syndrome. J Bone Joint Surg 53A: 160–162

Butler E D, Hamill J P, Seipel R S, DeLorimier A A 1960

Tumors of the hand. A ten-year survey and report of 437 cases. Am J Surg 100: 293–302

Butt W D 1962 Fractures of the hand. I. Description. Can Med Assoc J 86: 731–735

Button M 1979 Epithelioid sarcoma: a case report. J Hand Surg 4: 368–371

Bynum D K Jr, Gilbert J A 1988 Avulsion of the flexor digitorum profundus: anatomic and biomechanical considerations. J Hand Surg (Am) 13: 222–227

Bywaters E G L, Scott J T 1963 The natural history of vascular lesions in rheumatoid arthritis. J Chronic Dis 16: 905

Cabbabe E B 1985 Xeroradiography as an aid in planning resection of arteriovenous malformation of the upper extremities. J Hand Surg (Am) 10: 670–674

Caffee H H, Master N T 1984 Atherosclerosis of the forearm and hand. J Hand Surg (Am) 9: 193–196

Cahill B R, Palmer R E 1983 Quadrilateral space syndrome. J Hand Surg (Am) 8: 65–69

Cain J E Jr, Shepler T R, Wilson M R 1987 Hamatometacarpal fracture-dislocation: classification and treatment. J Hand Surg (Am) 12: 762–767

Caldwell E H, McCormack R M 1980 Acute radiation injury of the hands: report on a case with a twenty-one year follow-up. J Hand Surg 5: 568–571

Calin A, Ports J, Fries J F, Schurman D J 1977 Clinical history as a screening test for ankylosing spondylitis. J Am Med Assoc 237: 2613–2614

Calkins M S, Burkhalter W, Reyes F 1987 Traumatic segmental bone defects in the upper extremity. J Bone Joint Surg (Am) 69: 19–27

Callan J E, Wood V E 1975 Spontaneous resolution of an osteochondroma. J Bone Joint Surg 57A: 723

Campanacci M, Bacci G, Pagani P, Giunti A 1980 Multiple drug chemotherapy for the primary treatment of osteosarcoma of the extremities. J Bone Joint Surg 62B: 93–101

Campbell D C, Bryan R S, Cooney W P, Ilstrup D 1979 Mechanical cornpicker hand injuries. J Trauma 19: 678–681

Campbell R D, Lance E M, Chin Bor Yeoh 1964 Lunate and perilunar dislocations. J Bone Joint Surg 46B: 55–72

Campbell R D, Thompson C, Lance E M, Adler J B 1965 Indications for open reduction of lunate and perilunate dislocations of the carpal bones. J Bone Joint Surg 47A: 915–937

Canale S T, Ikard S T 1984 The orthopaedic implications of purpura fulminans. J Bone Joint Surg (Am) 66: 764–769

Canales F L, Newmeyer W L 3rd, Kilgore E S Jr 1989 The treatment of felons and paronychias. Hand Clin 5: 515–523

Canipe T L, Howell J A, Howell C M 1964 Subungual carcinoma. Plastic Reconstr Surg 33: 263–265

Cantor R M, Braunstein E M 1988 Diagnosis of dorsal and palmar rotation of the lunate on a frontal radiograph. J Hand Surg (Am) 13: 187–193

Capener N 1966 The vulnerability of the posterior interosseous nerve of the forearm. J Bone Joint Surg 48B: 770–783

Caplan A 1953 Certain unusual appearances in the chest of coal miners suffering from rheumatoid arthritis. Thorax 8: 29–37

Carducci A T 1981 Potential boutonniere deformity — its recognition and treatment. Orthopaedic Rev 10: 121–123

Carithers H A, Carithers C M, Edwards R O 1969 Cat scratch disease: its natural history. J American Med Assoc 207: 312–316

Carlson C S Jr, Curtis R M 1984 Steroid injection for flexor tenosynovitis. J Hand Surg (Am) 9: 286–287

Carneirio R S, Mann R J 1979 Occlusion of the ulnar artery associated with an anomalous muscle: a case report. J Hand Surg 4: 412–414

Carneiro R D S 1974 Aneurysm of the wrist. Plastic Reconstr Surg 54: 483–489

Carneiro R S, Okunski W J, Hefernan A H 1977 Detection of a relatively radiolucent foreign body in the hand by xerography. Plastic Reconstr Surg 59: 862–863

Carr D, Davis P 1985 Distal posterior interosseous nerve syndrome. J Hand Surg (Am) 10: 873–878

Carriquiry C E 1990 Versatile fasciocutaneous flaps based on the medial septocutaneous vessels of the arm. Plastic Reconstr Surg 86: 103–109

Carroll C 4th, Moore J R, Weiland A J 1987 Posttraumatic ulnar subluxation of the extensor tendons: a reconstructive technique. J Hand Surg (Am) 12: 227–231

Carroll M P, Montero C 1980 Rare anomalous muscle cause of carpal tunnel syndrome. Orthopaedic Rev 9: 83–85

Carroll R 1974 Ring injuries in the hand. Clin Orthopaedics 104: 175–182

Carroll R E 1953 Osteoid osteoma in the hand. J Bone Joint Surg 35A: 888–893

Carroll R E 1955 Epidermoid (epithelial) cyst of the hand. Am J Surg 85: 327–334

Carroll R E 1976 Squamous cell carcinoma of the nail bed. J Hand Surg 1: 92–97

Carroll R E 1987 Juvenile aponeurotic fibroma. Hand Clin 3: 219–224

Carroll R E, Berman A T 1972 Glomus tumors of the hand. Review of the literature and report of 28 cases. J Bone Joint Surg 54A: 691–703

Carroll R E, Carlson E 1989 Diagnosis and treatment of injury to the second and third carpometacarpal joints. J Hand Surg (Am) 14: 102–107

Carroll R E, Coyle M P Jr 1985 Dysfunction of the pisotriquetral joint: treatment by excision of the pisiform. J Hand Surg (Am) 10: 703–707

Carroll R E, Green D P 1975 Reconstruction of the hypoplastic digits. J Bone Joint Surg 57A: 727

Carroll R E, Hill N A 1969 Small joint arthrodesis in hand reconstruction. J Bone Joint Surg 51A: 1219–1221

Carroll R E, Hill N A 1970 Triceps transfer to restore elbow flexion. The study of fifteen patients with paralytic lesions and arthrogryposis. J Bone Joint Surg 52A: 239–244

Carroll R E, Hill N A 1973 Arthrodesis of the carpometacarpal joint of the thumb. J Bone Joint Surg 55B: 292–294

Carroll R E, Sinton W, Carcis A 1955 Acute calcium deposits in the hand. J Am Med Assoc 157: 422–426

Carter P R, Benton L J, Dysert P A 1986 Silicone rubber carpal implants: a study of the incidence of late osseous complications. J Hand Surg (Am) 11: 639–644

Carter S, Mersheimer W 1970 Infections of the hand. Orthopaedic Clin North Am 1: 455–466

Caudle R J, Stern P J 1987 Melorheostosis of the hand. A case report with long-term follow-up. J Bone Joint Surg (Am) 69: 1229–1231

Cervantes-Perez Col P, Toro-Perez Col A H, Rodriguez Jurado P 1980 Pulmonary involvement in rheumatoid arthritis. J Am Med Assoc 243: 1715–1719

Chait L A 1975 The treatment of burns by early tangential

excision and skin grafting. South African Med J 49: 1375–1379

Chalmers J 1978 Unusual causes of peripheral nerve compression. Hand 10: 168–175

Chalmers J 1981 Aneurysmal bone cysts of the phalanges. Hand 13: 296–300

Chan C W 1981 Intraosseous glomus tumor — case report. J Hand Surg 6: 368–369

Chan K M, Ma G F, Cheng J C, Leung P C 1984 The Krukenberg procedure: a method of treatment for unilateral anomalies of the upper limb in Chinese children. J Hand Surg (Am) 9: 548–551

Chang W H J, Thoms O J, White W L 1972 Avulsion injury of the long flexor tendons. Plastic Reconstr Surg 50: 260–264

Charters A C, Davis J W 1978 The roll-bar hand. J Trauma 18: 601–604

Chase R A 1968 The damaged index digit — a source of components to restore the crippled hand. J Bone Joint Surg 50A: 1152–1160

Chase R A 1973 Atlas of hand surgery. W B Sanders Co, Philadelphia

Chase R A 1985 Historical review of skin and soft tissue coverage of the upper extremity. Hand Clin 1: 599–608

Cheng J C, Chan K M, Ma G F, Leung P C 1984 Polydactyly of the thumb: a surgical plan based on ninety-five cases. J Hand Surg (Am) 9: 155–164

Cherup L L, Zachary L S, Gottlieb L J, Petti C A 1990 The radial forearm skin graft-fascial flap. Plastic Reconstr Surg 85: 898–902

Chicarilli Z N, Watson H K, Linberg R, Sasaki G 1986 Saddle deformity. Posttraumatic interosseous-lumbrical adhesions: review of eighty-seven cases. J Hand Surg (Am) 11: 210–218

Chick L R, Borah G B 1992 Treatment of hydrofluoric acid burns of the hand. Plastic Reconstr Surg (in press)

Chick L R, Lister G D 1991 Emergency management of thermal, electrical, and chemical burns. In: Kasdan M L (ed) Occupational hand and upper extremity injuries and diseases. Hanley & Belfus, Philadelphia

Chick L R, Lister G D, Souder L 1992 Early free flaps in the management of electrical burns. Plastic Reconstr Surg 89: 1013–1019

Childers J C 1980 Pyogenic arthritis due to Bacteroides fragilis infection. Orthopedics 3: 319–320

Chiu H Y, Chen M T 1984 Revascularization of digits after thirty-three hours of warm ischemia time: a case report. J Hand Surg (Am) 9A: 63–67

Cho K 1978 Entrapment occlusion of the ulnar artery in the hand. J Bone Joint Surg 60A: 841–843

Chow J A, Van Beek A L, Meyer D L, Johnson M C 1985 Surgical significance of the motor fascicular group of the ulnar nerve in the forearm. J Hand Surg (Am) 10: 867–872

Chow S P, Ip F K, Lau J H, Collins R J et al 1987 Mycobacterium marinum infection of the hand and wrist. Results of conservative treatment in twenty-four cases. J Bone Joint Surg (Am) 69: 1161–1168

Chow S P, Stroebel A B, Lau J H, Collins R J 1983 Mycobacterium marinum infection of the hand involving deep structures. J Hand Surg (Am) 8: 568–573

Chuinard R G, D'Ambrosia R D 1977 Human bite infections of the hand. J Bone Joint Surg 59A: 416–418

Chuinard R G, Friermood T G, Lipscomb P R 1979 The 'suicide' wrist: epidemiologic study of the injury. Orthopaedics 2: 499–502

Chun S, Palmer A K 1987 Chronic ulnar wrist pain secondary to partial rupture of the extensor carpi ulnaris tendon. J Hand Surg (Am) 12: 1032–1035

Ciano M, Burlin J R, Pardoe R, Mills R L, Hentz V R 1981 High-frequency electromagnetic radiation injury to the upper extremity: local and systemic effects. Ann Plastic Surg 7: 128–135

Claman H N 1877 New hope for neurofibromastosis — the mast cell connection. JAMA 258–283

Clare RA, Krenzelok EP 1988 Chemical burns secondary to elemental metal exposure. Am J Emerg Med 6: 355–357

Clay N R, Austin S 1988 Idiopathic thenar muscle hypertrophy. J Hand Surg (Br) 13: 100–101

Clayburgh R H, Beckenbaugh R D, Dobyns J H 1987 Carpal tunnel release in patients with diffuse peripheral neuropathy. J Hand Surg (Am)12: 380–383

Clayburgh R H, Wood M B, Cooney W P 3rd 1983 Nail bed repair and reconstruction by reverse dermal grafts. J Hand Surg (Am) 8: 594–598

Clayton M L 1965 Surgical treatment at the wrist in rheumatoid arthritis. J Bone Joint Surg 47A: 741–750

Cleary J E, Omer G E Jr 1985 Congenital proximal radio-ulnar synostosis. Natural history and functional assessment. J Bone Joint Surg (Am) 67: 539–545

Clendenin M B, Smith R J 1984 Fifth metacarpal/hamate arthrodesis for posttraumatic osteoarthritis. J Hand Surg (Am) 9: 374–378

Clifford R H, Kelly A P 1959 Diagnosis and treatment of tumors of the hand. Clin Orthopaedics 13: 204–212

Clippinger F W, Goldner J L, Roberts J M 1962 Use of the electromyogram in evaluating upper-extremity peripheral nerve lesions. J Bone Joint Surg 44A: 1047–1060

Cohen B E 1982 Local muscle flap coverage of the proximal ulna without functional loss. Plastic Reconstr Surg 70: 745–748

Cohen M, Ghosh L, Schafer M E 1987 Congenital embryonal rhabdomyosarcoma of the hand and Apert's syndrome. J Hand Surg (Am) 12: 614–617

Cohn B T, Shall L 1986 Idiopathic bilaterally symmetrical brachymetacarpia of the fourth and fifth metacarpals. J Hand Surg (Am) 11: 735–737

Coleman S S, Anson B J 1961 Arterial patterns in the hand based on a study of 650 specimens. Surg Gynecol Obstet 113: 409–424

Colen L, Bunkis J, Gordon L, Walton R 1985 Functional assessment of ray transfer for central digital loss. J Hand Surg (Am) 10: 232–237

Coles M, Smith M, Rankin E A 1989 An unusual case of dermatofibrosarcoma protuberans. J Hand Surg (Am) 14: 135–138

Coll GA 1987 Palmar dislocation of the scaphoid and lunate. J Hand Surg (Am) 12: 476–480

Colles A 1814 On fracture of the carpal extremity of the radius. Edin Med Surg J 10: 181 (reprinted in Clin Orth Rel Res (1972) 83: 3–5)

Colyer R A, Kappelman B 1981 Flexor pollicis longus tenodesis in tetraplegia at the sixth cervical level — a prospective evaluation of functional gain. J Bone Joint Surg 63A: 376–379

Committee on Injury Scaling. 1985 The abbreviated injury scale 1985 revision. American Association for Automotive Medicine, Morton Grove, IL

Comstock C P, Louis D S, Eckenrode J F 1988 Silicone wrist implant: long-term follow-up study. J Hand Surg (Am) 13: 201–205

Comtet J J, Herzberg G, Naasan I A 1989 Biomechanical basis of transfers for shoulder paralysis. Hand Clin 5: 1–14

Comtet J, Quicot L, Moyen B 1978 Compression of the deep palmar branch of the ulnar nerve by the arch of the adductor pollicis. Hand 10: 176–180

Conklin W T, Dabb R W, Danyo J J 1981 Microvascular salvage of the embolized hand. Orthopaedic Rev 10: 169–171

Constantz R, Bluestone R 1980 Diagnosis of the seronegative spondyloarthropathies: HL-A B27 testing as an aid to diagnosis. Contemp Orthopaedics 2: 141–147

Coon J, Bergan J, Bell J 1970 Hypothenar hammer syndrome: Post-traumatic digital ischemia. Surgery 68: 1122–1128

Cooney W P 3rd, Lucca M J, Chao E Y, Linscheid R L 1981 The kinesiology of the thumb trapeziometacarpal joint. J Bone Joint Surg (Am) 63: 1371–1381

Cooney W P 3rd, Wilson M R, Wood M B 1983 Intravascular fibrinolysis of small-vessel thrombosis. J Hand Surg (Am) 8: 131–138

Cooney W P 1988 Tendon transfer for median nerve palsy. Hand Clin 4: 155–165

Cooney W P, Dobyns J H, Linscheid R L 1990 Arthroscopy of the wrist: anatomy and classification of carpal instability. Arthroscopy 6: 133–140

Cooney W P, Garcia-Elias M, Dobyns J H, Linscheid R L 1989 Anatomy and mechanics of carpal instability. Surg Rounds Ortho: 15–24

Cooney W P, Linscheid R L, An K N 1984 Opposition of the thumb: an anatomic and biomechanical study of tendon transfers. J Hand Surg (Am) 9: 777–786

Cooney W P, Linscheid R L, Dobyns J H, Wood M B 1988 Scaphoid nonunion: role of anterior interpositional bone grafts. J Hand Surg (Am) 13: 635–650

Coonrad R W, Hooper W R 1973 Tennis elbow: its source, natural history, conservative and surgical management. J Bone Joint Surg 55A: 1177–1182

Copeland S A, Taylor I G 1979 Synovectomy of the elbow in rheumatoid arthritis. J Bone Joint Surg 61B: 69–74

Cornell S J 1981 Multiple glomus tumors in one digit. Hand 13: 301–302

Cosio M Q, Camp R A 1986 Percutaneous pinning of symptomatic scaphoid nonunions. J Hand Surg (Am) 11: 350–355

Costa H, Soutar D S 1988 The distally based island posterior interosseous flap. Br J Plastic Surg 41: 221–227

Cowen N J, Loftus J M 1978 Distraction augmentation manoplasty technique for lengthening digits of hands. Orthopaedic Rev 7: 45–53

Crabb D J M 1981 The value of plain radiographs in treating greasegun injuries. Hand 13: 39–42

Craigen M A, Chesney R B 1988 Metastatic adenocarcinoma of the carpus: a case report. J Hand Surg (Br) 13: 306–307

Craven P R, Green D P 1980 Cubital tunnel syndrome. Treatment by medial epicondylectomy. J Bone Joint Surg (Am) 62: 986–989

Crawford G P 1984 The molded polythene splint for mallet finger deformities. J Hand Surg (Am) 9: 231–237

Crawford G P, Offerman R J 1980 Pigmented villonodular synovitis in the hand. Hand 12: 282–287

Crawford G P, Taleisnik J 1983 Rotatory subluxation of the scaphoid after excision of dorsal carpal ganglion and wrist manipulation — a case report. J Hand Surg (Am) 8: 921–925

Creighton J J Jr, Peimer C A, Mindell E R, Boone D C et al 1985 Primary malignant tumors of the upper extremity: retrospective analysis of one hundred twenty-six cases. J Hand Surg (Am) 10: 805–814

Crick J C, Conners J J, Franco R S 1990 Irreducible palmar dislocation of the proximal interphalangeal joint with bilateral avulsion fractures. J Hand Surg (Am) 15: 460–463

Crick J C, Vandevelde A G 1986 Mycobacterium fortuitum midpalmar space abscess: a case report. J Hand Surg (Am) 11: 438–440

Cronin T D 1951 The cross-finger flap — a new method of repair. Ann Surg 17: 419–425

Crosby E B, Linscheid R L, Dobyns J H 1978 Scaphotrapezial trapezoidal arthrosis. J Hand Surg 3: 223–234

Crosby L A, Murphy R P 1988 Subperiosteal osteoid osteoma of the distal phalanx of the thumb. J Hand Surg (Am) 13: 923–925

Culver J E, Fleegler E J 1987 Osteoarthritis of the distal interphalangeal joint. Hand Clin 3: 385–403

Cunningham M W, Yousif N J, Matloub H S, Sanger J R et al 1985 Retardation of finger growth after injury to the flexor tendons. J Hand Surg (Am) 10: 115–117

Cuono C B, Watson H K 1979 The carpal boss: surgical treatment and etiological considerations. Plastic Reconstr Surg 63: 88–94

Curreri P W, Asch M J, Pruitt B A 1970 The treatment of chemical burns. J Trauma 10: 634

Curtin J, Kay N R M 1976 Hand injuries due to soccer. Hand 8: 93–95

Curtis R M 1953 Congenital arteriovenous fistulae of the hand. J Bone Joint Surg 35A: 917–928

Curtis R M 1957 Cross-finger pedicle flap in hand surgery. Ann Surg 145: 650

Curtis R M, Eversmann W W 1973 Internal neurolysis as an adjunct to the treatment of the carpal tunnel syndrome. J Bone Joint Surg 55A: 733–740

Curtis R M, Reid R L, Provost J M 1983 A staged technique for the repair of the traumatic boutonniere deformity. J Hand Surg (Am) 8: 167–171

Cusenz B J, Hallock G G 1986 Multiple anomalous tendons of the fourth dorsal compartment. J Hand Surg (Am) 11: 263–264

Cushing H 1916 Hereditary anchylosis of proximal phalangeal joints (symphalangism). Genetics 1: 90–106

Czitrom A A, Dobyns J H, Linscheid R L 1987 Ulnar variance in carpal instability. J Hand Surg (Am) 12: 205–208

Czitrom A A, Lister G D 1988 Measurement of grip strength in the diagnosis of wrist pain. J Hand Surg (Am) 13: 16–19

Dabezies E J, Schutte J P 1986 Fixation of metacarpal and phalangeal fractures with miniature plates and screws. J Hand Surg (Am) 11: 283–288

Dacey L J, Dow R W, McDaniel M D, Walsh D B, Zwolak R M, Cronenwett JL 1988 Cost-effectiveness of intra-arterial thrombolytic therapy. Arch Surg 123: 1218–1223

Dahlin D C 1987 Giant-cell-bearing lesions of bone of the hands. Hand Clin 3: 291–297

Dahners L E, Wood F M 1984 Anconeus epitrochlearis, a rare cause of cubital tunnel syndrome: a case report. J Hand Surg (Am) 9: 579–580

Dai S Y, Lin D X, Han Z, Zhoug SZ 1990 Transference of thoracodorsal nerve to musculocutaneous nerve or axillary nerve in old traumatic injury. J Hand Surg 15: 36–37

Dangles C J 1984 True aneurysm of a thumb digital artery. J Hand Surg (Am) 9: 444–445

Darrow J C Jr, Linscheid R L, Dobyns J H, Mann J M 3rd et al 1985 Distal ulnar recession for disorders of the distal radioulnar joint. J Hand Surg (Am) 10: 482–491

Davidson S F, Das S K, Smith E E 1989 Cellular schwannoma of the hand. J Hand Surg (Am) 14: 907–909

Davis T S, Graham W P, Blomain E W 1981 A ten-year experience with glomus tumors. Ann Plastic Surg 6: 297–299

Dawson W J 1989 Radius fracture after total wrist arthroplasty. J Hand Surg (Am) 14: 630–634

De Quervain F 1895 Ueber eine form von chronischer tendovaginitis. Correspondenz-Blatt F Schweizer Aerzte 25: 389–394

De Smet L, Vercauteren M 1984 Palmar dislocation of the proximal interphalangeal joint requiring open reduction: a case report. J Hand Surg (Am) 9: 717–718

DeBenedetto M R, Nappi J F, Ruff M E, Lubbers L M 1989 Doppler mapping in hypothenar syndrome: an alternative to angiography. J Hand Surg (Am) 14: 244–246

DeBoer P, Collinson P O 1981 The use of silver sulphadiazine occlusive dressings for fingertip injuries. J Bone Joint Surg 4: 545–547

Deenstra W 1988 Synovial hand infection from *Mycobacterium terrae*. J Hand Surg (Br) 13: 335–336

Defiebre B K 1978 Bowen's disease of the nail bed: a case representation and review of the literature. J Hand Surg 3: 184–186

DeHaan M R, Wong L B, Petersen D P 1987 Congenital anomaly of the thumb: aplasia of the flexor pollicis longus. J Hand Surg (Am) 12: 108–109

DeHaven K E, Wilde A H, O'Duffy J D 1972 Sporotrichosis arthritis and tenosynovitis. Report of a case cured by synovectomy and amphotericin B. J Bone Joint Surg 54A: 874–877

DeHertogh D, Ritland D, Green R 1988 Carpal tunnel syndrome due to gonococcal tenosynovitis. Ortho 2: 199–200

Dell P C 1979 Compression of the ulnar nerve at the wrist secondary to a rheumatoid synovial cyst: case report and review of the literature. J Hand Surg 4: 468–473

Dell P C 1985 Macrodactyly. Hand Clin 1: 511–524

Dell P C 1987 Distal radioulnar joint dysfunction. Hand Clin 3: 563–583

Dell P C, Brushart T M, Smith R J 1978 Treatment of trapeziometacarpal arthritis: results of resection arthroplasty. J Hand Surg 3: 243–249

Dell P C, Sheppard J E 1984 Vascularized bone grafts in the treatment of infected forearm nonunions. J Hand Surg (Am) 9: 653–658

Dellinger E P, Caplan E S, Leaver L D et al 1988 Duration of preventive antibiotic administration for open extremity fractures. Arch Surg 123: 333–339

Dellinger E P, Miller S D, Wertz M J, Grypma M, Droppert B, Anderson P A 1988 Risk of infection after open fracture of the arm or leg. Arch Surg 123: 1320–1327

Dellon A L 1978 The moving two-point discrimination test: clinical evaluation of the quickly adapting fiber/receptor system. J Hand Surg 3: 474–481

Dellon A L 1981 Evaluation of sensibility and reeducation of sensation in the hand. Williams & Wilkins, Baltimore

Dellon A L 1983 The extended palmar advancement flap. J Hand Surg (Am) 8: 190–194

Dellon A L 1984 Touch sensibility in the hand. J Hand Surg (Br) 9: 11–13

Dellon A L 1988 Operative technique for submuscular transposition of the ulnar nerve. Cont Ortho 16: 17–24

Dellon A L 1989 Review of treatment results for ulnar nerve entrapment at the elbow. J Hand Surg (Am) 14: 688–700

Dellon A L, Curtis R M, Edgerton M T 1974 Reeducation of sensation in the hand after nerve injury and repair. Plastic Reconstr Surg 53: 297–305

Dellon A L, Kallman C H 1983 Evaluation of functional sensation in the hand. J Hand Surg (Am) 8: 865–870

Dellon A L, Mackinnon S E 1984 The pronator quadratus muscle flap. J Hand Surg (Am) 9: 423–427

Dellon A L, Mackinnon S E 1986 Pain after radial sensory nerve grafting. J Hand Surg (Br) 11: 341–346

Dellon A L, Mackinnon S E 1986 Radial sensory nerve entrapment in the forearm. J Hand Surg (Am) 11: 199–205

Dellon A L, Mackinnon S E 1986 Treatment of the painful neuroma by neuroma resection and muscle implantation. Plastic Reconstr Surg 77: 427–438

Dellon A L, Mackinnon S E, Crosby P M 1987 Reliability of two-point discrimination measurements. J Hand Surg (Am) 12: 693–696

Dellon A L, Rayan G 1981 Congenital absence of the thenar muscles. Report of two cases. J Bone Joint Surg (Am) 63: 1014–1015

Dellon A L, Weiss S W, Mitch W E 1978 Bilateral extraosseous chondromas of the hand in a patient with chronic renal failure. J Hand Surg 3: 139–141

DeLuca F N, Cowen N J 1975 Median nerve compression complicating a tendon graft prosthesis. J Bone Joint Surg 57A: 553

Denman E 1979 Rupture of the extensor pollicis longus — a crush injury. Hand 11: 295–298

Denman E E 1978 The anatomy of the space of Guyon. Hand 10: 69–76

Dennis D A, Clayton M L, Ferlic D C, Patchett C E 1985 Bilateral traumatic dislocations of Volz total wrist arthroplasties: a case report. J Hand Surg (Am) 10: 503–504

Dennis D A, Ferlic D C, Clayton M L 1986 Volz total wrist arthroplasty in rheumatoid arthritis: a long-term review. J Hand Surg (Am) 11: 483–490

Derkash R S, Niebauer J J 1981 Entrapment of the posterior interosseous nerve by a fibrous band in the dorsal edge of the supinator muscle and erosion of a groove in the proximal radius. J Hand Surg 6: 524–526

Derkash R S, Niebauer J J Jr, Lane C S 1986 Long-term follow-up of metacarpal phalangeal arthroplasty with silicone Dacron prostheses. J Hand Surg (Am) 11: 553–558

Desai S S, Pearlman H S, Patel M R 1986 Clicking at the wrist due to fibroma in an anomalous lumbrical muscle: a case report and review of literature. J Hand Surg (Am) 11: 512–514

Dibbell D, Hedberg J, McGraw J, Rankin J, Souther S A 1979 Quantitative examination of the use of fluorescein in predicting viability of skin flaps. Ann Plastic Surg 3: 101–105

Dibell D G, Iverson R E et al 1970 Hydrofluoric acid burns of the hand. J Bone Joint Surg 52A: 931–936

Dick H M 1987 Malignant fibrous histiocytoma of the hand. Hand Clin 3: 263–268

Dick H M 1987 Synovial sarcoma of the hand. Hand Clin 3: 241–245

Dick H M, Angelides A C 1989 Malignant bone tumors of the hand. Hand Clin 5: 373–381

Dick T, Lamb D W, Douglas W B 1984 A wrist-powered hand prosthesis. J Bone Joint Surg (Br) 66: 742–744

Dickason W L, Barutt J P 1984 Investigation of an acute microwave-oven hand injury. J Hand Surg (Am) 9A: 132–135

DiFazio F, Mogan J 1989 Intravenous pyogenic granuloma of the hand. J Hand Surg 14A: 310–312

Dinham I M, Meggitt B F 1974 Trigger thumbs in children. J Bone Joint Surg 56B: 153–155

Dinham J M, Meggitt D F 1974 Trigger thumbs in children. J Bone Joint Surg 56B: 153

Dixon J H 1981 Non-tuberculous mycobacterial infection of the tendon sheaths in the hand. A report of six cases. J Bone Joint Surg (Br) 63B: 542–544

Dobyns J H 1985 Segmental digital transposition in congenital hand deformities. Hand Clin 1: 475–482

Dobyns J H 1987 Role of the physician in workers' compensation injuries. J Hand Surg (Am) 12: 826–829

Docken W P 1987 Clinical features and medical management of osteoarthritis at the hand and wrist. Hand Clin 3: 337–349

Dodds G A 3rd, Hale D, Jackson W T 1990 Incidence of anatomic variants in Guyon's canal. J Hand Surg (Am) 15: 352–355

Dodge L D, Brown R L, Niebauer J J, McCarroll H R Jr 1984 The treatment of mucous cysts: longterm follow-up in sixty-two cases. J Hand Surg 9A: 901–904

Doi K, Kuwata N, Sakai K, Tamaru K, Kawai S 1987 A reliable technique of free vascularized sural nerve grafting and preliminary results of clinical applications. J Hand Surg (Am) 12: 677–684

Dolphin J A 1965 Extensor tenotomy for chronic boutonniere deformity of the finger. J Bone Joint Surg 47A: 161–164

Donaldson W R, Millender L W 1978 Chronic fracture subluxation of the proximal interphalangeal joint. J Hand Surg 3: 149–153

Donovan T L, Chapman M W, Harrington K D, Nagel D A 1976 Serratia arthritis. Report of seven cases. J Bone Joint Surg 58A: 1009–1011

Dooley T W, Welsh C F, Puckett C L 1989 Noninvasive assessment of microvessels with the duplex scanner. J Hand Surg (Am) 14: 670–673

Dormandy J A, Barkley H 1979 Bilateral axillary artery aneurysms in a child. Br J Surg 66: 650

Dowd G S E 1986 Predicting stump healing following amputation for peripheral vascular disease using the transcutaneous oxygen monitor. Ann Roy Coll Surg 68: 31–35

Doyle J R 1988 Tendon xanthoma: a physical manifestation of hyperlipidemia. J Hand Surg (Am) 13: 238–241

Doyle J R, Blythe W 1975 The finger flexor tendon sheath and pulleys: anatomy and reconstruction. Symposium on tendon surgery in the hand. AAOS. Mosby, St Louis

Doyle L K, Ruby L K, Nalebuff E G, Belsky M R 1985 Osteoid osteoma of the hand. J Hand Surg (Am) 10: 408–410

Dray G J, Jablon M 1987 Clinical and radiologic features of primary osteoarthritis of the hand. Hand Clin 3: 351–369

Dray G J, Millender L H, Nalebuff E A, Philips C 1981 The surgical treatment of hand deformities in systemic lupus erythematosis. J Hand Surg 6: 339–345

Dray GJ 1989 The hand in systemic lupus erythematosus. Hand Clin 5: 145–155

Drewniany J J, Palmer A K, Flatt A E 1985 The

scaphotrapezial ligament complex: an anatomic and biomechanical study. J Hand Surg (Am) 10: 492–498

Dreyfuss U Y, Auslander L, Bialik V, Fishman J 1980 Ewing's sarcoma of the hand following recurrent trauma. A case report. Hand 12: 300–303

Dreyfuss U Y, Boome R S, Kranold D H 1986 Synovial sarcoma of the hand — literature study. J Hand Surg (Br) 11: 471–474

Dreyfuss U Y, Singer M 1985 Human bites of the hand: a study of one hundred six patients. J Hand Surg (Am) 10: 884–889

Dreyfuss U Y, Smith R J 1988 Sensory changes with prolonged double-cuff tourniquet time in hand surgery. J Hand Surg (Am) 13: 736–740

Dryer R, Buckwalter J, Flatt A, Bonfiglio M 1979 Ewing's sarcoma of the hand. J Hand Surg 4: 372–374

Duinslaeger L, Vierendeels T, Wylock P 1987 Vascular leiomyoma in the hand. J Hand Surg (Am) 12: 624–627

Duncan G J, Walker L G 1990 Herbert screw fixation of scaphoid fractures: indications and technique. Contemp Orthopaedics 21: 384–388

Dunlap J, Manske P R, McCarthy J A 1989 Perfusion of the abductor digiti quinti after transfer on a neurovascular pedicle. J Hand Surg (Am) 14: 992–995

Dupuytren G 1834 Permanent retraction of the fingers produced by an affliction of the palmar fascia. Lancet 2: 222

Earle A S, Vlastou C 1980 Crossed fingers and other tests of ulnar nerve motor function. J Hand Surg 5: 560–565

Earley M J 1989 The first web hand flap. J Hand Surg 14B: 65–69

Earley M J 1989 The second dorsal metacarpal artery neurovascular island flap. J Hand Surg (Br) 14: 434–440

Earley M J, Milner R H 1987 Dorsal metacarpal flaps. Br J Plastic Surg 40: 333–341

Eastridge C E 1972 Actinomycosis: a 24 year experience. Southern Med J 65: 839–843

Eaton R G, Akelman E, Eaton B H 1989 Fascial implant arthroplasty for treatment of radioscaphoid degenerative disease. J Hand Surg (Am) 14: 766–774

Eaton R G, Dobranski A I, Littler J W 1973 Marginal osteophyte excision in treatment of mucous cysts. J Bone Joint Surg 55A: 570–574

Eaton R G, Floyd W E 3rd 1988 Thumb metacarpophalangeal capsulodesis: an adjunct procedure to basal joint arthroplasty for collapse deformity of the first ray. J Hand Surg (Am) 13: 449–453

Eaton R G, Glickel S Z 1987 Trapeziometacarpal osteoarthritis. Staging as a rationale for treatment. Hand Clin 3: 455–471

Eaton R G, Glickel S Z, Littler J W 1985 Tendon interposition arthroplasty for degenerative arthritis of the trapeziometacarpal joint of the thumb. J Hand Surg (Am) 10: 645–654

Eaton R G, Lane L B, Littler J W, Keyser J J 1984 Ligament reconstruction for the painful thumb carpometacarpal joint: a long-term assessment. J Hand Surg (Am) 9: 692–699

Eaton R G, Littler J W 1973 Ligament reconstruction for the painful thumb carpometacarpal joint. J Bone Joint Surg 55A: 1655–1666

Eaton R G, Littler J W 1976 Joint injuries and their sequelae. Clin Plastic Surg 3: 85–98

Eaton R G, Malerich M M 1980 Volar plate arthroplasty of

the proximal interphalangeal joint: a review of ten years' experience. J Hand Surg 5: 260–268

Eckenrode J F, Louis D S, Greene T L 1986 Scaphoid-trapezium-trapezoid fusion in the treatment of chronic scapholunate instability. J Hand Surg (Am) 11: 497–502

Eckhardt W A, Palmer A K 1981 Recurrent dislocation of extensor carpi ulnaris tendon. J Hand Surg 6: 629–631

Edelman P A 1987 Chemical and electrical burns. In: Achauer B M (ed) Management of the burned patient. Appleton & Lange, Norwalk, C T, pp 183–202

Edgerton M T, Snyder C B, Webb W L 1965 Surgical treatment of congenital thumb deformities. J Bone Joint Surg 47A: 1453–1474

Edgerton M T, Tuerk D B I 1974 Macrodactyly (digital gigantism): its nature and treatment. In: Littler J W, Cramer L M, Smith J W (eds) Symposium on reconstructive hand surgery. C V Mosby Co, St Louis, pp 157–172

Egawa M, Asai T 1983 Fracture of the hook of the hamate: report of six cases and the suitability of computerized tomography. J Hand Surg (Am) 8: 393–398

Egleff D V, Verdan C 1983 Pollicization of the index finger for reconstruction of the congenitally hypoplastic or absent thumb. J Hand Surg (Am) 8: 839–848

Eguro H, Goldner J L 1973 Bilateral thrombosis of the ulnar arteries in the hands. Plastic Reconstr Surg 52: 573–578

Egyed B, Eory A, Veres T, Manninger J 1980 Measurement of electrical resistance after nerve injuries of the hand. Hand 12: 275–281

Ehrlich W, Dellon A L, Mackinnon S E 1986 Classical article: Cheiralgia paresthetica (entrapment of the radial nerve). (A translation in condensed form of Robert Wartenberg's original article published in 1932) J Hand Surg (Am) 11: 196–199

Eichenblat M, Wass A, Kessler I 1982 Synovectomy of the elbow in rheumatoid arthritis. J Bone Joint Surg 64A: 1074

Eichenholtz S N, Deangelis C 1965 Squamous cell carcinoma of nail bed. J Am Med Assoc 191: 102–104

Eiken O 1979 Implant arthroplasty of the scapho-trapezial joint. Scand J Plastic Reconstr Surg 13: 461–468

Eiken O, Jonsson K 1980 Carpal bone cysts. A clinical and radiographic study. Scand J Plastic Reconstr Surg 14: 285–290

Eiken O, Hagberg L, Lundborg G 1981 Evolving biologic concepts as applied to tendon surgery. Clin Plastic Surg 8: 1–12

Eisenbaum S L, Eversmann W W Jr 1985 Juvenile aponeurotic fibroma of the hand. J Hand Surg (Am) 10: 622–625

Ejeskar A 1988 Upper limb surgical rehabilitation in high-level tetraplegia. Hand Clin 4: 585–599

Ekerot L 1977 Postanesthetic ulnar neuropathy at the elbow. Scand J Plastic Reconstr Surg Hand Surg 11: 225–229

Ekerot L, Eiken O 1981 Tuberculosis of the hand. Scand J Plastic Reconstr Surg 15: 77–79

Ekerot L, Eiken O, Jonsson K, Lindstrom C 1981 Malignant hemangioendothelioma of metacarpal bones. Scand J Plastic Reconstr Surg 15: 73–76

Ellenhorn M J, Barceloux D G 1988 Medical toxicology: diagnosis and treatment of human poisoning. Elsevier, New York

Elliott R, Hoehn J, Stayman J W 1979 Management of the viable soft tissue cover in degloving injuries. Hand 11: 69–71

Ellison M R, Flatt A E, Kelly K I 1974 Ulnar drift of the finger in rheumatoid disease. J Bone Joint Surg 53A: 1061–1082

Ellison M R, Kelly K I, Flatt A E 1971 The results of surgical synovectomy of the digital joints in rheumatoid disease. J Bone Joint Surg 53A: 1041–1060

Ellstein J, Xeller C, Fromowitz F, Elias J M et al 1984 Soft tissue T cell lymphoma of the forearm: a case report. J Hand Surg (Am) 9: 346–350

Elsahy N I 1976 Doppler ultrasound detection of displaced neurovascular bundles in Dupuytren's contracture. Plastic Reconstr Surg 57: 104–105

Elstrom J A, Pankovich A M, Egwele R 1978 Extra-articular low-velocity gunshot fractures of the radius and ulna. J Bone Joint Surg 60A: 335–341

Elton R C 1975 Gunshot and fragment wounds of the hand. Contemp Surg 7: 13–18

Engber W D, Flatt A E 1977 Camptodactyly: an analysis of sixty-six patients and twenty-four operations. J Hand Surg 2: 216–224

Engber W D, Gmeiner J G 1980 Palmar cutaneous branch of the ulnar nerve. J Hand Surg 5: 26–29

Engdahl D E, Schacherer T G 1989 A new method of evaluating angulation of scaphoid nonunions. J Hand Surg (Am) 14: 1033–1034

Engel J, Salai M, Yaffe B, Tadmor R 1987 The role of three dimension computerized imaging in hand surgery. J Hand Surg (Br) 12: 349–352

Engel J, Zinneman H, Tsur H, Farin I 1978 Carpal tunnel syndrome due to carpal osteophyte. Hand 10: 283–284

Engkvist O, Johansson S H 1980 Perichondrial arthroplasty. Scand J Plastic Reconstr Surg 14: 71–87

Engkvist O, Lundborg U, Lundborg G 1979 Rupture of the extensor pollicis longus tendon after fracture of the lower end of the radius. A clinical and microangiographic study. Hand 11: 76–86

Engkvist O, Ohlsen L N 1979 Reconstruction of articular cartilage with free autologous perichondrial grafts: an experimental study in rabbits. Scand J Plastic Reconstr Surg 13: 269–274

Engkvist O, Skoog V, Pastacaldi P, Yormuk E, Juhlin R 1979 The cartilaginous potential of the perichondrium in rabbit ear and rib: a comparative study in vivo and vitro. Scand J Plastic Reconstr Surg 13: 275–280

Enna C 1978 Adenoid basal cell epithelioma involving a finger. Hand 10: 309–311

Enneking W F 1983 Musculoskeletal surgery. Churchill Livingstone, Edinburgh

Entin M A 1976 Syndactyly of upper limb. Clin Plastic Surg 3: 129–140

Enzinger F M 1970 Epithelioid sarcoma. Cancer 26: 1029–1040

Epstein L I, Bennett J E 1970 Syndactyly with ipsilateral chest deformity. Plastic Reconstr Surg 46: 236–240

Erb W H 1874 Uber eine eigenthumliche Localisation von Lahemengen im Plexus brachialis. Verhandl. d. Naturhist. Medical (Heidelberg) 2: 130

Ernst D, Hurlow R, Strachan C, Chandler S 1978 The assessment of digital vessel disease by dynamic hand scanning. Hand 10: 217–225

Ertel A N 1989 Flexor tendon ruptures in rheumatoid arthritis. Hand Clin 5: 177–190

Ertel A N, Millender L H, Nalebuff E, McKay D, Leslie B 1988 Flexor tendon ruptures in patients with rheumatoid arthritis. J Hand Surg (Am) 13: 860–866

Eversmann W W 1988 Tendon transfers for combined nerve injuries. Hand Clin 4: 187–199

Ewald F C, Scheinberg R D, Poss R, Thomas W H, Scott R D, Sledge C B 1980 Capitellocondylar total elbow arthroplasty. J Bone Joint Surg 62A: 1259–1263

Eyring E J, Longert A, Bass J C 1971 Synovectomy in juvenile rheumatoid arthritis. J Bone Joint Surg 53A: 638–651

Faciszewski T, Coleman D A 1989 Human bite wounds. Hand Clin 5: 561–569

Fahmy N R M, Noble J 1981 Ulnar nerve palsy as a complication of synovial osteochondromatosis of the elbow. Hand 13: 308–310

Fahrer M, Millroy P J 1981 Ulnar compression neuropathy due to an anomalous abductor digiti minimi — clinical and anatomic study. J Hand Surg 6: 266–268

Failla J M, Amadio P C 1988 Recognition and treatment of uncommon carpal fractures. Hand Clin 4: 469–476

Falconer D P 1988 Tendon transfers about the shoulder and elbow in the spinal cord injured patient. Hand Clin 4: 211–221

Fanconi G 1967 Familial constitutional panmyelocytopathy, Fanconi's anemia (FA). I. Clin Asp Semin Hematol 4: 233

Farmer C, Mann R 1966 Human bite infections of the hand. Southern Med J 59: 515–518

Farmer R, Gifford R, Hines E 1961 Raynaud's disease with sclerodactylia. A follow-up study of seventy-one patients. Circulation 23: 13–15

Farrell H F 1979 Pain and the pronator teres syndrome. Bull Hosp Joint Dis 37: 59–62

Fatti J F, Palmer A K, Mosher J F 1986 The long-term results of Swanson silicone rubber interpositional wrist arthroplasty. J Hand Surg (Am) 11: 166–175

Fayman M, Schein M, Braun S 1985 A foreign body related actinomycosis of a finger. J Hand Surg (Am) 10: 411–412

Fee N F, Dobranski A, Bisla R S 1977 Gas gangrene complicating open forearm fractures. Report of five cases. J Bone Joint Surg 59A: 135–138

Feldman F 1987 Primary bone tumors of the hand and carpus. Hand Clin 3: 269–289

Feldman R G, Travers P H, Chirico-Post J, Keyserling W M 1987 Risk assessment in electronic assembly workers: carpal tunnel syndrome. J Hand Surg (Am) 12: 849–855

Felty A R 1924 Chronic arthritis in the adult associated with splenomegaly and leukopenia. Bull Johns Hopkins Hosp 35: 16–20

Ferlic D C 1983 Pyoderma gangrenosum presenting as an acute suppurative hand infection — a case report. J Hand Surg (Am) 8: 573–575

Ferlic D C 1989 Boutonniere deformities in rheumatoid arthritis. Hand Clin 5: 215–222

Ferlic D C, Busbee G A, Clayton M L 1977 Degenerative arthritis of the carpometacarpal joint of the thumb: a clinical follow-up of eleven Neibauer prostheses. J Hand Surg 2: 212–215

Ferlic D C, Turner B D, Clayton M L 1983 Compression arthrodesis of the thumb. J Hand Surg (Am) 8: 207–210

Ferlic D C, Clayton M 1978 Flexor tenosynovectomy in the rheumatoid finger. J Hand Surg 3: 364–367

Ferlic C D, Morin P 1989 Idiopathic avascular necrosis of the scaphoid: Preiser's disease? J Hand Surg 14A: 13–16

Fernandez D L 1981 Irreducible radiocarpal fracture dislocation and radioulnar dissociation with entrapment of the ulnar nerve, artery and flexor profundus II–V — case report. J Hand Surg 6: 456–461

Fernandez D L 1984 A technique for anterior wedge-shaped grafts for scaphoid nonunions with carpal instability. J Hand Surg (Am) 9: 733–737

Fernandez D L 1990 Anterior bone grafting and conventional lag screw fixation to treat scaphoid nonunions. J Hand Surg (Am) 15: 140–147

Fernandez D L, Ghillani R 1987 External fixation of complex carpal dislocations: a preliminary report. J Hand Surg (Am) 12: 335–347

Fernandez G N 1988 Locking of a metacarpo-phalangeal joint caused by a haemangioma of the volar plate. J Hand Surg (Br) 13: 323–324

Ferraiouli E B 1968 Repair of the disrupted flexor mechanism of the hand. Asoc Med Puerto Rico Bol 60: 11–16

Ferrari B, Steffee A D 1986 Trapeziometacarpal total joint replacement using the Steffee prosthesis. J Bone Joint Surg (Am) 68: 1177–1184

Fess E E 1986 The need for reliability and validity in hand assessment instruments. J Hand Surg (Am) 11: 621–623

Field J H 1981 Posterior interosseous nerve palsy secondary to synovial chondromatosis of the elbow joint. J Hand Surg 6: 336–338

Field J H, Krag D O 1973 Congenital constricting bands and congenital amputation of the fingers: placental studies. J Bone Joint Surg 55A: 1035–1041

Figgie M P, Inglis A E, Sobel M, Bohn W W, Fisher D A 1990 Metacarpal-phalangeal joint arthroplasty of the rheumatoid thumb. J Hand Surg (Am) 15: 210–216

Figgie M P, Ranawat C S, Inglis A E, Sobel M, Figgie H E 3rd 1990 Trispherical total wrist arthroplasty in rheumatoid arthritis. J Hand Surg (Am) 15: 217–223

Finkelstein H 1930 Stenosing tendovaginitis at the radial styloid process. J Bone Joint Surg 12: 509–540

Finsterbush A, Husseini N, Rousso M 1981 Multifocal hemangioendothelioma of bones in the hand — a case report. J Hand Surg 6: 353–356

Fissette J, Onkelirx A, Fandi N 1981 Carpal and Guyon tunnel syndrome in burns at the wrist. J Hand Surg 6: 13–15

Fisson J M, Shea F W, Goldin W 1968 Lesions of the flexor carpi radialis tendon and sheath causing pain at the wrist. J Bone Joint Surg 50B: 359

Fitch R D, Urbaniak J R, Ruderman R 1984 Conjoined flexor and extensor pollicis longus tendons in the hypoplastic thumb. J Hand Surg (Am) 9: 417–419

Fitzgerald R H, Brewer N S, Dahlin D C 1976 Squamous cell carcinoma complicating chronic osteomyelitis. J Bone Joint Surg 58A: 1146–1148

Fitzpatrick D 1989 Arthroscopic surgery of the wrist. Can Oper Room Nurs J 7: 4, 6, 8–9

Fitzpatrick D J, Bullough P G 1977 Giant cell tumor of the lunate bone: a case report. J Hand Surg 2: 269–270

Flatt A E 1957 The thenar flap. J Bone Joint Surg 39B: 80–85

Flatt A E 1966 Closed and open fractures of the hand. Fundamentals of management. Postgrad Med 39: 17–26

Flatt A E 1972 Care of minor hand injuries, 3rd edn. C V Mosby, St Louis

Flatt A E 1977 The care of congenital hand anomalies. C V Mosby, St Louis

Flatt A E 1980 Digital artery sympathectomy. J Hand Surg 5: 550–556

Flatt A E 1983 Care of the arthritic hand, 4th edn. C V Mosby, St Louis

Flatt A E, Wood V 1970 Multiple dorsal rotation flaps from the hand for thumb web contractures. Plastic Reconstr Surg 45: 258–262

Flatt A E, Wood V E 1975 Rigid digits or symphalangism. Hand 7: 197–214

Fleegler E J 1987 Tumors involving the skin of the upper extremity. Hand Clin 3: 197–212

Fleegler E J, Marks K E, Sebek B A, Groppe C W, Belhobek G 1980 Osteosarcoma of the hand. Hand 12: 316–322

Fleischer A, McGrath M H 1984 Rheumatoid nodulosis of the hand. J Hand Surg (Am) 9: 404–411

Fletcher A G, Horn R C 1951 Giant cell tumors of tendon sheath origin. A consideration of bone involvement and report of two cases with extensive bone destruction. Ann Surg 133: 374–385

Flint M H 1966 Plastic injection moulding injury. Br J Plastic Surg 19: 70–78

Floyd T, Burger R S, Sciaroni C A 1990 Bilateral palmaris profundus causing bilateral carpal tunnel syndrome. J Hand Surg (Am) 15: 364–366

Floyd W E 3rd, Gebhardt M C, Emans J B 1987 Intra-articular entrapment of the median nerve after elbow dislocation in children. J Hand Surg (Am) 12: 704–707

Fluhr J E, Farrow A, Nelson S 1989 Vitamin B6 levels in patients with carpal tunnel syndrome. Arch Surg 124: 1329–1330

Forster R S, Fu F H 1985 Reflex sympathetic dystrophy in children: a case report and review of literature. Orthopedics 8: 475–476

Forsythe R L, Bajaj P, Engeron O, Shadid E A 1978 The treatment of squamous cell carcinoma of the hand. Hand 10: 104–108

Foucher G, Sammut D, Citron N 1990 Free vascularized toe-joint transfer in hand reconstruction: a series of 25 patients. Recon Microsurg 6: 201–208

Foucher G, van Genechten F, Merle N, Michon J 1984 A compound radial artery forearm flap in hand surgery: an original modification of the Chinese forearm flap. Br J Plastic Surg 37: 139–148

Frankel V H 1977 The Terry-Thomas sign. Clin Ortho 129: 321

Frantz C H, O'Rahilly R 1961 Congenital skeletal limb deficiencies. J Bone Joint Surg 43: 1202

Frassica F J, Amadio P C, Wold L E, Beabout J W 1988 Aneurysmal bone cyst: clinicopathologic features and treatment of ten cases involving the hand. J Hand Surg (Am) 13: 676–683

Frassica F J, Amadio P C, Wold L E, Dobyns J H, Linscheid R L 1989 Primary malignant bone tumors of the hand. J Hand Surg (Am) 14: 1022–1028

Freedlander E, Dickson W A, McGrouther D A 1986 The present role of the groin flap in hand trauma in the light of a long-term review. J Hand Surg (Br) 11: 187–190

Freehafer A A, Kelly C M, Peckham P H 1984 Tendon transfer for the restoration of upper limb function after a cervical spinal cord injury. J Hand Surg (Am) 9: 887–893

Freehafer A A, Peckham P H, Keith M W 1988 New concepts on treatment of the upper limb in the tetraplegic. Surgical restoration and functional neuromuscular stimulation. Hand Clin 4: 563–574

Freehafer A A, Peckham P H, Keith M W, Mendelson L S 1988 The brachioradialis: anatomy, properties, and value for tendon transfer in the tetraplegic. J Hand Surg (Am) 13: 99–104

Freehafer A A, Vonhaam E, Allen V 1974 Tendon transfers to improve grasp after injuries of the cervical spinal cord. J Bone Joint Surg 56A: 951–959

Freeland A E, Finley J S 1984 Displaced vertical fracture of the trapezium treated with a small cancellous lag screw. J Hand Surg (Am) 9: 843–845

Freeland A E, Finley J S 1986 Displaced dorsal oblique fracture of the hamate treated with a cortical mini lag screw. J Hand Surg (Am) 11: 656–658

Freeland A E, Jabaley M E, Burkhalter W E, Chaves A M 1984 Delayed primary bone grafting in the hand and wrist after traumatic bone loss. J Hand Surg (Am) 9A: 22–28

Freeland A E, Senter B S 1989 Septic arthritis and osteomyelitis. Hand Clin 5: 533–552

Freeman A M, Meland N B 1989 Angioleiomyomas of the extremities: report of a case and review of the Mayo clinic experience. Plastic Reconstr Surg 83: 328–331

Freeman B H, Hay E L 1985 Nonunion of the capitate: a case report. J Hand Surg (Am) 10: 187–190

Freeman E A, Sheldon J H 1938 Craniocarpotarsal dystrophy. Undescribed congenital malformations. Arch Dis Child 13: 277

Freiberg A, Mulholland R S, Levine R 1989 Nonoperative treatment of trigger fingers and thumbs. J Hand Surg (Am) 14: 553–558

Freiburg A, Manktelow R 1972 The Kutler repair for fingertip amputations. Plastic Reconstr Surg 50: 371–375

Frey M, Mandl H, Holle J 1980 Secondary operations after replantations. Chirurgia Plastica 5: 235–241

Froehlich J A, Akelman E, Herndon J H 1988 Extensor tendon injuries at the proximal interphalangeal joint. Hand Clin 4: 25–37

Frohse F, Frankel M 1908 Die Muskaln des Menschlichen Aunes. Bardelehen's Handbuch der Anatomie des Manschlichen. Fischer, Jena

Froimson A I 1971 Hand reconstruction in arthritis mutilans. J Bone Joint Surg 53A: 1377–1382

Froimson A I 1981 Osteotomy for digital deformity. J Hand Surg 6: 585–589

Froimson A I 1987 Benign solid tumors. Hand Clin 3: 213–217

Froimson A I 1987 Tendon interposition arthroplasty of carpometacarpal joint of the thumb. Hand Clin 3: 489–505

Froimson A I, Zahrawi F 1980 Treatment of compression neuropathy of the ulnar nerve at the elbow by epicondylectomy and neurolysis. J Hand Surg 5: 391–395

Froment M J 1915 La paralysie de l'adducteur du pouce et le signe de la prehension. Rev Neurol 28: 1236–1240

Fromont M J 1895 Anomalies musculaires multiples de la main. Absence du flechisseur propre du pouce. Absence des muscles de l'eminence thenar; lombricaux supplementaires. Bull Soc Anat Paris 70: 395–401

Frykman E B, Af Ekenstam F, Wadin K 1988 Triscaphoid arthrodesis and its complications. J Hand Surg (Am) 13: 844–849

Frykman G K, O'Brien B M, Morrison W A, MacLeod A M 1986 Functional evaluation of the hand and foot after one-stage toe-to-hand transfer. J Hand Surg (Am) 11: 9–17

Frykman G K, Taleisnik J, Peters G, Kaufman R et al 1986 Treatment of nonunited scaphoid fractures by pulsed electromagnetic field and cast. J Hand Surg (Am) 11: 344–349

Frykman G, Wood V 1978 Peripheral nerve hamartoma with macrodactyly in the hand: report of three cases and review of the literature. J Hand Surg 3: 307–312

Fryktman E 1980 Dislocation of the triquetrum. Scand J Plastic Reconstr Surg 14: 205–207

Frymoyer J W, Bland J 1973 Carpal tunnel syndrome in patients with myxedematous arthropathy. J Bone Joint Surg 55A: 78–82

Fuhs S E, Herndon J H 1979 Aneurysmal bone cysts involving the hand: a review and report of two cases. J Hand Surg 4: 160–164

Fultz C W, Lester D K, Hunter J M 1986 Single stage lengthening by intercalary bone graft in patients with congenital hand deformities. J Hand (Br) 11:40–46

Furnas D W 1985 Z-plasties and related procedures for the hand and upper limb. Hand Clin 1: 649–665

Furnas D W, Achauer B M 1983 Microsurgical transfer of the great toe to the radius to provide prehension after partial avulsion of the hand. J Hand Surg (Am) 8: 453–460

Furnas D, Spinner M 1978 The 'sign of horns' in the diagnosis of injury or disease of the extensor digitorum communis of the hand. Br J Plastic Surg 31: 263–265

Fyfe I S, MacFarlane A 1980 Pigmented villonodular synovitis of the hand. Hand 12: 179–188

Gaal A S, Doyle J R, Larsen I J 1988 Symphalangism in Hawaii: a study of three distinct ethnic pedigrees. J Hand Surg (Am) 13: 783–787

Gabbiani G, Majho G 1972 Dupuytren's contracture: fibroblast contraction? Am J Pathol 66: 131–138

Gainor B J 1985 Simultaneous dislocation of the hamate and pisiform: a case report. J Hand Surg (Am) 10: 88–90

Gaisford J C 1960 Tumors of the hand. Surg Clin North Am 40: 549

Gama C 1983 Extensor digitorum brevis manus: a report on 38 cases and a review of the literature. J Hand Surg (Am) 8: 578–582

Gamble J G, Mochizuki C, Rinsky L A 1989 Trapeziometacarpal abnormalities in Ehlers–Danlos syndrome. J Hand Surg (Am) 14: 89–94

Ganel A, Engel J, Luboshitz S, Melamed R, Rimon S 1981 Choline acetyltransferase nerve identification method in early and late nerve repair. Ann Plast Surg 6: 228–230

Gansel J, Waters R, Gellman H 1990 Transfer of the pronator teres tendon to the tendons of the flexor digitorum profundus in tetraplegia. J Bone Joint Surg (Am) 72: 427–432

Ganzhorn R W, Baliri G, Horowitz M 1981 Osteochondroma of the distal phalanx. J Hand Surg 6: 625–626

Garcia G, McQueen D 1981 Bilateral suprascapular nerve entrapment syndrome. Case report and review of the literature. J Bone Joint Surg 63A: 491–492

Garcia-Elias M 1987 Dorsal fractures of the triquetrum-avulsion or compression fractures? J Hand Surg (Am) 12: 266–268

Garcia-Elias M, An K N, Amadio P C, Cooney W P, Linscheid RL 1989 Reliability of carpal angle determinations. J Hand Surg (Am) 14: 1017–1021

Garcia-Elias M, An K N, Cooney W P 3rd, Linscheid R L, Chao E Y 1989 Stability of the transverse carpal arch: an experimental study. J Hand Surg (Am) 14: 277–282

Garcia-Elias M, Cooney W P, An K N, Linscheid R L, Chao EY 1989 Wrist kinematics after limited intercarpal arthrodesis. J Hand Surg (Am) 14: 791–799

Garcia-Elias M, Dobyns J H, Cooney W P 3rd, Linscheid RL 1989 Traumatic axial dislocations of the carpus. J Hand Surg (Am) 14: 446–457

Garcia-Elias M, Vall A, Salo J M, Lluch A L 1988 Carpal

alignment after different surgical approaches to the scaphoid: a comparative study. J Hand Surg (Am) 13: 604–612

Garden R S 1961 Tennis elbow. J Bone Joint Surg 43B: 100–106

Garfin S R, Mubarak S J, Evans K L, Hargens A R, Akeson W H 1981 Quantification of intracompartmental pressure and volume under plaster casts. J Bone Joint Surg 63A: 449–453

Garn S M, Rohmann C G, Silverman F N 1967 Radiographic standards for postnatal ossification and tooth calcification. Med Radiogr Photogr 43: 45–66

Garner R W, Mowat A G, Hazleman B L 1973 Wound healing after operations on patients with rheumatoid arthritis. J Bone Joint Surg 55B: 134–144

Garrett W E Jr, Seaber A V, Boswick J, Urbaniak J R, Goldner J L 1984 Recovery of skeletal muscle after laceration and repair. J Hand Surg (Am) 9: 683–692

Garrod A E 1875 Concerning pads upon the finger joints and their clinical relationships. Br Med J 1: 665

Gartsman G M, Kovach J C, Crouch C C, Noble P C, Bennett J B 1986 Carpal arch alteration after carpal tunnel release. J Hand Surg (Am) 11: 372–374

Gartsman G M, Ranawat C S 1984 Treatment of osteoid osteoma of the proximal phalanx by use of cryosurgery. J Hand Surg (Am) 9: 275–277

Gaul J S 1969 Radial innervated cross-finger flap from index to provide sensory pulp to injured thumbs. J Bone Joint Surg 51A: 1257–1263

Gaul J S Jr 1983 Electrical fascicle identification as an adjunct to nerve repair. J Hand Surg (Am) 8: 289–296

Gaul J S Jr 1986 Electrical fascicle identification as an adjunct to nerve repair. Hand Clin 2: 709–722

Gaul J S Jr 1987 A palmar-hinged flap for reconstruction of traumatic thumb defects. J Hand Surg (Am) 12: 415–421

Gebhardt M C, Mankin H J 1988 Osteosarcomas: a review and update — Part I. Surg Rounds Ortho 21–30

Gebhardt M C, Mankin H J 1988 Osteosarcomas: the treatment controversy — Part II. Surg Rounds Ortho 25–42

Gedda K O 1954 Studies on Bennett's fracture: anatomy, roentgenology, and therapy. Acta Chir Scand (suppl): 193: 5–108

Geister J H, Eversmann W W 1978 Closed system venography in the evaluation of upper extremity hemangiomas. J Hand Surg 3: 173–178

Gelberman R H, Aronson D, Weisman M H 1980 Carpal tunnel syndrome. J Bone Joint Surg 62A: 1181–1184

Gelberman R H, Bauman T, Menon J, Akeson W 1975 Ulnar variance in Kienbock's disease. J Bone Joint Surg 57A: 674–676

Gelberman R H, Blasingame J P 1981 The timed Allen test. J Trauma 21: 477–479

Gelberman R H, Gould R N, Hargens A R, Vande Berg J S 1983 Lacerations of the ulnar artery: hemodynamic, ultrastructural, and compliance changes in the dog. J Hand Surg (Am) 8: 306–309

Gelberman R H, Hergenroeder P T, Hargens A R, Lundburg G N, Akeson W H 1981 The carpal tunnel syndrome — study of carpal pressures. J Bone Joint Surg 63A: 380–383

Gelberman R H, Nunley J A, Koman L A, Gould J S et al 1982 The results of radial and ulnar arterial repair in the forearm. Experience in three medical centers. J Bone Joint Surg (Am) 64: 383–387

Gelberman R H, Panagis J S, Taleisnik J, Baumgaertner M

1983 The arterial anatomy of the human carpus. Part I. The extraosseous vascularity. J Hand Surg (Am) 8: 367–375

Gelberman R H, Verdeck W N, Brodhead W T 1975 Supraclavicular nerve-entrapment syndrome. J Bone Joint Surg 57A: 119

Gelberman R, Goldner J L 1978 Congenital arteriovenous fistulas of the hand. J Hand Surg 3: 451–454

Gelberman R, Posch J L, Jurist J M 1975 High-pressure injection injuries of the hand. J Bone Joint Surg 57A: 935–937

Gelberman R, Urbaniak J, Bright D, Levin L S 1978 Digital sensibility following replantation. J Hand Surg 3: 313–319

Gelberman T H, Menon J, Fronek A 1980 The peripheral pulse following arterial injury. J Trauma 20: 948–950

Geller E R, Gursel E 1986 A unique case of high-pressure injection injury of the hand. J Trauma 26: 483–485

Geller H S, Tofte R W, Cunningham B L 1983 *Aeromonas hydrophila* wound infection of the hand initially presenting as clostridial myonecrosis. J Hand Surg (Am) 8: 333–335

Gellis M, Pool R 1977 Two-point discrimination distances in the normal hand and forearm. Plastic Reconstr Surg 59: 57–63

Gellman H, Kan D, Gee V, Kuschner S H, Botte M J 1989 Analysis of pinch and grip strength after carpal tunnel release. J Hand Surg (Am) 14: 863–864

Gervis W H 1973 A review of excision of the trapezium for osteoarthritis of the trapezio-metacarpal joint after 25 years. J Bone Joint Surg 55B: 56

Ghiam G F, Bora F W 1978 Osteoid osteoma of the carpal bones. J Hand Surg 3: 280–283

Giannakis A, Papachristou G, Tiniakos G, Chrysafidis G, Hartofilakidis-Garofalidis G 1977 Osteoid osteoma of the terminal phalanges. Hand 9: 295–300

Gibson C T, Manske P R 1987 Isolated avulsion of a flexor digitorum superficialis tendon insertion. J Hand Surg (Am) 12: 601 602

Gifford D B, Patzakis M, Ivler D, Swezey L 1975 Septic arthritis due to *Pseudomonas* in heroin addicts. J Bone Joint Surg 57A: 631–635

Gilbert A 1982 Toe transfers for congenital hand defects. J Hand Surg 7: 118–124

Gilbert A 1985 Reconstruction of congenital hand defects with microvascular toe transfers. Hand Clin 1: 351–360

Gilbert A 1989 Congenital absence of the thumb and digits. J Hand Surg (Br) 14: 6–17

Gilbert A, Romana C, Ayatti R 1988 Tendon transfers for shoulder paralysis in children. Hand Clin 4: 633–642

Gilbert M S, Robinson A, Baez A, Gupta S et al 1988 Carpal tunnel syndrome in patients who are receiving long-term renal hemodialysis. J Bone Joint Surg (Am) 70: 1145–1153

Gilula L A 1979 Carpal injuries: analytic approach and case exercises. Am J Roentgenol 133: 509

Given K S, Puckett C L, Kleinert H E 1978 Ulnar artery thrombosis. Plastic Reconstr Surg 61: 405–411

Glass A G, Hoover R N 1989 The emerging epidemic of melanoma and squamous cell cancer. JAMA 262: 2097–2100

Glasson D W, Lovie M J 1988 The ulnar island flap in hand and forearm reconstruction. Br J Plastic Surg 41: 349–353

Glickel S Z 1988 Hand infections in patients with acquired immunodeficiency syndrome. J Hand Surg (Am) 13: 770–775

Godina M 1986 Arterial autografts in microvascular surgery. Plastic Reconstr Surg 78: 293–294

Godina M 1986 Early microsurgical reconstruction of complex trauma of the extremities. Plastic Reconstr Surg 78: 285–292

Godina M 1991 A thesis. Presernova Druzba, Ljubljana

Godina M, Bajec J, Baraga A 1986 Salvage of the mutilated upper extremity with temporary ectopic implantation of the undamaged part. Plastic Reconstr Surg 78: 295–299

Goldberg B J, Light T R, Blair S J 1989 Ulnar neuropathy at the elbow: results of medial epicondylectomy. J Hand Surg (Am) 14: 182–188

Goldberg B, Eversmann W W, Eitzen E M 1982 Invasive aspergillosis of the hand. J Hand Surg 7: 38–42

Goldberg B, Heller A P 1987 Dorsal dislocation of the triquetrum with rotary subluxation of the scaphoid. J Hand Surg (Am) 12: 119–122

Goldberg I, Amit S, Bahar A, Seelenfreund M 1981 Complete dislocation of the trapezium (multangulum majus). J Hand Surg 6: 193–195

Goldberg M J, Bartoshesky L E 1985 Congenital hand anomaly: etiology and associated malformations. Hand Clin 1: 405–415

Goldberg N H, Watson H K 1982 Composite toe (phalanx and epiphysis) transfers in the reconstruction of the aphalangic hand. J Hand Surg 7: 454–459

Goldner J L 1983 Pain: general review and selected problems affecting the upper extremity. J Hand Surg (Am) 8: 740–745

Goldner J L 1988 Surgical reconstruction of the upper extremity in cerebral palsy. Hand Clin 4: 223–265

Goldner R D, Fitch R D, Nunley J A, Aitken M S, Urbaniak J R 1987 Demographics and replantation. J Hand Surg (Am) 12: 961–965

Goldner R D, Stevanovic M V, Nunley J A, Urbaniak J R 1989 Digital replantation at the level of the distal interphalangeal joint and the distal phalanx. J Hand Surg 14: 214–220

Goldstein E J, Barones M F, Miller T A 1983 *Eikenella corrodens* in hand infections. J Hand Surg (Am) 8: 563–567

Goldstein E, Miller T, Citron D, Finegold S 1978 Infections following clenched-fist injury: a new perspective. J Hand Surg 3: 455–457

Goldstein E, Miller T, Citron D, Wield B, Finegold S 1979 Clenched-fist injuries: infection and empiric antibiotic selection. Contemp Orthopaedics 1: 30–33

Goldstein S A, Imbriglia J E 1986 Fibrous hamartoma of the wrist in infancy. J Hand Surg (Am) 11: 847–849

Goldstein S A, Sturim H S 1985 Intraosseous nerve transposition for treatment of painful neuromas. J Hand Surg (Am) 10: 270–274

Gonzalez R I 1985 The use of skin grafts in the treatment of Dupuytren's contracture. Hand Clin 1: 641–647

Goodman M I, Millender L H, Nalebuff E A, Philips C A 1980 Arthroplasty of the rheumatoid wrist with silicone rubber: an early evaluation. J Bone Joint Surg 5: 114–121

Goodman M, Shankman G B 1983 Palmar dislocation of the trapezoid — a case report. J Hand Surg (Am) 8: 606–609

Goodman M L, Shankman GB 1984 Update: palmar dislocation of the trapezoid — a case report. J Hand Surg (Am) 9A: 127–131

Gordon L, Buncke H J, Alpert B S, Wilson C, Kock R A 1985 Free vascularized osteocutaneous transplants from the groin for delayed primary closure in the management of loss of soft-tissue and bone in the hand and wrist. Report of two cases. J Bone Joint Surg (Am) 67: 958–964

Gordon L, Leitner D W, Buncke H J, Alpert B S 1985 Hand reconstruction for multiple amputations by double microsurgical toe transplantation. J Hand Surg (Am) 10: 218–225

Gordon L, Monsanto E H 1987 Acute vascular compromise after avulsion of the distal phalanx with the flexor digitorum profundus tendon. J Hand Surg (Am) 12: 259–261

Gordon S 1964 Dupuytren's contracture, plantar involvement. Br J Plastic Surg 17: 421–423

Gordon S L 1972 Scaphoid and lunate dislocation. J Bone Joint Surg 54A: 1769–1772

Gore D R 1971 Carpometacarpal dislocation producing compression of the deep branch of the ulnar nerve. J Bone Joint Surg 53A: 1387–1390

Gorkisch K, Boese-Landgraf J, Vaubel E 1984 Treatment and prevention of amputation neuromas in hand surgery. Plastic Reconstr Surg 73: 293–299

Gorsche T S, Wood M B 1988 Mutilating corn-picker injuries of the hand. J Hand Surg (Am) 13: 423–427

Gottschalk R G, Smith R T 1963 Chondrosarcoma of the hand. J Bone Joint Surg 45A: 141–150

Gozna E R, Harris W R 1979 Traumatic winging of the scapula. J Bone Joint Surg 61A: 1230–1233

Grace T G, Omer G E 1980 The management of upper extremity pit viper wounds. J Hand Surg 5: 168–177

Grad J B, Beasley R W 1985 Fingertip reconstruction. Hand Clin 1: 667–676

Graham T J, Stern P J, True M S 1990 Classification and treatment of postburn metacarpophalangeal joint extension contractures in children. J Hand Surg (Am) 15: 450–456

Graham W P III 1973 Variations of the motor branch of the median nerve at the wrist. Plastic Reconstr Surg 51: 90–91

Granberry W M, Bryan W 1978 Chondrosarcoma of the trapezium: a case report. J Hand Surg 3: 277–279

Granberry W M, Mangum G L 1980 The hand in the child with juvenile rheumatoid arthritis. J Hand Surg 5: 105–113

Grange W J 1978 Subperiosteal ganglion: a case report. J Bone Joint Surg 60B: 124–125

Grayson M J, Saldana M J 1987 Toxic shock syndrome complicating surgery of the hand. J Hand Surg (Am) 12: 1082–1084

Greco R J, Hartford C E, Haith L R et al 1988 Hydrofluoric acid-induced hypocalcemia. J Trauma 28: 1593–1596

Green D P 1984 Diagnostic and therapeutic value of carpal tunnel injection. J Hand Surg 9A: 850–854

Green D P 1985 The effect of avascular necrosis on Russe bone grafting for scaphoid nonunion. J Hand Surg 10A: 597–605

Green D P 1987 Proximal row carpectomy. Hand Clin 3: 163–168

Green D P, Dominguez O J 1979 A transpositional skin flap for release of volar contractures of a finger at the MP joint. Plastic Reconstr Surg 64: 516–520

Green D P, O'Brien E T 1978 Open reduction of carpal dislocations: indications and operative techniques. J Hand Surg 3: 250–265

Green D P, Terry G C 1973 Complex dislocation of the metacarpophalangeal joint. J Bone Joint Surg 55A: 1480–1486

Green J, Harzinder K, Leon-Barth C A, Hamm A 1989 Microwave hand injury. Contemp Orthopaedics 19: 564–566

Green S M, Posner M A 1985 Irreducible dorsal dislocations of the proximal interphalangeal joint. J Hand Surg (Am) 10: 85–87

Green W T, Mital M 1979 Congenital radio-ulnar synostosis: surgical treatment. J Bone Joint Surg 61A: 738–748

Greenberg B M, Cuadros C L, Panda M, May J W Jr 1988 St Clair Strange procedure: indications, technique, and long-term evaluation. J Hand Surg (Am) 13: 928–935

Greenberg B M, May J W Jr 1988 Great toe-to-hand transfer: role of the preoperative lateral arteriogram of foot. J Hand Surg (Am) 13: 411–414

Greene T L, Noellert R C, Belsole R J, Simpson L A 1989 Composite wiring of metacarpal and phalangeal fractures. J Hand Surg (Am) 14: 665–669

Greene T L, Strickland J W 1984 Fibroma of tendon sheath. J Hand Surg (Am) 9: 758–760

Grenga T E 1990 Intratendinous fibroma of flexor tendon. J Hand Surg (Am) 15: 92–93

Griffin A C, Gilula L A, Young V L, Strecker W B, Weeks P M 1988 Fracture of the dorsoulnar tubercle of the trapezium. J Hand Surg (Am) 13: 622–626

Griffin J M, Vasconez L O, Schatten W E 1978 Congenital arteriovenous malformations of the upper extremity. Plastic Reconstr Surg 62: 49–58

Griffiths J C 1964 Fractures at the base of the first metacarpal bone. J Bone Joint Surg 46B: 712

Grogono B J S 1973 Auger injuries. Injury 4: 247–257

Gropper P T 1983 Ulnar dimelia. J Hand Surg (Am) 8: 487–491

Gropper P T, Bowen V 1984 Cerclage wiring of metacarpal fractures. Clin Orthop 188: 203–207

Gropper P T, Pisesky W A, Bowen V, Clement P B 1983 Flexor tenosynovitis caused by Coccidioides immitis. J Hand Surg (Am) 8: 344–347

Gross M S, Gelberman R H 1985 Metacarpal rotational osteotomy. J Hand Surg (Am) 10: 105–108

Gross W, Louis D 1978 Doppler hemodynamic assessment of obscure symptomatology in the upper extremity. J Hand Surg 3: 467–473

Grossland S G, Nevisser R 1977 Complications of radial artery catheterization. Hand 9: 287–290

Gruber W 1870 Uber die Verbundung des Nervus medianus mit dem Nervus ulnaris am unterarme des Meuchen und der Saugethiere. Arch Anat Physiol Med Leipzig 37: 501–522

Grundberg A B 1977 Osteoid osteoma of the thumb. Report of a case. J Hand Surg 2: 266

Grundberg A B 1981 Intramedullary fixation for fractures of the hand. J Hand Surg 6: 568–573

Grundberg A B 1983 Carpal tunnel decompression in spite of normal electromyography. J Hand Surg (Am) 8: 348–349

Grundberg A B, Reagan D S 1985 Pathologic anatomy of the forearm: intersection syndrome. J Hand Surg (Am) 10: 299–302

Grundberg A B, Reagan D S 1987 Central slip tenotomy for chronic mallet finger deformity. J Hand Surg (Am) 12: 545–547

Grunert B K, Devine C A, Matloub H S, Sanger J R, Yousif N J 1988 Flashback after traumatic hand injuries: prognostic indicators. J Hand Surg (Am) 13: 125–127

Grunert B K, Devine C A, McCallum-Burke S, Matloub H S et al 1989 On-site work evaluations: desensitisation for avoidance reactions following severe hand injuries. J Hand Surg (Br) 14: 239–241

Grunert B K, Matloub H S, Sanger J R, Yousif N J 1990 Treatment of posttraumatic stress disorder after work-related hand trauma. J Hand Surg (Am) 15: 511–515

Guber S, Rudolph R 1978 The myofibroblast. Surg Obstet Gynecol 146: 641–649

Guides to evaluation of permanent impairment, 3rd edn. 1990 American Medical Association, Chicago, IL

Guimberteau J C, Goin J L, Panconi B, Schuhmacher B 1988 The reverse ulnar artery forearm island flap in hand surgery: 54 cases. Plastic Reconstr Surg 81: 925–932

Gunn A 1967 Electric fire burn. Br Med J 3: 764–766

Gunn C, Milbrandt W E 1976 Tennis elbow and the cervical spine. Can Med Assoc J 114: 803–809

Gunther S F 1985 Dorsal wrist pain and the occult scapholunate ganglion. J Hand Surg (Am) 10: 697–703

Gunther S F, Bruno P D 1985 Divergent dislocation of the carpometacarpal joints: a case report. J Hand Surg (Am) 10: 197–201

Gunther S F, Elliott R C 1976 *Mycobacterium kansasii* infection in the deep structures of the hand. Report of two cases. J Bone Joint Surg 58A: 140–142

Gunther S F, Elliott R C, Brand R L, Adams J P 1977 Experience with atypical mycobacterial infection in the deep structures of the hand. J Hand Surg 2: 90–96

Gunther S F, Gunther A G, Hoeg J M, Kruth H S 1986 Multiple flexor tendon xanthomas and contractures in the hands of a child with familial hypercholesterolemia. J Hand Surg (Am) 11: 588–593

Gunther S F, Levy C S 1989 Mycobacterial infections. Hand Clin 5: 591–598

Gupta A, Burke F D 1990 Correction of camptodactyly. Preliminary results of extensor indicis transfer. J Hand Surg (Br) 15: 168–170

Gupta S, Kumar A, Gupta I 1980 Giant cell tumor of the first metacarpal bone. Hand 12: 288–292

Gustilo R B, Anderson J T 1976 Prevention of infection in the treatment of one thousand and twenty-five open fractures of long bones. Retrospective and prospective analysis. J Bone Joint Surg 58A: 453–458

Gustilo R B, Gruninger R P, Davis T 1987 Classification of Type III (severe) open fractures relative to treatment and results. Orthopedics 10: 1781–1788

Guttman L 1956 The problem of treatment of pressure sores in spinal paraplegics. Br J Plastic Surg 8: 196–213

Guy R J 1990 The etiologies and mechanisms of nail bed injuries. Hand Clin 6: 9–19

Guyon F 1861 Note sur une disposition anatomique propre a la face anterieure de la region du poignet et non encore decrite. Bull Society Anat Paris 36: 184–186

Guzman-Stein G, Schubert W, Najarian D W, Press B H, Cunningham B L 1989 Composite in situ vein bypass for upper extremity revascularization. Plastic Reconstr Surg 83: 533–536

Gwathmey F W, House J H 1984 Clinical manifestations of congenital insensitivity of the hand and classification of syndromes. J Hand Surg (Am) 9: 863–869

Haber M H, Alter A H, Whellock M C 1965 Tumors of the hand. Surg Gynecol Obstet 121: 1073–1080

Haddad R I, Riordan D C 1967 Arthrodesis of the wrist. J Bone Joint Surg 49A: 950–954

Hadidi A T, Kaddah N T, Zaki M S, Sami A, Aal N A 1990 Congenital malformations of the hand. A study of the vascular pattern. J Hand Surg (Br)15: 171–180

Hagan H J, Hastings II 2nd 1988 Fusion of the thumb metacarpophalangeal joint to treat posttraumatic arthritis. J Hand Surg (Am) 13: 750–753

Hagert C G 1987 The distal radioulnar joint. Hand Clin 3: 41–50

Hagert C G, Lundborg G, Hansen T 1977 Entrapment of the posterior interosseous nerve. Scand J Plastic Reconstr Surg 11: 205–212

Haher T R, Devlin V J, Haher J N, Freeman B, Smith A G 1984 A case report of calcinosis universalis. J Hand Surg 9A: 243–245

Hajdu S J 1979 Pathology of soft tissue tumors. Lea & Febiger, Philadelphia

Hajj A A, Wood M B 1986 Stenosing tenosynovitis of the extensor carpi ulnaris. J Hand Surg (Am) 11: 519–520

Hakstian R W, Tubiana R 1968 Ulnar deviation of the fingers. J Bone Joint Surg 49A: 299–316

Hall R F Jr, Gleason T F, Kasa R F 1985 Simultaneous closed dislocations of the metacarpophalangeal joints of the index, long, and ring fingers: a case report. J Hand Surg (Am) 10: 81–85

Hallett J 1981 Entrapment of the median nerve after dislocation of the elbow: a case report. J Bone Joint Surg 63B: 408–412

Halpern A, Mochizuki R M 1980 Compartment syndrome of the interosseous muscles of the hand. Orthopaedic Rev 9: 121–127

Hamilton W C, Ramsey P L, Hanson S M, Schiff D C 1975 Osseous xanthoma and multiple hand tumors as a complication of hyperlipidemia. J Bone Joint Surg 57A: 551–553

Handle N, Winspur I, Hoehn R 1979 Coverage of a shoulder wound with a deltoid muscle flap. Ann Plastic Surg 3: 277–279

Hanel D P, Robson D B 1987 The image intensifier as an operating table. J Hand Surg (Am) 12: 322–323

Hankin F M, Hankin R C, Louis D S 1987 Malignant fibrous histiocytoma involving a digit. J Hand Surg (Am) 12: 83–86

Hankin F M, Janda D H 1989 Tendon and ligament attachments in relationship to growth plates in a child's hand. J Hand Surg (Br) 14: 315–318

Hankin F M, White S J, Braunstein E M, Louis D S 1986 Dynamic radiography evaluation of obscure wrist pain in the teenage patient. J Hand Surg (Am) 11: 805–809

Hansbrough J F, Zapata-Sirvent R, Dominic W et al 1985 Hydrocarbon contact injuries. J Trauma 25: 250–252

Hansen C A, Peterson T H 1987 Fracture of the thumb sesamoid bones. J Hand Surg (Am) 12: 269–270

Hansen P, Nielsen P T, Wahlin A B 1988 Pigmented villonodular synovitis of the extensor tendon sheaths in a child. J Hand Surg (Br) 13: 313–314

Hansford T, Bood H, Kent B, Lutz G 1986 Blood flow changes at the wrist in manual workers after preventive interventions. J Hand Surg (Am) 11: 503–508

Hanson P G, Standridge J, Jarrett F, Mali D 1977 Freshwater wound infections due to *Aeromonas hydrophila*. J Am Med Assoc 238: 1053–1054

Hardy A E 1981 Birth injuries of the brachial plexus. J Bone Joint Surg 63B: 98–101

Hardy D C, Totty W G, Carnes K M, Kyriakos M et al 1988 Arthrographic surface anatomy of the carpal triangular fibrocartilage complex. J Hand Surg (Am) 13: 823–829

Hardy D C, Totty W G, Reinus W R, Gilula L A 1987 Posteroanterior wrist radiography: importance of arm positioning. J Hand Surg (Am) 12: 504–508

Harrelson J M, Newmann M 1975 Hypertrophy of the flexor carpi ulnaris as a cause of ulnar nerve compression in the distal part of the forearm. J Bone Joint Surg 57A: 554–555

Harris C, Rutledge G L 1972 The functional anatomy of the extensor mechanism of the finger. J Bone Joint Surg 54A: 713–726

Harris C, Wood V 1978 Rollover injuries of the upper extremity. J Trauma 18: 605–607

Harris H, Joseph J 1949 Variation in the extension of the metacarpophalangeal and interphalangeal joints of the thumb. J Bone Joint Surg 31B: 547–559

Harrison D H 1977 The stiff proximal interphalangeal joint. Hand 9: 102–108

Harrison S H 1974 The Harrison Nicolle intramedullary peg. Follow-up study of 100 cases. Hand 6: 304–307

Harrison S H 1974 The tactile adherence test estimating loss of sensation after nerve injury. Hand 6: 148–149

Harrison S, Smith P, Maxwell D 1977 Stabilization of the first metacarpophalangeal and terminal joints of the thumb. Hand 9: 242–249

Hart J A L 1972 Extensor digitorum brevis manus. Hand 4: 265–267

Hart J A L 1973 Intraosseus lipoma. J Bone Joint Surg 55B: 624–632

Hart V L, Gaynor V 1941 Roentgenographic study of the carpal canal. J Bone Joint Surg 23: 382–383

Harter B T Jr, Harter K C 1986 High-pressure injection injuries. Hand Clin 2: 547–552

Hartrampf C R, Vasconez L O, Mathes S 1975 Construction of one good thumb from both parts of a congenitally bifid thumb. Plastic Reconstr Surg 54: 148–152

Hartz C R, Linscheid R L, Gramse R R, Daube J R 1981 The pronator teres syndrome: compressive neuropathy of the median nerve. J Bone Joint Surg 63A: 885–890

Harvey F J, Bosanquet J S 1981 Carpal tunnel syndrome caused by simple ganglion. Hand 13: 164–166

Harvey F J, Chu G, Harvey P M 1983 Surgical availability of the plantaris tendon J Hand Surg (Am) 8: 243–247

Harvey F J, Harvey P M, Horsley M W 1990 De Quervain's disease: surgical or nonsurgical treatment. J Hand Surg (Am) 15: 83–87

Harvey F J, Negrine J 1990 Synovial chondromatosis in the distal interphalangeal joint. J Hand Surg (Am) 15: 102–105

Hastings D E, Silver R L 1984 Intercarpal arthrodesis in the management of chronic carpal instability after trauma. J Hand Surg (Am) 9: 834–840

Hastings H 2nd, Carroll C 4th 1988 Treatment of closed articular fractures of the metacarpophalangeal and proximal interphalangeal joints. Hand Clin 4: 503–527

Hastings H 2nd, Davidson S 1988 Tendon transfers for ulnar nerve palsy. Evaluation of results and practical treatment considerations. Hand Clin 4: 167–178

Hastings H 2nd, Misamore G 1987 Compartment syndrome resulting from intravenous regional anesthesia. J Hand Surg (Am) 12: 559–562

Hauswald K R, Kasdan M L, Weis D L 1975 Vascular leiomyoma of the hand. Plastic Reconstr Surg 55: 89–91

Hay E L, Collawn S S, Middleton F G 1986 *Sporothrix* schenckii tenosynovitis: a case report. J Hand Surg (Am) 11: 431–434

Hayashi Y, Kojima T, Kohno T 1984 A case of cubital tunnel syndrome caused by the snapping of the medial head of the triceps brachii muscle. J Hand Surg (Am) 9A: 96–99

Hayes C 1978 Ulnar tunnel syndrome from giant cell tumor of tendon sheath: a case report. J Hand Surg 3: 187–188

Hayes J R, Mulholland R C, O'Connor B T 1969 Compression of the deep palmar branch of the ulnar nerve. J Bone Joint Surg 51B: 469–472

Hayter R G, Becton J L 1984 Fibrous dysplasia of a metacarpal; a case report. J Hand Surg (Am) 9: 587–589

Healey J H, Turnbull A D, Miedema B, Lane J M 1986 Acrometastases. A study of twenty-nine patients with osseous involvement of the hand and feet. J Bone Joint Surg (Am) 68: 743–746

Healy C, Mercer N S, Earley M J, Woodcock J 1990 Focusable Doppler ultrasound in mapping dorsal hand flaps. Br J Plastic Surg 43: 296–299

Heath R D 1972 The subclavian steal syndrome. Cause of symptoms in the arm. J Bone Joint Surg 54A: 1033–1039

Heberden W 1802 Commentaries on history and cure of disease. T Payne, London

Heckler F R, Jabaley M E 1986 Evolving concepts of median nerve decompression in the carpal tunnel. Hand Clin 2: 723–736

Heim U, Pfeiffer K M 1988 Internal fixation of small fractures, 3rd edn. Springer Verlag, Heidelberg

Heithoff S F, Millender L H, Nalebuff E A, Petruska A J Jr 1990 Medial epicondylectomy for the treatment of ulnar nerve compression at the elbow. J Hand Surg (Am) 15: 22–29

Helal B, Vernon-Roberts B 1976 Intraosseous ganglion of the pisiform bone. Hand 8: 150–154

Heller R, Becker J, Wasselle J et al 1991 Detection of submicroscopic lymph node metastases in patients with melanoma. Arch Surg 126: 1455–1460

Hellstrand P H 1989 Injuries caused by firewood splitting machines. Scand J Plastic Reconstr Surg Hand Surg 23: 51–54

Helm R H 1987 Hand function after injuries to the collateral ligaments of the metacarpophalangeal joint of the thumb. J Hand Surg (Br) 12: 252–255

Henard D C 1984 Giant cell tumor of the thumb metacarpal in an elderly patient: a case report. J Hand Surg (Am) 9: 343–345

Henderson H P, Reid D A C 1980 Long term follow up of neurovascular island flaps. Hand 12: 113–122

Henderson J J, Arafa M A 1987 Carpometacarpal dislocation. An easily missed diagnosis. J Bone Joint Surg 69B: 212–214

Henderson W R 1948 Clinical assessment of peripheral nerve injuries. Lancet i: 801–805

Hennessy M J, Mosher T F 1981 Mucormycosis infection of an upper extremity. J Hand Surg 6: 249–252

Henry A K 1973 Extensile exposure, 2nd edn. Churchill Livingstone, Edinburgh

Hentz V R, Brown M, Keoshian L A 1983 Upper limb reconstruction in quadriplegia: functional assessment and proposed treatment modifications. J Hand Surg (Am) 8: 119–131

Hentz V R, Hamlin C, Keoshian L A 1988 Surgical reconstruction in tetraplegia. Hand Clin 4: 601–607

Hentz V R, Marich K W, Dev P 1984 Preliminary study of the upper limb with the use of ultrasound transmission imaging. J Hand Surg (Am) 9: 188–193

Herbert J 1989 Internal fixation of the carpus with the Herbert bone screw system. J Hand Surg (Am) 14: 397–400

Herbin M L 1987 Work capacity evaluation for occupational hand injuries. J Hand Surg (Am) 12: 958–961

Herndon J H, Lanoue A M 1972 *Mycobacterium fortuitum*

infections involving the extremities. J Bone Joint Surg 54A: 1279–1282

Herndon J, Eaton R, Littler J W 1976 Management of painful neuromas in the hand. J Bone Joint Surg 58A: 369–373

Herrick R T, Godsil R D, Widener J H 1980 Lipofibromatous hamartoma of the radial nerve. A case report. J Hand Surg 5: 211–213

Heycock M H 1966 On the management of hand injuries caused by woodworking tools. Br J Plastic Surg 19: 58

Heymans M, Jardon-Jeghers C, Vanwijck R 1990 Hand metastases from urothelial tumor. J Hand Surg (Am) 15: 509–511

Heywood A E B 1969 Correction of the rheumatoid boutonniere deformity. J Bone Joint Surg 51A: 1309–1314

Hicks L M, Hunt J L, Baxter C R 1979 Liquid propane cold injury: a clinicopathologic and experimental study. J Trauma 19: 701–703

Hiersche D L, Waters R L 1985 Interphalangeal fixation of the thumb in Moberg's key grip procedure. J Hand Surg (Am) 10: 30–32

Hildreth D H, Breidenbach W C, Lister G D, Hodges A D 1989 Detection of submaximal effort by use of the rapid exchange grip. J Hand Surg (Am) 14: 742–745

Hill M B, Achauer B M, Martinez S 1984 Tar and asphalt burns. J Burn Care Rehabil 5: 271–274

Hill N A, Howard F M, Huffer B R 1985 The incomplete anterior interosseous nerve syndrome. J Hand Surg (Am) 10: 4–16

Hill N A, Hurst L C 1989 Dupuytren's contracture. Hand Clin 5: 349–357

Him F P, Casanova R, Vasconez L O 1985 Myocutaneous and fasciocutaneous flaps in the upper limb. Hand Clin 1: 759–768

Hindley C J, Metcalfe J W 1987 A colonic metastatic tumor in the hand. J Hand Surg (Am) 12: 803–805

Hing D N, Buncke H J, Alpert B S 1988 Use of the temporoparietal free fascial flap in the upper extremity. Plastic Reconstr Surg 81: 534–544

Hing D N, Buncke H J, Alpert B S, Gordon L 1985 Free flap coverage of the hand. Hand Clin 1: 741–758

Hirai M, Shinoya S 1979 Arterial obstruction of the upper limb in Buerger's disease: its incidence and primary lesion. Br J Surg 66: 124–129

Hirasawa Y, Sawamura H, Sakakida K 1979 Entrapment neuropathy due to bilateral epitrochleoanconeus muscles: a case report. J Hand Surg 4: 181–185

Hirotani H 1975 An unusual cause of ulnar nerve compression. Hand 7: 266–268

Hitchcock T F, Amadio P C 1989 Fungal infections. Hand Clin 5: 599–611

Hixson F P, Shafiroff B B, Werner F W, Palmer A K 1986 Digital tourniquets: a pressure study with clinical relevance. J Hand Surg (Am) 11: 865–868

Hixson M L, Stewart C 1990 Microvascular anatomy of the radioscapholunate ligament of the wrist. J Hand Surg (Am) 15: 279–282

Ho P K, Choban S J, Eshman S J, Dupuy T E 1987 Complex dorsal dislocation of the second carpometacarpal joint. J Hand Surg (Am) 12: 1074–1076

Ho P K, Jacobs J L, Clark G L 1985 Trapezium implant arthroplasty: evaluation of a semiconstrained implant. J Hand Surg (Am) 10: 654–660

Ho P K, Weiland A J, McClinton M A, Wilgis E F 1987 Aneurysms of the upper extremity. J Hand Surg (Am) 12: 39–46

Hoang P H, Mills C, Burke F D 1989 Triceps to biceps transfer for established brachial plexus palsy. J Bone Joint Surg (Br) 71: 268–271

Hobbs R A, Magnussen P A, Tonkin M A 1990 Palmar cutaneous branch of the median nerve. J Hand Surg 15A: 38–43

Hodgkinson D J, Shepard G H 1983 Muscle musculocutaneous and fasciocutaneous flaps in forearm reconstruction. Ann Plastic Surg 10: 400–407

Hoehn J 1978 Multiple fibrous xanthomas of tendon sheath. Hand 10: 306–308

Hofammann D Y, Ferlic D C, Clayton M L 1987 Arthroplasty of the basal joint of the thumb using a silicone prosthesis. Long-term follow-up. J Bone Joint Surg (Am) 69: 993–997

Hoffer M M, Braun R, Hsu J, Mitani M, Temes K 1981 Functional recovery and orthopaedic management of brachial plexus palsies. J Am Med Assoc 246: 2467–2470

Hoffer M M, Lehman M, Mitani M 1986 Long-term follow-up on tendon transfers to the extensors of the wrist and fingers in patients with cerebral palsy. J Hand Surg (Am) 11: 836–840

Hoffer M M, Lehman M, Mitani M 1989 Surgical indications in children with cerebral palsy. Hand Clin 5: 69–74

Hoffer M M, Zeitzew S 1988 Wrist fusion in cerebral palsy. J Hand Surg (Am) 13: 667–670

Holcomb H S III, Behrens F, Winn W C Jr, Hughes I M, McCue F C III 1981 *Prototheca wickerhamii* — an alga infecting the hand. J Hand Surg 6: 595–599

Holden C E A 1979 The pathology and prevention of Volkmann's ischaemic contracture. J Bone Joint Surg 61B: 296–300

Holdsworth B J 1985 Nerve tumours in the upper limb. A clinical review. J Hand Surg (Br) 10: 236–238

Holevich J 1965 Early skin grafting in the treatment of traumatic avulsion injuries of the hand and fingers. J Bone Joint Surg 47A: 944–957

Holst-Nielsen F, Jensen V 1984 Tardy posterior interosseous nerve palsy as a result of an unreduced radial head dislocation in Monteggia fractures: a report of two cases. J Hand Surg (Am) 9: 572–575

Holtzman R N, Mark M H, Patel M R, Wiener L M 1984 Ulnar nerve entrapment neuropathy in the forearm. J Hand Surg (Am) 9: 576–578

Hooper G 1978 Tooth fragment in a metacarpophalangeal joint. Hand 10: 215–216

Hooper G J 1987 An unusual variety of skier's thumb. J Hand Surg (Am) 12: 627–629

Hooper G, McMaster M J 1979 Stenosing tenovaginitis affecting the tendon of extensor digiti minimi at the wrist. Hand 11: 299–301

Hoopes J E, Graham W P 3rd, Shack R B 1985 Epithelioid sarcoma of the upper extremity. Plastic Reconstr Surg 75: 810–813

Hoover G H, Flatt A E, Weiss M W 1970 The hand in Apert's syndrome. J Bone Joint Surg 52A: 878–895

Hori M, Nakamura R, Inoue G, Imamura T et al 1987 Nonoperative treatment of camptodactyly. J Hand Surg (Am) 12: 1061–1065

Horii E, Garcia-Elias M, Bishop A T, Cooney W P et al 1990 Effect on force transmission across the carpus in procedures used to treat Kienbock's disease. J Hand Surg (Am) 15: 393–400

Horn J J 1951 The use of full thickness hand skin flaps in the reconstruction of injured fingers. Plastic Reconstr Surg 7: 463–481

Hoskin H D 1960 The versatile cross-finger flap. J Bone Joint Surg 42A: 261–277

Houpt P, Storm van Leeuwen J B, van den Bergen H A 1989 Intraneural lipofibroma of the median nerve. J Hand Surg (Am) 14: 706–709

House J H, Gwathmey F W, Fidler M O 1981 A dynamic approach to the thumb-in-palm deformity in cerebral palsy. Evaluation and results in fifty-six patients. J Bone Joint Surg 63A: 216–225

House J H, Gwathmey F W, Lundsgaard D K 1976 Restoration of strong grasp and lateral pinch in tetraplegia due to cervical spinal cord injury. J Hand Surg 1: 152–159

House J H, Shannon M A 1985 Restoration of strong grasp and lateral pinch in tetraplegia: a comparison of two methods of thumb control in each patient. J Hand Surg (Am) 10: 22–29

Howard F M 1961 Ulnar nerve palsy in wrist fractures. J Bone Joint Surg 43A: 1197–1201

Howard F M 1986 Compression neuropathies in the anterior forearm. Hand Clin 2: 737–745

Howard F M, Lassen K 1984 Giant cell tumor of the capitate. J Hand Surg (Am) 9: 272–274

Howard F, Thomas F, Wojcie E 1974 Rotatory subluxation of the navicular. Clin Ortho Rel Res 104: 134

Howard J B, Highgenboten C L, Nelson J D 1976 Residual effects of septic arthritis in infancy and childhood. J Am Med Assoc 236: 932–935

Huang T T, Blackwell S J, Lewis S R 1978 Hand deformities in patients with snakebite. Plastic Reconstr Surg 62: 32–36

Hubbard L F 1988 Metacarpophalangeal dislocations. Hand Clin 4: 39–44

Hubbard L F, Burton R I 1977 Malignant fibrous histiocytoma of the forearm. Report of a case and review of the literature. J Hand Surg 2: 292–296

Huber D F, Weis L D 1985 Metastatic carcinoma of the distal ulna from an occult pancreatic carcinoma. J Hand Surg (Am) 10: 725–727

Huber E 1921 Hilssoperation bei medianuslahmung. Deutsche Zeitschrift fur Chirurgie 162: 271–275

Hueston J T 1952 Pathology of the inter-digital pilonidal sinus. Aust NZ J Surg 21: 226–229

Hume M C, Gellman H, McKellop H, Brumfield R H Jr 1990 functional range of motion of the joints of the hand. J Hand Surg (Am) 15: 240–244

Hung L K, Cheng J C, McGuire L J, Tsao S Y 1988 Primary malignant lymphoma of the deep tissues of the hand. J Hand Surg (Am) 13: 683–686

Hung L K, Kinninmonth A W, Woo M L 1988 *Vibrio vulnificus* necrotizing fasciitis presenting with compartmental syndrome of the hand. J Hand Surg (Br) 13: 337–339

Hunt J R 1908 Occupation neuritis of the deep palmar branch of the ulnar nerve. J Neurol Mental Dis 35: 673–689

Hunter G A 1968 Chemical burns of the skin after contact with petrol. Br J Plastic Surg 21: 337–341

Hunter J M 1983 Staged flexor tendon reconstruction. J Hand Surg (Am) 8: 789–793

Hunter J M 1985 Tendon salvage and the active tendon implant: a perspective. Hand Clin 1: 181–186

Hunter J M, Cowen N J 1970 Fifth metacarpal fractures in a compensation clinic population. A report on one hundred and thirty-three cases. J Bone Joint Surg (Am) 52: 1159–1165

Hunter J M, Jaeger S H, Matsui T, Miyaji N 1983 The pseudosynovial sheath — its characteristics in a primate model. J Hand Surg (Am) 8: 461–470

Hurst L C, Amadio P C, Badalamente M A, Ellstein J L, Dattwyler R J 1987 *Mycobacterium marinum* infections of the hand. J Hand Surg (Am) 12: 428–435

Hurst L C, Badalamente M A, Blum D 1984 Carbon dioxide laser transection of rat peripheral nerves. J Hand Surg (Am) 9: 428–433

Hutton P, Kernohan J, Birch R 1981 An anomalous flexor digitorum superficialis indicis muscle presenting as carpal tunnel syndrome. Hand 13: 85–86

Huvos A G 1991 Bone Tumors, 2nd end. W B Saunders, Philadelphia

Ikeda A, Ugawa A, Kazihara Y, Hamada N 1988 Arterial patterns in the hand based on a three-dimensional analysis of 220 cadaver hands. J Hand Surg (Am) 13: 501–509

Ikuta Y 1985 Vascularized free flap transfer in the upper limb. Hand Clin 1: 297–309

Imbriglia J E, Boland D M 1984 An exercise-induced compartment syndrome of the dorsal forearm — a case report. J Hand Surg (Am) 9A: 142–143

Imbriglia J E, Broudy A S, Hagberg W C, McKernan D 1990 Proximal row carpectomy: clinical evaluation. J Hand Surg (Am) 15: 426–430

Imbriglia J E, Goldstein S A 1987 Intratendinous ruptures of the flexor digitorum profundus tendon of the small finger. J Hand Surg (Am) 12: 985–991

Incavo S J, Mogan J V, Hilfrank B C 1989 Extension splinting of palmar plate avulsion injuries of the proximal interphalangeal joint. J Hand Surg (Am) 14: 659–661

Inglis A E, Hamlin C, Sengelmann R P 1972 Reconstruction of the metacarpophalangeal joint of the thumb in rheumatoid arthritis. J Bone Joint Surg 54A: 704–712

Inglis A E, Jones E C 1977 Proximal row carpectomy for diseases of the proximal row. J Bone Joint Surg 59A: 460–463

Inglis A E, Pellicci P M 1980 Total elbow replacement. J Bone Joint Surg 62A: 1252–1258

Inglis A E, Ranawat C S, Straub L R 1971 Synovectomy and debridement of the elbow in rheumatoid arthritis. J Bone Joint Surg 53A: 652–662

Inoue G, Maeda N 1987 Irreducible palmar dislocation of the distal interphalangeal joint of the finger. J Hand Surg (Am) 12: 1077–1079

Ireland D C R, Takayama N, Flatt A E 1976 Poland's syndrome. A review of forty-three cases. J Bone Joint Surg 58A: 52–58

Ishizuki M 1988 Injury to collateral ligament of the metacarpophalangeal joint of a finger. J Hand Surg (Am) 13: 444–448

Ishizuki M, Isobe Y, Arai T, Nagatsuka Y, Tanabe K, Okumura S 1977 Osteochondromatosis of the finger joints. Hand 9: 198–200

Itoh Y, Horiuchi Y, Takahashi M, Uchinishi K, Yabe Y 1987 Extensor tendon involvement in Smith's and Galeazzi's fractures. J Hand Surg (Am) 12: 535–540

Iverson R E, Vistnes L M 1973 Coccidioidomycosis tenosynovitis in the hand. J Bone Joint Surg 55A: 413–417

Jabaley M E 1978 Personal observations on the role of the lumbrical muscles in carpal tunnel syndrome. J Hand Surg 3: 82–84

Jabaley M E, Freeland A E 1986 Rigid internal fixation in the hand: 104 cases. Plastic Reconstr Surg 77: 288–298

Jablon M, Horowitz A, Bernstein D A 1990 Magnetic

resonance imaging of a glomus tumor of the fingertip. J Hand Surg (Am) 15: 507–509

Jablon M, Rabin S I 1988 Late flexor pollicis longus tendon rupture due to retained glass fragments. J Hand Surg (Am) 13: 713–716

Jackson I T, Simpson R G 1979 Interpositional arthroplasty of the wrist in rheumatoid arthritis. Hand 11: 169–175

Jackson W T, Protas J M 1981 Snapping scapholunate subluxation. J Hand Surg 6: 590–594

Jain V K, Cestero R V M, Baum J 1979 Carpal tunnel syndrome in patients undergoing maintenance hemodialysis. J Am Med Assoc 242: 2868–2869

James J H, Morris A M 1977 The use of hand bags compared with a conventional dressing in the treatment of superficial burns of the hand. Chirurgia Plastica 4: 67–72

Janes P C, Mann R J 1987 Extracutaneous sporotrichosis. J Hand Surg (Am) 12: 441–445

Janzon L, Niechajev I A 1981 Wrist ganglia. Scand J Plastic Reconstr Surg 15: 53–56

Jarev A, Hirshowitz B 1978 A two stage cross arm flap for severe multiple degloving injury of the hand. Hand 10: 276–278

Jasmine M S, Packer J W, Edwards G S Jr 1988 Irreducible trans-scaphoid perilunate dislocation. J Hand Surg (Am) 13: 212–215

Jaworska M, Popiolek 1968 Genetic counselling in lobster-claw anomaly: discussion of variability of genetic influence in different families. Clin Pediatr 7: 396–399

Jazheimer E C, Morain W D, Brown F E 1981 Woodsplitter injuries of the hand. Plastic Reconstr Surg 68: 83–88

Jeffery A K 1971 Compression of the deep palmar branch of the ulnar nerve by an anomalous muscle. J Bone Joint Surg 53B: 718–723

Jelalian C, Mehrohof A, Cohen I K, Richardson J, Merritt W H 1985 Streptokinase in the treatment of acute arterial occlusion of the hand. J Hand Surg (Am) 10: 534–538

Jelenko C 1974 Chemicals that burn. J Trauma 14: 65–72

Jenkins A McL, Macpherson A I S, Nolan B, Housely E 1976 Peripheral aneurysms in Behcet's disease. Br J Surg 63: 199–202

Jensen B V, Christensen C 1990 An unusual combination of simultaneous fracture of the tuberosity of the trapezium and the hook of the hamate. J Hand Surg (Am) 15: 285–287

Jensen E G 1979 Osteoid osteoma of the capitate bone. Hand 11: 102–105

Jewusiak E M, Spence K, Sell K 1971 Solitary benign enchondroma of the long bones of the hand. J Bone Joint Surg 53A: 1587–1590

Johannson S H 1982 Nagelwallhildung durch Thenarlappen bei Kompletter Syndaktylie. Handchirurgie 14: 199–203

Johnson J, Omer G E Jr 1985 Congenital ulnar deficiency. Natural history and therapeutic implications. Hand Clin 1: 499–510

Johnson M K, Lawrence J F 1975 Metaplastic bone formation (myositis ossificans) in the soft tissue of the hand. Case report. J Bone Joint Surg 57A: 999–1000

Johnson R J, Bonfiglio M 1969 Lipofibromatous hamartoma of the median nerve. J Bone Joint Surg 51A: 984–990

Johnson R K, Spinner M, Shrewsbury M M 1979 Median nerve entrapment syndrome in the proximal forearm. J Hand Surg 4: 48–52

Johnson R P 1980 The acutely injured wrist and its residuals. Clin Orthop 149: 33

Johnston A D 1987 Aneurysmal bone cyst of the hand. Hand Clin 3: 299–310

Johnstone B R, Bennett C S 1989 Lawnmower injuries in children. Aust NZ J Surg 59: 713–718

Jokl P, Albright J A, Goodman A H 1971 Juxtacortical chondrosarcoma of the hand. J Bone Joint Surg 53A: 1370–1376

Jones B M, O'Brien C J 1985 Acute ischaemia of the hand resulting from elevation of a radial forearm flap. Br J Plastic Surg 38: 396–397

Jones F E 1986 Calcification simulating infection in congenital brachydactyly. J Hand Surg (Am) 11: 35–37

Jones J A, Pellegrini V D Jr 1989 Transverse fracture-dislocation of the trapezium. J Hand Surg (Am) 14: 481–485

Jones L A 1989 The assessment of hand function: a critical review of techniques. J Hand Surg (Am) 14: 221–228

Jones M W, Wahid I A 1988 *Mycobacterium marinum* infections of the hand and wrist. J Bone Joint Surg (Am) 70: 631–632

Jones M W, Wahid I A, Matthews J P 1988 Septic arthritis of the hand due to *Mycobacterium marinum*. J Hand Surg (Br) 13: 333–334

Jones N F, Conklin W T, Albo V C 1986 Primary invasive aspergillosis of the hand. J Hand Surg (Am) 11: 425–428

Jones N F, Imbriglia J E, Steen V D, Medsger T A 1987 Surgery for scleroderma of the hand. J Hand Surg (Am) 12: 391–400

Jones N F, Jupiter J B 1985 Irreducible palmar dislocation of the proximal interphalangeal joint associated with an epiphyseal fracture of the middle phalanx. J Hand Surg (Am) 10: 261–264

Jones N F, Ming N L 1988 Persistent median artery as a cause of pronator syndrome. J Hand Surg (Am) 13: 728–732

Joseph F R, Posner M A 1983 Glomus tumors of the wrist. J Hand Surg (Am) 8: 918 920

Joseph F R, Posner M A, Terzakis J A 1984 Compartment syndrome caused by a traumatized vascular hamartoma. J Hand Surg (Am) 9: 904–907

Joseph K N, Kalus A M, Sutherland A B 1981 Glass injuries of the hand in children. Hand 13: 113–119

Joshi B B 1972 Dorsolateral flap from same finger to relieve flexion contracture. Plastic Reconstr Surg 49: 186–189

Joshi B B 1974 A local dorsolateral island flap for restoration of sensation after avulsion injury of fingertip pulp. Plastic Reconstr Surg 54: 175–182

Jozsa L, Reffy A, Demel S, Balint J B 1989 Foreign bodies in tendons. J Hand Surg (Br) 14: 84–85

Jupiter J B, Koniuch M P, Smith R J 1985 The management of delayed union and nonunion of the metacarpals and phalanges. J Hand Surg (Am) 10: 457–466

Jupiter J B, Pess G M, Bour C J 1989 Results of flexor tendon tenolysis after replantation in the hand. J Hand Surg (Am) 14: 35–44

Justis E J Jr, Dart R C 1983 Chondrosarcoma of the hand with metastasis: a review of the literature and case report. J Hand Surg (Am) 8: 320–324

Justis E J, Moore S V, LaVelle D G 1987 Woodworking injuries: an epidemiologic survey of injuries sustained using woodworking machinery and hand tools. J Hand Surg (Am) 12: 890–895

Kaempffe F, Peimer C A 1990 Distraction for wrist arthroscopy. J Hand Surg (Am) 15: 520–521

Kaiser T E, Sim F H, Kelly P J 1981 Radial nerve palsy

associated with humeral fractures. Orthopedics
4: 1245–1251

Kambolis C, Bullough P G, Jaffe H I 1973 Ganglionic cystic
defects of bone. J Bone Joint Surg 55A: 496–505

Kanavel A B 1925 Infections of the hand. Lea & Febiger,
Philadelphia

Kanaya F, Gonzalez M, Park C M, Kutz J E et al 1990
Improvement in motor function after brachial plexus
surgery. J Hand Surg (Am) 15: 30–36

Kapff P D, Hocken D B, Simpson R H 1987 Elastofibroma
of the hand. J Bone Joint Surg (Br) 69: 468–469

Kaplan E B 1957 Dorsal dislocation of the
metacarpophalangeal joint of the index finger. J Bone Joint
Surg 39A: 1081–1086

Kaplan E B 1969 Muscular and tendinous variations of the
flexor superficialis of the fifth finger of the hand. Bull Hosp
Joint Dis 30: 59

Kaplan's functional and surgical anatomy of the hand. 3rd
edn. 1984 Spinner M (ed). J B Lippincott, Philadelphia

Kappel D A, Burech J G 1985 The cross-finger flap. An
established reconstructive procedure. Hand Clin
1: 677–683

Karev A 1979 Malignant histiocytoma of the arm in a four
year old boy. Hand 11: 106–108

Karev A 1984 The 'belt loop' technique for the
reconstruction of the pulleys in the first stage of flexor
tendon grafting. J Hand Surg 9A: 923–924

Karev A, Stahl S 1986 Treatment of painful nerve lesions in
the palm by 'rerouting' of the digital nerve. J Hand Surg
(Am) 11: 539–542

Karev A, Stahl S 1990 Spontaneous rupture of the biceps
muscle due to a concealed malignant fibrous histiocytoma.
J Hand Surg (Am) 15: 94–97

Karr M A, Aulicino P L, DuPuy T E, Gwathmey F W 1984
Osteochondromas of the hand in hereditary multiple
exostosis: report of a case presenting as a blocked proximal
interphalangeal joint. J Hand Surg (Am) 9: 264–268

Kartchner M M, Wilcox W C 1976 Thrombolysis of palmar
and digital arterial thrombosis by intra-arterial
thrombolysin. J Hand Surg 1: 67–74

Kato H, Ogino T, Minami A, Usui M 1989 Restoration of
sensibility in fingers repaired with free sensory flaps from
the toe. J Hand Surg (Am) 14: 49–54

Kato S, Ishii S, Ogino T, Shiono H 1983 Anomalous hands
with cleft formation between the fourth and fifth digits.
J Hand Surg (Am) 8: 909–913

Katsaros J, Schusterman M, Beppu M, Banis J C Jr, Acland
R D 1984 The lateral upper arm flap: anatomy and clinical
applications. Ann Plastic Surg 12: 489–500

Kaufman H D 1968 High-pressure injection injuries. Br J
Surg 55: 214–218

Kawabata H, Masada K, Aoki Y, Ono K 1986 Infantile
digital fibromatosis after web construction in syndactyly.
J Hand Surg (Am) 11: 741–743

Kawabata H, Tsuyuguchi Y, Kawai H, Yasui N 1984
Melorheostosis of the upper limb: a report of two cases.
J Hand Surg (Am) 9: 871–876

Kay S, Werntz J, Wolff T W 1989 Ring avulsion
injuries: classification and prognosis. J Hand Surg (Am)
14: 204–213

Kay Y, Masuda S, Ushijima M, Kojima T, Sugioka Y 1987
Pseudomalignant myositis ossificans occurring in the hand.
J Hand Surg (Am) 12: 634–638

Kaye J J 1990 *Vibrio vulnificus* infections in the hand. Report
of three patients. J Bone Joint Surg (Am) 72: 283–285

Kazayeri M, Gallo G 1979 Synovial sarcoma: a case report.
Orthopedics 2: 496–498

Keenan M A, Abrams R A, Garland D E, Waters R L 1987
Results of fractional lengthening of the finger flexors in
adults with upper extremity spasticity. J Hand Surg (Am)
12: 575–581

Keenan M A, Korchek J I, Botte M J, Smith C W, Garland
D E 1987 Results of transfer of the flexor digitorum
superficialis tendons to the flexor digitorum profundus
tendons in adults with acquired spasticity of the hand. J
Bone Joint Surg (Am) 69: 1127–1132

Keenan M A, Romanelli R R, Lunsford B R 1989 The use of
dynamic electromyography to evaluate motor control in the
hands of adults who have spasticity caused by brain injury.
J Bone Joint Surg (Am) 71: 120–126

Keenan M A, Todderud E P, Henderson R, Botte M 1987
Management of intrinsic spasticity in the hand with phenol
injection or neurectomy of the motor branch of the ulnar
nerve. J Hand Surg (Am) 12: 734–739

Keenan M A, Tomas E S, Stone L, Gersten L M 1990
Percutaneous phenol block of the musculocutaneous nerve
to control elbow flexor spasticity. J Hand Surg (Am)
15: 340–346

Keith J E Jr, Wilgis E F 1986 Kaposi's sarcoma in the hand of
an AIDS patient. J Hand Surg (Am) 11: 410–413

Keith M W, Peckham P H, Thrope G B, Stroh K C et al
1989 Implantable functional neuromuscular stimulation in
the tetraplegic hand. J Hand Surg (Am) 14: 524–530

Kelikian H, Doumanian A 1957 Congenital anomalies of the
hand. Part I. J Bone Joint Surg 39A: 1002–1019

Kelly C M, Freehafer A A, Peckham P H, Stroh K 1985
Postoperative results of opponensplasty and flexor tendon
transfer in patients with spinal cord injuries. J Hand Surg
(Am) 10: 890–894

Kelly E P, Stanley J K 1990 Arthroscopy of the wrist. J Hand
Surg (Br) 15: 236–242

Kelly G L 1973 Radial artery occlusion by a carpal ganglion.
Plastic Reconstr Surg 52: 191–193

Kelsey J L, Pastides H, Kreiger M, Harris C, Chernow R A
1980 Upper extremity disorders: a survey of their frequency
and impact in the United States. C V Mosby, St Louis

Kenan S, Graham S, Lewis M, Yabut S M Jr 1987
Intraosseous ganglion in the first metacarpal bone. J Hand
Surg (Am) 12: 471–473

Kenney J G, Morgan R F, McLaughlin R, Edgerton M T
1983 The 'fold-back' flexor ulnaris muscle flap for repair of
soft tissue losses about the elbow. Contemp Orthop
7: 63–66

Kent K W, Guise E R 1978 Metastatic tumors of the hand: a
report of six cases. J Hand Surg 3: 271–276

Kenzora J E 1978 Dialysis carpal tunnel syndrome.
Orthopaedics 1: 195–203

Kerin R 1958 Metastatic tumors of the hand. J Bone Joint
Surg 40A: 263

Kerin R 1983 Metastatic tumors of the hand. A review of the
literature. J Bone Joint Surg (Am) 65: 1331–1335

Kerin R 1987 The hand in metastatic disease. J Hand Surg
(Am) 12: 77–83

Kernohan J, Dakin P K, Quain J S, Helal B 1984 An
anomalous flexor digitorum superficialis indicis muscle in
association with a fibroma presenting as a stiff painful
finger. J Hand Surg (Br) 9: 335–336

Kernohan J, Dakin R P, Quain J S, Helal B 1984 An unusual
'giant' lipofibroma in the palm. J Hand Surg (Br)
9: 347–348

Kerr R 1986 Malignant fibrous histiocytoma of bone. Ortho 9: 910–913

Kessler F B, Epstein M J, Culver J E Jr, Prewitt J, Homsy C A 1984 Proplast stabilized stemless trapezium implant. J Hand Surg (Am) 9: 227–231

Kessler I 1979 A simplified technique to correct hyperextension deformity of the metacarpophalangeal joint of the thumb. J Bone Joint Surg 61A: 903–905

Kessler I, Baruch A, Hecht O 1977 Experience with distraction lengthening of digital rays in congenital anomalies. J Hand Surg 2: 394–401

Kessler R 1973 Aetiology and management of adduction contracture of the thumb in rheumatoid arthritis. Hand 5: 170–174

Ketchum L D 1985 Symposium on skin and soft tissue coverage of the upper extremity. Hand Clin 1: 597–776

Ketchum L D, Hixson F P 1987 Dermofasciectomy and full-thickness grafts in the treatment of Dupuytren's contracture. J Hand Surg (Am) 12: 659–664

Kettelkamp D B, Flatt A E, Moulds R 1971 Traumatic dislocation of the long finger extensor tendon. A clinical anatomical and biomechanical study. J Bone Joint Surg 53A: 229–240

Keyser J J, Littler J W, Eaton R G 1990 Surgical treatment of infections and lesions of the perionychium. Hand Clin 6: 137–153, discussion 155–157

Khuri S M 1986 Tension band arthrodesis in the hand. J Hand Surg (Am) 11: 41–45

Khuri S M, Ger E 1979 The ulnar clubhand — congenital ulnar deficiency. Ortho Rev 8: 149–153

Kiefhaber T R, Stern P J, Grood E S 1986 Lateral stability of the proximal interphalangeal joint. J Hand Surg (Am) 11: 661–669

Kienbock R 1910 Concerning traumatic malacia of the lunate and its consequences: degeneration and compression fractures (reprinted in Clin Orth Rel Res 149: 4–8, 1980)

Kienbock R 1910 Uber traumatische malacie des mondbeins und ihre folgezustande: entartungsformen und kompressionfrakturen. Fortschr Geb Rontgenstrahlen 16: 78

Kikuchi S, Macnab I, Moreau P 1981 Localisation of the level of symptomatic cervical disc degeneration. J Bone Joint Surg 63B: 272–277

Kilgore E S Jr 1983 Hand infections. J Hand Surg (Am) 8: 723–762

Kilgore E S, Graham W P 1968 Operative treatment of boutonniere deformity. Surgery 64: 999–1000

Kimura H, Kamura S, Akai M, Ohno T 1988 An unusual coronal fracture of the body of the hamate bone. J Hand Surg (Am) 13: 743–745

King G J, McMurtry R Y, Rubenstein J D, Gertzbein S D 1986 Kinematics of the distal radioulnar joint. J Hand Surg (Am) 11: 798–804

King G J, McMurtry R Y, Rubenstein J D, Ogston N G 1986 Computerized tomography of the distal radioulnar joint: correlation with ligamentous pathology in a cadaveric model. J Hand Surg (Am) 11: 711–717

Kirner J 1927 Doppelseitige Verkrummung des Kleinfingergrundgliedes als selbstandiges Krankheitsbild. Fortschr Rontgenstr 36: 804–806

Kirtley J A, Riddell D H, Stoney W S, Wright J K 1967 Cervicothoracic sympathectomy in neurovascular abnormalities of the upper extremity. Ann Surg 165: 869–879

Kirwan L A, Scott F A 1988 Roping injuries in the hand: mechanism of injury and functional results. Plastic Reconstr Surg 81: 54–61

Kisner W H 1976 Thumb neuroma: a hazard of ten pin bowling. Br J Plastic Surg 29: 225–226

Kisner W H 1980 Double sublimis tendon to fifth finger with absence of profundus. Plastic Reconstr Surg 65: 229–230

Kitayama Y, Tsukada S 1983 Patterns of arterial distribution in the duplicated thumb. Plastic Reconstr Surg 72: 535–542

Kitayama Y, Tsukada S, Ishikura N, Ide Y, Kojima M 1985 Rudimentary polydactyly: report of five cases. J Hand Surg (Am) 10: 382–385

Kleinert H E, Burget G C, Morgan J A, Kutz J E, Atasoy E 1973 Aneurysms of the hand. Arch Surg 106: 554–557

Kleinert H E, Cole N M, Wayne L, Harvey R, Kutz J E, Atasoy E 1973 Post-traumatic sympathetic dystrophy. Orth Clin North Am 4: 917–927

Kleinert H E, Hayes J E 1971 The ulnar tunnel syndrome. Plastic Reconstr Surg 47: 21–24

Kleinert H E, Jablon M, Tsai T 1980 An overview of replantation and results of 347 replants in 245 patients. J Trauma 20: 390–398

Kleinert H E, Kasdan M L 1965 Reconstruction of chronically subluxated proximal interphalangeal finger joint. J Bone Joint Surg 47A: 958–964

Kleinert H E, Kutz J E, Fishman I H, McCraw L H 1972 Etiology and treatment of the so-called mucous cyst of the finger. J Bone Joint Surg 54A: 1455–1458

Kleinert H E, McAlister C G, MacDonald C J, Kutz J E 1974 A critical evaluation of cross-finger flaps. J Trauma 14: 756–763

Kleinert H E, Putcha S M, Ashbell T S, Kutz J E 1967 The deformed fingernail, a frequent result of failure to repair nailbed injuries. J Trauma 7: 176–190

Kleinert H E, Volanitis G J 1965 Thrombosis of the palmar arterial arch and its tributaries: etiology and newer concepts in treatment. J Trauma 5: 446–457

Kleinert J M, Lister G D 1986 Silicone implants. Hand Clin 2: 271–290

Kleinman W B 1987 Management of chronic rotary subluxation of the scaphoid by scapho-trapezio-trapezoid arthrodesis. Rationale for the technique, postoperative changes in biomechanics, and results. Hand Clin 3: 113–133

Kleinman W B 1989 Long-term study of chronic scapho-lunate instability treated by scapho-trapezio-trapezoid arthrodesis. J Hand Surg (Am) 14: 429–445

Kleinman W B, Bishop A T 1989 Anterior intramuscular transposition of the ulnar nerve. J Hand Surg (Am) 14: 972–979

Kleinman W B, Carroll C 4th 1990 Scapho-trapezio-trapezoid arthrodesis for treatment of chronic static and dynamic scapho-lunate instability: a 10-year perspective on pitfalls and complications. J Hand Surg (Am) 15: 408–414

Kleinman W B, Petersen D P 1984 Oblique retinacular ligament reconstruction for chronic mallet finger deformity. J Hand Surg (Am) 9: 399–404

Kline S C, Moore J R, deMente S H 1990 Glomus tumor originating within a digital nerve. J Hand Surg (Am) 15: 98–101

Klug M S, Ketchum L D, Lipsey J H 1983 Symmetric hyperphalangism of the index finger in the palatodigital syndrome: a case report. J Hand Surg (Am) 8: 599–603

Klumpke A 1885 Contribution a l'etude des paralysies radiculaires du plexus brachial. Rev Med 5: 591–596

Kobayashi A, Ohmiya K, Iwakuma T, Mitsuyasu M 1976 Unusual congenital anomalies of the thumb extensors. Hand 8: 17–21

Kohnlein H E, Achinger R 1982 A new method of treatment of hydrofluoric acid burns of the extremities. Chir Plast 6: 297–305

Kojima T, Ide Y, Marumo E, Ishikawa E, Yamashita H 1976 Haemangioma of median nerve causing carpal tunnel syndrome. Hand 8: 62–65

Kojima T, Nagano T, Uchida M 1987 Periungual fibroma. J Hand Surg (Am) 12: 465–470

Koman L A, Bond M G, Carter R E, Poehling G G 1985 Evaluation of upper extremity vasculature with high-resolution ultrasound. J Hand Surg (Am) 10: 249–255

Koman L A, Nunley J A 1986 Thermoregulatory control after upper extremity replantation. J Hand Surg (Am) 11: 548–552

Koman L A, Nunley J A, Goldner J L, Seaber A V, Urbaniak J R 1984 Isolated cold stress testing in the assessment of symptoms in the upper extremity: preliminary communication. J Hand Surg (Am) 9: 305–313

Koman L A, Nunley J A, Wilkinson R H Jr, Urbaniak J R, Coleman R E 1983 Dynamic radionuclide imaging as a means of evaluating vascular perfusion of the upper extremity: a preliminary report. J Hand Surg (Am) 8: 424–434

Koman L A, Poehling G G, Price J L 1986 Thumb reconstruction — an algorithm. Ortho 9: 873–878

Koman L A, Poehling G G, Toby E B, Kammire G 1990 Chronic wrist pain: indications for wrist arthroscopy. Arthroscopy 6: 116–119

Koman L A, Urbaniak J R 1981 Ulnar artery insufficiency: a guide to treatment. J Hand Surg 6: 16–24

Koman L A, Urbaniak J R 1985 Ulnar artery thrombosis. Hand Clin 1: 311–325

Koman L A, Weiland A J, Moore J R 1985 Toe-to-hand transfer based on the medial plantar artery. J Hand Surg (Am) 10: 561–566

Koniuch M P, Peimer C A, VanGorder T, Moncada A 1987 Closed crush injury of the metacarpophalangeal joint. J Hand Surg (Am) 12: 750–757

Kopp J R 1985 Isolated palmar dislocation of the trapezoid. J Hand Surg (Am) 10: 91–93

Korkala O L, Antti-Poika I U 1989 Late treatment of scaphoid fractures by bone grafting and compression staple osteosynthesis. J Hand Surg (Am) 14: 491–495

Korn J A, Gilbert M S, Siffert R S, Jacobson J H 1975 Clostridium welchii arthritis. J Bone Joint Surg 57A: 555–557

Kornberg M, Aulicino P L 1985 Hand and wrist joint problems in patients with Ehlers–Danlos syndrome. J Hand Surg (Am) 10: 193–196

Kornberg M, Aulicino P L, DuPuy T E 1983 Bifid median nerve with three thenar branches — case report. J Hand Surg (Am) 8: 583–584

Koshima I, Soeda S, Takase T, Yamasaki M 1988 Free vascularized nail grafts. J Hand Surg (Am) 13: 29–32

Kowalski M F, Manske P R 1988 Arthrodesis of digital joints in children. J Hand Surg (Am) 13: 874–879

Kozin F, Genant C, Bekerman C, McCarty D J 1976 The reflex sympathetic dystrophy syndrome II. Roentgenographic and scintigraphic evidence of bilaterality and of periarticular accentuation. Am J Med 60: 332–338

Kozin F, McCarty D J, Genant H 1976 The reflex sympathetic dystrophy syndrome I. Clinical and histologic studies: evidence for bilaterality, response to corticosteroids and articular involvement. Am J Med 60: 321–331

Krag C, Rasmussen B 1975 The neurovascular island flap for defective sensibility of the thumb. J Bone Joint Surg 57B: 495–499

Krylov V S, Milanov N O, Borovikov A M, Trofimaov E I, Shiriaev A A 1985 Functional reconstruction of both hands by free transfer of combined second and third toes from both feet. Plastic Reconstr Surg 75: 584–589

Kuczynski K 1974 Carpometacarpal joint of the human thumb. J Anat 118: 119–126

Kuczynski K 1975 The thumb and the saddle. Hand 7: 120–122

Kudo H, Iwano K, Watanabe S 1980 Total replacement of the rheumatoid elbow with a hingeless prosthesis. J Bone Joint Surg 62A: 277–285

Kuhlmann J N, Boabighi A, Guero S, Mimoun M, Baux S 1988 Boutonniere deformity in Dupuytren's disease. J Hand Surg (Br) 13: 379–382

Kulick R G, DeFiore I C, Straub L R, Ranawat C S 1981 Long-term results of dorsal stabilization in the rheumatoid wrist. J Hand Surg 6: 272–280

Kumar S, James R 1985 Closed rupture of flexor profundus tendon in the palm. J Hand Surg (Br) 10: 193–194

Kumar V P, Satku K, Helm R, Pho R W 1988 Radial reconstruction in segmental defects of both forearm bones. J Bone Joint Surg (Br) 70: 815–817

Kummel B M, Zazanis G A 1973 Shoulder pain as the presenting complaint in carpal tunnel syndrome. Clin Orthopaedics Rel Res 92: 227–230

Kummel W 1895 Die Missbildungen der Extremitaten durch defeckt. Verwachsung and Uberzahl. Hefte 3. Bibliotheca Medica, Kassel

Kupfer K 1986 Palmar dislocation of scaphoid and lunate as a unit: case report with special reference to carpal instability and treatment. J Hand Surg (Am) 11: 130–134

Kuschner S H, Gelberman R H, Jennings C 1988 Ulnar nerve compression at the wrist. J Hand Surg (Am) 13: 577–580

Kusumi R K, Plouffe J F 1981 Gas in soft tissue of forearm in an 18-year-old emotionally disturbed diabetic. J Am Med Assoc 246: 679–680

Kutz J E, Singer R, Lindsay M 1985 Chronic exertional compartment syndrome of the forearm: a case report. J Hand Surg (Am) 10: 302–304

Labbate V A, Ehrlich E E 1976 Rheumatoid arthritis with unusual myositis resembling muscular dystrophy. J Bone Joint Surg 58A: 571–572

Labosky D A, Waggy C A 1986 Apparent weakness of median and ulnar motors in radial nerve palsy. J Hand Surg (Am) 11: 528–533

Lacey S H, Wilber R G, Peckham P H, Freehafer A A 1986 The posterior deltoid to triceps transfer: a clinical and biomechanical assessment. J Hand Surg (Am) 11: 542–547

Lafferty K A, Nelson E L, Demuth R J, Miller S H, Harrison M W 1986 Juvenile aponeurotic fibroma with disseminated fibrosarcoma. J Hand Surg (Am) 11: 737–740

Laforgia R, Specchiulli F, Mariani A 1990 Dorsal dislocation of the fifth carpometacarpal joint. J Hand Surg (Am) 15: 463–465

Lagier R, Chamay A 1984 Localized Sudeck's dystrophy and distal interphalangeal osteoarthritis of a finger: anatomicoradiologic study. J Hand Surg (Am) 9: 328–332

Laha R K, Dujovny M, DeCastro S C 1977 Entrapment of

median nerve by supracondylar process of the humerus. J Neurosurg 46: 252–255

Lai M F, Krishna B V, Pelly A D 1981 The brachioradialis myocutaneous flap. Br J Plastic Surg 34: 431–434

Lain T M 1969 The military brace syndrome: a report of sixteen cases of Erb's palsy occurring in military cadets. J Bone Joint Surg 51A: 557–560

Lamb D W 1977 Radial club hand. A continuing study of sixty-eight patients with one hundred and seventeen club hands. J Bone Joint Surg 59A: 1–13

Lamb D W 1983 Prosthetics in the upper extremity. J Hand Surg (Am) 8: 774–777

Lamb D W 1983 Upper limb dysplasia, form and function. J Roy Coll Surg Edinb 28: 203–213

Lamb D W, Castillo F D 1981 Phalangeal osteoid osteoma in the hand. Hand 13: 291–295

Lamb D W, Chan K M 1983 Surgical reconstruction of the upper limb in traumatic tetraplegia. A review of 41 patients. J Bone Joint Surg (Br) 65: 291–298

Lamb D W, Dick T D, Douglas W B 1988 A new prosthesis for the upper limb. J Bone Joint Surg (Br) 70: 140–144

Lamb D W, Kuczynski K 1981 The practice of hand surgery. Blackwell, Edinburgh

Lamb D W, Lamdry R M 1972 The hand in quadriplegia. Paraplegia 9: 204–212

Lamb D W, Wynne-Davies R, Whitmore J M 1983 Five-fingered hand associated with partial or complete tibial absence and pre-axial polydactyly. A kindred of 15 affected individuals in five generations. J Bone Joint Surg (Br) 65: 60–63

Lamberta F I, Ferlic D C, Clayton M L 1980 Volz total wrist arthroplasty in rheumatoid arthritis: a preliminary report. J Hand Surg 5: 245–252

Lamp J C, Graham J H, Urbach F, Burgoon C F 1964 Keratoacanthoma of the subungual region. A clinicopathological and therapeutic study. J Bone Joint Surg 46A: 1721–1731, 1752

Landi A, Brooks D, De Santis G 1983 Sarcoidosis of the hand — report of two cases. J Hand Surg (Am) 8: 197–200

Landi A, Copeland S 1979 Value of the Tinel sign in brachial plexus lesions. Ann Roy Coll Surg Engl 61: 470–471

Landi A, Copeland S A, Wynn, Parry C B, Jones S J 1980 The role of somatosensory evoked potentials and nerve conduction studies on the surgical management of brachial plexus injuries. J Bone Joint Surg 62B: 492–496

Landra A P 1979 The latissimus dorsi musculocutaneous flap used to resurface a defect on the upper arm and restore extension to the elbow. Br J Plastic Surg 32: 275–277

Lane C S 1977 Detecting occult fractures of the metacarpal head: the Brewerton view. J Hand Surg 2: 131–133

Langa V, Posner M A 1986 Unusual rupture of a flexor profundus tendon. J Hand Surg (Am) 11: 227–229

Langa V, Posner M A, Steiner G E 1987 Lipofibroma of the median nerve: a report of two cases. J Hand Surg (Br) 12: 221–223

Lanier V C 1981 The fillet flap principle. Orthopaedic Rev 10: 63–66

Lankford L L 1993 Reflex sympathetic dystrophy. In: Green D P (ed) Operative hand surgery. Churchill Livingstone, New York, pp 627–660

Lanz U 1977 Anatomical variations of the median nerve in the carpal tunnel. J Hand Surg 2: 44–53

Larossa D, Hamilton R 1971 Herpes simplex infections of the digits. Arch Surg 102: 600–603

Larsen R D, Takagishi N, Posch J L 1960 The pathogenesis of Dupuytren's contracture. J Bone Joint Surg 42A: 993–1007

Larsson S E, Lorentzon R, Boquist L 1975 Giant cell tumor of bone. J Bone Joint Surg 57A: 167–173

Larsson S E, Lorentzon R, Boquist L 1975 Malignant haemangioendothelioma of bone. J Bone Joint Surg 57A: 84–89

LaSalle W B, Strickland J W 1983 An evaluation of the two-stage flexor tendon reconstruction technique. J Hand Surg (Am) 8: 263–267

Lassa R, Shrewsbury M 1975 A variation in the path of the deep motor branch of the ulnar nerve at the wrist. J Bone Joint Surg 57A: 990–991

Lauri G, Santucci M, Ceruso M, Innocenti M 1990 Recurrent digital fibromatosis of childhood. J Hand Surg (Am) 15: 106–109

Lavey E B, Pearl R M 1981 Patent median artery as a cause of carpal tunnel syndrome. Ann Plastic Surg 7: 3236–3238

Lazaro L 1972 Carpal tunnel syndrome from an insect sting. J Bone Joint Surg 54A: 1095–1096

Learmonth J R 1919 A variation in the distribution of the radial branch of the musculo-spiral nerve. J Anat Physiol 53: 371–372

Learmonth J R 1942 A technique for transplanting the ulnar nerve. Surg Gynecol Obstet 75: 792–793

Leddy J P 1985 Avulsions of the flexor digitorum profundus. Hand Clin (1): 77–83

Leddy J P 1986 Infections of the upper extremity. J Hand Surg (Am) 11: 294–297

Leddy J P, Packer J W 1977 Avulsion of the profundus tendon insertion in athletes. J Hand Surg 2: 66–69

Lee B 1960 Dog bites and local infection with *Pasteurella septica*. Br Med J i: 1969–1976

Lee B S 1983 Desmoid tumor of the hand — case report and literature review. J Hand Surg (Am) 8: 95–97

Lee K E 1985 Tuberculosis presenting as carpal tunnel syndrome. J Hand Surg (Am) 10: 242–245

Lee M H 1963 Intra-articular and peri-articular fractures of the phalanges. J Bone Joint Surg 45B: 103–109

Leffert R D 1972 Lipomas of the upper extremity. J Bone Joint Surg 54A: 1262–1266

Leffert R D 1974 Brachial plexus injuries. New Engl J Med 291: 1059–1067

Leffert R D, Dorfman H D 1972 Antecubital cyst in rheumatoid arthritis — surgical findings. J Bone Joint Surg 53A: 1555–1557

Leffert R D, Pess G M 1988 Tendon transfers for brachial plexus injury. Hand Clin 4: 273–288

Legge J H, McFarlane R M 1980 Prediction of results of treatment of Dupuytren's disease. J Hand Surg 5: 608–616

Lemon R A, Engber W D 1985 Trigger wrist: a case report. J Hand Surg (Am) 10: 61–63

Leon P, Daly J M, Synnestvedt M et al 1991 The prognostic implications of microscopic satellites in patients with clinical stage I melanoma. Arch Surg 126: 1461–1468

Leonard L G 1982 Chemical burns: effect of prompt first aid. J Trauma 22: 420–422

LeQuang C 1989 Postirradiation lesions of the brachial plexus. Results of surgical treatment. Hand Clin 5: 23–32

Lesavoy M A, Meals R A 1984 Pay phone receiver cord injuries to the hand. J Hand Surg (Am) 9: 908–909

Leslie B M 1989 Rheumatoid extensor tendon ruptures. Hand Clin 5: 191–202

Leslie B M, Ericson W B Jr, Morehead J R 1990 Incidence of

a septum within the first dorsal compartment of the wrist. J Hand Surg (Am) 15: 88–91

Leslie I J 1980 Compression of the deep branch of the ulnar nerve due to edema of the hand. Hand 12: 271–272

Leslie I J, Dickson R A 1981 The fractured carpal scaphoid. J Bone Joint Surg 63B: 225–230

Leung P 1978 Tuberculosis of the hand. Hand 10: 285–291

Leung P C 1980 Transplantation of the second toe to the hand. A preliminary report of sixteen cases. J Bone Joint Surg (Am) 62: 990–996

Leung P C 1985 Thumb reconstruction using second-toe transfer. Hand Clin 1: 285–295

Lev–El A, Adar R, Rubinstein Z 1981 Axillary artery injury in erect dislocation of the shoulder. J Trauma 21: 323–325

Levein B A, Sirinek K R, Peterson H D, Pruitt B A 1979 Efficacy of tangential excision and immediate autografting of deep second-degree burns of the hand. J Trauma 19: 670–673

Levin S, Pearsall G, Ruderman R J 1978 Von Frey's method of measuring pressure sensibility in the hand: an engineering analysis of Weinstein–Semmes pressure aesthesiometer. J Hand Surg 3: 211–216

Levy M, Pauker M 1978 Carpal tunnel syndrome due to thrombosed persisting median artery. A case report. Hand 10: 65–68

Lewis M H 1978 Median nerve decompression after Colles' fracture. J Bone Joint Surg 60B: 195–196

Lewis R A, Adams J P, Gerber N L, Decker I L, Parsons D B 1978 The hand in mixed connective tissue disease. J Hand Surg 3: 217–222

Lewis R C, Nannini L H, Cocke W M 1981 Multifocal neurilemmomas of median and ulnar nerves of the same extremity — case report. J Hand Surg 6: 406–408

Lewis R C, Nordyke M D, Tenny J R 1986 The tenon method of small joint arthrodesis in the hand. J Hand Surg (Am) 11: 567–569

Li Z T, Liu K, Cao Y D 1989 The reverse flow ulnar artery island flap: 42 clinical cases. Br J Plastic Surg 42: 256–259

Lichter R L, Jacobson T 1975 Tardy palsy of the posterior interosseous nerve with a Monteggia fracture. J Bone Joint Surg 57A: 124–125

Lichtman D M 1988 The wrist and its disorders. W B Saunders, Philadelphia

Lichtman D M, Noble W H, Alexander C E 1984 Dynamic triquetrolunate instability. J Hand Surg 9: 185–189

Lichtman D M, Schneider J R, Swafford A R et al 1981 Ulnar midcarpal instability. Clinical and laboratory analysis. J Hand Surg 6: 515–523

Lichtman D, Johnson D, Mack G, Lack E 1978 Maduromycosis (*Allescheria boydii*) infection of the hand: a case report. J Bone Joint Surg 60A: 546–548

Light T R 1981 Buttress pinning techniques. Orthopaedic Rev 10: 49–55

Light T R, Ogden J A 1987 Metacarpal epiphyseal fractures. J Hand Surg (Am) 12: 460–464

Lillmars S A, Bush D C 1988 Flexor tendon rupture associated with an anomalous muscle. J Hand Surg (Am) 13: 115–119

Lilly C J, Magnell T D 1985 Severance of the thenar branch of the median nerve as a complication of carpal tunnel release. J Hand Surg (Am) 10: 399–402

Lin E, Engel J, Bubis J J, Herman O 1984 Aneurysmal bone cyst of the hamate bone. J Hand Surg (Am) 9: 847–850

Lin S D, Lai C S, Chiu C C 1984 Venous drainage in the reverse forearm flap. Plastic Reconstr Surg 74: 508–512

Lineaweaver W, Mathes S J 1988 Distal avulsion of the palmar plate of the interphalangeal joint of the thumb. J Hand Surg (Am) 13: 453–455

Linscheid R L 1979 Carpal tunnel syndrome secondary to ulnar bursa distention from the intercarpal joint: report of a case. J Hand Surg 4: 191–193

Linscheid R L 1985 Kienbock's disease. J Hand Surg 10A: 1–3

Linscheid R L 1987 Ulnar lengthening and shortening. Hand Clin 3: 69–79

Linscheid R L, Dobyns J H 1985 Radiolunate arthrodesis. J Hand Surg (Am) 10: 821–829

Linscheid R L, Dobyns J H, Beabout J W, Bryan R S 1972 Traumatic instability of the wrist. J Bone Joint Surg 54A: 1612–1632

Linscheid R L, Dobyns J H, Beckenbaugh R D, Cooney W P 3rd, Wood M B 1983 Instability patterns of the wrist. J Hand Surg (Am) 8: 682–686

Linscheid R, Dobyns J 1975 Common and uncommon infections of the hand. Orthopedic Clin North Am 6: 1063–1103

Linson M A 1980 Axillary artery thrombosis after fracture of the humerus. J Bone Joint Surg 62A: 1214–1215

Linson M A, Leffert R, Todd D P 1983 The treatment of upper extremity reflex sympathetic dystrophy with prolonged continuous stellate ganglion blockade. J Hand Surg (Am) 8: 153–159

Lipton H A, May J W Jr, Simon S R 1987 Preoperative and postoperative gait analyses of patients undergoing great toe-to-thumb transfer. J Hand Surg (Am) 12: 66–69

Liseki E J, Curl W W, Markey K L 1980 Hand and forearm infections caused by *Aeromonas hydrophila*. J Hand Surg 5: 605

Lister G 1978 Intraosseous wiring of the digital skeleton. J Hand Surg 3: 427–435

Lister G D 1979 Reconstruction of pulleys employing extensor retinaculum. J Hand Surg 4: 461–464

Lister G D 1981 The theory of the transposition flap and its practical application in the hand. Clin Plastic Surg 8: 115–128

Lister G D 1983 Incision and closure of the flexor sheath during primary tendon repair. Hand 15: 123–135

Lister G 1985 Indications and techniques for repair of the flexor tendon sheath. Hand Clin 1: 85–95

Lister G D 1985 Local flaps to the hand. Hand Clin 1: 621–640

Lister G D 1985 Pitfalls and complications of flexor tendon surgery. Hand Clin 1: 133–146

Lister G D 1988 Emergency free flaps. In: Green D P (ed) Operative hand surgery, 2nd edn. Churchill Livingstone, New York

Lister G D 1988 Microsurgical transfer of the second toe for congenital deficiency of the thumb. Plastic Reconstr Surg 82: 658–665

Lister G D 1990 Flexor tendon. In: McCarthy J G (ed) Plastic surgery. W B Saunders, Philadelphia, pp 4516–4564

Lister G D 1990 Microvascular free transfer of the nail. In: Strauch B, Vasconez L O, Hall-Findlay E J (eds) Grabb's Encyclopedia of flaps. Little Brown & Co, Boston, pp 898–901

Lister G 1991 Musculus lumbricalis pollicis. J Hand Surg 16A: 622–625

Lister G 1991 Pollex abductus in the hypoplastic and duplicated thumb. J Hand Surg 16A: 626–633

Lister G D 1991 Radial tunnel syndrome. In: Gelberman R H

(ed) Operative nerve repair and reconstruction. Lippincott, Philadelphia, pp 1023–1037

Lister G D 1991 Replantation. In: Smith J W, Aston S J (eds) Grabb & Smith's plastic surgery, 4th edn. Little, Brown and Company, Boston, pp 1079–1112

Lister G D 1991 The VY advancement flap. In: Foucher G (ed) Fingertip and nailbed injuries. Churchill Livingstone, New York, pp 52–61

Lister G D 1993 Free skin and composite flaps. In: Green D P (ed) Operative hand surgery, 3rd edn. Churchill Livingstone, New York, pp 1103–1158

Lister G D 1993 Skin Flaps. In: Green D P (ed) Operative hand surgery. Churchill Livingstone, New York, pp 1741–1822

Lister G D, Milward T M 1976 Skin contracture of the first web space. Transactions Sixth International Congress of Plastic and Reconstructive Surgery, Masson, Paris, pp 594–604

Lister G D, Smith R R 1976 Ideas and innovations. Protection of the radial artery in the resection of adherent ganglions of the wrist. Plastic Reconstr Surg 61: 127–129

Lister G, Scheker L 1988 Emergency free flaps to the upper extremity. J Hand Surg (Am) 13(1): 22–28

Lister G D, McGregor I A, Jackson I T 1973 Groin flap in hand injuries. Br J Accident Surg 4: 229–239

Lister G D, Kleinert H E, Kutz J E, Atasoy E 1977 Arthritis of the trapezial articulations treated by prosthetic replacement. Hand 9: 117–129

Lister G D, Kleinert H E, Kutz J E, Atasoy E 1977 Primary flexor tendon repair followed by immediate controlled mobilization. J Hand Surg 2: 441–455

Lister G D, Belsole R B, Kleinert H E 1979 The radial tunnel syndrome. J Hand Surg 4: 52–60

Lister G D, Kalisman M, Tsai T M 1983 Reconstruction of the hand with free microneurovascular toe-to-hand transfer: experience with 54 toe transfers. Plastic Reconstr Surg 71: 372–386

Littler J W 1976 On making a thumb: one hundred years of surgical effort. J Hand Surg 1: 35–51

Littler J W, Cooley S G E 1963 Opposition of the thumb and its restoration by abductor digiti quinti transfer. J Bone Joint Surg 45A: 1389–1396

Littler J W, Eaton R G 1967 Redistribution of forces in the correction of the boutonniere deformity. J Bone Joint Surg 49A: 1267–1274

Lloyd-Roberts G C, Lettin A W F 1970 Arthrogryposis multiplex congenita. J Bone Joint Surg 52B: 494–508

Loder R T, Robinson J H, Jackson W T, Allen D J 1988 A surface ultrastructure study of ganglia and digital mucous cysts. J Hand Surg (Am) 13: 758–762

Loebl D, Kirby S, Stephenson R, Cook E, Mealing H, Bailey J 1979 Psoriatic arthritis. J Am Med Assoc 242: 2447–2451

Logan S E, Alpert B S, Buncke H J 1988 Free serratus anterior muscle transplantation for hand reconstruction. Br J Plastic Surg 41: 639–643

Lombardi R M, Wood M B, Linscheid R L 1988 Symptomatic restrictive thumb-index flexor tenosynovitis: incidence of musculotendinous anomalies and results of treatment. J Hand Surg (Am) 13: 325–328

London P S 1961 Simplicity of approach to treatment of the injured hand. J Bone Joint Surg 43B: 454–464

Long P I, Espiniella J L 1978 Squamous cell carcinoma of the nail bed. J Am Med Assoc 239: 2154–2155

Long W T, Filler B C, Cox E 2nd, Stark H H 1988 Toxic

shock syndrome after a human bite to the hand. J Hand Surg (Am) 13: 957–959. (Comment in J Hand Surg (Am) 1989 14: 1036–1037.)

Lopez-Burbano L F, Cimorra G A, Gonzalez-Peirona E, Alfora J 1987 Malignant clear-cell hidradenoma. Plastic Reconstr Surg 80: 300–303

Lord R S A, Irani C N 1974 Assessment of arterial injury in limb trauma. J Trauma 14: 1042–1053

Lotem M, Fried A, Levy M, Solzi P, Najenson T, Nathan H 1971 Radial palsy following muscular effort. J Bone Joint Surg 53B: 500–506

Loth T S, McMillan M D 1988 Coronal dorsal hamate fractures. J Hand Surg (Am) 13: 616–618

Louis D S 1987 Cumulative trauma disorders. J Hand Surg (Am) 12: 823–825

Louis D S 1987 Incomplete release of the first dorsal compartment — a diagnostic test. J Hand Surg (Am) 12: 87–88

Louis D S 1987 Peripheral nerve tumours in the upper extremity. Hand Clin 3: 311–318

Louis D S, Buckwalter K A 1989 Magnetic resonance imaging of the collateral ligaments of the thumb. J Hand Surg (Am) 14: 739–741

Louis D S, Dick H M 1973 Ossifying lipofibroma of the median nerve. J Bone Joint Surg 55A: 1082–1084

Louis D S, Eckenrode J F 1986 Autogenous nerve pedicle graft in the forearm. J Hand Surg (Am) 11: 703–706

Louis D S, Greene T L, Jacobson K E, Rasmussen C et al 1984 Evaluation of normal values for stationary and moving two-point discrimination in the hand. J Hand Surg (Am) 9: 552–555

Louis D S, Hankin F M 1986 Arthrodesis of the wrist: past and present. J Hand Surg (Am) 11: 787–789

Louis D S, Hankin F M 1987 Symptomatic relief following carpal tunnel decompression with normal electroneuromyographic studies. Ortho 10: 434–436

Louis D S, Hankin F M, Greene T L, Dick H M 1985 Lipofibromas of the median nerve: long-term follow-up of four cases. J Hand Surg (Am) 10: 403–408

Louis D S, Hankin F M, Hankin R C, Brennan M, Greene T L 1986 Synovial cell sarcoma: a case report with a comment on 27 years of treatment. J Hand Surg (Am) 11: 578–581

Louis D S, Lamp M K, Greene T L 1985 The upper extremity and psychiatric illness. J Hand Surg (Am) 10: 687–693

Louis D S, Palmer A K, Burney R E 1980 Open treatment of digital tip injuries. J Am Med Assoc 244: 697–698

Louis D S, Silva J Jr 1979 Herpetic whitlow: herpetic infections of the digits. J Hand Surg 4: 90–94

Love G L, Melchior E 1985 *Mycobacterium terrae* tenosynovitis. J Hand Surg (Am) 10: 730–732

Love J G 1944 Glomus tumors: diagnosis and treatment. Mayo Clin Proc 19: 113–116

Lovie M J, Duncan G M, Glasson D W 1984 The ulnar artery forearm free flap. Br J Plastic Surg 37: 486–492

Lowen R M, Rodgers C M, Ketch L L, Phelps D B 1989 *Aeromonas hydrophila* infection complicating digital replantation and revascularization. J Hand Surg (Am) 14: 714–718

Lubahn J D 1988 Dorsal fracture dislocations of the proximal interphalangeal joint. Hand Clin 4: 15–24

Lubahn J D 1989 Mallet finger fractures: a comparison of open and closed technique. Hand Surg (Am) 14: 394–396

Lubahn J D, Carlier A, Lister G D 1985 The denervated first

dorsal interosseous muscle flap: a case report. J Hand Surg (Am) 10: 684–686

Lubahn J D, Koeneman J, Kosar K 1985 The digital tourniquet: how safe is it? J Hand Surg (Am) 10: 664–669

Lubahn J D, Lister G D 1983 Familial radial nerve entrapment syndrome: a case report and literature review. J Hand Surg (Am) 8: 297–299

Lubahn J D, Lister G D, Wolfe T 1984 Fasciectomy and Dupuytren's disease: a comparison between the open-palm technique and wound closure. J Hand Surg (Am) 9A: 53–58

Lucas G L, Bartlett D H 1981 *Pasteurella multocida* infection in the hand. Plastic Reconstr Surg 67: 49–53

Lucas G L, Sponsellar P D 1984 Synovial chondrometaplasia of the hand: case report and review of the literature. J Hand Surg (Am) 9: 269–272

Luce E A, Gottlieb S E 1984 'True' high-tension electrical injuries. Ann Plastic Surg 12: 321–326

Luce E A, Griffen W 1978 Shotgun injuries of the upper extremity. J Trauma 18: 487–492

Luck J U 1959 Dupuytren's contracture. J Bone Joint Surg 41A: 635–664

Lundborg G, Dahlin L B, Hansson H A, Kanje M, Necking L E 1990 Vibration exposure and peripheral nerve fiber damage. J Hand Surg (Am) 15: 346–351

Lutz G, Hansford T 1987 Cumulative trauma disorder controls: the ergonomics program at Ethicon, Inc. J Hand Surg (Am) 12: 863–866

MacCollum M S 1977 Dorsal wrist ganglions in children. J Hand Surgery 2: 325

MacDonell J A 1968 Age of fitting upper extremity prostheses in children. J Bone Joint Surg 40A: 655–662

MacDougal B, Weeks P M, Wray R C 1977 Median nerve compression and trigger finger in the mucopolysaccharidoses and related disease. Plastic Reconstr Surg 59: 260–263

Macht S D, Watson H K 1980 The Moberg volar advancement flap for digital reconstruction. J Hand Surg 5: 372–376

Mackay I, Simpson R G 1980 Closed rupture of extensor digitorum communis tendon following fracture of the radius. Hand 12: 214–216

MacKenzie E J, Shapiro S, Siegel J 1988 The economic impact of traumatic injuries. JAMA 260: 3290–3296

Mackinnon S E, Dellon A L 1985 The overlap pattern of the lateral antebrachial cutaneous nerve and the superficial branch of the radial nerve. J Hand Surg (Am) 10: 522–526

Mackinnon S E, Dellon A L 1985 Two-point discrimination tester. J Hand Surg (Am) 10: 906–907

Mackinnon S E, Dellon A L 1986 Experimental study of chronic nerve compression. Clinical implications. Hand Clin 2: 639–650

Mackinnon S E, Dellon A L 1988 A comparison of nerve regeneration across a sural nerve graft and a vascularized pseudosheath. J Hand Surg (Am) 13: 935–942

Mackinnon S E, Dellon A L 1988 Evaluation of microsurgical internal neurolysis in a primate median nerve model of chronic nerve compression. J Hand Surg (Am) 13: 345–351

Mackinnon S E, Gruss J S 1985 Soft tissue expanders in upper limb surgery. J Hand Surg (Am) 10: 749–754

Mackinnon S E, Holder L E 1984 The use of three-phase radionuclide bone scanning in the diagnosis of reflex sympathetic dystrophy. J Hand Surg (Am) 9: 556–563

Macnicol M 1978 Roentgenographic evidence of median nerve entrapment in a greenstick humeral fracture. J Bone Joint Surg 60A: 998–1000

Madelung V 1975 Die spontane subluxation der hand nach norne Verh Dtsch Ges Chir 7: 259, 1878. Arch Klin Chir 23: 395

Maeda K, Miura T, Komada T, Chiba A 1977 Anterior interosseous nerve paralysis. Report of 13 cases and review of Japanese literature. Hand 9: 165–171

Maeda M, Matsue T 1985 Camptodactyly caused by an abnormal lumbrical muscle. J Hand Surg 10B: 95–96

Magierski M, Sakiel S, Buczak B, Koisar J, Kepny A, Ciembroniewicz W 1979 Analysis of reasons and locations of burns on hands. Scand J Plastic Reconstr Surg 13: 141–142

Magnell T D, Pochron M D, Condit D P 1988 The intercalated tendon graft for treatment of extensor pollicis longus tendon rupture. J Hand Surg (Am) 13: 105–109

Magyar E, Talerman A, Feher M, Wouters H W 1974 Giant bone cyst in rheumatoid arthritis. J Bone Joint Surg 56B: 121–129

Mahaffey P J, Tanner N S, Evans H B, McGrouther D A 1985 The degloved hand: immediate complete restoration of skin cover with contralateral forearm free flap. Br J Plastic Surg 38: 101–106

Maher D P 1987 Granular cell tumor in the hand. J Hand Surg (Am) 12: 800–803

Mahoney J L 1987 Soft tissue chondromas in the hand. J Hand Surg (Am) 12: 317–320

Mahoney J, Naiberg J 1987 Toe transfer to the vessels of the reversed forearm flap. J Hand Surg (Am) 12: 62–65

Maisels D O 1962 Acrosyndactyly. Br J Plastic Surg 15: 166–172

Maisels D O 1970 Lobster-claw deformities of the hands and feet. Br J Plastic Surg 23: 269–282

Malerich M M, Baird R A, McMaster W, Erickson J M 1987 Permissible limits of flexor digitorum profundus tendon advancement — an anatomic study. J Hand Surg (Am) 12: 30–33

Maley E D, McDonald C J 1975 Bilateral subungual glomus tumors. Plastic Reconstr Surg 55: 488–489

Malfeyt G A M 1976 Burns of the dorsum of the hand treated by tangential excision. Br J Plastic Surg 29: 78–81

Malinowski R, Strate R G, Perry J F, Fischer R 1979 The management of human bite injuries of the hand. J Trauma 19: 655–659

Mancini L H, Fort L K 1989 Rehabilitation of the infected hand. Hand Clin 5: 635–641

Mancusi-Ungaro A, Corres J J, Di Spaltro F 1976 Case reports: median carpal tunnel syndrome following a vascular shunt procedure in the forearm. Plastic Reconstr Surg 57: 96–97

Mandel M 1978 Immune competence and diabetes mellitus: pyogenic human hand infections. J Hand Surg 3: 458–461

Mandel M, Dauchot P 1977 Radial artery cannulation in 1000 patients: precautions and complications. J Hand Surg 2: 482–485

Mankin HJ 1987 Principles of diagnosis and management of tumors of the hand. Hand Clin 3: 185–195

Manktelow R T 1988 Functioning microsurgical muscle transfer. Hand Clin 4: 289–296

Manktelow R T, Wainwright D J 1984 A technique of distraction osteosynthesis in the hand. J Hand Surg (Am) 9: 858–862

Mann R J 1989 Hand infections. Hand Clin 5: 515–667

Mann R J, Hoffeld T A, Farmer C B 1977 Human bites of the hand: twenty years of experience. J Hand Surg 2: 97–104

Mann R J, Peacock J M 1977 Hand infections in patients with diabetes mellitus. J Trauma 17: 376–380

Mannerfelt L 1966 Studies on the hand in ulnar nerve paralysis. A clinical and experimental investigation in normal and anomalous innervation. Acta Ortho Scand (suppl) 87

Mannerfelt L G 1988 Tendon transfers in surgery of the rheumatoid hand. Hand Clin 4: 309–316

Manske P 1976 Fracture of the hook of the hamate presenting as carpal tunnel syndrome. Hand 10: 181–183

Manske P R 1977 Compression of the radial nerve by the triceps muscle. Case report. J Bone Joint Surg 59A: 835–836

Manske P R 1985 Redirection of extensor pollicis longus in the treatment of spastic thumb-in-palm deformity. J Hand Surg (Am) 10: 553–560

Manske P R 1989 Treatment of duplicated thumb using a ligamentous/periosteal flap. J Hand Surg (Am) 14: 728–733

Manske P R, Lesker P A 1978 Avulsion of the ring finger flexor digitorum profundus tendon. Hand 10: 52–55

Manske P R, McCaroll H R Jr 1985 Index finger pollicization for a congenitally absent or nonfunctioning thumb. J Hand Surg (Am) 10: 606–613

Manske P, McCarroll H 1978 Abductor digiti minimi opponensplasty in congenital radial dysplasia. J Hand Surg 3: 552–559

Mantero R, Rossello M I, Grandis C 1989 Digital subtraction angiography in preoperative examination of congenital hand malformation. J Hand Surg (Am) 2: 351–352

Marck K W, Klasen H J 1986 Fracture-dislocation of the hamatometacarpal joint: a case report. J Hand Surg (Am) 11: 128–130

Marcus N A, Blair W F, Shuck J M, Omer G E 1980 Low-velocity gun-shot wounds to extremities. J Trauma 20: 1061–1064

Margileth A M 1968 Cat scratch disease. Pediatrics 42: 803–818

Margles S W 1988 Intra-articular fractures of the metacarpophalangeal and proximal interphalangeal joints. Hand Clin 4: 67–74

Markley J M 1977 The preservation of close two-point discrimination in the interdigital transfer of neurovascular island flaps. Plastic Reconstr Surg 59: 812–816

Markley J M Jr 1985 Island flaps of the hand. Hand Clin 1: 689–699

Marks M R, Gunther S F 1989 Efficacy of cortisone injection in treatment of trigger fingers and thumbs. J Hand Surg (Am) 14: 722–727

Marks T W, Bayne L G 1978 Polydactyly of the thumb: abnormal anatomy and treatment. J Hand Surg 3: 107–116

Marmor L 1972 Surgery of the rheumatoid elbow. Follow-up study on synovectomy combined with radial head excision. J Bone Joint Surg 54A: 573–578

Marmor L, Horner R L 1959 Metastasis to a phalanx simulating infection in a finger. Am J Surg 97: 236

Marshall J H, Sonsire J M, Nielsen P E, Nigogosyan G, Terzian J 1987 Digital angiography and osteoblastoma of the triquetrum. J Hand Surg (Am) 12: 256–258

Marten E 1979 Hand deformities in patients with snakebite. Plastic Reconstr Surg 64. 554

Martin D F, Tolo V T, Sellers D S, Weiland A J 1989 Radial nerve laceration and retraction associated with a supracondylar fracture of the humerus. J Hand Surg (Am) 14: 542–545

Martin R 1763 Tal om Nervers allmanna Egenskaper i Manniskans kroop. L Salvius, Stockholm

Martinez R E, Couchel S, Swartz W M, Smith M B 1989 Mycetoma of the hand. J Hand Surg (Am) 14: 909–912

Maruyama Y 1990 The reverse dorsal metacarpal flap. Br J Plastic Surg 43: 24–27

Masear V R, Hayes J M, Hyde A G 1986 An industrial cause of carpal tunnel syndrome. J Hand Surg (Am) 11: 222–227

Masear V R, Hill J J Jr, Cohen S M 1989 Ulnar compression neuropathy secondary to the anconeus epitrochlearis muscle. J Hand Surg (Am) 13: 720–724 (Comment in: J Hand Surg (Am) 1989 14: 917–919.)

Masear V R, Meyer R D, Pichora D R 1989 Surgical anatomy of the medial antebrachial cutaneous nerve. J Hand Surg (Am) 14: 267–271

Mason M L 1937 Tumors of the hand. Surg Gynecol Obstet 64: 129

Mass D P, Ciano M C, Tortosa R, Newmeyer W L, Kilgore E S Jr 1984 Treatment of painful hand neuromas by their transfer into bone. Plastic Reconstr Surg 74: 182–185

Mass D P, Tortosa R, Newmeyer W L, Kilgore E S Jr 1982 Compression of posterior interosseous nerve by a ganglion. Case report. J Hand Surg 7: 92–94

Match R M 1975 Radiation-induced brachial plexus paralysis. Arch Surg 110: 384–386

Match R M, Leffert R D 1987 Massive neurofibromatosis of the upper extremity with paralysis. J Hand Surg (Am) 12: 718–722

Matev I 1964 Transposition of the lateral slips of the aponeurosis of long-standing boutonniere deformity of the fingers. Br J Plastic Surg 17: 281–286

Matev I 1976 A radiological sign of entrapment of the median nerve in the elbow joint after posterior dislocation. J Bone Joint Surg 58B: 353–355

Matev I 1985 The osteocutaneous pedicle forearm flap. J Hand Surg (Br) 10: 179–182

Matev I B 1980 Tactile gnosis in free skin grafts in the hand. Br J Plastic Surg 33: 434–439

Matev I B 1980 Thumb reconstruction through metacarpal bone lengthening. J Hand Surg 5: 482–487

Matev I B 1989 The bone-lengthening method in hand reconstruction: twenty years' experience. J Hand Surg (Am) 14: 376–378

Matev J 1979 Thumb reconstruction in children through metacarpal lengthening. Plastic Reconstr Surg 64: 665–669

Mathes S J, Nahai F 1981 Classification of the vascular anatomy of muscles: experimental and clinical correlation. Plastic Reconstr Surg 67: 177–187

Mathes S J, Vasconez L O, Jurkiewicz M J 1977 Extension and further applications of the muscle flap transposition. Plastic Reconstr Surg 60: 6–13

Mathiowetz V, Rennells C, Donahoe L 1985 Effect of elbow position on grip and key pinch strength. J Hand Surg (Am) 10: 694–697

Mathiowetz V, Weber K, Volland G, Kashman N 1984 Reliability and validity of grip and pinch strength. J Hand Surg (Am) 9: 222–226

Matloubi R 1988 Transfer of sensory branches of radial nerve in hand surgery. J Hand Surg (Br) 13: 92–95

Matsen F A 1980 Compartmental syndromes. Grune & Stratton, New York

Matsen F A, Winquist R A, Krugmire R B 1980 Diagnosis

and management of compartmental syndromes. J Bone Joint Surg 62A: 286–291

Matthews P 1973 Ganglia of the flexor tendon sheaths in the hand. J Bone Joint Surg 55B: 612–617

Matthews R E, Gould J S, Kashlan M B 1981 Diffuse pigmented villonodular tenosynovitis of the ulnar bursa — a case report. J Bone Joint Surg 6: 64–69

Matthews R N, Morgan B D 1987 Multiple seagull flaps for digital contractures in electrical burns. Br J Plastic Surg 40: 47–51

Maxwell G P, Curtis R, Wilgis F 1979 Multiple digital glomus tumors. J Hand Surg 4: 363–367

May J W Jr, Atkinson R, Rosen H 1984 Traumatic arteriovenous fistula of the thumb after blunt trauma: a case report. J Hand Surg (Am) 9: 253–255

May J W Jr, Bartlett S P 1985 Great toe-to-hand free tissue transfer for thumb reconstruction. Hand Clin 1: 271–284

May J W Jr, Donelan M B, Toth B A, Wall J 1984 Thumb reconstruction in the burned hand by advancement pollicization of the second ray remnant. J Hand Surg (Am) 9: 484–489

May J W Jr, Rothkopf D M, Savage R C, Atkinson R 1989 Elective cross-hand transfer: a case report with a five year follow-up. J Hand Surg (Am) 14: 28–34

May J W, Bartlett S P 1981 Staged groin flap in reconstruction of the pediatric hand. J Hand Surg 6: 163–171

Mayfield J K, Johnson R P, Kilcoyne R K 1980 Carpal dislocations: pathomechanics and progressive perilunar instability. J Hand Surg 5: 226–241

Mayhall W S T, Tiley F T, Paluska D I 1981 Fracture of silastic radial-head prosthesis. Case report. J Bone Joint Surg 63A: 459–460

McCabe S J, Murray J F, Ruhnke H L, Rachlis A 1987 *Mycoplasma* infection of the hand acquired from a cat. J Hand Surg (Am) 12: 1085–1088

McCabe W P, Ditmars D M 1973 Soft tissue changes in the hands of drug addicts. Plastic Reconstr Surg 52: 538–540

McCarrol H R Jr, Manske P R 1982 Congenital absence of the thenar muscles (letter). J Bone Joint Surg (Am) 64: 153

McCarroll H R Jr 1985 Congenital flexion deformities of the thumb. Hand Clin 1: 567–575

McCash C R 1956 Cross-arm bridge flaps in the repair of flexion contractures of the finger. Br Plastic Surg 9: 25–33

McCollam S M, Corley F G, Green D P 1988 Posterior interosseous nerve palsy caused by ganglions of the proximal radioulnar joint. J Hand Surg (Am) 13: 725–728

McCormick T M, Burch B H 1979 Routine angiographic evaluation of neck and extremity injuries. J Trauma 19: 384–387

McCraw J B, Dibbell D G, Carraway J H 1977 Clinical definition of independent myocutaneous vascular territories. Plastic Reconstr Surg 60: 341–352

McCue F C, Honner R, Johnson M C, Gieck J H 1970 Athletic injuries of the proximal interphalangeal joint requiring surgical treatment. J Bone Joint Surg 52A: 937–956

McDonald I 1979 *Eikenella corrodens* infection of the hand. Hand 11: 224–227

McDowell C L, Hencreoth D 1977 Malignant fibrous histiocytoma of the hand. A case report. Journal of Hand Surgery (Am) 2: 297–298, 345

McDowell C L, Moberg E A, House J H 1986 The second international conference on surgical rehabilitation of the upper limb in tetraplegia. J Hand Surg 11A: 604–608

McDowell C L, Rago T A, Gonzalez SM 1989 Tetraplegia. Hand Clin 5: 343–349

McDowell C, Moberg E A, Smith A G 1979 International conference on surgical rehabilitation of the upper limb in tetraplegia. J Hand Surg 4: 387–390

McElfresh E C, Dobyns J H 1983 Intra-articular metacarpal head fractures. J Hand Surg (Am) 8: 383–393

McEvedy B V 1962 Simple ganglion. Br J Surg 49: 585–594

McFarland G B, Hoffer M M 1971 Paralysis of the intrinsic muscles of the hand secondary to lipoma in Guyon's canal. J Bone Joint Surg 53A: 375–376

McFarlane R M 1974 Patterns of diseased fascia in the fingers in Dupuytren's contracture. Plastic Reconstr Surg 54: 31–44

McFarlane R M 1983 The current status of Dupuytren's disease. J Hand Surg (Am) 8: 703–708

McFarlane R M, Curry G I, Evans H B 1983 Anomalies of the intrinsic muscles in camptodactyly. J Hand Surg (Am) 8: 531–544

McFarlane R M, Mayer J R, Hugill J V 1976 Further observations on the anatomy of the ulnar nerve at the wrist. Hand 8: 115–117

McGlynn J T, Smith R A, Bogumill G P 1988 Arthrodesis of small joints of the hand: a rapid and effective technique. J Hand Surg (Am) 13: 595–599

McGowan A J 1950 The results of transposition of the ulnar nerve for traumatic ulnar neuritis. J Bone Joint Surg 32B: 293–301

McGrath M H 1984 Local steroid therapy in the hand. J Hand Surg (Am) 9: 915–921

McGrath M H, Fleischer A 1989 The subcutaneous rheumatoid nodule. Hand Clin 5: 127–135

McGraw J M, Stern P J 1989 Flexion contracture of the thumb: a malignant etiology. J Hand Surg (Am) 14: 736–738

McGregor A D 1987 The Allen test — an investigation of its accuracy by fluorescein angiography. J Hand Surg (Br) 12: 82–85

McGregor A D 1987 The free radial forearm flap — the management of the secondary defect. Br J Plastic Surg 40: 83–85

McGregor I A, Glover L 1988 The E-flat hand. J Hand Surg (Am) 13: 692–693

McGregor I A, Jackson I T 1969 Sodium chlorate bomb injuries of the hand. Br J Plastic Surg 22: 16–29

McGregor I A, Morgan G 1973 Axial and random pattern flaps. Br J Plastic Surg 26: 202–213

McIntyre D I 1975 Subcoracoid neurovascular entrapment. Clin Orthopaedics 108: 27–30

McKain C W, Urban B J, Goldner J L 1983 The effects of intravenous regional guanethidine and reserpine — a controlled study. J Bone Joint Surg (Am) 65: 808–811

McKay D, Pascarelli E F, Eaton R G 1973 Infections and sloughs in the hands in drug addicts. J Bone Joint Surg 55A: 741–746

McLatchie G R, Davies J E, Caulley J H 1980 Injuries in karate — a case for medical control. J Trauma 20: 956–958

McMaster M 1972 The natural history of the rheumatoid metacarpophalangeal joint. J Bone Joint Surg 54B: 687–697

McMurtry R Y, Paley D, Marks P, Axelrod T 1990 A critical analysis of Swanson ulnar head replacement arthroplasty: rheumatoid versus nonrheumatoid. J Hand Surg (Am) 15: 224–231

Meagher S W 1987 Tool design for prevention of hand and wrist injuries. J Hand Surg (Am) 12: 855–857

Meals R A, Meuli H C 1985 Carpenter's nails, phonograph needles, piano wires, and safety pins: the history of operative fixation of metacarpal and phalangeal fractures. J Hand Surg (Am) 10: 144–150

Meals R A, Mirra J M, Bernstein A J 1989 Giant cell tumor of metacarpal treated by cryosurgery. J Hand Surg (Am) 14: 130–134

Meals R A, Shaner M 1983 Variations in digital sensory patterns: a study of the ulnar nerve–median nerve palmar communicating branch. J Hand Surg (Am) 8: 411–414

Medlar R C, Sprague H H 1979 Osteochondroma of the carpal scaphoid. J Hand Surg 4: 150–152

Mehrotra O N, Crabb D J M 1979 The pattern of hand injuries sustained in the overturning motor vehicle. Hand 11: 321–328

Meland N B, Lincenberg L S M, Cooney W P III, Wood M B, Hentz V R 1989 Experience with the island radial forearm flap in local hand coverage. J Trauma 29: 489–493

Melvin J L, Schuchmann J A, Lanese R R 1973 Diagnostic specificity of motor and sensory nerve conduction variables in the carpal tunnel syndrome. Arch Phys Med Rehab 54: 69–74

Mendelson L S, Peckham P H, Freehafer A A, Keith M W 1988 Intraoperative assessment of wrist extensor muscle force. J Hand Surg (Am) 13: 832–836

Menelaus M B 1976 Radial club hand with absence of the biceps muscle treated by centralisation of the ulna and triceps transfer. J Bone Joint Surg 58B: 488–491

Menon J 1983 Reconstruction of the metacarpophalangeal joint with autogenous metatarsal. J Hand Surg (Am) 8: 443–446

Menon J, Rankin D, Jacobson C 1988 Recurrent osteoblastoma of the carpal hamate. Ortho 11: 609–611

Menon J, Schoene H, Hohl J 1981 Trapeziometacarpal arthritis — results of tendon interpositional arthroplasty. J Hand Surg 6: 442–446

Menon J, Wood V E, Schoene H R, Frykman G K et al 1984 Isolated tears of the triangular fibrocartilage of the wrist: results of partial excision. J Hand Surg (Am) 9: 527–530

Mercer, Newman J H, Watt I 1984 Acute calcific periarthritis in a child. J Hand Surg (Br) 9: 351–352

Merkow R L, Bansal M, Inglis A E 1985 Giant cell reparative granuloma in the hand: report of three cases and review of the literature. J Hand Surg 10A: 733–739

Merle M, Foucher G, Dap F, Bour C 1989 Tendon transfers for treatment of the paralyzed hand following brachial plexus injury. Hand Clin 5: 33–41

Meyer F N, Pflaum B C 1987 Median nerve compression at the wrist caused by a reversed palmaris longus muscle. J Hand Surg (Am) 12: 369–371

Meyn M A, Roth A M 1980 Isolated dislocation of the trapezoid bone. J Hand Surg 5: 602–604

Mikhail I K 1964 Median nerve lipoma in the hand. J Bone Joint Surg 46B: 726

Mikkelsen O A 1976 Dupuytren's disease — a study of the pattern of distribution and stage of contracture in the hand. Hand 8: 265–271

Mikkelsen O A 1977 Knuckle pads in Dupuytren's disease. Hand 9: 301–305

Mikkelsen O T 1980 Arthrodesis of the wrist joint in rheumatoid arthritis. Hand 12: 149–153

Milberg P, Kleinert H E 1980 Giant cell tumor compression of the deep branch of the ulnar nerve. Ann Plastic Surg 4: 426–429

Millea T P, Hansen R H 1989 Snowblower injuries to the hand. J Trauma 29: 229–233

Millender L H, Nalebuff E A 1973 Arthrodesis of the rheumatoid wrist. J Bone Joint Surg 55A: 1026–1234

Millender L H, Nalebuff E A, Holdsworth D E 1973 Posterior interosseous nerve syndrome secondary to rheumatoid synovitis. J Bone Joint Surg 55A: 753–757

Millender L H, Nalebuff M D, Edward A, Holdsworth D E 1973 Posterior interosseous nerve syndrome secondary to rheumatoid synovitis. J Bone Joint Surg 55A: 753–757

Millender L H, Philips C 1978 Combined wrist arthrodesis and metacarpophalangeal joint arthroplasty in rheumatoid arthritis. Orthopedics 1: 43–48

Millender L, Nalebuff E, Dasdan E 1972 Aneurysms and thromboses of the ulnar artery in the hand. Arch Surg 105: 686–690

Miller A, Campbell D R, Gibbons G W, Pomposelli F B, Freeman D V, Jepsen S J, Lees R S, Isaacsohn J L, Purcell D, Bolduc M, LeGerfo F W 1989 Routine intraoperative angioscopy in lower extremity revascularization. Arch Surg 124: 604–608

Miller J K, Wenner S M, Kruger L M 1986 Ulnar deficiency. J Hand Surg (Am) 11: 822–829

Miller R J 1988 Dislocations and fracture dislocations of the metacarpophalangeal joint of the thumb. Hand Clin 4: 45–65

Miller-Breslow A, Millender L H, Feldon PG 1989 Treatment considerations in the complicated rheumatoid hand. Hand Clin 5: 279–289

Millesi H 1977 Surgical management of brachial plexus injuries. J Hand Surg 2: 367–379

Millesi H 1984 Brachial plexus injuries. Clin Plastic Surg 2: 115–120

Millesi H 1986 The nerve gap. Theory and clinical practice. Hand Clin 2: 651–663

Mills M B, Millender L H, Nalebuff E A 1976 Stiffness of the proximal interphalangeal joints in rheumatoid arthritis. The role of flexor tenosynovitis. J Bone Joint Surg 58A: 801–805

Mills W J, Whaley R, Fish W 1960 Frostbite: experience with rapid rewarming and ultrasonic therapy. Alaska Med 2: 1–3, 114–122

Milner R H, Sykes P J 1987 Diffuse cavernous haemangiomas of the upper limb. J Hand Surg (Br) 12: 199–200

Minami A, An K N, Cooney W P 3rd, Linscheid R L, Chao E Y 1985 Ligament stability of the metacarpophalangeal joint: a biomechanical study. J Hand Surg (Am) 10: 255–260

Minami A, Ogino T 1987 Carpal tunnel syndrome in patients undergoing hemodialysis. J Hand Surg (Am) 12: 93–97

Minami A, Ogino T, Hamada M 1989 Rupture of extensor tendons associated with a palmar perilunar dislocation. J Hand Surg (Am) 14: 843–847

Minami M, Ishii S 1987 Satisfactory elbow flexion in complete (preganglionic) brachial plexus injuries; produced by suture of the third and fourth intercostal nerves to musculocutaneous nerve. J Hand Surg 12: 1114–1118

Minami M, Yamazaki J, Chisaka N, Kato S et al 1987 Nonunion of the capitate. J Hand Surg (Am) 12: 1089–1091

Minami M, Yamazaki J, Ishii S 1984 Isolated dislocation of the pisiform: a case report and review of the literature. J Hand Surg (Am) 9A: 125–127

Minkin B I, Mills C L, Bullock D W, Burke F D 1987 *Mycobacterium kansasii* osteomyelitis of the scaphoid. J Hand Surg (Am) 12: 1092–1094

Mino D E, Palmer A K, Levinsohn E M 1983 The role of radiography and computerized tomography in the diagnosis of subluxation and dislocation of the distal radioulnar joint. J Hand Surg (Am) 8: 23–31

MitchellI G M, Morrison W A, Papadopoulos A et al 1985 A study of the extent and pathology of experimental avulsion injury in rabbit arteries and veins. Br J Plastic Surg 38: 278

Mitchell S W 1872 Injuries of nerves and their consequences. J B Lippincott, Philadelphia

Miura T 1973 Thumb reconstruction using radial innervated cross-finger pedicle graft. J Bone Joint Surg 55A: 563–569

Miura T 1976 Triphalangeal thumb. Plastic Reconstr Surg 58: 587–594

Miura T 1977 An appropriate treatment for post-operative Z-formed deformity of the duplicated thumb. J Hand Surg 2: 380–386

Miura T 1977 Congenital absence of the flexor pollicis longus. Hand 9: 272–274

Miura T 1981 Congenital hand anomalies, and their association with other congenital abnormalities. Hand 13: 267–270

Miura T 1988 Cleft hand involving only the ring and small fingers. J Hand Surg (Am) 13: 530–535

Miura T 1988 Congenital absence of the fourth metacarpal bone (congenital dysplasia of the ring finger). J Hand Surg (Am) 13: 93–96

Miura T, Komada T 1979 Simple method for reconstruction of the cleft hand with an adducted thumb. Plastic Reconstr Surg 64: 65–67

Miura T, Nakamura R, Imamura T 1987 Polydactyly of the hands and feet. J Hand Surg (Am) 12: 474–476

Miura T, Nakamura R, Suzuki M, Kanie J 1984 Congenital radio-ulnar synostosis. J Hand Surg (Br) 9: 153–155

Miura T, Nakamura R, Torii S 1986 Conservative treatment for a ruptured extensor tendon on the dorsum of the proximal phalanges of the thumb (mallet thumb). J Hand Surg 11: 229–233

Miura T, Torii S, Nakamura R 1986 Brachymetacarpia and brachyphalangia. J Hand Surg (Am) 11: 829–836

Moberg E 1958 Objective methods for determining the functional value of sensibility in the hand. J Bone Joint Surg 40B: 454–476

Moberg E 1960 Arthrodesis of finger joints. Surg Clin North Am 40: 465–470

Moberg E 1960 Examination of sensory loss by the ninhydrin printing test in Volkmann's contracture. Bull Hosp Joint Dis 21: 296–303

Moberg E 1964 Evaluation and management of nerve injuries in the hand. Surg Clin North Am 44: 1019

Mogan J V, Newberg A H, Davis P H 1981 Intraosseous ganglion of the lunate. J Hand Surg 6: 61–63

Mogensen B A, Mattsson H S 1980 Post-traumatic instability of the metacarpophalangeal joint of the thumb. Hand 12: 85–90

Mogensen B A, Mattsson H S 1980 Stenosing tendovaginitis of the third compartment of the hand. Scand J Plastic Reconstr Surg 14: 127–128

Moloney S R, Cabbabe E B, Shively R E, deMello D E 1986 Recurring digital fibroma of childhood. J Hand Surg (Am) 11: 584–587

Monballiu G 1981 Plexiform neurofibroma of the median nerve. Chirurgia Plastica 6: 141–145

Moneim M S 1988 Management of greater arc carpal fractures. Hand Clin 4: 457–467

Moneim M S, Omer G E 1986 Latissimus dorsi muscle transfer for restoration of elbow flexion after brachial plexus disruption. J Hand Surg (Am) 11: 135–139

Monroe P W, Floyd W E 1981 Chromohyphomycosis of the hand due to *Exophiala jeanselmei*, (*Phialophora jeanselmei*, *Phialophora gougerotii*) Case report and review. J Hand Surg 6: 370–373

Monsanto E H, Johnston A D, Dick H M 1986 Isolated blastomycotic osteomyelitis: a case simulating a malignant tumor of the distal radius. J Hand Surg (Am) 11: 896–898

Monzingo D W, Smith A A, McManus W F et al 1988 Chemical burns. J Trauma 28: 642–647

Moore J R, Curtis R M, Wilgis E F 1983 Osteocartilaginous lesions of the digits in children: an experience with 10 cases. J Hand Surg (Am) 8: 309–315

Moore J R, Tolo V T, Weiland A J 1985 Painful subluxation of the carpometacarpal joint of the thumb in Ehlers–Danlos syndrome. J Hand Surg (Am) 10: 661–663

Moore J R, Weiland A J 1985 Embolotherapy in the treatment of congenital arteriovenous malformations of the hand: a case report. J Hand Surg (Am) 10: 135–139

Moore J R, Weiland A J 1985 Gouty tenosynovitis in the hand. J Hand Surg (Am) 10: 291–295

Moore J R, Weiland A J, Curtis R M 1984 Localized nodular tenosynovitis: experience with 115 cases. J Hand Surg (Am) 9: 412–417

Moore J R, Weiland A J, Valdata L 1987 Independent index extension after extensor indicis proprius transfer. J Hand Surg (Am) 12: 232–236

Moore J R, Weiland A J, Valdata L 1987 Tendon ruptures in the rheumatoid hand: analysis of treatment and functional results in 60 patients. J Hand Surg (Am) 12: 9–14

Moore M R, Garfin S R, Hargens A R 1987 Wide tourniquets eliminate blood flow at low inflation pressures. J Hand Surg (Am) 12: 1006–1011

Morely G H 1964 Intraneural lipoma of the median nerve in the carpal tunnel. Report of a case. J Bone Joint Surg 46B: 734–735

Morgan L R, Stein F 1972 Method for a rapid and good thumb reconstruction. Plastic Reconstr Surg 50: 131–133

Morgan R F, Edgerton M T 1985 Tissue expansion in reconstructive hand surgery: case report. J Hand Surg (Am) 10: 754–757

Morgan R F, Nichter L S, Friedman H I, McCue F C 3rd 1984 Rodeo roping thumb injuries. J Hand Surg (Am) 9: 178–180

Morgan R F, Reisman N R, Wilgis E F 1983 Anatomic localization of sympathetic nerves in the hand. J Hand Surg (Am) 8: 283–288

Morgan R F, Wilgis E F 1986 Thermal changes in a rabbit ear model after sympathectomy. J Hand Surg (Am) 11: 120–124

Morgan W J, Leopold T, Evans R 1984 Foreign bodies in the hand. J Hand Surg (Br) 9: 194–196

Morgan W, Groves RJ 1984 Scapholunate dissociation from a fall on the elbow. J Hand Surg (Am) 9: 845–847

Morrey B F, Askew L, Chao E T 1981 Silastic prosthetic replacement for the radial head. J Bone Joint Surg 63A: 454–458

Morrey B F, Bryan R S, Dobyns I H, Linscheid R L 1981 Total elbow arthroplasty. A five year experience at the Mayo Clinic. J Bone Joint Surg 63A: 1050–1063

Morrison W A 1990 Microvascular nail transfer. Hand Clin 6: 69–76

Morrison W A, O'Brien B M, MacLeod A M 1980 Thumb reconstruction with a free neurovascular wrap-around flap from the big toe. J Hand Surg 5: 575

Morrison W A, O'Brien B M, MacLeod A M 1984 Ring finger transfer in reconstruction of transmetacarpal amputations. J Hand Surg (Am) 9A: 4–11

Morrison W, O'Brien B, MacLeod A 1978 Digital replantation and revascularization. A long-term review of one hundred cases. Hand 10: 125–134

Mosely L H, Finseth F 1977 Cigarette smoking: impairment of digital blood flow and wound healing in the hand. Hand 9: 97–100

Moses J M, Flatt A E, Cooper R R 1979 Annular constricting bands. J Bone Joint Surg 61A: 562–565

Mosher J F 1976 Multiple enchondromatosis of the hand. A case report. J Bone Joint Surg 58A: 717–719

Mosher J, Peckham A 1978 Osteoblastoma of the metacarpal: a case report. J Hand Surg 3: 358–360

Moskovich R, Posner M A 1988 Intratendinous aponeurotic fibroma. J Hand Surg (Am) 13: 563–566

Moss A L, Ibrahim N B 1985 Lymphangiosarcoma of the hand arising in a pre-existing non-irradiated lymphangioma. J Hand Surg (Br) 10: 239–242

Moss L D, Stueber K, Hafiz M A 1982 Congenital hemangioendothelioma of the hand — case report. J Hand Surg 7: 53–56

Mubarak S J, Owen C A, Hargens A R, Garetto L P, Enneking W F 1978 Acute compartment syndromes. Diagnosis and treatment with the aid of the wick catheter. J Bone Joint Surg 60A: 1091–1099

Mueller J J 1986 Carpometacarpal dislocations: report of five cases and review of the literature. J Hand Surg (Am) 11: 184–188

Muffly-Elsey D, Flinn-Wagner S 1987 Proposed screening tool for the detection of cumulative trauma disorders of the upper extremity. J Hand Surg (Am) 12: 931–935

Muhlbauer W, Herndl E, Stock W 1982 The forearm flap. Plastic Reconstr Surg 70: 336–342

Mulholland R C 1966 Nontraumatic progressive paralysis of the posterior interosseous nerve. J Bone Joint Surg 48B: 781–785

Muller W 1937 Die angeborenen Fehlbildugen der menschlichen Hand. Thieme, Leipzig

Mullis W F, Rosato E F, Butler C J, Mayer L J 1972 The glomus tumor. Surg Gynecol Obstet 135: 705–707

Mumford J, Morecraft R, Blair W F 1987 Anatomy of the thenar branch of the median nerve. J Hand Surg (Am) 12: 361–365

Murakami Y, Komiyama Y 1978 Hypoplasia of the trochlea and the medial epicondyle of the humerus associated with ulnar neuropathy. J Bone Joint Surg 60B: 225–227

Murphy A F, Wilson J N 1958 Tenosynovial osteochondroma in the hand. J Bone Joint Surg 40A: 1236

Murphy C P, Chuinard R G 1988 Management of the upper extremity in traumatic tetraplegia. Hand Clin 4: 201–209

Murray J A, Schlafly B 1986 Giant-cell tumors in the distal end of the radius. Treatment by resection and fibular autograft interpositional arthrodesis. J Bone Joint Surg (Am) 68: 687–694

Murray J A, Thaggard A, Wallace S, Benmenachem G 1979 Arteriography of osteoid osteoma: an aid in differentiation and management. Orthopedics 2: 359–365

Murray J F, Carman W, MacKenzie J K 1977 Transmetacarpal amputation of the index finger: a clinical assessment of hand strength and complications. J Hand Surg 2: 471–481

Mutz S B, Curl W 1977 Alveolar cell rhabdomyosarcoma of the hand. Case report with four year survival and no evidence of recurrence. J Hand Surg 2: 283–284

Naasan A, Quaba A A 1990 Successful transfer of two reverse forearm flaps despite disruption of both palmar arches. Br J Plastic Surg 43: 476–479

Nagano A, Tsuyama N, Ochiai N, Hara T, Takahashi M 1989 Direct nerve crossing with the intercostal nerve to treat avulsion injuries of the brachial plexus. J Hand Surg 14: 980–985

Nahas L F, Bennett J E 1981 Case reports: nocardiosis of the upper limb. Plastic Reconstr Surg 68: 593–595

Nakamura R, Hori M, Horii E, Miura T 1987 Reduction of the scaphoid fracture with DISI alignment. J Hand Surg (Am) 12: 1000–1005

Nakazato T, Ogino T 1986 Epiphyseal destruction of children's hands after frostbite: a report of two cases. J Hand Surg 11A: 289–292

Nalebuff E A 1968 Diagnosis classification and management of rheumatoid thumb deformities. Bull Hosp Joint Dis 29: 119–137

Nalebuff E A 1989 The rheumatoid swan-neck deformity. Hand Clin 5: 203–214

Nalebuff E A, Garrett J 1976 Opera glass hand in rheumatoid arthritis. J Hand Surg 1: 210–220

Nalebuff E A, Millender L H 1975 Surgical treatment of the boutonniere deformity in rheumatoid arthritis. Orthopedic Clin North Am 6: 753–763

Nalebuff E A, Millender L H 1975 Surgical treatment of the swan-neck deformity in rheumatoid arthritis. Orthopedic Clin North Am 6: 733–752

Nalebuff E A, Patel M R 1973 Flexor digitorum superficialis transfer for multiple extensor tendon ruptures in rheumatoid arthritis. Plastic Reconstr Surg 52: 530–533

Nalebuff E A, Smith R J 1979 Preservation of terminal branches of the median palmar cutaneous nerve in carpal tunnel surgery. Orthopaedics 2: 369–372

Narakas A 1981 Brachial plexus surgery. Orthop Clin North Am 12: 303–323

Narakas A O 1988 Paralytic disorders of the shoulder girdle. Hand Clin 4: 619–632

Nathan P A, Trung N B 1977 The Krukenberg operation: A modified technique avoiding skin grafts. J Hand Surg 2: 127

Nathan R, Lester B, Melone CP Jr 1987 The acutely injured wrist — an anatomic basis for operative treatment. Orthopaedic Rev 16: 80–95

Nather A, Pho R W H 1981 Carpal tunnel syndrome produced by an organising haematoma within the anomalous second lumbrical muscle. Hand 13: 87–91

Neblett C, Ehni G 1970 Medial epicondylectomy for ulnar palsy. J Neurosurg 32: 55–62

Neilson D, Dundas S, Page R E 1988 Carcinoma cuniculatum of the hand. J Hand Surg (Br) 13: 218–220

Neimkin R J, Jupiter J B 1985 Metastatic nontraumatic *Clostridium septicum* osteomyelitis. J Hand Surg (Am) 10: 281–284

Neimkin R J, Smith R J 1983 Double tourniquet with linked mercury manometers for hand surgery. J Hand Surg (Am) 8: 938–941

Nelson C L, Sawmiller S, Phalen G S 1984 Ganglions of the

wrist and hamartoma of the hand. J Hand Surg (Br) 9: 349–350

Nemoto K, Matsumoto N, Tazaki K, Horiuchi Y et al 1987 An experimental study on the 'double crush' hypothesis. J Hand Surg (AM) 12: 552–559 (An erratum appears in J Hand Surg (Am) 1987 12: 1011.)

Neu B R, Murray J F, MacKenzie J K 1985 Profundus tendon blockage: quadriga in finger amputations. J Hand Surg (Am) 10: 878–883

Neviaser R 1978 Closed tendon sheath irrigation for pyogenic flexor tenosynovitis. J Hand Surg 3: 462–466

Neviaser R 1979 Congenital hypoplasia of the thumb with absence of the extrinsic extensors, abductor pollicis longus and thenar muscles. J Hand Surg 4: 301–304

Neviaser R J 1983 Proximal row carpectomy for posttraumatic disorders of the carpus. J Hand Surg (Am) 8: 301–305

Neviaser R J 1989 Tenosynovitis. Hand Clin 5: 525–531

Neviaser R J, Adams J, May G 1976 Complications of arterial puncture in anticoagulated patients. J Bone Joint Surg 58A: 218–220

Neviaser R J, Butterfield W C, Wiechi D R 1972 The puffy hand of drug addiction. A study of the pathogenesis. J Bone Joint Surg 54A: 629–633

Neviaser R J, Newman W 1977 Dermal angiomyoma of the upper extremity. J Hand Surg 2: 271–274

Neviaser R J, Wilson J N 1972 Benign chondroblastoma in the finger. J Bone Joint Surg 54A1: 389–392

Newman E D, Harrington T M, Torretti D, Bush D C 1989 Suppurative extensor tenosynovitis caused by Staphylococcus aureus. J Hand Surg (Am) 14: 849–851

Newman J H, Goodfellow J W 1975 Fibrillation of head of radius as one cause of tennis elbow. Br Med J 1: 328–330

Newmeyer W L 3rd 1988 Management of sea urchin spines in the hand. J Hand Surg (Am) 13: 455–457

Nicholson C P, Grotting J C, Dimick A R 1987 Acute microwave injury to the hand. J Hand Surg (Am) 12: 446–449

Nicolai J P A, Hentenaar G 1981 Sensation in cross-finger flaps. Hand 13: 12–16

Nicolai J P, Schoch S L 1986 Polydactyly in the bible. J Hand Surg 11: 293

Nicolle F V 1973 Recent advances in the management of joint disease in the rheumatoid hand. Hand 5: 91

Nicolle F V, Dickson R A 1979 Surgery of the rheumatoid hand. Heinemann Medical Books, London

Nielsen J B 1977 Madelung's deformity: a follow-up study of 26 cases and a review of the literature. Acta Orthopaedica Scand 48: 379–384

Nielsen P T, Hedeboe J 1984 Posttraumatic scapholunate dissociation detected by wrist cineradiography. J Hand Surg (Am) 9A: 135–138

Nieman E A, Swann P G 1977 Karate injuries. Br Med J 223

Nirschl R P, Pettrone F A 1979 Tennis elbow. J Bone Joint Surg 61A: 823–839

Nissenbaum M 1984 Class IIA ring avulsion injuries: an absolute indication for microvascular repair. J Hand Surg (Am) 9: 810–815

Nitz A J, Dobner J J 1989 Upper extremity tourniquet effects in carpal tunnel release. J Hand Surg (Am) 14: 499–504

Noble J, Heathcote J G, Cohen H 1984 Diabetes mellitus in the aetiology of Dupuytren's disease. J Bone Joint Surg (Br) 66: 322–325

Norbeck D E Jr, Larson B, Blair S J, Demos T C 1987

Traumatic longitudinal disruption of the carpus. J Hand Surg (Am) 12: 509–514

North E R, Eaton R G 1983 Degenerative joint disease of the trapezium: a comparative radiographic and anatomic study. J Hand Surg (Am) 8: 160–166

North E R, Thomas S 1988 An anatomic guide for arthroscopic visualization of the wrist capsular ligaments. J Hand Surg (Am) 13: 815–822

Northmore-Ball, Heger H, Hunter G A 1980 The below-elbow myo-electric prosthesis with the hook and functional hand. J Bone Joint Surg (Br) 62: 363–367

Notta A 1850 Recherches sur une affection particulière des gaines tendineuses de la main, caracterisée par le developpement d'une nodosité sur le trajet des tendons flechisseurs des doigts et par l'empêchement de leurs movements. Arch Gen Med 24: 142–161

Nunley J A, Goldner R D, Koman L A, Gelberman R, Urbaniak J R 1987 Arterial stump pressure: a determinant of arterial patency? J Hand Surg (Am) 12: 245–249

Nunley J A, Spiegl P V, Goldner R D, Urbaniak J R 1987 Longitudinal epiphyseal growth after replantation and transplantation in children. J Hand Surg (Am) 12: 274–279

Nunley J A, Ubaniak J R 1980 Partial bony entrapment of the median nerve in a greenstick fracture of the ulna. J Hand Surg 5: 557–559

Nussbaum R, Sadler A H 1986 An isolated, closed, complex dislocation of the metacarpophalangeal joint of the long finger: a unique case. J Hand Surg (Am) 11: 558–561

Nuts J N, Flatt A E 1981 Congenital central hand deficit. J Hand Surg 6: 48–60

Nyquist S R, Stern P J 1984 Open radiocarpal fracture-dislocations. J Hand Surg (Am) 9: 707–710

O'Brien B, Gould J S, Morrison W A, Russell R C et al 1984 Free vascularized small joint transfer to the hand. J Hand Surg (Am) 9: 634–641

O'Donovan T M, Ruby L K 1989 The distal radioulnar joint in rheumatoid arthritis. Hand Clin 5: 249–256

O'Hara J J, Stone J H 1988 Ulnar neuropathy at the wrist associated with aberrant flexor carpi ulnaris insertion. J Hand Surg (Am) 13: 370–372

O'Hara J J, Stone J H 1990 An intratendinous epidermoid cyst after trauma. J Hand Surg (Am) 15: 477–479

O'Hara J P, Tegtmeyer C, Sweet D E, McCue F C 1975 Angiography in the diagnosis of osteoid osteoma of the hand. J Bone Joint Surg 57A: 163–166

O'Neil D, Sheppard J E 1989 Transient compartment syndrome of the forearm resulting from venous congestion from a tourniquet. J Hand Surg (Am) 14: 894–896

O'Reilly R J, Blatt G 1975 High-pressure injection injury. J Am Med Assoc 233: 533–534

O'Riain S 1973 New and simple test of nerve function in hand. Br Med J 3: 615–616

O'Rourke S K, Gaur S, Barton N 1989 Long-term outcome of articular fractures of the phalanges: an eleven year follow up. J Hand Surg (Br) 14B: 183–193

Ogden J A, Watson H K, Bohne W 1976 Ulnar dysmelia. J Bone Joint Surg 58A: 467–475

Ogiela D M, Peimer C A 1981 Acute gonococcal flexor tenosynovitis. Case report and literature review. J Hand Surg 6: 470–472

Ogilvie-Harris D J, Fornasier V L 1980 Pseudomalignant myositis ossificans: heterotopic new bone formation without a history of trauma. J Bone Joint Surg 62A: 1274–1283

Ogunro O 1983 Avulsion of flexor profundus, secondary to

enchondroma of the distal phalanx. J Hand Surg (Am) 8: 315–316

Ogunro O 1983 Fracture of the body of the hamate bone. J Hand Surg (Am) 8: 353–355

Ogura R, Inoue H, Tanabe G 1987 Anatomic and clinical studies of the extensor digitorum brevis manus. J Hand Surg (Am) 12: 100–107

Ohlsen L 1978 Cartilage regeneration from perichondrium. Experimental studies and clinical applications. Plastic Reconstr Surg 62: 507–513

Ohshio I, Ogino T, Miyake A 1986 Dislocation of the hamate associated with fracture of the trapezial ridge. J Hand Surg (Am) 11: 658–660

Ohtsuka H, Imagawa S 1985 Reconstruction of a posterior defect of the elbow joint using an extensor carpi radialis longus myocutaneous flap: case report. Br J Plastic Surg 38: 238–240

Omer G E 1988 Timing of tendon transfers in peripheral nerve injury. Hand Clin 4: 317–322

Omer G E Jr 1968 Evaluation and reconstruction of the forearm and hand after acute traumatic peripheral nerve injuries. J Bone Joint Surg 50A: 1454–1478

Omer G E Jr 1986 Acute management of peripheral nerve injuries. Hand Clin 2: 193–206

Onne L 1962 Recovery of sensibility and sudo-motor activity in the hand after nerve suture. Acta Chir Scand (suppl) 300: 1–69

Onukak E E 1980 Squamous cell carcinoma of the nail bed: a diagnostic and therapeutic problem. Br J Surg 67: 893–894

Ortiguela M E, Wood M B, Cahill D R 1987 Anatomy of the sural nerve complex. J Hand Surg (Am) 12: 1119–1123

Osborne G 1957 The surgical treatment of tardy ulnar neuritis. J Bone Joint Surg 39B: 782

Osborne G 1970 Decompression of ulnar nerve at elbow. Hand 2: 10–13

Oster L H, Blair W F, Steyers C M 1989 Large lipomas in the deep palmar space. J Hand Surg (Am) 14: 700–704

Oster L H, Blair W F, Steyers C M, Flatt A E 1989 Crossed intrinsic transfer. J Hand Surg (Am) 14: 963–971

Osterman A L 1990 Arthroscopic debridement of triangular fibrocartilage complex tears. Arthroscopy 6: 120–124

Osterman A L, Mikulics M 1988 Scaphoid nonunion. Hand Clin 4: 437–455

Ostrowski D M 1990 Locking of the metacarpophalangeal joint: a case report and literature review. Cont Ortho 21: 265–269

Pagalidis T, Kuczynski K, Laatnb D W 1981 Ligamentous stability of the base of the thumb. Hand 13: 29–35

Pahle J A, Raunio P 1969 Influence of wrist position on finger deviation in rheumatoid arthritis. J Bone Joint Surg 51B: 664–676

Pak T J, Martin G M, Magness J L, Kavanaugh G L 1970 Reflex sympathetic dystrophy, review of 140 cases. Minn Med 53: 507–512

Paletta F X 1981 Venous gangrene of the hand. Plastic Reconstr Surg 67: 67–69

Paletta F X, Senay L C 1981 Lipofibromatous hamartoma of median nerve and ulnar nerve: surgical treatment. Plastic Reconstr Surg 68: 915–926

Paley D, McMurtry R Y 1985 Median nerve compression test in carpal tunnel syndrome diagnosis. Ortho Rev 15: 41–45

Paley D, McMurtry R Y, Cruickshank B 1987 Pathologic conditions of the pisiform and pisitriquetral joint. J Hand Surg (Am) 12: 110–119

Palmer A K 1981 Trapezial ridge fractures. J Hand Surg 6: 561–564

Palmer A K 1986 Complications from tourniquet use. Hand Clin 2: 301–305

Palmer A K 1987 The distal radioulnar joint. Anatomy, biomechanics, and triangular fibrocartilage complex abnormalities. Hand Clin 3: 31–40

Palmer A K 1989 Triangular fibrocartilage complex lesions: a classification. J Hand Surg (Am) 14: 594–606

Palmer A K, Glisson R R, Werner F W 1984 Relationship between ulnar variance and triangular fibrocartilage complex thickness. J Hand Surg (Am) 9: 681–682

Palmer A K, Levinsohn E M, Kuzma G R 1983 Arthrography of the wrist. J Hand Surg (Am) 8: 15–23

Palmer A K, Linscheid R L 1978 Chronic recurrent dislocation of the proximal interphalangeal joint of the finger. J Hand Surg 3: 95–97

Palmer A K, Werner F W, Glisson R R, Murphy D J 1988 Partial excision of the triangular fibrocartilage complex. J Hand Surg (Am) 13: 391–394

Palmer A K, Werner F W, Murphy D, Glisson R 1985 Functional wrist motion; a biomechanical study. J Hand Surg (Am) 10: 39–46

Palmer A, Louis D 1978 Assessing ulnar instability of the metacarpophalangeal joint of the thumb. J Hand Surg 3: 542–546

Palmer R E 1984 Eosinophilic granuloma of the hand: case report. J Hand Surg (Am) 9: 283–285

Palmieri T J 1983 Subcutaneous hemangiomas of the hand. J Hand Surg (Am) 8: 201–204

Palmieri T J 1984 Chondrosarcoma of the hand. J Hand Surg (Am) 9: 332–338

Palmieri T J, Grand F M, Hay E L, Burke C 1987 Treatment of osteoarthritis in the hand and wrist. Nonoperative treatment. Hand Clin 3: 371–383

Panagis J S, Gelberman R H, Taleisnik J, Baumgaertner M 1983 The arterial anatomy of the human carpus. Part II. The intraosseous vascularity. J Hand Surg (Am) 8: 375–382

Panas J 1878 Sur une case pas connue de paralysie du neuf cubital. Arch Gen Med 2: 5–22

Pancoast H K 1932 Superior pulmonary sulcus tumor. J Am Med Assoc 99: 1391–1396

Papilion J D, DuPuy T E, Aulicino P L, Bergfield T G, Gwathmey F W 1988 Radiographic evaluation of the hook of the hamate: a new technique. J Hand Surg (Am) 13: 437–439

Paplanus S H, Payne C M 1988 Axillary lymphadenopathy 17 years after digital silicone implants: study with X-ray microanalysis. J Hand Surg (Am) 13: 399–400

Pardoe R, Minami R T, Sato R M, Schlesinger S L 1977 Phenol burns. Burns 3: 29–41

Parker M D, Irwin R S 1975 Mycobacterium kansasii tendinitis and fasciitis. J Bone Joint Surg 57A: 557–559

Parker R D, Froimson A I 1986 Neurogenic arthropathy of the hand and wrist. J Hand Surg (Am) 11: 706–710

Parkes A 1971 The 'lumbrical plus' finger. J Bone Joint Surg 53B: 236–239

Parks B J, Hamlin C 1986 Chronic sesamoiditis of the thumb: pathomechanics and treatment. J Hand Surg (Am) 11: 237–240

Parry C B, Salter M 1976 Sensory re-education after median nerve lesions. Hand 8: 250–257

Parsonage M J, Turner J W A 1948 Neuralgic amyotrophy: The shoulder-girdle syndrome. Lancet i: 973–978

Pasch A R, Bishara R A, Schuler J J, Lim L T, Meyer J P, Merlotti G, Barrett J A, Flanigan P 1986 Results of venous reconstruction after civilian vascular trauma. Arch Surg 121: 607–611

Patel C B, Tsai T M, Kleinert H E 1986 Hemangioma of the median nerve: a report of two cases. J Hand Surg (Am) 11: 76–79

Patel M R, Desai S S 1988 Anomalous muscles of the first dorsal compartment of the wrist. J Hand Surg (Am) 13: 829–831

Patel M R, Desai S S, Bassini-Lipson L 1986 Conservative management of chronic mallet finger. J Hand Surg (Am) 11: 570–573

Patel M R, Desai S S, Gordon S L 1986 Functional limb salvage with multimodality treatment in epithelioid sarcoma of the hand: a report of two cases. J Hand Surg (Am) 11: 265–269

Patel M R, Desai S S, Gordon S L, Nimberg G A et al 1987 Management of skeletal giant cell tumors of the phalanges of the hand. J Hand Surg (Am) 12: 70–77

Patel M R, Desai SS, Bassini-Lipson L, Namba T, Sahoo J 1989 Painful extensor digitorum brevis manus muscle. J Hand Surg (Am) 14: 674–678

Patel M R, Lipson L B, Desai SS 1986 Conservative treatment of mallet thumb. J Hand Surg (Am) 11: 45–47

Patel M R, Pearlman H S, Engler J, Wollowick B S 1977 Chondrosarcoma of the proximal phalanx of the finger. Review of the literature and report of a case. J Bone Joint Surg 59A: 401–403

Patel M R, Zinberg E M 1984 Pigmented villonodular synovitis of the wrist invading bone — report of a case. J Hand Surg (Am) 9: 854–858

Patel M, Silver J, Lipton D, Pearlman H 1979 Lipofibroma of the median nerve in the palm and digits of the hand. J Bone Joint Surg 61A: 393–397

Patel M, Srinivasion K, Pearlman H 1978 Malignant hemangioendothelioma in the hand. J Hand Surg 3: 585

Patel MR, Desai S 1989 Subungual keratoacanthoma in the hand. J Hand Surg (Am) 14: 139–142

Patterson R H, Helwing E L 1980 Subungual melanoma: a clinical pathological study. Cancer 46: 2074–2087

Patterson T J S 1961 Congenital ring-constrictions. Br J Plastic Surg 14: 1–31

Peacock K C, Hanna D P, Kirkpatrick K, Breidenbach W C et al 1988 Efficacy of perioperative cefamandole with postoperative cephalexin in the primary outpatient treatment of open wounds of the hand. J Hand Surg (Am) 13: 960–964

Peckham P H, Keith M W, Freehafer A A 1988 Restoration of functional control by electrical stimulation in the upper extremity of the quadriplegic patient. J Bone Joint Surg (Am) 70: 144–148

Pedowitz R A, Toutounghi F M 1988 Chronic exertional compartment syndrome of the forearm flexor muscles. J Hand Surg (Am) 13: 694–696

Peeples E, Boswick J A, Scott F A 1980 Wounds of the hand contaminated by human or animal saliva. J Trauma 20: 383–389

Peimer C A 1985 Combined reduction osteotomy for triphalangeal thumb. J Hand Surg (Am) 10: 376–381

Peimer C A, Medige J, Eckert B S, Wright J R, Howard C S 1986 Reactive synovitis after silicone arthroplasty. J Hand Surg (Am) 11: 624–638

Peimer C A, Putnam M D 1987 Proximal interphalangeal joint following traumatic arthritis. Hand Clin 3: 415–427

Peimer C A, Schiller A L, Mankin H J, Smith R J 1980 Multicentric giant cell tumor of bone. J Bone Joint Surg 62A: 652–656

Peimer C A, Schiller A L, Mankin H J, Smith R J 1980 Multicentric giant-cell tumors of bone. J Bone Joint Surg (Am) 62: 652–656

Peimer C A, Smith R J, Sirota R L, Cohen B E 1977 Epithelioid sarcoma of the hand and wrist: patterns of extension. J Hand Surg 2: 275–282

Peimer C A, Sullivan D J, Wild D R 1984 Palmar dislocation of the proximal interphalangeal joint. J Hand Surg (Am) 9A: 39–48

Peitner C A, Smith R J, Leffert R D 1981 Distraction in the primary treatment of metacarpal bone loss. J Hand Surg 6: 111–124

Peled I, Iosipovich Z, Rousso M, Wexler M R 1980 Hemangioma of the median nerve. J Hand Surg 5: 363–365

Pellegrini V D Jr 1988 Fractures at the base of the thumb. Hand Clin 4: 87–102

Pellegrini V D Jr, Burton R I 1986 Surgical management of basal joint arthritis of the thumb. Part I. Long-term results of silicone implant arthroplasty. J Hand Surg (Am) 11: 309–324

Pellegrini V D Jr, Tompkins A 1986 Management of subungual keratoacanthoma. J Hand Surg (Am) 11: 718–724

Pellegrini V D, Jr, Burton R I 1990 Osteoarthritis of the proximal interphalangeal joint of the joint: arthroplasty or fusion? J Hand Surg (Am) 15: 194– 209

Pellicci P M, Ranawat C S, Tsairis P, Bryan W I 1981 A prospective study of the progression of rheumatoid arthritis of the cervical spine. J Bone Joint Surg 63A: 342–350

Pensler J M, Steward R, Lewis S R, Herndon D N 1988 Reconstruction of the burned palm: full thickness versus split-thickness skin grafts — long-term follow-up. Plastic Reconstr Surg 81: 46–49

Perlman R, Jubelirer A, Schwarz J 1972 Histoplasmosis of the common palmar tendon sheath. J Bone Joint Surg 54A: 676–678

Pessa J E, Tsai T M, Li Y, Kleinert H E 1990 The repair of nail deformities with the nonvascularized nail bed graft: indications and results. J Hand Surg (Am) 15: 466–470

Petersen D P, Wong L B 1981 Nocardia infection of the hand. Case report. J Hand Surg 6: 502–505

Peterson P, Sacks S 1986 Fracture-dislocation of the base of the fifth metacarpal associated with injury to the deep motor branch of the ulnar nerve: a case report. J Hand Surg (Am) 11: 525–528

Pezehski C, Daneshbod K, Faghihi E 1980 Multiple hemangiomas of bone of upper extremity. Orthopaedic Rev 9: 67–69

Phalen G S 1951 Spontaneous compression of the median nerve at the wrist. J Am Med Assoc 145: 1128–1133

Phalen G S 1966 The carpal tunnel syndrome: 17 years experience in diagnosis and treatment of 654 hands. J Bone Joint Surg 48A: 211–228

Phalen G S 1981 The birth of a syndrome, or carpal tunnel revisited. J Hand Surg 6: 109–111

Phalen G S, McCormack L J, Gazale W J 1959 Giant cell tumor of tendon sheath (benign synovioma) in the hand. Evaluation of 56 cases. Clin Orthopedics 15: 140–151

Phelps D B, Buchler U, Boswick J A 1977 The diagnosis of factitious ulcer of the hand: a case report. J Hand Surg 2: 105–108

Phillips J H, Mackinnon S E, Murray J F, McMurtry R Y 1986 Exercise-induced chronic compartment syndrome of the first dorsal interosseous muscle of the hand: a case report. J Hand Surg (Am) 11: 124–127

Pho R W H 1979 Local composite neurovascular island flap for skin cover in pulp loss of the thumb. J Hand Surg 4: 11–16

Pho R W, Patterson M, Lee Y S 1988 Reconstruction and pathology in macrodactyly. J Hand Surg (Am) 13: 78–83

Pichora D R, McMurtry R Y, Bell M J 1989 Gamekeepers thumb: a prospective study of functional bracing. J Hand Surg (Am) 14: 567–573

Pike J, Arons M S 1990 Vibration Syndrome: a new test and rating system for disability compensation. Con Ortho 20: 303–308

Pike J, Patterson A, Arons MS 1988 Chemistry of cement burns: pathogenesis and treatment. J Burn Care Rehabil 9: 258–260

Pillet J 1983 Esthetic hand prostheses. J Hand Surg (Am) 8: 778–781

Pin P G, Semenkovich J W, Young V L, Bartell T et al 1988 Role of radionuclide imaging in the evaluation of wrist pain. J Hand Surg (Am) 13: 810–814

Pin P G, Young V L, Gilula L A, Weeks P M 1989 Management of chronic lunotriquetral ligament tears. J Hand Surg (Am) 14: 77–83

Pinstein M L, Scott R L, Sebes J I 1981 Tuberculous arthritis of the wrist: differential diagnosis and case report. Orthopaedics 4: 1016–1018

Pinzur M S 1985 Surgery to achieve dynamic motor balance in adult acquired spastic hemiplegia: a preliminary report. J Hand Surg (Am) 10: 547–553

Pinzur M S, Wehner J, Kett N, Trilla M 1988 Brachioradialis to finger extensor tendon transfer to achieve hand opening in acquired spasticity. J Hand Surg (Am) 13: 549–552

Poitevin L A 1988 Proximal compressions of the upper limb neurovascular bundle. An anatomic research study. Hand Clin 4: 575–584

Polivy K D, Millender L H, Newberg A, Philips C A 1985 Fractures of the hook of the hamate — a failure of clinical diagnosis. J Hand Surg (Am) 10: 101–104

Pollen A G 1968 The conservative treatment of Bennett's fracture-subluxation of the thumb metacarpal. J Bone Joint Surg (Br) 50: 91 –101

Pollock F H, Drake D, Bovill E G, Day L, Trafton P G 1981 Treatment of radial neuropathy associated with fractures of the humerus. J Bone Joint Surg 63A: 239–243

Popelka S, Vainio K 1974 Entrapment of the posterior interosseous branch of the radial nerve in rheumatoid arthritis. Acta Orthopaedica Scand 45: 370–372

Poplawski Z J, Wiley A M, Murray J F 1983 Post-traumatic dystrophy of the extremities. A clinical review and trial of treatment. J Bone Joint Surg 65A: 642–655

Poppen N K, Niebauer J J 1977 Recurring digital fibrous tumor of childhood. J Hand Surg 2: 256–257

Poppen N K, Norris T R, Buncke H J Jr 1983 Evaluation of sensibility and function with microsurgical free tissue transfer of the great toe to the hand for thumb reconstruction. J Hand Surg (Am) 8: 516–531

Poppen N, Niebauer J 1978 'Tie-in' trapezium prosthesis: long-term results. J Hand Surg 3: 445–450

Poppi M, Padovani R, Martinelli P, Pozzati E 1978 Fracture of the distal radius with ulnar nerve palsy. J Trauma 18: 276–278

Porter R W 1968 Functional assessment of transplanted skin in volar defects of the digits. J Bone Joint Surg 50A: 955–963

Posch J L 1956 Tumors of the hand. J Bone Joint Surg 38A: 517–540

Posner M 1979 Ray transposition for central digital loss. J Hand Surg 4: 242–257

Posner M A 1983 Flexor superficialis tendon transfers to the thumb — an alternative to the free tendon graft for treatment of chronic injuries within the digital sheath. J Hand Surg (Am) 8: 876–881

Posner M A, Ambrose L 1989 Boxer's knuckle — dorsal capsular rupture of the metacarpophalangeal joint of a finger. J Hand Surg (Am) 14: 229–236

Posner M A, Green S M 1984 Intraosseous ganglion of a phalanx. J Hand Surg (Am) 9: 280–282

Posner M A, Greenspan A 1988 Trispiral tomography for the evaluation of wrist problems. J Hand Surg (Am) 13: 175–181

Posner M A, Kapila D 1986 Chonic palmar dislocation of proximal interphalangeal joints. J Hand Surg (Am) 11: 253–258

Posner M A, Langa V, Ambrose L 1988 Intrinsic muscle advancement to treat chronic palmar instability of the metacarpophalangeal joint of the thumb. J Hand Surg (Am) 13: 110–115

Posner M A, Langa V, Green S M 1986 The locked metacarpophalangeal joint: diagnosis and treatment. J Hand Surg (Am) 11: 249–253

Posner M A, Smith R J 1971 The advancement pedicle flap for thumb injuries. J Bone Joint Surg 53A: 1618–1621

Potenza A D, Winslow D J 1961 Rhabdomyosarcoma of the hand. J Bone Joint Surg 43A: 700–708

Poznanski A K 1974 The hand in radiologic diagnosis. W B Saunders, Philadelphia

Poznanski A K, Pratt G B, Manson G, Weiss L 1969 Clinodactyly, camptodactyly, Kirner's deformity, and other crooked fingers. Radiology 93: 573–582

Press B H, Chiu D T, Cunninghan B L 1990 The rectus abdominis muscle in difficult problems of hand soft tissue reconstruction. Br J Plastic Surg 43: 419–425

Prince H, Ispahani P, Baker M 1988 A *Mycobacterium malmoense* infection of the hand presenting as carpal tunnel syndrome. J Hand Surg (Br) 13: 328–330

Pritchard R 1979 Semiconstrained elbow prosthesis. A clinical review of five years of experience. Orthopaedic Rev 8: 33–43

Pritchard R 1981 Long-term follow-up study: semi-constrained elbow prosthesis. Orthopedics 4: 151–155

Pritsch M, Engel J, Farin I 1981 Manipulation and external fixation of metacarpal fractures. J Bone Joint Surg 63A: 1289–1291

Pritsch M, Engel J, Horowitz A 1980 Cystic change in the wrist, causing carpal tunnel syndrome. Plastic Reconstr Surg 65: 494–495

Pruzansky M E, Remer S 1986 Abscesses of the hand associated with otopharyngeal infections in children. J Hand Surg (Am) 11: 844–846

Prystowsky S D, Herndon J H, Freeman R G 1975 Bronchogenic carcinoma metastatic to the hand. Cutis 16: 678–681

Puckett C L, Winters R R, Geter R K, Goelel D 1985 Studies of pathologic vasoconstriction (vasospasm) in microvascular surgery. J Hand Surg (Am) 10: 343–349

Pulvertaft R G 1964 Unusual tumours of the median nerve. Report of two cases. J Bone Joint Surg 46B. 731–733

Punnett L 1987 Upper extremity musculoskeletal disorders in hospital workers. J Hand Surg (Am) 12: 858–862

Quaba A A, Davison P M 1990 The distally-based dorsal hand flap. Br J Plastic Surg 43: 28–39

Quaba A A, Elliot D, Sommerlad B C 1988 Long term hand function without long finger extensors: a clinical study. J Hand Surg (Br) 13: 66–71

Rainer W G, Mayer J, Sadler T R, Dirks D 1973 Effect of graded compression on nerve conduction velocity. Arch Surg 107: 719–721

Raju S, Carner D V 1981 Brachial plexus compression: complication of delayed recognition of arterial injuries of the shoulder girdle. Arch Surg 116: 175–178

Rakower S, Shahgoli S, Wong S 1978 Doppler ultrasound and digital plethysmography to determine the need for sympathetic blockage after frostbite. J Trauma 18: 713–718

Ramirez Ruiz G, Combalia Aleu A, Valer Tito A, Bordas Sales J L, Rofes Capo S 1985 Simultaneous subluxation of the metacarpophalangeal joints of all four fingers: a case report. J Hand Surg (Am) 10: 78–80

Ramos H, Posch J L, Lie K K 1970 High-pressure injection injuries of the hand. Plastic Reconstr Surg 45: 221–226

Rana N A, Hancock D O, Taylor A R, Hill A G S 1973 Atlanto-axial subluxation in rheumatoid arthritis. J Bone Joint Surg 55B: 458–470

Rana N A, Hancock D O, Taylor A R, Hill A G S 1973 Upward translocation of the dens in rheumatoid arthritis. J Bone Joint Surg 55B: 471–477

Rana N A, Taylor A R 1973 Excision of the distal end of the ulna in rheumatoid arthritis. J Bone Joint Surg 55B: 96–105

Ranawat C S, DeFiore J, Straub L R 1975 Madelung's deformity: an end-result study of surgical treatment. J Bone Joint Surg 57A: 772

Ranawat C S, O'Leary P, Pellicci P, Tsairis P, Marchisello P, Dorr L 1979 Cervical spine fusion in rheumatoid arthritis. J Bone Joint Surg 61A: 1003–1010

Rangarathnam C S, Linscheid R L 1984 Infected mucous cyst of the finger. J Hand Surg 9A: 245–247

Rank B K 1978 Long-term results in epiphyseal transplants in congenital deformities of the hand. Plastic Reconstr Surg 61: 321–329

Rankin E A, Uwagie-Ero S 1986 Locking of the metacarpophalangeal joint. J Hand Surg (Am) 11: 868–871

Rasi H B, Mascardo T, Jinkdrak K 1980 Congenital fibrosarcoma of hand. Orthopaedic Rev 9: 49–54

Rask M R 1977 Suprascapular nerve entrapment: a report of two cases treated with suprascapular notch resection. Clin Orthopaedics 123: 73–75

Ratna S 1976 Case reports: hemangiopericytoma of the hand. Plastic Reconstr Surg 57: 746–748

Raturi U, Burkhalter W 1986 Gnathostomiasis externa: a case report. J Hand Surg (Am) 11: 751–753

Ravitch M M 1977 Poland's syndrome — a study of an eponym. Plastic Reconstr Surg 59: 508–512

Rawles J G Jr 1988 Dislocations and fracture-dislocations at the carpometacarpal joints of the fingers. Hand Clin 4: 103–112

Rayan G M 1984 Congenital hypoplastic thumb with absent thenar muscles: anomalous digital neurovascular bundle. J Hand Surg (Am) 9: 665–668

Rayan G M 1986 Wrist arthrodesis. J Hand Surg (Am) 11: 356–364

Rayan G M, Flournoy D J, Cahill S L 1984 Aerobic mouth flora of the rhesus monkey. J Hand Surg (Am) 12: 299–301

Rayan G M, Mullins P T 1987 Skin necrosis complicating mallet finger splinting and vascularity of the distal interphalangeal joint overlying skin. J Hand Surg (Am) 12: 548–552

Rayan G M, Putnam J L, Cahill S L, Flournoy D J 1988 *Eikenella corrodens* in human mouth flora. J Hand Surg (Am) 13: 953–956

Rayan GM, Brentlinger A, Purnell D, Garcia-Moral C A 1987 Functional assessment of bilateral wrist arthrodeses. J Hand Surg (Am) 12: 1020–1024

Rayhack J M, Belsole R J, Skelton W H Jr 1984 A strain recording model: analysis of transverse osteotomy fixation in small bones. J Hand Surg (Am) 9: 383–387

Raynaud A G M 1862 De l'asphyxie locale et de la gangrene symetrique des extremites. Rignoux, Paris

Rayner C R W 1981 The results of treatment of two hundred and seventy-three carcinomas of the hand. Hand 13: 183–186

Reading G 1980 Secretan's syndrome: hard edema of the dorsum of the hand. Plastic Reconstr Surg 65: 182–187

Reagan D S, Linscheid R L, Dobyns J H 1984 Lunotriquetral sprains. J Hand Surg (Am) 9: 502–512

Redler I, Williams J T 1967 Rupture of a collateral ligament of the proximal interphalangeal joint of the finger. J Bone Joint Surg 49A: 322–326

Reef T C, Brestin S G 1975 The extensor digitorum brevis manus and its clinical significance. J Bone Joint Surg 57A: 704–706

Rees M J, de Geus J J 1988 Immediate amputation stump coverage with forearm free flaps from the same limb. J Hand Surg (Am) 13: 287–292

Rees R, Shack R B, Withers E, Madden J, Franklin J, Lynch J B 1981 Management of the brown recluse spider bite. Plastic Reconstr Surg 68: 768–773

Reicher M A, Kellerhouse LE 1990 MRI of the wrist and hand. Raven Press, New York

Reid C D, Moss L H 1983 One-stage repair with vascularised tendon grafts in a dorsal hand injury using the 'Chinese' forearm flap. Br J Plastic Surg 36: 473–479

Reid D A C 1973 Escalator injuries of the hand. Injury 5: 47

Reid D A C 1980 The Gillies thumb lengthening operation. Hand 12: 123–129

Reid R L 1988 Radial nerve palsy. Hand Clin 4: 179–185

Reinisch J F, Winters R, Puckett C L 1984 The use of the osteocutaneous groin flap in gunshot wounds of the hand. J Hand Surg (Am) 9A: 12–17

Reinus W R, Hardy D C, Totty W G, Gilula L A 1987 Arthrographic evaluation of the carpal triangular fibrocartilage complex. J Hand Surg (Am) 12: 495–503

Reis N D 1980 Anomalous triceps tendon as a cause for snapping elbow and ulnar neuritis: a case report. J Hand Surg 5: 361–362

Reisman N R, Dellon A L 1983 The abductor digiti minimi muscle flap: a salvage technique for palmar wrist pain. Plastic Reconstr Surg 72: 859–863

Resnik C S, Miller B W, Gelberman R H, Resnick D 1983 Hand and wrist involvement in calcium pyrophosphate dihydrate crystal deposition disease. J Hand Surg (Am) 8: 856–863

Rettig A C, Strickland J W 1977 Glomus tumor of the digits. J Hand Surg 2: 261–265

Revol M P, Servant J M 1987 Classification of the main tenodesis technique used in hand surgery. Plastic Reconstr Surg 79: 237–242

Reyes F A 1989 Infections secondary to intravenous drug abuse. Hand Clin 5: 629–633

Reyes F A, Burkhalter W E 1988 The fascial radial flap. J Hand Surg (Am) 13: 432–437

Rhoades C E, Reckling F W 1983 Palmar dislocation of the trapezoid — case report. J Hand Surg (Am) 8: 85–88

Richards R R, Urbaniak J R 1984 Spontaneous retrocarpal radial artery thrombosis: a report of two cases. J Hand Surg (Am) 9: 823–827

Richman J A, Gelberman R H, Engber W D, Salamon P B, Bean D J 1987 Ganglions of the wrist and digits: results of treatment by aspiration and cyst wall puncture. J Hand Surg (Am) 12: 1041–1043

Richman J A, Gelberman R H, Rydevik B L, Hajek P C et al 1989 Carpal tunnel syndrome: morphologic changes after release of the transverse carpal ligament. J Hand Surg (Am) 14: 852–857

Riddell D H, Martin R S 1951 Glomus tumor to unusual size. Ann Surg 133: 401–403

Rieser T V, Waters R L 1986 Long-term follow-up of the Moberg key grip procedure. J Hand Surg (Am) 11: 724–728

Riester J, Mosher J F 1984 Osteoid osteoma of the capitate: a case report. J Hand Surg (Am) 9: 278–280

Riggs S A Jr, Cooney W P 3rd 1983 External fixation of complex hand and wrist fractures. J Trauma 23: 332–336

Riley D A, Lang D H 1984 Carbonic anhydrase activity of human peripheral nerves: a possible histochemical aid to nerve repair. J Hand Surg (Am) 9A: 112–120

Rinaldi E 1983 Neurilemmomas and neurofibromas of the upper limb. J Hand Surg (Am) 8: 590–593

Rinaldi E 1987 Autografts in the treatment of osseous defects in the forearm and hand. J Hand Surg (Am) 12: 282–286

Riordan D C 1955, 1963 Congenital absence of the radius. J Bone Joint Surg 37A: 1129–1140, 45A: 1783

Riordan D C 1978 Congenital absence of the ulna. In: Lovell W W, Winter R B (eds) Pediatric orthopedics. J B Lippincott, Philadelphia, pp 714–719

Riordan D C 1983 Tendon transfers in hand surgery. J Hand Surg (Am) 8: 748–753

Riordan D C, Fowler S B 1989 Arthroplasty of the metacarpophalangeal joints: review of resection-type arthroplasty. J Hand Surg (Am) 14: 368–371

Ritter M A, Inglis A E 1969 The extensor indicis proprius syndrome. J Bone Joint Surg 51A: 1645–1648

Ritts G D, Wood M B, Engber W D 1985 Nonoperative treatment of traumatic dislocations of the extensor digitorum tendons in patients without rheumatoid disorders. J Hand Surg (Am) 10: 714–716

Riveros M, Pack T 1951 The glomus tumor. Report of 20 cases. Ann Surg 133: 394–400

Robbins T H 1986 Nerve capping in the treatment of troublesome terminal neuromata. Br J Plastic Surg 39: 239–240

Robbs J, Baker L 1978 Major arterial trauma: review of experience with 267 injuries. Br J Surg 65: 532–538

Robert P 1936 Radiographie de l'articulation trapezometacarpienne. Les athroses de cette jointure. Bulletins et memoires de la Societe de Radiologie medicale de France 24: 687–690

Roberts B 1976 The acutely ischemic limb. Heart Lung 5: 273–276

Roberts P H, Price C H G 1977 Chondrosarcoma of the bones of the hand. J Bone Joint Surg 59B: 213–221

Robertson D C 1964 The fusion of interphalangeal joints. Can J Surg 7: 433–437

Robinson D W, Hardin C A 1955 Corn picker injuries. Am J Surg 89: 780–783

Robinson D, Aghasi M, Halperin N 1989 The treatment of carpal tunnel syndrome caused by hypertrophied lumbrical muscles. Case reports. Scand J Plastic Reconstr Surg Hand Surg 23: 149–151

Robinson R A 1945 Actinomycosis of the subcutaneous tissue of the forearm secondary to a human bite. J Am Med Assoc 142: 1049–1051

Robson M C, Heggers J P 1981 Evaluation of hand frostbite blister fluid as a clue to pathogenesis. J Hand Surg 6: 43–47

Rogers W D, Watson H K 1989 Radial styloid impingement after triscaphe arthrodesis. J Hand Surg (Am) 14: 297–301

Rogers W D, Watson H K 1990 Degenerative arthritis at the triscaphe joint. J Hand Surg (Am) 15: 232–235

Rohrich R J, Stevenson T R, Piepgrass W 1987 End-stage reflex sympathetic dystrophy. Plastic Reconstr Surg 79: 625–626

Rolando S 1910 Fracture de la base du premier metacarpien: et principalement sur une variete non encore decrite. Presse Medicale 33: 303

Roles N C, Maudsley R 1972 Radial tunnel syndrome: resistant tennis elbow as a nerve entrapment. J Bone Joint Surg 54B: 499–508

Rolfsen L 1970 Snapping triceps tendon with ulnar neuritis. Acta Orthopaedica Scand 41: 74–76

Romm S 1986 Henri-Francois Secretan. Hand Clin 2: 453–456

Roos D B 1966 Experience with first rib resection for thoracic outlet syndrome. Ann Surg 163: 354–358

Roos D B 1979 New concepts of thoracic outlet syndrome that explain etiology, symptoms, diagnosis, and treatment. Vasc Surg 13: 313–321

Rorabeck C H, Harris W R 1981 Factors affecting the prognosis of brachial plexus injuries. J Bone Joint Surg 63B: 404–407

Rose B A, Wood F M 1983 Metastatic bronchogenic carcinoma masquerading as a felon. J Hand Surg (Am) 8: 325–328

Rose E H 1983 Local arterialized island flap coverage of difficult hand defects preserving donor digit sensibility. Plastic Reconstr Surg 72: 848–858

Rose E H 1984 Reconstruction of central metacarpal ray defects of the hand with a free vascularized double metatarsal and metatarsophalangeal joint transfer. J Hand Surg (Am) 9A: 28–31

Rose E H, Kowalski T A 1985 Restoration of sensibility to anesthetic scarred digits with free vascularized nerve grafts from the dorsum of the foot. J Hand Surg (Am) 10: 514–521

Rose E H, Norris M S 1990 The versatile temporoparietal fascial flap; adaptability to a variety of composite defects. Plastic Reconstr Surg 85: 224–232

Rose J H, Belsky M R 1989 Psoriatic arthritis in the hand. Hand Clin 5: 137–144

Rosen, I, Werner C 1980 Neurophysiological investigation of posterior interosseous nerve entrapment causing lateral elbow pain. Electroencephalog Clin Neurophysiol 50: 125–133

Rosenfeld K, Bora F W, Lane J M 1973 Osteoid osteoma of the hamate. J Bone Joint Surg 55A: 1085–1087

Rosenfeld N, Kurzer A 1978 Acute flexor tenosynovitis

caused by gonococcal infection. A case report. Hand 10: 213–214

Rosenfeld N, Rascoff J H 1980 Tendon ruptures of the hand associated with renal dialysis. Plastic Reconstr Surg 65: 77–79

Rosenthal E A 1987 Tenosynovitis: tendon and nerve entrapment. Hand Clin 3: 585–609.

Ross G N, Baraff L J, Quismorio F P 1975 Serratia arthritis in heroin users. J Bone Joint Surg 57A: 1158–1160

Ross P M, Schwentker E P, Bryan H 1976 Mutilating lawnmower injuries in children. J Am Med Assoc 236: 408

Ross R 1979 Inhibition of myofibroblasts by skin grafts. Plastic Reconstr Surg 63: 473–481

Rosson J W, Walker G 1989 The natural history of ganglia in children. J Bone Joint Surg (Br) 71: 707–708

Roth J H, de Lorenzi C 1988 Displaced intra-articular coronal fracture of the body of the hamate treated with a Herbert screw. J Hand Surg (Am) 13: 619–621

Roth J H, Poehling G G 1990 Arthroscopic "-ectomy": surgery of the wrist. Arthroscopy 6: 141–147

Roth J H, Poehling G G, Whipple T L 1988 Arthroscopic surgery of the wrist. Instr Course Lect 37: 183–194

Rottler P D, Meystrik R, Puckett CL 1990 Microvascular angioscopy. Plastic Reconstr Surg 85: 397–403

Rousso M, Katz S, Khodadadi D 1976 Treatment of a case of macrodactyly of the thumb. Hand 8: 131–133

Rowland S A 1977 Case report: ten-year follow-up of lipofibroma of the median nerve in the palm. J Hand Surg 2: 316–317

Rowland S A 1978 Trigger finger due to neurilemmoma in the carpal tunnel. Hand 10: 229–301

Rowland S A 1986 Acute traumatic subluxation of the extensor carpi ulnaris tendon at the wrist. J Hand Surg (Am) 11: 809–811

Ruby L K, An K N, Linscheid R L, Cooney W P 3rd, Chao E Y 1987 The effect of scapholunate ligament section on scapholunate motion. J Hand Surg (Am) 12: 767–771

Ruby L K, Cooney W P 3rd, An K N, Linscheid R L, Chao E Y 1988 Relative motion of selected carpal bones: a kinematic analysis of the normal wrist. J Hand Surg (Am) 13: 1–10

Rushfort G F 1971 Two cases of subungual malignant melanoma. Br J Surg 58: 451

Rusko R A, Larsen R D 1981 Intraneural lipoma of the median nerve — case report and literature review. J Hand Surg 6: 388–391

Russe O 1960 Fracture of the carpal navicular. Diagnosis, nonoperative treatment and operative treatment. J Bone Joint Surg (Am) 42: 759

Russell R C, Van Beek A L, Wavak P, Zook E G 1981 Alternative hand flaps for amputations and digital defects. J Hand Surg 6: 399–405

Ryan J J, Hoopes J E, Jabaley M E 1974 Drug injection injuries of the hands and forearms in addicts. Plastic Reconstr Surg 53: 445–451

Rybka F J, Pratt F E 1979 Thumb reconstruction with a sensory flap from the dorsum of the index finger. Plastic Reconstr Surg 64: 141–144

Ryu J, Watson H K, Burgess R C 1985 Rheumatoid wrist reconstruction utilizing a fibrous nonunion and radiocarpal arthrodesis. J Hand Surg (Am) 10: 830–836

Sachagello C R, Ernst C B, Griffen W O 1974 The acutely ischemic upper extremity: selective management. Surgery 76: 1002–1009

Sadegbpour E, Noer H R, Mahinpour S 1981 Skull-C2 fusion in rheumatoid patients with atlantoaxial subluxation. Orthopedics 4: 1369–1374

Sadr B 1984 Sequential rupture of extensor tendons after a Colles fracture. J Hand Surg (Am) 9A: 144–145

Saferin E H, Posch J L 1976 Secretan's disease. Posttraumatic hard edema of the dorsum of the hand. Plastic Reconstr Surg 58: 703–707

Sahdev P, Jacobs L, Ellison L 1989 Extremity vascular injury from blunt trauma. Contemp Surg 35: 20–25

Saito H, Suzuki Y, Fujino K, Tajima T 1983 Free nail bed graft for treatment of nail bed injuries of the hand. J Hand Surg (Am) 8: 171–178

Sakurai M 1986 Use of bromphenol blue printing method for detecting sweat on the palm. J Hand Surg (Br) 11: 125–130

Saldana M J, McGuire R A 1986 Chronic painful subluxation of the metacarpal phalangeal joint extensor tendons. J Hand Surg (Am) 11: 420–423

Salgeback S 1977 Ulnar tunnel syndrome caused by anomalous muscles. Scand J Plastic Reconstr Surg 11: 255–258

Salibian A H, Anzel S H, Mallerich M M, Tesoro V E 1984 Microvascular reconstruction for close-range gunshot injuries to the distal forearm. J Hand Surg (Am) 9: 799–804

Salisbury R E, Dingeldein G P 1988 The burned hand and upper extremity. In: Green D P (ed) Operative hand surgery, 2nd edn. Churchill Livingstone, Edinburgh

Salisbury R E, Hunt J L, Warden G D, Pruitt B A 1973 Management of electrical burns of the upper extremity. Plastic Reconstr Surg 51: 648–652

Salisbury R E, Pruitt B A 1976 Burns of the upper extremity. W B Saunders, Philadelphia

Salisbury R E, Taylor J W, Levine N S 1976 Evaluation of digital escharotomy in burned hands. Plastic Reconstr Surg 58: 440–443

Salisbury R, McKeel D 1974 Ischemic necrosis of the intrinsic muscles of the hand after thermal injuries. J Bone Joint Surg 56A: 1701–1707

Salter R B, Harris W R 1963 Injuries involving the epiphyseal plate. J Bone Joint Surg 45A: 587–622

Salvi V 1969 Technique for the buttonhole deformity. Hand 1: 96–97

Samson R, Pasternak B M 1980 Traumatic arterial spasm — rarity or nonentity. J Trauma 20: 607–609

Sanders J O, Weiland A J, Moore J R 1986 Leiomyosarcoma of the forearm: treatment with wide local excision and a lateral arm flap. J Hand Surg (Am) 11: 906–910

Sanders R J, Roos D B 1989 The surgical anatomy of the scalene triangle. Cont Surg 35: 11–16

Sanders W E 1988 Evaluation of the humpback scaphoid by computed tomography in the longitudinal axial plane of the scaphoid. J Hand Surg (Am) 13: 182–187

Sands M J, McDonough M T, Cohen A M, Rutenberg H L, Elsner J W 1975 Fatal malignant degeneration in multiple neurofibromatosis. J Am Med Assoc 233: 1381–1382

Sandzen S C Jr 1985 Classification and functional management of congenital central defect of the hand. Hand Clin 1: 483–498

Sanger J R, Stampfl D A, Franson T R 1987 Recurrent granulomatous synovitis due to *Mycobacterium kansasii* in a renal transplant recipient. J Hand Surg (Am) 12: 436–441

Sanger J R, Yousif N J, Matloub H S 1989 *Aeromonas hydrophila* upper extremity infection. J Hand Surg (Am) 14: 719–721

Sanguinetti M V 1977 Reconstructive surgery of roller injuries of the hand. J Hand Surgery 2: 134–140

Saplys R, Mackinnon S E, Dellon A L 1987 The relationship between nerve entrapment versus neuroma complications and the misdiagnosis of de Quervain's disease. Cont Ortho 15: 51–56

Sarokhan A J, Eaton R G 1983 Volkmann's ischemia. J Hand Surg (Am) 8: 806–809

Sarrafian S K, Breihan J H 1990 Palmar dislocation of scaphoid and lunate as a unit. J Hand Surg (Am) 15: 134–139

Saveyev V, Zarevakhin I, Stepanov N 1977 Artery embolism of the upper limbs. Surgery 81: 367–375

Saydjari R, Abston S, Desai M H, Herndon D N 1986 Chemical burns. J Burn Care Rehabil 7: 404–408

Scavenius M, Fauner M, Walther-Larsen S, Buchwald C, Nielsen S L 1981 A quantitative Allen's test. Hand 13: 318–320

Schechter W, Meyer A, Schechter G, Giuliano A, Newmeyer W, Kilgore E 1982 Necrotizing fasciitis of the upper extremity. J Hand Surg 7: 15–20

Schecter W P, Markison R E, Jeffrey R B, Barton R M, Laing F 1989 Use of sonography in the early detection of suppurative flexor tenosynovitis. J Hand Surg (Am) 14: 307–310

Schecter W P, Wong D, Kilgore E S, Newmeyer W L, Howes E L, Clark G 1982 Peripartum pseudomalignant myositis ossificans of the finger. J Hand Surg 7: 44–46

Scheker L R, Kleinert H E, Hanel D P 1987 Lateral arm composite tissue transfer to ipsilateral hand defects. J Hand Surg (Am) 12: 665–672

Schenck R R 1986 Dynamic traction and early passive movement for fractures of the proximal interphalangeal joint. J Hand Surg (Am) 11: 850–858

Schenkar D L, Kleinert H E 1977 Desmoplastic fibroma of the hand. Plastic Reconstr Surg 59: 128–133

Scher C, Schun F D, Harvin J S 1973 High pressure paint gun injuries of the hand. Br J Plastic Surg 26: 167–171

Scherr D D, Dodd T A 1976 In vitro bacteriological evaluation of the effectiveness of antimicrobial irrigating solution. J Bone Joint Surg 58A: 119–122

Scherr D D, Dodd T A, Buckingham W W 1972 Prophylactic use of topical antibiotic irrigation in uninfected surgical wounds. A microbiological evaluation. J Bone Joint Surg 54A: 634–640

Scherr D D, Lichti E L, Lambert K L 1973 Tissue viability assessment with Doppler ultrasonic flowmeter in acute injuries of extremities. J Bone Joint Surg 55A: 157–161

Schiavon M, Mazzoleni F, Chiarelli A, Matano P 1988 Squamous cell carcinoma of the hand: fifty-five case reports. J Hand Surg (Am) 13: 401–404

Schiffman K L, Harris D C, Hooper G 1988 Hemangiopericytoma of the median nerve. J Hand Surg (Am) 13: 75–78.

Schlafly B, Lister G 1987 Median nerve compression secondary to bifid reversed palmaris longus. J Hand Surg (Am) 12: 371–373

Schlenker J D 1980 Important considerations in the design and construction of groin flaps. Ann Plastic Surg 5: 353–357

Schlenker J D, Atasoy E, Lyon J 1980 The abdominohypogastric flap — axial pattern flap for forearm coverage. Hand 12: 248–252

Schlenker J D, Averill R M 1980 The iliofemoral (groin) flap for hand and forearm coverage. Orthopaedic Rev 9: 57–63

Schlenker J D, Clark D D, Weckesser E C 1973 Calcinosis circumscripta of the hand in scleroderma. J Bone Joint Surg 55A: 1051–1056

Schlenker J D, Lister G D, Kleinert H E 1981 Three complications of untreated partial laceration of flexor tendons — entrapment, rupture and triggering. J Hand Surg 6: 392–396

Schmidt D R, Heckman J D 1983 Eikenella corrodens in human bite infections of the hand. J Trauma 23: 478–482

Schmidt P E, Hewitt R L 1980 Severe upper limb ischemia. Arch Surg 115: 1188–1191

Schmitz R L, Keeley J L 1957 Lipomas of the hand. Surgery 42: 696–700

Schneider L 1988 Tendon transfers in muscle and tendon loss. Hand Clin 4: 267–272

Schneider L H 1988 Fractures of the distal phalanx. Hand Clin 4: 537–547

Schneider L H, Hankin F M, Eisenberg T 1986 Surgery of Dupuytren's disease: a review of the open palm method. J Hand Surg (Am) 11: 23–27

Schneider L H, Rosenstein R G 1983 Restoration of extensor pollicis longus function by tendon transfer. Plastic Reconstr Surg 71: 533–537

Schneider L H, Wiltshire D 1983 Restoration of flexor pollicis longus function by flexor digitorum superficialis transfer. J Hand Surg (Am) 8: 98–101

Schneller S 1989 Medical considerations and perioperative care for rheumatoid surgery. Hand Clin 5: 115–126

Schoo M J, Scott F A, Boswick J A 1980 High pressure injection injuries of the hand. J Trauma 20: 229–238

Schuhl J F, Leroy B, Comtet J J 1985 Biodynamics of the wrist: radiologic approach to scapholunate instability. J Hand Surg (Am) 10: 1006–1008

Schuind F, Merle M, Dap F, Bour C, Michon J 1988 Hyperostotic macrodactyly. J Hand Surg (Am) 13: 544–548

Schuind F, Ventura M, Pasteels J L 1990 Idiopathic carpal tunnel syndrome: histologic study of flexor tendon synovium. J Hand Surg (Am) 15: 497–503

Schultz R J, Endler P M, Huddleston H D 1973 Anomalous median nerve and an anomalous muscle belly of the first lumbrical associated with carpal tunnel syndrome. J Bone Joint Surg 55A: 1744–1746

Schultz-Johnson K 1987 Assessment of upper extremity — injured persons' return to work potential. J Hand Surg (Am) 12: 950–957

Schumacker H B 1982 Frostbite. In: Flynn J E (ed) Hand surgery, 3rd edn. Williams & Wilkins, Baltimore, p 591

Schvarcz L W 1977 Congenital dermatofibrosarcoma protuberans of the hand. Hand 9: 182–185

Schwager R G, Smith J W, Goulian D 1975 Small deep forearm lacerations. Plastic Reconstr Surg 55: 190–194

Schwartz M G, Green S M, Coville F A 1990 Dorsal dislocation of the lunate with multiple extensor tendon ruptures. J Hand Surg (Am) 15: 132–133

Scott F A, German C, Boswick J A 1981 Haemophilus influenzae cellulitis of the hand. J Hand Surg 6: 506–509

Scott F A, Howar J W, Boswick J A 1981 Recovery of function following replantation and revascularization of amputated hand parts. J Trauma 21: 204–214

Scott M M, Mulligan P J 1980 Stabilizing severe phalangeal fractures. Hand 12: 44–50

Seckel B R 1986 Self-advancing silicone rubber splint for repair of split nail deformity. J Hand Surg (Am) 11: 143–144

Secretan H 1901 Hard edema and traumatic hyperplasia of the dorsum of the metacarpus. Rev Med Suisse Rom 21: 409

Seddon H J 1952 Carpal ganglion as a cause of paralysis of the deep branch of the ulnar nerve. J Bone Joint Surg 34B: 386–390

Seddon Sir H J 1972 Surgical disorders of peripheral nerves. Williams & Wilkins, Baltimore

Segmuller G 1973 Surgical stabilization of the skeleton of the hand. Williams & Wilkins, Baltimore

Seiler J G 3rd, Milek M A, Carpenter G K, Swiontkowski M F 1989 Intraoperative assessment of median nerve blood flow during carpal tunnel release with laser Doppler flowmetry. J Hand Surg (Am) 14: 986–991

Seimon L P 1972 Compound dislocation of the trapezium. J Bone Joint Surg 54A: 1297–1300

Seitz W H Jr 1989 Distraction osteogenesis of a congenital amputation at the elbow. J Hand Surg (Am) 14: 945–948

Seitz W H Jr, Froimson A I 1988 Management of malunited fractures of the metacarpal and phalangeal shafts. Hand Clin 4: 529–538

Seitz W H Jr, Gomez W, Putnam M D, Rosenwasser M P 1987 Management of severe hand trauma with a mini external fixateur. Orthopedics 10: 601–610

Semer N B, Goldberg N H, Cuono C B 1989 Upper extremity entrapment neuropathy and tourniquet use in patients undergoing hemodialysis. J Hand Surg (Am) 14: 897–900

Senrui H, Egawa T, Horiki A 1982 Anatomical findings in the hands of patients with Poland's syndrome. J Bone Joint Surg (Am) 64: 1079–1082

Seradge H, Kutz J A, Kleinert H E, Lister G D et al 1984 Perichondrial resurfacing arthroplasty in the hand. J Hand Surg 9: 880–886

Seradge H, Seradge E 1990 Median innervated hypothenar muscle: anomalous branch of median nerve in the carpal tunnel. J Hand Surg (Am) 15: 356–359

Seradge H, Sterbank P T, Seradge E, Owens W 1990 Segmental motion of the proximal carpal row: their global effect on wrist motion. J Hand Surg (Am) 15: 236–239

Serafin D, Puckett C L, McCarty G 1976 Successful treatment of acute vascular insufficiency in a hand by intra-arterial fibrinolysin, heparin and reserpine. Plastic Reconstr Surg 58: 506–509

Serra J M, Muirragui A, Tadjalli H 1985 Extensive distal subcutaneous metastases of a 'benign' giant cell tumor of the radius. Plastic Reconstr Surg 75: 263–267

Serra J M, Muirragui A, Tadjalli H 1985 Glomus tumor of the metacarpophalangeal joint: a case report. J Hand Surg (Am) 10: 142–143

Seyfer A E, Grammer N Y, Bogumill G P, Provost J M, Chandry U 1985 Upper extremity neuropathies after cardiac surgery. J Hand Surg (Am) 10: 16–19

Seyffarth H 1951 Primary myoses in the m. pronator teres as a cause of lesion of the n. medianus (the pronator syndrome). Acta Psych Scand suppl 74: 251

Shapiro J S 1970 A new factor in the etiology of ulnar drift. Clin Orthop 68: 32

Shapiro J S 1982 Wrist involvement in rheumatoid swan-neck deformity. J Hand Surg 7: 484

Sharrard W J W 1966 Posterior interosseous neuritis. J Bone Joint Surg 48B: 777–780

Sharrard W J W 1968 Injection injuries. J Bone Joint Surg 50B: 1

Shaw D T 1980 Tubed pedicle construction: the single pedicle abdominal tube and the acromiopectoral flap. Ann Plastic Surg 4: 219–223

Shaw J A 1987 Osteoid osteoma of the lunate. J Hand Surg (Am) 12: 128–130

Shaw J A, Mosher J F 1983 A giant-cell tumor in the hand presenting as an expansile diaphyseal lesion. Case report. J Bone Joint Surg 65: 692–695

Shepard G H 1980 High-energy, low-velocity, close-range shotgun wounds. J Trauma 20: 1065–1067

Shepard G H 1983 The use of lateral V–Y advancement flaps for fingertip reconstruction. J Hand Surg (Am) 8: 254–259

Shepard G H 1983 Treatment of nail bed avulsions with split-thickness nail bed grafts. J Hand Surg (Am) 8: 49–54

Shepard G H 1990 Management of acute nail bed avulsions. Hand Clin 6: 39–56

Shepard G H 1990 Nail grafts for reconstruction. Hand Clin 6: 79–102

Shereff M J, Posner M A, Gordo M H 1980 Upper extremity hypertrophy secondary to neurofibromatosis: a case report. J Hand Surg 5: 355–357

Sherlock D A 1987 Traumatic dorsoradial dislocation of the trapezium. J Hand Surg (Am) 12: 262–265

Shibata M, Tsai T M, Firrell J, Breidenbach W C 1988 Experimental comparison of vascularized and nonvascularized nerve grafting. J Hand Surg (Am) 13: 358–365

Shigematsu S, Abe M, Onomura T, Kinoshita M, Inoue T 1989 Arthrography of the normal and posttraumatic wrist. J Hand Surg (Am) 14: 410–412

Short W H, Palmer A K 1981 Amyloidosis and the carpal tunnel syndrome. Orthopaedic Rev 10: 89–94

Short W H, Watson H K 1982 Prediction of the spiral nerve in Dupuytren's contracture. J Hand Surg 7: 84–86

Shrewsburry M M, Johnson R K 1983 Form, function, and evolution of the distal phalanx. J Hand Surg (Am) 8: 475–479

Shrewsbury M, Johnson R K 1975 The fascia of the distal phalanx. J Bone Joint Surg 57A: 784–788

Shuck J M, Omer G E, Lewis C E 1972 Arterial obstruction due to intimal disruption in extremity fractures. J Trauma 12: 481–489

Shurr D G, Blair W F, Bassett G 1986 Electromyographic changes after carpal tunnel release. J Hand Surg (Am) 11: 876–880

Siegel D, Gebhardt M, Jupiter J B 1987 Spontaneous rupture of the extensor pollicis longus tendon. J Hand Surg (Am) 12: 1106–1109

Siegel R S, Steichten F M 1967 Cervicothoracic outlet syndrome. J Bone Joint Surg 49A: 1187–1192

Siegert J J, Cooney W P, Dobyns J H 1990 Management of simple camptodactyly. J Hand Surg (Br) 15: 181–189

Siemionow M, Lister G D 1987 Tendon ruptures and median nerve damage after Hamas total wrist arthroplasty. J Hand Surg (Am) 12: 374–377

Sieracki J C, Kelly A P 1959 Traumatic epidermoid cysts involving digital bones: epidermoid cysts of the distal phalanx. Arch Surg 78: 597–603

Sigurdsson J, Bjornsson A, Gudmundsson ST 1983 Formic acid burn — local and systemic effects. Burns 9: 358–361

Silver M A, Gelberman R H, Gellman H, Rhoades C E 1985 Carpal tunnel syndrome: associated abnormalities in ulnar nerve function and the effect of carpal tunnel release on these abnormalities. J Hand Surg (Am) 10: 710–713

Silverman I 1935 Epithelioma following chronic paronychia. Am J Surg 19: 141–142, 151

Silverman M E, Copeland A J Jr, Hurst J W 1970 The Holt–Oram syndrome: the long and the short of it. Am J Cardiol 25: 11–17

Silverstein B, Fine L, Stetson D 1987 Hand-wrist disorders among investment casting plant workers. J Hand Surg (Am) 12: 838–844

Silverton J S, Nahai F, Jurkiewicz M J 1978 The latissimus dorsi myocutaneous flap to replace a defect of the upper arm. Br J Plastic Surg 31: 29–31

Sim F H, Dahlin D C, Beabout J W 1975 Osteoid osteoma: diagnostic problems. J Bone Joint Surg 57A: 154–159

Sim F H, Dahlin D C, Ivins J C 1977 Extra-articular synovial chondromatosis. J Bone Joint Surg 59A: 492–495

Simmons B P 1985 Polydactyly. Hand Clin 1: 545–565

Simmons B P, McKenzie W D 1985 Symptomatic carpal coalition. J Hand Surg (Am) 10: 190–193

Simmons B P, Nutting J T 1989 Juvenile rheumatoid arthritis. Hand Clin 5: 157–168

Simmons B P, Southmayd W W, Riseborough E J 1983 Congenital radioulnar synostosis. J Hand Surg (Am) 8: 829–838

Simmons B P, Vasile R 1980 The clenched fist syndrome. J Hand Surg 5: 420–427

Simmons E H, Peteghem K V, Tramell T R 1980 Onchocerciasis of the flexor compartment of the forearm: a case report. J Hand Surg 5: 502–504

Simpson L A, Cruse C W 1981 Gasoline immersion injury. Plastic Reconstr Surg 67: 54–57

Simpson R G 1977 Delayed rupture of extensor pollicis longus tendon following closed injury. Hand 9: 160–161

Singer D I, O'Brien B M, Angel M F, Gumley G J 1989 Digital distraction lengthening followed by free vascularized epiphyseal joint transfer. J Hand Surg (Am) 14: 508–512

Singer R M, Gorosh J E 1990 Purpura fulminans. J Hand Surg (Am) 15: 172–175

Sirikulchayanonta V, Visuthikosol V, Tanphaichitra D, Prajaktham R 1989 Prototothecosis following hand injury. A case report. J Hand Surg (Br) 14: 88–90

Sjogren H 1933 A new conception of kerato conjunctivitis sicca. Acta Ophthal Kbh suppl 2: 1

Skerik S K, Flatt A E 1969 The anatomy of congenital radial dysplasia. Clin Orthopaedics 66: 125–143

Skoog T 1963 The pathogenesis and etiology of Dupuytren's contracture. Plastic Reconstr Surg 31: 258–267

Skoog T, Johansson S H 1976 The formation of articular cartilage from free perichondrial grafts. Plastic Reconstr Surg 57: 1–6

Small J O, Brennen M D 1988 The first dorsal metacarpal artery neurovascular island flap. J Hand Surg (Br) 13: 136–145

Small J O, Brennen M D 1990 The first dorsal metacarpal artery neurovascular island flap. Br J Plastic Surg 43: 17–23

Smith B L 1987 An inside look: hand injury-prevention program. J Hand Surg (Am) 12: 940–943

Smith D J Jr, Bendick P J, Madison S A 1984 Evaluation of vascular compromise in the injured extremity: a photoplethysmographic technique. J Hand Surg (Am) 9: 314–319

Smith D K, Cooney W P 3rd, An K N, Linscheid R L, Chao E Y 1989 The effects of simulated unstable scaphoid fractures on carpal motion. J Hand Surg (Am) 14: 283–291

Smith J A, Millender L H 1979 Treatment of recurrent giant cell tumor of the digit by phalangeal excision and toe phalanx transplant. A case report. J Hand Surg 4: 164–168

Smith J R, Asturias J 1968 Card injury of the hand: its characteristics and treatment. J Bone Joint Surg 50A: 1161–1170

Smith J, Ruby L K 1977 Nocardia asteroides thenar space infection: a case report. J Hand Surg 2: 109–110

Smith K F 1979 The thoracic outlet syndrome: a protocol of treatment. J Orthopaedic Sports Phys Therapy 2: 89–99

Smith M A 1980 The mechanism of acute ulnar instability of the metacarpophalangeal joint of the thumb. Hand 12: 225–230

Smith P 3rd, Wright T W, Wallace P F, Dell P C 1988 Excision of the hook of the hamate: a retrospective survey and review of the literature. J Hand Surg (Am) 13: 612–615

Smith R I, Kaplan E B 1967 Rheumatoid deformities at the metacarpophalangeal joints of the fingers. J Bone Joint Surg 49A: 31–47

Smith R J 1971 Anomalous muscle belly of the flexor digitorum superficialis causing carpal tunnel syndrome. J Bone Joint Surg 53A: 1215–1216

Smith R J 1971 Non-ischemic contractures of the intrinsic muscles of the hand. J Bone Joint Surg 53A: 1313–1331

Smith R J 1975 Factitious lymphedema of the hand. J Bone Joint Surg 57A: 89–94

Smith R J 1977 Post-traumatic instability of the metacarpophalangeal joint of the thumb. J Bone Joint Surg 59A: 14–21

Smith R J 1977 Tumors of the hand. Who is best qualified to treat tumors of the hand? J Hand Surg 2: 251–255

Smith R J 1983 Extensor carpi radialis brevis tendon transfer for thumb adduction — a study of power pinch. J Hand Surg 8: 4–15

Smith R J 1986 Indications for tendon transfers to the hand. Hand Clin 2: 235–237

Smith R J, Atkinson R E, Jupiter J B 1985 Silicone synovitis of the wrist. J Hand Surg (Am) 10: 47–60

Smith R J, Brushart T M 1985 Allograft bone for metacarpal reconstruction. J Hand Surg (Am) 10: 325–334

Smith R J, Gumley G J 1985 Metacarpal distraction lengthening. Hand Clin 1: 417–429

Smith R J, Kaplan E B 1968 Camptodactyly and similar atraumatic flexion deformities of the proximal interphalangeal joints of the fingers. J Bone Joint Surg 50A: 1187–1203

Smith R J, Lipke R W 1979 Treatment of congenital deformities of the hand and forearm. N Engl J Med 300: 402–407

Smith R J, Mankin H J 1977 Allograft replacement of distal radius for giant cell tumor. J Hand Surg 2: 299–309

Smith R J, Peimer C A 1977 Injuries to the metacarpal bones and joints. Adv Surg 11: 341–374

Sneddon J 1969–70 Sepsis in hand injuries. Hand 1–2: 58–62

Sneddon J 1970 The care of hand infections. Williams & Wilkins, Baltimore

Snow J W 1976 A method for reconstruction of the central slip of the extensor tendon of a finger. Plastic Reconstr Surg 57: 455–459

Snow J W 1985 Volar advancement skin flap to the fingertip. Hand Clin 1: 685–688

Snow J W, Littler J W 1969 Surgical treatment of cleft hand. Transactions of the Fourth International Congress of Plastic and Reconstructive Surgery 888–893. Excerpta Medica Foundation, Amsterdam

Snyder C C 1989 Animal bite wounds. Hand Clin 5: 571–590

Snyder C C, Straight R, Glenn J 1972 The snakebitten hand. Plastic Reconstr Surg 49: 275–282

Song R, Gao Y, Song Y, Yu Y, Song Y 1982 The forearm flap. Clin Plastic Surg 9: 21

Soucatos P N, Hartofilakidis-Gsrofalidis G C 1981 Dislocation of the triangular bone: report of a case. J Bone Joint Surg 63A: 1012–1014

Soutar D S, Tanner N S 1984 The radial forearm flap in the management of soft tissue injuries of the hand. Br J Plastic Surg 37: 18–26

Souter W A 1974 The problem of boutonniere deformity. Clin Orthopaedics 104: 116–133

Souter W A 1989 Planning treatment of the rheumatoid hand. Hand 11: 3

Southmayd W W, Millender L H, Nalebuff E A 1975 Rupture of the flexor tendons of the index finger after Colles' fracture. J Bone Joint Surg 57A: 562–563

Southwick G, Lister G D 1979 Actinomycosis of the hand: a case report. J Hand Surg 4: 360–362

Sowa D T, Holder L E, Patt P G, Weiland A J 1989 Application of magnetic resonance imaging to ischemic necrosis of the lunate J Hand Surg 14A: 1008–1016

Sowa D T, Moore J R, Weiland A J 1987 Extraskeletal osteochondromas of the wrist. J Hand Surg (Am) 12: 212–217

Specht E E, Konkin L A 1976 Juvenile aponeurotic fibroma. The cartilage analogue of fibromatosis. J Am Med Assoc 236: 626–628

Specht E E, Staheli L T 1977 Juvenile aponeurotic fibroma. J Hand Surg 2: 258–260

Spector D, Miller J, Viloria J 1979 Malignant fibrous histiocytoma. J Bone Joint Surg 61B: 190–193

Spiegel J D, Szabo R M 1988 A protocol for the treatment of severe infection of the hand. J Hand Surg (Am) 13: 254–259

Spinner M 1968 The arcade of Frohse: its relationship to posterior interosseous nerve paralysis. J Bone Joint Surg 50B: 809–812

Spinner M 1969 Fashioned transpositional flap for soft tissue adduction contracture of the thumb. Plastic Reconstr Surg 44: 345–348

Spinner M 1976 Cryptogenic infraclavicular brachial plexus neuritis. Bull Hosp Joint Dis 37: 98–104

Spinner M 1978 Injuries to the major branches of peripheral nerves of the forearm 2nd edn. W B Saunders Co, Philadelphia

Spinner M, Aiache A, Silver L, Barsky A S 1973 Impending ischemic contracture of the hand. Plastic Reconstr Surg 50: 341–349

Spinner M, Freundlich B D, Teicher J 1968 Posterior interosseous nerve palsy as a complication of Monteggia fractures in children. Clin Orthopaedics 58: 141–145

Spinner M, Kaplan E B 1976 The relationship of the ulnar nerve to the medial intermuscular septum in the arm and its clinical significance. Hand 8: 239–242

Spinner M, Olshansky K 1973 The extensor indicis proprius syndrome. Plastic Reconstr Surg 51: 134–138

Sponseller P D, Engber W D 1983 Double-entrapment radial tunnel syndrome. J Hand Surg (Am) 8: 420–423

Sprague H H, Howard F M 1988 The Herbert screw for treatment of the scaphoid fracture. Contemp Orthopaedics 16: 19–25

Spurling R G, Scoville W R 1944 Lateral rupture of the cervical intervertebral discs. Surg Gynecol Obstet 78: 350–357

Srinivasan H 1981 A simple method for assessing abduction of the thumb. J Hand Surg 6: 583–584

Srinivasan H 1983 Postural changes in thenar paralysis and their significance. J Hand Surg (Am) 8: 194–196

St Onge R A, Jackson I T 1977 An uncommon sequel to thumb trauma: epidermoid cyst. Hand 9: 52–56

Stackhouse T G, Weiland A J 1984 Extraosseous chondrosarcoma of the wrist: a case report. J Hand Surg (Am) 9: 338–342

Stahl S, Wolff T W 1988 Delayed rupture of the extensor pollicis longus tendon after nonunion of a fracture of the dorsal radial tubercle. J Hand Surg (Am) 13: 338–341

Stain S C, Yellin A E, Weaver F A, Pentecost M J 1989 Selective management of nonocclusive arterial injuries. Arch Surg 124: 1136–1141

Stambough J L, Bora F W Jr, DuShuttle R P 1986 Sarcoid flexor tenosynovitis of the finger: a case report. J Hand Surg (Am) 11: 436–438

Stark H H, Ashworth C R, Boyes J H 1961 Grease gun injuries of the hand. J Bone Joint Surg 43A: 485–491

Stark H H, Ashworth C R, Boyes J H 1967 Paint gun injuries of the hand. J Bone Joint Surg 49A: 637–647

Stark H H, Chao E K, Zemel N P, Rickard T A, Ashworth C R 1989 Fracture of the hook of the hamate. J Bone Joint Surg (Am) 71: 1202–1207

Stark H H, Jones F E, Jernstrom P 1971 Parosteal osteogenic sarcoma of a metacarpal bone. J Bone Joint Surg 53A: 147–153

Stark H H, Moore J F, Ashworth C R, Boyes J H 1977 Fusion of the first metacarpotrapezial joint for degenerative arthritis. J Bone Joint Surg 59A: 22–26

Steichen J B, Idler R S 1986 Results of central ray resection without bony transposition. J Hand Surg (Am) 11: 466–474

Steichen J B, Petersen D P 1984 Junctura tendinum between extensor digitorum communis and extensor pollicis longus. J Hand Surg (Am) 9: 674–676

Stein H, Horer D, Horesh Z 1984 The use of external fixators in the treatment and rehabilitation of compound limb injuries. Orthopedics 7: 707–714

Stelling F 1963 The upper extremity. In: Ferguson A B (ed) Orthopaedic surgery in infancy and childhood, vol 2. Williams & Wilkins, Baltimore, pp 304–308

Stener B 1962 Displacement of the ruptured ulnar collateral ligament of the MCP joint of the thumb. J Bone Joint Surg 44B: 869–879

Stern H S, Lloyd G J 1978 Metacarpal shortening. Hand 10: 202–204

Stern P J 1981 Stener lesion after lateral dislocation of the proximal interphalangeal joint — indication for open reduction. J Hand Surg 6: 602–604

Stern P J, Caudle R J 1988 Tendon transfers for elbow flexion. Hand Clin 4: 297–307

Stern P J, Gula D C 1986 Mycobacterium chelonei tenosynovitis of the hand: a case report. J Hand Surg (Am) 11: 596–599

Stern P J, Ho S 1987 Osteoarthritis of the proximal interphalangeal joint. Hand Clin 3: 405–413

Stern P J, Kastrup J J 1988 Complications and prognosis of treatment of mallet finger. J Hand Surg (Am) 13: 329–334

Stern P J, Lee A F 1985 Open dorsal dislocations of the proximal interphalangeal joint. J Hand Surg (Am) 10: 364–370

Stern P J, Neale H W, Graham T J, Warden G D 1987

Classification and treatment of postburn proximal interphalangeal joint flexion contractures in children. J Hand Surg (Am) 12: 450–457

Stern P J, Neale H W, Gregory R O, Kreilein J G 1982 Latissimus dorsi musculocutaneous flap for elbow flexion. J Hand Surg 7: 25–30

Stern P J, Phillips D 1986 Phalangeal osteochondroma: an unusual cause of swan-neck deformity. J Hand Surg (Am) 11: 70–73

Stern P J, Staneck J L, McDonough J J, Neale H W, Tyler G 1983 Established hand infections: a controlled, prospective study. J Hand Surg (Am) 8: 553–559

Stern P J, Vice M 1983 Compression of the deep branch of the ulnar nerve — a case report. J Hand Surg (Am) 8: 72–74

Stevanovic M V, Stark H H 1984 Dorsal dislocation of the fourth and fifth carpometacarpal joints and simultaneous dislocation of the metacarpophalangeal joint of the small finger: a case report. J Hand Surg (Am) 9: 714–716

Stevenson J H, Zuker R M 1986 Upper limb motor and sensory recovery after multiple proximal nerve injury in children: a long term review in five patients. Br J Plastic Surg 39: 109–113

Stewart J D 1986 Electrodiagnostic techniques in the evaluation of nerve compressions and injuries in the upper limb. Hand Clin 2: 677–687

Steyers C M, Blair W F 1989 Measuring ulnar variance: a comparison of techniques. J Hand Surg (Am) 14: 607–612

Still G F 1897 On a form of chronic joint disease in children. Med Chir Trans 80: 47–59

Still J M, Kleinert H E 1973 Anomalous muscles and nerve entrapment in the wrist and hand. Plastic Reconstr Surg 52: 394–400

Stilwell J H, Maisels D O 1981 Subungual Bowen's disease. Hand 13: 287–290

Stirrat C R 1989 Treatment of tenosynovitis in rheumatoid arthritis. Hand Clin 5: 169–175

Stone P A 1973 Hand burns caused by electric fires. Injury 4: 240–246

Stothard J, Caird D M 1981 Experience with arthrography of the first metacarpophalangeal joint. Hand 13: 257–266

Strachan J C H, Ellis B W 1971 The vulnerability of the posterior interosseous nerve during radial head resection. J Bone Joint Surg 53B: 320–323

Strahan J, Crockett D J 1969 Wringer injury. Injury 1: 57

Straub L R, Ranawat C S 1969 The wrist in rheumatoid arthritis. J Bone Joint Surg 51A: 1–20

Straub L R, Smith I W, Carpenter G K, Dietz G H 1961 The surgery of gout in the upper extremity. J Bone Joint Surg 43A: 731

Straub L R, Wilson E H 1956 Spontaneous rupture of extensor tendons in the hand associated with rheumatoid arthritis. J Bone Joint Surg 38A: 1208–1217

Strauch B 1975 Dorsal thumb flap for release of adduction contracture of the first web space. Bull Hos Joint Dis 36: 34–39

Strauch B, de Moura W 1990 Arterial system of the fingers. J Hand Surg (Am) 15: 148–154

Strauch B, Spinner M 1976 Congenital anomaly of the thumb: absent intrinsics and flexor pollicis longus. J Bone Joint Surg 58A: 115–118

Strauss A 1922 Lipoma of the tendon sheaths: with report of case and review of the literature. Surg Gynecol Obstet 35: 161

Strecker W B, Emanuel J P, Dailey L, Manske P R 1988 Comparison of pronator tenotomy and pronator rerouting in children with spastic cerebral palsy. J Hand Surg (Am) 13: 540–543

Strickland J W 1985 Flexor tendon repair. Hand Clin 1: 55–68

Strickland J W 1985 Flexor tenolysis. Hand Clin 1: 121–132

Strickland J W 1985 Results of flexor tendon surgery in zone II. Hand Clin 1: 167–179

Strickland J W 1989 Flexor tendon surgery. Part 2: Free tendon grafts and tenolysis. J Hand Surg (Br) 14: 368–382

Strickland J W, Bassett R L 1985 The isolated digital cord in Dupuytren's contracture: anatomy and clinical significance. J Hand Surg (Am) 10: 118–124

Strickland J W, Steichen J B 1977 Nerve tumors of the hand and forearm. J Hand Surg 2: 285–291

Stromberg B V 1985 Changing bacteriologic flora of hand infections. J Trauma 25: 530–533

Strong M L 1975 Chondromas of the tendon sheath of the hand. Report of a case and review of the literature. J Bone Joint Surg 57A: 1164–1165

Strong M L 1983 Bowen's disease in multiple nail beds — case report. J Hand Surg (Am) 8: 329–330

Stuchin S A, Kummer F J 1984 Stiffness of small–bone external fixation methods: an experimental study. J Hand Surg (Am) 9: 718–724

Sturim H S, Edmond J A 1980 Carpal tunnel compression syndrome secondary to a retracted flexor digitorum sublimis tendon. Plastic Reconstr Surg 66: 846–848

Sturn J T, Rothenberger D A, Strate R 1978 Brachial artery disruption following closed elbow dislocation. J Trauma 18: 364–366

Styf J, Forssblad P, Lundborg G 1987 Chronic compartment syndrome in the first dorsal interosseous muscle. J Hand Surg (Am) 12: 757–762

Su C T, Hoopes J E, Daniel R 1972 Congenital absence of the thenar muscles innervated by the median nerve. J Bone Joint Surg 54A: 1087–1090

Subin G D, Mallon W J, Urbaniak J R 1989 Diagnosis of ganglion in Guyon's canal by magnetic resonance imaging. J Hand Surg (Am) 14: 640–643

Sudeck P 1900 Uber die akute entzundliche Knochenatropie. Arch Klin Chir 11: 147

Sugiura I 1976 Desmoplastic fibroma. Case report and review of the literature. J Bone Joint Surg 58A: 126–130

Sugiura I 1976 Intra-osseous glomus tumor. J Bone Joint Surg 58B: 245–247

Sugiura Y 1976 'Poland's syndrome'. Clinicoroentgenographic study on 45 cases. Cong Anom 16: 17–28

Sullivan C R, Dahlin D C, Bryan R S 1956 Lipoma of the tendon sheath. J Bone Joint Surg 38A: 1275–1280

Sullivan W G, Scott F A, Boswick J A 1981 Rehabilitation following electrical injury to the upper extremity. Ann Plastic Surg 7: 347–353

Sunderland S 1978 Nerves and nerve injuries, 2nd edn. Churchill Livingstone, Edinburgh

Sunram F, Hippe P 1979 Radial nerve paralysis by congenital angioleiomyoma. Hand Chirurgia 11: 27–29

Suso S, Peidro L, Ramon R 1988 Tuberculous synovitis with 'rice bodies' presenting as carpal tunnel syndrome. J Hand Surg (Am) 13: 574–576

Suso S, Vicente P, Angles F 1985 Surgical treatment of the non-functional spastic hand. J Hand Surg (Br) 10: 54–56

Swafford A R, Lichtman D H 1982 Suprascapular nerve entrapment. Case report. J Hand Surg 7: 57–60

Swanson A B 1968 Restoration of hand function by the use of partial or total prosthetic replacement. J Bone Joint Surg 45A: 276–283

Swanson A B 1972 Disabling arthritis at the base of the thumb. J Bone Joint Surg 54A: 456–471

Swanson A B 1973 Flexible implant arthroplasty in the hand and extremities. C V Mosby, St Louis

Swanson A B 1976 A classification for congenital limb malformation. J Hand Surg 1: 8–22

Swanson A B, Boeve N R, Lumsden R M 1977 The prevention and treatment of amputation neuromata by silicone capping. J Hand Surg 2: 70–78

Swanson A B, de Groot Swanson G 1989 Evaluation and treatment of the upper extremity in the stroke patient. Hand Clin 5: 75–96

Swanson A B, Herndon J H 1977 Flexible (silicone) implant arthroplasty of the metacarpophalangeal joint of the thumb. J Bone Joint Surg 59A: 362–368

Swanson A B, Maupin B K, de Groot Swanson G, Ganzhorn R W, Moss S H 1985 Lunate implant resection arthroplasty: long-term results. J Hand Surg (Am) 10: 1013–1024

Swanson A B, Maupin B K, Gajjar N V, Swanson G D 1985 Flexible implant arthroplasty in the proximal interphalangeal joint of the hand. J Hand Surg (Am) 10: 796–805

Swanson A B, Swanson G D 1983 Osteoarthritis in the hand. J Hand Surg (Am) 8: 669–675

Swanson A B, Swanson G D, Tada K 1983 A classification for congenital limb malformation. J Hand Surg (Am) 8: 693-702

Swanson A B, Swanson G G, Maupin B K, Hynes D E, Jindal P 1989 Failed carpal bone arthroplasty: causes and treatment. J Hand Surg (Am) 14: 417–424

Swanson A B, Swanson G, Watermeier J I 1981 Trapezium implant arthroplasty — long-term evaluation of 150 cases. J Hand Surg 6: 125–141

Swanson A B, Tada K, Yonenobu K 1984 Ulnar ray deficiency: its various manifestations. J Hand Surg (Am) 9: 658–664

Swanson A F, Leonard J B, deGroot Swanson G 1986 Implant resection arthroplasty of the finger joints. Hand Clin 2: 107–117

Swanson E, Boyd J, Manktelow R T 1990 The radial forearm flap; reconstructive applications and donor site defects in 35 consecutive patients. Plastic Reconstr Surg 85: 258–266

Swanson E, Freiberg A, Salter D R 1990 Radial artery infections and aneurysms after catheterization. J Hand Surg (Am) 15: 166–171

Swartz W M 1984 Immediate reconstruction of the wrist and dorsum of the hand with a free osteocutaneous groin flap. J Hand Surg (Am) 9A: 18–21

Swiggett R, Ruby L K 1986 Median nerve compression neuropathy by the lacertus fibrosus: report of three cases. J Hand Surg (Am) 11: 700–703

Szabo R M, Chidgey L K 1989 Stress carpal tunnel pressures in patients with carpal tunnel syndrome and normal patients. J Hand Surg (Am) 14: 624–627

Szabo R M, Gelberman R H 1985 Operative treatment of cerebral palsy. Hand Clin 1: 525–543

Szabo R M, Gelberman R H 1987 The pathophysiology of nerve entrapment syndromes. J Hand Surg (Am) 12: 880–884

Szabo R M, Gelberman R H, Dimick M P 1984 Sensibility testing in patients with carpal tunnel syndrome. J Bone Joint Surg (Am) 66: 60–64

Tada K, Yonenobu K, Tsuyuguchi Y, Kawai H, Egawa T 1983 Duplication of the thumb. A retrospective review of two hundred and thirty-seven cases. J Bone Joint Surg (Am) 65: 584–598

Tajima T 1983 Considerations on the use of the tourniquet in surgery of the hand. J Hand Surg (Am) 8: 799–802

Tajima T 1985 Classification of thumb hypoplasia. Hand Clin 1: 577–594

Tajima T 1988 Treatment of post-traumatic contracture of the hand. J Hand Surg (Br) 13: 118–129

Takigawa K 1971 Carpal chondroma. J Bone Joint Surg 53A: 1601–1604

Takigawa K 1971 Chondroma of the bones of the hand. J Bone Joint Surg 53A: 1591–1600

Taleisnik J 1973 The palmar cutaneous branch of the median nerve and the approach to the carpal tunnel. J Bone Joint Surg 55A: 1212–1217

Taleisnik J 1985 The wrist. Churchill Livingstone, Edinburgh

Taleisnik J 1987 Combined radiocarpal arthrodesis and midcarpal (lunocapitate) arthroplasty for treatment of rheumatoid arthritis of the wrist. J Hand Surg (Am) 12: 1–8

Taleisnik J 1988 Clinical and technologic evaluation of ulnar wrist pain (editorial). J Hand Surg (Am) 13: 801–802

Taleisnik J 1989 Rheumatoid arthritis of the wrist. Hand Clin 5: 257–278

Taleisnik J, Gelberman R H, Miller B W, Szabo R M 1984 The extensor retinaculum of the wrist. J Hand Surg (Am) 9: 495–501

Taleisnik J, Watson H K 1984 Midcarpal instability caused by malunited fractures of the distal radius. J Hand Surg (Am) 9: 350–357

Tank M S, Lewis R C Jr, Coates P W 1983 The lateral antebrachial cutaneous nerve as a highly suitable autograft donor for the digital nerve. J Hand Surg (Am) 8: 942–945

Taweepoke P, Frame J D 1990 Acute ischaemia of the hand following accidental radial artery infusion of Depo-Medrone. J Hand Surg (Br) 15: 118–120

Taylor A R 1974 Ulnar nerve compression at the wrist in rheumatoid arthritis. J Bone Joint Surg 56B: 142–143

Taylor A R, Mukerjea S K, Rana N A 1976 Excision of the head of the radius in rheumatoid arthritis. J Bone Joint Surg 58B: 485–487

Taylor W, Pelmear P L 1975 Vibration white finger in industry. Academic Press Inc, San Diego, CA pp 21–30

Teisinger J 1972 Vascular disease disorders resulting from vibrating tools. J Med 14: 129–133

Telford L E D, McCann M B, MacCormack D H 1949 Dead hand in users of vibrating tools. Lancet i: 359

Terranova W A, Williams G S, Kuhlman T A, Morgan R F 1985 Acute phalangeal fractures due to undiagnosed sarcoidosis. J Hand Surg (Am) 10: 902–903

Terrill R Q, Groves R J, Cohen M B 1987 Two cases of chondroid syringoma of the hand. J Hand Surg (Am) 12: 1094–1097

Terrono A, Millender L 1989 Surgical treatment of the boutonniere rheumatoid thumb deformity. Hand Clin 5: 239–248

Terzis J K, Daniel R K, Williams H B, Spencer P S 1978 Benign fatty tumors of the peripheral nerves. Ann Plastic Surg 1: 193–216

Terzis J K, Dykes R E, Hakstian R W 1976

Electrophysiological recordings in peripheral nerve surgery: a review. J Hand Surg 1: 52–66

Terzis J K, Liberson W T, Levine R 1986 Obstetric brachial plexus palsy. Hand Clin 2: 773–786

Thakore HK 1985 Hand injury with paint–gun. J Hand Surg (Br) 10: 124-126

Thayer D T 1988 Distal interphalangeal joint injuries. Hand Clin 4: 1–4

Theander G, Carstam N 1974 Longitudinally bracketed diaphysis. Ann Radiologie 17: 355–360

Thiru R G, Ferlic D C, Clayton M L, McClure D C 1986 Arterial anatomy of the triangular fibrocartilage of the wrist and its surgical significance. J Hand Surg (Am) 11: 258–263

Thirupathi R G, Ferlic D C, Clayton M L 1983 Dorsal wrist synovectomy in rheumatoid arthritis — a long-term study. J Hand Surg (Am) 8: 848–856

Thompson L 1991 Postoperative care. In: Kasdan M L (ed) Occupational hand and upper extremity injuries and diseases. Hanley & Belfus, Philadelphia, pp 433–442

Thompson S E, Jacobs N F, Zacarias F, Rein M F, Shulman J A 1980 Gonococcal tenosynovitis — dermatitis and septic arthritis. Intravenous penicillin vs oral erythromycin. J Am Med Assoc 244: 1101–1102

Thomsen B 1977 Processus supracondyloidea humeri with concomitant compression of median nerve and ulnar nerve. Acta Orthopaedica Scand 48: 391–393

Thorne F L, Kroop R J 1983 Wound botulism: a life-threatening complication of hand injuries. Plastic Reconstr Surg 71: 548–551

Thorrens S, Tripple O H, Bergan J J 1966 Arteriosclerotic aneurysms of the hand. Arch Surg 92: 937–939

Timmons M J, Missotten F E, Poole M D, Davies D M 1986 Complications of radial forearm flap donor sites. Br J Plastic Surg 39: 176–178

Tinel J 1915 Le signe du 'Fourrnillement' dans les lesion des Neufs Peripheriques. Press Med 47: 388–389

Tinel J 1917 Nerve Wounds. Bailliere Tindal and Cox, London

Toby E B, Poehling G G, Koman A L 1989 Midcarpal arthroscopy. Surg Rounds Ortho: 23–27

Tonkin M A, Lister G D 1988 The palmaris brevis profundus. An anomalous muscle associated with ulnar nerve compression at the wrist. J Hand Surg (Am) 10: 862–864

Toranto I R 1989 Aneurysm of the median artery causing recurrent carpal tunnel syndrome and anatomic review. Plastic Reconstr Surg 84: 510–512

Tountas C P, Bihrle D M, MacDonald C J, Bergman R A 1987 Variations of the median nerve in the carpal canal. J Hand Surg (Am) 12: 708–712

Tranquilli-Leali E 1935 Ricostruzione dell'apice delle falangi ungueali mediante autoplastica volare peduncolata per scorrimento. Infort Traum Lavoro 1: 186–193

Trumble T 1987 Forearm compartment syndrome secondary to leukemic infiltrates. J Hand Surg (Am) 12: 563–565

Trumble T E, Bour C J, Smith R J, Glisson R R 1990 Kinematics of the ulnar carpus related to the volar intercalated segment instability pattern. J Hand Surg (Am) 15: 384–392

Trumble T E, Watson H K 1985 Posttraumatic sesamoid arthritis of the metacarpophalangeal joint of the thumb. J Hand Surg (Am) 10: 94–100

Trumble T, Bour C J, Smith R J, Edwards G S 1988

Intercarpal arthrodesis for static and dynamic volar intercalated segment instability. J Hand Surg (Am) 13: 384–390

Trumble T, Seaber A V, Urbaniak J R 1987 Patency after repair of forearm arterial injuries in animal models. J Hand Surg (Am) 12: 47–53

Tsai T M, Kalisman M, Burns J, Kleinert H E 1983 Restoration of elbow flexion by pectoralis major and pectoralis minor transfer. J Hand Surg (Am) 8: 186–190

Tsai T M, Manstein C, DuBou R, Wolff T W et al 1984 Primary microsurgical repair of ring avulsion amputation injuries. J Hand Surg (Am) 9A: 68–72

Tsai T M, Singer R 1984 Elective free vascularized double transfer of toe joint from second to proximal interphalangeal joint of index finger: a case report. J Hand Surg (Am) 9: 816–820

Tse D H W, Slabaugh P B, Carlson P A 1980 Injury to the axillary artery by a closed fracture of the clavicle. J Bone Joint Surg 62A: 1372–1376

Tsuchida Y, Kasai S, Kojima T 1976 Congenital absence of flexor pollicis longus and flexor pollicis brevis: a case report. Hand 8: 294–297

Tsuge K 1967 Treatment of macrodactyly. Plastic Reconstr Surg 39: 590–599

Tsuge K 1985 Treatment of macrodactyly. J Hand Surg (Am) 10: 968–969

Tsuyuguchi Y, Masada K, Kawabata H, Kawai H, Ono K 1985 Congenital clasped thumb: a review of forty-three cases. J Hand Surg (Am) 10: 613–618

Tubiana R, DuParc J 1961 Restoration of sensibility in the hand by neurovascular skin island transfer. J Bone Joint Surg 43B: 474–480

Tunon J B, Gonzalez F P 1977 Angiomatosis of the metacarpal skeleton. Hand 9: 88–91

Tupper J W 1969 Pollex abductus due to congenital malposition of the flexor pollicis longus. J Bone Joint Surg 51A: 1285–1290

Tupper J W 1989 The metacarpophalangeal volar plate arthroplasty. J Hand Surg (Am) 14: 371–375

Tupper J W, Booth D M 1976 Treatment of painful neuromas of nerves in the hand: a comparison of traditional and newer methods. J Hand Surg 1: 144–151

Turner J W A, Parsonage M J 1957 Neuralgic amyotrophy (paralytic brachial neuritis) with special reference to prognosis. Lancet ii: 209–212

Turner M S, Caird D M 1977 Anomalous muscles and ulnar nerve compression at the wrist. Hand 9: 140–141

Upton A R M, McComas A J 1973 The double crush and nerve entrapment syndromes. Lancet ii: 359–362

Upton J, Mulliken J B, Murray J E 1985 Classification and rationale for management of vascular anomalies in the upper extremity. J Hand Surg (Am) 10: 970–975

Upton J, Rogers C, Durham-Smith G, Swartz W M 1986 Clinical applications of free temporoparietal flaps in hand reconstruction. J Hand Surg (Am) 11: 475–483

Upton J, Sohn S A, Glowacki J 1981 Neocartilage derived from transplanted perichondrium: what is it? Plastic Reconstr Surg 68: 166–172

Upton J, Zuker R M 1991 Apert syndrome. Clin Plastic Surg 18: 217–235

Urbaniak J R 1985 Repair of the flexor pollicis longus. Hand Clin 1: 69–76

Urbaniak J R 1985 Wrap-around procedure for thumb reconstruction. Hand Clin 1: 259–269

Urbaniak J R, Evans J P, Bright D S 1981 Microvascular

management of ring avulsion injuries. J Hand Surg 6: 25–30

Urbaniak J R, Hayes M G 1981 Chronic boutonniere deformity: an anatomic reconstruction. J Hand Surg 6: 379–383

Uriburu I J F, Morchio F J, Marin J C 1976 Compression syndrome of the deep motor branch of the ulnar nerve (piso–hamate hiatus syndrome). J Bone Joint Surg 58A: 145–147

Uriburu I J F, Morchio F J, Mario J C 1976 Metastases of carcinoma of the larynx and thyroid gland to the phalanges of the hand. Report of two cases. J Bone Joint Surg 58A: 134–136

Urschel H C, Razzuk M A 1972 Management intelligence. Management of the thoracic outlet syndrome. New Engl J Med 286: 1140–1143

Usami F 1987 Bilateral congenital absence of the flexor pollicis longus with craniofacial abnormalities. J Hand Surg (Am) 12: 603–604

Vahvanen V, Tallroth K 1984 Arthrodesis of the wrist by internal fixation in rheumatoid arthritis: a follow-up study of forty-five consecutive cases. J Hand Surg (Am) 9: 531–536

Vahvanen V, Viljakka T 1986 Silicone rubber implant arthroplasty of the metacarpophalangeal joint in rheumatoid arthritis: a follow-up study of 32 patients. J Hand Surg (Am) 11: 333–339

Vainio K 1989 Vainio arthroplasty of the metacarpophalangeal joints in rheumatoid arthritis. J Hand Surg (Am) 14: 367–368

Van Alphen W A, Smith A R, ten Kate F J 1988 Maximum hypothermic ischemia in replants containing muscular tissue. J Hand Surg (Am) 13: 415–422

Van Beek A L 1986 Electrodiagnostic evaluation of peripheral nerve injuries. Hand Clin 2: 747–760

Van Beek A L, Kassan M A, Adson M H, Dale V 1990 Management of acute fingernail injuries. Hand Clin 6: 23–35

Van Beek A L, Kutz J E, Zook E 1978 Importance of the ribbon sign, indicating unsuitability of the vessel, in replanting a finger. Plastic Reconstr Surg 61: 32–35

Van Beek A, Zook E, Yaw P, Gardner R, Smith R, Glover J 1974 Nonclostridial gas-forming infections. Arch Surg 108: 552–557

Vance R, Gelberman R 1978 Acute ulnar neuropathy with fractures at the wrist. J Bone Joint Surg 60A: 962–965

Vander Grend R, Dell P C, Glowczewskie F, Leslie B, Ruby L K 1984 Intraosseous blood supply of the capitate and its correlation with aseptic necrosis. J Hand Surg (Am) 9: 677–683

Vanik R K, Weber R C, Matloub H S, Sanger J R, Gingrass R P 1984 The comparative strengths of internal fixation techniques. J Hand Surg (Am) 9: 216–221

Varian J P, Cleak D K 1980 Glomus tumors in the hand. Hand 12: 293–299

Vathana P 1984 Primary hemangiopericytoma of bone in the hand: a case report. J Hand Surg (Am) 9: 761–764

Veal J R, McCord W M 1936 Congenital abnormal arteriovenous anastomoses of the extremities with special reference to diagnosis by arteriography and by the oxygen saturation test. Arch Surg 33: 848–866

Veitch J M, Omer G E 1979 Case report: treatment of catbite injuries of the hand. J Trauma 19: 201–203

Vender M I, Watson H K, Wiener B D, Black D M 1987 Degenerative change in symptomatic scaphoid nonunion. J Hand Surg (Am) 12: 514–519

Verdan C 1960 Syndrome of the quadriga. Surg Clin North Am 40: 425–426

Verdan C 1968 The reconstruction of the thumb. Surg Clin North Am 48: 1033–1061

Vetter W L, Weiland A J, Arnett F C 1983 Factitious extension contracture of the elbow: case report. J Hand Surg (Am) 8: 277–279

Vicar A J 1988 Proximal interphalangeal joint dislocations without fractures. Hand Clin 4: 5–13

Vicar A J, Burton R I 1986 Surgical management of the rheumatoid wrist — fusion or arthroplasty. J Hand (Am) 11: 790–797

Vichare N A 1968 Spontaneous paralysis of the anterior interosseous nerve. J Bone Joint Surg 50B: 806–808

Viegas S F 1986 Trigger thumb of de Quervain's disease. J Hand Surg (Am) 11: 235–237

Viegas S F, Bean J W, Schram R A 1987 Transscaphoid fracture/dislocations treated with open reduction and Herbert screw internal fixation. J Hand Surg (Am) 12: 992–999

Viegas S F, Calhoun J H 1986 Lead poisoning from a gunshot wound to the hand. J Hand Surg (Am) 11: 729–732

Viegas S F, Evans E B, Calhoun J, Goodwillier S E 1985 Tumoral calcinosis: a case report and review of the literature. J Hand Surg 10A: 744–748

Viegas S F, O'Meara C 1986 Hand injuries from shrimp boat winches. J Trauma 26: 851–853

Viegas S F, Patterson R M, Peterson P D, Pogue D J 1990 Ulnar-sided perilunate instability: an anatomic and biomechanic study. J Hand Surg (Am) 15: 268–278

Viegas S F, Patterson R M, Peterson P D, Pogue D J et al 1990 Evaluation of the biomechanical efficacy of limited intercarpal fusions for the treatment of scapho-lunate dissociation. J Hand Surg (Am) 15: 120–128

Viegas S F, Rimoldi R, Patterson R 1989 Modified technique of intramedullary fixation for wrist arthrodesis. J Hand Surg (Am) 14: 618–623

Vlastou C, Earle A S, Blanchard J M 1985 A palmar cross-finger flap for coverage of thumb defects. J Hand Surg (Am) 10: 566–569

Volkmann R 1967 Die ischaemischen muskellahmugen und-kontrakturen. Centrabl F Chir (translation by Edgar Bick). Clin Orthopaedics 50: 5–6

Vorenkamp S E, Nelson T L 1987 Ulnar nerve entrapment due to heterotopic bone formation after a severe burn. J Hand Surg (Am) 12: 378–380

Walker L G 1989 Bennett's fracture. Surg Rounds Orthopaedics 3: 79–80

Walker L G, Lesavoy M A 1990 Traumatic rupture of the profundus tendon proximal to the lumbrical origin. J Hand Surg (Am) 15: 484–486

Walker L G, Simmons B P, Lovallo J L 1990 Pediatric herpetic hand infections. J Hand Surg (Am) 15: 176–180

Walker M A, Hurley C B, May J W Jr 1986 Radial nerve cross-finger flap differential nerve contribution in thumb reconstruction. J Hand Surg (Am) 11: 881–887

Wallace P, Fitzmorris C 1978 The S-H-A-F-T syndrome in the upper extremity. J Hand Surg 3: 492–494

Walsh R J 1970 Acrosyndactyly: a study of 27 patients. Clin Orthopaedics 71: 99–111

Wang W 1983 Keys to successful second toe-to-hand transfer: a review of 30 cases. J Hand Surg (Am) 8: 902–906

Ward J W, Pensler J M, Parry S W 1985 Pollicization for thumb reconstruction in severe pediatric hand burns. Plastic Reconstr Surg 76: 927–932

Ware J W 1977 Subungual malignant melanoma presenting as sub-acute paronychia following trauma. Hand 9: 49–51

Warrens A N, Heaton J M 1987 Thoracic outlet compression syndrome: the lack of reliability of its clinical assessment. Ann R Coll Surg Eng 69: 203–204

Wartenberg R 1932 Cheiralgia paresthetica (Isolierte Neuritis des Ramus Superficialis Nerve Radialis). Z Ges Neurol Psychiatr 141: 145–155

Wassel H D 1969 The results of surgery for polydactyly of the thumb. Clin Orthopaedics 64: 175–193

Waters R L, Stark L Z, Gubernick I, Bellman H, Barnes G 1990 Electromyographic analysis of brachioradialis to flexor pollicis longus tendon transfer in quadriplegia. J Hand Surg (Am) 15: 335–339

Waters R, Moore K R, Graboff S R, Paris K 1985 Brachioradialis to flexor pollicis longus tendon transfer for active lateral pinch in the tetraplegic. J Hand Surg (Am) 10: 385–391

Waters W R, Penn I, Ross H M 1967 Airless paint gun injuries of the hand. 39: 613–618

Watson A C, McGregor J C 1981 The simultaneous use of a groin flap and a tensor fascia latae myocutaneous flap to provide tissue cover for a completely degloved hand. Br J Plastic Surg 34: 349–352

Watson H K, Ashmead D 4th, Makhlouf M V 1988 Examination of the scaphoid. J Hand Surg (Am) 13: 657–660

Watson H K, Ballet F L 1984 The SLAC wrist: scapholunate advanced collapse pattern of degenerative arthritis. J Hand Surg (Am) 9: 358–365

Watson H K, Boyes J H 1967 Congenital angular deformity of the digits — delta phalanx. J Bone Joint Surg 49A: 333–338

Watson H K, Carlson L 1987 Treatment of reflex sympathetic dystrophy of the hand with an active 'stress loading' program. J Hand Surg (Am) 12: 779–785

Watson H K, Light T R, Johnson T R 1979 Checkrein resection for flexion contracture of the middle joint. J Hand Surg 4: 67–72

Watson H K, Lovallo J L 1987 Salvage of severe recurrent Dupuytren's contracture of the ring and small fingers. J Hand Surg (Am) 12: 287–289

Watson H K, Rogers W D 1989 Nonunion of the hook of the hamate: an argument for bone grafting the nonunion. J Hand Surg (Am) 14: 486–490

Watson H K, Rogers W D, Ashmead D 4th 1989 Reevaluation of the cause of the wrist ganglion. J Hand Surg (Am) 14: 812–817

Watson H K, Ryu J Y, Burgess R C 1986 Matched distal ulnar resection. J Hand Surg (Am) 11: 812–817

Watson H K, Ryu J, Akelman E 1986 Limited triscaphoid intercarpal arthrodesis for rotatory subluxation of the scaphoid. J Bone Joint Surg (Am) 68: 345–349

Watson H K, Ryu J, DiBella A 1985 An approach to Kienbock's disease: triscaphe arthrodesis. J Hand Surg 10A: 179–187

Watson N, Songcharoen G P 1985 Lead synovitis in the hand: a case report. J Hand Surg (Br) 10: 423–424

Weber E H 1835 Ueber den Tastsinn. Arch Anat Physiol Wissenischs Med 3: 152–160

Weckesser E C, Reed J R, Heiple K G 1968 Congenital clasped thumb (congenital flexion-adduction deformity of the thumb). J Bone Joint Surg 37A: 1417–1428

Weeks P 1978 A cause of wrist pain: non-specific tenosynovitis involving the flexor carpi radialis. Plastic Reconstr Surg 62: 263–266

Weeks P M 1965 Surgical correction of upper extremity deformities in arthrogrypotics. Plastic Reconstr Surg 36: 459–465

Weeks P M 1967 The chronic boutonniere deformity: a method of repair. Plastic Reconstr Surg 40: 248–251

Weeks P M 1981 Invited comment on three complications of untreated partial laceration of flexor tendons — entrapment, rupture and triggering. J Hand Surg 6: 396–398

Weeks P M, Vannier M W, Stevens W G, Gayou D, Gilula L A 1985 Three-dimensional imaging of the wrist. J Hand Surg (Am) 10: 32–39

Weeks P M, Young V L 1982 Ulnar artery thrombosis and ulnar nerve compression associated with an anomalous hypothenar muscle (case report). 69: 130–131

Wei F C, Chen H C, Chuang C C, Noordhoff M S 1986 Reconstruction of a hand, amputated at the metacarpophalangeal level, by means of combined second and third toes from each foot: a case report. J Hand Surg (Am) 11: 340–344

Wei F C, Chen H C, Chuang C C, Noordhoff M S 1988 Reconstruction of the thumb with a trimmed-toe transfer technique. Plastic Reconstr Surg 82: 506–515

Wei F C, Chen H C, Chuang C C, Noordhoff M S 1988 Simultaneous multiple toe transfers in hand reconstruction. Plastic Reconstr Surg 81: 366–377

Wei F C, Chuang C C, Chen H C, Tsai Y C, Noordhoff M S 1984 Ten-digit replantation. Plastic Reconstr Surg 74: 826–832

Wei F C, Colony L H, Chen H C, Chuang C C, Noordhoff M S 1989 Combined second and third toe transfer. Plastic Reconstr Surg 84: 651–661

Weil D J, Wood V E, Frykman G K 1989 A new class of ring avulsion injuries. J Hand Surg (Am) 14: 662–664

Weiland A J, Lister G D, Villarreal–Rios A 1976 Volar fracture dislocations of the second and third carpometacarpal joints associated with acute carpal tunnel syndrome. J Trauma 16: 672–675

Weiland A J, Lister G D, Villarreal-Rios A 1976 Volar fracture dislocations of the second and third carpometacarpal joints associated with acute carpal tunnel syndrome. J Trauma 16: 672–675

Welling R E, Cranley J J, Krause R J, Hafner C D 1981 Obliterative arterial disease of the upper extremity. Arch Surg 116: 1593–1596

Welsh C L 1980 The effect of vibration on digital blood flow. Br J Surg 67: 708–710

Wendt J R, Lamm R C, Altman D I, Cruz H G, Achauer B M 1986 An unusually aggressive Mycobacterium marinum hand infection. J Hand Surg (Am) 11: 753–755

Wenner S M, Johnson K 1987 Giant cell reparative granuloma of the hand. J Hand Surg (Am) 12: 1097–1101

Wenner S M, Johnson K A 1988 Transfer of the flexor carpi ulnaris to the radial wrist extensors in cerebral palsy. J Hand Surg (Am) 13: 231–233

Wenner S M, Saperia B S 1987 Proximal row carpectomy in arthrogrypotic wrist deformity. J Hand Surg (Am) 12: 523–525

Werner C 1979 Lateral elbow pain and posterior interosseous nerve entrapment. Acta Orthopaedica Scand 50: suppl 174

Werner R, Davidoff G, Jackson M D, Cremer S et al 1989 Factors affecting the sensitivity and specificity of the three-phase technetium bone scan in the diagnosis of reflex sympathetic dystrophy syndrome in the upper extremity. J Hand Surg (Am) 14: 520–523

Wexler M R, Yeschua R, Neuman Z 1975 Early treatment of burns of the hand by tangential excision and grafting. Plastic Reconstr Surg 54: 268–273

Whipple T L 1990 Precautions for arthroscopy of the wrist. Arthroscopy 6: 3–4

Whitaker L A 1973 Management of hand infections in the narcotic addict. Plastic Reconstr Surg 52: 384–389

White G M 1986 Ligamentous avulsion of the ulnar collateral ligament of the thumb of a child. J Hand Surg (Am) 11: 669–672

White G M, Weiland A J 1984 Symptomatic palmar tendon subluxation after surgical release for de Quervain's disease: a case report. J Hand Surg (Am) 9: 704–706

White G M, Weiland A J 1987 Madelung's deformity: treatment by osteotomy of the radius and Lauenstein procedure. J Hand Surg (Am) 12: 202–204

White R E Jr 1986 Resection of the distal ulna with and without implant arthroplasty in rheumatoid arthritis. J Hand Surg (Am) 11: 514–518

White S 1984 Anatomy of the palmar fascia on the ulnar border of the hand. J Hand Surg (Br) 9: 50–56

White S H, Goodfellow J W, Mowat A 1988 Posterior interosseous nerve palsy in rheumatoid arthritis. J Bone Joint Surg (Br) 70: 468–471

White S H, Goodfellow J W, Mowat L A 1988 Posterior interosseous nerve palsy in rheumatoid arthritis. J Bone Joint Surg (Br) 70: 468–471

Whitney T M, Buncke H J, Alpert B S, Buncke G M, Lineaweaver W C 1990 The serratus anterior free muscle flap: experience with 100 consecutive cases. Plastic Reconstr Surg 86: 481–490

Widenfalk B, Wallin J 1988 Recurrent herpes simplex virus infections in the adult hand. Scand J Plastic Reconstr Surg Hand Surg 22: 177–180

Widgerow A, Edinburg M, Biddulph S L 1987 An analysis of proximal phalangeal fractures. J Hand Surg (Am) 12: 134–139

Wilgis E F 1985 Digital sympathectomy for vascular insufficiency. Hand Clin 1: 361–367

Wilgis E F, Murphy R 1986 The significance of longitudinal excursion in peripheral nerves. Hand Clin 2: 761–766

Wilgis E, Jezic D, Stonesifer G, Classen J, Sekercan K 1974 The evaluation of small-vessel flow. J Bone Joint Surg 56A: 1199–1206

Wilhelm A 1976 Radialis kompressions syndrome. Handchirurgie 8: 113–116

Williams C S, Riordan D C 1973 Mycobacterium marinum (atypical acid-fast bacillus) infections of the hand. J Bone Joint Surg 55A: 1042–1050

Williams G D, Hoffman S, Schwartz I S 1984 Malignant transformation in a plexiform neurofibroma of the median nerve. J Hand Surg (Am) 9: 583–587

Williams H B, Jabaley M E 1986 The importance of internal anatomy of the peripheral nerves to nerve repair in the forearm and hand. Hand Clin 2: 689–707

Williams H J, Biddulph E C, Coleman S S, Ward I R 1977 Isolated subcutaneous nodules (pseudorheumatoid). J Bone Joint Surg 59A: 73–76

Williams J G P 1977 Surgical management of traumatic non-effective tenosynovitis of the wrist extensors. J Bone Joint Surg 59B: 408–410

Williams J L, Thomas C G 1968 Natural history of Peyronie's disease. Proc Roy Soc Med 61: 876–877

Wilson C S, Buncke H J, Alpert B S, Gordon L 1984 Composite metacarpophalangeal joint reconstruction in great toe-to-hand free tissue transfers. J Hand Surg (Am) 9: 645–649

Wilson D W 1973 Synovectomy of the elbow in rheumatoid arthritis. J Bone Joint Surg 55B: 106–111

Wilson J H 1972 Arthroplasty of the trapezio-metacarpal joint. Plastic Reconstr Surg 49: 143–148

Wilson K M, Jubert A V, Joseph J I 1989 Sweat gland carcinoma of the hand (malignant acrospiroma). J Hand Surg (Am) 14: 531–535

Wilson M R, Louis D S, Stevenson T R 1988 Poland's syndrome: variable expression and associated anomalies. J Hand Surg (Am) 13: 880–882

Wilson R L 1985 Flexor tendon grafting. Hand Clin 1: 97–107

Wilson R L, Carlblom E R 1989 The rheumatoid metacarpophalangeal joint. Hand Clin 5: 223–237

Wilson R L, Liechty B W 1986 Complications following small joint injuries. Hand Clin 2: 329–345

Winspur I 1985 Distant flaps. Hand Clin 1: 729–739

Winter W G, Larson R K, Honeggar M H, Jacobesen D, Pappagianis D M, Huntington R W 1975 Coccidioidal arthritis and its treatment. J Bone Joint Surg 57A: 1152–1157

Wirman J A, Sherman S, Sullivan M R 1981 Dermatofibrosarcoma protuberans arising on the hand. Hand 13: 187–190

Wise K S 1975 The anatomy of the metacarpophalangeal joints, with observations of the aetiology of ulnar drift. J Bone Joint Surg 578: 485–490

Wiss D 1979 Aberrant lumbrical muscles causing carpal tunnel syndrome. Orthopedics 2: 357–358

Wiss D A, Reid B S 1983 Painless osteoid osteoma of the fingers — report of three cases. J Hand Surg (Am) 8: 914–917

Wissiner H A, McClain E J, Boyes J H 1966 Turret exostosis. Ossifying hematoma of the phalanges. J Bone Joint Surg 48A: 105

Witczak J W, Masear V R, Meyer R D 1990 Triggering of the thumb with de Quervain's stenosing tendovaginitis. J Hand Surg (Am) 15: 265–268

Wittels N P, Donley J M, Burkhalter W E 1984 A functional treatment method for interphalangeal pyogenic arthritis. J Hand Surg (Am) 9: 894–898

Wolfe J S, Eyring E J 1974 Median nerve entrapment within a greenstick fracture. J Bone Joint Surg 56A: 1270–1272

Wolfe S J, Summerskill W H J, Davidson C S 1956 Thickening and contraction of the palmar fascia (Dupuytren's contracture) associated with alcoholism and hepatic cirrhosis. New Eng J Med 255: 559–563

Wolfort F G, Cochran T C, Filtzer H 1973 Immediate interossei decompression following crush injury of the hand. Arch Surg 106: 826–828

Wong J H, Xu S H, Skinner K A et al 1991 Prospective evaluation of the use of antigen-specific immune complexes in predicting the development of recurrent melanoma. Arch Surg 126: 1450–1454

Wood J 1864 On some varieties in human myology. Proc Roy Soc Lond 13: 299–303

Wood M B 1987 Upper extremity reconstruction by

vascularized bone transfers: results and complications. J Hand Surg (Am) 12: 422–427

Wood M B 1987 Wrist arthrodesis using dorsal radial bone graft. J Hand Surg (Am) 12: 208–212

Wood M B, Linscheid R L 1973 Abductor pollicis longus bursitis. Clin Orthopedics Rel Res 93: 293–296

Wood M R 1980 Hydrocortisone injections for carpal tunnel syndrome. Hand 12: 62–64

Wood V 1978 Polydactyly and the triphalangeal thumb. J Hand Surg 3: 436–444

Wood V E 1971 Treatment of central polydactyly. Clin Orthopaedics 74: 196–205

Wood V E 1976 Treatment of the triphalangeal thumb. Clin Orthop 120: 188–200

Wood V E 1980 Nerve compression following opponensplasty as a result of wrist anomalies. Report of a case. J Hand Surg 5: 279–280

Wood V E 1988 Different manifestations of hyperphalangism. J Hand Surg (Am) 13: 883–887

Wood V E 1988 The extensor carpi radialis intermedius tendon. J Hand Surg (Am) 13: 242–245

Wood V E, Boindi J 1990 Treatment of the windblown hand. J Hand Surg (Am) 15: 431–438

Wood V E, Flatt A E 1977 Congenital triangular bones in the hand. J Hand Surg 2: 179–193

Wood V E, Ichtertz D R, Yahiku H 1989 Soft tissue metacarpophalangeal reconstruction for treatment of rheumatoid hand deformity. J Hand Surg (Am) 14: 163–174

Wood V E, Mudge M K 1987 Treatment of neuromas about a major amputation stump. J Hand Surg (Am) 12: 302–306

Wood V E, Sandlin C 1983 The hand in the Pierre Robin syndrome. J Hand Surg (Am) 8: 273–276

Wood V E, Sauser D, Mudge D 1985 The treatment of hereditary multiple exostosis of the upper extremity. J Hand Surg (Am) 10: 505–513

Workman C E 1964 Metacarpal fracture. Missouri Med 61: 687–690

Wright C S, McMurtry R Y 1983 AO arthrodesis in the hand. J Hand Surg (Am) 8: 932–935

Wright I S 1945 The neurovascular syndrome produced by hyperabduction of the arms. Am Heart J 29: 1–19

Wright P E, Stewart M J 1985 Fascial arthroplasty of the elbow. In: Morrey B F (ed) The elbow and its disorders. W B Saunders Co, Philadelphia, p 530

Wu G, Johnson D E 1983 Perichondrial arthroplasty in the hand: a case report. J Hand Surg (Am) 8: 446–453

Wu K K, Collon D J, Guise E R 1980 Extraosseous chondrosarcoma. Report of five cases and review of the literature. J Bone Joint Surg 62A: 189–194

Wu K K, Frost H M, Guise E E 1983 A chondrosarcoma of the hand arising from an asymptomatic benign solitary enchondroma of 40 years' duration. J Hand Surg (Am) 8: 317–319

Wu K K, Kelly A P 1977 Periosteal (juxta-cortical) chondrosarcoma. Report of a case occurring in the hand. J Hand Surg 2: 314–315

Wu K K, Winkelman N Z, Guise E R 1980 Metastatic bronchogenic carcinoma to the finger simulating acute osteomyelitis. Orthopedics 3: 25–28

Wylock P, Jaeken R, Deraemaecker R 1983 Anthrax of the hand: case report. J Hand Surg (Am) 8: 576–578

Wynn Parry C B 1989 Orthotics and rehabilitation after extensive upper limb paralysis. Hand Clin 5: 97 105

Yamano T 1985 Replantation of the amputated distal part of the fingers. J Hand Surg (Am) 10: 211–218

Yamauchi S, Nomura S, Yoshimura M, Ueno T et al 1983 A clinical study of the order and speed of sensory recovery after digital replantation. J Hand Surg (Am) 8: 545

Yang G et al 1981 Forearm free skin flap transplantation. Natl Med J China 61: 139

Yao S, Gourmos C, Papathanasiou K, Irvine W 1972 A method for assessing ischemia of the hand and fingers. Surg Obstet Gynecol 135: 373–378

Yaremchuk M J, Elias L S, Graham R R, Wilgis E F 1984 Sweat gland carcinoma of the hand: two cases of malignant eccrine spiradenoma. J Hand Surg (Am) 9: 910–914

Yeschua R, Wexler M R, Neuman Z 1977 Cross-arm triangular flaps for correction of adduction contracture of the web space in the hand. Plastic Reconstr Surg 59: 859–861

Yoshimura M 1980 Toe-to-hand transfer. Plastic Reconstr Surg 66: 74–83

Yoshitake K 1975 Clinical and experimental studies of the congenital constriction band syndrome, with an emphasis on its etiology. J Bone Joint Surg 57A: 636–642

Youm Y, Flatt A 1980 Kinematics of the wrist. Clin Orthop 149: 21–32

Young S C, Freiberg A 1985 A case of an intratendinous ganglion. J Hand Surg (Am) 10: 723–724

Young V L, Pin P, Kraemer B A, Gould R B et al 1989 Fluctuation in grip and pinch strength among normal subjects. J Hand Surg (Am) 14: 125–129

Younger C P, DeFiore J C 1977 Rupture of flexor tendons to the fingers after a Colles fracture. Case report. J Bone Joint Surg 59A: 828–829

Yu Z J 1987 Reconstruction of a digitless hand. J Hand Surg (Am) 12: 722–726

Yuan R T, Cohen M J 1985 Candida albicans tenosynovitis of the hand. J Hand Surg (Am) 10: 719–722

Zadek I, Cohen H G 1953 Epidermoid cyst of the terminal phalanx of a finger with a review of literature. American Journal of Surgery 85: 771

Zahrawi F 1984 Acute compression ulnar neuropathy at Guyon's canal resulting from lipoma. J Hand Surg (Am) 9: 238–239

Zancolli E 1970 Arthritic ulnar drift. An operation for metacarpophalangeal dislocation before cartilage destruction. J Bone Joint Surg 52A: 1067

Zancolli E A 1957 Clawhand caused by paralysis of the intrinsic muscles. J Bone Joint Surg 39A: 1076–1081

Zancolli E A 1979 Structural and dynamic bases of hand surgery, 2nd edn. J B Lippincott Co, Philadelphia

Zancolli E A, Angrigiani C 1988 Posterior interosseous island forearm flap. J Hand Surg (Br) 13: 130–135

Zancolli E A, Goldner L J, Swanson A B 1983 Surgery of the spastic hand in cerebral palsy: report of the Committee on Spastic Hand Evaluation (International Federation of Societies for Surgery of the Hand). J Hand Surg (Am) 8: 766–772

Zancolli E A, Zancolli E R Jr 1988 Palliative surgical procedures in sequelae of obstetric palsy. Hand Clin 4: 643–669

Zancolli E, Zancolli E Jr 1985 Congenital ulnar drift of the fingers. Pathogenesis, classification, and surgical management. Hand Clin 1: 443–456

Zdeblick T A, Field GA, Shaffer J W 1988 Treatment of experimental frostbite with urokinase. J Hand Surg (Am) 13: 948–953

Zeichner D M, Hoehn J G 1981 Karate-induced hand injuries. Orthopaedic Rev 10: 127–131

Zeide M S, Wiessel S, Terry R 1978 Juvenile aponeurotic fibroma. Plastic Reconstr Surg 61: 922–923

Zemel N P, Balcomb T V, Stark H H, Ashworth C R et al 1987 Dupuytren's disease in women: evaluation of long-term results after operation. J Hand Surg (Am) 12: 1012–1016

Zemel N P, Start K K, Ashworth C R, Rickard T A, Anderson DR 1984 Treatment of selected patients with an ununited fracture of the proximal part of the scaphoid by excision of the fragment and insertion of a carved silicone-rubber spacer. J Bone Joint Surg (Am) 66: 510–517

Zielinski C J, Bora F W Jr 1984 *Vibrio* hand infections: a case report and review of the literature. J Hand Surg (Am) 9: 754–757

Zimmerman N B, Suhey P V, Clark G L, Wilgis E F 1989 Silicone interpositional arthroplasty of the distal interphalangeal joint. J Hand Surg (Am) 14: 882–887

Zimmy M L, Redler I 1984 Ultrastructure of solitary enchondromas. J Hand Surg (Br) 9: 95–97

Zinberg E M, Palmer A K, Coren A B, Levinsohn E M 1988 The triple-injection wrist arthrogram. J Hand Surg (Am) 13: 803–809

Zingaro E A, Kilgore E S 1988 Partial hand amputation following radial artery cannulation. Contemp Orthopaedics 16: 46–47

Zlatkin M B, Chao P C, Osterman A L, Schnall M D et al 1989 Chronic wrist pain: evaluation with high resolution MR imaging. Radiology 173: 723–729

Zook E G 1977 Extensive giant cell tumor of the finger. A case history. Orthopedics 2: 267–268

Zook E G 1985 Nail bed injuries. Hand Clin 1: 701–716

Zook E G 1990 Anatomy and physiology of the perionychium. Hand Clin 6: 1–7

Zook E G, Guy R J, Russell R C 1984 A study of nail bed injuries: causes, treatment, and prognosis. J Hand Surg (Am) 9: 247–252

Zook E G, Kucan J O, Guy R J 1988 Palmar wrist pain caused by ulnar nerve entrapment in the flexor carpi ulnaris tendon. J Hand Surg (Am) 13: 732–735

Zook E G, Miller M, Van Beek A L, Wavek P 1980 Successful treatment protocol for canine fang injuries. J Trauma 20: 243–247

Zook E G, Russell R C 1990 Reconstruction of a functional and esthetic nail. Hand Clin 6: 59–68

Zubowicz V N, Ishii C H 1987 Management of ganglion cysts of the hand by simple aspiration. J Hand Surg (Am) 12: 618–620

Zuker R M, Manktelow R T 1986 The dorsalis pedis free flap; technique of elevation, foot closure, and flap application. Plastic Reconstr Surg 77: 93–104

Zvetina J R, Foster J, Reves C V 1979 *Mycobacterium kansasii* infection of the elbow joint. J Bone Joint Surg 61A: 1090–1102

Zweifach S S, Hargens A R, Evans K L, Smith R K, Mubarak S J, Akeson W H 1980 Skeletal muscle necrosis in pressurized compartments associated with haemorrhagic hypotension. J Trauma 20: 941–947

Index

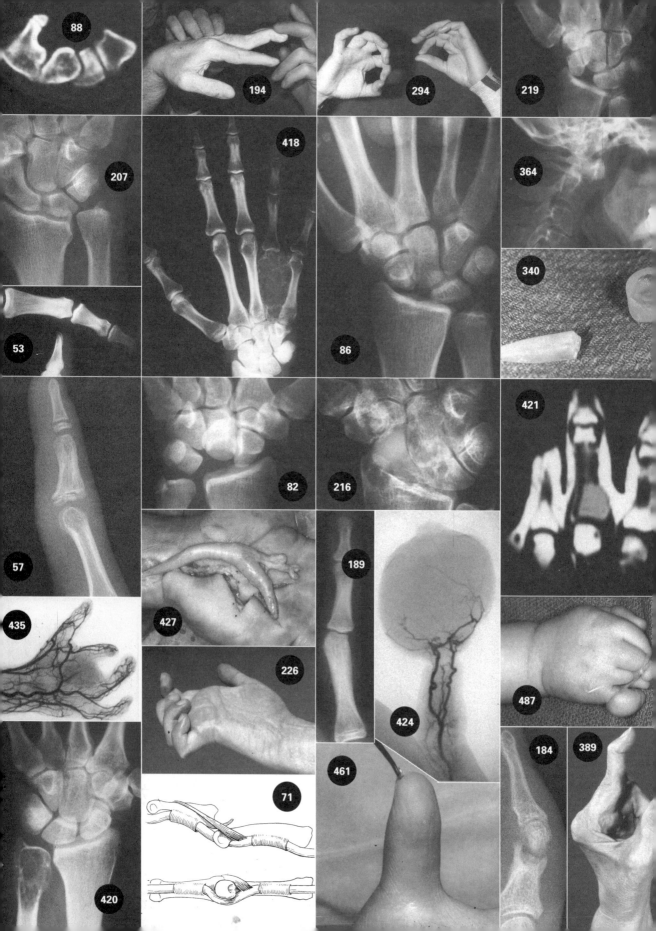